HINSHAW A.S.   FEETHAM S.L. & SHAVER J.L. (Eds)

Handbook of Clinical Nursing Research

HANDBOOK OF CLINICAL NURSING RESEARCH

DEDICATION

We dedicate this handbook to those before us with the vision, belief, and wisdom to advance a science of nursing and to the students and clinicians who will learn from this research. As well, we dedicate it to the faculties who will use this handbook as a basis for where we have come from, as a guide for future nursing research, and to inform practice and public policy. Our gratitude goes to the individuals and families who, while in our care, prompted us to generate the research questions that are the basis for nursing science, and to those who participated in our research as we worked to answer these questions.

ACKNOWLEDGMENTS

We thank our colleagues who enthusiastically accepted the challenge and became the chapter authors for this landmark book. We also acknowledge our partner section editors for working "shoulder-to-shoulder" with each of us to guide the production of this landmark publication. We acknowledge our students, clinicians and scientific colleagues, patients, and families, who constantly challenge the science and push the envelope of what we need to know. Every book of this magnitude has a cadre of support people and systems behind its production, some of whom remain invisible when our scholarship emerges in print. We are grateful, as they are the unsung heroes.

Special recognition goes to Sarah Kasprowicz, now a student at Rush Medical College, who was the conscientious, untiring linchpin in coordinating the compilation and ultimate completion of this handbook.

HANDBOOK

OF CLINICAL

NURSING

RESEARCH

Editors
Ada Sue Hinshaw
Suzanne L. Feetham
Joan L. F. Shaver

SAGE Publications
International Educational and Professional Publisher
Thousand Oaks London New Delhi

For information:

SAGE Publications, Inc.
2455 Teller Road
Thousand Oaks, California 91320
E-mail: order@sagepub.com

SAGE Publications Ltd.
6 Bonhill Street
London EC2A 4PU
United Kingdom

SAGE Publications India Pvt. Ltd.
M-32 Market
Greater Kailash I
New Delhi 110 048 India

Printed in the United States of America

Library of Congress Cataloging-in-Publication Data

Main entry under title:

Handbook of clinical nursing research / edited by Ada Sue Hinshaw,
Suzanne L. Feetham, Joan L. F. Shaver.
    p. cm.
  Includes bibliographical references and index.
  ISBN 0-8039-5784-X (cloth: acid-free paper)
  1. Nursing—Research—Handbooks, manuals, etc. I. Hinshaw, Ada
Sue. II. Feetham, Suzanne. III. Shaver, Joan.
  RT81.5 .H25 1999
  610.73'072—dc21   99-6034

99 00 01 02 03 10 9 8 7 6 5 4 3 2 1

Acquiring Editor:	Dan Ruth
Production Editor:	Astrid Virding
Editorial Assistant:	Nevair Kabakian
Typesetter/Designer:	Danielle Dillahunt
Indexer:	Will Ragsdale

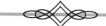

CONTENTS

PART IIH. ENVIRONMENTS FOR OPTIMIZING CLIENT OUTCOMES / 629

PREFACE

The vision for the *Handbook of Clinical Nursing Research* is to provide a foundational text outlining the state of the science for the discipline at the end of the 20th century. This time follows approximately the first decade of increased resources for nursing investigations, such as the establishment of the National Institute of Nursing Research. Such handbooks are common in many disciplines, but this is the first handbook for the nursing discipline. Although the anticipated effort was daunting, the editors felt the opportunities and potential contributions outweighed the challenges. The intent of this handbook is to address the current range of scientific progress in the discipline, explore the depth of knowledge to date, and provide specific direction to advance the science for nursing in the future.

For the past two decades, clinical nursing research has been the focus of the nursing scientific community. The goal was clear: to generate a body of knowledge that would guide nursing practice to optimize health for the individuals, families, and communities the profession serves. In the past 15 years, there has been an explosion of knowledge from these scientific endeavors, with concurrent advances in research-based practice. The *Handbook of Clinical Nursing Research* identifies the major areas in which there is significant depth in the research that can be reliably used to guide nursing practice, as well as providing a compendium of such knowledge.

The objectives for the handbook are to

- analyze major scientific areas that show substantiated research results that can guide nursing practice;
- synthesize knowledge in the identified areas of clinical nursing research, as well as addressing specific gaps in the science;
- stimulate further research through the understanding of the current state of the science for nursing research, including its strengths, weaknesses, and future directions; and
- provide a compendium of knowledge as a reference text for scholars and practitioners in nursing and other disciplines with similar interests and goals.

This first *Handbook of Clinical Nursing Research* is a landmark publication that will establish a baseline for the evolving science for the discipline. The text is intended for multiple audiences, including baccalaureate, master's, and doctoral students; faculties; clinicians; and professionals in other health disciplines with common issues.

The *Handbook of Clinical Nursing Research* provides overviews, synopses, and critiques of the state of the science in nursing in areas that have evolved to guide practice. The content is divided into two sections. Part I examines the theoretical and methodological issues, and Part II presents syntheses of defined areas of clinical nursing research. It is not intended that every aspect of nursing research be exhaustively covered. Several criteria were used to select the areas of clinical research: (a) an identified body of research exists related to a specific clinical content area, (b) the clinical research area is central to the practice of nursing, and (c) substantiated findings are evident that allow for reliable use in nursing practice. The clinical research areas are conceptualized and organized to cut across a number of traditional fields of practice.

In Part I of this handbook, a theoretical analysis of the core of the discipline, such as caring, is examined, and the methodological perspectives and issues in nursing research are addressed. The chapters focus on the unique philosophical perspectives of nursing science, and the developing infrastructures for the science. In Part II, the chapters synthesize the science in areas of clinical practice, including health needs of diverse racial and ethnic populations, clinical therapeutic strategies, families, health promotion and risk reduction across the life span, assessment and management of biobehavioral manifestations of health and illness, women's health, and health and illness in older adults. Research examining the environments for optimizing health outcomes is also synthesized. This handbook addresses the complexity and diversity of nursing and the populations it serves. The chapter authors speak to all areas of nursing practice, including the individual, family, community, developmental, life-span, health promotion, prevention, mental health, physical health, interdependence with the environment, and health systems.

Efforts to control the rapidly escalating costs of health care make it imperative that nursing care of the highest quality be accessible and delivered efficiently and economically. Because it is essential to quantify the benefits of nursing care, it is also imperative that nursing scientists provide the research-based evidence. It is science, with a promise of guiding practice for these ends, that stands to be recognized as "evidence." Nursing science has grown enormously in the past two decades in support of "evidence-based" practice, but several challenges remain, and these emerge as common themes in the analyses done by the authors in this handbook .

The themes evident throughout this text relate to the attention paid to (a) the perspective of theory generation or development; (b) diversity in populations studied; (c) methodological tactics, especially the progress of intervention research; and (d) interdisciplinary considerations.

From a perspective of theory development, there is an overriding emphasis on "individual" health rather than "public" or "population-based health" in nursing science. Although inroads are being made as we develop science related to community health, family health, and effective

delivery models and systems, to date this progress has been scant. The emphasis of nursing scientists on health promotion is laudable, but it does not outweigh the emphasis on health restoration in the face of disease or illness, which is the focus of most nursing scientists. Further, the authors point out that much more is known about the person and environmental elements that threaten or promote health than about how to influence human health behavior for sustained change in health status.

With respect to populations of study, a common theme in nursing science is a focus on vulnerable individuals and populations. In almost all realms of research analyzed, a focus on vulnerable or "at-risk" groups can be seen. It does stand to reason that science related to women's and infants' health has been prominent historically within nursing. Although earlier foci were on women and childbearing, a broader emphasis can now be seen: on women's health across the lifespan. Populations of growing emphasis include the very young (as we can now physiologically rescue very low birth weight infants), and, in accordance with demographic changes, the very old. A central value in nursing has long been to understand people and health across multiple ethnic, racial, age-related, socioeconomic, and geographic groups.

From a methodological standpoint, much of nursing science is descriptive and correlational in nature, and the authors frequently mention weaknesses in theory generation or testing. Cross-sectional, retrospective, and atheoretical designs have predominated. Prospective studies to explore causal relationships among variables according to theoretically derived postulates have been few. There is still slow progress on pushing descriptive research to tests of interventions. Therefore, there is still a relatively small, albeit increasing, literature related to intervention and outcomes research. That only a few sustained programs of research, under the direction of one or a group of investigators, can be detected in the literature affects this progress.

Another common observation across the nursing science arena is that nursing research is best described and often best facilitated from an interdisciplinary perspective. We in the nursing discipline embrace multiple methods and believe it is imperative to have interdisciplinary colleagues, communicate in interdisciplinary or crossdisciplinary venues, and consider those with whom we study as research partners. Our research also calls for collaborative research and service partnerships with communities. In the latter case, we are seeing advocates for community capacity building through research methods as a direction to be pursued.

Future Directions for Clinical Nursing Research

A number of exciting opportunities and challenges are evident when considering future directions for clinical nursing research. Following are our own ideas about a preferred future for nursing science, but first it is worth noting that there are several burgeoning health care foci affecting the health of individuals of all ages that are conspicuous by their absence in this *Handbook of Clinical Nursing Research*. Examples of these "gaps" include

- Advances in genetic knowledge and genetic therapeutics. Genetics is predicted to be the central science of health care. The Human Genome Project is adding dramatically to our understanding of the mechanisms of diagnosis, treatment, and prevention of disease. Nursing scientists can make major contributions in the application of genetics in health care. Nursing can provide leadership, especially in examining the ethical and social implications of these discoveries.

- Effects and use of the technological and telecommunications advances affecting nursing practice. These advances affect the diagnosis, treatment, and management of disease, as well as health promotion. Areas for research include telehealth systems and the use of technological advances in standardizing nursing taxonomies of diagnosis, interventions, and outcomes in national databases. The access to the amount and types of information through the Internet is unprecedented, and the examination of the effects on clinical decision making for professionals and the populations we serve is warranted.

- Explicit models and strategies for informing health and/or social policy through the findings of nursing research. A limited number of programs of nursing research have been sufficiently substantiated to be used in health policy formation. Also, nursing scientists need explicit preparation in models and strategies that will use the results of their research programs in informing health policy. The influence of research for the "public good" comes from linking research results to the derivation of adopted "best practices." The application of those practices by organized health care and the learning of best practices by students are essential. However, it is the translation of best practices into public policy that synchronizes access, quality, and cost that is most crucial to health care reformation through research. For the future, our goal is that the research of nursing scientists

becomes a critical driving force in the development of new health care policy.

- Study of mind/body interaction within multiple contexts. In research into "individual" or "personal" health, scientists have separated mind and body. Scientists have pursued normative data by which to judge health and illness status, with only limited examination of attributions for health status. They have also tended to use linear reasoning in a "causal" vein. In the future, we predict that nursing scientists will place more emphasis on seeking to understand mind/body reciprocity, seek to explain variability, and incorporate even wider considerations of "context." They will pursue ever more complex contingency models and use nonlinear, as well as linear, dynamic frameworks for characterizing phenomena, particularly the biologic aspect of biobehavioral phenomenon.

- Expansion of systems-level research to include integrated health care systems and communities. In the research into "public" or "community" health, the complexities of modeling health-related dynamics will grow. Research that is grounded in full participation of communities, beginning with problem identification, will become more commonplace. Health care delivery will become regional and based on the research of nursing scientists.

The challenges in pursuing the future directions of clinical nursing research are many. They include broadening the discipline's theoretical and methodological approaches in systematic inquiry, preparing nursing scientists in new interdisciplinary fields, synthesizing multiple knowledge perspectives, and pursuing a holistic framework or perspective for understanding the health and illness experiences of individuals, families, and communities.

This historic text, the *Handbook of Clinical Nursing Research*, provides a compendium of much of the current science in the discipline. If the handbook accomplishes the editors' goals, it will raise more questions than it answers, will stimulate the intellectual curiosity of colleagues in the nursing scientific community, and motivate all who use this text to greater investigative endeavors.

—Ada Sue Hinshaw
University of Michigan, Ann Arbor
—Suzanne L. Feetham
University of Illinois at Chicago
—Joan L. F. Shaver
University of Illinois at Chicago

PART

I

PHILOSOPHICAL, THEORETICAL, AND METHODOLOGICAL PERSPECTIVES AND ISSUES

Ada Sue Hinshaw

The four chapters in this section focus on the philosophical, theoretical, and methodological aspects of clinical nursing research, especially the philosophical and methodological perspectives and issues. From a theoretical frame, Swanson, through a literary meta-analysis, examines the concept of "caring" as developed in numerous nursing studies. The concept of caring is highlighted because of its pivotal role in providing effective, high-quality nursing, as well as its acknowledged core importance in supporting human dignity and sustaining humankind as people struggle with the experience of health and illness. After reviewing about 130 studies and publications, an inductively derived five-level framework for categorizing the studies and articles on caring was developed. The five levels are based on studies using qualitative and quantitative methodological approaches.

Jacox, Suppe, Campbell, and Stashinko, as well as Murdaugh's chapters, address the diversity of qualitative and quantitative methods used in nursing research. Both

chapters suggest that such diversity is a major strength for the evolving science of the discipline. Jacox and colleagues, in "Diversity in Philosophical Approaches," relate the methodological diversity to the various philosophical scientific perspectives. Ultimately, a philosophical approach that synthesizes the more traditional approaches is predicted to evolve. This chapter also addresses multiple sociopolitical factors that influence nursing science.

Adopting a different focus, Murdaugh, in "Relationship of Research Perspectives to Methodology," considers the importance of scientific pluralism and the value of resolving the qualitative-versus-quantitative debate in favor of such diversity. Several methods and strategies, such as triangulation, are discussed in regard to promoting the use of multiple methodological approaches in nursing research.

In another chapter, "Evolving Nursing Research Traditions: Influencing Factors," Hinshaw outlines a number of established and evolving research traditions which strengthen the science of the discipline and facilitate the endeavors of nurse investigators. Many of the factors influencing these nursing research traditions are considered.

This section of the *Handbook of Clinical Nursing Research* provides a philosophical, theoretical, and methodological context for understanding the scientific processes underlying the research addressed in Part II of the text.

1

DIVERSITY IN
PHILOSOPHICAL APPROACHES

Ada Jacox
Frederick Suppe
Jacquelyn Campbell
Elaine Stashinko

Nursing is characterized by great diversity. This is as true in the philosophical approaches taken to clinical nursing research as it is in other areas. Although there are some problems associated with diversity, such as nursing's occasional inability to agree on important issues, in general, nursing's diversity is a source of strength.

Nurse researchers have been educated in various sciences and intellectual perspectives and have had different experiences with patients. These and other differences in how nurse theorists and researchers view the world have produced a rich diversity of philosophical and research approaches. The diversity has enabled nurses to study human behavior in wellness and illness from a variety of perspectives and with multiple methods. Nursing research runs the gamut of sciences to include basic physiologic research, the study of clinical problems, and the study of patients and caregivers in organizations and communities. With such a broad scope of research interests, the need for breadth in research approaches is apparent.

There has been considerable debate within nursing about its philosophical, theoretical, and methodological

3

underpinnings. There has also been a significant amount of research undertaken by nurses who have been more or less attuned to the philosophical debates.

This intellectual debate and empirical work has resulted in several philosophical approaches to clinical nursing research. The major ones are (a) the postpositivist approach, arising out of logical positivism, and (b) the interpretive, humanistic, or naturalistic approach, which is concerned with understanding the meaning of an experience. A third approach, (c) the critical or emancipatory, combines elements of the first two to address how sociopolitical and cultural factors influence experiences (Ford-Gilboe, Campbell, & Berman, 1995).

Although there are other ways to characterize philosophical approaches, these three reflect contemporary modes of theory and research generally and in clinical nursing research. In describing these three approaches, it is important to underscore that philosophies and theories do not fall neatly into mutually exclusive categories. Instead, there is overlap in the assumptions, in the problems studied, in the methods used, and in the interpretation and implications for practice. Thus, whereas it is useful to classify approaches for the purpose of description, comparisons, and analysis, it is equally important to keep in mind that there are commonalities as well as differences among them. What is significant is that this kind of conscious consideration of nursing's intellectual work furthers the effort to develop a knowledge base that improves patient care.

Another major theme of this chapter is that, at least for the next decade, clinical nursing research will benefit by a preponderance of researchers focusing their efforts at the level of middle-range theory. This is in contrast, on the one hand, to the collection of facts isolated from any theoretical framework and, on the other hand, to global or grand theories, in which concepts are related at such a high level of abstraction and include so much that they are of little use in guiding research on specific clinical problems. Over 40 years ago, Robert K. Merton (1957) suggested the development of theories of the middle range to avoid the disadvantages of both grand theory and abstract empiricism. Middle-range theories include a limited number of variables and focus on a limited aspect of reality for the purpose of guiding research that addresses specific clinical problems and populations.

In the remainder of this chapter, we

discuss efforts during the past 30 years to develop nursing theory and research;

describe philosophical approaches to clinical nursing research, with attention to both their differences and commonalities;

describe middle-range theory and its usefulness in clinical nursing research;

show how the three philosophical approaches are used to study clinical problems, using examples from two areas of clinical nursing research: pain and violence against women; and

discuss factors in contemporary heath sciences and society that will have major impacts on clinical nursing research over the next decade.

In writing this chapter, we have considered several important issues: (a) How can the philosophically, theoretically, and methodologically diverse approaches to clinical nursing research be characterized? (b) How can the diversity of approaches be used to develop knowledge useful for practice (and how can nursing embrace and promote continued diversity)? (c) How can nurses develop and use knowledge about what works with most patients most of the time and in most settings, yet retain a focus on individualized care? (d) How can nursing increase the fit between present and future practice and the theories and research underlying nursing practice? and (e) How can nursing develop its own knowledge base and simultaneously participate in interdisciplinary research and theory development?

Historical Context for Development of Nursing Theory and Research

Following work in the 1950s and early 1960s to identify concepts underlying nursing practice, nurses began to propose theories and to focus on the development of theories as a way to relate the concepts. Prior to the 1960s, most nurses who were doctorally prepared were educated in schools of education. The initiation of the nurse-scientist program in the mid-1960s gave increased impetus to the effort to determine which knowledge from various sciences was most relevant to nursing and how nursing might best develop its own theory and research. Several national conferences were held during this time, including one series of three held in 1969 and 1970 and directed by Catherine M. Norris (1970, 1971, 1972) at the University of Kansas. The reports of these conferences indicated a focus on some specific theories, such as time and stress, chronicity, alienation, empathy, and general systems theory. The majority of the conference, however, focused on the *process* of theory development. Hildegard Peplau, Imogene King, and others at that conference were just beginning to develop global theories of nursing.

Since those early conferences, much has occurred to promote and shape nursing theory and research. This has included the development of global nursing theories by Martha Rogers, Imogene King, Sister Calista Roy, Dorothy Johnson, Margaret Neuman, Dorothea Orem, Myra Levine, Betty Neuman, and others. For the most part, these grand theories represented worldviews of nursing and identified major phenomena of concern to nurses. They provided broad perspectives regarding the nature of nursing, the person, and health and environment and emphasized the need to place investigation in a theoretical context. They helped to define nursing and nursing research. At the same time, because of their high level of abstraction, they were difficult to test and were not very useful in guiding specific clinical research.

During the 1970s and 1980s, there was a major increase in the amount of clinical nursing research conducted. Although several grand nursing theories were available, the great majority of nurse investigators drew their concepts and theories from other disciplines (Beck, 1985; Mood et al., 1988).

Nurses began to develop middle-range nursing theories in the 1980s. Those currently being used in practice and research include Mischel's (1990) theory of uncertainty in illness, Cox's (1982) interaction model of client health behavior, Morse and Johnson's (1991) illness constellation model, and Pender's (1996) model of health promotion and illness prevention. There was continued debate regarding the merits and weaknesses of quantitative and qualitative research, with many in the 1980s viewing them as in opposition.

The major factor contributing to the increased clinical research was the increase in the number of nurses earning master's and doctoral degrees, particularly doctorates in nursing. Over the past 30 years, there has been an enormous increase in the number of universities that award doctorates in nursing. In 1965, three universities awarded doctorates in nursing; by 1997, 66 universities did. The number of nurses with doctoral preparation increased dramatically, from approximately 500 in 1965 to approximately 18,000 in 1998 (Jacox, 1993).

Another indicator of the rapid growth in nursing research was the increase in research-based publications.

Nursing Research, the first nursing journal dedicated specifically to research, was first published in 1951. Beginning in 1983, the *Annual Review of Nursing Research* (*ARNR*) published critical summaries of areas of nursing research. The amount of research reported has been impressive in scope, and a number of *ARNR* chapters have been updated in subsequent reviews.

The program of federal support for nursing research moved from its unusual and peripheral location in the Manpower Division of the Health Resources Services Administration to the mainstream of health care research, the National Institutes of Health. Established as the Center for Nursing Research in 1985, it was elevated to institute status in 1993. This acknowledgment of the status of nursing research and the other indicators of progress in developing nursing's theoretical and research base as described above are evidence of nursing's growing strength as a research-based discipline. Nursing's scientific growth in the future will depend in great part on how well nurses understand both their history and the current sociopolitical context in which nursing operates. Following a characterization of the major current philosophical approaches used by nurse researchers, sociopolitical factors affecting contemporary nursing science are discussed.

Characterization of the Three Philosophical Approaches

The dominant philosophical approach in contemporary science is postpositivism. Following the Renaissance (about 400 years ago), there was much debate about what science is and how theories are developed. The dominant 17th-century worldview included the idea that the world was like a clock or simple machine and only God understood fully the laws by which it operated. The aim of science was to discover those laws and learn enough about them to achieve perfect predictability (Webster & Jacox, 1985). There was near consensus concerning the nature of the world, and the consensus continued until the 19th century. During that time, an intellectual bifurcation occurred that produced two competing worldviews. One was the philosophy of nature, which based its understanding of reality on the physical sciences, especially mathematical physics. The second was the philosophy of mind, which was concerned with the nature of human experience and represented by such traditions as German idealism, phenomenology, and existentialism. Positivism developed from the philosophy of nature in the 19th-century worldview, whereas the interpretive philosophical approach emerged from the philosophy of mind.

Postpositivist Approach

Although both traditions were developed, science was dominated by individuals focusing on physical reality and the philosophy of science. A group of philosophers gathered in Vienna in the 1930s and labeled themselves logical positivists. Logical positivists were concerned with formal logic and formalization issues. They rejected metaphysics because they believed that the only reality was physical reality and that the physical sciences were the only appropriate disciplines for study. They believed that theoretical and observational terms could be clearly separated and that less basic sciences could be reduced to more basic sciences.

The tenets of logical positivism evolved into the "received view" of science. This was a name given to a set of ideas that portrayed science and theories in a dogmatic, formalized, and precise way that did not adequately reflect the reality with which it was concerned (Suppe, 1977). There was much debate regarding the received view of science, and those who had developed it (Carnap, 1953) gradually qualified it to the point that it ceased to exist as an identifiable theory about the nature of science by the early 1960s. Although philosophers of science rejected this narrow view of science, it continued for some time to dominate what was thought to be science and theory in many disciplines, including sociology and nursing. Since the 1960s, a number of competing theories of science have been espoused (Feyerabend, 1975; Laudan, 1977; Suppe, 1989). Along with these alternatives, there have been simultaneous efforts to show how postpositivism differs from the positivist approach (Guba, 1990; Schumacher & Gortner, 1992).

The postpositivist approach is characterized by an effort to identify patterns and regularities to describe, explain, and predict phenomena. Truth can be discovered only imperfectly and probabilistically. The context or conditions under which patterns occur is important, and the need to control environmental influences to understand phenomena under study is emphasized (Ford-Gilboe et al., 1995).

The postpositivist approach encompasses the use of diverse types of data, including both sensory experiences and the perception of those experiences. Emphasis is placed on using a variety of forms of data to falsify hypotheses and provide support for specific theories. Application and triangulation of methods, as well as accumulated evidence, are used to develop, test, and revise theories or replace them with new ones.

The traditional postpositivist approach accepts the use of both quantitative and qualitative data in understanding phenomena. Considerable effort currently is being made to develop methods for summarizing and synthesizing the results of findings accumulated from a wide variety of sources and studies. These synthesizing techniques include meta-analysis, best evidence synthesis, and cross-design analysis. The debates among those attempting to synthesize research results reflect the continuing controversy among postpositivists regarding what can legitimately be counted as science. Some meta-analysts assert that only double-blind, randomized clinical trials count as science and should be included in meta-analyses. Others advocate the development of methods to synthesize the results of a variety of studies so that quasiexperimental and descriptive studies are included in meta-analyses. It is clear that the postpositivist tradition is much more flexible in its philosophical assumptions and methods than was positivism and that there is a wide range of ideas regarding how science should be "done" (conducted) and what constitutes a theory.

Interpretive, Humanistic, or Naturalistic Approach

The interpretive philosophical perspective encompasses the naturalistic, constructivist interpretive (Gioia & Pitre, 1990), and humanistic paradigms. It emerged from the 19th-century tradition of philosophy of mind and has been viewed since then by some as a (the) valid approach to science and theory development. The interpretive approach to science has had considerably less impact on health science research than has the postpositivist approach, although both are increasingly viewed as legitimate ways to conduct scientific research and to develop and test theories. According to Gioia and Pitre, the goal of the interpretive paradigm is to describe and explain in order to diagnose and understand. The goal of research in the interpretive paradigm is to generate descriptions and insights and reveal the individual meaning of events or experiences within different contexts. Thus, interpretive theory building tends to be more inductive in nature, and methods employed are typically qualitative (Gioia & Pitre, 1990; Guba, 1990). Meaning or truth is constructed in the course of the interaction between the researcher and the participant in a natural environment; that is, in a setting in which the participant feels comfortable.

Consistent with the goal of describing and understanding, stories of participants have been regarded as the best way of capturing the richness and diversity of subjective experience in interpretive research (Ford-Gilboe et al., 1995). Methodologically, the interpretivist aims to identify the variety of individual constructions that exist and bring them to as much consensus as possible. Thus, a hermeneutic, dialectic method is frequently employed whereby individual constructions are elicited and refined as accurately as possible and compared and contrasted dialectically to create a more informed and sophisticated representation of reality (Guba, 1990). Modes of inquiry include ethnography, phenomenology, grounded theory, and historical research.

▬ *Critical or Emancipatory Approach*

The third philosophical approach, the critical or emancipatory, encompasses critical theory, feminist research, Afrocentric (or other minority group ethnocentric approaches), action research, and poststructuralist investigations. This philosophical approach combines aspects of postpositivist and humanistic approaches and addresses how sociopolitical and cultural factors influence experience. It was first described and used in nursing in the 1980s, with critical and feminist methodology being used at about the same time (Allen, 1985; Allen, Benner, & Diekelmann, 1986; Chinn & Wheeler, 1985; MacPherson, 1985; Thompson, 1987). Although distinctions can and should be made among the specific emancipatory methods, they hold the same basic aims: elucidating historical, structural, and cultural biases and forces as well as seeking to make emancipatory change for the actual participants or the groups they represent as a result of or as part of the research process (Campbell & Bunting, 1991). These approaches are characterized by the use of quantitative and qualitative data and a variety of designs influenced by the methodological principles of nonhierarchical research arrangements and relations; partnerships with research participants; and attention to and competence with gender, ethnic, and cultural issues, dialogic interview techniques, and validation of the research enterprise (study or group of studies) in terms of amount of emancipatory change achieved (Lincoln's catalytic validity) (Bunting & Campbell, 1994; Ford-Gilboe et al., 1995; Guba, 1990).

The critical or emancipatory approach focuses not only on individual growth, change, and empowerment but also on the structures that keep people from making individual and family changes. Thus, it necessitates that nursing intervention research focus on system change as well as on individuals and families.

A researcher using the emancipatory approach would use quantitative or qualitative data or both in conjunction with participant involvement and whichever research design had the most potential for emancipatory outcomes for the particular group in the particular situation. The specific design or type of data gathered is less important in this philosophical approach than the amount of change engendered. Thus, if the desired end was policy change in a health insurance practice that disallowed a particular nursing intervention for HIV/AIDS patients in one particular state, the most persuasive case might be made by a combination of a statewide random sample survey demonstrating public support for the type of intervention, a phenomenological study of patients to demonstrate their sense of existing in an oppressive environment and to elicit their description of the effects of the intervention, and a clinical trial of the nursing intervention to demonstrate cost effectiveness and efficacy in reducing symptom distress and promoting a sense of well-being. The studies would be planned with AIDS patients, their advocates, and the nurses providing care, all as partners.

In emancipatory paradigms, clinicians practice by doing research. This idea is captured by Paulo Freire's (1970) concept of *praxis,* or the expert (or researcher or scientist) conducting work for the good of those the research is involved with while learning and working with those participants (patients) in the enterprise.

▬ *Commonalities Across the Perspectives*

Some nurse theorists and researchers (Leininger, 1994; Moccia, 1988; Parse, 1987) have viewed postpositivist and interpretive approaches as distinct paradigms, adopting assumptions that require the use of distinct quantitative methods for postpositivist and qualitative methods for interpretive. In their view, the assumptions of the two approaches are incompatible, and their use in combination is a compromise that produces less rigorous research. In fact, quantitative and qualitative approaches commonly have been combined in the social and behavioral sciences as well as in nursing. A common practice in the policy sciences, for example, has been to combine use of a large state or national database derived from survey research on a problem with one or more case studies of examples of the problem to increase understanding of the meaning of the survey data. Nurse researchers have long combined quantitative and qualitative approaches to study such diverse problems as pain (Jacox & Stewart, 1973) and renal dialysis (O'Brien, 1983).

During the past decade, many have acknowledged a need to move beyond debates over which approach is more appropriate, making it possible for nursing to understand that the choice of philosophical and methodological approaches is somewhat dependent on the problem to be addressed and that the approaches can be combined (Knafl, Pettengill, Bevis, & Kirchoff, 1988). The critical theory approach is explicit in its use of multiple methods, advocating the use of methods likely to be most effective in bringing about change in the problem addressed.

In a recent analysis of the three approaches, Ford-Gilboe et al. (1995) argue that they are not method specific but only provide a general approach to research. The methods cut across the approaches, and choice of the methods is made according to the purposes of the research. These researchers identify four issues that must be addressed in evaluating the quality of the research: (a) quality of the data, (b) investigator bias, (c) quality of the research process, and (d) usefulness of the study findings. They then describe how each of the approaches views and deals with the methodological issues.

Another issue important to consider is how the level of theory abstraction can influence the usefulness of the theory in guiding research.

Relation of Middle-Range Theory to the Three Philosophical Approaches

It has been characteristic of emerging psychosocial science disciplines to devote much attention to the role of theory as they pursue the legitimation of the discipline as a real science. A particular concern is what sorts of theory ought to be developed. When sociology fought these battles, Robert K. Merton (1957) introduced the term *middle-range theories,* as distinct from *grand theories* and *abstracted empiricism,* thereby focusing the debate on the relative importance of developing middle-range rather than grand theories in the legitimation of sociology as a scientific discipline. Nursing, too, has found Merton's distinction useful as it has waged its own battle for legitimation as a science.

Indeed, it is held by many that one aim of nursing science ought to be to develop middle-range theories suitable for guiding practice and for stimulating further research (Jacox, 1970; Lenz, Suppe, Gift, Pugh, & Milligan, 1995). Despite a rich body of nursing metatheory, little has been offered by way of precise characterization of middle-range theories. So, too, discussions of how middle-range theories are useful for guiding research and practice tend to be vague and imprecise.

Discussing middle-range theories, Merton (1968) tells us that they "lie between the minor but necessary working hypotheses and the all-inclusive efforts to develop a unified theory," that they "are intermediate to general theories too remote to account for what is observed and to those detailed orderly descriptions of particulars that are not generalized at all" (p. 68). Further, they involve abstractions but are close enough to observed data to permit empirical testing. On the basis of such comments, it is commonly claimed that middle-range theories are differentiated from grand theories by their scope and degree of abstraction.

However, those remarks are from Merton's heuristic introduction of the notion, and, if we look carefully at his official characterization of middle-range theories, we find that what actually distinguishes middle-range from grand theories for Merton is that the former are testable whereas the latter are not, where testability is characterized in terms of the logical positivistic, received-view analysis of theories:[1] Middle-range theories consist of limited sets of assumptions from which specific hypotheses are logically derived[2] and confirmed by empirical investigation.[3] This characterization not only presupposes some sort of division of scientific vocabulary into the theoretical and the observational and empirical but, more important for our purpose, that the theory contains correspondence rules—a kind of operational definition built into the axiomatized theory—that connect the theoretical and observational vocabularies to facilitate the logical derivation of empirical predictions.[4]

The positivistic received view does not show up in our characterization of the three main philosophical approaches guiding nursing research because the positivistic approach used by Merton has been repudiated by philosophers of science. Indeed, all three of the philosophical approaches reject the notion of a fixed observational or theoretical distinction and the idea that correspondence rules are proper parts of theories. Without these notions, the positivistic notion of testability absolutely collapses. As testability is presupposed in Merton's characterization of middle-range versus grand theories, so too does his characterization of the distinction collapse.

The question is whether Merton's middle-versus-grand-theory distinction can be divorced from its discredited positivistic underpinnings and reinterpreted in a manner applicable to the three contemporary approaches. For present purposes, a relativized notion will suffice: Of the three contemporary views, theory and observation/experiment tend to use the same descriptive vocabularies. We can distinguish theories that postulate relationships between the (quantitative or objectively coded qualitative) values of those descriptors and theories that do not. The three philosophical approaches differ in what they take to be appropriate values and the proper means for obtaining them, but they all share the insistence that theories be evaluated on the basis of data. We understand the notions *measure* or *objectively code* in accordance with whichever philosophical approach is being used.

So understood, a time-relative distinction can be drawn between those descriptive terms that now can be measured or objectively coded and those that cannot. At time *t,* a theory *T* is middle range if it postulates relationships between the (quantitative or objectively coded qualitative) values of its descriptors and if it is possible now to measure or objectively code those descriptors. We thus have a successor notion of middle-range theories that captures Merton's basic intuition but divorces it from its positivistic origins.

The question to be faced now is whether nurses should aspire to develop middle-range nursing theories so understood, and, if so, what proportion of theoretical efforts should be devoted to developing them. Little relevant guidance is offered by Merton's original reasons for championing middle-range theories, for Merton was advocating the development of middle-range theories as opposed to grand theories. In nursing, the development of grand theories was critical to the emergence of nursing as a legitimate scientific and academic research discipline, but now that nursing is well established, the production of grand theories is a diminishing research enterprise (Suppe, 1992), although concern with assessing the role and place of nursing in the larger health and human spheres surely will continue to be valued. Certain concepts, such as self-care, from the grand nursing theories also continue to have explanatory value and are included in middle-range nursing theories, thus contributing their uniqueness and value to nursing. Additionally, middle-

range theories can be deduced or derived from grand theories (e.g., Frey, 1995).

Insofar as researchers triage their research efforts and resources, it is increasingly a choice between what Merton called abstracted empiricism—the development of local-scope, specialized empirical correlations and statistically significant differences—and middle-range theory. It is often supposed that the generality of middle-range theories renders them clinically useless, but much abstracted empiricism research does not inform clinical practice very much either. The fact is that nursing interventions tend to vary widely in the extent of their research basis, and where there is such a basis it often is not only from nursing research.

One principal merit Merton claimed for middle-range theory was that it could be used to guide empirical inquiry (Merton, 1968). In the characterization of middle-range theories developed here, the crucial features are (a) postulating relationships between the (quantitative or objectively coded qualitative) values of its descriptors and (b) having the resources *now* to measure or objectively code those descriptors. Each of the three philosophical approaches gives further guidance to the development and use of descriptors to obtain relevant data.

Constructing middle-range theory thus involves sufficiently precise development of descriptors in accordance with an associated philosophy so as to make them measurable (if quantitative) or objectively codable (if qualitative) and identification of precise regularities between measured or objectively coded values for these descriptors. Properly done, the operationalization of descriptors themselves will often be middle-range theories.

In the present context, the decisive advantage of middle-range theories is that the three different philosophical approaches each can be used to develop the same descriptors for a common theory. Thus, the strengths of all three approaches can be exploited in the development of middle-range theory. In contrast, the lower level correlations and hypotheses of abstracted empiricism are always tied to the method and procedures of a single philosophical approach.

Of particular concern in clinical nursing research is documenting the efficacy of nursing interventions for diverse nursing diagnoses. As classified by the North American Nursing Diagnoses Association (NANDA) and the Nursing Interventions Classification (NIC), nursing diagnoses and interventions enjoy the generality of middle-range theory components yet are defined in terms of concrete descriptors of specific activities or presenting conditions. Claims about the efficacy of specific interventions for specific nursing diagnoses will thus typically take the form of middle-range theories, not simple empirical generalizations between activities and symptoms. That fact alone is sufficient pragmatic justification for an emphasis on the development of middle-range theory.

But interest in middle-range theory does not start there. As nursing has become a legitimated research domain, it has moved from a purely clinical discipline to one that combines clinical and basic scientific research whose principal focus is understanding. Nursing research has become nursing science, and middle-range theories, not the local generalizations of abstracted empiricism, provide the most potential for such understanding. Nursing science is both applied and basic, and that combination demands that the development of middle-range theories be a significant part of the effort.

The three philosophical approaches presented here differ not in the value they ascribe to middle-range theory but in the manner in which they go about developing descriptors, harnessing them to theories, and using them to collect data to evaluate and further develop such theories. The next section examines substantive differences in how these three philosophical approaches influence the development of descriptors, collection of data, and development of middle-range theory in two clinically relevant areas: *pain* and *violence against women.*

Illustration of the Three Philosophical Approaches in Nursing Research

One of the tensions among the philosophical approaches is seen in the definition and operationalization of the concepts of person and environment. In the postpositivist approach, the person is viewed as a holistic, active, sentient being in reciprocal interaction with the environment (Fawcett, 1993). Within clinical nursing research, in this approach the focus is on establishing normative data that can be generalized to other populations. A goal of the clinical researcher is to create a design that is, as much as possible, context free. Salient words in this clinical research approach include *power analysis, statistical significance, reliability and validity of measurement,* and *control of bias.* In contrast, in the naturalistic, interpretive approach, the person is viewed as a unitary human being in simultaneous interaction with the envi-

ronment. The emphasis in this philosophical approach is on the uniqueness of each individual and the experiential meaning of health within context. Researchers assume that appropriate designs will be context dependent and value laden. Salient words include *choice, patterns of behavior, values,* and *understanding.* In the critical or emancipatory approach, the person is viewed as a unitary human being integrally related to a sociopolitical community. The focus of emancipatory clinical nursing research is on change not only for the individual or normative groups but for the community. Key words congruent with this approach include *enlightenment* and *empowerment* (Henderson, 1995).

Every philosophical perspective reveals some truths and conceals some biases (Skrtic, 1990). As Newman (1994) states, "People working out of different paradigms see things differently and arrive at different conclusions, sometimes even with the same data" (p. 155). In promoting a multiapproach perspective, Gioia and Pitre (1990) assert that theory building ought to be viewed not as a search for *the* truth but as more of a search for comprehensiveness stemming from different worldviews. Within this mosaic of philosophical worldviews, nursing as a discipline is in the developmental stage of moving from control to community (Hegyvary, 1992). To advance nursing science and human care, it is necessary to transcend philosophical and methodological biases to see more clearly the potentials of nursing and its human care practice. The potential of the three philosophical perspectives to increase understanding of phenomena relevant to nursing practice is illustrated in the following two examples.

Clinical Research Example: Pain

Sickle cell anemia is a genetic disease that affects approximately 1 in 600 African Americans (Shapiro, 1993). The complexity and multidimensionality of the pain experience is emphasized in this population because the natural history of sickle-cell-related pain and patterns within and among individuals varies greatly. Some individuals with sickle cell disease experience no pain until adolescence or young adulthood, but for some children and adolescents the normal baseline is daily pain, with intermittent acute exacerbations (Platt, Thorington, & Brambilla, 1991; Shapiro, Dinges, Ohene-Frempong, & Orne, 1990). The hallmark of sickle cell pain is its extreme variability and unpredictability in timing, location, and intensity (Shapiro, 1993). We consider the problem of pain assessment and management in preschool children with sickle cell disease from the three philosophical approaches, any or all of which could contribute to a middle-range theory of pain management.

From a postpositivist perspective, the researcher would initially search the literature for an age-appropriate, reliable, and valid tool to assess pain, such as the African American version of the Oucher pain scale (Denyes & Villarruel, 1988; Villarruel & Denyes, 1991). A question to be studied might be, What risk factors predict sickle cell painful events in this age group? Patients from a hematology clinic might be stratified into high- or low-risk categories based on the presence or absence of painful events within the last year. In a prospective, longitudinal study, physiological, behavioral, and social-psychological risk factors would be empirically defined and measured in both groups over a 1-year period, controlling for any potentially confounding variables. Interviews about pain assessment and management techniques might be conducted with children and family members to elucidate or enrich the data but would not be the only method of inquiry. Within this philosophical perspective, emphasis is placed on empirical observations, methodological controls, and inferential data-analytic techniques studied through both quantitative and qualitative data and their analysis (Fawcett, 1993).

Questions addressed from an interpretive perspective might include, What is the meaning of the sickle cell disease experience to preschool children and their families? Or, using Leininger's theory of culture care diversity and universality, What is the meaning of this health experience to this cultural group? Parents might be asked to maintain a pain diary for a year and to record any pain observations, what they and the child were doing prior to the painful event, and what they did in response to the event. Diary data might be supplemented by open-ended interviews with family members, including the child, and perhaps by behavioral observation. The researcher would provide a detailed description of the participant's natural environment—the physical setting where the participant lives, works, or experiences significant events. Over time, the nurse researcher or clinician might identify a conceptual definition of the painful event to this family or culture and unique patterns of behavior surrounding painful events—triggers, choices and consequences, and coping strategies that work for this family or for this culture. Confirmation of the data findings and conclusions with the participants are important parts of the research process in this approach. Data generated from this study may not be generalizable to a larger population.

Questions arising from the critical or emancipatory perspective might include, What social ideologies and power imbalances exist with the life experiences of children and their families dealing with sickle cell disease? What culturally specific nursing interventions are most likely to relieve the pain? Several recent studies have documented the presence of biased pain assessments and inadequate analgesia in adult African Americans as compared to Whites (Blendon, Aiken, Freeman, & Corey, 1989; Cleeland et al., 1994). Similarly, the literature suggests that concerns about drug dependency and racial bias influence the professional's ability to make accurate assessments of pain in children with sickle cell disease (Morrison & Vedro, 1989). Thus, the research emphasis might be on emancipation of individual families or on exposing the ideology of professionals. An Afrocentric method of inquiry is an appropriate choice of method (Porter & Villarruel, 1993). An Afrocentric inquiry would center the study of this phenomenon in the particular cultural voice of the composite African American people, with an emphasis on understanding-related health care issues (pain assessment and management) within the context of the history of slavery and ongoing oppression. The study would be planned with preschool-age children with sickle cell disease, their family members, and nurses providing care, all participating in the research process with the researcher as partners. For an emancipatory theorist and researcher, lack of participant input into the study design would be a grievous error.

Clinical Research Example: Violence Against Women

From a postpositivist approach, the most highly valued way to study violence against women would be an experimental design or randomized clinical trial. That investigation would be based on preliminary risk factor identification by case control, survey, or correlational designs and on theoretical derivation and testing, with theory testing and structural modeling designs predicated on descriptive investigations.

Qualitative data might be collected early in the investigation or as an adjunct to a primarily quantitative study. Qualitative data most likely would be analyzed by content analysis to develop categories for further quantitative analysis, to develop items to better quantitatively operationalize a relatively new or little-understood concept, or to further substantiate preliminary, small-sample pilot studies designed to justify a population-based study or a full clinical trial (Ford-Gilboe et al., 1995; Knafl et al., 1988). The most highly valued, gold-standard premises in postpositivist research are true experimental design (or randomized clinical trial), to establish internal validity and population-based random sampling, preferably national, to support external validity. Nursing research in this approach would identify risk factors for violence against women and for depression and other physical and mental sequelae of abuse. They might then use random assignment to standard interventions (e.g., referral to psychiatry or social work) or to a more comprehensive nursing intervention comprising lethality assessment, safety planning, and counseling (Campbell & Humphreys, 1993).

The effects of the intervention would be measured by including a combination of physiological (e.g., injury, stress-related physical problems, immune system), psychological (e.g., depression, self-esteem, self-efficacy), interpersonal (e.g., social support), and behavioral (e.g., self-care) outcomes to reflect the holistic nature of nursing concerns. The research, or nursing outcome studies, would be enhanced by process evaluation components with qualitative data. This aspect of research is important because the nursing intervention may involve responding to individual client concerns rather than following a detailed and highly standardized intervention protocol.

Research on battered women from the naturalistic approach would investigate in depth the physical, emotional, spiritual, and behavioral responses of women to being abused. Such studies would be directed at the entire context of women's experiences to better understand seemingly contradictory circumstances and behaviors, ambivalent feelings, the complex interactional processes between women and their partners, and women and their children and other family members and friends. Ethnonursing studies of abused women might try to determine caring behaviors that have been helpful to battered women as well as meanings of violence and health effects of battering within and across cultures. Longitudinal naturalistic and/or interpretive inquiries would be done to elucidate these processes over time. The researcher taking this approach might use a grounded theory to determine the processes by which women experience and respond to abuse (Landenberger, 1989; Wuest, 1994) or use naturalistic inquiry to elucidate how battered women and their children care for each other (Humphreys, 1991).

Interpretive design research, except for ethnography and ethnonursing, generally has not dealt overtly with culture and ethnicity. In fact, other methodologies from this perspective often have resulted in a selection of all White or almost all White samples because of small sample sizes and concerns for homogeneity.

Nursing studies from an empowerment or critical perspective might include collection of both quantitative and qualitative data, innovative implementation of experimental designs, and process evaluation with participants and practitioners as equal partners in the enterprise (Connell, Kubisch, Schorr, & Weiss, 1995; Gondolf, Yllö, & Campbell, 1997). In this model of intervention testing research, the researcher would take the role of a colearner, advocate, and translator of research to practitioners and practice realities to academicians, as well as facilitator of the program or practice setting to demonstrate its strengths and to discover what needs to be improved or discarded. Research in this perspective would be aimed at changing the systems that tend to contribute to women's victimization. This would include publishing how nursing practice should change, based on research. Explicit empowerment research would address that change as an overt part of the research process.

Critical or empowerment research would address the kinds of policy changes that are needed in the health care system. One such study might be to analyze the effects of mandatory reporting of abuse by health care professionals, a policy that is being initiated in the military and in California and is being considered in other states. From an empowerment perspective, such an investigation would involve the battered women themselves to help identify appropriate outcome measures and the means to keep women safe during the research process. It would include practicing nurses and other health care professionals as partners in the research process to better anticipate the pragmatic problems of such research. There are many important health, practice setting (e.g., patient satisfaction, autonomy, and confidentiality), and safety outcomes for women who are affected by this policy that nursing could fully consider in this kind of investigation. The results would be used to inform legislators and advocates as well as health care professionals about the prevention of violence and the progress of care for abused women.

Sociopolitical Influences on Contemporary Nursing Science

Just as the past 30 years have been a period of ferment in nursing theory and research, they have also been a time of major and sometimes revolutionary change in the health care system. In considering how nursing research may make the greatest progress over the next decade, it is useful to consider the social context in which nursing research is and will be conducted.

Some of the major factors that will influence health care research over the next decade are

continued allocation of the lion's share of the research dollar to postpositivist research;

increased proportion of funding from the private sector;

increased emphasis on interdisciplinary research;

continued recognition of the limited science base for health care practices, with corresponding efforts to rationalize care and emphasize what is effective in producing desirable patient outcomes; and

increased ability to manage large data sets and to synthesize results of multiple studies using a diversity of research designs.

Recognition of these factors influencing health care research should help to shape the philosophical approaches taken in clinical nursing research.

Although there has been an increase in the amount of federal research dollars allocated to alternative approaches in health care research, the amount allocated has been minuscule in comparison to that allocated to traditional biomedical science. Within traditional science, major emphasis continues to be placed on the physiological, biochemical, and molecular sciences, with a few institutes in the NIH gradually increasing their budgets for the behavioral sciences. In the National Institute of Nursing Research (1997), there has been a recent tendency to emphasize traditional biomedical approaches and problems more strongly and to move away from the broader nursing focus on families, self-care, and classification and study of nursing phenomena that characterized the institute's (center's) early research programs. This emphasis on biomedical research is not likely to change dramatically over the next decade, and careful thought must be given to how nursing can move forward with diverse philosophical approaches in this funding climate. One way is to understand the commonalities in the diversity and learn how to frame the problems and their solutions so that they can be recognized as areas of importance that merit funding.

Two important factors related to health research are the many agencies within the federal government that support research and the gradual change in the proportion

of research funded by private sources rather than by the federal government. Although the NIH is considered to be the mainstream of the federal health research enterprise, there are many other organizational entities within the federal government that support health care research and research training. These include the Agency for Health Care Policy and Research (AHCPR), the Centers for Disease Control (CDC), the Department of Veterans Affairs (VA), and others. Additionally, there has been an increase in the amount of support for health research from the private sector, including foundations and industry. Depending on the ideologies of the policy makers and proposal reviewers in these private organizations, various philosophical approaches will be more or less congruent with their funding priorities and practices. The implication for nursing of the diversity in funding sources and priorities is that a diversity of philosophical approaches should increase the overall opportunities for success in achieving needed financial support for nursing research. For some time to come, for example, a postpositivist approach will be required throughout much of the NIH and other federal research programs, although the National Institute for Nursing Research (when first established), the Office of Alternative Medicine, and other NIH entities have funded some interpretive studies. In contrast, some private foundations fund programs that are more consistent with a critical approach, in that they encourage innovation, use of multiple methods, and working closely with the target population in an effort to improve conditions for various vulnerable inner-city and other groups with limited power bases.

A third major factor influencing health research is its increasingly interdisciplinary nature. This mirrors the increase in interdisciplinary practice, as evidenced by the use of clinical protocols, clinical pathways, benchmarking, clinical algorithms, clinical practice guidelines, and other efforts to specify more precisely what care should be given to a patient with a specific condition over time. These pathways and guidelines often do not distinguish among the various types of providers who deliver the care.

Interdisciplinary protocols, pathways, and guidelines raise two issues of importance for the development of scientific knowledge for practice: how to address the problem of providing standardized care in most situations while simultaneously acknowledging the need for individualization in care. Both generalizability and individuality are necessary in science and in practice. The 17th-century philosophers believed that it was possible to develop laws of science that could achieve perfect predictability of behavior. Subsequent philosophers and scientists have recognized the multiple biochemical, physical, psychological, sociocultural, and environmental factors that interact to influence human behavior and that make the precise prediction, or even the retrospective explanation, of the behavior of a specific individual in a specific set of circumstances difficult. Although research can provide the ability to make generalizations about human behavior, the nurse must use professional judgment to consider how these generalizations apply to a specific patient. For example, through research we know the dosages of morphine that generally provide relief to patients in pain. Because of physiologic differences in response to morphine, the development of tolerance, attitudes toward the use of opiates, and multiple other physiological and sociocultural factors, an evidence-based drug table of morphine dosages can provide only the appropriate range of dosage. The clinician must use this guideline and assessment of an individual patient to determine what works best in this particular situation. Additionally, interpretive research could provide insights in understanding the meaning of pain and how that may influence patients' responses to morphine and other drugs. Viewing philosophical approaches to research as complementary rather than as opposing should help to clarify how to identify the commonalities in an illness experience and, at the same time, understand the unique meaning of health-related experiences to individual patients. The need is to understand how to use different philosophical approaches to develop better knowledge for improving patient care.

The second issue raised by interdisciplinary practice and research is how nurse researchers can contribute to the interdisciplinary fund of knowledge yet preserve nursing's identity in science. There has been considerable discussion in the nursing literature regarding the extent to which nursing theory and research are unique and to what extent nursing theory borrows from and is related to theories of other disciplines. The substantial overlap in the practice of health care disciplines has implications for the body of knowledge underlying the practice of those disciplines.

It is possible to be interdisciplinary and yet preserve nursing's identity by taking care that nursing's perspective is emphasized in interdisciplinary research and practice and that the totality of the theory and research is brought back into nursing. An example of this is the U.S. Agency for Health Care Policy and Research's *Management of Cancer Pain: Clinical Practice Guidelines No. 9*

(Jacox et al., 1994). The guidelines were developed by an interdisciplinary group of researchers and clinicians who focused not on who does what with patients but on what knowledge is available to guide the best pain management practices. Nurses contributed to the development of the guidelines by focusing on those areas of practice of greatest concern to nurses, which included assessment; the use of both pharmacological and non-pharmacological approaches; and concern with patient teaching, discharge planning, and quality improvement programs. Although the nursing perspective is clearly represented in the cancer pain guidelines, it is not explicitly identified as nursing research, theory, or practice. Rather, it is included as part of an interdisciplinary body of knowledge that underlies the practice of health professionals. It is likely that, without substantial nursing input, the guidelines would have been more narrowly focused on the pharmacological and physiological aspects of care. Although some nurses will be interested in other aspects of pain management, such as radiation and neurosurgical techniques, theory and research in these areas are not generally of prime interest to nurses. It should be possible for nurses to participate in interdisciplinary research and theory development not by insisting on uniqueness and use of a different language but by emphasizing the core dimensions of nursing.

When nurses engage in interdisciplinary research, there is a need to be sure that the nursing perspective is represented and visible and that the results of the interdisciplinary research are brought back into nursing through its publications. Often when interdisciplinary or team research is conducted, members of the various disciplines represented take those parts of the research that have the most interest and relevance for their discipline and publish them in their disciplinary journals. The broader overview of the research may be published in interdisciplinary journals or in sophisticated lay journals aimed at broader audiences, but the more detailed aspects of the research and the detailed data analyses are published in the disciplinary journals. Thus, it is important that nurses involved in interdisciplinary research publish in interdisciplinary journals as part of the research team and that they also publish in nursing journals.

Another set of factors that will influence the focus of clinical research in the next decade is the increased awareness of how little health care practice is actually based on science. Estimates of the amount of medical practice based on science range from 1% to 20% (Perry, quoted in Subcommittee on Education and Health, 1989).

The research done over the past 20 years by John Wennberg (1988) and others, showing the tremendous variations in medical practice for patients with, presumably, the same conditions, and the work of David Eddy (1994), showing the lack of a science base for much of medical practice, emphasize the weaknesses in the science base for medicine. The need to use resources more cost-effectively in health care, combined with recognition of the amount of uncertainty that underlies practice, has given rise to what has been called the effectiveness/outcomes initiative in health care research. This initiative challenges health care professionals to develop and refine more effective methods of achieving desirable patient outcomes, such as reduced illness, increased comfort, reduced complications, and improvement in patients' understanding of their condition and treatment. In a sense, clinical and health services researchers across disciplines are now consciously and politically focused on what nursing has been trying to do for the past 30 or more years—develop a scientific knowledge base for practice.

A factor that will influence nursing research in the near future is the increasing ability to collect and manage large data sets. The revolutionary developments in computer technology have made it possible to collect and analyze data on a scale never before possible. Both the public and private health care sectors are rapidly developing their capacity to collect and use data to monitor health care and to understand better how multiple factors influence health care delivery, costs, and patient outcomes. Efforts are under way to learn how to merge various databases across public and private sectors and to understand the subsequent implications. Increasingly, attempts are made to standardize the kind of health care data collected, to merge clinical and administrative databases, and to use databases on an ongoing basis to manage patient outcomes.

The availability of large and complex databases and the capacity to relate them to each other will make it possible to combine data from multiple sources. How they are combined and what data are used can best be guided by nursing theories that identify phenomena of importance to nursing care. The ability to relate nursing problems and interventions to nursing-sensitive patient outcomes will be dependent on ensuring that nursing-relevant data are included in the databases (American Nurses Association, 1995). Just as nursing theory can guide the data elements to be included, the availability of large, complex data sets relevant to nursing should enable more rapid testing and revision of specific nursing theo-

ries. Although there are many factors in the present sociopolitical environment that will influence nursing theory, research, and practice, those discussed above are some of the key factors.

Implications for Clinical Nursing Research

In concordance with others, we advocate diversity and plurality in nursing philosophy, science, research methods, and practice (Meleis, 1991). As Shaw (1993) states,

> Not only is adoption of a specific perspective unlikely in a discipline that understands multidimensional, complex human behavior, but theoretical consensus is quite unlikely in a discipline that values the role of perceptions, uniqueness, and individuality in health and illness. (p. 1652)

Focusing less on homogeneity and more on the creative diversity of multiple philosophical approaches may enhance the scientific value of nursing research and result in new methods to address the health needs of all people (Ford-Gilboe et al., 1995).

Nursing can use the philosophical diversity to develop a more comprehensive knowledge base, increase nurses' understanding of health problems, and promote understanding of how to effect desired changes in preventing or managing health problems. Through the increased use of middle-range theory to guide research, nurses can produce results useful in a variety of clinical populations and settings. Middle-range theories are sufficiently abstract to extend beyond a specific place, time, or population, yet specific enough and sufficiently close to empirical data to guide research and interventions.

There are many factors in the current sociopolitical environment that support the need for diverse philosophical approaches in the conduct of clinical nursing research. There is increased awareness of the lack of research underlying the management of many health problems, with calls for evidence-based practice. This is accompanied by greater acceptance by consumers and health care providers of alternatives to traditional, biomedically based care.

A sensitivity to these and other factors, as described, will enable nurses to use and contribute to the knowledge underlying the practice of health professionals generally while simultaneously paying particular attention to the visibility of the nursing perspective in multidisciplinary research and practice.

Notes

1. See, for example, Merton (1968), pp. 50-53, 56-62, and especially the Summary on pp. 68-69. On page 60, he tells us that the most

thoroughgoing and detailed analysis of the nature of middle-range theories is Zeterberg (1965), which is an expansion of an earlier 1961 article in German.

2. The notion of logical derivation here is that of deductive derivation within an axiomatic system and should not be confused with the analogical sorts of derivations discussed in Walker and Avant (1995), which is the more common usage of *derivation* in nursing science.

3. See Merton (1968), p. 68.

4. See pages 6-114 of Suppe (1977) for detailed characterizations of the positivistic received view and the objections that led to its rejection.

References

Allen, D. G. (1985). Nursing research and social control: Alternative models of science that emphasize understanding and emancipation. *Image: Journal of Nursing Scholarship, 17,* 58-64.

Allen, D. G., Benner, P., & Diekelmann, N. L. (1986). Three paradigms for nursing research: Methodological implications. In P. Chinn (Ed.), *Nursing research methodology: Issues and implementation* (pp. 59-65). Rockville, MD: Aspen.

American Nurses Association. (1995). *An emerging framework: Data system advances for clinical nursing practice.* Washington, DC: American Nurses Publishing.

Beck, C. T. (1985). Theoretical frameworks cited in *Nursing Research* from January, 1974–June, 1985. *Nurse Educator, 10*(6), 36-38.

Blendon, R. J., Aiken, L. H., Freeman, H. E., & Corey, C. R. (1989). Access to medical care for Black and White Americans: A matter of continuing concern. *Journal of the American Medical Association, 261,* 278-81.

Bunting, S., & Campbell, J. C. (1994). Through a feminist lens: A model to guide nursing reseach. In P. Chinn (Ed.), *Advances in methods of inquiry for nursing* (pp. 75-87). Gaithersburg, MD: Aspen.

Campbell, J. C., & Bunting, S. (1991). Voices and paradigms: Perspectives on critical and feminist theory in nursing. *Advances in Nursing Science, 13,* 1-15.

Campbell, J. C., & Humphreys, J. (1993). *Nursing care of survivors of family violence.* St. Louis, MO: Mosby.

Carnap, R. (1953). Testability and meaning. In H. Feigl & M. Brodbeck (Eds.), *Readings in the philosophy of science* (pp. 47-92). New York: Appleton-Century-Crofts.

Chinn, P., & Wheeler, C. (1985). Feminism and nursing: Can nursing afford to remain aloof from the women's movement? *Nursing Outlook, 33,* 74-77.

Cleeland, C. S., Gonin, R., Hatfield, A. K., Edmonson, J. H., Blum, R. H., Stewart, J. A., & Pandya, K. J. (1994). Pain and pain treatment in outpatients with metastatic cancer: The Eastern Cooperative Oncology Group's Outpatient Pain Study. *New England Journal of Medicine, 330,* 592-596.

Connell, J. P., Kubisch, A. C., Schorr, L. B., & Weiss, C. H. (1995). *New approaches to evaluating community initiatives.* Washington, DC: Aspen Institute.

Cox, C. L. (1982). An interaction model of client health behavior: A theoretical prescription for nursing. *Advances in Nursing Science, 5*(1), 41-56.

Denyes, M., & Villarruel, A. (1988, July). *Measurement of pain in Afro-American and Hispanic children.* Paper presented at the First International Symposium on Pediatric Pain, Seattle, WA.

Eddy, D. L. (1994). Variations in physician practice: The role of uncertainty. *Health Affairs, 3*(2), 74-89.

Fawcett, J. (1993). From a plethora of paradigms to parsimony in world views. *Nurse Science Quarterly, 6*(2), 56-58.

Feyerabend, P. (1975). *Against method.* New York: Schocken.

Ford-Gilboe, M., Campbell, J., & Berman, H. (1995). Stories and numbers: Co-existence without compromise. *Advances in Nursing Science, 18,* 14-26.

Freire, P. (1970). *Pedagogy of the oppressed.* New York: Seabury Press.

Frey, M. (1995). Toward a theory of families, children and chronic illness. In M. A. Frey & C. Sieloff (Eds.), *Advancing King's systems framework and theory of nursing* (pp. 109-125). Thousand Oaks, CA: Sage.

Gioia, D. A., & Pitre, E. (1990). Multiparadigm perspectives on theory building. *Academy of Management Review, 15,* 584-602.

Gondolf, E., Yllö, K., & Campbell, J. (1997). Collaboration between researchers and advocates. In G. Kantor & J. Jasinski (Eds.), *Out of the darkness: Contemporary perspectives on family violence.* Thousand Oaks, CA: Sage.

Guba, E. G. (Ed.). (1990). *The paradigm dialog.* Newbury Park, CA: Sage.

Hegyvary, S. (1992). From truth to relativism: Paradigms for doctoral education. In *Proceedings of the 1992 Annual Forum on Doctoral Nursing Education. Nursing as a human science: Prevailing paradigms and their implications for preparing nurse scientists* (pp. 1-13). Baltimore: University of Maryland at Baltimore.

Henderson, D. (1995). Consciousness raising in participatory research: Method and methodology for emancipatory nursing inquiry. *Advances in Nursing Science, 17,* 58-69.

Humphreys, J. C. (1991). The children of battered women: Worries about their mothers. *Pediatric Nursing, 17,* 343-345, 354.

Jacox, A. (1970). Issues in theory construction. In C. M. Norris (Ed.), *Proceedings: First Nursing Theory Conference* (pp. 111-113). Kansas City: University of Kansas Medical Center.

Jacox, A. (1993). Estimates of the supply and demand for doctorally prepared nurses. *Nursing Outlook, 41,* 43-45.

Jacox, A., Carr, D. B., Payne, R., Berde, C. B., Brietbart, W., Cain, J. M., Chapman, C. R., Cleeland, C. S., Ferrell, B. R., Finley, R. S., Hester, N. O., Hill, C. S., Leak, W. D., Lipman, A. G., Logan, C. L., McGarvey, C. L., Miaskowski, C. A., Mulder, D. S., Paice, J. A., Shapiro, B. S., Silberstein, E. B., Smith, R. S., Stover, J., Tsou, C. V., Vecchiarelli, L., & Weissman, D. E. (1994). *Management of cancer pain: Clinical practice guidelines No. 9* (AHCPR Pub. No. 94-0592). Rockville, MD: Agency for Health

Care Policy and Research, Public Health Service, U.S. Department of Health and Human Services.

Jacox, A., & Stewart, M. G. (1973). *Psychosocial contingencies of the pain experience.* Iowa City: College of Nursing, University of Iowa.

Knafl, K., Pettengill, M., Bevis, M., & Kirchoff, K. (1988). Blending qualitative and quantitative approaches to instrument development and data collection. *Journal of Professional Nursing, 88,* 30-37.

Landenberger, K. (1989). A process of entrapment in recovery from an abusive relationship. *Issues in Mental Health Nursing, 3,* 309-327.

Laudan, L. (1977). *Progress and its problems.* Berkeley: University of California Press.

Leininger, M. (1994). Evaluation criteria and critique of qualitative research studies. In J. M. Morse (Ed.), *Critical issues in qualitative research studies* (pp. 95-115). Thousand Oaks, CA: Sage.

Lenz, E. R., Suppe, E., Gift, A. G., Pugh, L. C., & Milligan, R. A. (1995). Collaborative development of middle-range nursing theories: Toward a theory of unpleasant symptoms. *Advances in Nursing Science, 17*(3), 1-13.

MacPherson, J. (1985). Osteoporosis and menopause: A feminist analysis of the social construction of a syndrome. *Advances in Nursing Science, 7,* 11-12.

Meleis, A. I. (1991). *Theoretical nursing: Development and progress* (2nd ed.). Philadelphia, PA: Lippincott.

Merton, R. K. (1957). *Social theory and social structure.* Glencoe, IL: Free Press.

Merton, R. K. (1968). On sociological theories of the middle range. In R. K. Merton (Ed.), *Social theory and social structure* (2nd ed., pp. 39-72). New York: Free Press.

Mischel, M. H. (1990). Reconceptualization of the uncertainty in illness theory. *Image, 22*(4), 256-62.

Moccia, P. (1988). A critique of compromise: Beyond the methods debate. *Advances in Nursing Science, 10,* 1-9.

Mood, L. E., Wilson, M. E., Smith, R., Schwartz, R., Tittle, M., & Van Cott, M. L. (1988). Analysis of a decade of nursing practice research, 1977-1986. *Nursing Research, 37,* 374-379.

Morrison, R., & Vedro, D. (1989). Pain management in the child with sickle cell disease. *Pediatric Nursing, 15,* 595-599.

Morse, J. M., & Johnson, H. K. (1991). *The illness experience: Dimensions of suffering.* Newbury Park, CA: Sage.

National Institute for Nursing Research. (1997). *Extramural research programming: Areas of science.* Retrieved November 24, 1998 from the World Wide Web: http://www.nih.gov/ninr/function.htm

Newman, M. A. (1994). Theory for nursing practice. *Nursing Science Quarterly, 7,* 153-157.

Norris, C. M. (Ed.). (1970). *Proceedings: First Nursing Theory Conference.* Kansas City: University of Kansas Medical Center.

Norris, C. M. (Ed.). (1971). *Proceedings: Second Nursing Theory Conference.* Kansas City: University of Kansas Medical Center.

Norris, C. M. (Ed.). (1972). *Proceedings: Third Nursing Theory Conference.* Kansas City: University of Kansas Medical Center.

O'Brien, M. E. (1983). *The courage to survive: The life career of the chronic dialysis patient.* New York: Grune & Stratton.

Parse, R. R. (1987). *Nursing science: Major paradigms, theories and critiques.* Philadelphia: W. B. Saunders.

Pender, N. (1996). *Health promotion in nursing practice* (3rd ed.). Stanford, CT: Appleton & Lange.

Platt, O. S., Thorington, B. D., & Brambilla, D. J. (1991). Pain in sickle cell disease: Rates and risk factors. *New England Journal of Medicine, 325,* 11-16.

Porter, C., & Villarruel, A. M. (1993). Nursing research with African-American and Hispanic people: Guidelines for action. *Nursing Outlook, 41,* 59-67.

Schumacher, K., & Gortner, S. (1992). (Mis)conceptions and reconceptions about traditional science. *Advances in Nursing Science, 14,* 1-11.

Shapiro, B. (1993). Management of painful episodes in sickle cell disease. In N. Schechter, C. Berde, & M. Yaster (Eds.), *Pain in infants, children, and adolescents* (pp. 385-409). Baltimore, MD: Williams & Wilkins.

Shapiro, B., Dinges, D. F., Ohene-Frempong, K., & Orne, M. T. (1990). Recording of crisis pain in sickle cell disease. In D. Tyler & E. Krane (Eds.), *Advances in pain research and therapy* (pp. 313-321). New York: Roden.

Shaw, M. C. (1993). The discipline of nursing: Historical roots, current perspectives, future directions. *Journal of Advanced Nursing, 18,* 1651-1656.

Skrtic, T. (1990). Social accommodation: Toward a dialogical discourse in educational inquiry. In E. G. Guba (Ed.), *The paradigm dialog* (pp. 125-135). Newbury Park, CA: Sage.

Subcommittee on Education and Health, Joint Economic Committee, U.S. Congress. (1989). *Medical alert* (Staff Report S.PRT, pp. 101-151). Washington, DC: Government Printing Office.

Suppe, F. (1977). *The structure of scientific theories* (2nd ed.). Chicago: University of Chicago Press.

Suppe, F. (1989). *The semantic conception of theories and scientific realism.* Urbana: University of Illinois Press.

Suppe, F. (1992). Paradigms, socialization and nursing science. In *Proceedings of the 1992 Annual Forum on Nursing Doctoral Education. Nursing as a human science: Prevailing paradigms and their implications for preparing nurse scientists* (pp. 17-34). Baltimore: University of Maryland at Baltimore.

Thompson, J. L. (1987). Critical scholarship: The critique of domination in nursing. *Advances in Nursing Science, 10,* 27-38.

Villarruel, A., & Denyes, M. (1991). Pain assessment in children: Theoretical and empirical validity. *Advances in Nursing Science, 14,* 32-41.

Walker, L., & Avant, K. (1995). *Strategies for theory construction in nursing* (3rd ed.). Norwalk, CT: Appleton & Lange.

Webster, G., & Jacox, A. (1985). Toward the liberation of nursing theory. In J. McCloskey & H. Grace (Eds.), *Contemporary issues in nursing* (2nd ed.). Boston: Blackwell Scientific.

Wennberg, J. C. (1988, Spring). Improving the medical decision-making process. *Health Affairs, 7*(1), 99-106.

Wuest, J., 1994. A feminist approach to concept analysis. *Western Journal of Nursing Research, 16*(5), 577-586.

Zeterberg, H. J. (1965). *On theory and verification in sociology* (3rd ed.). Totawa, NJ: Bedminster.

2

EVOLVING NURSING RESEARCH TRADITIONS
Influencing Factors

Ada Sue Hinshaw

Nursing knowledge and research has expanded rapidly in the past several decades. The profession's commitment to the development of systematically generated knowledge to guide nursing practice has been the driving force for the growth of nursing research coupled with a strengthened national infrastructure and set of resources to support such knowledge generation. Several basic characteristics of the discipline have supported the commitment to a strong, focused, scientifically based body of knowledge for nursing practice:

- definition of the science of nursing as a "human" science, reflecting the human aspects of dealing with health and illnesses;
- strong emphasis on understanding and explaining the actual practice of nursing to achieve optimal outcomes for patients, families, and communities;
- commitment to develop knowledge to empower clients, nurses, and the discipline; and
- High value placed on understanding the client or consumer's experiences for the purpose of optimizing health care and health promotion (adapted from Meleis, 1992).

Major shifts in health care during the mid-1990s have also enhanced the importance of nursing knowledge and practice, given the contribution that nursing can make to the health of the American public. These shifts include the strong emphasis on health promotion and community-based care, with which nursing has a long history; the drastic increase in the number of individuals and families living with chronic illnesses, which draws on nursing's experience with long-term care issues; and the heightened need for knowledgeable, well-prepared

19

professionals to provide care for clients in hospitals with ever-increasing intense and complex requirements.

A number of nursing research traditions have rapidly matured during this era of expanding nursing knowledge. Multiple factors have contributed to the research traditions coming to fruition. Laudan defines research traditions in a narrow sense to include only the methods of scientific inquiry used within a discipline (Gorenberg, 1983). The concept of *research traditions* is used more broadly in this chapter to refer to established and evolving patterns of behavior that are characteristic of and "accepted" expectations within the discipline of nursing (Hinshaw, 1996). This is in keeping with the general definition of the term *tradition,* that is, an established custom or practice that has the effect of an unwritten or generally accepted law.

The purpose of this chapter is to examine the "accepted" research traditions that have evolved in the recent history of the discipline of nursing and to consider future developing traditions. These nursing research traditions are examined within the context of the factors that have facilitated their growth.

First, the national infrastructure and resource factors that have supported the rapid expansion of nursing knowledge and research as well as the evolution of the nursing research traditions are addressed. Second, nursing research traditions are considered in relation to the specific factors influencing their evolution. Third, future directions for new nursing research traditions that are needed are discussed.

National Infrastructure and Resource Factors

A number of national infrastructure and resource factors have influenced the rapid growth of nursing research and research traditions in the past decades. The major factor was the establishment of the National Center for Nursing Research (NCNR) in April 1986 and its redesignation as the National Institute of Nursing Research (NINR) in 1993 (Hinshaw & Merritt, 1988; Merritt, 1986). However, this hallmark event could not have occurred without several other events having been accomplished. Several national professional organizational factors were critical in the development of nursing research and the NINR: the development of a community of nurse scholars within the profession, an understanding

and commitment to nursing research by the broader nursing profession, and a unified commitment by the major nursing professional organizations for political action. Furthermore, the profession could not have been optimally productive with the resources and facilitation provided by the NINR without the strong nursing research and clinical specialist infrastructures that had been developed by the Division of Nursing (DN), Health Services Resources Agency (HSRA), Department of Health and Human Services (DHHS), United States Government since its inception in 1952 (Gortner, 1973).

National professional organizational factors. Several major professional organizational factors influenced the creation of the major national resource for nursing research, the NINR. One factor that evolved over several decades is the development of a community of nursing scholars with a strong commitment to the generation of a knowledge base for nursing practice and the translation of that knowledge to practitioners to promote evidence-based practice. This community development was facilitated by the position statements and ever-increasing numbers of scientific conferences and seminar activities of organizations such as the American Nurses Association's (ANA's) Cabinet and Council of Nursing Research and Sigma Theta Tau International. Sigma Theta Tau International conferences especially emphasized the partnership required between clinical nursing leaders and researchers in transferring research findings into professional practice. Such endeavors provided the forum for scientific debate and dialogue, critique of the research studies being conducted, and stimulation of new directions for nursing research.

The research conferences provided the structure for the development of a scientific community that allowed for collegial support among the nurse scientists who were pioneering the early research programs. The scientific community also facilitated the definition and importance of nursing research. Scholars in the discipline, such as Gortner (1983; Gortner & Schultz, 1988), addressed the important characteristics of a scientific community and thus helped make explicit what needed to be developed. Vital scientific community characteristics such as collegiality, communality, and constructive competition have evolved. Collegiality refers to the intellectual and colleague support for conducting, disseminating, and applying research among scholars. Communality involves the constructive review and critique of colleagues' scientific endeavors with the intent of enhancing the quality and accuracy of the science as well as generating new ideas for further study. Constructive competition acknowledges the natural advancement and ownership of scientific ideas by various scientists and urges sensitivity in handling the competition among researchers in a constructive manner to further nursing science as well as individual careers (Hinshaw, 1992). The scholarly communities have been formally established at the university or local level, the regional level (e.g., Eastern Nursing Research Society, Midwest Nursing Research Society, Southern Nursing Research Society, and the Western Nursing Research Society) and the national level, with, for example, the early ANA Council of Nurse Researchers conferences, and internationally by the multicountry research conferences sponsored by Sigma Theta Tau, the International Council of Nurses (ICN), ANA, and a number of specialty organizations (Stevenson, 1987).

The ANA initiated several organizational structures that advanced and facilitated nursing research:

- The Cabinet and Council of Nursing Research have changed in structure over the years but the basic purpose remains unchanged: the promotion and facilitation of nursing research to provide a knowledge base for the practice of the profession. Their endeavors have resulted in position statements such as the "ANA Blueprint for Nursing Research" (1962) and the two policy statements "Directions for Nursing Research: Toward the 21st Century," published in 1985 and updated in 1997. These policy statements have provided important direction for the research programs of the members of the scientific community. The 1985 policy statement outlined 11 areas for nursing research, ranging from promoting health and well-being, to minimizing the negative consequences of treatment on individuals and families with acute and/or chronic health problems, to designing and testing different models for health care delivery. The 1997 directions statement reaffirmed the professions' commitment to clinical nursing research and cited the increased need to focus on health care and patient outcomes, balancing quality of care issues with costs. In addition, the Cabinet and Council activities have heightened the visibility of nursing research with professional practitioners and policy makers in terms of the importance of nursing research.

- The first scientific journal for the discipline, *Nursing Research,* was established in 1952 through the American Journal of Nursing Company that is the publishing arm of the ANA. This publication provided a critical communication forum for the discipline and specifically the scientific community.

- The ANA Political Action Committee was formed. It consists of an organizational coordinating body, policy advisory body, and a grassroots network of professionals in the legislative districts of the country. The purpose of this organization is to communicate and exert influence on national political policy makers about important health and nursing issues. This organizational network has been critical in informing both congresspersons and practicing nurses about nursing research and its value to the public's health.

A number of other organizations have also established such political action structures to inform and shape the decisions of policy makers; for example, the American Association of Colleges of Nursing (AACN), the National League for Nursing (NLN), the American Organization of Nurse Executives (AONE), the National Organization of Nurse Practitioners (NONP), the Oncology Nursing Society (ONS), and the American Association of Critical Care Nurses (AACN). Each of the organizations has focused on nursing research and its impact on the health of the public as part of its agenda, which greatly enhanced the visibility of nursing research.

These organizational structures have led to a greater understanding and commitment to nursing research by the broader nursing profession. The major general nursing organizations unified to form the Tri-Council. Originally, the organizations included the ANA, the American Association of Colleges of Nursing (AACN), and the NLN. Later, the Tri-Council expanded to include the American Organization of Nurse Executives (AONE) but retained its organizational title. The purpose of the Tri-Council has been consistent: to study issues and concerns of common interest across the organizations and provide concrete unified plans, positions, and actions for such issues. The Tri-Council adopts common policies on political actions of interest to nursing and health care so that nursing speaks with a unified voice to Congress and other policy makers. The opportunity to create a National Institute of Nursing (earlier called the National Center for Nursing Research) at the National Institutes of Health was such a common interest, and it required extensive political action.

With the professional nursing association structures in place to enhance the visibility and importance of research for practice, the profession was able to take advantage of a breakthrough opportunity to develop a national structure to support and advance the science of the discipline. This opportunity consisted of a congressperson, Representative Edward Madigan (R-Illinois), who wished to sponsor a National Institute of Nursing (NIN) as part of the National Institutes of Health (NIH). The Tri-Council agreed to lead this initiative, with the ANA Cabinet on Nursing Research heavily involved. All of the organizational legislative offices and political action networks were committed to this endeavor. Nursing research and its critical importance to nursing practice of all types was an issue all the organizations could support and facilitate. Working with Congress and the various professional organizations in a strong unified stance for nursing research, the profession was successful in moving nursing research into the mainstream of health care research at the NIH (Merritt, 1986).

The establishment of nursing research within the NIH was crucial for the development of the scientific base of the discipline within a strong, enriched, interdisciplinary environment that was financially stable. This move recognized nursing research as an important area of science and health care that needed to be a federal responsibility and initiative with stronger support and resources. In essence, this was a national legitimization of nursing research as a critical field of health science.

Federal resources for building nursing research. The dramatic growth in nursing research that occurred with the establishment of the NCNR/NINR in 1986 built on the strong foundations developed by the Division of Nursing (DN) at HRSA. From 1955 on, a research and research training section with allocated federal funds existed at the DN (Gortner & Nahm, 1977; Salmon, 1997). A number of federal award programs were provided to support the evolution of nursing research, including developing faculty to conduct research, establishing the core infrastructures in schools of nursing such as offices or centers for nursing research, enhancing the doctoral programs in nursing, and building the pool of clinical specialists and nurse scientists needed to generate nursing knowledge.

Three DN award programs facilitated the development of faculty in schools of nursing:

- The Faculty Research Development Grant (FaRDeg) program, initiated in 1959, provided resources to increase faculty skills for participating in research and supported small studies (Batey, 1978).
- The Research Development Grant program (RDG) was the second institutional program to promote research in nursing. These awards built on the prior faculty development and focused on the generation of

research studies and infrastructures to sustain research productivity in schools of nursing such as offices or centers for nursing research. Batey's (1978) classic evaluation of this program, "Research Development in University Schools of Nursing," illustrated the importance of such infrastructures in increasing and maintaining research productivity as evident through successful extramural funding and publications of faculty.

- The Enhancement of Doctoral Programs in Nursing program was a third set of awards provided to advance the research programs of faculty in schools offering doctoral preparation in nursing. The intent was to further advance faculty research programs, the scientific environment, and the mentored experiences of individuals enrolled in such programs (Salmon, 1997).

The DN, through the research branch, also offered support for nurses seeking doctoral preparation in nursing or in other related disciplines. Several different types of research training awards were provided:

- The Special Research Fellowship program for doctoral study was an award offered to support individual nurses seeking doctoral preparation. It was made available in 1955 as part of the initial federal funding of nursing research (Gortner & Nahm, 1977).
- The Nurse Scientist Program, initiated in 1962, provided institutional grants for research training to schools of nursing that developed collaborative educational arrangements with selected biological and behavioral science departments of their universities. Under this program, the nurse fellows studied and received their earned doctorates from the interdisciplinary departments such as physiology, sociology, psychology and anthropology. The intent of the program was for these individuals to return to schools of nursing to serve as faculty for the evolving doctoral programs in the discipline (Batey, 1978).
- The National Research Service Award Programs (NRSA) provided and continues to fund individual and institutional grants for the support of doctoral and postdoctoral preparation. This broad program offered federal support for the preparation of scientists in multiple disciplines, including nursing. Due to limited resources, the DN primarily funded individual fellowships for doctoral preparation. The increased funding of institutional NRSA training grants and for postdoctoral preparation occurred with the establishment of the NCNR/NINR and the influx of additional funds (Hinshaw, 1992).

TABLE 2.1 National Nursing Research Agenda

Phase I (1989-1994)	Phase II (1995-1999)
Prevention and care of low birth weight infants and mothers	Community-based nursing models
Prevention and care of individuals with human immunodeficiency virus (HIV) infection	Effectiveness of nursing interventions in HIV/AIDS
Long-term care of older persons	Cognitive impairment
Symptom management: Acute pain	Living with chronic illness
Information systems: Improvement of patient care	Biobehavioral factors related to immunocompetence
Health promotion of children and adolescents	

These programs generated the cadre of nurse investigators who assumed the faculty leadership positions in schools of nursing and developed beginning research programs to generate knowledge for the discipline. Without this pool of prepared researchers, the NINR's award programs to support the conduct of clinical nursing research would have been far less productive. Because the cadre of nurse scientists existed, the NINR support and resources could be effectively used to advance the science required for nursing practice.

For a number of years, the DN has also supported the preparation of clinical nurse specialists through the Professional Nurse Training Program. This has facilitated the development of a pool of clinical experts who are vital in generating strong, relevant nursing research and in transferring the findings of nursing investigations into practice. This was another critical foundation for the conduct and use of nursing research.

Establishment of the National Institute of Nursing Research

On April 16, 1986, the National Center for Nursing Research (NCNR) was established within the National Institutes of Health (NIH), after 2 years of legislative processes that resulted in a compromise from a National Institute of Nursing to a National Center for Nursing Research. The legislatively stated purpose of the NCNR/NINR is "the conduct and support of, and dissemination of information respecting, basic and clinical nursing research, training, and other programs in patient care research" (Health Research Extension Act of 1985). McBride (1987) suggested that the "placement of an institute of nursing in the NIH would greatly improve both

communication about the largest health care profession to other disciplines and the flow of information about NIH priorities to nursing and would ultimately bring nurses into the setting of national research priorities" (p. 2). The NCNR was redesignated the National Institute of Nursing Research (NINR) in June 1993, using unified organizational political action strategies similar to those used from 1984 to 1986. In addition, a formal process supporting the redesignation was generated by the NIH and the DHHS Executive Branch.

The mission of the NINR is to facilitate national programs of nursing research and promote excellence in the knowledge base developed for the profession. Essentially, the organization serves as the focal point for federal support of nursing research and research training (Health Research Extension Act of 1985). The NINR mission is consistent with the broader National Institutes of Health mission, which is to improve the health of the American public by advancing knowledge pertaining to human health and disease processes.

In the initial years, several leadership initiatives of the NINR staff greatly enhanced the development of excellence in the evolving science for nursing practice. These initiatives included identifying nursing research priorities with the scientific community, developing a trajectory for research training and career development, increasing collaborative interdisciplinary research endeavors, and enhancing international research expansion for the nursing discipline (Hinshaw, 1990; Hinshaw, Heinrich, & Bloch, 1988).

The National Nursing Research Agenda (NNRA) consisted, from 1989 to 1999, of the nursing research priorities developed with the nursing scientific community that partially guided the first 10 years of major research programming and funding by the NINR (Hinshaw, Heinrich, & Bloch, 1988). Two phases of the NNRA were developed, identifying major public health issues and concerns that nursing could influence given a solid base of research (Bloch, 1990). The priorities were organized within those two phases (Table 2.1).

These priorities focused the clinical nursing research endeavors of the nurse scientists and targeted the growing but still limited funding resources available to support nursing research. Focusing on selected priorities promoted depth in the specific clinical areas of study. Historically, due to the lack of resources, nursing research tended to be scattered, with a limited number of studies related to a particular area of study. Focusing on an identified priority and providing funds for research in that area resulted in multiple studies and substantiated results across investigations, thus building depth in the science.

Developing a research training and career development trajectory expanded the discipline's concept of scientific education to a life-long learning commitment, as well as establishing a series of grant awards for funding such a trajectory. The trajectory extended from predoctoral programs to postdoctoral study to mid-career study to a senior investigative stage. Grant awards were established to facilitate each of the stages on the trajectory, with special attention in the initial years of the NINR to the use of the National Service Research Awards, both individual and institutional for predoctoral and postdoctoral study. Over time, mid-career awards and senior fellowships were also established to support continued career development in the later stages.

Taking advantage of the rich interdisciplinary milieu at the NIH and within research universities, the NINR actively initiated grant programs that facilitated interdisciplinary perspectives in the extramurally funded nursing research awards. By providing funding for interdisciplinary collaboration, the nurse researchers were able to form strong networks with other relevant disciplines within the universities, enhancing the development of clinical nursing research. Clinical nursing research addresses complex health care issues that often require multiple perspectives and disciplinary expertise. Incorporating a strong interdisciplinary perspective for nursing research promoted an enriched approach to clinical interventions, outcomes, and to understanding the environmental and organizational context of care. In the early 1990s, an intramural research program was established at the NINR to conduct basic and clinical nursing research within the rich, interdisciplinary context of the NIH intramural scientific community.

One major NINR initiative was to enhance the development of an international nursing research community to advance the study of nursing phenomena across national and cultural boundaries and to enhance the di-

versity of ideas across the multiple, national nursing research communities. The NINR facilitated the development of one of the first formal sets of international nursing research priorities for the global nursing community. The institute cosponsored a major nursing research task force with the International Council of Nurses in 1990, which published a formal set of priorities. These priorities were later adopted by the ICN as part of its mission and responsibilities. The priorities were broad and process oriented in nature:

- promote depth in the knowledge base for nursing practice,
- recognize nursing research as an integral aspect of nursing practice and education across the countries,
- facilitate cross-cultural research,
- assure preparation of nurse researchers for faculty positions on master's and doctoral programs and for positions in clinical research, and
- Encourage all national nurse associations to establish ethical research standards (NCNR/ICN, 1990).

These NINR initiatives and the funding infrastructure in the federal government have influenced the development and evolution of several of the research traditions of the discipline.

Nursing Research Traditions

Several nursing research traditions have evolved and stabilized in the past decade due to several factors: maturity of the scientific community, availability of increased funding for research and research training, and the maturity of schools of nursing within the university and college systems. Other research traditions are still relatively new and require attention by the discipline. Among the more stable traditions are the development of long-term individual research programs and the research infrastructures to support them, acknowledgment of the need for postdoctoral study for nurse researchers, establishment of nursing research priorities to guide the use of limited scientific resources and investigator endeavors, and a strong methodological tradition for diversity or scientific pluralism.

Research programs. Establishing a program of research is an accepted expectation of nurse scientists and thus an established research tradition. By definition, "a research program is a series of projects comprising an area of study undertaken by an individual investigator" (Hinshaw, 1989, p. 168). These are long-term programs in which the investigator builds on his or her earlier results and experiences.

One of the major factors in stabilizing this research tradition is the growth in funding through the NINR and other sources to support multiple phases of a research program. Many investigators have diversified the funding sources for their research to include support from multiple NIH institutes and private foundations. Another major factor is the growth in the number of faculty who are doctorally prepared and can choose long-term, active research careers rather than being drawn into administrative positions because of professional leadership needs.

The second phase of this research tradition, institutional research programs, is currently developing. Characteristically, institutional programs involve a cadre of nurse researchers investigating a common area of interest, such as consequences of serious illnesses, cognitive functioning, or woman's health. The investigators form a subcommunity focused on a particular public health issue and reinforce and extend each other's scientific endeavors. Most of the institutional research programs are formalized as a "center of excellence" of some type. This is an important research infrastructure, which usually provides core funding, research staff, and consultative expertise, as well as an opportunity for scientific dialogue and critique. Such centers of excellence may exist in academic or service settings. Among the current doctoral programs in nursing, 43% have formal or informal centers of excellence in their schools of nursing (Hinshaw & Berlin, 1997).

Postdoctoral study for nurse researchers. Postdoctoral education is the "window of opportunity" for a nurse scientist to construct a solid foundation for a long-term research career (Hinshaw, 1992; Lev, Souder, & Topp, 1989). This opportunity allows an individual to have the time, space, resources, and intellectual support system for planning the first phase of his or her research program with a strong mentor. In postdoctoral study, the first stage of an investigator's research program can be piloted or implemented at a point when the individual is not balancing the multiple roles involved with academic or professional positions (Hinshaw, 1991). Postdoctoral study is important for the discipline to ensure well-prepared scientists who are committed to the preparation needed to stay on the cutting edge of a particular field of study.

Postdoctoral study has become a tradition since the inception of the NINR and the initiative that provided a career trajectory for nurse researchers with sources of funding for the different stages (Ketefian & Redman, 1994). In a sense, this research tradition is still evolving; the number of individuals in postdoctoral study is limited. However, the discipline is in agreement that such study is a critical component of preparing for a scientific career. The issues are funding and geographic access to appropriate, prepared mentors. Different models for postdoctoral preparation, criteria for programs, selection of faculty mentors, and other issues are still evolving, usually highly individualized to the goals and needs of the postdoctoral fellow. A major factor detracting from this tradition is the age of prospective postdoctoral fellows. As the average assistant professor in academia is 46.5 years of age, this means an individual is considering postdoctoral study either prior to or during this period. It is difficult at this age, with multiple position opportunities at much higher salaries, to consider postdoctoral study for 1 to 2 years (Hinshaw & Ketefian, 1996).

Nursing research priorities. The concept of identifying nursing research priorities dates back a number of decades. The early priorities were process in nature and laid the foundation for the more substantive, content-oriented priorities that have been apparent in the past 25 years. One of the first formal sets of priorities that focused on clinical nursing research issues was the Delphi Survey of Priorities in Clinical Nursing Research, conducted by Lindemann (1975) in the mid-1970s. These priorities focused on quality of care in nursing practice. Since that time, a series of formal research agendas or position statements on the future directions and priorities for nursing research has been developed; for example, the research policy statements of the Cabinet and Council of the ANA (ANA, 1985, 1997), and the nursing administration research directions by AONE (Fralic, 1991; Lynn & Cobb, 1994). One of the best-known sets of formal nursing research priorities is the National Nursing Research Agenda, which was developed by the nursing research community and the NINR staff.

Why set nursing research priorities? First, facilitating excellence in the science base for nursing has necessitated focusing limited resources on the generation of knowledge and conduct of research. To develop depth in the science—that is, solid, substantiated bodies of knowledge around critical areas of research for the discipline—priorities need to be explicit. The intent is to focus resources and evolve a series of studies in the identified areas of importance. Thus, the research would yield substantiated knowledge that could then be disseminated and applied in nursing practice. Otherwise, because nursing research boundaries are so broad, the knowledge generated could be quite scattered and diffuse. In addition, a critical mass of researchers could be trained and supported to conduct studies in an area of common interest—which builds the body of experts needed in relation to critical, important societal health issues of concern to the profession.

Second, setting nursing research priorities facilitates long-range strategic planning for the nursing research community. As a relatively young scientific discipline with limited institutional as well as national resources, nursing research needs time to build research programs and to respond to conducting research in a particular area of priority. Setting research priorities as part of strategic planning for the discipline's scientific programs allows the community as a "whole" to establish specific directions and allows the individual members of the scientific group to respond within a "doable" timeframe.

The tradition of establishing nursing research priorities has continued with, for example, a new formal agenda purposed by the ANA Council of Nurse Researchers Executive Committee in 1997 in the updated policy statement titled *Directions for Nursing Research: Toward the Twenty-First Century.* New priorities are evident from the NINR in terms of the program announcements that are published, calling for grant applications in a specific area. A number of other countries have identified formal nursing research priorities—for instance, the Nordic countries (Hinshaw, Boontong, Chipiro-Mupepi, Hamerin, & Jillings, 1997).

Methodological tradition for diversity. Nursing's current research tradition of methodological diversity or scientific pluralism has been adopted after extensive debate. Through the late 1980s, a number of methodological debates were evident in the literature: use of qualitative versus quantitative methods in research, descriptive versus intervention or prescriptive approaches, different philosophical approaches to research methods with a focus on which was correct, and others (e.g., Gorenberg, 1983; Hinshaw, 1998). In the late 1980s, scholars began to suggest that a diversity of methodologies was more realistic. The important issue is the research question being asked and the state of the science available from which to study the question. In addition, two major scholars, Meleis (1987) and Stevenson (1988), were encouraging nurse researchers to be less invested in methodological arguments and focus instead on the actual substantive clinical questions that needed to be studied.

Simultaneously, the NINR was established (as the NCNR), and the National Nursing Research Agenda was developed, with funding support provided for clinical nursing research studies focused on substantive, important questions. These factors influenced the consideration of the methodological issues within the context of the clinical nursing research questions and state of the science. Generally, this set of circumstances has resulted in a discipline that uses and values multiple methodologies, often merging several types of methods in one study.

Research Traditions for the Future

Several future research traditions are in the early stages of evolution. These include research programs that integrate the biological and behavioral aspects of nursing science, research programs with greater generalizability for the science, research programs focused on intervention studies, research training programs for "fast-tracking" career development, and research programs whose purpose is testing models for the use of results in practice or for informing health policy (see Chapter 12, this volume).

Integrating the biological and behavioral aspects of nursing science. The importance of integrating the biological and behavioral aspects of nursing science is based on the discipline's holistic approach to health and illness for individuals and families. Shaver's (1985) classic article, titled "A Biopsychosocial View of Human Health," outlines the philosophical premises and conceptualization for merging the multiple sciences (biological and behavioral) in understanding individuals' and families' responses to health and illness. This is a unique perspective that nursing contributes to the health sciences. This perspective was further developed by Cowan, Heinrich, Lucas, Sigmon, and Hinshaw (1993) during a visiting scholar experience at the NINR in the early 1990s. In their article, "Integration of Biological and Nursing Sciences: A 10-Year Plan to Enhance Research and Training," a strategic plan was delineated for the long-term development of federal resources and awards needed to facilitate the integration of these sciences for the nursing discipline.

The merger of the biological and behavioral aspects of nursing science is an evolving research tradition. The review of clinical nursing science provided in this text gives an excellent overview of the degree to which such integration has progressed. In a limited number of research programs, biological and social science parameters are used to measure particular symptoms such as sleep or fatigue. In addition, a recent review of the articles reported in *Nursing Research,* from 1996 through spring 1998, indicates that relatively few of the studies used a biobehavioral approach to the topics under investigation (Hinshaw, 1998). A similar review, published in *Nursing Research* in 1991 by Abraham, Chalifoux, and Evers, did not acknowledge any studies with an integrated biologic and behavioral focus. Even though more studies now use a biobehavioral measurement of the concepts in nursing, almost no studies are evident that conceptualize biological and behavioral ideas in an explicit theoretical framework and study the relationships among such concepts (Hinshaw, 1998). Thus, some progress is evident in integrating the biological and behavioral aspects of nursing science, but this tradition is relatively new for the discipline.

Generalizability of nursing science. Achieving generalizability for nursing science is a tradition that is in the early stages. Ten to 15 years of stronger resources for nursing research through the NINR and other funding sources has not provided enough support for multiple studies within the scientists' research programs. Not all nurse researchers focus on replication in some manner in the later stages of their investigations but are focused on extending the theoretical explanations for a particular phenomena. Both of these perspectives are important. However, a greater focus on generalizability is important if the evolving science is to be considered reliable and usable in nursing practice and in informing health policy.

An excellent model for a research program that is generalizable is Brooten and her colleagues', such as Naylor, investigation of the effectiveness of systematic early discharge from the hospital with community follow-up by advanced practice nurses (Brooten & Naylor, 1995). Studying critical quality and cost outcomes, this research program has shown positive quality outcomes and decreased costs for multiple populations receiving such systematic transition care. The systematic transition intervention and outcome relationships have been studied in multiple populations such as very low birth weight infants, women experiencing cesarean sections, elderly individuals discharged from the hospital, pregnant women hospitalized with diabetes, and women experiencing hysterectomies. The consistency of the relationships among the systematic transition care intervention

and the quality and cost outcomes shown across multiple populations makes them particularly valuable in influencing both nursing practice and health policy. Only a limited number of research programs have achieved this level of generalizability for nursing science. Thus, this research tradition is in its early development.

Intervention research programs. A shift to intervention studies is evident within the research programs of the discipline. In 1991, Abraham and his colleagues noted a limited number of intervention studies reported in the nursing research journals. However, a recent similar review shows a much stronger trend toward studies that cite either an experimental or causal modeling design used to test specific stated relationships among certain interventions and outcomes or among multiple concepts theorized to influence certain other concepts (Hinshaw, 1998). This research tradition toward intervention studies or suggesting how certain variables affect others is not based on the old positivistic tradition but, rather, on the perspective that given multiple conditions, it is still important to understand the influence of certain nursing interventions in terms of the probability of specific outcomes occurring (see Chapter 4, this volume). How else will the discipline reach the stage of prescription of interventions with a relatively reliable sense of predicting the outcomes? Nursing practice requires such capability from the discipline's knowledge base but within a qualitative perspective that provides the richness of the context surrounding the understanding of such relationships. Thus, the research tradition for intervention studies advances in a framework of many qualifiers.

"Fast-tracking" research career development. A research tradition that is just evolving is the concept of fast-tracking individuals through their nursing research career development. The basic concern is that with the current pattern, individuals are completing doctoral or postdoctoral study and starting new assistant professor positions in academia at about 46.5 years of age, approximately 10 years behind other biological and behavioral scientists (Hinshaw & Ketefian, 1996). This poses real difficulties to the individuals and to the discipline. It takes approximately 7 to 10 years, at least, to have a fully developed research program with usable results for shaping practice and informing health policy. This leaves less than a decade for mentoring new scientists and assuming leadership in national health policy debates. Thus, there is a short span for developing science for the discipline and an even shorter span for preparing the next genera-

tion and providing leadership in the profession and in health care for interdisciplinary health policy arguments.

This career development shortchanges the profession and the science of nursing, as well as placing major stress on the individuals evolving through this pattern. Strategies need to be developed to fast-track individuals through the educational programs. The concern with this approach to nursing education is the possibility of curtailing individuals' clinical experience. Precautions need to be taken that the individuals receive quality, carefully chosen clinical experiences. Early incentives for investing in a career in nursing research also need to be developed and tested. Program models for combining "fast-tracking careers and balancing family roles and responsibilities also need to be planned and evaluated" (Hinshaw & Ketefian, 1996).

Informing nursing practice and health policy. Nursing research has a long history of the development of models and processes for research use (White, Leske, & Pearcy, 1995). Many of the professional journals publish articles that apply the findings of research to practice, and journals have been developed just for articles that showcase the use of findings in nursing practice—for example, *Applied Nursing Research.* The value of and commitment to the importance of using nursing research findings in practice is well established (e.g., Stetler, 1994). However, the tradition and infrastructures are less well developed. A number of articles show concern with the alleged gap between research and practice (e.g., Bostrom & Wise, 1994; Briones & Bruya, 1990). There are a number of success stories in individual hospitals where research has been integrated into practice with specific clinical issues (e.g., Langner & Wolf, 1996), but there is no solid tradition or expectation for using research within all agencies or professional roles, and limited infrastructure and incentives within hospitals and other health care organizations exist to ensure such use. Structures and processes for incorporating research into various practice arenas must be developed, and incentives for using research findings in practice need to be planned and evaluated. Crane (1995) suggests that this process must be a partnership among the nurse researchers and leaders in the clinical arenas. According to Crane, a merger of clinical and research expertise from nursing leaders in the academic and practice agencies would provide the strongest plan and infrastructure.

Informing health policy through nursing research is an important evolving research tradition for the discipline. The research programs of the discipline are expected to lead to changes in nursing practice based on desirable outcomes and, on a more expansive level, provide perspective and information for informing health policy.

These are changing times in terms of the health care needs of the public. As Callahan (1985) and others have predicted, the era of chronic illness and the long-term toll that is inherent in managing and caring for individuals under such conditions has arrived. Also, it has become increasingly evident that promoting health and preventing disease is preferable to struggling with the human, social, and financial costs inherent in illness. Prevention and health promotion will require enhancing or adapting certain lifestyle behaviors. Current health care includes a strong emphasis on the importance of promoting independence in maintaining health and facilitating appropriate self-care for individuals and families experiencing illness.

Disciplines such as nursing that focus on the issues of chronic illness, health promotion, independence in health, and the care of the acutely ill are central to shaping health care policy because these are heavily emphasized values for the future. The science generated by the discipline is timely and relevant. Thus, nursing and its science base can be expected to be strategically placed to inform health policy.

Summary

Nursing research has advanced dramatically during the past decade. Research traditions have been established and are still evolving for both the science and the scientists of the discipline. Nurse investigators are generating knowledge related to critical public health issues that the profession can influence and that optimize the health and well-being of individuals, families, and communities. They have established programs of research and are committed to a trajectory or lifetime of career development, insuring that their science will be cutting edge. Strong infrastructures have been established, ranging from institutional offices and centers for nursing research and centers of excellence to the National Institute for Nursing Research within the mainstream of federal research funding for health science.

As far as the discipline has advanced, there are still many challenges ahead. A number of traditions are still evolving for nursing research: for example, integrating the biological and behavioral aspects of the discipline's science, increasing the ability to understand the relationship of clinical interventions to desired outcomes, and informing practice and health policy through nursing research. These evolving traditions, as well as those yet unidentified, pose many opportunities for scientific dialogue and for broadening nursing's horizons. Interdisciplinary and international collaboration offer many possibilities for understanding the complexities and cultural base of nursing research and practice. The opportunities and challenges for the next decade promise as dramatic a growth pattern as the recent past in terms of the evolution of nursing research traditions.

References

Abraham, I. L., Chalifoux, A. L., & Evers, G.C.M. (1991). *Conditions, interventions, and outcomes: A quantitative analysis of nursing research (1981-1990).* Proceedings of a Conference Sponsored by the National Center for Nursing Research, Patient Outcomes Research: Examining the Effectiveness of Nursing Practice, DHHS, PHS, NIH Pub. No. 93-3411. September 11-13.

American Nurses Association. (1962). ANA blueprint for research in nursing. *American Journal of Nursing, 62*(8), 69-71.

American Nurses Association. (1985). *Directions for nursing research: Toward the twenty-first century.* Kansas City, MO: Author.

American Nurses Association. (1997). *Directions for nursing research: Toward the twenty-first century* (Rev. ed.) Kansas City, MO: Author.

Batey, M. V. (1978). *Research development in university schools of nursing: Organizational structure and process variables related to research goal attainment.* Washington, DC: U.S. Department of Health, Education, and Welfare.

Bloch, D. (1990). Strategies for setting and implementing the National Center for Nursing Research priorities. *Applied Nursing Research, 3*(1), 2-6.

Bostrom, J., & Wise, L. (1994). Closing the gap between research and practice. *Journal of Nursing Administration, 24*(5), 22-27.

Briones, T., & Bruya, M. A. (1990). The professional imperative: research utilization in the search for scientifically based nursing practice. *Focus on Critical Care, 17*(1), 78-81.

Brooten, D., & Naylor, M. D. (1995). Nurses' effect on changing patient outcomes. *Image: The Journal of Nursing Scholarship, 27*(2), 95-99.

Callahan, D. (1985). Ethics and health care: The next 20 years. *American Journal of Hospital Pharmacy, 42,* 1053-1057.

Cowan, M. J., Heinrich, J., Lucas, M., Sigmon, H., & Hinshaw, A. S. (1993). Integration of biological and nursing sciences: A 10-year plan to enhance research and training. *Research in Nursing and Health, 16*(1), 3-9.

Crane, J. (1995). The future of research utilization. *Nursing Clinics of North America, 30*(3), 565-577.

Fralic, F. F. (1991). New directions for nursing administration research. *Journal of Nursing Administration, 21*(10), 10-11.

Gorenberg, B. (1983). The research tradition of nursing: An emerging issue. *Nursing Research, 32*(6), 347-349.

Gortner, S. R. (1973). Research in nursing: The federal interest and grant program. *American Journal of Nursing, 73*(6), 1052-1055.

Gortner, S. R. (1983). The history and philosophy of nursing science and research. *Advances in Nursing Science, 5*(1), 1-8.

Gortner, S. R., & Nahm, H. (1977). An overview of nursing research in the United States. *Nursing Research, 26*(1), 10-33.

Gortner, S. R., & Schultz, P. R. (1988). Approaches to nursing science methods. *Image: The Journal of Nursing Scholarship, 20*(1), 22-27.

Health Research Extension Act of 1985, Subpart 3—National Center for Nursing Research Pub. L. No. 99-158, Nov 20, 1985. 99 STAT. 867-869.

Hinshaw, A. S. (1989). Nursing science: The challenge to develop knowledge. *Nursing Science Quarterly, 2*(4), 162-171.

Hinshaw, A. S. (1990). National Center for Nursing Research: A commitment to excellence in science. In J. C. McCloskey & H. K. Grace (Eds.), *Current issues in nursing* (pp. 357-362). St. Louis, MO: Mosby.

Hinshaw, A. S. (1991). The federal imperative in funding post-doctoral education: Indices of quality. In *Proceedings for the 1991 forum on doctoral education in nursing. Postdoctoral education in nursing science: Purpose, process, outcome* (pp. 81-108). Amelia Island: University of Florida Press.

Hinshaw, A. S. (1992). Nursing research: Weaving the past and the future. In L. Aiken & C. Fagin (Eds.), *Charting nursing's future: Agenda for the 1990s* (pp. 485-503). Philadelphia, PA: Lippincott.

Hinshaw, A. S. (1996). Research traditions: A decade of progress. *Journal of Professional Nursing, 12*(2), 68.

Hinshaw, A. S. (1998). Methodological innovations in knowledge development. *Priorities in nursing science beyond the year 2000: Which way Europe?* Proceedings: Workgroup of European Nurse Researchers, Helsinki, Finland, July 1-9, 1998.

Hinshaw, A. S., & Berlin, L. (1997, January). *The future for quality doctoral nursing programs.* Paper presented at the AACN Doctoral Conference, Sanibel Island, FL.

Hinshaw, A. S., Boontong, T., Chipiro-Mupepi, S., Hamerin, E., & Jillings, C. R. (1997, June). Sharing health care challenges: Nursing research priorities for the next century. *Sharing the health challenge.* International Council of Nurses, Vancouver, Canada.

Hinshaw, A. S., Heinrich, J., & Bloch, D. (1988). Evolving clinical nursing research priorities: A national endeavor. *Journal of Professional Nursing, 4*(6), 398, 458-459.

Hinshaw, A. S., & Ketefian, S. (1996). A missing research tradition. *Journal of Professional Nursing, 12*(4), 196.

Hinshaw, A. S., & Merritt, D. H. (1988). Moving nursing research to NIH. In *Perspectives in nursing 1987-1989,* (pp. 93-103). New York: National League for Nursing.

Ketefian, S., & Redman, R. W. (1994). The changing face of graduate education. In J. C. McCloskey & H. K. Grace (Eds.), *Current issues in nursing* (pp. 188-195). St. Louis, MO: Mosby.

Langner, S. R., & Wolf, Z. R. (1996). Integrating research into acute care settings: Reflections of two nurse researchers. *Nursing Administration Quarterly, 20*(4), 41-51.

Lev, E., Souder, E., & Topp, R. (1989). The postdoctoral fellowship experience. *Image: The Journal of Nursing Scholarship, 22*(2), 116-120.

Lindeman, C. A. (1975). Delphi survey of priorities in clinical nursing research. *Nursing Research, 24*(6), 434-441.

Lynn, M. R., & Cobb, B. K. (1994). Changes in nursing administration research priorities: A sign of the times. *Journal of Nursing Administration, 24*(4S), 12-18.

McBride, A. (1987). The National Center for Nursing Research. *Social Policy Report, 2*(2), 1-11.

Meleis, A. F. (1987). Revisions in knowledge development: A passion for substance. *Scholarly Inquiry for Nursing Practice, 1*(1), 5-19.

Meleis, A. I. (1992). Directions for nursing theory development in the 21st century. *Nursing Science Quarterly, 5*(3), 112-117.

Merritt, D. H. (1986). The National Center for Nursing Research. *Image: The Journal of Nursing Scholarship, 18*(3), 84-85.

National Center for Nursing Research/International Council of Nurses. (1990, April 30-May 2). *Nursing research worldwide.* Report of the Task Force on International Nursing Research, Geneva, Switzerland.

Salmon, M. E. (1997). Division of Nursing, U.S. Public Health Service—50 years. *Image: The Journal of Nursing Scholarship, 29*(4), 302-303.

Shaver, J. F. (1985). A biopsychosocial view of human health. *Nursing Outlook, 33*(4), 186-191.

Stetler, C. (1994). Refinement of the Stetler/Marram model for application of research findings to practice. *Nursing Outlook, 42*(1), 15-25.

Stevenson, J. S. (1987). Forging a research discipline. *Nursing Research, 36*(1), 60-64.

Stevenson, J. S. (1988). Nursing knowledge development: Into era II. *Journal of Professional Nursing, 4*(3), 152-162.

White, J. M., Leske, J. S., & Pearcy, J. M. (1995). Models and processes of research utilization. *Nursing Clinics of North America, 30*(3), 409-420.

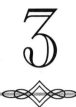

WHAT IS KNOWN ABOUT CARING IN NURSING SCIENCE

A Literary Meta-Analysis

Kristen M. Swanson

ver the past two decades, there has been an escalating interest in the concept of caring, as evidenced in nursing dissertations, publications, investigations, theory debates, curriculum revolutions, conference agendas, and the making of professional policy. At the forefront of these activities are noted nurse theorists and philosophers such as Watson (1985, 1988a), Leininger (1981, 1988), Benner (1984), Benner and Wrubel (1989), Gaut (1983), Boykin (1994), Boykin and Schoenhofer (1993), Gadow (1980, 1984) and Roach (1984). These scholars remind the profession of the importance of studying caring because of its pivotal role in the practice of effective nursing as well as its centrality to preserving human dignity and sustaining humankind.

In the early 1990s, based on a review of the publications of 26 nursing authors, Morse and her colleagues (Morse, Bottorf, Neander, & Solberg, 1991, Morse, Solberg, Neander, Bottorf, & Johnson, 1990) suggested that there were at least five conceptualizations of caring extant in then-current nursing discourse. They concluded that caring had been studied as a: human trait, moral imperative, affect, interpersonal relationship, and nursing therapeutic. As this 1997 review of the caring literature was initiated, it became apparent that nursing dialogue about caring could still best be characterized as a modern-day "Tower of Babble." There were many publications, some data based, some theory based, but few that built on the work of previous investigators. Hence, the *purpose* of this chapter is to summarize a literary meta-analysis of published nursing research on the concept of caring and to propose a framework that adequately integrates the current state of substantive knowledge about caring in nursing. Also, throughout this chapter, issues pertaining to syntax (methodology) are addressed.

At the Wingspread Caring Conference, sponsored by the Robert Wood Johnson Foundation and the American Academy of Nursing, summary papers of the importance of caring were offered by Watson (1990) and Leininger (1990), the philosophic and moral underpinnings were examined by Gadow (1990) and Benner (1990), and state-of-the-art papers were delivered by Stevenson (1990) and Tripp-Riemer (Tripp-Riemer & Cohen, 1990). Tripp-Riemer focused on programs of qualitative inquiry pertaining to caring. Stevenson's paper was an extensive review of quantitative studies of therapeutic nursing interventions: She equated the term *nursing care* with clinical interventions. The Wingspread Caring Conference is of historical import to nursing science for several reasons: (a) by virtue of its occurrence, it provided concrete evidence that key professional gatekeepers in the discipline valued the concept of caring to the extent that resources were devoted to scholarly debate of the importance of role of caring in building knowledge for the discipline, profession, and society; (b) it brought together nurse scholars (from empirical, interpretive, and critical postmodern perspectives), consumers and practitioners (individuals invited because of key familiarity with practicing, receiving, or recognizing the need for caring), and nurse leaders (i.e., from the National Institutes of Health [at that time the National Center for Nursing Research], the Academy of Nursing, and other professional nursing organizations). Since that time, the visibility of caring in key nursing documents has become more and more commonplace (for example, the recently revised American Nurses Association Social Policy Statement and current National League for Nursing standards for curriculum evaluation).

This chapter differs somewhat from each of those summaries offered at the Wingspread conference in that it does not deal with the *philosophic underpinnings* or *importance* of caring to the discipline (the importance is assumed); it reviews *both* quantitative and qualitative published studies and attempts to pull together conclusions about what is known. Furthermore, unlike Stevenson's equating of "nursing care" with "nurse caring," the view taken by this author is that not all of nursing care (practice) necessarily equates with nurse caring (a *way* of practicing). Although many intervention studies (e.g.,

pain management, pre-op teaching) may be conceptually pulled together under the rubric of caring, unless those studies were published as conceptually grounded in caring, they have not been included in this chapter.

Methods

Literature reviewed was primarily limited to published, data-based investigations of the concept of caring. Included were interpretive and empiric-analytic investigations of caring. Noticeably lacking is a review of studies that offer a more critical (in the postmodern sense) and/or historic perspective on caring. International publications (English-language only) were retrieved via a computer search of recent nursing literature supplemented with additional studies referenced in those retrieved articles. Having not addressed unpublished theses and dissertations, this chapter is further limited.

Approximately 130 publications (articles, chapters, or books) were reviewed, the preponderance of which were published between 1980 and 1996. Most reviewed investigations focused explicitly on the concept of caring. In those investigations, data were obtained in many ways: from patient charts, observations of practice, and surveys or interviews of patients, families, nurses, students, teachers and other health care professionals. Research participants were observed or queried about their experiences, expectations, preferences, observations, meanings, and/or expressions of caring. Relationships investigated included nurse-colleagues, nurse-patient/family, student-teacher, student-student, student-patients, healthcare provider-patient/family, and family caregiver-family member. Several articles reviewed actually focused on concepts related to caring (e.g., expert practice or excellence in nursing, reassurance, nursing support, use of nursing intuition, comfort, family caregiving, etc.). These related concepts were included because the researchers' findings ultimately unearthed additional information about the concept of caring (e.g., caring may have been included as a descriptive or essential component of the related concept).

After reading at least half of the articles, a framework for categorizing *findings* from the studies reviewed was inductively derived. Focusing on each study's findings rather than its stated purpose ultimately made more sense. As has oftentimes been this author's experience with qualitative inquiry, the question with which the researchers started out may prove not quite the right direction to have been heading, given what is inductively learned about the phenomenon as it is explored (Swanson-Kauffman, 1986b; Swanson-Kauffman & Schonwald, 1988). In other words, where qualitative inquiry oftentimes takes investigators is not where they thought they were heading—rather, it is where the phenomenon examined takes them. Hence, realizing that findings take pragmatic precedence over questions, *research findings* were categorized into the five hierarchical levels of capacities, commitments/concerns, conditions, caring actions, and consequences.

In Level I, characteristics of persons with the *capacity* for caring are identified. Of interest in Level I findings are questions about whether these traits and characteristics are inherent (nature) or if they may be environmentally enhanced or diminished (nurture). Level II, *concerns/commitments,* focuses on the beliefs or values that undergird caring actions. Categorized in Level III are *conditions.* These are patient-, nurse-, or organization-related circumstances that enhance or diminish the likelihood that caring transactions will take place. Level IV (the bulk of qualitative and quantitative nursing inquiry about caring) describes *caring actions,* behaviors, or therapeutic interventions. Finally, Level V focuses on the positive and negative *consequences* of caring. These are both the intentional and the unintentional outcomes of caring for provider and/or recipient. Also in Level IV, caring actions, inductive findings about the enactment of caring, are categorized under Swanson's five caring categories (Swanson, 1990, 1991, 1993; Swanson-Kauffman, 1986a, 1988), thus providing both a conceptual framework for caring actions and empirical support for the generalizability of Swanson's middle-range theory of caring.

Glaser and Strauss (1967) described two possible levels of theory produced through qualitative inquiry. Theories of the first type, substantive, were considered to be very localized knowledge that is closely tied to the situation, context, or life experience of the limited number of participants included in the investigator's sample. The criteria for "truth" in studies of the substantive-theory-producing type were that the findings made sense to the people who participated in the investigation and that the researcher rigorously recreated what those participants had in common. Theories of the second type, formal, were considered more general, universal, or abstract and were better understood as descriptions of the structure of a given phenomena, life process, social construction, or concept. Formal theories were not yielded by single, intense, small-*n* studies; rather, they were the

accumulation of a series of investigations about a similar phenomenon. This series could be the work of a given investigator across a variety of samples and settings (for example, later in this chapter see the discussion of Beck's investigations of caring in academia) or the sum product of a series of investigators working on unearthing the essence of a given phenomena or concept. (This literary meta-analysis might in itself be an example of such.)

The five levels of caring knowledge are considered hierarchical not in order of import but in order of level of assumption. For example, an observational study of caring actions (Level IV) assumes that the individual or group studied had the capacity for caring (Level I), the commitment to act in a caring manner (Level II), and the conditions in place supportive of caring practices (Level III). Although, for any number of sound reasons, an investigator observing practice may not always administer a "caring capacity inventory" (assuming such an empirical device existed) to the practitioner ahead of time, it is not uncommon for an investigator wishing to study the occurrence of caring to query supervisors and peers for a known-to-be-caring nurse (e.g., as a criteria for recruitment) and to keep careful field notes about what else was going on during the period of observation (to deal with potential Level III historical competing variables). Similarly, if an organizational researcher observed that two separate long-term care facilities differed quite noticeably in contentment level of clients and their families, cleanliness of facilities, and staff retention patterns, the investigator might want to explore potential antecedents to these desirable (Level V) outcomes. The investigator might know personnel at both institutions and feel comfortable assuming that both facilities hire personnel who have the capacity (Level I) for caring and who are committed (Level II) to "doing good." Hence, the investigator may decide to target inquiry at the Level III conditions in place that may or may not support the occurrence of caring, as well as the Level IV caring actions themselves. In both of these examples offered, it is possible that the pragmatic investigators assumed too much and that failure to carefully measure the a priori assumed levels of caring may lead to making faulty or unnecessarily weak conclusions.

Level I: The Capacity for Caring

Findings about the characteristics of caring persons were rarely derived from questions directly addressing an individual's capacity to care. Results classified as Level I were more often produced by qualitative investigators posing such broad questions as "What constitutes caring in this critical care setting?" or "What is the experience of participating in a caring encounter for nurses, patients, students, families, and so on?" Typically, these studies yielded two kinds of information: what the nurse *does* and how the nurse *is*. Findings categorized under capacity are from those study results that interpret how a caring person *is*.

Listed in Table 3.1 are findings from 21 studies that yielded information about caring capacities. These data were derived from inductive studies employing open-ended questions posed via interviews or written questionnaires. Data were analyzed using a variety of qualitative methods (phenomenology, grounded theory, inductive content analysis). These studies span the years from 1986 to 1996 and involved a total of 718 participants (262 nurses, 174 patients and/or families, 33 healthcare providers, and 249 nursing students). Findings from these qualitative investigations suggest that the caring nurse is compassionate, empathic, knowledgeable, confident, and reflective.

Benner and Wrubel (1989), strongly influenced by the work of Heidigger (1962), postulated that the origins of concern and caring are at the essence of being, a claim that human wholeness is characterized by the capacity for concern, loving, and caring. Similarly, Boykin and Schoenhofer (1993), drawing heavily from the writings of Mayeroff (1971) and Roach (1984), view caring as a human mode of being, a mode that remains with the nurse from moment to moment, hence rendering it possible to enhance the personhood of both client and nurse in any given nursing situation.

Ray (1987) interviewed eight American critical care nurses and Clarke and Wheeler (1992) interviewed six British nurses. In both of these phenomenologic investigations, questions were raised as to whether the capacity for caring is innate, taught, or due to having been cared for. Benner's (1984) phenomenologic investigation of excellence in nursing practice demonstrated that the ability to practice expert caring is enhanced with experience. Suspecting a link between developmental readiness and caring capacity, Soldwisch (1993) hypothesized a positive association between ego stage development and capacity for empathy and congruence. Based on a survey design study of 33 nursing students, she upheld both hy-

pothesized relationships ($p < .03$) and provided evidence that the capacity to care effectively may be linked to maturational readiness.

Future directions for Level I inquiry. Similar to the next four levels, knowledge production on the capacity for caring has been quite small, local, and rarely builds on previous studies. The series of substantive investigations has involved small samples, single settings, or limited types of practice (e.g., critical care nurses). Table 3.1 suggests a structure for the capacities of caring providers, but it needs to be tested for utility. Further investigations are needed to develop research measures with which to quantify caring capacity, explore the origins of caring capacity, examine the effects of nurturing and experience on caring capacity, and examine the relationship between the capacity for caring and the actual occurrence of caring practice. Pragmatically, it is very possible that Level I knowledge about the capacity of individuals (or groups) for caring may most logically be the purview of other disciplines (e.g., developmental psychology, sociology, anthropology), and it would make perfect sense for nurse investigators to build on or adopt outright tools, methods, or theories that adequately deal with this basic level of inquiry about the capacity for caring.

Level II: Concerns/Commitments

Benner and Wrubel (1989) define concern as

a way of being involved in one's own world in which people and things matter to one. It describes a phenomenological relationship in which the world is apprehended directly in terms of meaning for the self. Concern is the reason why people act. (p. 408)

Their basic claim is that when something matters to a person, that individual will pay attention to it. What concerns people helps them figure out where their commitments lie.

Level II findings categorized as concerns/commitments were derived from those research studies that focused on the beliefs or values that underlie nurse caring. Watson (1988b) and Noddings (1984) suggest that the source of a provider's values may be his or her compas-

TABLE 3.1 Capacities of Caring Persons

First Author, Year (Participants)	Caring Capacities				
	Compassionate	*Empathic*	*Knowledgable*	*Positive*	*Reflective*
Bäck-Pettersson, 1993 (32 nurses)	compassionate		competent	courageous	
Beck, 1991 (47 students)	compassionate, dedicated	understanding, empathic	competent	confident	conscience, moral awareness
Beck, 1996 (37 students)	emotional warmth	understanding		has personality	open, willing to share
Clayton, 1991 (70 families)	compassionate	concerned	knowledgable	courageous	balanced, moral
Coulon, 1996 (156 students)	dedicated	aware, perceptive, intuitive	knowledgable, competent, skillful	cheerful, enabling personal qualities	visionary
Davies, 1990 (1 nurse, 10 cases)	giving of self, connecting			self-worth, self-esteem	looks inward, accepts and acknowledges own responses
Dietrich, 1992 (5 nurses)		aware of others' needs, sensitive	knowledgable		
Donoghue, 1993 (82 nurses)		sympathetic, can take another's perspective, empathic	knowledgable, skillful		
Drew, 1986 (35 patients)				self-reliant, adaptive, flexible	quiet, calm, patient
Euswas, 1993 (30 patients, 32 nurses)	benevolent		competent		constantly present in awareness of self
Fareed, 1996 (8 patients)		showing concern, being "in tune"	knowledgable, skillful	pleasant, cheerful attitude	
Girot, 1993 (10 nurses)		concerned, empathic	appropriately cautious, knows own limits	good self-concept	reflective
Halldorsdottir, 1990 (9 students)	committed	concerned	competent	positiveness	
Jensen, 1992 (16 nurses)	compassionate	concerned	knowledgable	courageous	reflective
Kahn, 1988 (25 nurses)	compassionate	empathic			
Miller, 1992 (16 nurses)	loving, involved			feels good within self	
Montgomery, 1992 (35 nurses)	unconditional love, involved, able to pull from abundance	receptive to patient experience			able to transcend ego
Poole, 1994 (5 patients)	patient	understanding		good mood	genuine
Propst, 1994 (9 patients)	warm	understanding		positive manner	
Ray, 1987 (8 nurses)		understanding	achieves mastery, competent	confident	
Williams, 1992 (17 parents, 33 health care providers)	have a caring heart		knowledgable		

sionate loving essence or possibly adoption of professional values. That is to say, caring could be an act of love, a call to duty, or perhaps both. Similarly, Davies and O'Berle (1990), having closely examined one nurse's supportive encounters with 10 patients, described how having either a global value of the importance of caring or a specific valuing of a given person was essential to motivate the nurse to engage in supportive patient care. Likewise, Boykin and Schoenhofer (1993) claim that "the values and assumptions of nursing as caring can assist the nurse to engage fully in nursing situations with persons where caring is difficult to discover" (p. 37).

Kahn and Steeves (1988) interpreted data from 25 nursing students in a master's degree program in their hermeneutic investigation of the ideologic concepts and principles that nurses bring with them to encounters with patients. Values that undergird practices included professional identity, seeing persons as unique beings, being compassionate and empathic, and believing that relationships should be therapeutic. Conversely, Kahn and Steeves concluded that a commitment to objectivity oftentimes hampered caring practices.

Summarized in Table 3.2 are the results of 18 qualitative investigations that yielded information about the values and beliefs to which nurses are committed. Included in these studies were a total of 582 participants (231 students, 309 nurses, 30 patients, and 12 family caregivers). Although it may not have been the stated purpose of many of these investigators to summarize nursing values, their findings (at least in part) are best understood as descriptors of "*why* the nurse does." As outlined in Table 3.2 (and very similar to Kahn and Steeves's conclusions), caring in nursing is based on commitments to recognize the dignity and worth of each person, focus on the needs of the other, connect with the other, do the right thing, and remain present to the nurse's self.

The cultural origins of concerns/commitments were addressed in Spangler's (1993) ethnonursing investigation of acute care American nurses from two culturally distinct backgrounds. The 22 Anglo-Americans interviewed believed in patients receiving education, being self-caring, and acting in compliance with care recommendations. They expected nurses to be autonomous and in control of situations. The 26 Filipino-American nurses valued serious dedication to work, attentiveness to patients' physical comfort (especially cleanliness), and the importance of patience and respect for elders and those in charge. Spangler concluded that Anglo-American nurses reflected Western values of self-reliance, mastery of nature, and primacy of scientific knowledge. The Filipino-

American nurses reflected more Eastern values of the importance of cleanliness, group orientation, social acceptance, and respect for authority.

The potential for conflict when a nurse's practice falls short of self-expectations was highlighted in Morrison's (1989, 1990) study of 25 charge level nurses. Using repertory grid-techniques, he asked each participant to generate his or her own list of constructs that characterize ideal nurses. Each nurse was then asked to rate him- or herself on each construct. Potential scores ranged from 0 to 48, and actual scores ranged from 1 to 26, with a mean score of 10.96. Morrison postulated that this gap between the view of self as "carer" and the "ideal carer" could lead to inner conflict wherein the provider might feel never quite good enough.

Last, Forrest's (1988) phenomenologic investigation of 17 hospital staff nurses demonstrated that their caring actions were affected not just by beliefs but also by their experiences, self-appraisal, and feelings about their work. Unfortunately, as will be discussed under *conditions,* not all nursing contexts are supportive of practicing in accordance with one's capacities or commitments.

Future directions for Level II inquiry. Knowledge building pertaining to Level II commitments and concerns calls for nursing investigations that rigorously bridge the standards for inquiry in ethics with insights into the everyday experiences of nurses in practice. Care must be taken not to prematurely close on the relevance of classic tenets (e.g., beneficence, justice, autonomy) of biomedical ethics to nursing practice, but nurse investigators are well advised to carefully consider the concerns and commitments that nurses employed in diverse settings (from the bedside to the national political arena) bring to their practice of caring. In addition, from a postmodern critical perspective, nurses must continue to address how the concerns and commitments that the profession holds may serve to inadvertently oppress both its practitioners and care recipients.

Level III: Conditions

Klausner (1971) suggested that any transaction will be affected by the demands, constraints, or resources brought to or evolving from the situation. Findings categorized under *conditions* were most often derived from questions about what affects caring, enhances caring interactions, or inhibits the occurrence of caring. Nurse and patient experiences, backgrounds and/or personalities, society, organizations, health status, and disease complications were all identified as influencing whether or not caring transpired.

Conditions that affect nurse caring could be as powerful and pervasive as homophobic, heterosexist biases (Powell-Cope, 1994) or as happenstance as everyday hassles such as weather or late delivery of supplies. Also important to the occurrence or perceptions of caring are the legal restrictions placed on practitioners. For example, Spangler (1993) noted that in addition to cultural influences on Filipino-American nurses, visa restrictions (real or perceived) might also account for the tendency of Filipino-American nurses to act in an extremely duty-conscious, dedicated, authority-honoring manner. Legal restrictions (e.g., limitations of licensure) might also account for some circumstances in which patients hold providers accountable for not adequately relieving their pain or completely addressing their immediate concerns.

It would be impossible to account for all conditions that might affect an unfolding nurse-client transaction. However, in Tables 3.3, 3.4, and 3.5, some of the patient- (Table 3.3), nurse- (Table 3.4), or organization- (Table 3.5) related conditions are outlined that may enhance or diminish the occurrence of caring actions. Findings in Table 3.3 were derived from 14 investigations involving 676 participants (177 students, 202 nurses, 72 patients/ families, and 225 healthcare providers). The majority of findings were derived from qualitative analyses of written or verbal accounts. One exception is Baer and Lowery's (1987) discriminant analysis of coded and quantified written student narratives of least- versus most-liked patient care situations. Typical studies that produced findings categorized under patient-related conditions focused on providers' preferences for "types" of patients they most liked. It is probably not safe to assume that liking a patient or the enjoyment of caring for a certain kind of patient automatically leads to caring actions (or the converse), but it is highly likely that attraction has at least some part to play in the actions that unfold in the nurse-patient encounter. Patient-related conditions that may influence the occurrence of caring include patient communication, personality, health problems, care needs, relationship with nurse, appearance, and "other."

As will be demonstrated a bit later in this chapter, giving time is frequently referred to as an action that indicates nurse caring. Two investigations provide evidence that patient-related conditions have a key part in soliciting nursing time. Halloran's (1985) exploration of nursing workload involved examining 2,560 patient records. These were the records of every patient admitted to a 279-bed acute care community hospital over a 4-month period. Charts were examined for nursing workload (dependent variable), nursing diagnosis, medical diagnosis, and patient demographics. It was found that 53.2% of the variance in nursing workload was accounted for by the patient's *nursing*-related condition as measured by the index of frequency of each nursing diagnosis. Medical diagnostic-related conditions accounted for 26.3% of the workload variance. When nursing workload was regressed on all independent variables, combined nursing and medical diagnostic indexes accounted for 60% of the variation in daily nursing. Swan, Benjamin, and Brown (1992) also examined the amount of time it took to provide care. They compared 20 patients with AIDS to 29 patient without AIDS on the variable "daily direct nursing care hours." They documented that patients with AIDS required 6.5 hr per day of direct nursing care; the comparison group took 5.43 hr. Interestingly, both exceeded the state's definitive criteria for a skilled nursing facility, which was 3 hr of direct care per day. Together, Halloran's and Swan and colleagues' studies provide evidence that caring—taken in its simplest sense, time—is directly related to patients' needs for supportive or substitutive care.

Table 3.4, nurse-related conditions that affect caring, is based on a total sample of 728 participants (322 nurses, 17 patients/parents, 33 healthcare providers, 258 students, and 98 observations of nursing practice). Once again, the majority of studies leading to the descriptions of nurse conditions affecting caring were derived from qualitative inquiry. Notable exceptions include Weiss's (1984) study of 240 students, wherein 120 males and 120 females were asked to view videotapes of nursing practice and identify instances and antecedents of nurse caring. Incorporated in Table 3.4 are results of Weiss's inquiry.

Young, Koch, and Preston (1989) viewed lack of understanding as a constraint to rural nurses adequately meeting the care needs of persons with AIDS. They offered a 1-day workshop in which they relayed information about HIV/AIDS and provided opportunities to deal with feelings and attitudes toward homosexuality and fears about caring for clients with AIDS. Before the workshop, immediately after, and 3 months after the workshop, participants completed investigator-developed surveys of their knowledge, attitudes, fears, and willingness to care for clients with AIDS. Two hundred nurses attended the workshop, 143 completed the first two surveys, and 56 completed the third survey. On every

TABLE 3.2 Concerns and Commitments

First Author, Year (Participants)	Concerns and Commitments				
	Recognize Dignity and Worth of Each Person	Focus on the Other's Experience	Connect With the Other	Do the Right Thing	Be Present to the Self
Beck, 1991 (47 students)	value others		allow participation in another's experiences		value self
Coulon, 1996 (156 students)	recognize each patient as a person	holistic approach to care		care without prejudice, maintain quality standards	consider nurse's own health
Davies, 1990 (1 nurse)	value inherent worth of other	do whatever has to be done to help the other	establish rapport; give of self	lend a hand; work on behalf of patient	find meaning; preserve own integrity
Donoghue, 1993 (82 nurses)				avoid hurting others	(–) seeing nursing as just a job
Euswas, 1993 (30 patients, 32 nurses)			realize intersubjective connectedness		must be mindfully present and aware
Forrest, 1988 (17 nurses)					protect self; focus on feeling good about own work
Hughes, 1992 (10 students)		faculty must place high priority on meeting needs of students			
Kahn, 1988 (25 nurses)	see persons as unique individuals		build therapeutic relationships		(–) need to maintain objectivity; practice in accordance with professional identity
Kosowski, 1995 (18 students)				vow to never be noncaring	
McNamara, 1995 (5 nurses)	value uniqueness of each person	value spiritual and psychological needs	must establish nurse-patient relationship		
Miller, 1992 (16 nurses)	respect patient dignity; treat patient as you would like to be treated	concentrate on patient, even when rushed			have to feel good within yourself
Montgomery, 1992 (35 nurses)		willingly focus on patient, not self; do not try to own patient's experience	allow for sacredness and interconnected-ness of human life; allow self to become part of patient's experience; be willing to fall in love		
Nelms, 1996 (5 nurses)	seek to create place where other's being can be preserved		feeling for patient leads to more fully feeling self		call to care = call to conscience = call to authenticity
Parker, 1994 (45 nurses)	right to be treated as a person; respect for privacy and modesty	care for whole person; think about how patient feels	feel for patient; earn and keep patient trust; value compassion	guard patient's welfare and well-being; know you are responsible; give 100%; willingly fight for patient; be accountable	know yourself; aim for inner harmony

TABLE 3.2 *Continued*

First Author, Year (Participants)	Concerns and Commitments				
	Recognize Dignity and Worth of Each Person	*Focus on the Other's Experience*	*Connect With the Other*	*Do the Right Thing*	*Be Present to the Self*
Powell-Cope, 1994 (12 FCGs)	must be willing to see gay partner or caregiver as significant other	phenomenologic orientation to strive to know another's experience	HCP must willingly enter a negotiated relationship with FCG	shed prejudice	must willingly confront own sexuality or homophobia
Ray, 1987 (8 nurses)	consider "what if it were me or my family member?"	value understanding the other; value and support patient or family choice	value trust; giving and receiving leads to bonding	make patient feel safe; make right decision; weigh in economics	deal with conflicting values
Spangler, 1993 (48 nurses)	Filipino Americans respect elders	(–) Anglo-Americans expect compliance		Anglo-Americans value patient education and self-care; Filipino Americans value cleanliness and physical comfort	Anglo-Americans value autonomy, control; Filipino Americans value patience, duty, and respect for authority
Swanson, 1990 (19 parents or HCPs)			attaching is part of care provision	avoid bad outcomes for others; manage responsibilities	avoid bad outcomes for self

NOTE: FCG = family caregiver; HCP = health care provider; (–) = condition that negatively affects caring.

measure, significant improvements (compared to pre-workshop) were found at the immediate and 3 months postmeasurement times ($p < .01$). Although this study is limited by design, instrumentation, and attrition, it does suggest that knowledge and an opportunity to deal openly with fears may enhance practice in situations in which nurses feel threatened.

Nurse-related conditions that affect caring may be personal (personality, family history) or professional (education, experience) in origin. Conditions may be further broken down into resources, demands, and constraints. An example of a nurse who is "primed" to acting in a caring fashion is one who has the personal resources of a strong, caring family upbringing and who is self-reflective, has limited personal constraints (e.g., is neither tired nor detached) and limited personal demands (e.g., not imbalanced or overburdened), has professional resources such as years of experience and ease with technology, has limited professional constraints (e.g., inadequate psychosocial skills or feeling constricted in how much he or she can disclose to a patient), and experiences minimal professional demands (e.g., feeling overstretched and morally conflicted). As Watson (1988a) has suggested, just as each patient's causal past will affect each caring transaction, so, too, will each nurse's per-

sonal and professional demands, constraints, and resources affect the capacity to act in a caring manner.

Outlined in Table 3.5 are the organization-related conditions that will affect caring. This table is based on a total sample of 543 participants (216 nurses, 65 administrators, 37 patients/family caregivers, 33 healthcare providers, and 192 individuals affiliated with a given hospital [includes providers and clients]). To date, Ray (1984, 1989) has published most extensively about characteristics of caring organizations. She strongly emphasizes that what constitutes caring for any individual frequently comes down to his or her role within the organization. Organizationally based factors affecting the occurrence of caring actions include role- and personnel-related demands, constraints, and resources; technologic possibilities and limitations; administrative support, decisions, and expectations; and worksite or practice conditions.

Future directions for Level III inquiry. This discussion of Level III conditions has been limited to nurse, patient, and organizational conditions that support the likelihood of caring actions occurring. Staying within this perspective, measures are clearly needed with which to quantify conditions that may serve as competing variables when

TABLE 3.3 Patient-Related Conditions That Affect Caring

First Author, Year (Participants)	Conditions: Patient Related					
	Communication	Personality	Health Problems	Care Needs	Nurse-Patient Relationship	Other
Baer, 1987 (140 students)		cheerful; accepts illness	has pain	ambulatory; needs nursing assistance	at least half of the reasons to like or dislike patient care are due to relationship	tidy; attractive; male
Beck, 1996 (37 students)	(–) verbally abusive	(–) combative; (–) distorted self-evaluation	(–) unpredictable			
Boyd, 1989 (15 RN students)		victimized; vulnerable	uncertainty in outcomes, treatment diagnoses, distressed	helpless		
Cohen, 1992 (23 nurses)	patient's gratitude	(–) patient or family is hard to deal with	patients becoming well; (–) patient's dying	physiologic emergencies; psychosocial needs		
Cohen, 1994 (38 nurses)	patient gratitude; (–) patient or family yelling at nurse	(–) patient anger	patients surviving; (–) losing patients	able to be comforted; (–) no cure available; (–) pain can't be relieved		
Euswas, 1993 (30 patients, 32 nurses)		vulnerable		needs nursing assistance		
Forrest, 1988 (17 nurses)	(±) what patient says	(–) hard-to-care-for patient			(–) disagreements with patient	
Green-Hernandez, 1991 (12 nurses)	patient or family responds favorably					
Jenny, 1996 (20 patients)			physically and emotionally distressed			
Kahn, 1988 (25 nurses)	(–) unwilling to communicate	alert, personable outgoing; (–) poor self-image; (–) patient's actions cause problems	many psychosocial problems; dire circumstances	relies on nurse	"fits" with nurse's personality; reciprocated friendship	
Leners, 1993 (40 nurses)			sicker patients bring out stronger use of nurse's intuition	nurse is more likely to use intuition in intense relationship		

TABLE 3.3 *Continued*

First Author, Year (Participants)	Conditions: Patient Related					
	Communication	Personality	Health Problems	Care Needs	Nurse-Patient Relationship	Other
Peteet, 1992 (192 HCPs)	honest about feelings and desires	spirited; courageous; has will to live; sense of humor; (–) unattractive in personality		has involved family; (–) unusually demanding	HCP able to identify with patient; patient interested in staff member's life	(–) unattractive appearance; (–) patient has VIP status
Poole, 1994 (5 patients)			physiologic concerns	needs physical care, information, and coordination of services	reciprocity; contact occurs	
Williams, 1992 (17 parents, 33 HCPs)	(–) patient or family directly resists support	(–) manifest anger; (–) denial			(–) patient or family openly clashes with staff	

NOTE: (–) = condition that negatively affects caring; (±) = depending on what patient says, could positively or negatively affect caring; HCP = health care provider.

attempting to investigate links between caring actions and their outcomes. However, there are distinct limits to restricting the measure of environmental conditions to the organizational level. Inquiry pertaining to Level III conditions calls for investigators who carefully consider the unit of analysis as larger than the classic individual nurse-individual patient dyad (practicing within an identified inpatient or community setting) and who recognize the wisdom that can be obtained from the study of aggregates. A more complete understanding of the conditions that affect the practice of caring calls for large-scale studies involving the examination of economic trends, cultural expectations, national policy outcomes, and sociopolitical constructions of what it is to be healthy, who is a patient, and what the criteria and qualifications of providers (nurses included) must be to meet the health care needs of society.

Level IV: Caring Actions

Quantitative inquiry. There have been two main ways of studying caring actions. The first, similar to the previous three levels, involves qualitative analysis of verbal text generated from nurse or client discourse about what caring means to them. The second thrust of caring action

investigations involves the use of caring behavior inventories that direct nurses, patients, or students to rank nurse caring behaviors on a least to most important scale. Tables 3.6 and 3.7 briefly summarize research findings pertaining to most highly ranked nurse caring behaviors according to nurses (Table 3.6) and patients (Table 3.7). Table 3.8 focuses specifically on studies that have employed Larson's (1984, 1986, 1987) CARE-Q sort and that published patient- or nurse-ranked behaviors according to Larson's theoretically generated subscales.

Caring behavior ranking studies have employed four different measures. Larson's original CARE-Q sort is the most widely used. It involves 50 nurse caring behaviors and six subscales. Items and subscales were initially generated from the literature. Respondents are directed to sort nurse caring behaviors along a quasinormal distribution ranging from (1) most to (7) least important. Cronin and Harrison's (1988) Caring Behaviors Assessment (CBA) includes 63 behaviors drawn from Watson's (1985) Carative Factors. Items are portrayed on a five-point Likert-type scale. Wolf (1986) generated the Caring Behavior Inventory (CBI) based on the literature and expert input. The original CBI consists of 75 caring words or phrases arranged on a four-point Likert-type scale. Lastly, Gardner and Wheeler's (1981, 1987) Supportive Nursing Behaviors Checklist (SNBC) consists of 67 behaviors derived from the literature and expert input. Items are arranged along a seven-point Likert-type scale.

TABLE 3.4 Nurse-Related Conditions That Affect Caring

First Author, Year (Participants)	Resources		Constraints		Demands	
	Personal	*Professional*	*Personal*	*Professional*	*Personal*	*Professional*
Brown, 1989 (25 nurses)				(–) lacks communication, conflict management, or family-centered care skills		
Clarke, 1992 (6 nurses)		talking and sharing with others	(–) tiredness; (–) unrecognized for their efforts	(–) frustrations; (–) witnessing patients who can't be cured	(–) personal problems	(–) feeling overstretched and too busy; (–) night duty
Cohen, 1992 (23 nurses)	life experience sensitizes and creates empathy	being able to offer comfort; witnessing miracles and patients surviving	(–) work evokes old unresolved issues from nurse's life		(–) difficulties balancing work and home	
Cohen, 1994 (38 nurses)	having learned from patients about personal priorities	witnessing survivals due to technological advances; learning new skills; getting through tough times		(–) having inadequate psychosocial skills; (–) witnessing death, suffering; (–) leaving patients at end of shift who are not well	(–) bringing work problems home	(–) balancing many different roles
Donoghue, 1993 (82 nurses)	caring family upbringing; personal experiences with death and illness; personal satisfaction from caring	education; more than 1 year experience; observing positive and negative role models				
Forrest, 1988 (17 nurses)	own experiences; self-appraisal; coping abilities	learning caring at school; feeling good about work	(–) personal stress			(–) dilemmas; (–) conflicts
Green-Hernandez, 1991 (12 nurses)	caring for self	education; professional practice; technical competency				
Kahn, 1988 (25 nurses)		can make the temporal investment needed to do the job	(–) tiredness; (–) animosity; (–) inability to get along with patient	(–) temporal limits		(–) can only "spread self so thin"
Kosowski, 1995 (18 students)	life-learning as background to book-learning	role-modeling; reversing (after seeing bad care modeled); experience leads to awareness				

TABLE 3.4 *Continued*

| First Author, Year (Participants) | Conditions: Nurse Related | | | | | |
| | Resources | | Constraints | | Demands | |
	Personal	*Professional*	*Personal*	*Professional*	*Personal*	*Professional*
Leners, 1993 (40 nurses)	nurse well-being; self-perception	experience with sensing, identifying, listening to intuition; intense patient relationship				
O'Berle, 1992 (1 nurse, 10 cases)	maintains wholeness; deals with stress; self-appraises; assesses personal costs of caring	feels good about own work				
Parker, 1994 (45 nurses)	experiencing inner harmony	ability to give knowledgable care; being accountable for patient's welfare and well-being	(–) not feeling respected for knowledge; (–) distrust bureaucratic motives	(–) being unable to tell patient the whole truth; (–) not able to practice according to values		(–) too many tasks; (–) going along with treatments nurse disagrees with
Ray, 1987 (8 nurses)		being comfortable enough with tehchnology to focus on patient				conflict between use of high-tech care and right to die
Solberg, 1991 (98 observations)			(–) detached	(–) believes infants feel no pain; (–) misses nonverbal cues		
Weiss, 1984 (240 students)		females attuned to verbal and nonverbal caring; males attuned to technical competency				
Williams, 1992 (17 parents, 33 HCPs)			(–) personal inabilities; (–) costs of being involved	(–) not seeing parents as experienced in care of own children		(–) too-intense work; (–) conflict with parents

NOTE: (–) = condition that negatively affects caring; HCPs = healthcare providers.

Because Larson's CARE-Q is the most widely used caring behavior measure, Tables 3.6 and 3.7 use Larson's items as the basis for comparison. When other caring measures were employed by investigators, I looked for items similar in meaning to those in the CARE-Q and included them in the comparison. Sometimes, the wordings of the alternative measure were slightly different; hence, noted in the legends under Tables 3.6 and 3.7 are those judgments I made as to which items seemed comparable.

TABLE 3.5 Organization-Related Conditions That Affect Caring

First Author Year (Participants)	Conditions: Organization Related			
	Personnel or Role-Related	*Technology*	*Administration*	*Work or Practice Conditions*
Brown, 1989 (25 nurses)			(–) no inservice to support parent care; (–) no rewards for parent care	(–) practice standards do not make nurse accountable for care of parents
Cohen, 1994 (38 nurses)	sense of community; peer support, respect; (–) poor teamwork; (–) peers critical, dominating, jealous	learning new technical, psychosocial, or cultural skills; (–) poor equipment; (–) learning the hard way	encourage development; (–) controlling, unwilling to share authority; (–) limited financial or human resources	(–) too little time to accomplish all that is required; (–) witnessing poor care; (–) when care seems futile
Cohen, 1992 (23 nurses)	peer recognition; (–) difficulties with medical staff; (–) peer conflict			(–) poor staffing, overworked and inadequate time; (–) unexpected crisis
Cooper, 1993 (9 nurses)		technology can enhance competent care or (–) detract nurse away from patient and to machines		
Dietrich, 1992 (5 nurses)			promotes communication; visible and available; easy to talk to; allows time to vent concerns; offers recognition; clear organizational mission	(–) overwhelming workload; (–) lack of time, space, interactions, help, or clear expectations
Duffy, 1995 (56 nurses)			communicates; creates open, trusting unit culture; share self; invest in staff	
Fareed, 1996 (8 patients)				reassuring environment is pleasant, unthreatening, and not rigid
Forrest, 1988 (12 nurses)	teamwork; fellow staff support		supportive unit supervisors; (–) difficult nurse administrators	(–) poor physical environment; (–) lack of time
Leners, 1993 (40 nurses)		intuition is used more if there is less equipment to rely on		intuition is used more if there are fewer others and fewer distractions
Powell-Cope, 1994 (12 FCGs)			policies must allow FCGs easier access to HCPs	
Ray, 1984 (192 HCPs, patients, Ad)	information shared; strong communication; high interactions	practical and technical skills essential; technology available, maintained, upgraded	economic welfare considered; coordinating activities and time	
Ray, 1989 (65 Ad)	team effort; work divided by roles; care concerns and expressions differ by role	in intensive care and emergency room, use of technology is a way to be caring	sustain economic viability of organization; garner resources to support care; support patient and nurse; make politically wise decisions	in different units there are differing care concerns (i.e., legal, technical, spiritual, etc.)
Ray, 1987 (8 nurses)		comfort with technology enables focus on patient and family		
Williams, 1992 (17 P, 33 HCPs)	(–) politics of nurse-physician communication; (–) inexperience		(–) inconsistent staffing patterns; (–) cumbersome bureaucracy	(–) lack of staff; (–) lack of time; (–) too-intense workloads

NOTE: HCPs = healthcare providers; P = parents; Ad = administrators; FCGs = family caregivers; (–) = condition that negatively affects caring.

TABLE 3.6 Nurses' Most Highly Rated Nurse Caring Behaviors

	Nurses' Most Highly Rated Nurse Caring Behaviors											
Caring Behavior Item (Items are abbreviated)	vonEssen,[a] 1994 (19 nurses)	Gooding, 1993 (46 nurses)	Keane, 1987 (26 nurses)	Komorita, 1991 (110 nurses)	Larson, 1986 (57 nurses)	Mayer, 1987 (28 nurses)	Mangold, 1991[b] (30 nurses)	Mangold, 1991[b] (30 students)	Gardner, 1981[c] (74 nurses)	Wolf, 1986 (97 nurses)	N/Possible N (Not all scales published comparable items)	Percentage of Possible Subjects
Listens to the patient	1	1	4.5	1	1	1	1	1	3	1	517/517	100%
Allows expression of feelings		2		2	3	2			2	4 "patience"	412/457	90%
Touches when comforting is needed				4	2	4				2 "comforts"	292/383	76%
Is perceptive of the patient's needs	4	4		5		5					203/286	71%
Realizes patient knows self best		3		3		3					184/286	64%
Gets to know patient as a person		5			4				1 "shows interest in patient as person"		177/360	49%
Gives the patient treatments and medications on time	2		4.5							5 "responsible"	142/383	37%
Tells patient what is important to know	4									3 "honesty"	116/383	30%
Talks to the patient					5						57/286	20%
Knows when to call doctor			1								26/286	9%
Puts patient first no matter what			3								26/286	9%
Gives good physical care			2								26/286	9%
Knows how to give shots and manage equipment	3										19/286	7%

NOTE: vonEssen, Larson, Gooding, Mayer = oncology nurses; Keane = rehabilitation nurses; Wolf = mostly adult care nurses; Gardner = medical-surgical and psychiatric nurses; Mangold = faculty and senior nursing students; Komorita = advanced practice nurses and faculty. Measures: Larson's CARE-Q used by Larson, vonEssen, Gooding, Keane, Mayer, Komorita, Mangold, total n = 346; Gardner and Wheeler's SNBC used by Gardner, n = 74; Wolf's CBI used by Wolf, n = 97. Math for combining samples: CARE-Q, SNBC, and CBI users, total n = 517; CARE-Q users minus Mangold sample plus CBI and SNBC users, total n = 457; CARE-Q users minus Mangold sample plus CBI and SNBC users, total n = 383; CARE-Q users minus Mangold sample plus CBI users, total n = 286; CARE-Q users minus Mangold sample plus SNBC users, total n = 360; CBI and SNBC users, total n = 171.
a. All references are cited by first author's name only.
b. Mangold only listed top chosen item.
c. Gardner only listed top three chosen items.

TABLE 3.7 Patients' Most Highly Rated Nurse Caring Behaviors

| | Patients' Most Highly Rated Nurse Caring Behaviors | | | | | | | | | |
Caring Behavior Item (Items are abbreviated)	vonEssen,[a] 1994 (19 patients)	Gooding, 1993 (42 patients)	Keane, 1987 (26 patients)	Larson, 1984 (57 patients)	Mayer, 1986 (54 patients)	Cronin, 1988 (22 patients)	Mullins, 1996 (46 patients)	Gardner, 1981, 1987 (119 patients)	N/possible N (Not all scales published comparable items)	Percentage of Possible Subjects
Helps me to feel confident adequate care was provided				1[b]		1[b]	2[b]	1	187/187	100%
Knows how to give shots and manage equipment		1	3	1	1	3	3		247/266	93%
Gets to know patient as a person							1[c]	3[d]	165/187	88%
Puts patient first no matter what			2		4	2[e]	4[e]	5[f]	267/385	69%
Treats me with respect							5		46/68	68%
Is cheerful					2			2[g]	173/317	55%
Knows when to call doctor		4	1	2		5			147/266	55%
Gives quick response to patient's call		2		3					99/198	50%
Is honest with patient	1							4	138/317	44%
Gives good physical care			5	4					83/198	42%
Gives the patient treatments and meds on time		3	4	5				X[h]	125/317	39%
Anticipates that first times are the hardest	4				5				73/198	37%
Knows how to handle equipment						4			22/68	32%
Encourages patient to ask questions					3				54/198	27%
Is perceptive of patient's needs		5						X	42/317	13%

Tells patient what is important to know	2		19/198	10%
Listens to patient	5		19/198	10%
Helps patient clarify his or her thinking	3	X	19/317	6%

NOTE: vonEssen, Gooding, Larson, Mayer = oncology patients; Keane = rehabilitation patients; Cronin = patients who had a myocardial infarction; Mullins = patients with HIV/AIDS; Gardner = medical-surgical and psychiatric adult patients. Measures: Larson's CARE-Q used by Larson, vonEssen, Gooding, Keane, Mayer, total n = 198; Cronin and Harrison's CBA used by Cronin, Mullin, total n = 68; Gardner and Wheeler's SNBC used by Gardner, n = 119. Math for combining samples: CARE-Q, SNBC, and CBA users, total n = 385; CARE-Q and CBA users, total n = 317; CARE-Q and SNBC users, total n = 266; SNBC and CBA users, total n = 187.

a. All references are cited by first author's name only.
b. "Knows what they're doing" (actual wording of researcher's questionnaire).
c. "Treat me as an individual."
d. "Showed interest in me."
e. "Makes me feel someone is there if I need them."
f. "Showed interest in my welfare."
g. "Was friendly."
h. X = SNBC has a similar item but not rated in top 5.

TABLE 3.8 Larson's CARE-Q Subscale Rankings for Nurses and Patients

| CARE-Q Subscale | Nurse Subscale Rankings | | | | | | | Patient Subscale Rankings | | | | |
	Mangold 1991 30 Nurses	Mangold 1991 28 Students	Mayer 1986 28 Nurses	Larson 1986 57 Nurses	vonEssen 1994 19 Nurses	Average of Nurse Ranking	Overall Nurse Rank	Mayer 1986 54 Patients	Larson 1984 57 Patients	vonEssen 1994 19 Patients	Average of Patient Rankings	Overall Patient Rank
Accessible	2	5	5	3	1	3.2	3	1	2	4	2.3	1
Explains	5	2	4	6	6	4.6	6	6	5	3	4.7	4
Anticipates	3	4	1	2	3	2.6	2	4	3	1	2.7	2
Comforts	6	1	2	1	2	2.4	1	3	4	2	3.0	3
Monitors and follows through	4	3	6	5	4	4.4	5	2	1	5	2.7	2
Trusting relationship	1	6	3	4	5	3.8	4	5	5	6	5.3	5

Table 3.6 focuses on nurses' most highly ranked caring behaviors. It is based on a combined sample of 517 nurses. Eight of the samples used Larson's CARE-Q, one sample used Gardner and Wheeler's SNBC, and another used Wolf's CBI. Listed are the top five endorsed caring behavior items per sample. Exceptions are Mangold (1991), who published only the top endorsed behavior, and Gardner and Wheeler, who published only the top three endorsed items. Across all samples, "Listens to the patient" falls within the top five endorsed behaviors. Likewise, 90% of the combined possible sample endorsed "Allows expression of feelings." Seventy-six percent endorsed touching to comfort, 71% favored being perceptive of patient needs, 64% realized the patient knew him- or herself best. These behaviors, which were endorsed as being in the top five-ranked nurse caring behaviors by more than 50% of the total sample, provide strong support for the fact that nurses believe it is important to know the patient well and to offer touch to comfort. Similar to the claim of Tanner, Benner, Chesla, and Gordon (1993), knowing the patient contextually is considered central to providing effective nursing care. Also, nurse touching based on striving to know the patient's feelings and experiences may account for why nurses claim their touching to comfort is therapeutic.

Table 3.7 outlines the five most highly ranked nurse caring behaviors endorsed by a combined sample of 385 patients drawn from eight separate studies. Once again, Larson's CARE-Q is used as the basis for comparison, as it was used in five of the studies. Two studies used Cronin and Harrison's CBA, and one used Gardner and

Wheeler's SNBC. Items were not quite as comparable across these three measures. Hence the most highly ranked behavior, "Helps me to feel confident adequate care was provided," was only applicable to samples using the CBA and SNBC. This item, along with the second most highly ranked item (93%), "Knows how to give shots and manage equipment," suggest that what patients value most highly is that the nurse is technically competent. The next four most highly endorsed items indicate that the patient wants the nurse to value, know, respect, and relate to them in a positive manner. The last two items endorsed by at least 50% of the combined samples suggest that patients want nurses to respond quickly when called and to know enough to call their doctor when necessary. Clearly, patients want nurses to be competent, focused on their evolving needs, and aware of when it is necessary to garner additional medical support.

It is fascinating to note the apparent divergent values between nurses and patients. Whereas 100% of the nurses value listening, only 10% of the patients ranked it in their top five behaviors. Likewise, whereas at least 93% of the patients endorsed the importance of technical skill, only 7% of nurses ranked "Knows how to give shots and manage equipment" in their top five behaviors. The origins of these discrepancies are compelling. Perhaps the gap lies in the fact that behaviors (not meanings) were solicited. Gaut (1983) stated that "whether certain actions will count as caring is dependent on what the action is, the intent of the doer, and the context in which it is done" (p. 317). It may be that both patients and nurses ultimately intend to ensure that safe, individualized care is offered, but nurses are challenged by the acts of getting to know each patient's personal needs for safe care, whereas patients are challenged by how the foreign, highly technical equipment surrounding them will be safely used to meet their personal needs.

In Table 3.8 are those studies that published subscale rankings using the Larson CARE-Q. The two overall most highly endorsed grouping of behaviors by nurses are the Comforts and Anticipates subscales. Patients most highly endorsed the Accessible subscale. There was a tie for patients' second most endorsed: Anticipates, and Monitors and Follows Through. Subscale level rankings would suggest that both nurses and patients value accessibility. However, nurses remain challenged to comfort, and patients desire that the nurses anticipate, monitor, and follow through with meeting their needs. Conceivably, nurses view accessibility, anticipating, monitoring, and following through as means to a goal of comforting.

Last of all, it must be noted that recently Larson and Ferketich (1993) and Wolf, Giardino, Osborne, and Ambrose (1994) have psychometrically revised their measures. Larson's scale has been factor analyzed and is now a 39-item visual analogue scale called the CARE/SAT (Caring Satisfaction Scale). Based on factor analysis of the revised original scale submitted to 268 hospitalized adults, three subscales were generated: Assistive, Benign Neglect, and Enabling. Surprisingly, the item "Listens to the patient" did not meet requirements for retention. It would be of interest to see if factor analysis of the same revised original scale submitted to nurses would produce similar results. In contrast, Wolf and colleagues did submit the CBI to a conveniently recruited sample of 278 patients and 263 nurses. Factor analysis yielded a 42-item, four-point Likert-type measure with five factors: respectful deference to the other, assurance of human presence, positive connectedness, professional knowledge and skill, and attentiveness to the other's experience.

Item level examination of the revised CBI suggests that Wolf and her colleagues (1994) have quantitatively arrived at a factor structure quite compatible with Swanson's (1990, 1991, 1993; Swanson-Kauffman, 1986a, 1988) phenomenologically derived five caring categories. Swanson initially derived her categories through phenomenologic inquiry into the caring desires of women who miscarried. She subsequently revised those categories, based on a study of what it is like to provide caring according to 19 care providers (parents or professionals) in a newborn intensive care unit. Last, the cate-

gories were reexamined for their relevance according to eight at-risk new mothers who had received an intensive long-term public health nursing intervention (Swanson, 1991). Each of Swanson's five caring categories is more fully discussed in the next section. Wolf's *attentiveness* parallels Swanson's *knowing*; *human presence* is akin to *being with*; *professional knowledge and skill* is like *doing for*; *respectful deference* echoes *enabling*; and *positive connectedness* has much in common with *maintaining belief*. The similarities between Wolf's and Swanson's findings are at least in part attributable to the fact that their factors or categories were derived from mixed samples of providers and recipients of caring.

Qualitative inquiry. Initial classification of the qualitatively derived caring actions resulted in a grid of 20 groupings of actions by 67 investigations. This involved a total sample of 2,314 participants (632 nurses, 607 patients/ families, 564 students, 259 healthcare providers [including nurses], 131 family caregivers, 98 practice observations, and 23 patient charts). Further examination of the 20 action groups led me to realize the utility of using the five caring categories I had previously derived through studies in three separate perinatal contexts. In the end, this effort led to two outcomes: a conceptually based framework for classifying caring actions that were inductively derived across many separate investigations, and validation for the generalizability of Swanson's middle-range theory of caring beyond the clinical contexts from which it was originally generated.

Swanson (1991) defines caring as "a nurturing way of relating to a valued other toward whom one feels a personal sense of commitment and responsibility" (p. 162). Similar to the overall framework for this chapter, alluded to in this definition are capacity (capability of valuing another), commitments (personal sense of commitment), role-related condition (responsibility), actions (way of relating), and consequences (nurturing). Categories identified by Swanson and used as an outline for Table 3.9 include *maintaining belief* (sustaining faith in the other's capacity to get through an event or transition and face a future with meaning), *knowing* (striving to understand an event as it has meaning in the life of the other), *being with* (being emotionally present to the other), *doing for* (doing for others what they would do for themselves if it were at all possible), and *enabling* (facilitating the other's passage through life transitions and unfamiliar events). Each of these categories involves subcategories that are italicized in Table 3.9.

TABLE 3.9 Inductively Derived Caring Action, Arranged by Swanson's (1990, 1991, 1993; Swanson-Kauffman, 1986a, 1988) Caring Categories

References[a]		*References*[a]	

Maintaining belief

Believing in or holding in esteem

1. Holistically viewing the other
   Recognizing personhood — 15,55
   Acknowledging uniqueness — 15
   Acknowledging the other — 15,49
   Confirming mind, body, and soul — 55
   Viewing as whole person — 34,36,45,48,50,55,59
   (Noncaring) Failing to see uniqueness — 31
2. Unconditionally regarding the other — 19,42,65
3. Respecting the other — 8,33,38,43,46,48,57,60,69

Helping find meaning[b]

1. Affirming experience
   Affirming meaning — 2,19
   Creating memories — 46
   Focusing on living, acknowledging dying — 26
2. Finding peace
   Alleviating guilt — 62
   Considering religious and spiritual needs — 17,49

Offering realistic optimism

1. Having a positive attitude — 57,58,59
2. Offering encouragement
   Realistic encouraging — 6,19,42,50,57,59
   Bolstering — 4,43
   Asserting optimism — 30
   Reassuring — 1,6,35,73

Offering a hope-filled attitude

1. Instilling and sustaining realistic hope — 43,50,57,58
   Seeing future possibilities — 40
2. Aiming for success
   Affirming the other's goals and potential — 39,59
   Promotes autonomous self-care — 44,69
   Holding high standards for the other — 16

"Going the distance"

1. Caring beyond expectations
   Risk-taking, courageous — 43
   Going beyond the basics — 14,24,36,50,59
2. Hanging in there no matter what
   Staying with until death or well-being — 55,70
   Giving off-duty time — 17,50

Knowing

Avoiding assumptions

1. Being open to the other's reality
   Accepting/open-minded — 27,61,65
   Being open, receptive — 40,52
2. Being nonjudgmental — 1,27,40
3. Checking back and checking out — 50,59,66
4. (Noncaring) distorting, minimizing — 32,39

Assesssing thoroughly

1. Assessing needs — 6,12,13,19,20,31,50,55,66,70,71
2. Assessing skills and capabilities — 1,13,27,40,48,58,71

Seeking cues

1. Monitoring vigilantly — 13,14,17,47
   Keeping watch — 13,14,69,73
2. Sensing concerns — 25,27
   Aware of emotional needs — 49
   Responding to stress — 29,40
3. Picking up cues, being sensitive — 32,33,68
   Tuning into the nonverbal — 50,60

Centering on the one cared for

1. Attending to the other
   Focusing on the other, not self — 52
   Conveying and gaining interest — 41,50
   Concerned — 37,42
   Individualized/ family-centered care — 19,23,34,35,42,46,50,58,62,70,72
2. Take the other's perspective — 15,36
   Perceiving/intuiting the other's reality — 53,70,73
3. Listening — 6,11,16,27,36,46,57,65
4. (Noncaring) Focusing away from the other
   Feeling negative about the other — 13,32,39,64
   Performing routinely/ task-oriented — 42,44,46
   Ignoring, neglect, being unavailable — 12,17,32,37,39,43,48,66

Engaging the self of both

1. Revealing or sharing self — 3,5,42,50,51,60,61
   Using self or putting self on the line — 17,32,47
   Being genuine/innermost self — 53,57
2. Becoming involved — 32,33,36,52,71
   Interpersonal interacting — 19,30
   Identifying with patient, "This could be me" — 20
3. Doing more than just a job — 39,64

TABLE 3.9 *Continued*

	References[a]		*References*[a]

Being with

Being there

1. Being present/there/with — 20,30,33,36,51,59,63,71,73
   Supportive/reassuring presence — 13,23
   Mindfully present — 29,38
   Physically present — 58
   Authentic/genuine presencing — 4,5,6,7,11,16,18,19,46,50,53,57,60
2. Connecting with the other — 2,5,15,19,26,32,45,50,51
   Intersubjective connecting — 29,52

Not burdening

1. Being responsible
   Considerate/kind/patient — 6,16,57,60,69
   Negotiated mutuality/respectful distance — 12,37
   Professional relationship with personal touch — 38,50
   (Noncaring) Intrusive/interfering — 39,60
2. Building trust — 16,27,29,30,37,43,48,50,60
3. Preserving self — 8,15,62

Conveying availability

1. Reaching out
   Touching to make a connection — 9,65
   Offering help — 52
2. Following up/following through — 6,24
3. Being accessible or available — 27,35,58,72
   Constant presence — 59

Enduring with

1. Ongoing relationship
   Nurse is part of patient's family — 60,70
   Involved, extended relationship — 15,19,37,63,71
   Friends, colleagues, comrades — 12,24,27,36,39,42,44,48,57,59,62
   Bonded, engaged, affiliated — 6,14,19,62
2. Investing time
   Persistent, timeless, ever changing — 39,50,53
   Spending time — 13,15,17,30,34,36,44,51,57,61,65,72

Sharing feelings

1. Loving
   Demonstrating love or fondness — 38,39,43
   Affection, tenderness — 44,48
   Warm attentiveness, pleasantness — 35,59
   Closeness — 33
   Commitment/compassion — 16,37,38,62,66
2. Feeling together
   Sharing/sharing feelings/beliefs — 1,6,7,31,33,35,45,50
   Reciprocal sharing/mutuality — 4,5,14,40,61,62
   Laughing/crying together — 5,11,16,40,50,53
   Social touching to "lighten up" — 9
   Expressive caring/responding — 13,27

Doing for

Comforting

1. Relieving pain and suffering
   Pain relief — 13,17,23,35,48,59,62
   Alleviating suffering — 43
   Satiating hunger — 23
2. Comforting/easing discomfort — 17,27,32,35,41,42,55,68
   Touching to comfort — 6,9,11,32,33,35,36,44,45,50,59,62

Performing competently and skillfully

1. Technically skilled — 13,14,23,25,36,37,45,48,51,59,60
2. Knowledgable performance — 6,19,24,32,33,35,36,45,46,60,71,72
3. Meeting needs — 17,23,29,44,46,50,59,60

Preserving dignity

1. Doing with — 24,29,63
2. Preserving the other's self
   Promoting autonomy/self-esteem — 10,13
   Dignity-preserving acts — 46,50,55
   Avoiding rudeness or belittling — 38,64
   Carrying the load for the other — 27

Anticipating

1. Being ready
   Anticipating/working in harmony — 10,32,50

Prepared/organized — 16,24,66
2. Rapidly responding
   Handling surprises or emergencies — 20
   Swift/spur-of-the-moment response — 43,48,50,52
3. Attending to many things at once
   Creative/overcoming barriers — 12,16,45,60
   Flexible — 8,12,48
   Setting priorities/balancing time, energy — 20,29

Protecting

1. Guarding safety/privacy
   Emotional, physical protection — 17,32,46,49,62,70,73
2. Modifying the environment
   Controlling/modifying environment — 17,23,69
   Teaching others how to respond — 1
   Making wise organizational choices — 63
3. Negotiating the system
   Coordinating resources/systems — 19,26,31,38,47,49,50,51,57,60,65,70,72,73
4. Advocating for — 23,42,43,44,45,46,55,71

(continued)

TABLE 3.9   *Continued*

	References[a]		*References*[a]
Enabling			
Informing/explaining		*Supporting/allowing*	
1. Telling it like it is		1. Providing support	23,31,36,42,46,49,72
Being honest/telling the		Nurturing, consoling	14,31,48
whole truth	1,27,41,70	Enhancing self-esteem	16,17
Responding objectively	40	2. (Noncaring) Controlling	12,38
2. Informing, explaining,	6,13,16,26,30,31,33,34,35,	*Focusing*	
coaching	41,46,50,57,58,62,70,72	1. Focusing, orienting	9,26
3. Communicating	1,12,16,24,29,30,36,40,44,46,	2. Focusing on specific concerns	
	47,49,62	Enhancing maternal-infant	
4. Many teaching,		attachment	59
communicating styles	8	Enhancing coping	2,73
Modeling	24,40	Resolving fears/tension	23,52,62
Supervising, overseeing	10,31	*Generating alternatives/*	
Using self as interactive		*thinking it through*	
tool	43	1. Assisting with self-care	
Providing opportunities		decisions	19,48,65,70
for practice	40	2. Empowering/increasing	
Validating/giving feedback		self-efficacy	11,19,26,57,65,73
1. Confirming/affirming	27,40,43,46,48	3. Counseling/problem solving	16,35
2. Normalizing	11,73		

a. Numbers refer to references in the Appendix.
b. New subcategory not previously published by Swanson.

Future directions for Level IV inquiry. Conceptually caring actions have a lot in common (*universality,* according to Leininger, 1988), but their actual expression will be as different as the individuals involved and the reasons for caring (Leininger's *diversality*). For example, what it takes to enable a single mother with breast cancer to live a quality life versus what it would take to support an elderly person with Alzheimer's to remain with family caregivers would both involve the enabling subcategories of informing/explaining, supporting/allowing, focusing, generating alternatives/thinking it through, and validating/giving feedback. However, the actual content of any of those enabling activities would be based on both knowing the specific client(s) and anticipating the challenges inherent in the relevant disease trajectories. Hence, the implication for designing caring-based intervention studies is that although the investigator may choose a caring framework for the clinical therapeutic, the actual content of the intervention would have to be drawn from knowledge of the health problem, its related symptomatology, and typical human responses to the disease's illness and healing trajectory. The clearest limitation to the study of Level IV caring actions is the lack of controlled clinical trials wherein protocols for caring-based therapeutic interventions are defined, applied, carefully monitored, and tested for effectiveness in promoting healthy outcomes.

Level V: Caring Consequences

Beck (1991, 1992a, 1992b, 1993, 1994) has conducted a program of research examining the experience and outcomes of caring within the academic setting. In her 1994 publication, Beck draws all of her studies together and succinctly and creatively reduces her multiple interpretive studies of caring within academia to the following statement: "Caring is centered in authentic presencing where selfless sharing and fortifying support flourish and lead to uplifting consequences" (p. 115). She further states, "once fortified from being cared-for [people] will, in turn, be better able to nurture their own ability to care for others" (p. 108). Hence, Beck offers phenomenologic validation to the claims of Watson (1988a) that participation in a caring transaction leads to the betterment of both provider and recipient.

Unfortunately, quantitative findings about the consequences of caring are minimal. This fact reflects the limited amount of investigators who have attempted to explicitly link caring-based therapeutic interventions to outcomes. Three exceptions to this claim were found. In the first study, Latham (1996) examined the associations among patient background variables (self-esteem and desire for behavioral and informational control), nurse caring (spiritual caring, supportive caring, physical caring, interpretive caring, and sensitive caring) and patient outcomes (appraisals, psychological distress, coping strategies and effectiveness). Nurse caring, supportive, was operationalized using Gardner and Wheeler's (1981) SNBC (described under "Level IV: Caring Actions"). The other four dimensions of nurse caring were measured using Latham's Holistic Caring Inventory (HCI). The HCI, based on Howard's (1975) holistic dimension of humanistic caring theory, is a 39-item, four-point Likert-type measure. All HCI subscale internal consistencies exceed .90. Whereas study participants reported experiencing minimal amounts of interpretive, spiritual, and supportive caring, they perceived moderate amounts of physical and sensitive caring. There was a weak (beta weight = .22) but statistically significant ($p \leq .05$) association between desire for cognitive control and perception of receiving supportive caring. Forty percent of the overall variance in coping effectiveness was accounted for by the combined variables of supportive and sensitive caring, problem and emotion-focused coping, and decreased psychological distress. Post-hoc analysis yielded additional information about caring. Those with lower self-esteem perceived more threat (measured as primary cognitive appraisal) from interactions with nurses ($p \leq .05$). Compared to older patients, younger patients were more likely to rate supportive caring behaviors as important ($p \leq .001$). Younger patients also viewed nurses as providing more supportive ($p \leq .001$) and physical caring ($p \leq .01$). Last, those with moderate (versus minimal or no) pain perceived more supportive and physical nurse caring ($p \leq .05$). In summary, Latham's investigation demonstrated that (a) certain patient conditions (self-esteem, age, and pain level) are associated with perceptions of nurses as caring and (b) sensitive and supportive nurse caring contributes to patients' overall coping effectiveness.

In a second quantitative investigation of caring consequences, Duffy (1992) examined the associations between nurse caring and patient satisfaction, health status, length of stay, and health care costs for 86 randomly selected patients. Duffy's Caring Assessment Tool (CAT) was used to quantify nurse caring (10 items, five-point Likert-type scale). The only statistically significant association demonstrated was between the CAT and patient satisfaction, as measured using a 100 mm visual analogue scale ($r = .46$, $p \leq .001$). Caring accounted for 19% of the overall variance in patient satisfaction. The third investigation of caring consequences was also conducted by Duffy (1993). To evaluate the effects of nurse administrators' caring, she developed a measure, based on Watson's (1985) carative factors, known as the CAT-A (94

items, five-point Likert-type scale). Fifty-six nurses participated in Duffy's examination of the relationships between perceptions of administrator nurse caring and staff nurse job satisfaction and turnover rates. The CAT-A had high internal consistency (Cronbach's alpha = 0.99). Mean overall perception of administrator caring was 339.84 and ranged from 196 to 470 (possible range 94 to 470). The association between the CAT-A and turnover was nonsignificant, but there was a significant association ($r = .36$) with the one-item rating of job satisfaction ($p = .007$).

Summarized in Table 3.10 are 30 relatively recent (1986 to 1996) qualitative studies in which potential outcomes of caring were interpreted. The studies used a total sample of 1,185 participants (420 nurses, 203 patients/families, 358 students, 12 family caregivers, and 192 healthcare providers [including nurses]). Consequences of caring for the one cared for (most often patient or student) were multiple indicators of enhanced well-being, including positive effects on self-esteem, mood, self-efficacy, satisfaction with care, and physical healing. It appears that oftentimes caring is credited with freeing up inner strengths and healing potential. Social benefits of participating in a caring relationship are that the recipient feels he or she can count on the provider, is less dependent, and is better able to navigate the healthcare system.

The second part of Table 3.10 summarizes the consequences of caring for the one caring (e.g., the nurse). Practicing in a caring manner leads to the nurse's well-being, both personally and professionally. Personal outcomes of caring include feeling important, accomplished, purposeful, aware, integrated, whole, and confirmed. Professionally practicing caring leads to enhanced intuition, empathy, clinical judgment, capacity for caring, and work satisfaction. Social outcomes of caring for nurses include feeling connected both to their patients and to their colleagues.

Also very briefly outlined in Table 3.10 are some potential consequences of noncaring. Patients who experience noncaring feel humiliated, out of control, despaired, frightened, and alienated. Sadly, bad memories of the noncaring episode linger. Finally, of greatest concern is the suggestion that participating in a noncaring encounter may lead to prolongation of physical healing. Noncaring also takes its toll on nurses, resulting in nurses becoming worn down, robotlike, depressed, hardened, and frightened.

Future directions for Level V inquiry. It is essential that nurse investigators take seriously the need to document

TABLE 3.10 Consequences of Caring and Noncaring for Clients and Nurses

Consequences of Caring	References[a]	Consequences of Noncaring	References[a]
Client[b] outcomes of caring		**Client outcomes of noncaring**	
Emotional-spiritual		*Emotional-spiritual*	
Enhanced self-esteem/-worth	3,5,6,37,50	Humiliated	64
Enhanced knowledge, coping	37,49,57,65,67,71	Frightened	64
Increased well-being/quality of life	19,61	Out of control	64
Feeling reassured/confident/good	4,6,67	Despair/helplessness	38
Gained control/independence	19,30	Alienation	38
Empowered, sustained, confident	6,19,65	Vulnerability	38
Positive mental attitude/uplifting		Lingering bad memories	37
consequences	7,67		
Satisfaction with care/expectations met	42,67		
Relaxed/happy/merriment	5,50		
Enhanced dignity/personhood	49,61,67		
Fostered spiritual freedom	38		
Enhanced growth and development	5,37,57		
Gratitude/feeling cared-for	4,37,42,67		
Feeling more caring toward others	3,4		
Physical		*Physical*	
Enhanced healing	14,22,42,47,67	Decreased healing	38
Feeling safe	49		
Life saved	14		
Decreased costs/length of stay	49,65		
Supports current energy	38		
Nurse knows patients' capacities	71		
Increased physical comfort	42		
Better coordination of care	65		
Social			
Meaningful reciprocal relationship	14,19,61		
Family empowered/less dependent	19		
Trust/someone to count on	50,65,67		
Enhanced relationship between patient			
and FCG	58		
Decreased alienation from HCDS	58		
Nurse outcomes of caring		**Nurse outcomes of noncaring**	
Emotional-spiritual		*Emotional-spiritual*	
Sense of accomplishment, self-satisfaction	28,49,50,52,56	Hardened, oblivious, robot-like	8
Sense of importance/purpose to own life	8,56	Depressed, frightened	8
Experiencing gratitude	21,22,56	Worn down	52
Preserved integrity/well-being	45,54		
Fulfillment/confirmation/wholeness	15,49,52		
Enhanced self-perception/self-esteem	5,45,54		
Uplifting consequences/self-			
transformation	5,7		
Learning about self/living own			
philosophy	5,8,15		
Respect for life/aware of			
own mortality	8		
Looking inward	54		
Professional			
Enhanced intuition/clinical judgement	45,47,71		
Increased skills and knowledge	21,45,71		
Mobilizes more caring	7,54		
Enhanced empathy/fewer assumptions	8		
Satisfaction with/love of nursing	49,50,65		
Social			
Sense of collegiality	49		
Connecting	52		
Relationship with patient	5,15,56,65		

NOTE: FCG = family caregiver; HCDS = healthcare delivery system.
a. Numbers refer to references in the Appendix.
b. "Client" can refer to a patient, a family, or a student.

the consequences of caring. The term *consequences* is deliberately chosen for two reasons. First, it draws attention to the thought pattern that underlies the thinking of clinical investigators (i.e., the occurrence of "y" is consequent to the earlier occurrence of "x"), and second, it highlights both the intended and unintended outcomes and potential side effects of caring actions. This chapter only highlights "good" from caring and "bad" from noncaring; it does not address the power differences assumed within a caring framework and the personal costs of caring.

Nurse researchers working in a clinical arena need to expand (some may say constrict) their thinking to consider caring as a commodity that may be measured, rigorously applied, and tested for its effectiveness in promoting healing, recovery, or optimal well-being. Such inquiry calls for nurse investigators who value the importance of caring and have clinical insight into the caring needs of a specific clinical group; the resources to design caring-based, clinically relevant controlled studies; and clarity about the intended and potentially unintended measurable consequences of caring protocols. Upon completion of such investigations, nurse scientists need to enter into dialogue about the universal mechanisms by which caring affects well-being. Such conceptual or philosophic debate should highlight the basic structure of caring, its antecedents, and its consequences.

Caring Relationships

Alluded to throughout this chapter has been the fact that some relationships may be considered caring and others are rendered noncaring. Ray (1995) critically dealt with the concern that for so many studies the range of responses is very narrow and skewed toward positive perceptions when examining patient perceptions of nurse caring or satisfaction with nursing care. Ray questioned whether clients answered positively due to having low expectations, respondent bias, or fear of negative sanctions for speaking frankly. Alternatively, she questioned if the issue lay in concept measurement error; that is, examining caring as though it occurred along a normal distribution versus viewing it as an expected given and measuring it as a norm-referenced criterion (e.g., *safe caring* should be expected at 100% and any deviance from that norm should be the focus of measurement).

Halldorsdottir (1991) interviewed nine patients and nine students about potential modes of being with another person. She proposed a creative framework consisting of five possible ways of characterizing nurse-patient relationships. Type 1, "biocidic" relationships, are defined as life destroying: They are "acid-edged," lead to anger, despair, and alienation, with the ultimate effects of diminishing healing and well-being, leaving the participants vulnerable and haunted by unforgettable bad memories. Type 2, "biostatic" relationships, are life restraining, wherein nurses coldly treat patients as a "nuisance," leading them to believe that the nurse does not care and is blind to them and their situation. Type 3, "biopassive" relationships, are defined as "life-neutral." The relationship is basically apathetic or detached, there is no person-to-person acknowledgment, and lives or energy levels are neither enhanced or diminished. Type 4, "bioactive" relationships, are life sustaining. This is the classic professional nurse-patient relationship, characterized as benevolent, kind, and concerned. The result of this encounter is that energy levels are sustained and good will ensues. Type 5, "biogenic" relationships, involves being fully present, with healing love flowing. Personhood is mutually acknowledged, care is negotiated, and professional intimacy (creative distance with respect and compassion) ensues. This relationship fosters spiritual freedom (Halldorsdottir, 1991).

Tieing together the deliberations of Ray (1995) with the findings of Halldorsdottir (1991), it is possible that most nurse-patient interactions fall between Types 3 (the "at least" or normative criterion) and 5 (perhaps the "extra credit" expectation). Type 3 relationships might characterize the transaction between a task-oriented nurse (e.g., the "med-nurse" who in a 30-second interaction safely administers 10:00 a.m. medications). A Type 4 interaction might characterize most nurse-patient interactions in which effective psychosocially and physiologically oriented therapeutic interventions transpire (e.g., an ongoing relationship between a school nurse and the group of "regulars" who stop by the health clinic). Type 5 interactions might be those exquisite moments of intimate connection—the occasions in which both nurse and patient feel transformed (even if only for the day) for having made it through a challenging time together (e.g., a midwife's and a couple's exhilaration at bringing forth a new life). Nurse-patient interactions that do not meet the Type 3 criterion would fall into the noncaring or possibly malpractice or abusive range (Type 2 = neglect; Type 1 = direct abuse).

Conclusions

Over the past few decades, the discipline of nursing has entertained considerable discourse about what constitutes appropriate methods for studying nursing phenomena. Historically, this discourse has been labeled the "qualitative-quantitative debate." It is beyond the scope of this chapter to deal with the limitations of such either-or discussion; however, this debate cannot go unacknowledged in summarizing the state of scientific knowledge about caring. Clearly, scientists interested in the concept of caring have by and large stuck with the more interpretive methods of knowledge building. The challenge remains for the discipline to allow for the coexistence of multiple paradigms for inquiry about caring. It is time to build on the rich descriptions and interpretations of caring that have been reviewed through this literary meta-analysis. From a strictly pragmatic stance, caring thoughts, theories, and concepts need to be translated into useful measures and testable protocols that are employed in replicable, generalizable research designs.

In this chapter, an attempt has been made to bring clarity to discourse about the concept of caring in nursing. It has been suggested that disciplinary conversations might best be characterized as having five levels of discussion. When referring to the concept *caring*, there is a need to be clear about whether the discourse is about the capacity for caring, the concerns and commitments that underlie caring, conditions that inhibit or enhance caring, caring actions, or the consequences of caring. Also proposed and supported throughout this chapter was a theoretical framework for categorizing therapeutic, caring interventions, based on Swanson's middle range theory of caring.

It is safe to say that collectively (across the discipline), at an interpretive level, much is known about caring. There remain, however, minimal quantitative empirical studies. Disciplinary challenges that lie ahead include the production of psychometrically sound measures for examining each level of caring; careful examination of associations within, between, and among the five caring levels; and a commitment to framing nursing intervention studies (caring actions) under the language of caring, hence providing a measurable and conceptually congruent framework to tie together the sound science underlying the practice of essential and effective professional nurse caring.

Appendix: Studies quoted
in Tables 3.9 and 3.10

Reference	Year	Author(s)	Participants	Reference	Year	Author(s)	Participants
1	1984	Aamodt, Grassl-Herwehe, Farell, and Hutter	8 children	17	1991	Chipman	26 students
2	1993	Bäck-Pettersson and Jensen	32 nurses	18	1992	Clarke and Wheeler	6 nurses
3	1991	Beck	47 students	19	1991	Clayton, Murray, Hornes, and Greene	70 families
4	1992a	Beck	53 students	20	1994	Cohen, Haberman, and Steeves	38 nurses
5	1992b	Beck	36 students	21	1994	Cohen, Haberman, Steeves, and Deatrick	38 nurses
6	1993	Beck	22 students	22	1992	Cohen and Sarter	23 nurses
7	1994	Beck	136 students, 17 faculty	23	1994	Collins, McCoy, Sale, and Weber	36 patients
8	1996	Beck	37 students	24	1996	Coulon, Krause, and Andersen	156 students
9	1993	Bottorf	8 patients	25	1993	Cooper	9 nurses
10	1987	Bowers	27 elders, 33 FCGs	26	1990	Davies and O'Berle	1 nurse, 10 cases
11	1989	Boyd and Munhall	15 nurses	27	1992	Dietrich	5 nurses
12	1989	Brown and Ritchie	25 nurses	28	1993	Donoghue	107 nurses
13	1986	Brown	50 patients	29	1993	Euswas	32 nurses,
14	1993	Burfitt, Greiner, Miers, Kinney, and Branyon	13 patients	30	1996	Fareed	30 patients
15	1994	Burns	8 nurses				8 patients
				31	1988	Flaherty	12 grandmothers
16	1988	Bush	14 students	32	1993	Finn	3 patients

Reference	Year	Author(s)	Participants	Reference	Year	Author(s)	Participants
33	1988	Forrest	17 nurses	52	1992	Montgomery	35 nurses
34	1993	Girot	10 nurses	53	1996	Nelms	5 nurses
35	1987	Gardner and Wheeler	110 patients	54	1992	O'Berle and Davies	1 nurse, 10 cases
36	1991	Green-Hernandez	12 nurses	55	1994	Parker	45 nurses
37	1990	Halldorsdottir	9 students	56	1992	Peteet, Rose, Medeiros, Walsh-Burke, and Rieker	192 HCPs
38	1991	Halldorsdottir	9 patients, 9 students	57	1994	Poole and Rowat	5 patients
39	1988	Hinds	25 patients	58	1994	Powell-Cope	12 FCGs
40	1992	Hughes	10 students	59	1994	Propst, Schenk, and Clairain	9 patients
41	1973	Irwin and Meier	20 HCPs, 20 FCGs	60	1996	Raudonis and Kirschling	9 FCGs
42	1996	Jenny and Logan	20 patients	61	1993	Raudonis	14 patients
43	1992	Jensen, Bäck-Pettersson, and Segesten	16 nurses	62	1987	Ray	8 nurses
44	1988	Kahn and Steeves	25 nurses	63	1984	Ray	192 HCPs
45	1995	Kosowski	18 students	64	1986	Riemen	10 patients
46	1991	Lemmer	28 parents	65	1992	Schroeder and Maeve	29 patients
47	1993	Leners	40 nurses	66	1991	Sherwood	10 patients
48	1996	Lovgren, Engstrom, and Norberg	80 patients, 12 family members	67	1993	Sherwood	10 patients
				68	1991	Solberg and Morse	98 observations
49	1995	McNamara	5 nurses	69	1993	Spangler	48 nurses
50	1992	Miller, Haber, and Byrne	15 patients, 16 nurses	70	1994	Steeves, Cohen, and Wise	38 nurses
51	1996	Milne and McWilliam	14 HCPs, 6 patients	71	1993	Tanner, Benner, Chesla, and Gordon	130 nurses
				72	1992	Williams	17 FCGs, 33 HCPs
				73	1994	Winters, Miller, Maracich, Compton, and Haberman	23 patient charts

NOTE: FCGs = family caregivers; HCPs = health care providers.

References

Aamodt, A. M., Grassl-Herwehe, S., Farell, F., & Hutter, J. (1984). The child's view of chemically induced alopecia. In M. M. Leininger (Ed.), *Care: The essence of nursing* (pp. 217-234). Thorofare, NJ: Slack.

Bäck-Pettersson, S. K., & Jensen, K. P. (1993). "She dares": An essential characteristic of the excellent Swedish nurse. In D. Gaut (Ed.), *A global agenda for caring* (pp. 257-265). New York: National League for Nursing.

Baer, E. D., & Lowery, B. J. (1987). Patient and situational factors that affect nursing students' like or dislike of caring for patients. *Nursing Research, 36*(5), 298-302.

Beck, C. T. (1991). How students perceive faculty caring: A phenomenological study. *Nursing Educator, 16,* 18-22.

Beck, C. T. (1992a). Caring among nursing students. *Nursing Educator, 17,* 22-27.

Beck, C. T. (1992b). Caring between nursing students and physically/mentally handicapped children: A phenomenological study. *Journal of Nursing Education, 31*(8), 361-366.

Beck, C. T. (1993). Caring relationships between nursing students and their patients. *Nurse Educator, 18*(5), 28-32.

Beck, C. T. (1994). Researching experiences of living caring. In A. Boykin (Ed.), *Living a caring-based program.* New York: National League for Nursing.

Beck, C. T. (1996). Nursing students' experiences caring for cognitively impaired elderly people. *Journal of Advanced Nursing, 23*(5), 992-998.

Benner, P. (1984). *From novice to expert.* Menlo Park, CA: Addison-Wesley.

Benner, P. J. (1990). The moral dimension of caring. In J. S. Stevenson & T. Tripp Reimer (Eds.), *Knowledge about care and caring: State of the art and future developments* (pp. 5-17). Washington, DC: American Academy of Nursing.

Benner, P., & Wrubel, J. (1989). *The primacy of caring.* Menlo Park, CA: Addison-Wesley.

Bottorf, J. L. (1993). The use and meaning of touch in caring for patients with cancer. *Oncology Nursing Forum, 20*(10), 1531-1538.

Bowers, B. J. (1987). Intergenerational caregiving: Adult caregiveers and their aging parents. *Advances in Nursing Science, 9*(2), 20-31.

Boyd, C. O., & Munhall, P. L. (1989). A qualitative investigation of reassurance. *Holistic Nursing Practice, 4*(1), 61-69.

Boykin, A. (1994). *Living a caring-based curriculum.* New York: National League for Nursing.

Boykin, A., & Schoenhofer, S. (1993). *Nursing as caring: A model for transforming practice.* New York: National League for Nursing.

Brown, L. (1986). The experience of care: Patients' perspectives. *Topics in Clinical Nursing, 8*(2), 56-62.

Brown, J., & Ritchie, J. A. (1989). Nurses' perceptions of their relationships with parents. *Maternal Child Nursing Journal, 18*(2), 79-96.

Burfitt, S. N., Greiner, D. S., Miers, L. J., Kinney, M. R., & Branyon, M. E. (1993). Professional nurse caring as perceived by critically ill patients: A phenomenologic study. *American Journal of Critical Care, 2*(6), 489-499.

Burns, M. (1994). Creating a safe passage: The meaning of engagement for nurses caring for children and their families. *Issues in Comprehensive Pediatric Nursing, 17,* 211-221.

Bush, H. A. (1988). The caring teacher of nursing. In M. M. Leininger (Ed.), *Care: Discovery and uses in clinical and community nursing* (pp. 169-187). Detroit: Wayne State University Press.

Chipman, Y. (1991). Caring: Its meaning and place in the practice of nursing. *Journal of Nursing Education, 30*(4), 171-175.

Clarke, J. B., & Wheeler, S. J. (1992). A view of the phenomenon of caring in nursing practice. *Journal of Advanced Nursing, 7,* 1283-1290.

Clayton, G. M., Murray, J. P., Hornes, S. D., & Greene, P. S. (1991). Connecting: A catalyst for caring. In P. Chinn (Ed.), *Anthology on caring* (pp. 155-168). New York: National League for Nursing.

Cohen, M. Z., Haberman, M. R., & Steeves, R. (1994). The meaning of oncology nursing. *Oncology Nursing Forum, 21*(8 supp.), 5-8.

Cohen, M. Z., Haberman, M. R., Steeves, R., & Deatrick, J. A. (1994). Rewards and difficulties of oncology nursing. *Oncology Nursing Forum, 21*(8 supp.), 9-17.

Cohen, M. Z., & Sarter, B. (1992). Love and work: Oncology nurses' view of the meaning of their work. *Oncology Nursing Forum, 19*(10), 1481-1486.

Collins, B. A., McCoy, S. A., Sale, S., & Weber, S. E. (1994). Descriptions of comfort by substance using and non-using postpartum women. *Journal of Obstetric and Gynecologic and Neonatal Nursing, 23*(4), 293-300.

Coulon, L., Krause, K. L., & Anderson, M. (1996). The pursuit of excellence in nursing care: What does it mean? *Journal of Advanced Nursing, 24*(4), 817-826.

Cooper, M. C. (1993). The intersection of technology and care in the ICU. *Advances in Nursing Science, 15*(3), 23-32.

Cronin, S. N., & Harrison, B. (1988). Importance of nurse caring behaviors as perceived by patients after myocardial infarctions. *Heart and Lung, 17*(4), 374-380.

Davies, B., & O'Berle, K. (1990). Dimensions of the supportive role of the nurse in palliative care. *Oncology Nursing Forum, 17*(1), 87-94.

Dietrich, L. (1992). The caring nursing environment. In D. A. Gaut (Ed.), *The presence of caring in nursing* (pp. 69-87). New York: National League for Nursing.

Donoghue, J. (1993). Humanistic care and nurses' experience. In D. Gaut (Ed.), *A global agenda for caring* (pp. 267-279). New York: National League for Nursing.

Drew, N. (1986). Exclusion and confirmation: A phenomenology of patients' experiences with caregivers. *Image: The Journal of Nursing Scholarship, 18*(2), 39-43.

Duffy, J. R. (1992). Impact of nurse caring on patient outcomes. In D. A. Gaut (Ed.), *The presence of caring in nursing* (pp. 113-136). New York: National League for Nursing.

Duffy, J. R. (1993). Caring behaviors of nurse managers: Relationships to staff nurse satisfaction and retention. In D. Gaut (Ed.), *A global agenda for caring* (pp. 365-377). New York: National League for Nursing.

Euswas, P. (1993). The actualized caring moment: A grounded theory of caring in nursing practice. In D. Gaut (Ed.), *A global agenda for caring* (pp. 309-326). New York: National League for Nursing.

Fareed, A. (1996). The experience of reassurance: Patient's perspectives. *Journal of Advanced Nursing, 23*(2), 272-279.

Flaherty, M. J. (1988). Seven caring functions of Black grandmothers in adolescent mothering. *MCN Journal, 17*(3), 191-207.

Finn, J. (1993). Caring in birthing: Experiences of professional nursing and generic care. In D. Gaut (Ed.), *A global agenda for caring* (pp. 63-79). New York: National League for Nursing.

Forrest, D. (1988). The experience of caring. *Journal of Advanced Nursing, 14,* 815-823.

Gadow, S. (1980). Existential advocacy: Philosophical foundation of nursing. In S. Spicker & S. Gadow (Eds.), *Nursing images and ideals* (pp. 86-101). New York: Springer.

Gadow, S. (1984). Touch and technology: Two paradigms of patient care. *Journal of Religion and Health, 23*(1), 63-69.

Gadow, S. (1990). The advocacy covenant: Care as clinical subjectivity. In J. S. Stevenson & T. Tripp Riemer (Eds.), *Knowledge about care and caring: State of the art and future developments* (pp. 33-40). Washington, DC: American Academy of Nursing.

Gardner, K. G., & Wheeler, E. (1981). Patients' and staff nurses' perceptions of supportive nursing behaviors: A preliminary analysis. In M. M. Leininger (Ed.), *Caring: An essential human need* (pp. 109-113). Thorofare, NJ: Slack.

Gardner, K. G., & Wheeler, E. (1987). Patient's perceptions of support. *Western Journal of Nursing Research, 9*(1), 115-131.

Gaut, D. (1983). Development of a theoretically adequate description of caring. *Western Journal of Nursing Research, 5,* 313-324.

Girot, E. A. (1993). Assessment of competence in clinical practice: A phenomenological approach. *Journal of Advanced Nursing, 18,* 114-119.

Glaser, B. G., & Strauss, A. L. (1967). *The discovery of grounded theory: Strategies for qualitative research.* New York: Aldine.

Gooding, B. A., Sloan, M., & Gagnon, L. (1993). Important nurse caring behaviors: Perceptions of oncology patients and nurses. *Canadian Journal of Nursing Research, 25*(3), 65-76.

Green-Hernandez, C. (1991). A phenomenological investigation of caring as a lived experience in nursing. In P. Chinn (Ed.), *Anthology on caring* (pp. 111-131). New York: National League for Nursing.

Halldorsdottir, S. (1990). The essential structure of a caring and uncaring encounter with a teacher: The perspective of the nursing student. In M. M. Leininger & J. Watson (Eds.), *The caring experience in education* (pp. 95-108). New York: National League for Nursing.

Halldorsdottir, S. (1991). Five basic modes of being with another. In D. Gaut & M. M. Leininger (Eds.), *Caring: The compassionate healer* (pp. 37-49). New York: National League for Nursing.

Halloran, E. J. (1985). Nursing workload, medical diagnostic related group, and nursing diagnosis. *Research in Nursing and Health, 8,* 421-433.

Heidigger, M. (1962). *Being and time* (J. Macquarrie & E. Roninson, Trans.). New York: Harper & Row.

Hinds, P. S. (1988). The relationship of nurses' caring behaviors with hopefulness and healthcare outcomes in adolescents. *Archives of Psychiatric Nursing, 2*(1), 21-29.

Howard, J. (1975). Humanization and dehumanization of health care: A conceptual view. In J. Howard & A. Strauss (Eds.), *Humanizing health care* (pp. 57-102). New York: John Wiley.

Hughes, L. (1992). Faculty-student interaction and the faculty perceived climate for caring. *Advances in Nursing Science, 14*(3), 60-71.

Irwin, B., & Meier, J. (1973). Supportive measures for relatives of the fatally ill. *Communicating Nursing Research, 6,* 119-128.

Jenny, J., & Logan, J. (1996). Caring and comfort metaphors used by patients in critical care. *Image: The Journal of Nursing Scholarship, 28*(4), 349-352.

Jensen, K. P., Bäck-Pettersson, S. R., & Segesten, K. M. (1992). The caring moment and the green-thumb phenomenon amongst Swedish nurses. *Nursing Science Quarterly, 6*(2), 98-104.

Kahn, D. L., & Steeves, R. H. (1988). Caring and practice: Construction of the nurse's world. *Scholarly Inquiry for Nursing Practice, 2*(3), 201-216.

Keane, S. M., & Chastain, B. (1987). Caring: Nurse-patient perceptions. *Rehabilitation Nursing, 12*(4), 182-185.

Klausner, S. Z. (1971). *On man and his environment.* San Francisco, CA: Jossey-Bass.

Komorita, N. I., Doehring, K. M., & Hirchert, P. W. (1991). Perceptions of caring by nurse educators. *Journal of Nursing Education, 30*(1), 23-29.

Kosowski, M.M.R. (1995). Clinical learning experiences and professional nurse caring: A critical phenomenological study of female baccalaureate nursing students. *Journal of Nursing Education, 34*(5), 235-242.

Larson, P. J. (1984). Important nurse caring behaviors perceived by patients with cancer. *Oncology Nursing Forum, 11*(6), 46-50.

Larson, P. J. (1986). Cancer nurses' perceptions of caring. *Cancer Nursing, 9*(2), 86-91.

Larson, P. J. (1987). Comparison of cancer patients and professional nurses' perceptions of important nurse caring behaviors. *Heart and Lung, 12*(2), 187-193.

Larson, P. J., & Ferketich, S. L. (1993). Patient satisfaction with nurse caring during hospitalization. *Western Journal of Nursing Research, 15*(6), 690-707.

Latham, C. P. (1996). Predictors of patient outcomes following interaction with nurses. *Western Journal of Nursing Research, 18*(5), 548-564.

Leininger, M. M. (1981). The phenomenon of caring: Importance of research and theoretical considerations. In M. M. Leininger (Ed.), *Caring: An essential human need.* Thorofare, NJ: Slack.

Leininger, M. M. (1988, November). Leininger's theory of nursing: Cultural care diversity and universality. *Nursing Science Quarterly, 1*(4), 152-160.

Leininger, M. M. (1990). Historic and epistemologic dimensions of care and caring with future directions. In J. S. Stevenson & T. Tripp Riemer (Eds.), *Knowledge about care and caring: State of the art and future developments* (pp. 19-31). Washington, DC: American Academy of Nursing.

Lemmer, C. M. (1991). Parental perceptions of caring following perinatal bereavement. *Western Journal of Nursing Research, 13*(4), 475-493.

Leners, D. W. (1993). Nursing intuition: The deep connection. In D. Gaut (Ed.), *A global agenda for caring* (pp. 223-240). New York: National League for Nursing.

Lovgren, G., Engstrom, B., & Norberg, A. (1996). Patient's narratives concerning good and bad caring. *Scandinavian Journal of Caring Sciences, 10,* 151-156.

Mangold, A. M. (1991). Senior nursing students' and professional nurses' perceptions of effective caring behaviors: A comparative study. *Journal of Nursing Education, 30*(3), 134-139.

Mayer, D. K. (1986). Cancer patients' and families' perceptions of nurses' caring behaviors. *Topics in Clinical Nursing, 8*(2), 63-69.

Mayeroff, M. (1971). *On caring.* New York: Harper & Row.

McNamara, S. A. (1995). Perioperative nurses' perceptions of caring practices. *Association of Operating Room Nurses Journal, 61*(2), 377-388.

Miller, B. K., Haber, J., & Byrne, M. W. (1992). The experience of caring in the acute care setting: Patient and nurse perspectives. In D. A. Gaut (Ed.), *The presence of caring in nursing* (pp. 137-156). New York: National League for Nursing.

Milne, H. A., & McWilliam, C. L. (1996). Considering nursing resource as caring time. *Journal of Advanced Nursing, 23*(4), 810-819.

Montgomery, C. L. (1992). The spiritual connection: Nurses' perception of the experience of caring. In D. A. Gaut (Ed.), *The presence of caring in nursing* (pp. 39-52). New York: National League for Nursing.

Morrison, P. (1989). Nursing and caring: A personal construct theory study of some nurses' self-perceptions. *Journal of Advanced Nursing, 44,* 421-426.

Morrison, P. (1990). An example of the use of repertory grid techniques in assessing nurses' self-perceptions in caring. *Nurse Education Today, 10,* 253-259.

Morse, J. M., Bottorf, J., Neander, W., & Solberg, S. (1991). Comparative analysis and conceptualizations and theories of caring. *Image: The Journal of Nursing Scholarship, 23*(2), 119-126.

Morse, J. M., Solberg, S. M., Neander, W. L., Bottorf, J. L., & Johnson, J. L. (1990). Concepts of caring and caring as a concept. *Advances in Nursing Science, 13*(1), 14.

Mullins, I. L. (1996). Nurse caring behaviors for persons with Acquired Immune Deficiency Syndrome/Human Immunodeficiency Virus. *Applied Nursing Research, 9*(1), 18-23.

Nelms, T. P. (1996). Living a caring presence in nursing: A Heideggerian hermeneutic analysis. *Journal of Advanced Nursing, 24*(2), 368-374.

Noddings, N. (1984). *Caring: A feminine approach to ethics and moral education.* Berkeley: University of California Press.

O'Berle, K., & Davies, B. (1992). Support and caring: Exploring the concepts. *Oncology Nursing Forum, 19*(5), 763-767.

Parker, M. E. (1994). Living nursing's values in nursing practice. In D. A. Gaut & A. Boykin (Eds.), *Caring as healing: Renewal through hope* (pp. 48-65). New York: National League for Nursing.

Peteet, J. R., Rose, D. M., Medeiros, C., Walsh-Burke, K., & Rieker, P. (1992). Relationships with patients: Can a clinician be a friend? *Psychiatry, 55,* 223-229.

Poole, G., & Rowat, K. (1994). Elderly clients' perceptions of caring of a home-care nurse. *Journal of Advanced Nursing, 20,* 422-429.

Powell-Cope, G. M. (1994). Family caregiving of people with AIDS: Negotiating partnerships with healthcare providers. *Nursing Research, 43*(6), 324-330.

Propst, M. G., Schenk, L. K., & Clairain, S. (1994). Caring as perceived during the birth experience. In D. A. Gaut & A. Boykin (Eds.), *Caring as healing: Renewal through hope* (pp. 252-264). New York: National League for Nursing.

Raudonis, B. M. (1993). The meaning and impact of empathetic relationships in hospice nursing. *Cancer Nursing, 16*(4), 304-309.

Raudonis, B. M., & Kirschling, J. M. (1996). Family caregivers' perspectives on hospice nursing care. *Journal of Palliative Care, 12*(2), 14-19.

Ray, L. D. (1995). Caring in clinical intervention research: Design and measurement issues [Abstract]. *Communicating Nursing Research, 28*(3), 282.

Ray, M. A. (1984). The development of a classification system of institutional caring. In M. M. Leininger (Ed.), *Care: The essence of nursing and health* (pp. 95-111). Thorofare, NJ: Slack.

Ray, M. A. (1987). Technological caring: A new model in critical care. *Dimensions of Critical Care Nursing, 6*(3), 166-173.

Ray, M. A. (1989). The theory of bureaucratic caring for nursing practice in the organizational culture. *Nursing Administration Quarterly, 13*(2), 31-42.

Riemen, D. J. (1986). Non-caring and caring in the clinical setting: Patients' descriptions. *Topics in Clinical Nursing, 8*(2), 30-36.

Roach, S. (1984). *Caring: The human mode of being: Implications for nursing—perspectives in caring* (Monograph 1). Toronto: Faculty of Nursing, University of Toronto.

Schroeder, C., & Maeve, M. K. (1992). Nursing care partnerships at the Denver Nursing Project in Human Caring: An application and extension of caring theory in practice. *Advances in Nursing Science, 15*(2), 25-38.

Sherwood, G. (1993). A qualitative analysis of patient responses to caring: A moral and economic imperative. In D. Gaut (Ed.), *A global agenda for caring* (pp. 243-255). New York: National League for Nursing.

Sherwood, G. (1991). Expressions of nurses' caring: The role of the compassionate healer. In D. A. Gaut & M. M. Leininger (Eds.), *Caring: The compassionate healer* (pp. 79-87). New York: National League for Nursing.

Solberg, S., & Morse, J. M. (1991). The comforting behaviors of caregivers toward distressed postoperative neonates. *Issues in Comprehensive Pediatric Nursing, 14,* 79-92.

Soldwisch, S. S. (1993). Care, caritas, and ego development. In D. Gaut (Ed.), *A global agenda for caring* (pp. 293-307). New York: National League for Nursing.

Spangler, Z. (1993). Generic and professional care of Anglo-American and Filipino-American nurses. In D. Gaut (Ed.), *A global agenda for caring* (pp. 47-61). New York: National League for Nursing.

Steeves, R., Cohen, M. Z., & Wise, C. T. (1994). An analysis of critical incidents describing the essence of oncology nursing. *Oncology Nursing Forum, 21*(8 supp.), 19-25.

Stevenson, J. S. (1990). Quantitative care research: Review of content, process, product. In J. S. Stevenson & T. Tripp Riemer (Eds.), *Knowledge about care and caring: State of the art and future developments.* Washington, DC: American Academy of Nursing.

Swan, J. H., Benjamin, A. E., & Brown, A. (1992). Skilled nursing facility care for persons with AIDS: Comparison with other patients. *American Journal of Public Health, 82*(3), 453-455.

Swanson, K. M. (1990). Providing care in the NICU: Sometimes an act of love. *Advances in Nursing Science, 13*(1), 60-73.

Swanson, K. M. (1991). Empirical development of a middle-range theory of caring. *Nursing Research, 40*(3), 161-166.

Swanson, K. M. (1993). Nursing as informed caring for the well-being of others. *Image: The Journal of Nursing Scholarship, 25*(4), 352-357.

Swanson-Kauffman, K. M. (1986a). Caring in the instance of unexpected early pregnancy loss. *Topics in Clinical Nursing, 8*(2), 37-46.

Swanson-Kauffman, K. M. (1986b). A combined qualitative research methodology for nursing research. *Advances in Nursing Science, 8*(3), 58-69.

Swanson-Kauffman, K.M. (1988). The caring needs of women who miscarried. In M. M. Leininger (Ed.), *Care: Discovery and uses in clinical and community nursing* (pp. 55-70). Detroit: Wayne State University Press.

Swanson-Kauffman, K. M., & Schonwald, E. (1988). Phenomenology. In B. Sarter (Ed.), *Paths to knowledge: Innovative research methods for nursing* (pp. 97-105). New York: National League for Nursing.

Tanner, C. A., Benner, P., Chesla, C., & Gordon, D. R. (1993). The phenomenon of knowing the patient. *Image: The Journal of Nursing Scholarship, 25*(4), 273-280.

Tripp-Riemer, T., & Cohen, M. Z. (1990). Qualitative approaches to care: A critical review. In J. S. Stevenson & T. Tripp Riemer (Eds.), *Knowledge about care and caring: State of the art and future developments* (pp. 83-96). Washington, DC: American Academy of Nursing.

vonEssen, L., Burstrom, L., & Sjoden, P. O. (1994). Perceptions of caring behaviors and patient anxiety and depression in cancer patient-staff dyads. *Scandinavian Journal of Caring Science, 8*(4), 205-212.

Watson, M. J. (1985). *Nursing: The philosophy and science of caring.* Boulder: Colorado Associated University Press.

Watson, M. J. (1988a). *Nursing: Human science and human care.* New York: National League for Nursing.

Watson, M. J. (1988b). Response to "Caring practice: Construction of the nurses' world." *Scholarly Inquiry for Nursing Practice, 2*(3), 217-221.

Watson, M. J. (1990). Human caring: A public agenda. In J. S. Stevenson & T. Tripp Riemer (Eds.), *Knowledge about care and caring: State of the art and future developments* (pp. 41-48). Washington, DC: American Academy of Nursing.

Weiss, C. J. (1984). Gender-related perceptions of caring in the nurse-patient relationship. In M. M. Leininger (Ed.), *Care: The essence of nursing and health* (pp. 161-181). Thorofare, NJ: Slack.

Williams, H.A. (1992). Comparing the perception of support by parents of children with cancer and by health professionals. *Journal of Pediatric Oncology, 9*(4), 180-186.

Winters, G., Miller, C., Maracich, L., Compton, K., & Haberman, M. R. (1994). Provisional practice: The nature of psychosocial bone marrow transplant nursing. *Oncology Nursing Forum, 21*(7), 1147-1154.

Wolf, Z. R. (1986). The caring concept and nurses' identified caring behaviors. *Topics in Clinical Nursing, 8*(2), 84-93.

Wolf, Z. R., Giardino, E. R., Osborne, P. A., & Ambrose, M. S. (1994). Dimensions of nurse caring. *Image: The Journal of Nursing Scholarship, 26*(2), 107-111.

Young, E. W., Koch, P. B., & Preston, D. B. (1989). AIDS and homosexuality: A longitudinal study of knowledge and attitude change among rural nurses. *Public Health Nursing, 6*(4), 189-196.

RELATIONSHIP OF RESEARCH PERSPECTIVES TO METHODOLOGY

Carolyn L. Murdaugh

Introduction

The selection of a mode of inquiry to address a research question is a major decision for the nurse scientist. Appropriate research methods for building nursing science continue to be debated in the nursing literature, and differing views are offered by nurse theorists and scientists. Methodological preferences go beyond the specific questions to be answered, as qualitative and quantitative research methods are based on different views of reality. Although the research methods are derived from the research questions, the philosophical perspective of the nurse scientist will, more often than not, influence the types of research questions generated (Bryman, 1984). This chapter provides an overview of the major paradigms that currently guide the two commonly preferred research methods chosen to investigate problems in nursing: empiricism, which emphasizes quantitative methods, and phenomenology, which stresses qualitative methods. A brief historical perspective is provided to make it possible for the reader to understand the use of these methods in nursing research. The paradigms on which each of the methodologies is based are succinctly reviewed, as well as their strengths and weaknesses for building nursing science. Triangulation, or the integration of the two major methods to accommodate differing paradigms, is the most recent trend advocated by many nurse scientists. Opposing views related to methods triangulation are reviewed as well. The chapter concludes with a review of recommendations offered by nurse scientists and theorists for resolving the methods debate.

Current Worldviews and Research Approaches

Historical Perspective

Several authors believe that nursing has conformed to the research tradition or paradigm of the scientific method in its quest for recognition as a science (Goren-berg, 1983; Norris, 1982, 1993; Watson, 1981). However, embracement of the scientific method as the major research approach was more likely, due to doctoral preparation of our first nurse scholars in disciplines other than nursing. These early nurse scientists brought with them a commitment to their disciplines' research traditions for studying problems (Gortner, 1983; Munhall, 1993). Psychology, sociology, anthropology, biology, and epidemiology offered a wide array of research approaches. Logical positivism overshadowed other approaches to building nursing science and was judged to be the superior method. The dominance of the medical model in nursing and its use of empiricism no doubt initially curtailed the emergence of other paradigms and research approaches (Playle, 1995). The unquestionable success of the scientific method in gaining control over phenomena in the natural sciences was also a factor. Because nurse scientists who adopted empiricism were the founders of nursing doctoral programs and the editors and reviewers of research manuscripts, the positivistic paradigm continued to prevail in the development of nursing science. Another reason for embracing the accepted scientific method was the nurse scientist's reliance on funding agencies that had traditionally supported biomedical research. These agencies evaluated (and continue to evaluate) a grant proposal's merit on conventional criteria that had met the test of time for the established disciplines. Thus, prospective grantees aimed for scientifically designed, controlled studies that paid attention to such things as sampling, power, psychometrics, and biostatistics.

Empiricism

Empiricism, also referred to as logical positivism or traditional scientific inquiry, remains the prevailing paradigm or research tradition for the biomedically focused disciplines and nursing, although to a lesser extent since the 1980s. Empiricism is defined as a philosophy that emphasizes observation as the source of knowledge, with a logical analysis of the meaning of the observations (Ayer, 1959). An underlying assumption is that the world is structured by lawlike regularities that can be identified and manipulated. The basic axioms or beliefs of the positivistic paradigm have been summarized (Allen, Benner, & Dickelmann, 1995; Duffy, 1987; Guba, 1990; Lincoln & Guba, 1985; Wolfer, 1993). First, there is a single reality that can be reduced to its simplest form. In other words, the whole can be broken down into measurable parts that can be studied independently of one another. Second, the relationship of the knower (investigator) and the known (subject) is independent to maintain objectivity, constituting a discrete dualism. Third, generalizations that are both time and context free are possible and highly valued. Fourth, every action can be explained as a result of a cause that precedes it temporally. Last, inquiry is value free, due to precision, objectivity, and control. The aim of inquiry within this paradigm is to produce scientific knowledge that leads to causal explanations that can explain, predict, and control the physical world. The methodological principles of the empirical view incorporate objective observations, accurate measurement, qualification of variables, control of extraneous and intervening variables, biostatistical models, quasiexperimental or experimental methods whenever possible, and verification through replication (Wolfer, 1993).

Within the logical positivistic philosophy, quantitative approaches that focus on deductive verification constitute the research strategies. The randomized controlled trial (RCT) is considered the gold standard with which to measure cause and effect. However, other accepted empirical methods include observational studies, prospective cohort studies, case-controlled studies, retrospective case-controlled studies, cross-sectional studies, surveillance, and consecutive cases (D'Agostino & Kwan, 1995; Moses, 1995). In nursing research texts, methods described under the quantitative umbrella include exploratory, descriptive case studies and surveys and correlational, quasiexperimental, and experimental research methods (see Burns & Grove, 1987, as an example).

Empiricism enables the investigator to make objective, systematic observations by controlling or manipulating factors that may influence the observations (Norbeck, 1987). *Rigor* is the term commonly used to describe quantitative methods, as precision and exactness are needed to answer the research question. For example, if a physiologic concept such as blood pressure is the subject matter, rigorous designs to test interventions to reduce blood pressure and precise measurement of changes in blood pressure are necessary. Reliability and validity of measurement are also characteristics of quantitative methods, as accurate, sensitive, measurable concepts are necessary to quantitative methods. For example, lack of progress in describing and predicting a patient's health-related quality of life has been attributed in part to the validity and lack of sensitivity of many of the instruments measuring this construct. Theory-building and theory-testing techniques such as causal modeling are useful analytical tools in quantitative methods, as they assist in describing and explaining relationships among nursing phenomena (Budd & McKeehan, 1995).

Many nurse scientists and theorists continue to defend the tenets of positivism because countless questions that need to be answered in nursing are consistent with the empirical-analytic view (Gortner, 1983; Norbeck, 1987; Wolfer, 1993). Complex patient problems can often be studied only if broken into parts. Controlled conditions also permit findings to be generalized to similar groups to enable practicing nurses to be able to predict and prescribe. Generating and testing predictive models for persons at risk for developing coronary artery disease, acquiring HIV disease, developing caregiver burden, committing elder abuse, and so on require well-designed longitudinal studies with systematic objective measures. Quantitative studies are also the methods of choice to test interventions that may decrease or eliminate risk factors for diseases, prevent abuse, alleviate discomfort, decrease complications, minimize stress, and promote self-care or well-being.

Schumacher and Gortner (1992) have examined three major critiques of the scientific method in light of shifts in philosophy. Their views reflect the assertions of postpositivistic science (Phillips, 1988). First, the reliance of traditional science on theory-neutral observations is no longer accepted, as this doctrine has been challenged and rejected by contemporary postpositivistic philosophers. The doctrine that observation is the absolute source of knowledge has been replaced by the view that knowledge sources are imperfect. Science progresses as errors in current knowledge are eliminated through successive theory testing. Second, the privilege granted to quantitative data in justifying knowledge has been broadened to verification of knowledge on the merits of all of the evidence. Replacing the term *observation* with *evidence* expands the sources and types of information that can be collected to support a knowledge claim. This shift broadens the types of data that are obtained. Third, the idea that in traditional science one searches for universal laws to predict and explain phenomena is now considered ambiguous and simplistic. However, generalizability is still highly valued and sought in spite of the inability to generalize universally. Schumacher and Gortner (1992) argue for the necessity of causality in nursing science in spite of the complexity of patient care because of its relevance for clinical practice. In summary, they emphasize that traditional science is not static, as some authors have described in the literature. Instead, the philosophy continues to unfold as scientists attempt to make it germane to clinical science without abolishing its major canons.

Naturalism

As nursing began to be defined as a human science, a second worldview or paradigm gained acceptance: the *naturalistic* or *interpretative* paradigm, also known as the *constructivist* or *phenomenological* view. Human science stresses the lived experience and declares that this experience cannot be adequately described with traditional science (Giorgi, 1970). A shift to this worldview was a result of an abandonment of the medical model to one that focused on holism (Munhall, 1993). The change in focus led to an exploration of research methods that were more compatible with holism and a human science. Within the naturalistic view, research is conducted in the natural setting or context. In contrast to the empirical view, the knower interacts with the known. The researcher becomes the data collection instrument, instead of paper-and-pencil tests or technology. The naturalistic paradigm has been described as the other end of the continuum of reality, as one moves from the science of the body to the domain of the mind, or from the physical sciences to the interpretative or human sciences (Wolfer, 1993). Basic axioms of this philosophical view have been detailed by Lincoln and Guba (1985). First, multiple constructed realities exist and can only be studied holistically. Second, the knower and the known interact to influence one another. Third, the aim of inquiry is to describe the individual case, the lived experience. No attempt is made to control or manipulate the individual or phenomenon being investigated, as understanding of the human experience, not generalization, is the goal. Last, inquiry is value bound, as it is influenced by the values and choices of the investigator. Table 4.1 compares the differences in the empirical and naturalistic paradigms.

The phenomenological movement has been reviewed in detailed in the nursing literature (Cohen, 1987; Oiler Boyd, 1993; Reeder, 1985) and will not be expanded here, as it is not the focus of this chapter. Other paradigms have also contributed to the philosophical foundations of qualitative research, including critical social theory (Allen, 1985), feminism (Campbell & Bunting, 1991; Chinn, 1985), historicism (Lauden, 1981), and the simultaneity worldview (Parse, 1992). Newman (1992) offers a clear review of the prevailing paradigms in nursing.

Qualitative research strategies are employed in the naturalistic paradigm, as the primary ways of knowing require access to the thoughts and feelings of persons to describe human events and behavior (Coward, 1990). To

TABLE 4.1 A Comparison of the Two Major Paradigms in Nursing[a]

	Empirical	*Humanistic*
Purpose	Verification	Discovery
Nature of reality	Single reality, quantifiable parts	Multiple realities, holistic
Nature of relationships	Objective, independent	Interactive, interdependent
Nature of truth	Context free, generalizability	Context bound, uniqueness

a. The comparisons have been greatly simplified so that they may be described in this format.

understand the lived experience, the investigator must have sustained contact with persons in their natural environments and maintain flexibility as data collection progresses. Data are collected in the form of observations, field notes, interviews, videotapes, photographs, and so on. Analysis of data results in a descriptive picture of the lived experience that has been inductively derived.

Qualitative research approaches include grounded theory, ethnography, phenomenology, and historical methods. Grounded theory is described as a method by which to derive theory from data systematically obtained from social research (Glaser & Strauss, 1967). The purpose of the grounded theory approach is to build theory inductively from the study of the phenomenon it represents. In an ethnographic approach, patterns of culture are observed and analyzed. Ethnographic approaches describe and analyze patterns of people in their own environments. Thus the central element in ethnography is culture. Phenomenological approaches describe the experiences of individuals as they are lived. In phenomenology, these descriptions are termed *lived experiences.* Reality is considered subjective in phenomenology. Instead, this approach explores individuals' perceptions or the meaning of experiences that are unique to them. Historical methods examine events of the past to expand our understanding of our profession and to interpret nursing and its contributions so they can be transmitted to those entering nursing as well as to persons outside of nursing. Historical methods, or historiography, analyze records,

artifacts, and other sources of data to describe and analyze historical events or persons.

In qualitative research approaches, the ways in which people make sense of their realities are explored through interviews initiated by broad questions that ask "What is it like?" or "How does it feel?" or "What is the experience of?" Or broad statements such as "Tell me about ____." may initiate the interview process. The various qualitative methods have devised differing analysis methods. However, a nonnumerical approach is the common analytical theme. Grounded theory methods incorporate Glaser and Strauss's (1967) method of constant comparative analysis; Colaizzi (1978) and van Kamm's (1966) methods of analysis have been applied to phenomenology methods. Analysis of ethnographic data follows the traditions outlined in anthropology (Spradley, 1979). In historical research, data must be interpreted to determine what actually occurred as accurately as possible. Table 4.2 provides an overview of the differences in quantitative and qualitative research approaches.

Some nurse scientists have attempted to apply the characteristic of rigor found in quantitative methods in attempts to make qualitative methods acceptable by the traditional scientific community. For example, the concepts of reliability, validity, and objectivity have been introduced into qualitative methods (Hutchinson & Wilson, 1992; Swanson-Kauffman, 1986). Lincoln and Guba (1985) have moved beyond attempts to apply these criteria and have devised new standards to establish the trust-

TABLE 4.2 Differences in the Two Major Research Approaches in Nursing[a]

	Quantitative	*Qualitative*
Setting	Controlled	Natural
Instrument	Objective measurement, observation	Investigator
Method	Deductive	Inductive
Sampling	Representative	Theoretical
Analysis	Hypothesis testing, statistical inferences	Uncovering meaning, lived experience

a. These comparisons have been simplified so that salient differences may be depicted.

worthiness of naturalistic approaches that include credibility, transferability, dependability, and confirmability. Other investigators believe the application of analogous criteria such as reliability and validity is inconsistent with the paradigm underlying qualitative methods and such efforts should be discarded (Sandelowski, 1995a). The quality of the research lies in the power of the language, which provides discovery and understanding (Buchanan, 1992).

Qualitative methods may result in descriptions and interpretations that provide meaning and understanding of the nature of human experience. A focus on individual experience and the context of that experience is considered a major strength of these methods, as these experiences enable nurses to understand daily living and practical concerns (Taylor, 1994). Reeder (1985) believes an understanding of the lived experience illuminates the nursing questions that need to be addressed.

Proposals to Accommodate Differing Paradigms

The Issue

Adoption of two conflicting paradigms in nursing has resulted in a polarization between qualitative and quantitative research strategies. One view maintains that the two perspectives must be kept separate, as each represents dissimilar frameworks for conceptualizing the nature of knowing. An opposing view posits that the paradigms can peacefully coexist, and the two methods can be combined in a single study. Each of these views is presented in more detail under the triangulation section to help readers better understand the ongoing debate in nursing.

Several nurse scientists and theorists argue that because qualitative and quantitative methods are based on fundamentally incompatible paradigms, they can not be combined (Lincoln & Guba, 1985; Moccia, 1988; Munhall, 1982, 1989; Watson, 1981; Wolfer, 1993). Phillips (1988) states that combining the two research methods is "logically fallacious" (p. 4). He asserts that the differing underlying paradigm assumptions are not complementary and cannot be blended to produce valid findings. Contrasting views of reality and diverse data collection and analytic techniques do not necessarily produce greater understanding. Leininger (1992) agrees with Phillips's stance and, as a purist, maintains that it is im-

possible to combine the axioms of both paradigms in a single study. Phillips (1988) suggests that attempts to combine the two methods may reflect the inadequacy of current research approaches and point to the need for new modes of inquiry to build nursing science.

Triangulation

The term *triangulation* was first used in navigation to describe the techniques employed when two known data points were applied to plot a third. Today, triangulation is defined as a research strategy that combines different theoretical perspectives, different data sources, different investigators, or different methods within a single study. Triangulation's major purpose is considered to be confirmation when multiple measures (methodological triangulation) are used in an attempt to obtain convergence on a single concept. Methods triangulation takes two forms: within methods and across methods (Jick, 1979). Within-methods triangulation refers to the use of similar data collection strategies to measure a concept within one study. For example, two or more quantitative methods may be used in the same study, or multiple qualitative data collection methods may be combined with the same study. Across-methods triangulation refers to the use of two different data collection strategies in the same study. Combining qualitative and quantitative approaches in the same study is considered across-methods triangulation. Campbell and Fiske's (1959) multitrait multimethod was an early application of triangulation for confirmation purposes. Triangulation results in a more comprehensive description of the topic under investigation; thus the method increases the trustworthiness of the data (Brietmayer, Ayres, & Knafl, 1993). Denzin (1970) extended the term to include the use of multiple investigators, multiple theories, and multiple analytic techniques to confirm one's findings. Fielding and Fielding (1986) expanded the meaning of triangulation to obtain completeness, either theoretical or substantive. In other words, multiple methods, data sources, and investigators are all combined in a single study as each aspect is thought to contribute elements that aid in understanding the phenomenon under study. This type of triangulation has been labeled multiple triangulation (Denzin, 1989). Operational definitions have been devised for theory, data, methods, investigator, and analysis triangulation to facilitate investigators to judge the achievement of triangulation (Kimchi, Polivka, & Stevenson, 1991).

Sandelowski (1995b) argues that triangulation has been misapplied in the qualitative domain and that the differences between the qualitative and quantitative modes of inquiry have been portrayed as inconsequential or unimportant. She cautions against the use of triangulation as a means to theoretical or substantive completeness (multiple triangulation) rather than for its rightful purpose as a confirmation strategy for convergent validity (methodological triangulation). Others remind us that the choice of a research strategy is more than a technical one (Moccia, 1988). Selection of research strategies must be consistent with the researcher's definition of reality, as the two paradigms reflect different realities (open versus closed) and require different methods of inquiry (Parse, Coyne, & Smith, 1985).

Supporters for triangulation are as numerous as dissenters. Proponents of combining qualitative and quantitative methods take a more pragmatic position, as they consider methodological triangulation essential to more accurately study the complexity of human phenomena (Steckler, McLeary, Goodman, Bird, & McCormick, 1992; Tripp-Reimer, 1985). Hinds and Young (1987) believe that methodological triangulation promotes the likelihood of uncovering multiple dimensions of the reality of a theoretical phenomenon as each method contributes unique knowledge.

Several nurse scientists offer suggestions to reconcile paradigm differences so that qualitative and quantitative methods can be combined through triangulation. However, others see the reconciliation as merely peacekeeping instead of facing the issues in the debate. Morse (1991) believes the key issue in applying methodological triangulation is that the study must be driven by theory either inductively or deductively derived, but not by both in the same study, as qualitative and quantitative methods cannot be weighted equally. If qualitative methods are the dominant approach in a study, the quantitative methods are complementary. According to Myers and Haase (1989), qualitative and quantitative approaches share a common goal and can be combined in the same study as long as the investigator recognizes the assumptions and values of both paradigms when integrating the two approaches and does not merely mix the two methods without attention to the paradigmatic assumptions. Other scientists argue that the qualitative-quantitative distinction is one of data collection methods, analysis, and interpretation, and the linkage between a specific paradigm and a certain method is not an inherent requirement (Goodwin & Goodwin, 1984; Morse, 1991; Reichardt & Cook, 1979). Goodwin and Goodwin (1984) contend that although certain methods are usually linked to certain

paradigms, the dichotomy is artificial, and either data collection method is appropriate within a paradigm. Others believe that the use of either method is based on the question that is being asked and not the linkage between the philosophy and the methodology (Dzurec, 1989; Porter, 1989).

Multiple analysis issues are raised in the application of triangulation (Mitchell, 1986). First, although there is no shortage of articles that describe or discuss issues about triangulation, guidelines and step-by-step procedures for using the method are lacking. Difficulties are inherent when attempting to merge numerical and textual data. Issues related to the weighting of the data have not been resolved, as well as the interpretation of disparate results that may be obtained with dissimilar data collection strategies. Combining concepts that have been operationally defined with concepts that are discovered in the qualitative data is another concern. Sampling has also been identified as another issue of concern when combining the two methods (Floyd, 1993). Decisions about weighting the contribution of the various methods in the interpretation of the results are complex and ambiguous. Most authors agree that the data from the two methods should be analyzed separately, initially. However, to date, no new analytical solutions have been offered.

Critical Multiplism

Critical multiplism is offered as a research strategy in which qualitative and quantitative methods are reconciled within a third model of scientific inquiry. Critical multiplism is considered an example of postpositivistic thinking in which triangulation has been extended to include multiple theories and multiple analyses as well as multiple methodologies (Cook, 1985). The strategy expands both the multitrait, multimethod approach (Campbell & Fiske, 1959) and across-methods triangulation (Denzin, 1989). Coward (1990) believes that critical multiplism leads to the identification and testing of significant nursing problems, as one makes careful choices among multiple options. Thoughtful, multiple perspectives are executed to define research goals; to decide research questions, methods, and analysis; and to interpret results. An underlying assumption is that no one mode of inquiry should be relied on solely. Critical multiplism also incorporates multiple stakeholders to develop the research questions, as well as multiple data collection and analysis methods. As a strategy, critical multiplism promotes a critical analysis and open scrutiny of multiple perspectives to select research questions and methods that are complementary (Coward, 1990). However, critical multiplism is not a set of techniques, and no guidelines are available, as guidelines are considered in opposition to the strategy, which operates through consensus (Cook, 1983). Last, the same difficulties encountered when applying methods triangulation discussed earlier in the chapter are also noted in this approach.

Scientific Pluralism

A bipolar framework is offered by Kim (1993) that delineates alternative linkages among philosophy, theory, and method as a way to distinguish different positions within scientific pluralism. The bipolar dimensions are (a) philosophy and theory and (b) methodology. Each dimension encompasses three possible levels of differentiation to provide for linkages between the two dimensions. For example, philosophy and theory encompass a realistic or relativistic philosophical orientation; inductive or deductive theory-generation level; and descriptive, explanatory, or prescriptive knowledge-type level. The methodology dimension includes an etic or emic reality orientation level, a quantity or quality reality-type level, and a controlled or naturalistic field orientation level. The proposed framework provides a strategy to describe multiple paths to knowledge in finer detail than ordinarily portrayed. Use of the framework enables an investigator to describe his or her research within all the levels of the two dimensions. The framework is also somewhat artificial in that alternative linkages are not realistic options in reconciling differences in assumptions and worldviews. However, scientific pluralism is a possible solution, as more than one path to knowledge is acknowledged.

In summary, the debate in nursing continues as to which paradigm should guide the methodology chosen by nurse scientists, as well as which methodology is preferable to answer research questions of concern for nursing. As noted, more and more scientists and theorists are crusading for the naturalistic paradigm-based on the premise that nursing is a human science; others are campaigning for using both methods in studies, based on the proposition that one methodology does not provide a complete picture due to the complexity of human phenomena. Triangulation, critical multiplism, and frameworks to link theories and methods have been proposed as potential strategies to accept the qualitative-quantitative dualism. A potentially achievable solution must be more comprehensive than an either/or stance yet must maintain the integrity of both paradigms.

Conclusions

What has been learned from this overview of the basic philosophies on which the two major methodologies in nursing are founded? First, the traditional empiricist paradigm with its accompanying quantitative methods is not considered adequate to investigate all the research problems for nursing. This argument is founded on the definition of nursing as a human science. A philosophy that encompasses humanism and individual interpretation of experiences cannot be studied only with traditional scientific methods. Over 20 years ago, Silva (1977) stated that the time had come to question a singular approach to the study of nursing knowledge. This statement remains timely, as scientists are now seriously pursuing methods that appreciate the assumptions underlying a humanistic, holistic science. Thus, methods that reflect the definition of nursing as a human science other than the traditional science approaches must be valued and applied to build nursing science.

Second, the qualitative-quantitative controversy is more than a methods debate. It represents contrasting worldviews in the development of nursing science. Differences in choice of philosophies and methodologies rests on fundamental differences that will not be settled in the near future. Paradigms structure the questions to be asked and the methods of inquiry within a discipline (Kuhn, 1970). Thus, an openness to multiple paradigms as well as to the evolution of multiple paradigms for the conduct of research is essential as nursing expands its research tradition (Dzurec, 1989). The development of nursing science is too embryonic to place closure on any type of methodology. All paths to knowledge need to be explored, which means that qualitative and quantitative methods must both be valued and seen as worthwhile in building nursing science.

Tolerance for a diversity of philosophies and methods should be supported instead of casting one against the other. As Schwandt (1990) states, no one path of inquiry should be elevated to "the status of an orthodoxy" (p. 276). The multifaceted nature and complexity of nursing can accommodate multiple paradigms, and a singular paradigm or methodology approach imposes limitations on the questions that can be answered. This does not mean that nurse scientists must be pluralists. It is simplistic to think that everyone should hold multiple philosophical beliefs, just as it is naive to think that all nurse scientists should become experts in all methodologies. The basic beliefs of nurse scientists guide their choice of paradigms and methods that guide their work. However, scientific pluralism, defined here as an appreciation of multiple philosophies and multiple methodologies to develop and test nursing science, is critical.

One example of scientific pluralism, the antecedent-sequence position in which the two worldviews are substantiated, offers promise for nursing (Munhall, 1993). Discovery questions, also termed *first-order activities of science*, incorporate qualitative methods to answer the "what" questions. First-order activities are a prelude to second-order activities, which encompass quantitative methods for validation. The qualitative-quantitative dichotomy becomes a continuum, in which qualitative methods are appropriate for discovering and developing theory and quantitative methods come into use when theory is tested. However, the continuum is circular, not linear, as investigators move back and forth between qualitative and quantitative methods. Munhall's proposed antecedent-sequence position is not new and will not be accepted by scientists and theorists who adhere to either/or positions. What is new is the attention to what Lincoln (1992) calls philosophical and paradigmatic flexibility to choose methods based on the kinds of problems being investigated. The qualitative-quantitative continuum allows for the development and testing of prescriptive theories to guide practice, if we believe that nursing's role is to provide interventions (Gortner, 1990). Johnson's (1991) discussion of the failure to recognize the difference in the science of nursing that deals with generalizations and the art of nursing that deals with the application of these generalizations is compatible with nursing's role in the development of prescriptive theory. The qualitative-quantitative continuum is supported by Schultz and Meleis (1988), who state that hypotheses that are tested may originate from subjective knowledge.

No matter the method, the knowledge generated must be credible to the nursing scientific community. The criteria for judging the credibility of one's findings should be congruent with the designs and methods employed in the research. For example, trustworthiness criteria have been suggested to evaluate the believability of qualitatively generated results (Brink, 1989; Lincoln & Guba, 1985). For quantitative results, numerous criteria are available to evaluate rigor, including objectivity, reliability, validity, generalizability, control, and so on (Acton, Irvin, & Hopkins, 1991; Campbell & Stanley, 1963; Hinshaw, 1979; Zeller & Carmines, 1980). Feinstein (1988) points out that although individuals or groups of people cannot be studied the same way molecules or animals can, nonexperimental studies must have the same high standards as the methods in other branches of science.

Investigators need to pay more attention to the scientific quality of evidence and less to the method that should be used to generate evidence. Kaplan (1964) made this point quite clear when he stated that the question is not whether everyone is using the same method but whether anything gets done by the method used. In other words, we need to ask how effective the methods are for facilitating the development of nursing science.

Summary

This chapter has discussed the two major research philosophies that guide the two major research methods used in nursing research. An understanding of the worldviews underlying these methods is necessary to appreciate the ongoing methods debate in the development of nursing science. Proposed solutions to accommodate multiple paradigms are described, including triangulation, critical multiplism, and scientific pluralism. The chapter concludes with suggested ways to curtail the methods debate. Tolerance for diversity is emphasized.

References

Acton, G. J., Irvin, B. L., & Hopkins, B. A. (1991). Theory testing research: Building the science. *Advances in Nursing Science, 14*(1), 52-61.

Allen, D. (1985). Nursing research and social control: Alternative models of science that emphasize understanding and emancipation. *Image: The Journal of Nursing Scholarship, 17,* 58-64.

Allen, D., Benner, P., & Dickelmann, N. L. (1995). Three paradigms for nursing research: Methodological implications. In P. Chinn (Ed.), *Nursing research methodology: Issues and implementation* (pp. 23-28). Rockville, MD: Aspen.

Ayer, A. J. (1959). *Logical positivism.* New York: Free Press.

Brietmayer, B. J., Ayres, L., & Knafl, K. A. (1993). Triangulation in qualitative research: Evaluation of completeness and confirmation purposes. *Image: The Journal of Nursing Scholarship, 25*(3), 237-243.

Brink, P. J. (1989). Issues in reliability and validity. In J. M. Morse (Ed.), *Qualitative nursing research: A contemporary dialogue* (pp. 149-168). Rockville, MD: Aspen.

Bryman, A. (1984). The debate about quantitative and qualitative research: A question of method or epistemology? *British Journal of Sociology, 35*(1), 75-92.

Buchanan, D. R. (1992). An uneasy alliance: Combining qualitative and quantitative research methods. *Health Education Quarterly, 19*(1), 117-135.

Budd, K. W., & McKeehan, K. M. (1995). Causal modeling: Heuristic and analytic path to nursing knowledge. In P. L. Chinn (Ed.), *Nursing research methodology: Issues and implementation* (2nd ed., pp. 121-132). Gaithersburg, MD: Aspen.

Burns, N., & Grove, S. K. (1987). *The practice of nursing research: Conduct, critique and utilization.* Philadelphia: W. B. Saunders.

Campbell, D. T., & Fiske, D. W. (1959). Convergent and discriminant validation by the multi-trait–multi-method matrix. *Psychological Bulletin, 56,* 81-105.

Campbell, D. T., & Stanley, J. C. (1963). *Experimental and quasi-experimental designs for research.* Chicago: Rand McNally.

Campbell, J. C., & Bunting, S. (1991). Voices and paradigms: Perspectives on critical and feminist theory in nursing. *Advances in Nursing Science, 13*(3), 1-15.

Chinn, P. (1985). Debunking myths in nursing theory and research. *Image: The Journal of Nursing Scholarship, 17*(2), 45-49.

Cohen, M. Z. (1987). A historical overview of the phenomenological movement. *Image: The Journal of Nursing Scholarship, 19*(1), 31-34.

Colaizzi, P. (1978). Psychological research as the phenomenologist views it. In R. S. Valle & M. King (Eds.), *Existential phenomenological alternatives for psychology.* New York: Oxford University Press.

Cook, T. (1983). Quasi-experimentation: Its ontology, epistomology, and methodology. In G. Morgan (Ed.), *Beyond method: Strategies for social research* (pp. 21-62). Beverly Hills, CA: Sage.

Cook, T. (1985). Postpositivist critical multiplism. In R. Shotland & M. Mark (Eds.), *Social science and social policy* (pp. 21-61). Beverly Hills, CA: Sage.

Coward, D. D. (1990). Critical multiplism: A research strategy for nursing science. *Image: The Journal of Nursing Scholarship, 22*(3), 163-167.

D'Agostino, R. B., & Kwan, H. (1995). Measuring effectiveness: What to expect without a randomized control group. *Medical Care, 33*(4 Suppl.), AS95-AS105.

Denzin, N. K. (1970). *Sociological methods: A source book.* Chicago: Aldine.

Denzin, N. K. (1989). *The research act* (3rd ed.). New York: McGraw-Hill.

Duffy, M. E. (1987). Methodological triangulation: A vehicle for merging quantitative and qualitative research methods. *Image: The Journal of Nursing Scholarship, 19*(3), 130-133.

Dzurec, L. C. (1989). The necessity for and evolution of multiple paradigms for nursing research: A poststructuralist perspective. *Advances in Nursing Science, 11*(4), 69-77.

Feinstein, A. R. (1988). Scientific standards in epidemiologic studies of the menace of daily life. *Science, 242,* 1257-1263.

Fielding, N. G., & Fielding, J. L. (1986). *Linking data.* Beverly Hills, CA: Sage.

Floyd, J. A. (1993). The use of across-method triangulation in the study of sleep concerns in healthy older adults. *Advances in Nursing Science, 16*(2), 70-80.

Giorgi, A. (1970). *Psychology as a human science.* New York: Harper & Rowe.

Glaser, B., & Strauss, A. (1967). *The discovery of grounded theory.* Chicago: Aldine.

Goodwin, L. D., & Goodwin, W. L. (1984). Qualitative vs. quantitative research or qualitative and quantitative research? *Nursing Research, 33*(6), 378-380.

Gorenberg, B. (1983). The research tradition of nursing: An emerging issue. *Nursing Research, 32*(6), 347-349.

Gortner, S. R. (1983). The history and philosophy of nursing science and research. *Advances in Nursing Science, 6,* 1-8.

Gortner, S. R. (1990). Nursing values and science: Toward a science philosophy. *Image: The Journal of Nursing Science, 22*(2), 101-105.

Guba, E. G. (1990). The alternative paradigm dialogue. In E. G. Guba (Ed.), *The paradigm dialogue* (pp. 17-30). Beverly Hills, CA: Sage.

Hinds, P. S., & Young, K. L. (1987). A triangulation of methods and paradigms to study nurse-given wellness care. *Nursing Research, 36*(3) 195-198.

Hinshaw, A. S. (1979). Planning for logical consistency among three theoretical structures. *Western Journal of Nursing Research, 1*(3), 319-324.

Hutchinson, S., & Wilson, H. S. (1992). Validity threats in scheduled semistructured research interviews. *Nursing Research, 41*(2), 117-119.

Jick, T. D. (1979). Mixing qualitative and quantitative methods: Triangulation in action. *Administrative Science Quarterly, 24,* 602-611.

Johnson, J. L. (1991). Nursing science: Basic, applied, or practical? Implications for the art of nursing. *Advances in Nursing Science, 14*(1), 7-16.

Kaplan, A. (1964). *The conduct of inquiry.* San Francisco, CA: Chandler.

Kim, H. S. (1993). Identifying alterative linkages among philosophy, theory and method in nursing science. *Journal of Advanced Nursing, 18,* 793-800.

Kimchi, J., Polivka, B., & Stevenson, J. S. (1991). Triangulation: Operational definitions. *Nursing Research, 40*(6), 364-366.

Kuhn, T. S. (1970). *The structure of scientific revolutions.* Chicago: University of Chicago Press.

Lauden, L. A. (1981). Problem solving approach to scientific progress. In I. Hacking (Ed.), *Scientific revolutions.* Oxford, UK: Oxford University Press.

Leininger, M. (1992). Current issues, problems, and trends to advance qualitative paradigmatic research methods for the future. *Qualitative Health Research, 2,* 392-415.

Lincoln, Y. S. (1992). Sympathetic connections between qualitative methods and health research. *Qualitative Health Research, 2*(4), 375-391.

Lincoln, Y. S., & Guba, E. G. (1985). *Naturalistic inquiry.* Beverly Hills, CA: Sage.

Mitchell, E. S. (1986). Multiple triangulation: A methodology for nursing science. *Advances in Nursing Science, 8*(3), 18-26.

Moccia, P. (1988). A critique of compromise: Beyond the methods debate. *Advances in Nursing Science, 10*(4), 1-9.

Morse, J. M. (1991). Approaches to qualitative-quantitative methodological triangulation. *Nursing Research, 40*(1), 120-123.

Moses, L. E. (1995). Measuring effects without randomization trials? Options, problems, challenges. *Medical Care, 33*(4 Suppl.), AS8-AS14.

Munhall, P. L. (1982). Nursing philosophy and nursing research: In apposition or opposition? *Nursing Research, 31*(3), 176-181.

Munhall, P. L. (1989). Philosophical ponderings on qualitative methods in nursing. *Nursing Science Quarterly, 2*(1), 20-28.

Munhall, P. L. (1993). Epistomology in nursing. In P. L. Munhall & C. Oiler Boyd (Eds.), *Nursing research: A qualitative perspective* (Pub. No. 19-2535, pp. 39-65). New York: National League for Nursing.

Myers, S. T., & Haase, J. E. (1989). Guidelines for integration of quantitative and qualitative approaches. *Nursing research, 38*(5), 299-301.

Newman, M. A. (1992). Prevailing paradigms in nursing. *Nursing Outlook, 40*(1), 10-32.

Norbeck, J. D. (1987). In defense of empiricism. *Image: The Journal of Nursing Scholarship, 19*(1), 28-30.

Norris, C. M. (1982). *Concept clarification in nursing.* Rockville, MD: Aspen.

Norris, C. M. (1993). A glance back in time: Toward a science of nursing. *Nursing Forum, 28*(3), 18-26.

Oiler Boyd, C. (1993). Philosophical foundations of qualitative research. In P. L. Munhall & C. Oiler Boyd (Eds.), *Nursing research: A qualitative perspective* (Pub. No. 19-2535, pp. 66-94). New York: National League for Nursing.

Parse, R. R. (1992). Human becoming: Parse's theory of nursing. *Nursing Science Quarterly, 5,* 35-42.

Parse, R. R., Coyne, A. B., & Smith, M. J. (1985). *Nursing research: Qualitative methods.* Bowie, MD: Brady Communications.

Phillips, J. R. (1988). Research blenders. *Nursing Science Quarterly, 1,* 4-5.

Playle, J. F. (1995). Humanism and positivism in nursing: Contradictions and conflicts. *Journal of Advanced Nursing, 22,* 979-984.

Porter, E. L. (1989). The qualitative-quantitative dualism. *Image: The Journal of Nursing Scholarship, 21*(2), 98-102.

Reeder, F. (1985). Hermeneutics. In B. Sarter (Ed.), *Paths to knowledge: Innovative research methods for nursing* (pp. 193-238). New York: National League for Nursing.

Reichardt, C., & Cook, T. (Eds.). (1979). *Qualitative and quantitative methods in evaluation research.* Beverly Hills, CA: Sage.

Sandelowski, M. (1995a). On the aesthetics of qualitative research. *Image: The Journal of Nursing Scholarship, 27*(3), 205-209.

Sandelowski, M. (1995b). Triangles and crystals: On the geometry of qualitative research. *Research in Nursing and Health, 18,* 569-574.

Schultz, P. R., & Meleis, A. I. (1988). Nursing epistemology: Traditions, insights, questions. *Image: The Journal of Nursing Scholarship, 20*(4), 217-221.

Schumacher, K. L., & Gortner, S. R. (1992). (Mis)conceptions and reconceptions about traditional science. *Advances in Nursing Science, 14*(4), 1-11.

Schwandt, T. R. (1990). Paths to inquiry in the social disciplines. In E. G. Guba (Ed.), *The paradigm dialogue* (pp. 258-276). Newbury Park, CA: Sage.

Silva, M. C. (1977). Philosophy, science, theory: Interrelationships and implications for nursing research. *Image: The Journal of Nursing Scholarship, 9*(3), 59-63.

Spradley, J. P. (1979). *The ethnographic interview.* New York: Holt, Rinehart & Winston.

Steckler, A., McLeary, K. R., Goodman, R. M., Bird, S. T., & McCormick, L. (1992). Toward integrating qualitative and quantitative methods: An introduction. *Health Education Quarterly, 19*(1), 1-8.

Swanson-Kauffman, K. M. (1986). A combined qualitative methodology for nursing research. *Advances in Nursing Science, 8*(3), 58-69.

Taylor R. (1994). *Being human: Ordinariness in nursing.* Melbourne: Churchill Livingstone.

Tripp-Reimer, T. (1985). Combining qualitative and quantitative methodologies. In M. M. Leininger (Ed.), *Qualitative research methods in nursing* (pp. 179-194). Orlando, FL: Grune & Stratton.

Van Kamm, A. L. (1966). *Existential foundations of psychology* (Vol. 3). Pittsburgh, PA: Duquesne University Press.

Watson, J. (1981). Nursing's scientific quest. *Nursing Outlook, 29*(7), 413-416.

Wolfer, J. (1993). Aspects of "reality" and ways of knowing in nursing: In search of an integrating paradigm. *Image: The Journal of Nursing Scholarship, 25*(2), 141-146.

Zeller, R. A., & Carmines, E. G. (1980). *Measurement in the social sciences.* Cambridge, UK: Cambridge University Press.

PART
IIA

CRITICAL HEALTH NEEDS OF COMMUNITIES AND VULNERABLE POPULATIONS

Clinical Nursing Research for Vulnerable Populations

Toni Tripp-Reimer

Vulnerable populations are those at high relative risk for physical, psychological or social problems and/or those with decreased access to health services based on their economic, ethnic, geographic, or social circumstances. In 1994, Hall, Stevens, and Meleis contended that the "future of nursing depends on the ability of the discipline to reach out to diverse communities and to meet the health needs of those most vulnerable" (p. 23). As we approach the new millenium, their statement is an even stronger imperative. Yet, there are tensions within the discipline of nursing that deter us from adequately addressing the needs of vulnerable populations.

In *At Risk in America: The Health and Health Care Needs of Vulnerable Populations in the United States*, Lu Ann Aday (1993) points out that "both the origins and remedies of vulnerability are rooted in the bonds of human communities" (p. 1). The intricate relationship that links vulnerability to community provides a mandate for nursing research and practice. But although community-focused approaches are widely lauded in nursing, they do not yet form the primary foundational perspective for the discipline. A key (but often hidden) factor thwarting the community-focused approach is that its underlying values do not compete well with values underlying the more individualistic approach that is more pronounced and highly favored in nursing education and practice. Aday (1997) elaborates this tension between the community perspective values (reciprocity, interdependence, and mutual benefit) and the market perspective values (autonomy, independence, and private interest). These dialectics merit open discussion and debate within nursing.

The cult of the individual has driven nursing education and practice for at least the past quarter century. It is, in large part, responsible for the relative lack of nursing initiatives with vulnerable populations. It has also been cited as a key factor contributing to racism in nursing (Barbee, 1993). If nursing is to realistically and fully address the health of vulnerable populations, the tension in the discipline between community-focused and individual-focused care must be addressed.

Since this section was originally conceptualized in 1994, there has been a relatively dramatic increase in the nursing literature concerning the issue of vulnerability. Several special issues of journals have been dedicated to related research (*Advances in Nursing Science*, March 1994; *Family and Community Health*, January 1997; and *Nursing Research,* March/April 1998). Considerable work has been generated concerning the conceptualization of vulnerability and its related processes of racism, marginalization, oppression, isolation, stigmatization, and anomie. Further, there has been an increase in participatory action research and community empowerment. These developments, in addition to the recent and increasing dialogue contrasting primary health care and primary care as well as community-based nursing and community health nursing, are heartening (Barnes et al., 1995; Shoultz & Hatcher, 1997; Zotti, Brown, & Stotts, 1996).

The four chapters in this section were developed in the context of this dialogue. In "Community-Focused Interventions and Outcome Strategies," Magilvy, Brown, and Moritz provide an orientation that grounds the other chapters in this section. They identify three primary perspectives that form the foundation guiding community research and practice. Primary health care (as distinct from primary care) provides the theoretical foundation. They draw on the Alma Alta definition of primary health care that emphasizes accessible, affordable, and acceptable services; integrated health care; multiple entry points; a variety of providers; partnership with clients; and client participation in decision making. Epidemiology is identified as the foundational methodology to enhance community-focused research; action research

(based on critical theory) is identified as the foundational process. Magilvy et al. address both general and specific design issues in community research; for example, offering the term *transferability* in addressing issues of generalizability and replicability. After noting the relatively small number of community studies, they provide selected exemplars of community-focused interventions and outcome research.

In the chapter "Cultural Interventions for Ethnic Groups of Color," Tripp-Reimer addresses intervention research for ethnic groups in the United States. She delineates the historical evolution of nursing research with ethnic groups of color and points out that an academic rather than an action approach has predominated. She further contends that the construct of *culture* has often been used as a cover term to obscure the deeper, more sinister issues of individual and institutional racism and poverty or economic disparities. Tripp-Reimer presents a model of culturally relevant research that depicts the predominance of descriptive cultural research and a relative lack of research focusing on testing and evaluating culturally focused interventions. She provides a synthesis of extant intervention-focused research and finds several commonalities in the results, such as the consistent positive results achieved through lay community health workers, the importance of social marketing strategies, and the pivotal issues of language and communication.

In the chapter, "Research With Immigrants and Refugees," Lispon and Meleis address this special segment of culturally diverse populations. They develop the constructs of transition and vulnerability as particularly relevant for this population. In reviewing the research, they note that although few intervention studies have been reported, there is a growing body of clinical guidelines. In addressing the research design, they note the need for special consideration of issues of recruitment, instrumentation, language differences, and theoretical frameworks. They caution that research must be examined for the potential of stereotyping or further marginalizing immigrants.

"The Sampler Quilt" deals with the health of rural communities. Weinert and Burman use the metaphor of the sampler quilt as a heuristic device to help the reader understand the construct of rurality. They highlight its diverse and multidimensional nature. After reviewing the extant literature, they conclude that the research on rural health is significantly restricted and does not yet provide meaningful guidance for clinical practice. Finally, they offer several mechanisms to ameliorate this situation.

Taken together, these chapters highlight several common themes:

- the complex and multidimensional nature of community focused health;
- consideration of philosophical and theoretical differences in conducting community-focused versus individually focused research;
- the importance of action research, with its goal of community empowerment and social change; and
- relatively small but increasing literature related to implementation, intervention, and outcomes research.

Community-focused interventions are pivotal in increasing access to care and improving the health of vulnerable populations.

References

Aday, L. A. (1993). *At risk in America: The health and health care needs of vulnerable populations in the United States.* San Francisco: Jossey-Bass.

Aday, L. A. (1997). Vulnerable populations: A community-oriented perspective. *Family and Community Health, 19*(4), 1-18.

Barbee, E. L. (1993). Racism in U.S. nursing. *Medical Anthropology Quarterly, 7,* 346-362.

Barnes, D., Cribes, C., Juarbe, T., Nelson, M., Proctor, S., Sawyer, L., Shaul, M., & Meleis, A. I. (1995). Primary health care and primary care: A confusion of philosophies. *Nursing Outlook, 43,* 7-16.

Hall, J. M., Stevens, P. E., & Meleis, A. I. (1994). Marginalization: A guiding concept for valuing diversity in nursing knowledge development. *Advances in Nursing Science, 16*(4), 23-41.

Shoultz, J., & Hatcher, P. A. (1997). Looking beyond primary care to primary health care: An approach to community-based action. *Nursing Outlook, 45,* 23-26.

Zotti, M. E., Brown, P., & Stotts, R. C. (1996). Community-based nursing vs. community health nursing: What does it all mean? *Nursing Outlook, 44,* 211-217.

THE SAMPLER QUILT
A Metaphor of Rural Communities

Clarann Weinert
Mary E. Burman

The quilt has been an integral component of everyday American life, not only as a means of warding off the cold, but as a way of passing on the "story of life." Over the past two centuries, quilts have been the most universal form of needlework produced by all women, of all socioeconomic levels, all ethnic groups, and all cultural groups in our country (Cross, 1993). One can engender personal memories of quilts—the one on grandma's bed, quilts at a county fair, or perhaps women working and visiting when you accompanied your mother to the "quilting circle." Today, quilting has moved from a necessity of life to an art form. Hundreds of patterns can be found, and one pattern familiar to many is the Sampler, which is a medley of patterns combined to form a quilt (McClun & Nownes, 1993). A Sampler quilt contains a variety of colors, fabrics, and stitches. Each square is unique, yet when stitched together, the squares form a unified whole. The Sampler quilt, through the images of bright prints, muted solid colors, and various textures and shapes, provides a metaphor of rural communities.

Nurse scholars are presented with the challenge of refining rural health science and grappling with issues such as "What is rural?" "Is there such a thing as rural?" "Is rural Wyoming the same as rural Missouri?" "Is a rural agricultural community the same as a small town with a tourism economy?" and "If unique rural characteristics exist, can these be operationally defined and measured so as to allow for rural/urban empirical comparisons?" Intellectually, we know that rural is not a single dimension. Yet, authors often do not define or adequately describe the rural population under study. Standard definitions of urban/rural or metropolitan/nonmetropolitan gloss over the richness of the multiple dimensions of rural life. Furthermore, the use of these dichotomous definitions can misrepresent and misclassify persons (Hewitt, 1992).

Perhaps the metaphor of the Sampler quilt can help as a heuristic device. The squares of the Sampler can be thought of as regions or rural clusters in the United States. In the Sampler quilt, each pattern forms a square, yet the textures, shapes, and colors of the fabric in each square are unique. For example, one consideration in describing rural areas is sociocultural background. Rural dwellers in the Southeast are predominately African American with a history of poverty, poor education, and discrimination. For rural areas in the western United States, primary occupations such as ranching, farming, or mining are factors that strongly influence particular groups of rural dwellers. Because of the interplay of these kinds of factors, no one quilt square is exactly like the other. What are the colors or fabric designs that define the specific health and social needs for a particular group or segment of the rural population? Are there universal subcultural values—pieces of fabric that are common to each square of the quilt? Are the rural subcultural values identified by Long and Weinert (1989), such as independence, self-reliance, and use of informal health care providers, demonstrated for dwellers in a large, sparsely populated area, applicable to all rural areas?

If nursing is to understand the needs of rural dwellers, advance rural health science, and be a critical factor in development of rural health delivery systems, we must appreciate the secrets of the Sampler quilt. The construct *rural* is like the Sampler quilt: Each square is made of many pieces. Across squares, there are pieces that are alike and some that are unique. Each square is a work of art unto itself, but only when the squares are stitched together can the overall pattern of the quilt be fully appreciated and understood.

Focus and Background

The focus of this chapter is on (a) a description of rural community health profiles and health care services, (b) an examination of the conceptual bases of rural nursing and a critique of the state of the science, (c) a discussion of issues for clinical nursing research, and (d) recommendations for needed research relevant to rural nursing practice and the expansion of the rural nursing knowledge base. Several publications, primarily by nurse scientists and clinicians, provide rich in-depth reviews of rural research. It is not the intent to re-review or critique the content or research findings in these documents but rather to draw them to the attention of the reader and to use segments of content as background for the discussion presented in this chapter.

In the *Annual Review of Nursing Research* (Weinert & Burman, 1994), we focused on health status, health perceptions and beliefs, and health-seeking behaviors of rural dwellers. Four major types of rural health care research were reviewed: (a) studies specifically examining rural and urban differences; (b) health and health-related phenomena in a rural area; (c) articles that focused on a concept such as chronic illness, where rurality was one of several demographic variables; and (d) studies of typical rural populations such as farmers and ranchers, migrants, or Native Americans. Rural research is of widely differing sophistication and ranges from highly structured, data-based studies to individual case studies and anecdotal reports. Likewise, we found a range of types of publications on rural research, from professional journals and narrow regional publications to federal documents. Thus the review of research relevant to rural nursing research and practice is not as clean-cut and concise as reviews of more delineated topics.

The American Nurses Association Rural/Frontier Task Force prepared a white paper titled *Rural/Frontier Nursing: The Challenge to Grow* (American Nurses Association, 1996). In this paper, key questions were addressed such as, "What services are really needed by rural clients?" "Where are the service gaps?" "What services do rural nurses provide most cost effectively?" and "What academic and experiential preparation is needed to provide quality rural nursing care?" The publication is designed to stimulate comprehensive planning at the local, state, regional, and national levels by nurses in rural education, clinical practice, research, and policy. The document contains a wealth of information on rural demographics, characteristics of rural consumers, health services, and rural nursing.

A review of the literature on rural elders is contained in the publication *Advances in Gerontological Nursing* (Weinert & Burman, 1996). The focus of this chapter is on describing the rural context, examining the availability and accessibility of health care for rural elders, and discussing issues for gerontological nursing related to research, practice, and education. We noted that rural nurses have a long history of caring and activism directed at meeting the health care needs of rural elders and that the ideas put forth in *Nursing's Agenda for Health Care Reform* (American Nurses Association, 1992), calling for the enhancement of access to quality services in convenient and familiar locations, are particularly appropriate for rural elders.

The National Institute of Nursing Research (NINR) convened a priority expert panel (PEP) to develop a report titled *Community-based Health Care: Nursing Strategies* (U.S. Department of Health and Human Services, 1995). The basis for this publication, which addressed community-based strategies for rural and underserved urban populations, is a realization that changes in the United States population and health care system are generating an increased interest in the diversity, boundaries, characteristics, and complexity of communities. The panel defined the concepts of primary health care and community-based health care and described the rural-urban continuum. The document contains an extensive and in-depth exploration of rural health and health needs, a review of the state of the science on community-based approaches to rural health issues, identification of research needs and opportunities, and research recommendations. The panel reviewed a number of existing models of rural health care and cited examples of community-based interventions that have been completed or are ongoing.

These four publications represent a list of nursing and non-nursing publications that have come out in the past 8 years and that are focused specifically on rural health needs and health care delivery in rural settings (see also Anderson, 1993; Bull, Howard, & Bane, 1991; Bushy, 1991a, 1991b; Coward, Bull, Kukulka, & Galliher, 1994; Krout, 1994; Straub & Walzer, 1992; Winstead-Fry, Tiffany, & Shippee-Rice, 1992). Most of these documents includes a rather extensive review of the literature, a discussion of the state of the science, and a rich bibliography. These publications stand as immensely valuable resources for those exploring rural nursing research and practice issues.

Rural Communities

Health Profiles

In the late 1980s, Patton (1989) identified the need to develop profiles of rural dwellers, their health status, and the accessibility and availability of health services along the continuum of frontier communities to larger rural cities. Development of profiles requires careful consideration of the individual shapes and colors of the fabric in each Sampler square to avoid the pitfalls of generali-

zation and failure to fully consider the unique characteristics of the community or rural subpopulation under study.

Rural residents generally are considered to be poorer and in poorer health (American Nurses Association, 1996). Summer (1991) indicated that rural residents have a higher incidence of maternal and infant mortality; chronic illness and disability; and morbidity due to diabetes, cancer, hypertension, and heart and lung disease, as compared to their urban counterparts. However, when Coward, McLaughlin, Duncan, and Bull (1994) examined six key sociodemographic variables, the discrepancies between rural and urban elders did not always place the rural elderly at a disadvantage. These authors concluded that the health of rural elders does differ from that of urban elders; however, these differences are not found on all indicators of health, nor are the rural elders always at greater risk.

The inconsistency of findings in relation to rural health is common. Suicide rates among farm populations have been reported to be higher than other populations (Stallones, 1990), yet suicide rates for rural men in Colorado were lower than for metropolitan residents (Stallones & Cook, 1992). Eggebeen and Lichter (1993) reported that, although rural residents consistently rate their physical health as poorer and are somewhat less happy than nonrural dwellers, the overall health and well-being of rural middle-aged and older adults appear to be better than their urban counterparts. Thorson and Powell (1992) reported that rural elders in Nebraska were generally in good health and able to care for themselves. According to McManus and Newacheck (1989), pregnant rural women tend to begin prenatal care later in pregnancy and make fewer than the recommended clinic visits. Yet, in a study conducted in Washington State, poor birth outcomes were no more likely among rural residents than urban ones, despite the fact that the rural women received less prenatal care (Larson, Hart, & Rosenblatt, 1992).

Actual health and illness differences between urban and rural dwellers can be demonstrated. Specific to the rural setting are injuries sustained from agricultural activities, exposure to toxic agents, motor vehicle accidents, and firearms (McGinnis & Foege, 1993). The most common cause of injury for children and adolescents living or working on farms is farm machinery and tractor rollovers, which account for one half of deaths (Wright, 1993). Machinery running in enclosed spaces may cause carbon monoxide poisoning. Harvesting equipment can cause crushing or amputation injuries and power-take-off equipment (farm or ranch equipment that uses moving belts or conveyor-type systems) can twist a worker around a shaft, causing suffocation, scalping, and avulsion injuries (Wright, 1993). Farm machinery tend to produce high noise levels and hearing loss is common among farm workers. In Wisconsin, 50% of the men had hearing loss affecting communication by age 50 (Karlovich, Wiley, Tweed, & Jensen, 1988). However, farm accidents may not be random incidents. According to a study in North Dakota (Geller, Ludtke, & Stratton, 1990), farm operators at high risk for accidents were younger and had a higher debt-to-asset ratio. Likewise, one out of four farmers cut corners on safety to save money.

Rural life is generally perceived as safer and healthier, yet the dynamics related to domestic violence are often intensified in rural areas (Goeckermann, Hamberger, & Barber, 1994). In addition to domestic violence, motor vehicle accidents are a serious concern. According to a study by Baker, Whitfield, and O'Neill (1987), the 15 counties with the highest death rates had sparse populations (two or fewer persons per square mile). Baker et al. attributed these mortality rates to high-speed driving, variations in road conditions, lack of use of seat belts, types of vehicles, and limited emergency care.

Other health issues observed by rural health care providers are high use of smokeless tobacco, vehicular accidents associated with alcohol misuse, and unintentional firearms injuries. However, conclusive statistical data are lacking. More adequate and accurate data should be forthcoming from research-based intervention programs designed to reduce injury and disease among agricultural workers (Myers, 1992).

▒ Health Care Services

A critical component of the health profile for rural communities is the availability, accessibility, and acceptability of the health care delivery system. In general, rural areas are thought to have fewer and a more restricted range of health care services (Hassinger, Hicks, & Godino, 1993; Krout, 1994). However, Gillanders and Buss (1993), in a study of 1,000 rural elderly in Ohio, found that concerns over access to health care appear to be more perceptual than real.

The availability of providers has been a significant issue in the rural health care literature. Approximately one third of all nonmetropolitan residents lived in Primary Care Health Professional Shortage Areas (American Nurses Association, 1996). Moreover, 92% of counties classified as nurse shortage counties were in rural areas (Stratton, Ludtke, Juhl, Dunkin, & Geller, 1993). These shortages affect rural residents of all ages. For example, rural children have less access to pediatric care, greater travel times to providers, and lower likelihood of having well-child visits (Goodman, Barff, & Fisher, 1992; Levey, Curry, & Levey, 1988).

Insurance coverage is an issue for some rural communities. Rural residents have less access to Medicaid, are more likely to be uninsured or underinsured and to have purchased private insurance outside the workplace, and are less likely to have insurance through their employer (Frenzen, 1993; Summer, 1991). Interestingly, farmers have been thought to be more likely to be uninsured or underinsured compared to other populations. However, in Minnesota, only 10% of the farmers in the study were uninsured, compared to over 25% nationally (Kralewski, Liu, & Shapiro, 1992).

Small hospitals have been a traditional source of care in rural areas since the Hill-Burton Act in the 1940s. Currently, issues of availability of acute care facilities are being examined relative to the steady closure of rural facilities (Fleming, Williamson, Hicks, & Rife, 1995; McKay & Coventry, 1995). Rural hospitals are often a primary employer and a critical element in a community's infrastructure. Having a hospital provides a competitive edge, and historically communities have fought over the site of the local hospital (Berry & Seavey, 1994). However, it is not uncommon for families to look elsewhere even when a local facility could provide the needed care. Berry and Seavey (1994) observed that in high-income rural communities more people sought care in urban hospitals, but in low-income communities the population was a captive market that sought care locally. Use of health care services is influenced also by rural residents' attitudes, values, and health beliefs. For example, attitudes and beliefs about mental health, the use of alcohol and drugs, and lack of anonymity may prevent rural dwellers from seeking professional help (Wagenfield, Murray, Mohatt, & DeBruyn, 1994).

Clearly, for some living in more isolated areas, distance to health care is an issue. In a study of Montana families managing cancer, those living in more isolated areas drove 214 miles round-trip for appointments at one of the five cancer treatment centers in the state (Bender, Weinert, Faulkner, & Quimby, 1991). Relocation to larger cities to obtain specialized care was identified in this study as an issue for some rural residents. Families often traveled long distances out of state for diagnosis, initial treatment, and follow-up care. For some, this relocation was of a significant duration. Other families temporarily relocated to an in-state treatment center, taking up residence with family and friends or living in recreation vehicles in the parking lot of the health care facility. For other families, relocation took place on a weekly basis, as they drove to a treatment center and stayed a day or two and then returned, often long distances to their homes, just to face the trip again in a week.

Factors associated with the decisions made in seeking cancer treatment included travel time, time lost from work, cost of lodging, patient and family comfort, specialized care not covered by insurance, and lack of health insurance altogether (Curtiss, 1993). Travel time was lengthened by harsh weather and poor road conditions. Families commented on the financial cost of lost work days for a spouse, the need to find someone to tend to the chores on the farm or ranch, and the physical strain of traveling on the family (Bender et al., 1991). They also noted the hidden costs of loss of social support when needing to leave their own community. Treatment at faraway centers compounds coping with cancer and its treatment (Curtiss, 1993). A diagnosis of cancer is profound, and people report feeling isolated, abandoned, and distanced from their family and friends.

Clearly, the issue of rural health is not a simple one. Caution must be taken when attempting to make general statements regarding rural health status. Health care needs are affected by differences in the distribution of income, education, race, age, and marital status in rural and urban areas (U.S. Department of Health and Human Services, 1995). Likewise, characteristics of the rural health care delivery system, as well as rural subcultural values that may influence the use of health care facilities, cannot be overlooked in health care delivery to rural dwellers. The caveat of needing to know the unique characteristics for each locale and subgroup cannot be stressed too strongly.

Many of the health problems and access issues of rural residents could be resolved by an adequate supply of community-based primary health care providers (American Nurses Association, 1996). Master's-prepared advanced practice nurses and bachelor's-prepared registered nurses have the expertise to deliver high-quality, client-centered care for rural populations, resulting in healthier communities. Nurses need to be adept at mobilizing community resources through coalition building and sensitivity to unique rural values and beliefs. Further, although rural nurses are subject to the exigencies of their environment, they have a window of opportunity through the processes of state- and local-level health care reform to further encourage change that is directed by nursing rather than entirely dependent on the goodwill of external agencies and institutions.

Conceptual Bases of Rural Nursing

Several schools of thought have dominated our thinking about rural communities, rural health, and rural health care. Undoubtedly, elements of truth can be found for each of these perspectives. First is the notion that rural communities and rural dwellers are disadvantaged and/or impoverished. This has been an effective mechanism to draw attention to the needs of rural areas and obtain financial resources for health care or research. However, this notion also blurs the rich diversity of rural areas. Second, rural life is perceived to be bucolic and pastoral. Indeed, according to the *American Heritage Dictionary,* useful synonyms for rural include "bucolic," "rustic," "pastoral," and "sylvan." Rural is specifically associated with farming and ranching. The image that comes to mind is of "rocking chairs, rolling farm fields, and lots of grandchildren squealing with wiggly puppies" (Weinert & Burman, 1996). As with the other notion of disadvantage and impoverishment, the bucolic and pastoral school of thought masks the diversity of rural areas and does not allow for an accurate assessment of health needs. Finally, rural dwellers are viewed as being hardy, independent, and more willing to use informal than formal means of support (Krout, 1994). Research by Weinert and Long (1987) and Magilvy, Congdon, and Martinez (1994) certainly supports this notion. What is missing is the comparison with urban counterparts, who may be equally hardy, independent, and self-reliant, perhaps in a different sense.

At this point, nursing is in the beginning stages of formulating a conceptual basis for rural nursing practice. Overall, the body of rural nursing knowledge is limited (Weinert & Burman, 1994). Even with the addition of research from other disciplines, the knowledge base is seriously fragmented, especially in relation to guiding nursing practice. However, several areas of emerging theory development or clusters of studies that are focused on a specific topic and/or rural subpopulation are discussed. This is not intended to be a comprehensive review (see Weinert & Burman, 1994, for such a review). Instead, the intention is to provide an overview of the state of the science in rural nursing research.

Health Beliefs

Several nurse researchers have explored the health beliefs and health-seeking behavior of rural dwellers. Weinert and Long have identified key rural concepts in their research in rural Montana: work and health beliefs, outside/insider, and oldtimer/newcomer (Long & Weinert, 1989; Weinert & Long, 1987, 1990, 1991). Rural dwellers in this sparsely populated rural area define health as the ability to do work, be productive, and do usual tasks. Rural dwellers are thought to be self-reliant and more likely to use informal sources of help, resisting assistance from those perceived as outsiders.

Some evaluation of the tenets of this theory has been conducted. Lee (1989) found that rural residents, in comparison with their urban counterparts, were more likely to associate health with the ability to work, function, and perform daily tasks. Davis and colleagues (1991) reported similar findings for older adults in rural areas. Maintaining independence was fundamental to the quality of life of older adults in Colorado (Magilvy et al., 1994). Counts and Boyle (1987) also found a high value placed on independence and self-reliance. Hardiness, self-sufficiency, and independence contribute to the competence of older adults living in rural areas; however, they may also lead to delays in seeking care (Lee, 1993).

Not all research findings have supported the initial propositions by Weinert and Long. Despite a hypothesized propensity to use informal sources of help, rural dwellers may not have informal resources to rely upon. Schultz (1990) found that for rural elders discharged from the hospital, friends and relatives were providing considerably less informal support for assistance with activities of daily living than were family and friends of the urban elderly in her study. In families experiencing multiple sclerosis (MS), rural men whose wives had MS reported less social support, fewer social network resources, and less support from neighbors than did rural woman whose husbands had the disease (Weinert & Long, 1993). Rural women had smaller networks and less affirmation support but longer duration of relationships and greater contact with support members than urban women (Pass, 1991). Moreover, family hardiness, a broader concept than individual hardiness, which incorporates confidence along with commitment, challenge, and control, was higher in urban families when compared with rural families (Dunkin, Holzwarth, & Stratton, 1993).

Older Adults

A growing body of research focuses on the health and health behaviors of older rural residents; there is more limited research in nursing on other age groups in rural areas. Older adults living in nonmetropolitan areas reported less stress than those living in metropolitan areas (Preston & Crawford, 1990). Only a small percentage of rural elders were in poor or frail health (Preston & Mansfield, 1984). McCulloch (1991) also found that older rural women generally had positive perceptions of their own health, despite the presence of chronic illnesses. In contrast, Johnson, Waldo, and Johnson (1993) reported high levels of stress and fair to poor health in their rural elder sample.

Rural elders exercise and eat a balanced diet to maintain their health (Davis et al., 1991). Social support facilitates health-promoting behaviors (Riffle, Yoho, & Sams, 1989). Rural elders are concerned about their health, although this may not translate into changing to a more healthy lifestyle (Dellasega, Brown, & White, 1995). Johnson (1991) reported that many positive health practices, such as adequate nutrition, sleep, exercise, and safe driving, were used infrequently and inconsistently by rural elders. In addition, rural elders tended not to consult health care professionals before using over-the-counter drugs (OTCs) and used more OTCs than urban elders (Johnson & Moore, 1988; Moore & Johnson, 1993). Diet and weight problems, medications and their side effects, fears, and lack of support significantly affect the management of hypertension in rural elders (Whetstone & Reid, 1991).

Women's Health

The well-being of rural women has been examined by several nurse researchers. Well-being, judged on amount of stress, life satisfaction, and degree of exhaustion, did not differ significantly between urban and rural women (Mansfield, Preston, & Crawford, 1988). Stress was predicted by other factors, such as health status and the presence of young children in the home. Bigbee (1988, 1990) reported similar findings: Stress and illness occurrence did not differ between rural and urban women. However, rural women tended to identify more environmentally related stresses, urban women reported more financial stressors (Bigbee, 1987).

Despite few differences in overall well-being, Edwards, Parker, Burks, West, and Adams (1991) found higher cardiovascular risks in rural women than urban women. Rural women who performed breast self-examination (BSE) were more likely to perceive benefits from BSE, saw fewer barriers to BSE, and had higher motivation scores (Gray, 1990). Urban women were more likely to smoke; rural women were more likely to wear seat belts (Mansfield, Preston, & Crawford, 1989).

Home Care

Magilvy and colleagues explored the home care of rural elders in Colorado (Congdon & Magilvy, 1995; Magilvy et al., 1994). Two "circles of care" support the frail elder in a rural setting: the circle of formal care and the circle of family and friends (Magilvy et al., 1994). Family is an essential source of support for many rural residents, not only in sickness, but in promotion of healthy lifestyles (Crawford & Preston, 1991). These two circles were often blended with nurses and other health care professionals as a part of the informal circle of care. This blending of informal and formal care is consistent with the proposition by Long and Weinert (1989) that rural nurses experience lack of anonymity and greater role diffusion than urban nurses. Discharge planning and professional networking contribute to the continuity of the circle of formal care. However, gaps could not always be prevented due to missed opportunities for referral, payment issues, or lack of services in the rural area. Rural dwellers who cared for a loved one with cancer also identified gaps in formal resources, especially those living in frontier areas (Buehler & Lee, 1992).

The findings from work with urban elders help to extend the concept of self-reliance from that of "shunning" professional services to, at least in some cases, actively seeking and using these services to maintain the independence of family members (Magilvy & Lakomy, 1991). However, frail rural elders were not always comfortable with professional care, although they felt it was necessary at times. Some felt it promoted dependence and delayed the attainment of independence (Magilvy et al., 1994).

Nursing Practice Issues

Researchers at the University of North Dakota have explored the recruitment, retention, and job satisfaction of rural nurses (Dunkin, Juhl, Stratton, Geller, & Ludtke, 1992; Movassaghi, Kindig, Juhl, & Geller, 1992; Strat-

ton, Gibbens, Dunkin, & Juhl, 1993; Stratton, Juhl, & Dunkin, 1992). Movassaghi and colleagues (1992) found significant differences in the educational background, salaries, and distribution of nurses between rural and urban areas. For example, nurses working in rural areas had lower salaries than those working in urban areas. Many barriers face nursing administrators in their attempts to recruit and retain rural nurses, and subsequently they use a variety of recruitment and retention strategies (Stratton, Juhl, et al., 1992). For rural nurses, job satisfaction is only one component of employment longevity. The majority of the respondents planned to stay in their current jobs for more than 5 years; however, they expressed dissatisfaction with specific aspects of their jobs (Dunkin, Juhl, et al., 1992).

Fuszard, Green, Kujala, and Talley (1994a, 1994b) have explored the structural and nursing practice variables of rural magnet hospitals. The nurses identified pride in excellence of patient care, ability to continue personal and professional growth, involvement in student education, and recruitment and retention of nurses as vital to the success of their hospitals.

Delivery of Rural Health Services

A rather large body of health services research exists, focusing on the issues of health care delivery in the era of health care reform, HMO penetration, managed care, mergers, and other reform strategies. However, most of this research is "outside" of nursing and is beyond the purview of this discussion. However, the impact of these health care delivery factors cannot be minimized when considering the health status and health care needs of rural communities. This knowledge, giving insight into the financing and organization of health care and the delivery of health care services, clearly has relevance to nursing research and practice in rural areas.

Several studies in the area of health services use have been done in nursing. Home-based services for rural residents tend to be small, with large service areas. Directors of these programs identify many needs, including personal and respite care (Burman, Steffes, & Weinert, 1994). To meet the needs of rural residents and maintain the financial viability of the rural home health care agency, patient referrals must be actively sought. However, the "spirit" of community health nurses has changed from a focus on caring and community service to an emphasis on reimbursement (Congdon & Magilvy, 1995). Heavy documentation requirements have led to lower productivity, job satisfaction, and quality of care, as well as higher nursing turnover.

Many nurses have called for the use of nursing centers in rural areas to enhance access of care (Barger, 1991; Dahl, Gustafson, & McCullagh, 1993). Hueston and Murry (1992) described a successful three-tier model of obstetrical care, using nurse midwives as the foundation of the system. Rural residents receiving care at nursing centers were satisfied with the care (Giltinan & Murray, 1992; Ramsey, Edwards, Lenz, Odom, & Brown, 1993).

Community-Based Nursing Strategies

The makeup of rural health care may be somewhat different than that for larger cities and urban areas. For example, rural areas have smaller hospitals or no hospitals, and many nurses work in long-term care and public health. Therefore, although community-based care is an important issue for all settings, it is especially appropriate for rural areas. A number of community-based strategies targeting health promotion, disease prevention, and supportive and restorative care are identified and reviewed in the report prepared by the NINR PEP panel (U.S. Department of Health and Human Services, 1995). For example, Ferketich, Phillips, and Verran (1990) evaluated a comprehensive, multilevel, community health nursing model with rural Hispanics. Buckwalter, Smith, Zevenberg, and Russell (1991) have examined mechanisms to reach rural elders in Iowa experiencing mental health problems, through the Elderly Outreach Program. Outreach, referral, and treatment are incorporated into this program. Community-based nursing interventions need to employ creative strategies to be successful. Jenkins (1991) described a community wellness program that used county extension agents as community catalysts to bring residents together to identify community needs and solutions.

The members of the NINR PEP panel concluded that a significant portion of the research in rural health has been largely descriptive and epidemiological, often conducted with the goal of describing health status and the distribution and use of health services and of examining issues of formal and informal care. The panel reiterated the need for both qualitative and quantitative studies to identify and develop outcome measures for community-based interventions. It encouraged studies to explore the ways that community members can be involved in planning, developing, implementing, and assessing health services. This panel also noted that the meaning of health

and the health and illness experiences of rural populations across the country and across the lifespan are still poorly understood (U.S. Department of Health and Human Services, 1995).

Methodological Issues

What is rural research? This may seem like an academic question, but it is a continual dilemma when reviewing the literature in this area. Conceptual clarity, careful measurement, and attention to differences within and between specific rural areas are critical to the furtherance of rural science. Is a study rural because the people in the sample come from a small town of less than 2,500 people? Not necessarily, although this assumption clearly has been made in the arena of rural research broadly and rural nursing research more specifically. In many cases, because a study is conducted in Idaho or Missouri, it is assumed to be rural. This debate is made difficult by the widely varying definitions of rural (Hewitt, 1992). However, to further the knowledge development in this area, the question of what constitutes rural research needs to be addressed. We argue that simply because a study has a rural sample or focuses on a rural topic (e.g., migrant or farm health) does not automatically make the study a rural one. As noted above, what has been left out of a lot of research is clearly identifying and addressing contextual variables that lead to the diversity of rural areas. For example, a study of urinary incontinence (UI) in Centennial, Wyoming (population 100) is not a rural study. However, studying the contextual factors of Centennial and how they affect UI or access to care in relation to UI is more likely a rural study.

Two predominant types of research have been done: (a) within rural descriptions (e.g., health problems and availability of health care resources in a specific rural community, county, or state) and (b) comparisons between urban and rural areas (e.g., comparisons between an urban area and a rural area in types of health problems). Both of these have the potential to contribute to rural nursing research. However, many of the studies remain isolated, rurality is poorly defined, and the implications for rural nursing are not clearly explicated.

Numerous examples can be found of the "within rural"-type study. For example, Burman, Steffes, and Weinert (1994) examined the size, structure, and service area of rural home health care agencies and hospices in Montana. No comparisons were made with urban areas, and the study was limited to a specific rural area—a sparsely populated Rocky Mountain state. As noted above, the challenge in this type of research is to make the connection to rurality and to clearly make the connection to rural nursing science. Tough questions need to be asked. Why is it important to study home health agencies and hospices in rural Montana? Is a study rural because the agencies happen to be located in small towns? Is the topic unique to rural areas?

In the broad arena of rural research, many examples can be found in which comparisons between urban and rural areas on various aspects of health or health care are made. Fewer of these types of studies exist in nursing. The challenge in this kind of research is to make relevant comparisons and meaningful categorizations or measurement of "rural" and "urban." Often, dichotomous classifications of metropolitan/nonmetropolitan or urban/rural are used to make comparisons. Using these classifications can result in as much within-group variance as between-group variance (Coward, McLaughlin, et al., 1994). In addition, conclusions may be quite different, depending on what classification scheme is used (Hewitt, 1992). Many researchers have proposed examining rural along a continuum incorporating population, economic, occupational, and access factors (Cordes, 1987; Coward, McLaughlin, et al., 1994; Ide, 1992; Krout, 1994). The Montana State University Rurality Index is one such example; it uses a continuum of rurality based on access and population variables (Weinert & Boik, 1995). Depending on the focus of the research, other factors may need to be incorporated in the definition and measurement of the degree of rurality, such as economic base or sociocultural characteristics.

Recommendations

At this point, nursing research focusing on rural health and health care is significantly restricted and does not necessarily provide meaningful guidance to nurse researchers and nurse clinicians in rural areas. Mechanisms to enhance research are needed. For example, we recommend mentoring programs that link new and established nurse researchers, pre- and postdoctoral programs focusing on rural nursing, and the use of computer technology to link underserved areas with large universities so that isolated nurses can have access to research

resources such as libraries or other nurse researchers (Weinert & Burman, 1996). Rural nursing research should focus on the following: (a) advancing the development and testing of emerging nursing theory; (b) careful operationalization and measurement of rurality; (c) care in avoiding generalizations about rural dwellers; (d) targeting research on specific topics with replication studies and multisite and collaborative studies; (e) developing well-designed studies to explore rural and urban differences; (f) evaluating, adapting, and developing of measures that are valid, reliable, and sensitive to rural issues; and (g) exploring innovative methods to capture the picture of rural life and rural health needs (Weinert & Burman, 1994).

The link between theory and research must be strengthened in rural research, especially in the area of rural context. The contextual factors that distinguish one rural area from another need to be identified, as well as the factors that are similar for all or most rural areas. Multisite, multi-investigator, and/or multidisciplinary research would be helpful in this regard. Secondary analysis, also, is a research methodology that would be useful in elucidating the rural context. Nurse researchers and other researchers have large data sets available that could be used to explore contextual variables for a broad range of rural research questions. To fully use these resources, new ways to communicate ongoing research are needed. Efforts by the Sigma Theta Tau International Virginia Henderson Library to archive conference proceedings and to establish a data bank of concepts and verified conceptual relationships are examples of ways to enhance investigator collaboration.

Another critical area identified by the PEP panel focusing on community-based health care is the need for more intervention and evaluation research using community-based nursing strategies (U.S. Department of Health and Human Services). Intervention strategies that work in rural areas (e.g., the use of computer technology and various outreach strategies) need to be identified. There must be recognition that these can be expensive investigations and that adequate financial and supportive resources need to be available.

Conclusions and Summary

Based on this review and others, nursing has only just begun to describe the squares of the rural quilt and has not come close to adequately describing the color, texture, and pattern for most of the squares, let alone describing the entire Sampler quilt. We know a little bit about the health beliefs of rural dwellers. Similarly, processes of home care of frail rural elders has begun to be described. However, for both of these areas, studies have used samples from the same or similar rural subpopulations, and replication with other subpopulations and empirical testing of the relational statements is needed (Weinert & Burman, 1994). The nursing research on older adults and women in rural areas has inconsistencies. Finally, we have scattered research in nursing practice issues and the delivery of rural nursing services.

The challenge for nurses doing rural research is a close examination of the rural context. "Recognizing the enormous complexity and diversity of the general features of rural environments is possibly the most poorly understood fundamental factor" in understanding rural communities (Berry & Seavey, 1994, p. 34). This context has not been well specified or measured in much of the rural nursing research. Without further careful consideration of the contextual factors, determining whether the study is actually "rural" can be difficult. Likewise, generalizing the findings to other rural areas is difficult, a clear understanding of rural and urban differences is blurred, and conducting appropriate and meaningful rural nursing research to enhance the rural nursing knowledge base and support rural nursing practice is hampered.

References

American Nurses Association. (1992). *Nursing's agenda for health care reform.* Washington, DC: American Nurses Publishing.

American Nurses Association. (1996). *Rural/frontier nursing: The challenge to grow.* Washington, DC: Author.

Anderson, J. (1993). Rural nursing. *Nursing Clinics of North America, 28,* 121-226.

Baker, S., Whitfield, R., & O'Neill, B. (1987). Geographic variations in mortality from motor vehicle crashes. *New England Journal of Medicine, 316,* 1384-1387.

Barger, S. (1991). The nursing center: A model for rural practice. *Nursing & Health Care, 12,* 290-294.

Bender, L., Weinert, C., Faulkner, L., & Quimby, R. (1991). *Montana families living with cancer.* Bozeman: Montana State University Press.

Berry, D., & Seavey, J. (1994). Assuring access to rural health services: The case for revitalizing small rural hospitals. *Health Care Management Review, 19*(2), 32-42.

Bigbee, J. (1987). Stressful life events among women: A rural-urban comparison. *Journal of Rural Health, 3,* 39-51.

Bigbee, J. (1988). Rurality, stress and illness among women: A pilot study. *Health Care for Women International, 9,* 43-61.

Bigbee, J. (1990). Stressful life events and illness occurrence in rural versus urban women. *Journal of Community Health Nursing, 7,* 105-113.

Buckwalter, K., Smith, M., Zevenberg, P., & Russell, D. (1991). Mental health services of the rural elderly outreach program. *The Gerontologist, 31,* 408-412.

Buehler, J., & Lee, H. (1992). Exploration of home care resources for rural families with cancer. *Cancer Nursing, 15,* 299-308.

Bull, C., Howard, D., & Bane, S. (1991). *Challenges and solutions to the provision of programs and services to rural elders.* Kansas City: University of Missouri–Kansas City Press.

Burman, M., Steffes, M., & Weinert, C. (1994). Cancer home care in Montana. *Home Health Care Services Quarterly, 4,* 37-42.

Bushy, A. (1991a). *Rural nursing* (Vol. 1). Newbury Park, CA: Sage.

Bushy, A. (1991b). *Rural nursing* (Vol. 2). Newbury Park, CA: Sage.

Congdon, J., & Magilvy, J. (1995). The changing spirit of rural community nursing: Documentation burden. *Public Health Nursing, 12*(1), 18-24.

Cordes, S. (1987). The changing rural environment and the relationship between health services and rural development. *Health Services Research, 23,* 757-784.

Counts, M., & Boyle, J. (1987). Nursing, health, and policy within a community context. *Advances of Nursing Science, 9*(3), 12-23.

Coward, R., Bull, C., Kukulka, G., & Galliher, J. (1994). *Health services for rural elders.* New York: Springer.

Coward, R., McLaughlin, D., Duncan, R., & Bull, C. (1994). An overview of health and aging in rural America. In R. Coward, N. Bull, G. Kukulka, & J. Galliher (Eds.), *Health services for rural elders* (pp. 1-32). New York: Springer.

Crawford, C., & Preston, D. (1991). Differences in specific sources of social support for four healthy behaviors. In A. Bushy (Ed.), *Rural nursing* (Vol. 1, pp. 215-227). Newbury Park, CA: Sage.

Cross, M. (1993). *Treasures in the trunk.* Nashville, TN: Rutledge Hill.

Curtiss, C. (1993). Trends and issues for cancer care in rural communities. *Nursing Clinics of North America, 28,* 241-251.

Dahl, S., Gustafson, C., & McCullagh, M. (1993). Collaborating to develop a community-based health service for rural homeless persons. *Journal of Nursing Administration, 23*(4), 41-45.

Davis, D., Henderson, M., Boothe, A., Douglas, M., Faria, S., Kennedy, D., Kitchense, E., & Weaver, M. (1991). An interactive perspective on the health beliefs and practices of rural elders. *Journal of Gerontological Nursing, 17*(5), 11-16.

Dellasega, C., Brown, R., & White, A. (1995). Cholesterol-related behaviors in rural elderly persons. *Journal of Gerontological Nursing, 21*(5), 6-12.

Dunkin, J., Holzwarth, C., & Stratton, T. (1993). Assessment of rural family hardiness: A foundation for intervention. In S. Feetham, S. Meister, J. Bell, & C. Gillis (Eds.), *The nursing of families* (pp. 247-255). Newbury Park, CA: Sage.

Dunkin, J., Juhl, N., Stratton, T., Geller, J., & Ludtke, R. (1992). Job satisfaction and retention of rural community health nurses in North Dakota. *Journal of Rural Health, 8,* 268-275.

Edwards, K., Parker, D., Burks, C., West, A., & Adams, M. (1991). Cardiovascular risk: Among Black and White rural-urban low income women. *Association of Black Nursing Faculty Journal, 2,* 72-76.

Eggebeen, D., & Lichter, D. (1993). Health and well-being among rural Americans: Variations across the life course. *Journal of Rural Health, 9,* 86-98.

Ferketich, S., Phillips, L., & Verran, J. (1990). *Multilevel nursing practice model for rural Hispanics* (Agency for Health Care Policy and Research Grant No. R18-HS0680). Rockville, MD: Agency for Health Care Policy and Research.

Fleming, S., Williamson, H., Hicks, L., & Rife, I. (1995). *Hospital and Health Services Administration, 40,* 247-262.

Frenzen, P. (1993). Health insurance coverage in U.S. urban and rural areas. *Journal of Rural Health, 9,* 204-213.

Fuszard, B., Green, E., Kujala, E., & Talley, B. (1994a). Rural magnet hospitals of excellence (Part 1). *Journal of Nursing Administration, 24*(1), 21-26.

Fuszard, B., Green, E., Kujala, E., & Talley, B. (1994b). Rural magnet hospitals of excellence (Part 2). *Journal of Nursing Administration, 24*(2), 35-41.

Geller, J., Ludtke, R., & Stratton, T. (1990). Nonfatal farm injuries in North Dakota: A sociological analysis. *Journal of Rural Health, 6,* 185-196.

Gillanders, W., & Buss, T. (1993). Access to medical care among the elderly in rural northeastern Ohio. *Journal of Family Practice, 37*(4), 349-355.

Giltinan, J., & Murray, K. (1992). Meeting the health care needs of rural elderly: Client satisfaction with a university-sponsored nursing center. *Journal of Rural Health, 8,* 305-309.

Goeckermann, C., Hamberger, L., & Barber, K. (1994, September). Issues of domestic violence unique to rural areas. *Wisconsin Medical Journal, 93*(4), 473-479.

Goodman, D., Barff, R., & Fisher, E. (1992). Geographic barriers to child health services in rural northern New England: 1980-1989. *Journal of Rural Health, 8,* 106-112.

Gray, M. (1990). Factors related to practice of breast self-examination in rural women. *Cancer Nursing, 13,* 100-107.

Hassinger, E., Hicks, L., & Godino, V. (1993). A literature review of health issues of the rural elderly. *Journal of Rural Health, 9,* 68-75.

Hewitt, M. (1992). Defining "rural" areas: Impact on health care policy and research. In W. Gesler & T. Ricketts (Eds.), *Health in rural North America* (pp. 25-54). New Brunswick, NJ: Rutgers University Press.

Hueston, W., & Murry, M. (1992). A three-tier model for the delivery of rural obstetrical care using a nurse midwife and family physician copractice. *Journal of Rural Health, 8,* 283-289.

Ide, B. (1992, 4th quarter). A process model of rural nursing. *Texas Journal of Rural Health,* pp. 30-34.

Jenkins, S. (1991). Community wellness: A group empowerment model. *Journal of Health Care for the Poor and Underserved, 1,* 388-404.

Johnson, J. (1991). Health-care practices of the rural aged. *Journal of Gerontological Nursing, 17,* 15-19.

Johnson, J., & Moore, J. (1988). Drug-taking practices of the rural elderly. *Applied Nursing Research, 1,* 128-131.

Johnson, J., Waldo, M., & Johnson, R. (1993). Stress and perceived health status in the rural elderly. *Journal of Gerontological Nursing, 19*(9), 24-29.

Karlovich, R., Wiley, T., Tweed, T., & Jensen, D. (1988). Hearing sensitivity in farmers. *Public Health Reports, 103,* 61-71.

Kralewski, J., Liu, Y., Shapiro, J. (1992). A descriptive analysis of health insurance coverage among farm families in Minnesota. *Journal of Rural Health, 8,* 178-184.

Krout, J. (Ed.). (1994). *Providing community-based services to the rural elderly.* Thousand Oaks, CA: Sage.

Larson, E., Hart, G., & Rosenblatt, R. (1992). Rural residence and poor birth outcome in Washington State. *Journal of Rural Health, 8,* 162-170.

Lee, H. (1989). *Quantitative validation of health perceptions of rural persons.* Unpublished manuscript, Montana State University, College of Nursing, Bozeman, MT.

Lee, H. (1993). Health perceptions of middle, new middle, and older rural adults. *Family and Community Health, 16,* 19-27.

Levey, L., Curry, J., & Levey, S. (1988). Rural-urban differences in access to Iowa child health services. *Journal of Rural Health, 4,* 59-72.

Long, K., & Weinert, C. (1989). Rural nursing: Developing the theory base. *Scholarly Inquiry for Nursing Practice, 3*(2), 113-127.

Magilvy, J., Congdon, J., & Martinez, R. (1994). Circles of care: Home care and community support for rural older adults. *Advances in Nursing Science, 16*(3), 22-33.

Magilvy, J., & Lakomy, J. (1991). Transitions of older adults to home. *Home Health Care Services Quarterly, 12*(4), 59-70.

Mansfield, P., Preston, D., & Crawford, C. (1988). Rural-urban differences in women's psychological well-being. *Health Care for Women International, 9,* 289-304.

Mansfield, P., Preston, D., & Crawford, C. (1989). The health behaviors of rural women: Comparisons with an urban sample. *Health Values, 16*(6), 12-20.

McClun, D., & Nownes, L. (1993). *Quilts, quilts, and more quilts.* Lafayette, CA: C & T.

McCulloch, B. (1991). Health and health maintenance profiles of older rural women, 1976-1986. In A. Bushy (Ed.), *Rural nursing* (Vol. 1, pp. 281-298). Newbury Park, CA: Sage.

McGinnis, J., & Foege, W. (1993). Actual causes of death in the United States. *Journal of the American Medical Association, 270,* 2207-2212.

McKay, N., & Coventry, J. (1995). Access implication of rural hospital closures and conversions. *Hospital & Health Services Administration, 40,* 227-246.

McManus, M., & Newacheck, P. (1989). Rural maternal, child, and adolescent health. *Health Services Research, 23,* 807-848.

Moore, J., & Johnson, J. (1993). Over-the-counter drug use by the rural elderly. *Geriatric Nursing, 14,* 190-191.

Movassaghi, H., Kindig, D., Juhl, N., & Geller, J. (1992). Nursing supply and characteristics in the nonmetropolitan areas of the United States: Findings from the 1988 National Sample Survey of Registered Nurses. *Journal of Rural Health, 8,* 276-282.

Myers, M. (1992). *Papers and proceedings of the surgeon general's Conference on Agricultural Safety and Health: Public Law 101-517: April 30–May 3, 1991* (DHHS Pub. No. 92-105). Washington, DC: U.S. Government Printing Office.

Pass, C. (1991). Social support and sex role orientation: A comparison of rural and urban pregnant women. In A. Bushy (Ed.), *Rural nursing* (Vol. 1, pp. 146-157). Newbury Park, CA: Sage.

Patton, L. (1989). Setting the rural health services research agenda: The congressional perspective. *Health Services Research, 23*(6), 1005-1051.

Preston, D., & Crawford, C. (1990). A study of community differences in stress among the elderly: Implications for community health nursing. *Public Health Nursing, 7,* 229-235.

Preston, D., & Mansfield, P. (1984). An exploration of stressful life events, illness, and coping among the rural elderly. *The Gerontologist, 24,* 490-494.

Ramsey, R., Edwards, J., Lenz, C., Odom, J., & Brown, B. (1993). Types of health problems and satisfaction with services in a rural nurse-managed clinic. *Community Health Nursing, 10,* 161-176.

Riffle, K., Yoho, J., & Sams, J. (1989). Health-promoting behaviors, perceived social support, and self-reported health of Appalachian elderly. *Public Health Nursing, 6,* 204-211.

Schultz, A. (1990). Rural/urban differences in health care need of the elderly after hospital discharge to home. *Dissertation Abstracts International, 52*(11), 5761B. (University Microfilms No. DA92-04799)

Stallones, L. (1990). Suicide mortality among Kentucky farmers: 1979-1985. *Suicide and Life Threatening Behavior, 20,* 156-163.

Stallones, L., & Cook, M. (1992). Suicide rated in Colorado from 1980 to 1989: Metropolitan, nonmetropolitan, and farm comparisons. *Journal of Rural Health, 8,* 139-142.

Stratton, T., Gibbens, B., Dunkin, J., & Juhl, N. (1993). How states respond to the rural nursing shortage. *Nursing & Health Care, 14,* 238-243.

Stratton, T., Juhl, N., & Dunkin, J. (1992). Recruitment and retention of registered nurses in rural hospitals and skilled nursing facilities: A comparison of strategies and barriers. *Nursing Administration Quarterly, 16*(4), 49-56.

Stratton, T., Ludtke, R., Juhl, N., Dunkin, J., & Geller, J. (1993). *A demographic analysis of nurse shortage counties: Implications for rural nursing policy.* Grand Forks, ND: University of North Dakota Rural Health Research Center.

Straub, L., & Walzer, N. (Eds.). (1992). *Rural health care: Innovation in a changing environment.* Westport, CT: Praeger.

Summer, L. (1991). *Limited access: Health care for the rural poor.* Washington, DC: Center on Budget and Policy Priorities.

Thorson, J., & Powell, F. (1992). Rural and urban elderly construe health differently. *Journal of Psychology, 126*(2), 251-260.

U.S. Department of Health and Human Services. (1995). *Community-based health care: Nursing strategies* (NINR Pub. No. 95-3917). Bethesda, MD: Author.

Wagenfield, M., Murray, D., Mohatt, D., & DeBruyn, J. (1994). *Mental health and rural America: 1980-1993* (NIH Pub. No. 94-3500). Washington, DC: U.S. Government Printing Office.

Weinert, C., & Boik, R. (1995). MSU Rurality Index: Development and evaluation. *Research in Nursing and Health, 18,* 453-464.

Weinert, C., & Burman, M. (1994). Rural health and health-seeking behaviors. *Annual Review of Nursing Research, 12,* 65-92.

Weinert, C., & Burman, M. (1996). Nursing of rural elders: Myth and reality. *Advances in Gerontological Nursing, 1,* 57-80.

Weinert, C., & Long, K. (1987). Understanding the health care needs of rural families. *Journal of Family Relations, 36,* 450-455.

Weinert, C., & Long, K. (1990). Rural families and health care: Refining the knowledge base. *Marriage and Family Review, 15,* 57-75.

Weinert, C., & Long, K. (1991). The theory and research base for rural nursing practice. In A. Bushy (Ed.), *Rural health nursing* (Vol. 1, pp. 21-38). Newbury Park, CA: Sage.

Weinert, C., & Long, K. (1993). Support systems for the spouses of chronically ill persons in rural areas. *Family and Community Health, 15,* 46-54.

Whetstone, W., & Reid, J. (1991). Health promotion of older adults: Perceived barriers. *Journal of Advanced Nursing, 16,* 1343-1349.

Winstead-Fry, P., Tiffany, J., & Shippee-Rice, R. (Eds.). (1992). *Rural health nursing.* New York: National League for Nursing Press.

Wright, K. (1993). Management of agricultural injuries and illnesses. *Nursing Clinics of North America, 28,* 253-266.

RESEARCH WITH IMMIGRANTS AND REFUGEES

Juliene G. Lipson
Afaf I. Meleis

Overview

This chapter reviews the nursing research literature on immigrant and refugee health that has implications for clinical practice. We focus on people who were born in another country and came to the United States, and on their children and grandchildren, rather than on second- or third-generation immigrants, who would be more appropriately placed in a chapter on diverse ethnic groups (e.g., Tripp-Reimer's 1983 field study of the use of health care among 328 urban Greek immigrants in Ohio who, despite long-standing residence in the United States, retained such ethnomedical beliefs and practices as *mati-asma,* or the evil eye, over four generations).

The first section describes types of immigrants, migration and health, transitions, and health. Six sources of vulnerability in immigrants and refugees provide a context for the next section, on nursing research, which is organized in terms of the following categories: earlier literature reviews, transitions and health, culture and health, barriers to care, nursing interventions, and research methods. For the most part, we include only published studies, mainly those dealing with immigrants and refugees to the United States.

Theoretical Orientation and Definitions

Types of Immigrants

The literature conceptually blurs "immigration" (movement of persons from one country to another with intention of permanent residence) and "migration" (movement within the same country), often using the

87

terms interchangeably. The U.S. Immigration and Naturalization Service defines an immigrant as a nonresident alien admitted for permanent residence. Several categories have been applied to immigrants in the United States:

Citizens by naturalization after 5 years as legal permanent residents.

Legal permanent residents possess "green cards": They are entitled to work and to most public benefits, but they cannot vote and must follow specific travel guidelines outside the United States. Pending legislation is likely to change their privileges.

Conditional residents married to U.S. citizens less than 2 years.

Permanent residents who applied through the 1986 *Legalization [amnesty] Program* if they were in the United States without legal status since 1982.

Spouses and children of immigrants in the legalization program (*Family Unity Program*).

Permanent residents who applied through the *Diversity Program (lottery)* from specified countries.

Asylees and refugees who have a well-founded fear of persecution based on race, religion, nationality, social group, or political opinion in their homelands. (Refugees applied for protection prior to coming to the United States; asylees applied for refugee status once in the United States).

Undocumented immigrants (a term we prefer to the more pejorative "illegal aliens") who are in the United States without papers demonstrating legal admittance for permanent residence; they include people with expired visitor's visas or false documents and those who have been smuggled into or came into the country secretly.

The history of immigration to the United States is beyond the scope of this chapter, but it is important to note that each major wave of immigration has been followed by a surge of xenophobia and/or racism. The first quotas by country were enacted in 1921, with 55% of all admissions restricted to northern and western Europe. National origin quotas were abolished in 1965. In 1948, Congress enacted the Displaced Persons Act, the first law to admit people fleeing from persecution. New immigration legislation is being enacted currently. However, national politics and global "hot spots" strongly influence the numbers and priority level of those admitted to the United States and the privileges of those already here. Persons of highest priority are those in immediate danger of loss of life or those who are political prisoners

referred to the United Nations High Commissioner on Refugees (UNHCR) or a U.S. Embassy, followed by immediate relatives of persons lawfully admitted as permanent resident aliens, refugees, or asylees. In FY 1997, people of special concern were from Bosnia, Burma, Cuba, Iran, Laos, the former Soviet Union, and Vietnam (U.S. Committee for Refugees, 1996).

▬ *Migration and Health*

Migration is a stressful experience requiring accommodation, adaptation, or coping (Coelho & Ahmed, 1980). Stress is an intervening variable that can appreciably increase the risk of adverse health outcomes (Cassell, 1974) such as hypertension, cancer, and heart disease (Hull, 1979; McKinlay, 1975). Recent data shows that, overall, foreign-born persons in the United States are healthier than the U.S.-born population. In virtually every measure of health status and sociodemographic variable, the most recent immigrants are healthier than those who have lived in the United States for 10 years or longer, and the latter group is healthier than the U.S.-born population. That this advantage decreases with increased time in the United States suggests either that immigrants had or acquired physical conditions or behaviors that put them at risk in the host country or that their access to health care has been limited (Stephens, Foote, Hendershot, & Schoenborn, 1994).

Recently, migration researchers have argued against single cause-and-effect relationships in health status in favor of addressing "a more detailed description of the dynamics of adaptation which so many public health studies of migration have been avoiding" (Kasl & Berkman, 1983, p. 86). However, there is no single comprehensive theoretical framework of migration and health; the literature is scattered and characterized by diverse theoretical frameworks, such as psychoanalytic, epidemiological, or sociocultural approaches. The complexity of this relationship requires a multifactoral model. Ethnographic or longitudinal studies that address many variables in social and historical context can depict this complexity, but cultural specificity may interfere with a comprehensive theoretical framework.

Theories of acculturative stress are useful in characterizing the situation of immigrants and refugees once they arrive in the host country. Williams and Berry (1991) describe the source of acculturative stressors as the process of acculturation, which often results in a particular set of stress behaviors that include anxiety, depression, feelings of marginality and alienation, heightened psychosomatic symptoms, and identity confusion. Acculturative stress may reduce physical, psychological, and social health. This model acknowledges that although mental problems often arise during acculturation, they are not inevitable; rather, acculturation can enhance one's life chances and mental health or virtually destroy one's ability to carry on.

Most studies of refugee and immigrant health focus on psychiatric issues, such as post-traumatic stress disorder (PTSD) and depression, with Southeast Asians having been studied most frequently. Much of the research focuses on the pathogenic influence of migration, often using the Cornell Medical Index, Social Readjustment Rating Scale, Hopkins Symptom Checklist (the SCL-90), Zung Depression Scale, and Vietnamese Depression Scale as tools to measure psychological adaptation.

Marjorie Muecke's (1992a) thought-provoking essay criticizes the two major paradigms underlying the literature. The first views refugees as a poverty-stricken and political class of excess people (rather than individuals), and the second objectifies refugees as a medical phenomenon. This paradigm underlies the study of contagious or "rare" tropical diseases based on a concern about protecting citizens or on the observation of frequently intractable medical problems, and this literature has "reduced the persona of refugees to physical bodies in need of repair" (p. 520). Muecke suggests two alternative paradigms, based on critical and feminist thought, that argue against essentialist and positivist biomedical interpretation. She encourages viewing refugees as being resilient, instead of focusing on refugee health or healthy refugees. She states that refugees provide a vivid example of the "human capacity to survive despite the greatest of losses and assaults on human identity and dignity" (p. 520).

Transitions and Health

Immigrants' experiences with health and illness reflect their process of resettlement in the host country. Thus, transition theory could be essential in describing, explaining, and understanding an immigrant's experience (Meleis, 1991, 1995). Transitions are periods in which change is perceived by a person or by others in the environment to be occurring in that person or the environment (Chick & Meleis, 1986). During periods of transition there are losses of support networks, possessions, and meaningful attachments; there is a sense of disequilibrium and uncertainty about the future (Schumacher & Meleis, 1994).

Immigrants must deal with endings that precede their immigration and beginnings—a new society, new values, new norms, and new sets of expectations. Most of the time, home- and host-country expectations are simultaneous, and they often conflict. Transitions also create identity issues, and emerging identities require a process. This state of being uprooted makes immigrants more vulnerable, particularly in societies that do not provide facilitators to help people establish new roots. Transitions are also characterized by periods of grief and mourning or euphoria, which are significant to understanding responses at different stages of the transition process.

Responses to health and illness may also be triggered or mediated by the frequency of transitions or by the degree to which issues with previous transitions are resolved or unresolved. Further, the transition experience and responses to it are influenced by whether the transition is by choice, by force, preplanned, or sudden. Therefore, because of war or disaster, refugees may react to immigration in a substantially different manner than do immigrants who chose their new country in search of a better life.

Transition theory reveals the experiences of immigrants and explains their responses, which may help identify stages, critical periods of vulnerability, and critical points for intervention. Transition can also be considered an organizing framework for the mission of nursing, a discipline concerned with "the process and the experiences of human beings undergoing transitions where health and perceived well-being is the outcome" (Meleis & Trangenstein, 1994, p. 257). The advantage of this framework is that it emphasizes multidimensional and longitudinal processes that can be applied cross-culturally across the lifespan.

Vulnerability: Definition and Sources

Vulnerable populations are exposed to risks or damage and experience, or demonstrate a sense of being unprotected from such risks or damage. Vulnerability incorporates both personal and environmental phenomena. Therefore, vulnerable individuals are also those who confront cultural, interpersonal, or economic conditions posing threats that may compromise them physically or mentally (Stevens, Hall, & Meleis, 1992).

Immigrants and refugees share stressors with other groups who are in transition, as well as with those who are poor and/or the target of social and/or political bias. They differ from these other groups in that they rarely share a single situation or social status; that is, they vary widely in culture or nationality, age, gender, health and hardiness, and socioeconomic status. For example, age is a variable. Many mainstream elderly are socially isolated, and a language barrier may magnify this source of vulnerability. Immigrants and refugees often suffer from downward socioeconomic mobility, or their education may be limited or not prepare them for work in the United States. Discussed below are five categories of factors that contribute to vulnerability and are especially pertinent to immigrants and refugees: the immigration process and experience, host country factors, cultural and occupational transition, acculturation and ethnic identity, and factors in the health care system.

Immigration Process and Experiences

Refugee research usually separates the processes of flight and settlement (Kunz, 1973). Although fewer authors focus on the antecedents than on the consequences of migration, it is theoretically important to differentiate immigrants and refugees because the "combination of circumstances of motivation—movements without destinations, lack of control of destinations, and fear of political persecution—is cumulative and interactive, producing . . . uniformities of refugee behavior that cannot be compared with those of immigrants" (Liu & Cheung, 1985, p. 491). Stein (1986) argues for a common refugee experience that produces particular refugee behavior and argues against treating specific refugee situations as being unique, atypical, or individual historical events. He cites Kunz's (1973) kinetic model of migration, which characterizes immigrants as being "pulled" to their new destinations, attracted by opportunities and a new life. Refugees, on the other hand, are "pushed" out; given a choice, they would not have left.

Time influences vulnerability. Stein (1986) outlines four major phases of adjustment that take about 10 years in all. Sluzki's (1979) classic article outlines stages of the migration process: (a) preparatory stage, (b) the act of migration, (c) period of overcompensation, (d) period of decompensation, and (e) transgenerational phenomena. Of particular import to nurses is his description of family clashes between generations and their preventive and therapeutic implications.

Host Country Factors: Bias, Jobs and Politics

Williams and Berry (1991) cite the nature of the larger society, acceptance of the particular group, and

tolerance as factors affecting acculturative stress. The current backlash against immigrants, exploited by too many politicians in the past few years, tends to portray newcomers as a drag on the economy. In a climate of recession and high unemployment, new arrivals are seen as competing for scarce jobs and worsening local and state budget problems by requiring tax-supported services. Contrary to popular perceptions, however, in San Francisco, the proportion of legal immigrants receiving public assistance at the time of the 1990 Census was only 1.7% above all households (Ness & Nakao, 1997). A 1994 California State Senate study found that the foreign born who arrived between 1980 and 1990 were not much more likely than the average Californian to be on public assistance (4.8% vs. 4.1%), even though their median household income is much lower ($22,300 vs. $34,900). Because recent immigrants are younger, fewer of them draw social security benefits than do long-term Californians. Moreover, they mainly vie with other immigrants for jobs that entail tough work for low pay.

Occupational and financial difficulties are rampant among newer immigrant and refugee populations. In general, refugees who were professionals in their own countries rarely regain their former social status. For example, physicians may be unable to pass the licensing examination because of limited financial resources, English problems, or outdated training. Some families, on the other hand, improve their economic situation in the United States because everyone in the family works hard at two or more jobs.

Ethnic Identity and Acculturation

A variety of group and individual characteristics influence the acculturative transition, including mode of acculturation (marginalized, integrated, or assimilating); phase of acculturation; socioeconomic status; social support; the existence of an ethnic community; age; and individual appraisal of the acculturating situation, coping, attitudes, and contact (Williams & Berry, 1991). For example, age and educational level influence language acquisition, one of the most significant factors for acculturation and integration into the host society. Families experience intergenerational conflict when children acculturate more quickly than their parents.

Factors in Health Care

The health care system has several barriers that limit access to immigrants and refugees—money or lack of health insurance being a major one. Some refugee populations had access to Medicaid, but, increasingly, fewer physicians accept it, and conversion of Medicaid to HMOs or managed care has effectively blocked access to many immigrants.

Language is another major barrier to access, not only in health provider-client interactions but in finding appropriate services, making appointments, and understanding the need for follow-up. Lack of transportation and child care are barriers that are common to the poor of any background, as are clinic structure and hours, which are often the same as immigrants' and refugees' working hours or require long waits that preclude lunch-hour appointments.

Another barrier is that dominant-culture health providers rarely understand immigrants' and refugees' experiences, explanatory frameworks of illness, or communication patterns. Examples are victims of torture or war who experience PTSD or different ways of describing the body (e.g., telling a health provider that "my heart is squeezed" [Lipson, 1992]). There is a need for research-based elementary education for health providers to help them better understand and care for their immigrant and refugee clients.

Nursing Research on Immigrant and Refugee Health

Previous Literature Reviews

Muecke (1990) complied a bibliography and an overview of the nursing research on refugees (Muecke, 1992b). In 1989, she found 86 research studies by nurses on refugees, none conducted before 1981. Seventy-nine percent were studies of Indochinese; the nursing literature was dispersed, but it focused mainly on maternal-child and public health, and much of the research remained unpublished in master's theses or conference proceedings.

By 1996, the published nursing research showed more topics and different populations, but the situation was similar to what Muecke described in her earlier reviews—the research was mainly clinically generated and qualitative, and studies of refugees outnumbered those on immigrants. The largest refugee groups have been in the United States from 15 to 20 years, so research concerns have shifted from communicable diseases, parasites, and acute medical needs to mental health issues.

Some authors have done more specific literature reviews. Kulig (1990) reviewed the research on Southeast Asian refugee women and found that the majority of studies focused on women's childbearing role, essentially defining women only in terms of their reproductive capacity and emphasizing their related cultural beliefs and the implications for the health care delivery system. Meleis, Lipson, Muecke, and Smith (1998) reviewed the literature on immigrant and refugee women in general. Laurence (1992a, 1992b) reviewed the mental health effects and treatment of victims of torture, a situation experienced by a significant proportion of some refugee populations.

Transitions and Health: The Social Context

A number of nursing studies describe stressful experiences inherent in the immigration transition, a few focus on leaving the homeland, and many involve adjustment issues in the host country following resettlement. Most are qualitative studies, and a few of them also include instruments that measure emotional distress or stress level.

Past losses, trauma. The most compelling theme associated with leaving their homeland for Southeast Asian women was separation from family members through war, escape, death, or abandonment; time had not eased their pain (Fox, Cowell, & Johnson, 1995). The investigators encourage nurses to be aware of the trauma and violence experienced by most refugees during war and escape and the signs of post-traumatic stress disorder and suggest intervention programs that encourage social support networks, family viability, and ethnic community development. Polish immigrants also experienced losses that disrupted their lives (Aroian, 1990), as did Afghan refugees, who also continued to suffer from traumatic escapes or observations of atrocities (Lipson, 1993). Stressors associated with resettlement and integration include work, role changes or conflict, ethnic identity issues, family and parenting issues, and social support. Iranian immigrants (Lipson, 1992) faced occupational and financial difficulties, loss of status, reduced social support, ethnic bias, differences in values, and interpersonal child-rearing styles. Afghan refugees experienced issues with social support, cultural conflict, language and economic problems, and stress associated with family adjustment (Lipson, 1991). Added to traumatic refugee flight sequella, these difficulties were expressed in psychosomatic symptoms and high stress scores on the Health Opinion Survey, a tool that elicits psychosomatic indications of stress.

The immigrant transition for women immigrants and refugees has been the topic of several studies that focus on family roles and work. In addition to dead-end, low-status, and low-prestige occupations such as domestic work, hotel maid, grocery store attendant, or fast-food clerk, immigrant women often work triple shifts in their daily lives (Lipson & Miller, 1994). For economic reasons, many take two jobs and, in addition, are homemakers and care for other relatives. In this regard, there has been little examination of workplace conditions in jobs held predominantly by women.

Demographic changes based on immigration and increased women's career opportunities in immigrant populations have created increasingly heterogeneous populations in U.S. nursing schools, particularly in urban areas. Johnston's (1989) study of a New York baccalaureate school of nursing with an extremely ethnically and linguistically diverse student population found that language was the major variable predictive of success on the NCLEX-RN, a stronger effect than grades or standardized test scores.

During transitions, immigrant women have numerous unrecognized roles, such as maintaining ethnic continuity and being culture brokers. Their families typically expect them to maintain their culture of origin, help family members maintain it, and, at the same time, help family members integrate into the educational and social systems of society. Major stressors for Jordanian new immigrant women (Hattar-Pollara & Meleis, 1995b) were finding jobs and schools for children, loss of social status, and inadequate English, which caused loneliness and social isolation. Those who had been in the United States longer attempted to maintain their ethnic identity in an environment with a different value system and were stressed by feeling like foreigners and the challenge of adjusting to the rapid pace of U.S. life and other differences in U.S. society.

Parenting adolescents is a major issue for immigrants. Jordanian mothers (Hattar-Pollara & Meleis, 1995a) needed to modify their traditional parenting approaches to avoid a bad reputation and loss of honor. The mothers reported such emotional difficulties as worry, despair, guilt, confusion, and fear of loss of respect in juggling to maintain a balance between two cultures. Their vigilance showed their lack of trust in their adolescents and in American society. Some were concerned about too-restrictive discipline; others advocated for their adolescents, mediating between them and their fathers.

Kulig (1994) used the case of "Theary, a Cambodian woman," to illustrate differences in perceptions of events according to cultural understandings. She described the consequences of community shunning based on Theary's having divorced abusive and neglectful husbands and having given birth to many children, which led the community to perceive her as being promiscuous. Kulig makes recommendations for community health nurses working with refugee women.

Elderly Afghan refugees also experience difficulties related to isolation. Omidian and Lipson (1992) highlighted the situation of elderly Afghan refugees in California, who speak little or no English and experience culture conflict and family role changes much more acutely than do younger family members. Acculturating grandchildren may be unable to speak their parents' language adequately, and that acculturation may result in their not being accorded sufficient respect. Elderly women, in particular, are often alone all day, unable to take public transportation and afraid of getting lost, while family members are off at work or at school.

Few nursing studies view the transition experience from a longitudinal perspective, but some cross-sectional studies use time in the United States as a variable to examine its influence on other variables. Meleis, Lipson, and Paul (1992) used several measures of health and ethnic identity in interviews with Egyptians, Yemenis, Iranians, Armenians, and Arabs to show that the five groups illustrated significant differences in ethnic identity and health variables. Longer time in the United States was related both to weaker home country identity and total symptoms.

Lynam (1985) found that women who had immigrated to Canada from nine different countries experienced isolation based on a lack of a mutual basis of understanding or shared needs with others. Women's sources of support included kin, "insiders" (from religious or ethnic community), and "outsiders" (agencies, service providers). Although they used different strategies to obtain support in each area, over time, they moved through kin and insiders and finally to outsiders. However, few women made much use of outside resources because of unfamiliarity with availability or appropriateness, which suggests that health providers should examine how women access resources to understand their integration process and how to help them link with appropriate resources.

Family Planning, Pregnancy, and Childbearing

An early study by Dempsey and Gesse (1983) with Haitian refugees highlighted the importance of research on childbearing beliefs and practices, noting that in Miami's county hospital, approximately one in five deliveries in 1980 was to a Haitian woman. This study used an assessment tool to develop a cultural profile of the refugee Haitian childbearing client to derive culturally appropriate nursing goals and interventions. They found that participants perceived pregnancy in ways similar to their American counterparts, but their responses also emphasized the need for accurate culture-specific assessment of each client to provide appropriate health care.

Judith Kulig's (1995) ethnographic studies of Cambodian refugees in Canada and the United States focused on the relationship between resettlement and Cambodian women's role and status changes and their childbearing interests and use of family planning. With regard to their views of sexuality, Kulig (1995) noted that pregnancy is accepted as inevitable and that Cambodian women receive very little information before marriage (except being told not to run away) in the belief that less knowledge will prevent behavior that will lead to premarital pregnancy. In addition, family honor is linked to a daughter's chaste behavior. The refugee camp experience had an impact on women's behavior, and camps spawned rumors about deleterious side effects associated with family planning methods. These beliefs have implications for teaching about family planning in a population that shows resistance to sexuality information.

A study of the health needs of pregnant women waiting in a Buffalo, New York shelter for asylum processing to Canada (Kahler, Sobata, Hines, & Griswold, 1996) found an unexpectedly low rate of hepatitis B and expected low immunization rates for tetanus and measles. Two thirds of the sample were from Somalia, a new group of refugees to North America, and all had experienced female genital mutilation, which prevented three from undergoing a pelvic examination. The majority of women had experienced violence, and three were pregnant as a result of rape in transit.

Korean immigrant women's beliefs, practices, and experiences of childbirth are influenced by their holistic view of health, which is attributed to regular lifestyle, nourishment, good environment, sound thinking, lack of stress and good stress management, family harmony, and faith in God (Park & Peterson, 1991). Most women used prenatal care, took vitamins, and ate well, but very few used such preventive practices as Pap smear or breast self-examination. Specific postpartum practices included rest, eating brown seaweed soup, and avoiding cold water or food.

Child and Adolescent Health

The earliest and most sustained clinical work with Southeast Asian refugees, out of which has come several studies, was done in San Diego, California, by Sheila Pickwell. She examined 400 elementary-school-aged Vietnamese, Laotian, Hmong, and Cambodian refugee children between 1977 and 1981 (Pickwell, 1982) and found that these recent arrivals had inadequate immunizations, dental disease, head lice or scabies, chronic otitus media, musculoskeletal problems, and intestinal parasites. She suggests learning as much as possible about the refugee experiences and cultures of these groups and using translators appropriately. This early research focus on physical health conditions has evolved into an emphasis on adjustment and mental health issues.

Comparative studies of two immigrant groups are both valuable and relatively rare. Thomas and DeSantis (1995) compared Cuban and Haitian immigrant woman on their concepts of child health and illness and of child-rearing beliefs and practices. With regard to infant feeding, although both groups believed that breast was better than bottle, 40% of the Haitian mothers expressed the fear that breast milk causes intestinal parasites or transmits mother's sickness to the infant. Despite their positive attitudes toward breast feeding, however, only about half of each group breast-fed their infants. Cuban mothers weaned their babies from the breast much earlier than Haitian mothers, but much later from the bottle. The authors emphasize that health providers' knowledge of cultural beliefs is very important, but, at least for Haitian mothers, the strength of socioeconomic and political stresses in the Haitian ethnic community (e.g., parenting alone, work, financial obligations, lack of education and marketable skills) may outweigh cultural factors.

In a second article on child-rearing beliefs, DeSantis and Thomas (1994) note that health care providers' failure to recognize the influence of culture on child development may lead to inappropriate expectations and mislabeling of children as developmentally slow. Both Cuban and Haitian children would be considered lagging developmentally when compared with measurements on the personal-social dimension of the Denver Development Test and expectations of American society. The authors suggest culture-specific implications for transcultural nursing care based on the concept of culture brokerage.

Health providers should learn how their immigrant and refugee clients seek health care for their children. Middle Eastern immigrant parents, for example, use a variety of resources when seeking help for children's health, including family in the Middle East. May (1992) examined the social networks of 73 immigrant parents from Egypt, Palestine, and Yemen and learned that these parents' perceptions of social support were lower than in the normative American sample. Percentage of network members living near the parent increased with years in the United States, and percentage of network members outside the United States correlated with less time in the United States.

Cambodian adolescents in America are at high risk for physical, psychosomatic, and drug-related problems (Frye & McGill, 1993). Communicating with the Cambodian community about and with teens is a challenge because of fundamental differences in American and Cambodian perceptions about parental roles and causation and treatment of illness. Frye and McGill suggest culturally congruent intervention strategies based on the dominant Cambodian cultural theme of equilibrium in treatment of illness, management of stress, and patterns of parenting.

In another study of Cambodian adolescents, Muecke and Sassi (1992) compared anxiety symptoms among teens in a Thailand refugee transit camp and high school students permanently resettled in Washington State. The U.S. teens showed higher levels of anxiety, which these authors attribute in part to the unusually optimistic perspective of adolescents in temporary asylum who were preparing for imminent resettlement to the United States. The U.S. group was confronting an often poor match between old habits and the demands of the new environment. This diachronic approach is one of few nursing studies that address the transition process at different points in health education and interventions—we need knowledge of women's beliefs and practices. Kulig's (1988) ethnographic study of Cambodian women and a traditional healer in a western Canadian city focused on beliefs and practices related to menstruation (e.g., the importance of blood flowing freely), conception (e.g., need for a cool body for conception and women having a predestined number of children), and herbal medicine use for menstruation and to prevent or facilitate pregnancy.

Lipson, Hosseini, Kabir, Omidian, and Edmonston's (1995) Afghan refugee community health assessment described cultural and immigration influences on women's access to health care, approach toward preventive care, control of information regarding sexuality, and the sensitive topic of spousal abuse. Despite a strong cultural emphasis on modesty, 60% of the sample had had a recent clinical breast examination. Although 60% of the women rarely or never examine their own breasts, 13% do it monthly. However, Afghan women know very little about their bodies and how they work. Older and more traditional women typically have little formal education, and very few women talk about this topic because "menstruation and other topics about women's bodies are 'haram' [sinful], especially among rural women" (p. 284). Of particular concern is some Afghan parents' refusal to allow their daughters to take sex education in American high schools. Lack of knowledge puts adolescents and young women at increased risk for pregnancy and sexually transmitted diseases.

▬ General Cultural Perceptions of Health or Illness

The greatest number of nursing studies describes health beliefs and folk medicine, using exploratory approaches, and several researchers based solid clinical articles on these studies. Folk medicine practices among Hmong refugees were explored through informal interviewing over 15 months with four Hmong participants and an American anthropology student fluent in the Hmong language. Cheon-Klessig, Camilleri, McElmurry, and Ohlson (1988) describe the use of traditional herbal medicine and Hmong shamans, as well as problems associated with use of the American health care system and, in particular, the unacceptability of surgery and blood tests.

Boyle's (1989, 1991) ethnographic study of health-promoting beliefs and practices of Salvadoran refugees found that well-being was enhanced by complex constellations of family, supportive friends, religious affiliations, and work opportunities. Informants emphasized the importance of fresh air, sleep, and good nutritional practices for health promotion.

The concept of health was explored with a group of older Hispanic immigrants from several Latin American countries who had been in the United States an average of 13 years. Ailinger and Causey (1995) elicited definitions of health, characteristics of a healthy person, contributions to health, and health maintenance activities. The concept of health included six major themes: an integration of physical, emotional, and spiritual aspects; mental health; feeling well; enjoying independence; using self-care; and family orientation.

Luna (1994) interviewed key informants among Lebanese Muslim immigrants in a Midwest city, most of whom had lived in the United States less than 10 years. Their meanings and experiences of care were influenced by worldview, social structure, and cultural context in the hospital, clinic, and home. She found similar themes of care in the three contexts, which reflected care as a religious obligation in Islam, care as equal-but-different gender role responsibilities, and care as individual and collective meanings of honor. She used Leininger's (1988) Theory of Cultural Care Diversity and Universality as the conceptual framework to frame nursing decisions and actions to achieve culturally congruent nursing care.

Chronic Health Conditions

Palinkas and Pickwell (1995) use four case studies of Cambodian refugees in San Diego to illustrate problems with the concept of acculturation as it is currently used in epidemiology as a risk factor for chronic disease. To make the concept theoretically and clinically meaningful, they suggest that (a) the perspectives of acculturation-as-process and acculturation-as-structure should be integrated; (b) acculturation should be viewed as both individual and group experiences of conflict and negotiation between two belief or behavior systems; (c) it should be measured longitudinally and as narrative; and (d) rather than being viewed as simply a health risk, acculturation can promote health by increasing access to care, adopting healthier behaviors, and decreasing risky ones.

There have been few nursing studies of HIV/AIDS among immigrants. Gallagher (1992) used a case study to explore the complexities of the immigration process as it relates to HIV infection. She suggests that understanding the immigration process will help nurses identify and refer illegal residents who are HIV infected to appropriate social-service agencies, thereby providing more comprehensive care to patients and their families.

Neves-Arruda, Larson, and Meleis (1992) interviewed 10 Hispanic immigrant cancer patients undergoing treatment to elicit the meaning of comfort. Characteristics of comfort included feeling normal, functioning and feeling integrated, feeling safe, feeling nurtured, feeling in control, and *comodo,* with particular emphasis on integration, meaning a sense of inner peace. Comfort needs included nurturing, familiar environment, safety, quality of life, normalcy, and *animo.* The investigators found that providers of comfort included self, family, health care providers, and God. This study underscores the importance of comfort to cancer patients, shows how it is influenced by culture, and suggests that nurses should take this influence into account in care.

Chinese immigrant women to Canada with diabetes were interviewed by Anderson (1991) to examine the existential experience of chronic illness. Thirteen spoke only Cantonese, and the majority had lived with diabetes for over nine years. A case history illustrated what it is like for non-English-speaking women to live with a chronic disease in which the diagnosis means drastic changes in lifestyle and definition of self. All the women experienced feelings of being devalued, which were heightened by the migration experience and the concomitant experiences of marginality in a foreign culture. Anderson urges nurses to consider the contextual conditions of distress rather than focusing on such microfactors as the disease itself or compliance with treatment.

In a follow-up study based on interviews of 196 Euro-Canadian and Chinese-Canadian women living with diabetes, Anderson, Blue, Holbrook, and Ng (1993) explored how the participants experience and manage their illness in their day-to-day lives and what factors influence daily management (diet, exercise, medication, and blood testing). Using a feminist perspective to interpret the data, they described Chinese women as having less education and more blue-collar jobs and as fearing job loss if they told their coworkers and employers about their diabetes. In other words, their life circumstances prevented some from properly managing their illness. Difficulty with access to health facilities and inadequate communication and resources from health professionals to help them understand their diabetes added to the burden of living with a chronic illness. Anderson, Blue, et al. point out that the social context of a patient's illness is not always recognized by health professionals.

In the same study, Anderson, Wiggins, et al. (1995) hypothesized that women's patterns of diabetes management would be associated with ethnicity and/or fluency in English, and they also examined the extent of desired professional care, awareness of biomedical knowledge, and satisfaction with family and friends' support. They found that diabetes management is complex and that the way in which women manage their illness is not reducible to their ethnicity but rather depends on their life context and access to resources. They state that management of diabetes must be understood within the mediating circumstances of a woman's life.

Arab-American patients (N = 102) with chronic conditions were interviewed in San Francisco to describe their illness and help-seeking behavior (Reizian & Meleis, 1987). As part of the interview, they were read an Arabic version of the Cornell Medical Index (CMI); only six participants chose to be interviewed in English. The participants reported the highest number of symptoms in the digestive and cardiovascular systems. Participants also reported many symptoms relating to level of sensitivity and a sense of inadequacy. When the CMI results were compared to other populations, symptom frequency and patterns were most similar to those in Vietnamese refugees. Of these 102 Arab immigrants, 46% complained of pain, located mainly in the chest, stomach, shoulder, or back. Reizian and Meleis (1986) characterize their responses to pain as constellations including other symptoms. These patients described even localized pain as related to the entire body, life, functioning, and activities of work and daily living. Arab Americans use analogies and metaphors in describing pain, such as likening burning pain to flame or fire. Nurses need to learn about cultural patterns of pain and symptom expression to better care for their patients.

Mental Health

Flaskerud and Anh's (1988) study of the mental health needs of Vietnamese refugees included a medical record review of 81 patients of two Los Angeles County mental health centers. Compared with other patients, Vietnamese had more frequent diagnoses of depression and adjustment disorder than other patients and averaged 3.74 somatic and 3.73 psychological complaints per person. Interviews of such key informants as clinical providers and clergy knowledgeable about Vietnamese in their agencies identified the most frequent problems as depression, schizophrenia and other psychotic disorders, family problems, somatization, nightmares, and PTSD. Based on these findings, the authors suggest that Vietnamese clients need help in adjustment, mental health education, and problems in living.

Mental health problems have frequently been identified among Cambodian refugees. A study of family management of culturally defined illness among 120 Cambodian informants in California and Massachusetts identified *koucharang* (a culture-bound syndrome defined as thinking too much) in response to violence experienced in Cambodia (Frye & D'Avanzo, 1994). Characterized by flashbacks and nightmares resurrecting terrifying memories, "thinking too much" causes headaches, chest pain, palpitations, or shortness of breath. More participants in California attributed this syndrome to haunting memories of the Khmer Rouge regime, but more Massachusetts participants attributed it to financial difficulties (this cohort was poorer and had more dependent children). Families managed this illness through withdrawal and sheltering. Withdrawal means suppressing sad thoughts or even thinking about suicide, but some used alcohol to numb themselves. Sheltering the afflicted family member was done by encouragement, talking to him or her "softly or sweetly," or making the person laugh.

Similar patterns of PTSD and depression are seen in other refugee populations from the most violent political regimes. Based on ethnographic research, including interviews of 90 Afghans and their health providers in California, Lipson (1993) described traumatic experiences before leaving Afghanistan (imprisonment of self or family members, observing atrocities, loss of family members) or during transit (being robbed, refugee camp hardships, seclusion of women). Continuing stressors include current events in Afghanistan, survivor guilt, culture conflict, and adjustment problems. Mental health professionals should elicit their refugee clients' immigration history, circumstances of flight and first asylum, and who and what was lost to put symptoms of depression, anxiety, and PTSD into context.

The social context of symptoms, however, is broader than immigration history and current life circumstances. Lipson and Omidian (1996) describe the transnational context of mental health issues, noting that ongoing events in Afghanistan strongly affect Afghans in California. The atrocities they physically left behind are mentally compounded by the news they hear, such as information about the continuing violence or the death of a family member. Afghans cope with the effects of news by aggressively seeking it out, by avoiding it or protecting vulnerable family members, or by taking such actions as sending money to relatives in Afghanistan or engaging in political activism in the United States.

Based on one of few cross-sectional studies using a large sample (N = 2,180), Chung and Kagawa-Singer (1993) examined data from the California Southeast Asian Mental Health Needs Assessment Study to determine whether premigration experiences affect psychological distress (depression and anxiety) over the long term and whether there are group differences in predictors of psychological distress among Vietnamese, Cambodians, and Lao. They found that even after 5 years, premigration stressors (transit events, years in refugee camps, number of family deaths) were still strong predictors of depression and anxiety, but postmigration stressors also predicted distress. They found group differences in postmigration predictors, such as low family income in Vietnamese, smaller family size in Cambodians, and receiving public assistance in Lao samples.

In another cross-sectional study using instruments, Franks and Faux (1990) interviewed 212 Chinese, Vietnamese, Portugese, and Latin American immigrant woman in a Canadian city. They examined levels of depression and relationships between depression, selected demographics, stress, mastery, and social support. They found a strong association between depression and resettlement and between mental illness and the refugee experience, particularly among those who were exposed to persecution and endured many years of camp life.

❖ Structural Barriers

Language is a major barrier to health care access. Many health care agencies rely on family members or miscellaneous staff for interpretation, which is usually ineffective and can result in gross misinterpretation. Even with trained staff interpreters, short appointment times inhibit provider/client understanding. Hatton and Webb's (1993) study of interpreters in a county health department revealed three styles of interpretation among nurses, interpreters, and clients. The "interpreter as voice box" attempted word-for-word translations of both clients' and providers' messages to "eliminate biases," but interpreters found it difficult to disregard their own sense of how to handle the situation. With "interpreter as excluder," the interpreter literally "took over," and nurses felt left out of the interaction. Both nurses and interpreters preferred "interpreter as collaborator," in which nurses and interpreters were colleagues; control changed hands depending on the topic, and the interpreter was able to serve as culture broker.

Inadequate health agency financial and personnel resources pose structural barriers for immigrant and refugee clients, particularly those who use the public health care system and have no health insurance or means to pay for health care. Immigrants' impact on the health care system was examined by DeSantis and Halberstein (1992), who interviewed 20 administrators and staff in South Florida agencies serving large immigrant populations and 201 immigrant clients served by these facilities. They also reviewed public documents relating to population trends, immigration policies, and health planning studies. Health agency personnel cited language and

communication barriers as reasons for patient dissatisfaction and decreased compliance. They noted insufficient funding, nursing and staff shortages, rapid personnel turnover, lack of space, unorganized referral systems, and insurance and immunization irregularities. Patients complained of long waiting periods and crowded conditions, organizational "red tape," negative staff attitudes, language, and transportation problems. Recommendations include hiring translators and working with traditional healers; increasing maternal-child and prenatal care services; providing nutritional, mental health, and preventive services for patients; and increasing health care protective services and staff education for staff.

Undocumented immigrants, the subject of recent negative public opinion, face additional structural barriers. Aroian's (1993) interviews with illegal Irish immigrants in Boston revealed difficulties and distress associated with being undocumented, although some did not have such experiences. The difficulties included finding satisfactory work, being exploited by employers, feelings of uncertainty about the future, restrictions on freedom of movement (e.g., to return to Ireland to visit family), and feelings of vulnerability and fear of being caught and deported. A disadvantage of illegal status is that jobs available to undocumented immigrants do not typically provide such benefits as health insurance.

Immigrant or refugee community assessments reveal the structural barriers faced by people who live in these communities. Laffrey, Meleis, Lipson, Solomon, and Omidian (1989) described an approach to identifying health needs and services for immigrant groups characterized by geographic and cultural diversity, such as Arab immigrants in San Francisco. This approach used four methods: community forums to identify important health issues, key informant interviews, social indicators based on the U.S. Census, and a member survey in three Arab social groups. The combination of methods contributed a more complete picture of Arab community health needs and overcame the weaknesses of each, such as small and convenience samples, anecdotal information from health professionals, and use of indirect data for social indicators.

A community assessment of Northern California Afghans included an exploratory telephone interview, seven community meetings, and a survey of 196 Afghan families through in-person interviews in Dari or Pashto (Lipson, Omidian, & Paul, 1995). This assessment revealed large gaps between identified community health problems and resources. Mental health problems were the most prominent concerns in this community, but few had sought help from the mental health care system because of language and financial barriers and the paucity of licensed Afghan mental health providers. Sixty-five percent had dental problems, and unmet dental needs were significantly related to insurance or financial problems or language barriers. Afghans desired health education on stress, heart health, nutrition, raising adolescents, and aging in the United States by means of TV, videos (many older women are illiterate), and lectures in Dari and Pashto.

A more subtle barrier to culturally competent care is health providers' lack of knowledge about cultural characteristics and typical needs of their immigrant or refugee patient populations. Lipson, Reizian, and Meleis (1987) examined the medical records of 106 patients with Arabic surnames who sought care in emergency, outpatient, and inpatient units of two hospitals. The study sought to examine help-seeking behavior and culturally related care needs, but the results reveal more about the charting habits of health care providers than about their Arab-American patients. An example of misinformation or missing information was country of origin; for example, 16% noted merely Arab or Arabian, and the chart of one woman described her variously as Arabic, Persian, Egyptian, and Hispanic. Notes on problems related to immigration or culture shock, use of folk or home remedies, or communication issues were nearly nonexistent.

Interventions and Nursing Therapeutics

There are very few studies of nursing interventions with immigrants and refugees, but there is a growing body of clinical guidelines (e.g., Lipson & Meleis, 1985). The existing literature mainly describes programs and their development, which will support the next step of testing the effectiveness of these models. The main program types are culturally appropriate health education and health promotion and those that bolster social support in vulnerable groups, focusing on maternal-child and mental health issues.

Madeleine Leininger and her students focus on the meanings of care in some immigrant populations for the purpose of enhancing culturally congruent nursing care. Leininger's (1988) Theory of Cultural Care Diversity and Universality was the basis of Luna's (1994) ethnonursing study of urban Lebanese Muslim immigrants who had been in the United States less than 10 years. The meanings and experiences of care were influenced by worldview, social structure, and cultural context in the hospital, clinic, and home. Care was viewed as a religious obligation in Islam, encompassed equal but different gender role responsibilities, and involved individual and collective meanings of honor.

Maternal-child. Based on her earlier study of maternal-infant health beliefs and infant feeding processes, Rossiter (1992, 1994) developed a language- and culture-specific health education program to promote breast-feeding among Vietnamese in Australia. She used an experimental design to test the effectiveness of the program with 182 Vietnamese pregnant women. Although the program significantly improved knowledge, attitudes, and planned and actual breast-feeding behavior, the effects on subjects were short lived and had diminished by the time the infants were 6 months old.

Mattson and Lew (1992) used the Southern California Southeast Asian Health Project (SEAHP) to evaluate client satisfaction with services and to obtain additional data about women's childbearing health practices. Four community workers fluent in Cambodian or Laotian interviewed recently delivered clients and learned that the majority of women were satisfied with SEAHP's services, particularly the interpretation and education in native languages. The program appears to be meeting the prenatal health care needs of Southeast Asians and ensuring access to and use of health services. Mattson (1995) describes strategies for providing perinatal care to Southeast Asians in the United States and Canada based on their history, current lifestyle, health problems, and traditional healing beliefs and practices pertaining to childbearing.

DeSantis and Thomas (1992) surveyed 30 Haitian mothers in Florida to learn what they thought about the value of health education received while seeking preventive health care for infants and preschool children in community health settings. Nearly all had sought well-child care for their children, and 66% received health education during the visits. The mothers considered nurses best for health teaching but mentioned such blocks to effective health education as providers who do not speak Haitian Creole and long clinic waiting periods. Participants preferred health teaching through radio and clinic lectures, and they wanted teaching to be understandable and practical, to reinforce parenting abilities, and to allow time for questions.

In the *De Madres a Madres* program, a community health nurse trained inner-city Hispanic volunteer mothers to become advocates for healthy pregnancies. The volunteers offered information to women in their own communities in a culturally acceptable language and milieu (Mahon, McFarlane, & Golden, 1991), based on the premise that culturally relevant social support and advocacy, coupled with community resource information, would enable pregnant women to transcend barriers to early prenatal care. Fourteen volunteer mothers from several Hispanic groups completed 8 hours of training on the importance of early prenatal care, resources for pregnant women, how to identify women at risk, and effective listening and social support skills. After the first year, more than 2,000 at-risk women had received information from a volunteer mother.

Mental health. Based on extensive research and clinical work among Southeast Asian refugees, Pickwell (1989) notes that adjustment difficulties are increasingly manifested in psychotic episodes, substance abuse, and other antisocial behaviors. She describes a family nurse practitioner-faculty-student clinical experience designed to provide community and home health services to Southeast Asian refugees with psychiatric diagnoses. Pickwell and colleagues' (Pickwell, 1981, 1982, 1994, 1996; Pickwell, Schimelpfening, & Palinkas, 1994) articles on cultural competence in primary care in Southeast Asian pediatric and other populations are some of the clearest and most useful in the nursing literature.

Cambodians are among the most traumatized of refugees. Because years of somatic therapies, psychotherapy and antidepressants, acupuncture, and traditional healing methods had not helped women with somatic symptoms related to PTSD, Shepard and Faust (1993) developed the Cambodian women's support group in the Refugee Clinic at San Francisco General Hospital. Rather than asking women to share their traumas, which would have been intrusive, the group focused on psychological strengths (they are survivors), helping them get to know each other, and building their concentration so they could begin to enter American society through their own community. Weekly 2-hour groups, facilitated by Shepard and a Cambodian health worker, included English as a Second Language, crafts, and stress-reduction training. Relaxation training used a Khmer language audiotape with guided visualization. The women's severe anxiety, sleep disorders, nightmares, and early waking began to decrease, and many of them began to fall asleep as soon as the tape began. To address the women's unresolved grief, Buddhist monks were hired to do group ceremonies to honor their dead loved ones. Outcomes included a 50% reduction in the number of clinic visits, group members' more positive affect, fewer complaints, and speaking broken English.

A particularly valuable adjunct to treatment of immigrants and refugees is culture brokering (Jezewski,

1993). Budman, Lipson, and Meleis (1992) describe the case of an adolescent Iraqi hospitalized in a California psychiatric unit to illustrate cross-cultural diagnostic and treatment issues. They show how a flexible therapist, teamwork, and intense involvement of an Arabic-speaking cultural consultant led to the adolescent's successful assessment and management. As a culture broker, the consultant participated in family meetings and team conferences and helped staff differentiate between normal cultural characteristics and pathology. As a clinician, she could help educate the parents about psychiatric treatment and psychotropic medications.

General health education. Shadick (1993) described the development and implementation of a transcultural health education program for the Hmong, using a pluralistic model of education that addresses both the implicit and explicit conditions of learning and education. The author suggests that a clinical nurse specialist (CNS) developing such a program must have expert knowledge of the target population's health beliefs, values, and practices as well as knowledge of their language, level of literacy, and traditional teaching-learning styles.

Videotapes are particularly effective for health education in illiterate or low-literacy populations. Clabots and Dolphin (1992) worked with the Multilingual Health Care Coalition in Rhode Island to produce videotapes to circumvent illiteracy in English and/or the mother tongue because the health agencies and a large proportion of each community group owned VCRs. Coalition members selected and prioritized the following topics: introduction to primary care, the hospital, hepatitis B, tuberculosis, sexually transmitted diseases, prenatal care, well-newborn care, discharge instructions for new mothers, and lead poisoning. Coalition and community members provided input into word choice, translatability of particular terms and concepts, and cultural issues. Tapes were narrated in English, Spanish, Portuguese, Cambodian, Hmong, Laotian, and Vietnamese. Following distribution of 378 tapes, recipients were asked to complete an evaluation survey rating the content and quality of the tapes.

Methods

Meleis (1991) suggests that whatever research design is chosen to study immigrants, it must be mediated through being from the cultural group, collaborating with others from that culture, and immersing oneself in that culture. It is also critical to work in cooperation with immigrant and refugee communities to assure that any research is relevant and valid.

Three general resources are pertinent to nursing research with immigrants and refugees. Marin and Marin's (1991) monograph on research issues with Hispanic populations covers such topics as group definition, enhancing research participation, development and adaptation of instruments, translation of instruments, and potential problems in interpreting data. Porter and Villarruel (1993) describe guidelines for designing, conducting, and critiquing research with African American and Hispanic people. Their critical questions include whether the conceptual framework is relevant to the population, whether various groups of a heterogeneous sample are identified, whether instruments are specifically developed for the population, and the race and ethnicity of the research team.

Sawyer et al. (1995) review the literature and outline issues associated with matching researcher with participants as a strategy for developing culturally competent research. They discuss which variables to match (e.g., ethnicity, race, gender, language), when to match, and feasibility issues. Because in some cases matching may be too complex to implement, the authors suggest that researchers reflect on their knowledge of the cultural group, their cultural sensitivity, and how collaboration is used during each phase of the research topic.

Recruitment, Sampling, and Rapport Issues

Lipson and Meleis (1989) use the example of Middle Eastern immigrants to the United States to describe such methodological issues as sampling difficulties in the absence of identifiable ethnic communities, immigrants' mistrust of research and researchers, reciprocity, consent, "non-termination," and culturally appropriate interviewing. They suggest that researchers provide limited health-related services and information to address reciprocity and increase trust through a personal approach, sharing food, and triangulating qualitative and quantitative approaches.

Lynam and Anderson (1986) cover similar issues, but they focus on women. Omidian and Lipson (1996) describe community involvement issues in attempting to launch a health education project in the Afghan refugee community; these issues include balancing funders' expectations with cultural/political community realities, "reciprocity," and mobilizing a community that is politically and ethnically divided.

A rich article by DeSantis (1990) describes ethical, moral, and legal issues in qualitative research with populations at risk, using the example of undocumented Haitian immigrants. Access to subjects is based on trust, and researchers must rely on nonprobability sampling through community gatekeepers and snowball methods; studies should be designed in consultation with the gatekeepers. Interdisciplinary team research and working through interviewers from the community creates trust and eases problems of recruitment, language, and keeping track of mobile Haitians. A major research issue with undocumented immigrants is confidentiality and anonymity, particularly the danger of the Immigration and Naturalization Service subpoenaing research records. DeSantis cautions readers to think about how research results are used, particularly by public officials and powerful but resentful persons from other ethnic groups, to manipulate the entrants or public sentiment about them.

Instrumentation Issues

Tools and instruments developed for European-American samples may be inappropriate for some immigrant and refugee groups. Aroian (1990) criticizes the use of "life change checklists," static outcome measures to rate psychological functioning unrelated to the sources of distress, and viewing migration only as risk. Aroian and Patsdaughter (1989) used triangulation of data in a multiple-method approach to test the validity of cross-cultural use of a standardized instrument to measure psychological distress. With 25 adult Polish immigrants who spoke and read English, they used the Brief Symptom Index (BSI), a paper-and-pencil self-report instrument, in-depth interviews, and micro-macro-level observations. They found that the translated BSI was relatively valid except for the psychoticism, paranoid, and interpersonal sensitivity subscales. Invalidity could be explained through information gathered by other methods. Aroian and Patsdaughter discuss the importance of decentered instrument translation for cross-cultural use as well as the need for multiple-method assessment in both clinical practice with ethnic populations and cross-cultural research.

Chung and Kagawa-Singer's (1995) exploratory study of symptom expression among Vietnamese, Chinese-Vietnamese, Cambodian, and Lao refugees was based on the premise that the manifestation of distress is greatly influenced by cultural background. They examined whether the BSI, developed in a Western population, was sensitive enough to capture culturally framed expressions of distress. Factor analyses found a single robust factor that included items from the depression, anxiety, somatic, and psychosocial dysfunction subscales in a pattern that strongly resembles "neurasthenia" rather than three separate factors as in the original measure. Neurasthenia has been found by other researchers to be an Asian cultural idiom of distress. The authors discuss clinical and research implications of this study.

Community Involvement and Participation

Urrutia-Rojas and Aday (1991) demonstrated the utility of Aday's framework for studying access to medical care in a Hispanic immigrant and refugee community through a description of the study design and findings. This framework is useful for organizing community-assessment data-gathering activities, can easily be used in public health nursing education or practice, and illustrates the potential for practitioner-academic partnerships.

Thompson's (1991) beautiful study of participatory feminist research focused on psychosocial and cultural adjustment among Khmer (Cambodian) women, with a focus on symbolic traditions. In addition to participant observation, life history, and trauma history interviews, the author, a Khmer interpreter, and a community health nurse brought Khmer women together in a support group that met for 3 hours biweekly to talk about their everyday health concerns. After dealing with the women's immediate needs, the group members described their dreams to reconfirm their stories of women's strength and resistance to oppression. Thompson's commitment to dialogic research meant that she and the other two facilitators shared their own dreams and life issues with the Khmer women. She concludes as follows: "In attempting to do feminist participatory research, we also found a form for scholarly work that makes nursing research come alive. It is a form of scholarship in which the living and the practice of feminism come together" (p. 46).

Discussion and Conclusions

Summary

Most of the nursing studies of immigrants and refugees we reviewed are qualitative studies and surveys that combined interviews with instruments and tools. The majority present descriptive data; very few propose or test

nursing interventions. A good approach is Rossiter's (1992, 1994) work, in which her study of Vietnamese women's beliefs about infant feeding led to designing and testing a breast-feeding education program based on the findings. Similarly, in conjunction with the research component of the Mid-East Study of Immigrant Health and Adjustment Project, we worked with Arab-American women leaders to develop a series of women's health education workshops (Meleis, Omidian, & Lipson, 1993).

The results of the qualitative studies illustrate the importance of considering the broader social context in which immigrants and refugees live in the country of resettlement. Several point out that past traumas, resettlement issues, jobs and poverty, and ethnic discrimination have a stronger impact on the health and health seeking of immigrants and refugees than do cultural characteristics. This broader context extends internationally, where connection with family members in the homeland must be considered (e.g., May's 1992 finding that Middle Eastern immigrant parents sought advice and help from family members in the Middle East; Lipson & Omidian's 1996 description of the impact of news in Afghanistan on the everyday mental health of Afghan refugees).

Another important theme is determining immigrants' own perceptions of their health issues and care needs before planning services; that is, the "need, appropriateness and effectiveness of health teaching to identify alternative sources of health education not necessarily associated with the medical care system" (DeSantis & Thomas, 1992, p. 87). Seeking input and developing partnerships should also extend to research. We must ask if research questions are of interest or meaning to the group itself, which is critical to cooperation and utility of findings.

Research Gaps and Issues

Methods and Designs

Longitudinal and long-term studies. Most nursing research on immigrants and refugees is a cross-sectional or one-time effort. Considering that immigration is a transition that includes pre-immigration, arrival, settling in, post-immigration, integration, and acculturation, we need research studies that capture the nature of the process and the responses that reflect the particular context. Following participants over time to see how a longer stay in the United States affects health, health habits, and use of care may help uncover critical points for preventive and therapeutic interventions. In addition, immigrant and refugee communities change considerably over time, as Lipson found in 10 years of ethnographic work with the Afghan community. Muecke and Sassi (1992) point out that almost all refugee research is carried out in the country of final resettlement rather than in countries of origin or temporary resettlement, which obscures the scope of the refugee experience. Their diachronic study of Cambodian teens in transit in Thailand and in Washington State attempts to address this gap.

Defining the group, sampling, and recruitment. Most small or qualitative studies used *nonprobability sampling.* Small samples are appropriate for answering some research questions but not others. Designing appropriate sampling strategies requires careful attention to issues of recruitment, and recruiting probability samples depends on locating a critical mass of immigrants from which a sample can be drawn. It may be impossible to rely on contiguous communities and Census data. Not all immigrants live in a geographical community, and the Census data is far from accurate, often undernumerating immigrants. For example, the 1990 Census' widely distributed short form specified only racial categories and Hispanics. Many Arab immigrants simply checked "white." Others who filled out the longer form may have checked "white" instead of identifying themselves with an all-inclusive "Arab" category of people from many countries.

Another barrier to appropriate sampling is the federal government's designation of four minority groups for research and community programs (African Americans, Hispanics, Native Americans, and Asians/Pacific Islanders), which may encourage researchers to lump together immigrant populations who otherwise differ culturally and in their immigration patterns (e.g., Filipinos and Cambodians). This designation also attracts proposals from nurse researchers with little preparation to study cultural differences and who have neither the time nor the inclination to define groups more narrowly. However, defining a population in terms of its national origin, although scientifically more appropriate, may be of less significance for policy proposals because of small numbers of country-specific immigrants. In our experience, the federal government is less interested in funding studies of specific unique groups (e.g., Afghans or Arabs) unless a strong case is made for the generalizability of the findings to other immigrant or refugee groups.

Sampling assumptions need careful attention. In choosing a study group, questions about homogeneity and heterogeneity should be addressed. Questions to consider include region of origin, socioeconomic status, work patterns, level of integration, the point in the transition process, gender, and the host country's attitude and responses to different subgroups of immigrants within the study group.

To enhance recruitment of study participants, researchers should address critical questions related to community involvement and reciprocity. Some minority communities object to research findings that either provide them with negligible benefits or further stereotype or stigmatize them. Therefore, we must address the extent to which the research questions reflect the needs of the community and the level of involvement of community members in the whole research process.

Instrumentation. Most of the qualitative studies, although they provided rich findings, were based on interview protocols designed specifically for the particular group and/or one-time study. Developing culturally appropriate interview protocols is time consuming and may be of limited use. Using specifically designed interview protocols also limits the potential for comparison between sets of data, which may be essential for supporting policies that enhance the quality of life of refugees and immigrants.

Attention to appropriate instrumentation may increase cost effectiveness as well as supporting validity. Instead of relying on one-time interview protocols, identifying key instrumentation questions may lead to the development of cumulative knowledge and wisdom. Examples of methodological questions are, How can one develop norms for a particular group to be used for comparison with other groups? What methods of data gathering are most effective? How does one uncover patterns of "social desirability" responses? Are Likert-type scales likely to elicit more valid data in some groups than others?

We need cumulative answers to questions related to the phenomenon of "real" data and the timing, trust, and reciprocity issues in uncovering such data. In our study of Middle Eastern immigrants, for example, the real data came out during casual conversations before the interview and during the long good-bye ritual at the door, and some participatants later admitted to not telling the truth in response to structured questions (Lipson & Meleis, 1989).

Language. Researchers should analyze questions related to language used in interviews and researcher role in translating and interpreting the data. Most of the larger cross-sectional studies mentioned in this chapter did not discuss the language of the interview nor issues of translation and interpretation. Similarly, there are issues inherent in the fit between the linguistic framework of the clinician and/or researcher and the patients or participants. What is the influence of culture on the meaning and validity of the instruments? For example, U.S. norms consider a Cornell Medical Index question, "I am sensitive," to be a "symptom" in the psychological section, but Iranian immigrants of both genders view being sensitive as a positive personal characteristic and will answer affirmatively (Meleis, Lipson, & Paul, 1992). Translation should be based on both content and meaning in cultural context. For example, a researcher testing the validity of a Spanish version of the CES-D learned that the statement "I enjoyed life" connoted being a "loose woman" to Mexican women.

Theoretical Appropriateness

Meleis (1992) identified caring, feminism, and self-care as theoretical perspectives used in research related to diversity. Luna (1994), for example, described patterns of caring among Lebanese Muslim immigrants, using Leininger's caring framework to define her research questions and data analyis. Anderson's (1985) participatory methodology uncovered a pattern in which immigrants in Canada sought help from the health care system for physical needs but only from family members for mental health needs. The feminist perspective provided a framework for interpreting help-seeking patterns within the context of how women are treated within their immigrant community and the larger society in which the existing health care system lacks cultural understanding and cannot meet their mental health care needs. Similarly, Thompson (1991) used a feminist archetypal theory to describe the meaning of the dreams of Khmer refugee women. Through participants' involvement in data collection and analysis, four themes were found that reflect the history of women's refugee experiences and culture: a preoccupation with violence and safety, communication with the spirits of relatives, sexuality and relationships with men, and premonitions about good and bad luck.

One other prevailing theoretical approach in the studies mentioned in this chapter is derived from cultural heritage, values, norms, and beliefs as a framework for methodology and data analysis. One limitation of this approach may be potential omission of the environmental and societal variables that affect the health and health care of immigrants. Another limitation is that the nursing perspective is rarely used to identify study phenomena. Clinical phenomena dealt with by nurses, such as comfort, safety, restlessness, sleeplessness, and others, have rarely been the focus of research with immigrants and refugees.

Future Research

Health care for minorities, including immigrants and refugees, is a worldwide imperative. Development of culturally appropriate interventions and increasing access to culturally competent care should be based on cumulative knowledge that is theoretically sound and methodologically valid. This requires local, state, and federal commitment to fund innovative projects to address methodological and recruitment issues in studying immigrants and refugees in studies that combine qualitative and quantative methods (Meleis, 1996). Future research should capture the transition experience of immigrants, provide opportunities for comparison, and address the issues surrounding language, accuracy, sympolic interpretation, and competence in uncovering meanings with cultural context.

Future research should also recognize such neglected immigrants as South Americans, Africans, Eastern Europeans, and Middle Easterners, as well as battered women, the elderly, or the disabled in immigrant studies. A major need is developing and testing nursing interventions to decrease structural barriers in accessing health care, such as language, nonbiomedical treatment modalities, and use of indigenous healers, among others. Another major need is developing understanding of culturally appropriate health promotive behaviors.

Finally, critical assessment of research on immigrants and refugees requires using some criteria for rigor. In addition to the rigor criteria proposed by Hall and Stevens (1991) and Meleis (1996), immigrant research must be examined for the potential of stereotyping or further marginalizing immigrants in their new country.

References

Ailinger, R., & Causey, M. (1995). Health concept of older Hispanic immigrants. *Western Journal of Nursing Research, 17,* 605-613.

Anderson, J. (1985). Perspectives on the health of immigrant women: A feminist analysis. *Advances in Nursing Science, 8*(1), 61-76.

Anderson, J. (1991). Immigrant women speak of chronic illness: The social construction of the devalued self. *Journal of Advanced Nursing, 16,* 710-717.

Anderson, J., Blue, C., Holbrook, A., & Ng, M. (1993). On chronic illness: Immigrant women in Canada's work force—a feminist perspective. *Canadian Journal of Nursing Research, 25*(2), 7-22.

Anderson, J., Wiggins, S., Rajwani, R., Holbrook, A., Blue, C., & Ng, M. (1995). Living with chronic illness: Chinese Canadian women with diabetes—exploring factors that influence management. *Social Science and Medicine, 41,* 181-195.

Aroian, K. (1990). A model of psychological adaptation to migration and resettlement. *Nursing Research, 39,* 5-10.

Aroian, K. (1993). Mental health risks and problems encountered by illegal immigrants. *Issues in Mental Health Nursing, 14,* 379-397.

Aroian, K., & Patsdaughter, C. (1989). Multiple-method, cross-cultural assessment of psychological distress. *Image: The Journal of Nursing Scholarship, 21,* 90-93.

Boyle, J. (1989). Constructs of health promotion and wellness in a Salvadoran population. *Public Health Nursing, 6,* 129-134.

Boyle, J. (1991). Transcultural nursing care of Central American refugees. *Imprint, 38,* 73-74, 76, 79.

Budman, C., Lipson, J., & Meleis, A. (1992). The cultural consultant in mental health care: The case of an Arab adolescent. *American Journal of Orthopsychiatry, 62,* 359.

Cassell, J. (1974). Psychosocial processes and "stress": Theoretical formulation. *International Journal of Health Services, 4,* 471-481.

Cheon-Klessig, Y., Camilleri, D., McElmurry, B., & Ohlson, V. (1988). Folk medicine in the health practice of Hmong refugees. *Western Journal of Nursing Research, 10,* 647-660.

Chick, N., & Meleis, A. (1986). Transitions: A nursing concern. In P. Chinn (Ed.), *Nursing research methodology: Issues and implementation* (pp. 237-257). Rockville, MD: Aspen.

Chung, R., & Kagawa-Singer, M. (1993). Predictors of psychological distress among Southeast Asian refugees. *Social Science and Medicine, 36,* 631-639.

Chung, R., & Kagawa-Singer, M. (1995). Interpretation of symptom presentation and distress: A Southeast Asian refugee example. *Journal of Nervous and Mental Disease, 183,* 639-648.

Clabots, R., & Dolphin, D. (1992). The multilingual videotape project: Community involvement in a unique health education program. *Public Health Reports, 107,* 75-80.

Coelho, C., & Ahmed, P. (Eds.). (1980). *Uprooting and development.* New York: Plenum.

Dempsey, P., & Gesse, T. (1983). The childbearing Haitian refugee: Cultural applications to clinical nursing. *Public Health Reports, 98,* 261-267.

DeSantis, L. (1990). Fieldwork with undocumented aliens and other populations at risk. *Western Journal of Nursing Research, 12,* 359-372.

DeSantis, L., & Halberstein, R. (1992). The effects of immigration on the health care system of South Florida. *Human Organization, 51,* 223-234.

DeSantis, L., & Thomas, J. (1992). Health education and the immigrant Haitian mother: Cultural insights for community health nurses. *Public Health Nursing, 9,* 87-96.

DeSantis, L., & Thomas, J. (1994). Childhood independence: Views of Cuban and Haitian immigrant mothers. *Journal of Pediatric Nursing, 9,* 258-267.

Flaskerud, J., & Anh, N. (1988). Mental health needs of Vietnamese refugees. *Hospital and Community Psychiatry, 39,* 435-437.

Fox, P., Cowell, J., & Johnson, M. (1995). Effects of family disruption on Southeast Asian refugee women. *International Nursing Review, 42*(1), 27-30, 26.

Franks, F., & Faux, S. (1990). Depression, stress, mastery and social resources in four ethnocultural women's groups. *Research in Nursing and Health, 13,* 283-292.

Frye, B., & D'Avanzo, C. (1994). Themes in managing culturally defined illness in the Cambodian refugee family. *Journal of Community Health Nursing, 11,* 89-98.

Frye, B., & McGill, D. (1993). Cambodian refugee adolescents: Cultural factors and mental health nursing. *Journal of Child and Adolescent Psychiatric and Mental Health Nursing, 6*(4), 24-31.

Gallagher, M., A. (1992). Human immunodeficiency virus and immigration status in the United States. *Journal of the Association of Nurses in AIDS Care, 3*(2), 32-35.

Hall, J., & Stevens, P. (1991). Rigor in feminist research. *Advances in Nursing Science, 13*(3), 16-19.

Hattar-Pollara, M., & Meleis, A. (1995a). Parenting their adolescents: The experiences of Jordanian immigrant women in California. *Health Care for Women International, 16,* 195-211.

Hattar-Pollara, M., & Meleis, A. (1995b). The stress of immigration and the daily lived experiences of Jordanian immigrant women in the United States. *Western Journal of Nursing Research, 17,* 521-539.

Hatton, D., & Webb, T. (1993). Information transmission in bilingual, bicultural contexts: A field study of community health nurses and interpreters. *Journal of Community Health Nursing, 10,* 137-147.

Hull, D. (1979). Migration, adaptation and illness: A review. *Social Science and Medicine, 13A,* 25-36.

Jezewski, M. (1993). Culture brokering as a model for advocacy. *Nursing and Health Care, 14,* 78-85.

Johnston, J. (1989). Changing demographics in New York State: Implications for nursing education and practice. *Journal of the New York State Nurses Association, 20*(2), 7-8, 13-15.

Kahler, L., Sobata, C., Hines, C., & Griswold, K. (1996). Pregnant woman at risk: An evaluation of the health status of refugee women in Buffalo, New York. *Health Care for Women International, 17,* 15-23.

Kasl, S., & Berkman, L. (1983). Health consequences of the experience of migration. *Annual Review of Public Health, 4,* 69-90.

Kulig, J. (1988). Conception and birth control use: Cambodian refugee women's beliefs and practices. *Journal of Community Health Nursing, 5,* 235-246.

Kulig, J. (1990). A review of the health status of Southeast Asian refugee women. *Health Care for Women International, 11,* 49-63.

Kulig, J. (1994). "Those with unheard voices": The plight of a Cambodian refugee woman. *Journal of Community Health Nursing, 11,* 99-107.

Kulig, J. (1995). Cambodian refugees' family planning knowledge and use. *Journal of Advanced Nursing, 22,* 150-157.

Kunz, E. (1973). The refugee in flight: Kinetic models and forms of displacement. *International Migration Review, 7,* 125-146.

Laffrey, S., Meleis, A., Lipson, J., Solomon, M., & Omidian, P. (1989). Assessing health care needs of Arab immigrants. *Social Science in Medicine, 29*(7), 877-883.

Laurence, R. (1992a). Part I: Torture and mental health: A review of the literature. *Issues in Mental Health Nursing, 13,* 301-310.

Laurence, R. (1992b). Part II: The treatment of torture survivors: A review of the literature. *Issues in Mental Health Nursing, 13,* 311-320.

Leininger, M. (1988). Leininger's theory of nursing: Cultural care diversity and universality. *Nursing Science Quarterly, 1*(4), 152-160.

Lipson, J. (1991). Afghan refugee health: Some findings and suggestions. *Qualitative Health Research, 1,* 349-369.

Lipson, J. (1992). Iranian immigrants: Health and adjustment. *Western Journal of Nursing Research, 14,* 10-29

Lipson, J. (1993). Afghan refugees in California: Mental health issues. *Issues in Mental Health Nursing, 14,* 411-423.

Lipson, J., Hosseini, T., Kabir, S., Omidian, P., & Edmonston, F. (1995). Health issues among Afghan women in California. *Health Care for Women International, 16,* 279-286.

Lipson, J., & Meleis, A. (1985). Culturally appropriate care: The case of immigrants. *Topics in Clinical Nursing, 7,* 48-56.

Lipson, J., & Meleis A. (1989). Methodological issues in research with immigrants. *Medical Anthropology, 12,* 103-115.

Lipson, J., & Miller, S. (1994). Changing roles of Afghan refugee women in the U.S. *Health Care for Women International, 14,* 171-180.

Lipson, J., & Omidian, P. (1996). Health and the transnational connection: Afghan refugees in the United States. In A. Rynearson & J. Phillips (Eds.), *Selected papers on refugee issues: IV* (pp. 2-17). Arlington, VA: American Anthropological Association.

Lipson, J., Omidian, P., & Paul, S. (1995). Afghan health education project: A community survey. *Public Health Nursing, 12,* 143-150.

Lipson, J., Reizian, A., & Meleis, A. (1987). Arab-American patients: A medical record review. *Social Science and Medicine, 24,* 101-107.

Liu, W., & Cheung, F. (1985). Research concerns associated with the study of Southeast Asian refugees. In T. Owan (Ed.), *Southeast Asian mental health: Treatment, prevention, services.* Washington, DC: National Institutes of Mental Health.

Luna, L. (1994, Winter). Care and cultural context of Lebanese Muslim immigrants: Using Leininger's theory. *Journal of Transcultural Nursing, 5*(2), 12-20.

Lynam, M. J. (1985). Support networks developed by immigrant women. *Social Science and Medicine, 31,* 327-333.

Lynam, M., & Anderson, J. (1986). Generating knowledge for nursing practice: Methodological issues in studying immigrant women. In P. Chinn (Ed.), *Nursing research methodology: Issues and implementation* (pp. 259-274). Rockville, MD: Aspen.

Mahon, J., McFarlane, J., & Golden, K. (1991). *De madres a madres:* A community partnership for health. *Public Health Nursing, 8,* 15-19.

Marin, G., & Marin, B. (1991). *Research with Hispanic populations.* Beverly Hills, CA: Sage.

Mattson, S. (1995) Culturally sensitive perinatal care for Southeast Asians. *Journal of Obstetric, Gynecologic, and Neonatal Nursing, 24*(4), 335-341.

Mattson, S., & Lew, L. (1992). Culturally sensitive prenatal care for Southeast Asians. *Journal of Obstetric, Gynecologic, and Neonatal Nursing, 21,* 48-54.

May, K. (1992). Middle Eastern immigrant parents' social networks and help-seeking for child health care. *Journal of Advanced Nursing, 17,* 905-912.

McKinlay, J. (1975). Some issues associated with migration, health status, and the use of human services. *Journal of Chronic Disease, 28,* 579-592.

Meleis, A. (1991). Between two cultures: Identity, roles and health. *Health Care for Women International, 12,* 365-377.

Meleis, A. (1992). Cultural diversity research. In *Communicating nursing research: Silver threads, 25 years of nursing excellence* (pp. 151-173). Boulder, CO: Western Institute of Nursing.

Meleis, A. (1995). Immigrant women in borderless societies: Marginalised and empowered. *Asian Journal of Nursing Studies, 2*(4), 39-47.

Meleis, A. (1996). Culturally competent scholarship: Substance and rigor. *Advances in Nursing Science, 19*(2), 1-16.

Meleis, A., Lipson, J., Muecke, M., & Smith, G. (1998). *Immigrant women and their health: An olive paper* [Monograph]. Indianapolis, IN: Sigma Theta Tau International.

Meleis, A., Lipson, J., & Paul, S. (1992). Ethnicity and health among five Middle Eastern immigrant groups. *Nursing Research, 41,* 98-103.

Meleis, A., Omidian, P., & Lipson, J. (1993). Women's health status in the United States: An immigrant women's project. In J. Beverly, K. McElmurry, F. Norr, & R. S. Parker (Eds.), *Women's health and development: A global challenge* (pp. 163-181). Boston: Jones and Bartlett.

Meleis, A., & Trangenstein, P. (1994). Facilitating transitions: Redefinitions of a nursing mission. *Nursing Outlook, 42,* 255-259.

Muecke, M. (1990). *Bibliography: Nursing research and practice with refugees* (Southeast Asian Refugee Studies, Occasional Papers, No. 10). Minneapolis, MN: Southeast Asian Refugee Studies Project, University of Minnesota.

Muecke, M. (1992a). New paradigms for refugee health problems. *Social Science and Medicine, 35,* 515-523.

Muecke, M. (1992b). Nursing research with refugees: A review and guide. *Western Journal of Nursing Research, 14,* 703-720.

Muecke, M., & Sassi, L. (1992). Anxiety among Cambodian refugee adolescents in transit and in resettlement. *Western Journal of Nursing Research, 14,* 267-291.

Ness, C., & Nakao, A. (1997, January 24). Study shows immigrant no big drain on welfare. *San Francisco Examiner,* p. 2.

Neves-Arruda, E., Larson, P., & Meleis, A. (1992). Comfort: Immigrant Hispanic cancer patients' views. *Cancer Nursing, 15,* 387-394.

Omidian, P., & Lipson, J. (1992). Elderly Afghan refugees: Tradition and transition in Northern California. In P. DeVoe (Ed.), *Refugee issues papers* (pp. 27-39). Washington, DC: American Anthropological Association.

Omidian, P. A., & Lipson, J. (1996). Ethnic coalitions and public health: Delights and dilemmas with the Afghan Health Education Project in Northern California. *Human Organization, 55,* 355-360.

Palinkas, L., & Pickwell, S. (1995). Acculturation as a risk factor for chronic disease among Cambodian refugees in the United States. *Social Science and Medicine, 40,* 1643-1653.

Park, K., & Peterson, L. (1991). Beliefs, practices, and experiences of Korean women in relation to childbirth. *Health Care for Women International, 12,* 261-269.

Pickwell, S. (1981). School health screening of Indochinese refugee children. *Journal of School Health, 51,* 102-105.

Pickwell, S. (1982). Primary health care for Indochinese refugee children. *Pediatric Nursing, 8*(2), 104-107.

Pickwell, S. (1989). The incorporation of family primary care for southeast Asian refugees in community-based mental health facility. *Archives of Psychiatric Nursing, 3*(3), 173-177.

Pickwell, S. (1994). Family nurse practitioner faculty clinical practice with undocumented migrants. *Family and Community Health, 16,* 32-38.

Pickwell, S. (1996). Providing health care to refugees. *Advanced Practice Nursing Quarterly, 2*(2), 39-44.

Pickwell, S., Schimelpfening, S., & Palinkas, L. (1994). "Betelmania": Betel quid chewing by Cambodian women in the United States and its potential health effects. *Western Journal of Medicine, 160,* 326-330.

Porter, C., & Villaruel, A. (1993). Nursing research with African American and Hispanic people: Guidelines for action. *Nursing Outlook, 41*(2), 59-67.

Reizian, A., & Meleis, A. (1986). Arab-Americans' perception of and responses to pain. *Critical Care Nursing, 6*(6), 30-37.

Reizian, A., & Meleis, M. (1987). Symptoms reported by Arab-American patients on the Cornell Medical Index. *Western Journal of Nursing Research, 9,* 368-384.

Rossiter, J. (1992). Maternal-infant health beliefs and infant feeding practices: The perception and experience of immigrant Vietnamese women in Sydney. *Contemporary Nurse, 1,* 79-82.

Rossiter, J. (1994). The effect of a culture-specific education program to promote breast-feeding among Vietnamese women in Sydney. *International Journal of Nursing Studies, 31,* 369-79.

Sawyer, L., Regev, H., Proctor, S., Nelson, M., Messias, D., Barnes, D., & Meleis, A. (1995). Matching versus cultural competence in research: Mythological considerations. *Research in Nursing & Health, 18,* 557-567.

Schumacher, K., & Meleis, A. (1994). Transitions: A central concept in nursing. *Image: The Journal of Nursing Scholarship, 26,* 119-1127.

Shadick, K. M. (1993). Development of a transcultural health education program for the Hmong. *Clinical Nurse Specialist, 7*(2), 48-53.

Shepard, J., & Faust, S. (1993). Refugee health care and the problem of suffering. *Bioethics Forum, 9,* 3-7.

Sluzki, C. (1979). Migration and family conflict. *Family Process, 18,* 379-390.

Stein, B. (1986). The experience of being a refugee: Insights from the research literature. In C. Williams & J. Westermeyer (Eds.), *Refugee mental health in resettlement countries* (pp. 3-23). Washington, DC: Hemisphere.

Stephens, E., Foote, K., Hendershot, G., & Schoenborn, C. (1994). Health of the foreign-born population: United States, 1989-90. *Advance Data, 14*(214), 1-12.

Stevens, P., Hall, J., & Meleis, A. (1992). Examining vulnerability of women clerical workers from five ethnic/racial groups. *Western Journal of Nursing Research, 14,* 754-774.

Thomas, J., & DeSantis, L. (1995). Feeding and weaning practices of Cuban and Haitian immigrant mothers. *Journal of Transcultural Nursing, 6,* 34-42.

Thompson, J. (1991). Exploring gender and culture with Khmer refugee women: Reflections on participatory feminist research. *Advances in Nursing Science, 13*(3), 30-48.

Tripp-Reimer, T. (1983). Retention of a folk-healing practice (*matiasma*) among four generations of urban Greek immigrants. *Nursing Research, 32,* 97-101.

Urrutia-Rojas, X., & Aday, L. (1991). A framework for community assessment: Designing and conducting a survey in a Hispanic immigrant and refugee community. *Public Health Nursing, 8,* 20-26.

U.S. Committee for Refugees. (1996). *Refugee Reports, 17*(12), 7.

Williams, C., & Berry, J. (1991). Primary prevention of acculturative stress among refugees. *American Psychologist, 46,* 632-641.

CULTURAL INTERVENTIONS
FOR ETHNIC GROUPS
OF COLOR

Toni Tripp-Reimer

Since at least the early 1960s, the disparity in health status and access to care that exists between White and minority populations in the United States has been a recognized problem. Research has consistently documented that on almost any measure, minorities have poorer health than do Whites. In 1985, the Secretary's Task Force on Black and Minority Health (U.S. Department of Health and Human Services, 1985-1986) published an eight-volume synthesis that highlighted the long-standing and persistent burden of death, disease, and disability experienced by individuals from the four federally defined ethnic groups of color (Black, Hispanic, Native American, and Asian). The report indicated that six specific health areas accounted for more than 80% of the higher annual proportion of minority deaths: cardiovascular and cerebrovascular diseases; cancer; chemical dependency, diabetes; homicide, suicide, unintentional injuries; and infant mortality and low birth weight. A decade later, in *Healthy People 2000: Mid-*

course Review and 1995 Revisions, Shalala (USDHHS, 1996) noted that minority groups continue to experience disproportionately worse health outcomes than Anglos. In fact, there is considerable evidence of increasing health disparities between White and minority groups (Lillie-Blanton, Parsons, Gayle, & Dievler, 1996; Williams, Lavizzo-Mourey, & Warren, 1994). Multiple factors have been identified as contributing to this situation, including poverty, issues of access to and use of health care, issues of individual and institutional racism, lifestyle choices, and a lack of cultural competence and appropriateness by health providers or programs.

The issue of whether to cast target population in terms of race, ethnicity, minority group status, culture, or people of color is sometimes a linguistic diversion and other times a meaningful distinction that has been extensively elaborated elsewhere (Tripp-Reimer & Fox, 1990; Tripp-Reimer & Lauer, 1987). All of these are multivocal terms that have connotative meanings based on the context, audience, and sender. Each term has its own history and accompanying mental associations. For example, the term *minority* accurately depicts a statistical relationship, but it also carries associated sociological meanings related to issues of power, control, and access to resources. Culture may be viewed as a set of values, beliefs, and rules of behavior that are shared by a group, but the size and characteristics of the group may vary from small, relatively homogeneous, isolated groups studied by early anthropologists to much broader groups that sometimes transcend continental boundaries (e.g., corporate culture). *Ethnicity* usually refers to a group identity based on race, language, religion, national or geographic origin, or symbolic identification, but recently this term has been restricted by some to "White" (European) ethnic groups such as Greek, Polish, or Czech. People of Color (sometimes Ethnic Groups of Color) is a phrase used by the federal government to denote four populations considered to be at particular risk due to a history of discrimination. These groups are identified as African American, Hispanic, Native American, and Asian/Pacific Islander, although the specific terms and their denoted constituencies have been modified over the past 50 years. For example, African Americans have been variously termed Negro/Colored in the 1940s and 1950s, Afro-American in the 1960s, and Black in the 1970s and 1980s. Finally, the term *race* was originally introduced and then discarded by the biological sciences. Although the term "race" is today considered a nonscientific term that has no meaning in terms of biology, race and racism have considerable meaning as social constructs. In this chapter, the terms employed by specific authors will be used as they were written; in other cases, the term *ethnic group* will be used in its broader form.

It is exceptionally difficult to describe or comprehend the extent to which ethnocentrism and White privilege have been woven into the fabric of our health care system. Most current health delivery systems (including those of nursing) are based on models developed for the general (read: "White middle-class") population.

Against this backdrop of health inequities, the discipline of nursing has had an uneven record. Historically, nursing was a pioneering discipline in innovative interventions, and because of its greater access to minority populations, it arguably could have the greatest impact of all health disciplines. Yet, currently nursing is less active and less visible than many other professions in addressing health disparities. Despite a few nursing figures and projects that are striking in their contributions, nursing generally falls far behind other disciplines (notably psychology and counselor education) in research investigating effective intervention strategies with minority populations.

Cultural competence has been defined as a "set of congruent behaviors, attitudes, and policies that come together in a system, agency, or amongst professionals and enables that system, agency, or those professionals to work effectively in cross-cultural situations" (Cross, Bazron, Dennis, & Isaacs, 1989, p. 4). The term "cultural competence" has come to widely reflect the need to extend beyond awareness and sensitivity (which often lose power after the assessment phase), and to plan, implement, and evaluate interventions on the basis of cultural factors. The mandate in nursing is evident in recent publications by the American Academy of Nursing (Lenburg et al., 1995; Meleis, Isenberg, Loerner, Lacy, & Stern, 1995). The components of cultural competence include awareness of and sensitivity to cultural differences; knowledge of cultural values, beliefs, and behaviors; and skill in working with culturally diverse populations.

This chapter contains an integrated review of clinical nursing research related to the four federally defined ethnic groups of color. Following a brief historical overview, the theoretical perspectives and constructs that have been most influential in guiding this area of nursing research are identified and a model for culturally relevant clinical research is presented. Subsequently, a synthesis of nursing science related to effective interventions specifically targeting ethnic groups will be delineated. Finally, a summary with recommendations for future research in this area is suggested.

Historical Perspectives

The history of nursing's attention in improving the health of minority patients has been sporadic and irregular and has largely reflected the social trends of a particular period. Early literature concerning the health of groups representing various cultures entered the nursing literature around the turn of the century as public health nurses described various ethnic and immigrant groups. However, the intent of nursing practice thus described was to promote assimilation into the American "melting pot" (Dougherty & Tripp-Reimer, 1985). On the whole, however, the social and cultural aspects of patient care were largely ignored in the first half of the century, as nursing emphasized disease pathology and nursing procedures.

Shortly after World War II, a new approach emerged, known as comprehensive care of the patient (or nursing the whole patient). With this broader focus, perspectives from the social sciences gained increased importance. This trend was fostered through mid-century reform in nursing spearheaded by the Brown Report (Brown, 1948) and supported by nursing educators and organizations (particularly the NLN), as well as social scientists affiliated with schools of nursing (such as MacGregor, 1960). Largely, however, the tone of the writing related to what nurses need to know about patients to provide good nursing care; it identified patient characteristics that nurses should understand so that misunderstandings and conflicts would not occur (see, for example, Brown, 1964). Descriptive investigations and discussions focused on topics such as communication issues, interpersonal relations, spiritual goals, role of social problems in patient problems, and even such specific issues as the need for translation and more flexible visitation schedules (Brown, 1961, 1964). However, the purpose of most articles was to sensitize nurses to patient characteristics rather than to develop effective nursing interventions.

A very different impetus came from the advancing Civil Rights social movement. The passage of the desegregation laws of the 1950s and the Civil Rights Act in 1964 stimulated dialogue. As this topic was being discussed in the broader social arena, it provided an impetus for nurses to reflect on their own history and social mandate. However, the highly significant contributions of ethnic nurses of color to this effort have largely been ignored in the literature.

In the mid-1960s, important health and social programs were initiated in response to the Civil Rights Movement and the antipoverty programs of the Kennedy-Johnson administrations. Two prominent programs enacted as a result of Congressional legislation were the community mental health centers (1963) and the neighborhood health centers (1965). These two programs had similar community-focused mandates, including a high degree of community voice, participation, and control; a guiding philosophy that health is a right, not a privilege; a belief in the importance of continuity of care and family-centered care; and a goal of equal access to quality health care. The idea of a team of health professionals was operationalized in these arenas, as were powerful models of the expanded role of the nurse. New health worker positions and roles were developed; most notably,

the community health worker (CHW). The CHWs (also called neighborhood health aides) were recruited largely from the ranks of those receiving public assistance; they received health and social service training and served as community advocates and liaisons. The 1966 session of Congress expanded the initial Neighborhood Health Centers program, funded through the Office of Economic Opportunity; by the beginning of 1970, 53 neighborhood health centers, each designed to serve up to 30,000 persons, were funded in 25 states (Office of Economic Opportunity, 1968). Unfortunately, after initial periods of funding, federal support did not continue, and local communities were often unable to sustain the centers for financial and political reasons.

During this period, nursing devised several exciting and excellent model programs. Storlie (1970) described a variety of programs targeting minority and vulnerable populations and identified specific strategies to foster more effective nursing approaches. Similarly, 22 innovative projects involving the expanded role of community health nurses are described in Warner's (1978) *Innovations in Community Health Nursing*; these include the Frontier Nursing Service, a Navajo service delivery system, midwifery in the Mississippi Delta, inner-city heath services in New York City and Miami, and rural mobile health clinics. Probably most prominent among the model programs was the "Mom and Tots Center" in Detroit, described by Milio (1967, 1970). These programs and initiatives from the 1960s and early 1970s are similar in many respects to those currently being proposed as innovative programs.

In 1970, two remarkable books were published that offered nursing two different paths for addressing minority health. In the first, *9226 Kercheval: The Storefront That Did Not Burn,* Nancy Milio described the community action program that evolved into a neighborhood health center in Detroit's Lower Southeast Side. During the 1967 Detroit riots, the storefront clinic was untouched, although stores surrounding it were destroyed. Milio chronicled the complex issues involved in establishing and attempting to sustain this model program in the context of strong racial tensions and a fitful federal and community funding base. This path was that of community-based social activism.

The second path was formalized by Leininger (1970) in *Nursing and Anthropology: Two Worlds to Blend.* This book took a more academic tone in describing the importance of incorporating cultural concepts from anthropology into the discipline of nursing. The field of medical anthropology had recently been formed and was a relatively popular area of doctoral study for nurses during the 1960s and 1970s. Content from anthropology that was emphasized included cultural variation in values, folk illness and treatments, folk healers, ethnic diversity in family structure, and acculturation issues. Specific recommendations for culturally sensitive nursing included becoming aware of personal biases, increasing knowledge about communication patterns and culturally defined systems of illness causation and treatment, and incorporating folk healers and healing into patient care. However, there was a considerable gap between the ethnographic data provided by anthropologists and nurse-anthropologists and its use in clinical interventions. Nurses were widely exhorted to consider the cultural variable, yet culturally specific treatment modalities were rarely articulated. During the next 15 years, the research by nurses on cultural topics tended to be descriptive or exploratory studies of various cultural groups, with particular emphasis on values, beliefs, and behaviors embedded in culture. This was so much the case that in 1985, when Tripp-Reimer and Dougherty wrote an integrated research review article for the *Annual Review of Nursing Research,* the literature available was almost wholly descriptive.

In both research and nursing education, nursing clearly took the academic path, an approach emphasizing specific cultural characteristics over the social activist approach. In the ensuing years, the "culture" of the patient has been used as a cover term, often serving to obscure the deeper, more sinister issues of individual or institutional racism and poverty or economic disparities.

Conceptual and Theoretical Perspectives

Theoretical grounding on issues of culture and ethnicity in nursing developed through three primary approaches: theoretical models, concept development, and models for practice. Theoretical models have been devised in an attempt to communicate about the domain of culture and nursing. Two macro models that have been devised include Leininger's (1984) Sunrise Model depicting the Theory of Culture Care Diversity and Universality and Dobson's (1991) Transcultural Health Visiting Schema. Leininger's model, for example, presents an ar-

ray of cultural domains for assessment and understanding and, further, notes that possible nursing interventions may include cultural care preservation and maintenance, cultural care accommodation and negotiation, and cultural care repatterning or restructuring. However, although these models are useful in helping clinicians cognitively frame an approach to culturally diverse clients, they are too abstract to have direct clinical utility.

A second approach to theory development has been at the level of construct and concept refinement. This approach largely represents a synthesis of concepts initially developed in anthropology and extended to specific application in nursing. For example, Tripp-Reimer (1985) elucidated the ways in which anthropological concepts influenced or contributed to the metaparadigm elements in nursing (humans, environment, health, and nursing action). The elaboration of the construct of culture expanded the way nursing conceptualized the environment, issues of ethnocentrism and cultural relativity influenced the construct of human, the emic-etic/illness-disease distinction broadened nursing's view of health, and the construct of culture broker increased options for nursing action.

The third approach includes a variety of models devised for use in clinical practice (generally through the nursing process). Overwhelmingly, these models have been focused on the area of assessment and are represented by Affonso's (1979) Framework for Cultural Assessment, Bloch's (1983) Assessment Guide for Ethnic/Culture Variations, Leininger's (1977) Culturological Assessment Domains, Tripp-Reimer's (1984) Cultural Assessment, Tripp-Reimer, Brink, and Saunder's (1984) Process Approach, Brownlee's (1978) Cross-Cultural Guide for Communities, Paxton, Ramirez, and Walloch's (1976) Holistic Assessment, Orque's (1983) Ethnic-Cultural System, Fong's (1985) Confer Model, and Giger and Davidhizer's (1991) Assessment Model for Six Cultural Phenomena. Models for intervention have been fewer and less developed. Some of these include Leininger's (1984) cultural preservation, accommodation, or repatterning and Tripp-Reimer and Brink's (1985) process of cultural brokerage.

On the whole, these theoretical and conceptual approaches to the topic have addressed the assessment portion of the nursing process. They are highly appropriate for contextual grounding and for obtaining data to use in planning interventions. Few, if any, have direct clinical application with regard to selecting or tailoring nursing interventions or evaluating patient outcomes. Further, a strong empha-

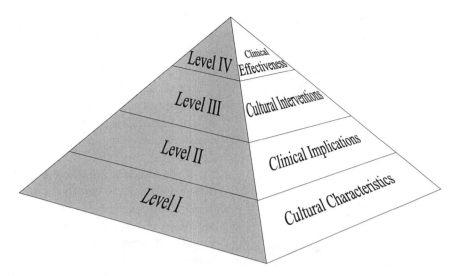

Figure 7.1 Pyramid of Culturally Relevant Nursing Research

sis on the more exotic and esoteric aspects of culture has obscured the deeper dimensions of diversity. We have not been successful at constructing midrange theories to understand why specific interventions may be particularly successful in certain clinical situations.

Figure 7.1 depicts a model designed to aid consideration of the clinical relevance of various types of culturally related nursing research. The model is a pyramid with levels ranging from the bottom, Level I, depicting descriptive research, to the top, Level IV, representing effectiveness research. These levels can be linked with phases of nursing process: The first two tiers link with assessment, the third with intervention, and the fourth with outcomes and effectiveness. The pyramid was chosen as the model frame for three reasons: First, the lower levels serve as the necessary foundation for the higher levels; second, the apex level (effectiveness) is the ultimate goal of nursing; and finally, the pyramid represents the current relative proportions of extant research in the discipline.

Level I: Cultural characteristics. This tier represents wholly descriptive research that takes one of two forms: (a) ethnographic investigations of the cultural characteristics of particular groups, typically values, beliefs, social structure, and patterns of behavior. These descriptions are conducted by nurses or anthropologists or other social scientists. (b) Epidemiological investigations may be made of particular risk factors or behaviors that pro-

mote or reduce wellness. In nursing, this level most often has focused on the delineation of folk beliefs and practices related to health (e.g., folk illnesses such as *susto, mal ojo, matiasma*), lay practices (e.g., folk treatments such as herbal treatments, dermabrasion, or cupping), and folk specialists (e.g., *curanderos,* root doctors).

Level II: Clinical implications. At this level, clinical implications are identified or proposed as a result of descriptive cultural research. Investigations at this level identify cultural characteristics that merit consideration in the planning and delivery of nursing care; however, the recommendations are presented in a general sense. For example, there is a frequent recommendation that the patient's beliefs (Explanatory Model) about an illness should be considered in the plan of care. This level also includes research that describes characteristics of the nurse that affect the clinical situation, such as racism (Barbee, 1993), open-versus closed-mindedness (Bonaparte, 1979; Ruiz, 1981), or ethnocentrism (Tripp-Reimer, 1982).

Level III: Culturally specific interventions. At this level, specific modifications for practice are recommended. These may be directed at initiating new or modifying existing interventions or programs, increasing patient access to care, or modifying staff attitudes and behaviors. At this level, the nurse is asked to take action in terms of modifying current interventions.

Level IV: Effectiveness of cultural interventions. At this level, the effectiveness of modified interventions is tested as it relates to specified patient outcomes (such as increased utilization, improved health, increased knowledge, or satisfaction). Both the specific changed professional behavior and the desired patient outcome are identified in these investigations.

State of the Science of Clinical Nursing Research

The vast majority of culturally relevant nursing research represents Levels I and II in the model described above. Although that content identifies important consideration for nursing, it does not provide direct guidance for clinical interventions. Therefore, the synthesis of nursing research to guide clinical nursing practice will be limited primarily to that of published articles from Levels III or IV. This synthesis will provide an overview of culturally relevant nursing interventions in specific clinical areas.

General Community Health Interventions

A large community-based program, the Urban Women's Health Advocacy Training Project, was a nursing intervention planned jointly by a university-based school of nursing in community partnership (McElmurry, Swider, Grimes, Dan, Irvin, & Lourenco, 1987). The purpose was to develop and test nursing interventions for training community health advocates. Young (17- to 21-year-old) Hispanic and Black trainees participated in an 8-week program emphasizing women's health education, health advocacy skills, and career awareness. The project was viewed as a means to increase access to and use of health care. A secondary goal was to increase employment opportunities for young women. The trainees served as liaisons between health care experts and women in the community. The success of the program was mixed. A majority of young women trainees returned to high school or college, but trainees identified areas of concern including the paucity of role models for persons wishing to be health advocates and the lack of employment opportunities deriving from the training (the lack of employment was linked to the health agencies' tendency to place volunteers in health advocacy positions). As a re-

sult, the benefits of health advocacy training were evaluated as more personal than career related. The authors frankly addressed the issue that preparing these women for the role of health advocates was training them for a job not valued (at least not monetarily) by society, thus further entrenching them in their societal position. The investigators proposed that future programs might focus on older women or find institutionalized mechanisms for paying health advocates.

Boyle, Szymanski, and Szymanski (1992) described a collaborative project between nursing investigators and members of Navajo culture to develop culturally appropriate community nursing. The project linked professional nursing staff (experts in health content) with the cultural experts from the tribal community (a Navajo LPN and aide) who provided knowledge about the Navajo. The authors provided several examples of methods the project used to improve home health care for Navajo clients. These included strategies to overcome language barriers: teaching staff members basic Navajo phrases, developing patient education programs in the Navajo language and recording them on audiotapes, and a deliberate use of pictures and diagrams consistent with Navajo culture. Because the investigators viewed that use of indigenous staff members as of primary importance to the collaboration, they strongly endorsed the importance of recruitment of indigenous nurses, LPNs, and aides.

A third broad-based intervention involved a community nursing intervention applied in rural Arizona communities with a high concentration of Mexican Americans (May, Mendelson, & Ferketich, 1995). The large project tested the effectiveness of three interventions in improving the health of community residents using three broad approaches: (a) personalized preventive nursing, which provided clinic services and community health nurse home visits by the clinic nurse; (b) developing and delivering a system of community health outreach by community health nurses and *promotoras* (trained indigenous lay health workers); and (c) community empowerment, which fostered community identification of heath problems, resources, and solutions, assisted by community health nurses and promotoras. May et al.'s 1995 report focused on the latter intervention, which was implemented through two health fairs. The issue of language as a barrier was featured in the evaluation; the investigators noted that there had been insufficient health literature available in Spanish, and problems resulted because many volunteers were not bilingual.

Health Promotion and Prevention Area

Perinatal Interventions

Several nursing intervention studies have targeted various groups. Two programs targeting Hispanic women were *de Madres a Madres* (from mothers to mothers) (Mahon, McFarlane, & Golden, 1991) and the Hispanic Outreach Worker Program (Bray & Edwards, 1994). The former was initiated in Houston, Texas among Mexican American women; it delivered culturally relevant social support and community resource information to high-risk women before they entered the health care system. The premise of this project was that this intervention would enable pregnant women to transcend barriers to early prenatal care. A single community health nurse (CHN) was responsible for program implementation. She identified 31 key community leaders for support and endorsement, and solicited from them the names of potential volunteer mothers. The CHN trained 14 volunteer mothers during an 8-hour training session. The volunteer mothers planned and implemented several communitywide events to share information, including an information booth at community functions, a brochure (which included community resources), and a video about the program. A small purse mirror with community resource numbers was given to all mothers visited by the volunteers. After the first year of the program, over 2,000 at-risk mothers had received information from volunteer mothers.

The second project (Bray & Edwards, 1994) was initiated by a Chicago county health department, which instituted a program of intensified home visits using bilingual, bicultural community outreach workers under the supervision of nurses. Three outreach workers received 3 weeks of formal training from an interdisciplinary team, followed by clinical observation and skills training. The outreach workers made home visits concentrating on improving families' skills and knowledge in infant and child care, basic nutrition, and referral and linkage to community resources. The program resulted in an increased number of women receiving services, earlier registering for prenatal care and the WIC program, and increased numbers of infants receiving WIC services and regular medical supervision. The outreach workers were viewed as peers by the families, making acceptance

and credibility easier to achieve and interventions more effective.

In African American communities, two intervention projects have been completed. The first was conducted by Norbeck, DeJoseph, and Smith (1996), who followed a randomized trail of an empirically driven social support intervention to prevent low birth weight (LBW) among African American women's infants. Based on prior research, the woman were identified as at risk for LBW due to inadequate social support if they lacked support from their mothers or male partners. A culturally relevant intervention, developed from focus group recommendations, was designed to provide support that would usually be provided by the woman's mother or male partner. It consisted of four standardized face-to-face sessions at 2-week intervals, with telephone contact in the intervening weeks. The rate of LBW was 9.1% in the experimental group versus 22.4% in the control group.

A community-based intervention for African Americans in Chicago has also been reported as an interagency home visiting program: Resources, Education and Care in the Home (REACH) (Barnes-Boyd, Norr, & Nacion, 1986, 1996). This program consisted of teams of a nurse and a community resident trained as maternal-child health advocates who visit women in inner-city Chicago for the first year of the newborn's life. Areas identified for additional home education included home safety, skin care, and early identification and treatment of upper respiratory infections.

Similar programs were successfully employed with Southeast Asian immigrants (Mattson & Lew, 1991) through the Southeast Asian Health Project (SEAHP), which included outreach work by community outreach workers (targeting preventive perinatal care). Initial contacts included door-to-door canvassing, posters and brochures in local markets, ads in refugee papers, meetings at Buddhist temples, and referrals, as well as development of resource materials and oral classes. SEAHP also provided classes to professional staff related to health practices and beliefs of Southeast Asians (especially childbearing women).

A large-scale community-based approach to prenatal and postpartum care targeting Hawaiian, Filipino, and Japanese women living on the island of Hawaii was initiated in 1990. The *Malama Na Wahine Hapai* (Caring for Pregnant Women) program has been well described (Affonso, 1995; Affonso, Mayberry, Graham, Shibuya, & Kunimoto, 1992, 1993; Affonso, Mayberry, Inaba, Robinson,

& Matsuno, 1995; Affonso, Mayberry, Shibuya, et al., 1993). Following formal needs assessment, focus groups for each ethnic group were initiated to identify unique stressors, cultural mores and health care needs for women in the three groups. As a result, a complex set of nursing interventions were developed: (a) the Neighborhood Women's Health Watch, an organization of community women with previous childbearing experience who fostered health promotion by locating and recruiting pregnant women into the program and also aided in monitoring these women in the local communities. One of its innovative recruitment strategies was advertising an "irregular menses service," which led to pregnancy diagnosis. (b) Aspects of cultural healing systems were incorporated by providing culturally sensitive rituals and practices designed to promote positive interpersonal relationships between pregnant women and their significant others. This intervention helped the women maintain a sense of meaning and mastery over their relationships during pregnancy and after birth by reconciling interpersonal conflicts through rituals or culturally appropriate mediations that offer conflict resolution. (c) Health stations were established in small towns to provide flexible on-site perinatal services to increase access in rural areas. (d) A buddy system was initiated to link women with lay community outreach workers. Buddies (chosen by the pregnant woman from her network) assisted with transportation, meal planning, and health education. (e) An incentive system (built on the Hawaiian tradition of giving gifts to express gratitude, affection, and respect for women's efforts at health promotion) was operationalized as a system of vouchers whereby women could purchase food at local grocery stores. Overall, this program illustrates how cultural elements (social networks, ritual mediating systems, customs) can serve as the foundation (or delivery mechanism).

A final clinical intervention that was an innovative community recruitment strategy for prenatal health promotion was conducted thorough a community baby shower for Native American women residing in Detroit, in which student nurses provided health information. As part of the intervention, a Native American spiritual leader began the shower with a traditional blessing (Duffy, Bonino, Gallup, & Pontseele, 1994).

AIDS Prevention

Research on interventions to reduce AIDS risk has been prominent in the recent health literature. Two major programs of nursing research are well established in this literature. The first, headed by Nyamathi and Flaskerud in California, demonstrates the development of an extensive program of clinical nursing research related to AIDS prevention among Black and Latino women in California. Beginning with investigations of women's knowledge, attitudes, and current practices (Flaskerud & Calvillo, 1991; Flaskerud & Nyamathi, 1989; Flaskerud & Rush, 1989; Koniak-Griffin, Nyamathi, Vasquez, & Russo, 1994; Nyamathi, Bennett, Leake, Lewis, & Flaskerud, 1993) the investigators noted that women maintained traditional ideas concerning illness causation and treatment and had incorporated lay theories of AIDS risk, prevention, and treatment into them. Further, they found that although some traditional practices served to minimize AIDS, others (such as the use of laxatives to treat AIDS, exhibited by Black women) could serve to worsen disease progression. They reported that the groups of women differed in their risk patterns, as highly acculturated Latino women demonstrated most prevalent IV drug use, whereas non-IV drug use and high-risk sexual activity was most prevalent for African American women (these examples are illustrative only). Subsequently, they designed (Nyamathi & Shin, 1990) and tested AIDS counseling interventions (Nyamathi, Flaskerud, Bennett, Leake, & Lewis, 1994; Nyamathi, Leake, Flaskerud, Lewis, & Bennett, 1993). In designing the interventions, the investigators incorporated four strategies to increase cultural sensitivity: using the language preferred by the participant, employing visual messages, developing culturally congruent health education content, and selecting educators at ease with sexual topics. Further, they tested whether a specialized program (targeting risk reduction skills and increased self-esteem and control) would be more effective than a traditional program based on AIDS education and community resources. Both intervention groups demonstrated a significant increase in knowledge and a reduction in a number of high-risk behaviors related to unprotected sex.

A second program of research testing AIDS interventions for African American and Latino male and female adolescents has been conducted by John and Loretta Sweet Jemmott (1991, 1992). They found that using a culturally sensitive social cognitive intervention based on the Theory of Reasoned Action was effective in decreasing HIV risk behaviors (Jemmott, Jemmott, & Fong, 1992) and that social-cognitive interventions were more effective than educational (information) interventions alone (Jemmott, Jemmott, Spears, Hewitt, & Cruz-Collins, 1992). Once they demonstrated the efficacy of this type of intervention, they investigated further dimensions of efficacy. They found, for example, that matching the race and gender of the facilitator with the target population did not result in improved results (Jemmott & Jemmott, 1996). However, they reasoned that this lack of effect might be the result of an otherwise culturally sensitive program (in terms of language, teaching modality, and content).

The development of programs using culturally relevant content (as elicited through focus groups) (Schinke, Orlandi, Schilling, & Parms, 1992) have been described. Further, using a program implemented in Botswana, Norr, McElmurry, Moeti, and Tlou (1992) described the kinds of modifications needed when programs are taken to international sites. They discuss how their program was strengthened because it relied on the established indigenous social structure. After conducting community and cultural assessments, the AIDS program used peer education and support groups led by trained community women coordinated by a nurse. This approach was employed because women are considered the key to health and family issues in Botswana.

Cancer Screening

Several lines of investigation have been used to document issues related to cancer screening among various ethnic groups. The majority of these have focused on screening rates (epidemiological) and barriers to screening. Factors that have been found to relate to African American women's lower rates of breast cancer screening behaviors include having other health factors of greater concern than breast cancer, fear of finding cancer (and its social consequences), cost (given competing priorities), a tradition of health seeking for problems (not prevention), and accuracy of knowledge about cancer cause and treatment (Duke, Gordon-Sosby, Reynolds, & Gram, 1994; Nemcek, 1989, 1990; Tessaro, Eng, & Smith, 1994).

Barriers identified for Hispanic (Mexican American) women include structural barriers (lack of knowledge of care facilities and language), lack of knowledge related to signs of cancer, and modesty concerns (Longman, Saint-Germain, & Modiano, 1992; Sugarek, Deyo, & Holmes, 1988), as well as values of *familismo* (which gives primacy to family over individual needs) and *personalismo* (related to lack of engaged, caring behaviors on the part of physicians) (Sennott-Miller, 1994). Additionally, Gonzalez (1990) noted that for low-income Mexican American women's breast self-examinations, self-efficacy was a more salient factor than barriers or

social support. For Chinese women, modesty, lack of need for preventive screening if living a "balanced life," and fears of exploitation were cited as factors diminishing participation in screening for breast or cervical cancer (Hoeman, Ku, & Ohl, 1996). The belief that there is no cure for cancer was also a belief that corresponded with lack of screening among African American men for colorectal cancer (Powe, 1995).

Despite considerable epidemiological information concerning the lower rates of participation in cancer screening by minority persons and the clear identification of barriers, only recently have clinical nursing interventions to increase participation been reported. Three projects have targeted Mexican American women's cancer screening behaviors: the first uses value-expectancy theory to frame an intervention that decreases perceived difficulty in adopting and maintaining behavior (Sennott-Miller, 1994); the second, *Su Vida, Su Salud* (Your Life, Your Health), is a community program to increase screening through the use of role models whose story is featured in media and through community volunteers who give social reinforcement at the local level (Suarez, Nichols, Pulley, Brady, & McAlister, 1993). The third project focuses on recruiting and training minority women to serve as lay health educators to deliver preventive health care information to their peers. These lay health educators have three primary functions: to serve as mediators between minority women and health agencies, to establish a social network, and to offer social support. The ongoing cancer screening intervention was developed by the Arizona Disease Prevention Center and targets Mexican American and Yaqui Indian women (Brownstein, Cheal, Ackermann, Bassford, & Campos-Outcalt, 1992). Two additional projects have targeted Native American women. The first found that health education programs to increase cancer screening among women need to address structures of care and authority as well as providerpatient communication. Health messages need to be wellness oriented and employ traditional methods of education, such as the talking circle, role modeling, and storytelling (Strickland, Chrisman, Yallup, Powell, & Squeoch, 1996). The second intervention positively evaluated the use of talking circles among rural and urban Native Americans in California after this strategy was initiated in four of eight American Indian clinics (Hodge, Fredericks, & Rodriguez, 1996).

Boehm, Schlenk, Funnell, Parzuchowski, and Powell (1995) reported the results of an educational and screening program for prostate cancer designed to increase knowledge and self-efficacy in African American men. Several culturally congruent strategies were employed by this team, including setting the program in churches and relying on African American males both to provide the content and to serve as models in sharing their experiences with prostate cancer and screening. Topics (such as fear of loss of sexuality and lack of trust in the health system) were brought to the discussion groups based on thematic results from prior focus groups. A final project, initiated with the African American community in Pittsburgh, pilot tested four interventions to increase awareness, provide education and early detection opportunities, and overcome barriers. The initial conclusions were that constant presence, cultural sensitivity, and repetition are necessary to overcome the barriers to cancer screening in this community (Robinson, Kimmel, & Yasco, 1995).

Smoking Cessation

Four culture-specific smoking cessation interventions for ethnic groups have been reported by nurse investigators. The first two are large-scale projects mounted by interdisciplinary teams. In the first, Stillman, Bone, Rand, Levine, and Becker (1993) reported results of a church-based smoking cessation program predominantly for African Americans in Baltimore. Employing strategies indicating equal partnership, this intervention, "Heart, Body and Soul," used lay volunteers recommended by pastors to deliver the information and support interventions. Notably, the investigators found that the churches individualized the intervention to make it most suitable to its specific congregation. The second project also used an "indigenous" approach, having trained lay adult Southeast Asian men to deliver the smoking cessation intervention (Chen et al., 1993). They found that an effective combination resulted from health educators identifying scientifically valid health messages and ethnic leaders identifying the mechanisms for delivering the message. For Southeast Asian groups, this resulted in culturally compatible interventions of printing health messages on wall calendars and having community leaders and physicians appear as speakers on videotaped "health commercials." A subsequent project by Wewers, a co-investigator on the previous project, and Ahijevych (Ahijevych & Wewers, 1993) investigated the effects of a low-intensity smoking cessation intervention among African American women. This project compared the results of a low-intensity intervention with a one-time advice-only intervention and a wait list control group. The low-intensity

intervention consisted of weekly mailings of printed materials selected on the basis of their salience as indicated in focus groups with 30 African American women and follow-up phone contacts to provide clarification and encouragement from an African American lay facilitator who had quit through a structured worksite program and had been an ex-smoker for 3 years. Unfortunately, the study design was compromised, as the facilitator was only able to contact 13 of the 20 women in the low-intervention group once and two additional women twice. As a result, the lack of significant findings is predictable. This approach merits further exploration with a more rigorous implementation standard. Finally, Pletsch (1991, 1994) first reported epidemiological findings concerning Hispanic women's prevalence of cigarette smoking and environmental tobacco smoke exposure using the national Hispanic Health and Nutrition Examination Survey (H-HANES) data; she reported that smoking cessation intervention needed to be developed, in particular for Puerto Rican women of childbearing age, and subsequently described "Smoke Free Madres," a smoking cessation study for pregnant Latinas in three cities (Pletsch, Howe, & Tenney, 1995).

Mental Health

In mental health more than in any other specialty area, nursing practice is perhaps most confounded by cultural features. This occurs because of the greater degree of subjectivity of many psychiatric diagnoses and because of the greater degree of cultural overlay in presenting symptoms. Further, the greater stigma often associated with issues of mental disorder among many minority populations delays health seeking. This situation is confounded by the serious issues of practitioner bias in diagnosis that can result from a number of variables, including inappropriate assessment measures for many minority clients, inappropriate interpretation of client behavior, dissonance between practitioner-client communication styles, and a stereotyped approach that biases the diagnostic procedures. This leads, for example, to the well-documented overrepresentation of African Americans as schizophrenic (when diagnosis is made by a White therapist); Euro-Americans are more likely to be diagnosed as having a depressive disorder. Barbee (1992) further discusses the diagnostic biases in research on depression among African American women that result from a contextualization of clinical data.

Flaskerud has addressed many clinical issues in mental health nursing. In 1982, she addressed adapting services for ethnic clients and identified key principles: (a) that comprehensive (holistic) care is preferred to efficiently address multiple health and social problems, (b) that social concerns and problems (time off from work, transportation problems, baby-sitting problems) may need as much intervention as traditional issues in mental health nursing; and (c) the importance of community participation in the planning and publicizing of services. Other elements included use of therapies particularly suited to clients (e.g., brief therapy and support groups rather than insight therapy), use of paraprofessionals, and modifying typical therapist interaction style (to include social amenities such as tea and willingness to accept gifts).

In 1987, Flaskerud proposed a culturally relevant therapy modality for Filipinos and Vietnamese: Somatopsychic Therapy. This approach assumed that the therapists would be bicultural and bilingual and used the term *counseling* to avoid the stigma of the terms *psychiatric* or *mental.* The unique features of this modality included a physical assessment with attention to somatic complaints (in addition to more routine psychiatric and functional assessments). Further, the use of medicines (either psychoactive or OTC) was incorporated as an expected aspect of treatment. The therapeutic approach was problem focused, active, and directive. Family and community support networks were incorporated into the treatment plan.

In 1986, Flaskerud proposed a model of nine major components of a culturally compatible approach in mental health nursing: (a) therapists share the client's culture (ethnic background); (b) therapists share the language or language style of clients (including aspects of self-disclosure and expressive styles); (c) the service is located within the client community; (d) hours and appointments are flexible; (e) referral services are provided for social, economic, legal, and medical problems; (f) family is used in therapy; (g) brief approaches (crisis, situation, or problem focused) are used; (h) there is use of and referrals to clergy and traditional healers; and (i) consumers are involved in determining, publicizing, and evaluating services. Using this framework, Flaskerud empirically investigated the effects of culturally compatible interventions on the utilization of mental health services by minority clients (Mexican American, Anglo, Vietnamese, and Filipino). She found that the most salient features related to extending length of treatment were ethnic and language

match of client and therapist and agency location within the ethnic community. Subsequent investigations by nonnurses found similar results for the test of cultural responsiveness. Specifically, in Los Angeles County, of the thousands of Asian, African, and Mexican clients, Flaskerud found that ethnic match was related to treatment length for all groups and ethnic match was relevant for treatment outcomes for Mexican Americans (Sue, Fujino, Hu, Takeuchi, & Zane, 1991).

A second ethnic-specific (*Ntu*) therapy was described by Campinha-Bacote (1991). Originally described by Phillips in an unpublished paper in 1988, Ntu is based on an Afrocentric worldview (Phillips, 1990). Principles derived from this approach emphasize the seven principles of Kwanza: unity, self-determination, collectivism, economic cooperation, purpose, creativity, and faith. Specific features in the therapeutic milieu include particular attention to the agency environment (e.g., having familiar [ethnic] posters, music, and pictures of heroic persons such as Martin Luther King) and emphasizing the expressive arts in therapy (e.g., ethnomusic therapy).

Barbee (1992) described a program of the National Black Women's Health Project's system of self-help groups. She clearly explained that this was not a therapy group but noted that the group focus on empowerment through self-help and unlearning oppression provided an active coping strategy that may have depression-protective functions. Barbee's point highlights the fact that because many groups stigmatize psychiatric disorder and treatment, there may need to be an effort to advertise or present therapeutic programs as educational rather than psychiatric.

Undoubtedly, the most comprehensive mental health program is the interdisciplinary, 16-year-old project initiated as the Miami Health Ecology Project by anthropologist Hazel Weidman in association with nurse Clarissa Scott and others. This effort originated as an ethnographic project documenting health beliefs and behaviors of five ethnic groups in Miami (Bahamian, Cuban, Haitian, Puerto Rican, and U.S. Black). Subsequently, the project evolved into a community-based mental health program in which seven teams (each working with discrete ethnic communities) served neighborhoods in miniclinics and centralized aftercare facilities. The teams relied on community paraprofessionals who acted as neighborhood workers and "culture brokers." The efficacy of this approach was documented: it had a high case load, low no-show and drop-out rates, high client satisfaction, high goal attainment, and low recidivism (Lefley & Bestman, 1991).

Intervention programs for addictive behaviors have been infrequently described in the nursing literature and evaluated even more rarely. This is rather surprising, given the state of the science in other disciplines. In summarizing data on intervention programs for Native Americans, Silk-Walker, Walker, and Kivlahan (1988) noted that most successful programs for Native Americans include elements of traditional religion and activities to increase Indian identification and promote self-image. These are generally integrated with selected portions of more standard 12-step programs (such as Alcoholics Anonymous). However, they note the lack of controlled studies to document efficacy. These conclusions can be echoed for all other ethnic groups in the United States. A notable exception is Project Hope, a government-funded perinatal addiction treatment program for low-income, predominantly Black, single women. This multidisciplinary treatment program uses a variety of interventions to address the multiple and multidimensional needs of the target population (Nardi & Rooda, 1996). The intensive outpatient addiction treatment includes a therapeutic nursery; individual, group, and 12-step therapy; poetry group; parenting group outreach services; home visits; and primary health care services for clients and families for a period of 3 years. Unique features include daily journaling and directed use of poetry and music. A key feature was the attention to the mother-child relationship and the focus both on the mother and on support for her valuing her child and their relationship. A most interesting point is that the staff noted that some aspects of the program were culture bound (type of acceptable parental discipline), and they describe how they worked within this dissonance. Women participated in the program for an average of 8 months, and 46% left after reaching their individual goals (primarily, staying sober). The program was evaluated as successful when compared with other programs' reported completion and sobriety rates.

Interventions With Chronic Disorders

The issues that accompany clinical nursing with culturally diverse patients having chronic disorders are multilevel. Aspects of symptom presentation, lay belief, illness-related stigma, issues of family control, decision making, and dependence, as well as treatment issues, abound. For nurses, several key issues surround the interventions related to patient education, such as medica-

tion management, diet, and exercise. The following section describes particularly notable efforts related to diabetes and hypertension.

Diabetes

In Canada, Hagey (1984, 1989) described two particularly successful approaches for diabetes health education. In the first, she describes the Native Diabetes Program and the development of stories and the use of metaphors by Ojibway and Cree leaders. The story "Nanabush and the Pale Stranger" was developed to provide an explanation for diabetes, as well as a model for dealing with the illness. Hagey advocated the use of culturally relevant metaphors as a strategy for making meaningful and tolerable that which is feared and avoided, making health information understandable and useful by providing resolution to conflicting systems of beliefs.

The use of folk tales or metaphorical narratives to transmit health concepts was presented by a Seminole tribal physician and adapted by nurses providing diabetes nursing education. Seminole folk tales were adapted, based on initiation stories, origin stories, or animal stories (for Seminoles), and stories were delivered by tribal women. Both of these projects were also presented with all participants seated in a circle to demonstrate the principles of equality and the value in sharing rather than imparting information.

In the second program, Hagey (1989) developed the program "belonging" in concert with tribal leaders. A Native diabetes program was developed for urban Natives in Canada. Key elements of this program included the development of Native-oriented material and community center programming that would help Native peoples with diabetes make positive health decisions and aid in their learning to cope with diabetes. The program developed several metaphors that tapped culturally relevant domains. It also incorporated what was called the "indirect approach," which she contended could best be used by Native persons. Components of the indirect approach include the educator self-presenting as sharing rather than as being an authority; not requiring direct or immediate responses from audience members; establishing ties through relatives, friends, or common locations; use of indirect referencing (e.g., addressing the topic toward "someone who has such a problem might do the following" rather than using a directive approach); incorporating humor during serious discussion to provide a balanced communication; and avoiding confrontation. Although these strategies were proposed as being too subtle for most practitioners, they are quite similar to those proposed for working with Appalachians (Tripp-Reimer, 1982). Consequently, it may rest with the nurse to determine a personal level of competence with this approach and its applicability to the target population. Subsequently, a program modeled on the principles described by Hagey was implemented between five tribal groups in southern Alberta and the regional medical center (MacDonald, Shah, & Campbell, 1990).

Another community-level intervention for diabetes education involved extensive planning with local tribal leaders among the Northern Ute (Tom-Orme, 1988). Multiple strategies implemented included patient and family education, provider education, development of clinical protocols, and increased tribal awareness of diabetes. Lay community health workers were initially employed to assist with transportation of patients and language interpretation between clinic staff and patients; however, their roles evolved into patient educators and cultural liaisons. Strategies to increase community awareness included presenting a culturally acceptable 75-slide educational program on diabetes, public service announcements aired on local Ute radio programs, and placing newspaper articles in local papers. Evaluation during the fifth year of the project demonstrated positive changes in blood glucose control and blood pressure, a fivefold increase in diabetes clinic attendance, and the tribal request to add monthly nutrition education programs. Although there was not a change in the rate of end-stage renal disease, this indicator may be too distal to serve as a good measure of program effectiveness in a five-year period.

As a counterpoint, the single concept approach to diet instruction (eat less sugar, be more active) is more effective with Native Americans than the diet exchange concept (Stegmayer, Lovrien, Smith, Keller, & Gohdes, 1988).

One diabetes education program has also reported outcomes for low-income Hispanic diabetics. It involved collaboration between a neighborhood health center and a school of nursing in the Southwest (Schwab & Simmons, 1989). They devised a project offering two workshops to low-income Mexican American diabetics. The collaboration process used participatory management and incorporated features of Hispanic culture. The workshops were presented in Spanish and included didactic presentation, discussion, and demonstrations. For example, the topic of food preparation included cooking demonstrations. Although there was no formal program evaluation, anecdotal responses were very positive and indicated some changes in diet and exercise patterns.

Hypertension

Culturally congruent hypertension screening and management programs have been described in nursing literature. Bray and Edwards (1991) developed a program that trained and employed Hispanic lay outreach workers, who canvassed Hispanic neighborhoods for blood pressure screening and referral. The outreach workers also provided health education in the home using bilingual health education materials that were left with the clients. This portion of the program was viewed as effective on the basis of subsequent follow-up. A 10-week weight control group was also developed in response to lay requests and was evaluated as moderately successful.

Two projects described by Eva Smith (1989, 1992) delivered hypertension-related health programs to African Americans through Black churches. The underlying assumption of these projects is that the church can serve as a natural support unit to aid in promoting health. In the first project, Smith (1989) reported that having a blood pressure screening service at the church did not, by itself, improve adherence or blood pressure control. In the second project, Smith (1992) prepared six registered nurses from six inner-city Black churches as educational experts who implemented a formal health education intervention. Although the participants demonstrated increased knowledge following the program, they did not show changes in self-reported blood pressure readings and sodium intake after 3 months. The investigator acknowledged that the 3-month period and the self-report data may have contributed to the lack of behavioral effect.

Synthesis of Cultural Intervention Nursing Research

One of the most notable features of the current state of the science related to cultural interventions in nursing is the consistent support for the principles that guided the implementation of the neighborhood health centers in the 1960s as described in the historical overview. These principles mandate, foremost, the involvement of community leaders in the identification of community health needs and in the planning, delivery, and evaluation of health services. They also include locating services within the targeted community to maximize access, offering a broad array of health and social services to increase efficiency and continuity, maintaining a consistent staff, having expanded hours of operation, and emphasizing family and community involvement in the health of individuals. The agency environment will, optimally, be consistent with that of community members with regard to colors, posters/pictures, music, and seating arrangements.

Another common effective approach across clinical areas was the training of and collaboration with lay community outreach workers. Use of these paraprofessionals is often the key to establishing direct cultural links because the CHWs serve as liaisons, bridging biomedicine and the ethnic community. Because they know the language and accepted patterns of behavior, their services are received more readily by the targeted community. Working in collaboration with nurses, the CHWs offer a cost-effective and culturally acceptable approach to delivering health care to underserved populations.

Effective social marketing strategies to publicize health programs and recruit participants or patients include tapping the established social structures and modes of communication. This involves identifying and working through the key social institutions (e.g., Black churches and barber shops) and indigenous leaders or roles (e.g., Black church mothers, Navajo female clan elders, Chinese male clan elders) within each community. Dissemination of information is most effective when delivered through established channels (e.g., Hispanic broadcast radio, ethnic newspapers).

Issues of interpersonal communication have been shown to dramatically affect the acceptability of health programs. The most important aspect here is language. Communication in the language of the client is crucial to effective care. This may occur through bilingual professional staff, lay workers, paid or unpaid translators, or use of special services such as the AT&T Language Line. Other linguistic issues include selecting a direct versus an indirect approach and a confrontive versus a collaborative style. Although the research is clear that matching staff and patient for language is crucial, there are conflicting reports concerning the advantage of matching staff and patients by ethnicity. However, having staff emphasize respect for all persons and maintaining client dignity is imperative. The incorporation of ritual (sharing food, initiating a project with a prayer, or giving symbolic gifts) may also aid in establishing an effective milieu.

In developing health education programs, the content, the teaching modality, and the persons providing information all merit consideration. A common issue with regard to content is that health professionals provide too much detail regarding pathophysiology and too little regarding the daily management of illnesses. It is important to assess patient beliefs and current practices concerning a condition and use that information as a foundation from which to build health education programs. If the health program is broadly implemented, important information from community members can be gleaned in focus groups prior to initiation of the program to target those areas of greatest concern for the target group. Cultural information can be well incorporated here as it relates to the area of health education. For example, if the intervention is nutritional counseling, inclusion of common foods, methods of preparation, and typical units of food measurement are necessary. Effective strategies related to teaching modalities include expanding traditional teaching approaches to incorporate diversity in learning styles. Several specific approaches have demonstrated efficacy, including use of cultural themes and imagery, metaphors, storytelling, or pictures (e.g., *fotonovelas*) to convey health messages; reconfiguration of group structure (e.g., talking circles); and inclusion of target community members as role models or coleaders.

A final important point of consideration is that no single model (either community based or individually focused) fits all ethnic communities or all individuals within a community. Similarly, in using any of these strategies at an individual level, it is important to assess that person's level of ethnic affiliation and acculturation prior to implementation.

Recommendations

In reviewing the state of the science, it is clear that the overwhelming majority of research has been at Levels I and II of the Pyramid of Clinical Relevance (Figure 7.1). This work has often been conducted by nurse-anthropologists or those identified as transcultural nurses. This descriptive work is very important in providing a foundation for practice, but it is not sufficient. Other disciplines (medicine, psychology, public health) have taken the lead in developing cultural interventions for health promotion (e.g., cancer screening, cigarette smoking) and for illness management (e.g., diabetes, hypertension, asthma). They have also figured much more prominently in devising strategies for teaching cultural competence skills (e.g., microtraining approaches). It is time that nursing reestablishes itself as a leader in the planning, delivery, and evaluation of culturally focused interventions.

Over the past 7 years, the National Institute of Nursing Research has provided considerable support to culturally focused projects just now coming to fruition. It is imperative that the results of these projects be widely disseminated. The most fruitful contributions have emanated from nurse scientists with programs of research focusing on particular clinical issues. This approach serves as an exemplar for the discipline.

There are several important areas of cultural intervention and effectiveness research in which nursing could make particularly strong contributions. These include testing innovative health delivery and education programs related to prevention or illness management, determining the ways in which cultural beliefs are linked with actual health behaviors, testing culturally congruent strategies for effective behavioral change, and testing strategies to more effectively tap the natural therapeutic networks within communities. Finally, although considerable effort is given to developing culturally sensitive and competent training programs for nurses, very few of these programs have been evaluated. More study is clearly warranted on methods that are effective in changing the behavior of health practitioners in general and nurses in particular.

References

Affonso, D. (1979). Framework for cultural assessment. In A. L. Clark (Ed.), *Childbearing: A nursing perspective* (2nd ed., pp. 107-119). Philadelphia: F. A. Davis.

Affonso, D. D. (1995). *Malama Na Wahine Hapai*—Community partnerships for prenatal care. *Professional Psychology: Research and Practice, 26*(2), 115-116.

Affonso, D. D., Mayberry, L. J., Graham, K., Shibuya, J., Kunimoto, J., & Kuramoto, M. (1992). Adaptation themes for prenatal care delivered by public health nurses. *Public Health Nursing, 9*(3), 172-176.

Affonso, D. D., Mayberry, L. J., Graham, K., Shibuya, J., & Kunimoto, J. (1993). Prenatal and postpartum care in Hawaii: A community-based approach. *Journal of Obstetric, Gynecologic and Neonatal Nursing, 22*(4), 320-325.

Affonso, D. D., Mayberry, L. J., Inaba, A., Robinson, E., & Matsuno, R. (1995). Neighborhood women's health watch: Partners in community care. *Advanced Practice Nursing Quarterly, 1*(3), 34-40.

Affonso, D. D., Mayberry, L. J., Shibuya, J., Kunimoto, J., Graham, K. Y., & Sheptak, S. (1993). Themes of stressors for childbearing women on the island of Hawaii. *Family & Community Health, 16*(2), 9-19.

Ahijevych, K., & Wewers, M. E. (1993). Factors associated with nicotine dependence among African American women cigarette smokers. *Research in Nursing and Health, 16*, 283-292.

Barbee, E. L. (1992). African American women and depression: A review and critique of the literature. *Archives of Psychiatric Nursing, 6*(5), 257-265.

Barbee, E. L. (1993). Racism in U.S. nursing. *Medical Anthropology Quarterly, 7*(4), 346-362.

Barnes-Boyd, C., Norr, K. F., & Nacion, K. W. (1986, March). *Reachfutures: A community-based approach to improve health of inner city minority mothers and infants.* Paper presented at the Midwest Nurses Research Society annual conference, Omaha, NE.

Barnes-Boyd, C., Norr, N. F., & Nacion, K. W. (1996). Evaluation of an interagency home visiting program to reduce postneonatal mortality in disadvantaged communities. *Public Health Nursing, 13*(3), 201-208.

Bloch, B. (1983). Bloch's assessment guide for ethnic/culture variations. In M. S. Orque & B. Bloch (Eds.), *Ethnic nursing care: A multi-cultural approach* (pp. 49-75). St. Louis, MO: C. V. Mosby.

Boehm, S., Schlenk, E. A., Funnell, M. M., Parzuchowski, J., & Powell, I. J. (1995). Prostate cancer in African American men: Increasing knowledge and self-efficacy. *Journal of Community Health Nursing, 12*(3), 161-169.

Bonaparte, B. (1979). Ego-defensiveness, open-closed mindedness, and nurses' attitudes toward culturally different patients. *Nursing Research, 28,* 166-172.

Boyle, J. S., Szymanski, M. T., & Szymanski, M. E. (1992). Improving home health care for the Navajo. *Nursing Connections, 5*(4), 3-13.

Bray, M. L., & Edwards, L. H. (1991). Prevalence of hypertension risk factors among Hispanic Americans. *Public Health Nursing, 8*(4), 276-280.

Bray, M. L., & Edwards, L. H. (1994). A primary health care approach using Hispanic outreach workers as nurse extenders. *Public Health Nursing, 11*(1), 7-11.

Brown, E. L. (1948). *Nursing for the future: A report prepared by the National Nursing Council.* New York: Russell Sage Foundation.

Brown, E. L. (1961). *Newer dimensions of patient care I: The use of the physical and social environment of the general hospital for therapeutic purposes.* New York: Russell Sage Foundation.

Brown, E. L. (1964). *Newer dimensions of patient care III: Patients as people.* New York: Russell Sage Foundation.

Brownlee, A. T. (1978). *Community, culture and care: A cross-cultural guide for health workers.* St. Louis, MO: C. V. Mosby.

Brownstein, J. N., Cheal, N., Ackermann, S. P., Bassford, T. L., & Campos-Outcalt, D. (1992). Breast and cervical cancer screening in minority populations: A model for using lay health educators. *Journal of Cancer Education, 7*(4), 321-326.

Campinha-Bacote, J. (1991). Community mental health services for the underserved: A culturally specific model. *Archives of Psychiatric Nursing, 5*(4), 229-235.

Chen, Jr., M. S., Guthrie, R., Moeschberger, M., Wewers, M. E., Anderson, J., Kuun, P., & Nguyen, H. (1993). Lessons learned and baseline data from initiating smoking cessation research with Southeast Asian adults. *Pacific Islander Journal of Health, 1*(1), 196-216.

Cross, T. L., Bazron, B. J., Dennis, K. W., & Isaacs, M. R. (1989). *Towards a culturally competent system of care: A monograph on effective services for minority children who are severely emotionally disturbed.* Washington, DC: Child and Adolescent Service System Program (CASSP), CASSP Technical Assistance Center, Georgetown University Child Development Center.

Dobson, S. M. (1991). *Transcultural nursing: A contemporary imperative.* London: Scutari.

Dougherty, M., & Tripp-Reimer, T. (1985). The interface of nursing and anthropology. *Annual Review of Anthropology, 14,* 219-241.

Duffy, S. A., Bonino, K., Gallup, L., & Pontseele, R. (1994). Community baby shower as a transcultural nursing intervention. *Journal of Transcultural Nursing, 5*(2), 38-41.

Duke, S. S., Gordon-Sosby, K., Reynolds, K. D., & Gram, I. T. (1994). A study of breast cancer detection practices and beliefs in Black women attending public health clinics. *Health Education Research, 9*(3), 331-342.

Flaskerud, J. H. (1982). Community mental health nursing: Its unique role in the delivery of services to ethnic minorities. *Perspectives in Psychiatric Care, 20*(1), 37-43.

Flaskerud, J. H. (1986). The effects of culture-compatible intervention on the utilization of mental health services by minority clients. *Community Mental Health Journal, 22*(2), 127-141.

Flaskerud, J. H. (1987). A proposed protocol for culturally relevant nursing psychotherapy. *Clinical Nurse Specialist, 1*(4), 150-157.

Flaskerud, J. H., & Calvillo, E. R. (1991). Beliefs about AIDS, health, and illness among low-income Latino women. *Research in Nursing and Health, 14,* 431-438.

Flaskerud, J. H., & Nyamathi, A. M. (1989). Black and Latina women's AIDS related knowledge, attitudes, and practices. *Research in Nursing and Health, 12*(6), 339-346.

Flaskerud, J. H., & Rush, C. E. (1989). AIDS and traditional health beliefs and practices of Black women. *Nursing Research, 38*(4), 210-215.

Fong, C. M. (1985). Ethnicity and nursing practice. *Topics in Clinical Nursing, 7*(3), 1-10.

Giger, J. N., & Davidhizer, R. E. (1991). *Transcultural nursing: Assessment and intervention.* St. Louis, MO: Mosby.

Gonzalez, J. T. (1990). Factors relating to frequency of breast self-examination among low-income Mexican American women: Implications for nursing practice. *Cancer Nursing, 13*(3), 134-142.

Hagey, R. (1984). The phenomenon, the explanations and the responses: Metaphors surrounding diabetes in urban Canadian Indians. *Social Science Medicine, 18*(3), 265-272.

Hagey, R. (1989). The native diabetes program: Rhetorical process and praxis. *Medical Anthropology, 12*(1), 7-33.

Hodge, F. S., Fredericks, L., & Rodriguez, B. (1996). American Indian women's talking circle. A cervical cancer screening and prevention project. *Cancer, 78*(Suppl. 7), 1592-1597.

Hoeman, S. P., Ku, Y. L., & Ohl, D. R. (1996). Health beliefs and early detection among Chinese women. *Western Journal of Nursing Research, 18*(5), 518-533.

Jemmott, J. B. III, & Jemmott, L. S. (1996). Strategies to reduce the risk of HIV infection, sexually transmitted diseases, and pregnancy among African American adolescents. In R. J. Resnick & R. H. Rozensky (Eds.), *Health psychology through the life span: Practice and research opportunities* (pp. 395-422). Washington, DC: American Psychological Association.

Jemmott, J. B. III, Jemmott, L. S., & Fong, G. T. (1992). Reductions in HIV risk-associated sexual behaviors among Black male adolescents: Effect of an AIDS prevention intervention. *American Journal of Public Health, 82*(3), 372-377.

Jemmott, J. B. III, Jemmott, L. W., Spears, H., Hewitt, N., & Cruz-Collins, M. (1992). Self-efficacy, hedonistic expectancies, and condom-use intentions among inner-city black adolescent women: A social cognitive approach to AIDS risk behavior. *Journal of Adolescent Health, 13*(6), 512-519.

Jemmott, L. S., & Jemmott, J. B. III. (1991). Applying the theory of reasoned action to AIDS risk behavior: Condom use among Black women. *Nursing Research, 40*(4), 228-234.

Jemmott, L. S., & Jemmott, J. B. III. (1992). Increasing condom-use intentions among sexually active Black adolescent women. *Nursing Research, 41*(5), 273-279.

Koniak-Griffin, D., Nyamathi, A., Vasquez, R., & Russo, A. A. (1994). Risk-taking behaviors and AIDS knowledge: Experience and beliefs of minority adolescent mothers. *Health Education Research, 9*(4), 449-463.

Lefley, H. P., & Bestman, E. W. (1991). Public-academic linkages for culturally sensitive community mental health. *Community Mental Health Journal, 27*(6), 473-488.

Leininger, M. M. (1970). *Nursing and anthropology: Two worlds to blend.* New York: Wiley.

Leininger, M. (1977). Culturological assessment domains for nursing practices. In M. Leininger (Ed.), *Transcultural nursing: Concepts, theories and practices* (pp. 86-87). New York: John Wiley.

Leininger, M. M. (1984). Southern rural Black and White American lifeways with focus on care and health phenomena. In M. M. Leininger (Ed.), *Care: The essence of nursing* (pp. 133-159). Thorofare, NJ: SLACK.

Lenburg, C. B., Lipson, J. G., Demi, A. S., Blaney, D. R., Stern, P. N., Schultz, P. R., & Gage, L. (1995). *Promoting cultural competence in and through nursing education: A critical review and comprehensive plan for action.* Washington, DC: American Academy of Nursing.

Lillie-Blanton, M., Parsons, P. E., Gayle, H., & Dievler, A. (1996). Racial differences in health: Not just Black and White, but shades of gray. *Annual Review of Public Health, 17,* 411-448.

Longman, A. J., Saint-Germain, M. A., & Modiano, M. (1992). Use of breast cancer screening by older Hispanic women. *Public Health Nursing, 9*(2), 118-124.

MacDonald, F., Shah, W. M., & Campbell, N. M. (1990). Developing the strength to fight diabetes: Assessing the education needs of native Indians with diabetes mellitus. *Beta Release, 14*(1), 13-16.

MacGregor, F.M.C. (1960). *Social science in nursing: Applications for the improvement of patient care.* New York: Russell Sage Foundation.

Mahon, J., McFarlane, J., & Golden, K. (1991). *De madres a madres:* A community partnership for health. *Public Health Nursing, 8*(1), 15-19.

Mattson, S., & Lew, L. (1991). Culturally sensitive prenatal care for southeast Asians. *Journal of Obstetric, Gynecologic and Neonatal Nursing, 21*(1), 48-54.

May, K. M., Mendelson, C., & Ferketich, S. (1995). Community empowerment in rural health care. *Public Health Nursing, 12*(1), 25-30.

McElmurry, B. J., Swider, S. M., Grimes, M. J., Dan, A. J., Irvin, Y. S., & Lourenco, S. V. (1987). Health advocacy for young, low-income, inner-city women. *Advances in Nursing Science, 9*(4), 62-75.

Meleis, A. I., Isenberg, M., Loerner, J. E., Lacey, B., & Stern, P. N. (1995). *Diversity, marginalization, and culturally competent health care: Issues in knowledge development.* Washington, DC: American Academy of Nursing.

Milio, N. (1967, June). Project in a Negro ghetto. *American Journal of Nursing, 67,* 1006-1010.

Milio, N. (1970). *9226 Kercheval: The storefront that did not burn.* Ann Arbor: University of Michigan Press.

Nardi, D. A., & Rooda, L. A. (1996). The use of a multicultural conceptual model in perinatal addiction treatment. *Journal of National Black Nurses Association, 8*(2), 68-78.

Nemcek, M. A. (1989). Factors influencing Black women's breast self-examination practice. *Cancer Nursing, 12*(6), 339-343.

Nemcek, M. A. (1990). Health beliefs and breast self-examination among Black women. *Health Values: Achieving High Level Wellness, 14*(5), 41-52.

Norbeck, J. S., DeJoseph, J. F., & Smith, R. T. (1996). A randomized trial of an empirically-derived social support intervention to prevent low birthweight among African American women. *Social Science & Medicine, 43*(6), 947-954.

Norr, K. F., McElmurry, B. J., Moeti, M., & Tlou, S. D. (1992). AIDS prevention for women: A community-based approach. *Nursing Outlook, 40*(6), 250-256.

Nyamathi, A., Bennett, C., Leake, B., Lewis, C., & Flaskerud, J. (1993). AIDS-related knowledge, perceptions, and behaviors among impoverished minority women. *American Journal of Public Health, 83*(1), 65-71.

Nyamathi, A. M., Flaskerud, J., Bennett, C., Leake, B., & Lewis, C. (1994). Evaluation of two AIDS education programs for impoverished Latina women. *AIDS Education and Prevention, 6*(4), 296-309.

Nyamathi, A. M., Leake, B., Flaskerud, J., Lewis, C., & Bennett, C. (1993). Outcomes of specialized and traditional AIDS counseling programs for impoverished women of color. *Research in Nursing and Health, 16*(1), 11-21.

Nyamathi, A., & Shin, D. M. (1990). Designing a culturally sensitive AIDS educational program for Black and Hispanic women of childbearing age. *NAACOGS Clinical Issues in Perinatal & Women's Health Nursing, 1*(1), 86-98.

Office of Economic Opportunity. (1968, March). *The comprehensive neighborhood health services program: Guidelines.* Washington, DC: Office of Economic Opportunity, Health Services Office, Community Action Program.

Orque, M. (1983). Orque's ethnic/cultural system: A framework for ethnic nursing care. In M. S. Orque & B. Bloch (Eds.), *Ethnic nursing care: A multi-cultural approach* (pp. 5-48). St. Louis, MO: C. V. Mosby.

Paxton, P., Ramirez, M. C., & Walloch, E. C. (1976). Nursing assessment and intervention. In M. F. Branch & P. P. Paxton (Eds.), *Providing safe nursing care for ethnic people of color* (pp. 148-191). New York: Appleton-Century-Croft.

Phillips, F. B. (1990). NTU psychotherapy: An Afrocentric approach. *Journal of Black Psychology, 17,* 55-74.

Pletsch, P. K. (1991). Prevalence of cigarette smoking in Hispanic women of childbearing age. *Nursing Research, 40*(2), 103-106.

Pletsch, P. K. (1994). Environmental tobacco smoke exposure among Hispanic women of reproductive age. *Public Health Nursing, 11*(4), 229-235.

Pletsch, P. K., Howe, C., & Tenney, M. (1995). Recruitment of minority subjects for intervention research. *Image: The Journal of Nursing Scholarship, 27*(3), 211-215.

Powe, B. D. (1995). Fatalism among elderly African Americans: Effects on colorectal cancer screening. *Cancer Nursing, 18*(5), 385-392.

Robinson, K. D., Kimmel, E. A., & Yasco, J. M. (1995). Reaching out to the African American community through innovative strategies. *Oncology Nursing Forum, 22*(9), 1383-1391.

Ruiz, M. (1981). Open-closed mindedness, intolerance of ambiguity and nursing faculty attitudes toward culturally different patients. *Nursing Research, 30,* 177-181.

Schinke, S. P., Orlandi, M. A., Schilling, R. F., & Parms, C. (1992). Feasibility of interactive videodisk technology to teach minority youth about preventing HIV infection. *Public Health Reports, 107*(3), 323-330.

Schwab, T., & Simmons, R. (1989). Collaboration in action. *Nursing Connections, 2*(1), 35-42.

Sennott-Miller, L. (1994). Using theory to plan appropriate interventions: Cancer prevention for older Hispanic and non-Hispanic White women. *Journal of Advanced Nursing, 20,* 809-814.

Silk-Walker, P., Walker, R. D., & Kivlahan, D. (1988). Alcoholism, alcohol abuse, and health in American Indians and Alaska natives. *American Indian and Alaska Native Mental Health Research, Journal of the National Center, 1,* 65-93.

Smith, E. D. (1989). The role of black churches in supporting compliance with antihypertension regimens. *Public Health Nursing, 6*(4), 212-217.

Smith, E. D. (1992). Hypertension management with church-based education: A pilot study. *Journal of National Black Nurses Association, 6*(1), 19-28.

Stegmayer, P., Lovrien, F. C., Smith, M., Keller, T., & Gohdes, D. M. (1988). Designing a diabetes nutrition education program for a Native American community. *Diabetes Educator, 14*(1), 64-66.

Stillman, F. A., Bone, L. R., Rand, C., Levine, D. M., & Becker, D. M. (1993). Heart, body, and soul: A church-based smoking-cessation program for urban African Americans. *Preventive Medicine, 22,* 335-349.

Storlie, F. (1970). *Nursing and the social conscience.* New York: Appleton-Century-Crofts.

Strickland, C. J., Chrisman, N. J., Yallup, M., Powell, K., & Squeoch, M. D. (1996). Walking the journey of womanhood: Yakama Indian women and Papanicolau (Pap) test screening. *Public Health Nursing, 13*(2), 141-150.

Suarez, L., Nichols, D. C., Pulley, L., Brady, C. A., & McAlister, A. (1993). Local health departments implement a theory-based model to increase breast and cervical cancer screening. *Public Health Reports, 108*(4), 477-482.

Sue, S., Fujino, D. C., Hu, L., Takeuchi, D. T., & Zane, N.W.S. (1991). Community mental health services for ethnic minority groups: A test of the cultural responsiveness hypothesis. *Journal of Consulting and Clinical Psychology, 59*(4), 533-540.

Sugarek, N. J., Deyo, R. A., & Holmes, B. C. (1988). Locus of control and beliefs about cancer in a multi-ethnic clinic population. *Oncology Nursing Forum, 15*(4), 481-486.

Tessaro, I., Eng, E., & Smith, J. (1994). Breast cancer screening in older African-American women: Qualitative research findings. *American Journal of Health Promotion, 8*(4), 286-293.

Tom-Orme, L. (1988). Chronic disease and the social matrix: A native American diabetes intervention. *Recent Advances in Nursing, 22,* 89-109.

Tripp-Reimer, T. (1982). Barriers to health care: Variations in interpretation of Appalachian client behavior by Appalachian and non-Appalachian health care professionals. *Western Journal of Nursing Research, 4*(2), 179-191.

Tripp-Reimer, T. (1984). Cultural assessment. In J. Bellack & P. Bamford (Eds.), *Nursing assessment: A multidimensional approach* (pp. 226-246). Monterey, CA: Wadsworth Health Sciences.

Tripp-Reimer, T. (1985). Expanding four essential concepts in nursing theory: The contribution of anthropology. In J. McCloskey & H. Grace (Eds.), *Current issues in nursing* (pp. 91-103). London: Blackwell.

Tripp-Reimer, T., & Brink, P. (1985). Cultural brokerage. In G. Bulechek & J. McCloskey (Eds.), *Nursing interventions: Treatments for nursing diagnoses* (pp. 352-364). Philadelphia: W. B. Saunders.

Tripp-Reimer, T., Brink, P., & Saunders, J. (1984). Cultural assessment: Content and process. *Nursing Outlook, 32,* 78-82.

Tripp-Reimer, T., & Dougherty, M. (1985). Cross-cultural nursing research. *Annual Review of Nursing Research, 3,* 77-104.

Tripp-Reimer, T., & Fox, S. S. (1990). Beyond the concept of culture: Or, how knowing the cultural formula does not predict clinical success. In J. McCloskey & H. Grace (Eds.), *Current issues in nursing* (3rd ed., pp. 542-547). London: Blackwell Scientific.

Tripp-Reimer, T., & Lauer, G. (1987). Ethnicity and families with chronic illness. In L. Wright & M. Leahey (Eds.), *Families and chronic illness* (pp. 77-100). Philadelphia: Springhouse.

U.S. Department of Health and Human Services. (1985-1986). *Secretary's task force on Black and minority health* (vols. I-VIII). Washington, DC: U.S. Government Printing Office.

U.S. Department of Health and Human Services. (1996). *Healthy people 2000: Midcourse review and 1995 revisions.* Washington, DC: U.S. Government Printing Office.

Warner, A. R. (1978). *Innovations in community health nursing: Health care delivery in Shatage areas.* St. Louis, MO: C. V. Mosby.

Williams, D. R., Lavizzo-Mourey, R., & Warren, R. C. (1994). The concept of race and health status in America. *Public Health Reports, 109*(1), 26-41.

COMMUNITY-FOCUSED INTERVENTIONS AND OUTCOMES STRATEGIES

Joan K. Magilvy
Nancy J. Brown
Patricia Moritz

Traditionally and currently, nursing as a discipline has been in a pivotal role to assist in the development and maintenance of healthier communities. From the activities of our historical foremothers, Nightingale, Wald, Doc, Barton, and many others, to our contemporary colleagues leading the march to community-focused care, nurses have long identified the community as a client of nursing practice, theory, and research. One of the primary professional disciplines involved in community-focused care, nursing is not working in isolation of other professional disciplines. In fact, the success of community interventions depends on the involvement of a variety of health care and other professionals interacting with the cross section of people, cultures, and environments represented in the community. Porter-O'Grady (1997), advocating for nursing leadership to play a major role in developing models and designs for community health, noted that the future of health care depends on the degree to which health professions join in partnership with ethnic communities and community political and social leaders. Nurses working cooperatively with other professional groups such as educators, social workers, recreation leaders, clergy, and law enforcement, as well as a wide range of health care professionals, ensure the success of community-focused interventions and promote interdisciplinary collaborative practice to develop healthier communities.

Although the recent trend to increased community-based health care is not new to nursing, the health of the community is less often emphasized and understood in our discipline than is the health of individuals and families. Many nursing theories avoid the notion of community as the client of nursing practice, but the growing national and international emphasis on community-focused primary health care demands that nursing address this issue (McCarthy et al., 1991).

Health, as applied to a community, must be conceptualized very broadly to fit the diversity of people living and working there. People characterized by multiple ages, ethnicities and cultures, health and illness states, socioeconomic status, occupations, education levels, and housing situations comprise the greater community and define the overall health of that community. To build healthier communities, a new vision of health care is required with a community-based focus toward achievement of human potential, connectedness, and sense of community (O'Malley, 1997). People are beginning to recognize that "health has more to do with factors affecting the broader community than individual lifestyle habits. Whether or not people have livable wages, safe streets, affordable housing, good schools, and a clean and green environment affects the community's health" (Flynn, 1997, p. 1).

Community is an elusive term applied to cities, towns, villages, large urban centers, counties, schools, churches, neighborhoods, barrios, worksites, prisons, and even nations. Community is a multifaceted level of nursing client reflecting a population or collective of individuals. Special populations within a community, including people who are identified as underserved, vulnerable, at-risk, or physically or mentally ill, have traditionally been of particular interest to nursing. Nurses, when focusing on the community as client, include community members as significant actors in activities associated with assessing health needs and with planning, implementing, or evaluating community health strategies. It is the involvement and interaction of community members that enable a synergy of purpose that leads to community-focused health strategies relevant to community needs.

Community-focused interventions and outcomes may be categorized in several ways, depending upon the unit of analysis or target of care delivered in community settings: individuals and families living in the commu-

nity; aggregates, collectives, or segments of populations; communitywide programs; and interventions aimed at the entire community as an entity. In this chapter, *intervention* is defined as deliberate actions carried out by nurses; these actions are selected based on clinical judgment and targeted at the population or community level of client. They are also referred to as community-focused interventions (National Institute of Nursing Research, 1992).

Many nurse scientists refer to classic work by Donabedian (1985) in defining outcomes: changes, either favorable or adverse, in the actual or potential health status of persons, groups, or communities, that can be attributed to prior or concurrent care (Donabedian, 1980). The definitions of outcomes have shifted over time from the more commonly used "four D's": death, disease, disability, and discomfort, to a combination of generic measures such as mortality and morbidity (Hegevary, 1991). Also included in current definitions are disease-specific measures, such as blood glucose level, and patient or client-focused measures, such as satisfaction, functional status, and quality of life (Moritz, 1995). Overall, the major emphasis is on determining clinical results and measuring benefits of nursing practice (Jones, Jennings, Moritz, & Moss, 1997).

Intervening and evaluating quality of health care and well-being at the community level requires inclusion of the broadest range of influencing factors (i.e., health care institutions, schools, religious institutions, social and recreational institutions, economic, cultural, historical, and environmental variables). Development of intervention and outcome strategies must involve the full engagement and participation of community stakeholders, interdisciplinary colleagues, and power brokers who influence the availability of resources necessary to accomplish the goals. Relevance of health strategies to the target community is considered an important factor to successful implementation and evaluation. These factors are considered integral to community-focused nursing practice and research.

The goal of this chapter is to evaluate and synthesize the state of the science related to intervention and evaluation strategies with the community as client. An overview of three pertinent theoretical and conceptual frameworks guiding community-focused practice and research is followed by a discussion of issues that demonstrate the complexity and multifaceted nature of this kind of practice and research. The remainder of the chapter presents several examples of community-focused interventions and outcomes research conducted by nurse scientists and others to highlight the state of the science and provide a basis for recommendations for advancing the science.

Theoretical Perspectives

A variety of theoretical and conceptual approaches have been used in health care practice and research focused on the community or population as client. The principal approaches originated in public health science, community health nursing, community medicine, and sociopolitical sciences. Three primary perspectives have been selected from the multitude of theories and frameworks, based on the belief that these perspectives form a foundation supporting community-focused practice and research.

Primary Health Care: A Foundational Framework

Primary Health Care (PHC) is the principal theoretical approach used worldwide in nursing and interdisciplinary health care practice focused on the community as client. Although definitions of PHC differ, the essential components identified at the 1978 World Health Organization (WHO) Conference at Alma Ata can be found in most descriptions: (a) essential health care focused on primary, secondary, and tertiary prevention in addressing community health needs; (b) integrated health care providing for comprehensive, coordinated, and continuous services to individuals and families; (c) highly accessible health care; (d) multiple entry points and a variety of providers; (e) a partnership between clients (ranging from individuals to the community) and providers that fosters client participation in decision making, strengthens self-care and coping abilities, and promotes growth and change; (f) practiced in the context of family and community; (g) acceptable to the community, promotes community participation at a cost the community can afford (World Health Organization, 1978). A partnership is a necessary component of PHC that facilitates community involvement in nursing and health care interventions at the community level. Partnership is an active process that occurs between health professionals and community stakeholders. Ideally, in forming a community partnership, health professionals join with community members in a mutual project with shared control and direction (Courtney, 1995; Courtney, Ballard, Fauver, Gariota, & Holland, 1996). The underlying assumption is that the

health of the community is directly influenced by interactions among community residents, health professionals, researchers, policy makers, and power brokers. In 1995, the National Institute of Nursing Research (NINR) published a priority-setting document that identifies the coinvolvement of clients and communities as a major element of community-based health care. Nurses, in partnership with clients (the community and its residents), assess the community's health, assist the community in determining health priorities, design and implement health care programs, encourage full community participation, and evaluate outcomes (NINR, 1995).

Epidemiology: A Foundational Methodology

Another model used in community and public health practice is epidemiology, the study of "how various states of health are distributed in the population and what environmental conditions, life-styles, or other circumstances are associated with the presence or absence of disease" (Valanis, 1992, p. 3). Epidemiology is a scientific methodology that is useful in examining the impact of public health control measures, prevention programs, clinical interventions, and health services on the health status of a population (Timmreck, 1994). The primary goals of epidemiology are prevention and the control of disease in populations, resulting in an emphasis on the concept of levels of prevention (Leavell & Clark, 1965). Primary prevention involves halting an occurrence of disease before it happens; secondary prevention is aimed at screening and early detection of health problems; and tertiary prevention is focused on blocking the progression of a disability, condition, or disorder to prevent the need for more advanced care. A variety of research studies and designs are commonly used in epidemiology, ranging from observational to experimental studies and from descriptive to analytical designs. Analytical studies may make comparisons between large aggregates of people (ecological studies) or may relate exposure and disease in the same individuals (relational studies). Many other designs are used in epidemiology to explore multiple causes and effects of health and illness in a population, allowing forecasting, planning, and testing of appropriate population-level interventions. A very quantitative science, epidemiology provides numbers and trends to reflect the health status of a population and is an essential but insufficient tool when used alone in community-focused practice and research. Although this methodology is not used as frequently in nursing research, increased use of this powerful analytic tool would enhance community-focused practice and research.

Action Research: A Foundational Process

Nurses in community-focused practice have traditionally worked with underserved, at-risk, vulnerable, and marginal populations. Intensified by social and political trends, limited economic resources, and health policy, our work with these groups continues. According to Stevens and Hall (1992), "inequitable access to health care resources, economic impoverishment, and unsafe physical surroundings inhibit health behaviors and threaten the safety and well-being" of communities across the United States (p. 2). Nurses and communities can become empowered to recognize social, economic, and political environmental influences on community health and intervene at the community level to effect change and gain control over threatening conditions. Action research, built upon a foundation of critical theories, provides a possible process framework for community-focused interventions and outcomes research. Noting a lack of conceptual clarity and theoretical frameworks to guide nursing practice with communities, Stevens and Hall suggested critical theories as a logical conceptual base for emancipatory practice addressing problems of health care access, economic inequities, environmental issues, and other realities of community life and health.

Although no single critical theory exists, the critical theory perspective originated and gained academic support in the 1920s in Germany. Many schools of thought have contributed to the development of the critical approach, including the Frankfurt School, Marxism, liberation scholarship of developing countries and minority populations, feminist theory, and others (e.g., Freire, 1970; Habermas, 1971). Stemming from resistance movements around the world, the many perspectives of critical theories center around liberation from oppression. Oppression is defined in various ways by people oppressed by a variety of cultural, historical, political, economic, and social conditions. Each liberation movement developed its own critical theory, critiquing the status quo and developing strategies to change the conditions and struggles of everyday life; thus the liberation process was a dialectic of action and reflection (Stevens & Hall, 1992).

The global significance of critical theory, the relationship with oppressed and underserved groups, and full participation and ownership by people within these groups makes a critical theory and action research approach congruent with a primary health care framework and useful for nurses planning, implementing, and evaluating intervention strategies at a community level. Flynn (1984) reflected that primary health care is based on the premise that to produce change in community health involves a community action to create its preferred future. She proposed an action research framework as the way to effect community-generated and -initiated change.

Stringer (1996) defined community-based action research as "a collaborative approach to inquiry that provides people with a means to take systematic action to resolve specific problems . . . favoring consensual and participatory procedures that enable people a) to investigate systematically their problems and issues, b) to formulate powerful and sophisticated accounts of their situations, and c) to devise plans to deal with the problems at hand" (p. 15). This strategy involves the collective mutual participation of all players—the community members; nurses and other health professionals; political, social, and environmental professionals; and others—in a noncompetitive and nonexploitive manner.

Acknowledging the state of the art and science of community-focused practice and the emerging scientific and sociopolitical trends in the United States and worldwide, the theoretical perspectives of primary health care, epidemiology, and action research provide a logical and appropriate foundation for practice and research with the community as client. Nurse scientists may choose to work within one of these or other perspectives, but we believe that a combination of perspectives may provide a more integrated approach necessary to handle an extremely complex practice and research environment. Numerous issues grounded in the realities of communities and populations may impede success in this setting.

Issues Affecting Community-Focused Practice and Research

Prior to discussion of the state of the science in community-focused interventions and outcomes research, several pertinent issues must be addressed. This discussion is focused on issues affecting the nature of the population and setting of community intervention studies, the nature of research questions and designs posed by nurse scientists, and the apparent chasm between scientific integrity and community needs and values.

▄▄▄ *Complexity and Multifaceted Nature of Community Health*

In communities, interaction exists among numerous health, social, economic, and environmental factors on multiple levels from individual to population. Although they do not completely overlap, these interacting factors affect and determine the health of the community at large. The issue is one of complexity in that health is itself multifaceted and cannot be served or studied in isolation. Inclusion of multiple factors and levels of analysis is necessary when planning and conducting community-focused research. Likewise, community-focused research draws strength from the knowledge developed in a variety of academic and professional disciplines, indicating a need for an interdisciplinary, collaborative approach. Recognizing the breadth of our science, the holistic nature of our practice, and the close contact of nurses with communities, it is logical and appropriate for nurse scientists to initiate and lead these research efforts.

The unit of analysis in community-focused research may be the entire community; a population; or segments, groups, or collectives. However, some would believe that nursing science must focus primarily on the individual, family, and small-group levels of analysis; others would argue that community health nursing research would appropriately focus on larger units of analysis or include multiple levels. What then is the responsibility of nursing science in community-focused studies? For the purposes of discussion in this chapter, our focus will remain at the more macrolevel of nursing client—the community, population, or broad segments of population. Recognizing that the responsibility of nursing science could well include multiple levels of analysis, the organization of this book includes numerous chapters on specific health and illness conditions, developmental levels, and client groups. The state of the science related to community-focused interventions and outcomes research is at a somewhat early phase of development, and many conceptual and design issues need to be analyzed. Therefore, this discussion will include identification and examination of several pertinent issues and provide possible paths toward resolution.

Some would argue that nursing research should emphasize only health problems that are amenable to nurs-

ing interventions and that can be measured by nursing-sensitive outcomes. However, in community-focused studies, expertise and knowledge developed by a variety of disciplinary perspectives must come into play. The variables identified and measured may be within the domains of nursing, social work, epidemiology, community medicine, anthropology, sociology, political science, and others. Another question that might be posed is, Does nursing science have a unique contribution to offer community-focused research? The multidisciplinary nature of community interventions might mask individual disciplinary uniqueness.

The core knowledge base of nursing science has long been a blending of theoretical knowledge from a variety of biological or life sciences perspectives, from social and behavioral sciences and from philosophy and the humanities, as well as having a strong grounding in nursing theory and practice. Community health nursing has a foundation in public health sciences, sociology, anthropology, and political science, as well as nursing theory and practice. Nursing science has emerged as a champion of multiple paradigms and methodologies, including quantitative, qualitative, and combined approaches. This stance puts nursing science in a strong position to address the multifaceted, multidimensional nature of community-focused health interventions. We may not have a singular contribution, but the acknowledged expertise of nurse scientists with qualitative research, the strong familiarity of community nurses with the human condition of people in the collective or population, and our understanding of human experiences in communities provide a strong rationale for our unique contributions.

Further complicating community-focused research is the cost and design of these studies. To include the many relevant variables, multiple levels of interventions and analysis, longer time required for completion, and the need to involve community stakeholders, complex planning, designs, and implementation are required. In addition, a systems perspective adds strength to community-focused research (Gruenewald, Treno, Taff, & Klitzner, 1997) by organizing the complexity of factors and levels of analysis needed to complete such studies successfully. It is crucial that researchers identify and address these issues practically. The NINR's (1995) recent publication on community-based research illustrates and reinforces the complexity of this type of research and provides some recommendations for the types of studies needed. Especially highlighted in this publication is the need to target research on rural and urban minority populations. Funding of these studies will most likely need to come from a variety of public, private, local, and national resources. A variety of foundations target specific underserved or vulnerable groups and emphasize development of partnerships between communities and health care systems. Research on these partnerships is limited and a fertile area for study.

Cultural Issues

Community health nurses have always worked with diverse populations, including diversity in ethnicity, culture, race, age, gender, sexual orientation, and geographic location. Research with culturally diverse populations requires attention to several issues, identified in a recent workshop on health behavior research with minority populations (Becker et al., 1992). Five tenets recommended by this group were that researchers must (a) respect the racial, cultural, and ethnic values of the group with whom they are working; (b) know the community; (c) be culturally competent; (d) ensure that the research benefits the community; and (e) involve community participants in the development, implementation, and evaluation, as well as sharing the results with the community.

Being culturally competent means that researchers must integrate an understanding of the community's worldview into all phases of the research study (Becker et al., 1992). The term *cultural competence* is one of many descriptors for this notion; also used are terms such as *cultural congruence, cultural sensitivity,* and *cultural relevance* (Martinez, 1995). Related to this concept is the issue of whether the researcher must be a member of the cultural or ethnic group studied. Insider-outsider status is a concept that has been recognized as significant in a number of areas of inquiry, with both advantages and disadvantages cited. Research teams would be strengthened by inclusion of members of both groups to enable development of "real life knowledge of the experiences of non-dominant cultures," their values, language, mores, and experiences (Zambrana, Hernandez, Dunkel-Schetter, & Scrimshaw, 1991, p. 226). Qualitative research approaches would facilitate development of cultural knowledge and sensitivity and, combined with other quantitative or epidemiological approaches, would enrich the credibility and transferability of findings (Lincoln & Guba, 1985). In addition, use of an action research and critical theories perspective would inform the development of culturally appropriate research strategies to address many of these issues.

Local Relevance and Participation

Consistent with principles of primary health care, the involvement of community members and other stakeholders in the development, implementation, and evaluation of community-focused interventions and research is essential. The project must have local relevance and be acceptable and accessible to the community. Formation of a partnership between health professionals, researchers, and client(s) is an active process with shared control and direction. As part of the Health of the Public Program supported by several private foundations, a workgroup on community health assessment produced a guidebook helpful to professionals working at the community level (Bor, Chambers, Inui, & Showstack, 1995). Researchers were cautioned to attend to building relationships and acknowledging ethical responsibilities. "Ten Commandments of Community-Based Research" were offered:

> Thou shalt not define, design, nor commit community research without consulting the community.
>
> As ye value outcomes, so shall ye value processes.
>
> When faced with a choice between community objectives and the satisfaction of intellectual curiosity, thou shalt hold community objectives to be the higher good.
>
> Thou shalt not covet the community's data.
>
> Thou shalt not commit analysis of community data without community input.
>
> Thou shalt not bear false witness to, or about, members of the community.
>
> Thou shalt not release community research findings before the community is consulted.
>
> Thou shalt train and hire community people to perform community research functions.
>
> Thou shalt not violate confidentiality.
>
> Thou shalt freely confess thyself to be biased and thine hypotheses and methodologies so likewise. (L. Brown, 1995)

The ten commandments provide guidelines for ethical conduct of science in communities; however, developing and maintaining community partnerships is essential and requires time and effort. Institutions or researchers need to make the necessary commitments to ensure a real partnership rather than a partnership of convenience or expediency (Annese, 1995). Development of a partnership is a process used frequently in community nursing practice and research (NINR, 1995). Courtney and colleagues (1996) describe the necessity of making changes in traditional roles, transforming professionals from "chief actors" and clients from "passive recipients" to full partners.

General Design and Methodological Issues

Compared with a research environment in which subjects are individuals, controls are relatively uncomplicated, and probability sampling is readily achievable, community-focused studies require consideration of a variety of different design strategies. The theoretical framework of primary health care emphasizes the inclusion of community stakeholders in planning, designing, and conducting community-focused research. Multiple actors will be engaged in implementing community assessments, interventions, impact evaluations, and maintenance of community linkages, adding to the complexity of this type of research. To address selected community health problems identified by community members or through community needs assessments (e.g., teen pregnancy, HIV infection, access to health care services) requires the use of multiple simultaneous interventions. The research would therefore require multiple, complex design approaches, such as population-based epidemiology, survey research methods, and qualitative ethnography. A team of scientists, public health experts, and community members is necessary to inform, participate in, and monitor the community intervention and to evaluate its impact.

The complexity of this task is evidenced by the limited literature on designing and implementing this type of research. Literature abounds on the importance of community involvement in community-focused interventions research, but literature on methodological approaches to evaluating the impact of these interventions is limited. Acknowledging the depth of nursing expertise in using multiple research methodologies, it is important for nurse scientists to take leadership in designing, planning, and conducting studies of this type. The design and implementation of community-focused research thus requires a variety of strategies, and numerous methodological issues can be identified. In the following discussion, a sampling of several major research design and implementation issues is presented.

Design Issues

As in any other type of investigation, research questions drive the methods, but how does this play out at the community level? The research questions in many com-

munity-level studies concern health needs; effectiveness of potential health-related interventions; effect and quality of these interventions on a population, community, or collective; and transfer of effective interventions to other community settings. Designs bridge qualitative and quantitative perspectives. Using experimental, quasiexperimental, ethnographic, epidemiologic, action research, and case studies, community-focused researchers conduct studies that will lead to more definitive analyses and potential comparisons across settings in cases.

Generalizability and Replicability

Generalizability issues may present difficulty in community-focused research. The unique nature of each community may preclude generalizability to other communities; thus the term *transferability* is suggested as an alternative. The notion of transferability is that the researcher describes methodology and findings in sufficient depth that the reader may make informed decisions about transferring that knowledge to other settings and samples (Lincoln & Guba, 1985). Although one community study would not be sufficient, multiple community studies would provide rich information on which to base transferability decisions. Transferability can be enhanced by careful attention to the specification of all aspects of the research design, such as employing careful field notes, activity logs, and decision trails (Lincoln & Guba, 1985). True replication of studies may not be possible for the same reasons of unique community needs and culture; however, using information and experience gained in previous work would facilitate repeating a study in a new site, making modifications appropriate to, and in consultation with, the new community. If the intervention strategy or model being introduced and examined is specified in detail and benchmarks are determined for implementation stages, repeatability is enhanced. Defining the unique characteristics of the intervention strategy ensure that the influence of the whole and possibly the parts can be measured and repeated. Such specification also enhances the achievement of sufficient strength in the independent variable for its effect to be determined at the aggregate level of analysis. By repeating the interventions in multiple sites, one can increase the ability to transfer the knowledge to additional communities.

Some have indicated that inclusion of community members as nonresearchers sets up an unacceptable contamination in a study. A number of strategies can be used; for example, use of advisory or liaison groups to inform the research and intervention process. Development of subunits of the research team members would also ensure that decision makers and intervention implementers are separated from those who collect data. In a complex community-based prenatal home visitation study conducted with involvement of community member and public health nurses, Olds (1992) and Olds and Kitzman (1993) contracted with a separate research organization to carry out all data collection to address this issue.

Why then should scarce research dollars be used for studies located in one community that may not yield broadly generalizable findings? The answer lies in the ability of the researchers to analyze and interpret data in such a manner that a rich description and understanding of the population, interventions used, implementation process, and the identification of outcomes are provided. This depth would facilitate adaptation of intervention strategies, instruments, and evaluation methods for use in other settings or in future multisite studies. Qualitative research approaches that uncover community values, lifestyles, and environmental contexts can assist with developing thick descriptions, meaning, and critical theories useful for interventions and outcomes research. Therefore, although it is not always generalizable to multiple other populations, community-focused research clearly has value for application beyond the communities studied.

Unit of Analysis

An issue that often arises in community-focused studies relates to the determination of the appropriate unit of analysis for the study—individual to population. In some research, although the individual may be the unit of analysis for data collection, the findings may be applied to the aggregate. To make meaningful comparisons among data, variables must be of the same unit or level of analysis. This situation often creates problems for the researcher because community-level data are not always easy to identify and collect. The temptation is to use data collected from individuals to compare to community-level indexes, resulting in improper comparisons. Data collected from individuals must be collapsed or aggregated into community-level data for accurate comparisons to be made. Variables that are statistically related at the individual level may show little or no relationship when aggregated into larger units as a result of a loss of variability in the data and/or the greatly reduced sample size.

Nurse researchers have explored another relevant problem of unit of analysis. Verran, Gerber, and Milton

(1995) suggested four criteria for examination of data collected at the individual level to assure that data can be aggregated to the group level. Content validity, representativeness, reliability, and validity of the aggregated scores were proposed as indicators of group phenomena. A need for further work in this area is indicated.

Comparison Groups

Comparison groups are useful in many research designs; how is this strategy employed in community-focused research? In communities with many segments of the population, subsampling may be necessary, or multisite studies can contribute comparison samples to evaluate interventions. In a recent study, Ferketich and colleagues (May, Mendelson, & Ferketich, 1995) tested a multilevel community-based nursing intervention to improve the health of rural Hispanics and White, non-Hispanic persons in several small rural communities. The model was based upon three parts: (a) preventive care for individuals and families delivered through nurse-managed clinics, (b) outreach education and follow-up with teams of community health nurses and *promotoras* (lay health workers), and (c) community empowerment activities. One strength of this study was the ability to implement and evaluate locally relevant interventions in each community as well as to compare results across communities, extending the applicability of findings.

In another study, community nurse researchers conducted two separate community analysis studies, identifying racism as a problem in each of the communities, one a rural town and the other a small community near a major metropolitan area (Supples & Smith, 1995). The researchers, comparing findings across communities, were able to describe similarities and differences in the expression of racism, again strengthening the applicability of their research.

In a third study, Affonso, Mayberry, Graham, Shibuya, and Kunimoto (1992, 1993) used contemporaneous state-level data to form a comparison group in the evaluation of outcomes of a culturally sensitive, community-based prenatal intervention strategy. The state-level data vary, but most states maintain sufficiently detailed databases to allow researchers to consider them for use in studies where the unit of analysis is at the community level. Ease of access to these databases varies by state, related to changes over time and changes in leadership in the relevant state agency. When added to data from other comparison groups, the use of state-level data increases the strength of the findings.

Needs Assessments

In community-focused research, interventions are built upon needs identified by community stakeholders; for example, the community's perception of community health status or the need for health care services. Researchers sensitive to community culture work closely with community members to assess problems and strengths; identify and prioritize needs; and plan appropriate, locally relevant interventions (Healthcare Forum, 1994; Stoner, Magilvy, & Schultz, 1992). Conduct of needs assessments is a crucial step in interventions and outcomes research. Congruent with primary health care principles, community needs assessments promote deeper understanding of the community's perspective on health and development of community ownership of planned interventions. Community needs assessments using combined research designs such as epidemiological, survey, and ethnographic approaches have been useful in community analysis studies of rural and urban communities. Examples include the University of Colorado Health Sciences Center School of Nursing's Project GENESIS studies (Barton, Smith, Brown, & Supples, 1993; Magilvy, McMahon, Bachman, Roark, & Evenson, 1987; Schultz & Magilvy, 1988) and the University of Indiana School of Nursing's Healthy Communities/Cities programs (Flynn, Rider, & Bailey, 1992; Rains & Wiles-Ray, 1995; Zagoras & Norris, 1994).

Secondary analysis of data or use of large data sets available from local, state, or national databases might provide useful comparisons of needs assessments in different communities. In a recent needs assessment of communities surrounding a major Superfund cleanup site (described in the State of the Science section later), primary data were collected qualitatively through the use of focus groups and interviews with key and primary informants in each community (Barton & Brown, 1997; N. J. Brown, Barton, & Bjork, 1996; N. J. Brown, Barton, & Clark, 1997). The focus of the interviews was the community's perception of the health risks associated with living near a nuclear weapons cleanup site. Following analysis of the primary data, the nurse scientists compared results to local, county, and statewide morbidity and mortality data to determine the extent to which people's perceptions of risk were verified in the secondary

data. The comparison opportunity provided through use of secondary data analysis lent support to the validity of the qualitatively derived primary data.

Implementation Phases

The close involvement of community stakeholders in community-focused research and the development process of the intervention and identification of outcomes suggests the use of some elements of an action research framework. This research would require a phased approach, with the first phase dedicated to entering the community and initiating the involvement of community members. Next, needs assessments are conducted, with coparticipation of community members and researchers (as previously discussed). Following identification or selection of one or more problems to be addressed, the interventions and anticipated outcomes are planned and specified. During this somewhat time-consuming but important phase, both community members and researchers engage in a process of exploration and decision making. Careful recording of all actions and events is required throughout these beginning phases to document the process and increase the potential for transferability to other communities.

In the fourth phase, implementation begins with ongoing participation and input from community members. In this phase, traditional researchers would recognize the beginning of the actual research (although community-focused researchers have been engaged in research all along). Finally, the interventions are implemented, and process and outcomes research is carried out. This process is not linear and involves ongoing dialogue with key participants or stakeholders and multiple feedback loops.

Internal Validity Issues

An important step in moving from intervention to research is identification of *benchmarks*, markers that indicate the accomplishment of various elements of the intervention. The benchmarks may be viewed as indicators that the process is leading to full implementation of the intervention. The next steps would entail identifying indicators of the previously determined outcomes and appropriate measures. When testing interventions and treatments in a community, it is important to specify the interventions, to determine anticipated effects, to show when interventions are in place, and to consider how to measure the effects. Specification of the intervention is achieved at the onset of study design and is crucial to the integrity of the study as well as data analysis. Determining the anticipated effects of an intervention can be achieved by pilot studies in localized geographic areas or other samples smaller than whole communities. In this case, the proposed study should be on a small scale, perhaps a single town or county. Showing when the intervention is in place requires dissecting the intervention into its component parts (benchmarks) and determining ways to identify when the parts are in place in the community. Benchmarks could assist with evaluating diffusion of the intervention (Rogers, 1995). Milton, Verran, Gerber, and Fleury (1995) described this process for acute care; however, the same process could easily be used for community-level research because in both cases the focus is on the intervention and its subcomponents. Measuring the effect of the intervention at the community level can be accomplished by using measures that are specific to the problem at which the intervention is aimed. It is important that the intervention is sufficiently strong to be evident in aggregated data. Pilot work could assist in clarifying this issue.

A factor important in intervention research with communities is knowing if the planned intervention is sufficient or whether modifications or other strategies will be needed to meet the community's objectives for the intervention. Designs that include cross-sectional and longitudinal approaches can be helpful in monitoring the influence of intervention implementation on planned outcome measures.

Measurement Issues

From a measurement perspective, few community-level assessment instruments appropriate for examining health and social issues at the aggregate level are available. Problems in measurement are similar to problems inherent in any type of clinical research; for example, unit of analysis issues, use of clinical diagnostic tools for outcomes assessments, and psychometric issues. In community-focused research, some instruments exist for community or aggregate assessment (e.g., the PRECEED model of Green, Kreuter, Deeds, & Partridge, 1980, and APEX, from the National Association of County Health Officials, 1991). More limited are instruments appropriate for outcomes assessment and evaluation. Rohrer (1996) described the Health Assessment Survey, designed for use with rural and urban populations; however,

psychometric properties and usefulness for outcome measurement were not clearly explicated. Numerous frameworks exist for the study of community needs, but the development of appropriate, psychometrically sound instruments useful in community-focused research is required.

Access to health care is an important factor in community-level interventions and important to measure (Institute of Medicine, 1993). Anderson and Davidson (1996) identified six types of access: potential, realized, equitable, inequitable, effective, and efficient. Each is measured in terms of factors that hinder or facilitate the use of health services. It is frequently assumed that community-level interventions provide access to their target populations, but that is only known if access is measured. This is accomplished by identifying specific community targets of the intervention, developing strategies to reach them, and measuring the effects.

Measurement of the impact of community-level interventions requires the consideration of the full complexity of quality evaluation strategies. Such interventions are initiated through community involvement that must be documented and categorized for later analysis. Interactions between community factors and the community intervention may be expected to occur and thus should be considered in design and measurement. A combined qualitative-quantitative design with measures and data points appropriate to the intervention and to the community will most likely provide the richest data for analysis. The structure, processes, content, and expected outcomes of the community intervention should be systematically documented and analyzed and intervening factors considered and documented as they are identified. Outcomes can be assessed through several approaches: (a) use of generic outcomes such as morbidity and general functional status that are easily applied across a population; (b) condition-specific outcomes such as clinical or functional status for a particular diagnosis that easily links to care delivery but are less easily linked to entire populations without substantial investment; and (c) sentinel or adverse events such as emergency room usage, suicide, or low birth weights. Such measures can be designed specifically for the community study or adapted from those described in the literature.

Wilkin, Hallam, and Doggett (1992) have provided a lengthy discussion of measures useful in primary health care. Their discussion of multidimensional measures provides some guidance when considering which outcome measures to use at the community level. These measures are applied at the individual level and can yield profiles of individuals that can be aggregated into profiles at the community level. Verran and colleagues (1995) discussed aggregating individual-level data to the group level. Measures that can be universally applied would be beneficial but are not feasible given the range of health problems and varying degrees of severity occurring in a community. Multidimensional measures give the investigator the advantage of incorporating physical, psychological, and social components in a single instrument. Multidimensional measures are of three general types: those that are general purpose, such as the Medical Outcomes Study (MOS) Short Form Health Survey; those designed specifically for primary health care, such as the Duke-University of North Carolina Health Profile; and those devised as global health indexes used in service planning, resource allocation, and evaluation, such as the Quality of Wellbeing Scale (Wilkin et al., 1992).

Sampling Issues

In community-focused research, sampling can be accomplished at the aggregate or individual level, depending on the methods and analyses planned. However, in community-focused research, where community stakeholders are involved in planning, conducting, and evaluating interventions, specific sampling issues of privacy, insider knowledge, dual participation, and sample recruitment and selection emerge. Communities are public places, in which people may know each other well and privacy may be compromised. This issue is especially relevant to rural communities or small neighborhoods. Researchers may be insiders themselves, leading to possible coercion or loss of objectivity.

The gold standard for clinical research is the randomized clinical trial with probability sampling. Is this possible in community-focused studies? Although clinical trials are used primarily in research with individuals, some strategies from these studies may be useful. Probability sampling techniques such as stratified random sampling and cluster sampling can be used in large populations; for example, in telephone and mailed surveys. However, when a subjective perspective is needed, qualitative research methods are most appropriate, and nonprobability approaches such as purposive, snowball, or convenience sampling strategies would be employed. Quota sampling might also be used to increase the likelihood of achieving appropriate distribution of persons with specific characteristics, such as ethnic minority

groups. Studies with combined designs would, therefore, use multiple sampling techniques.

Creative sample recruitment strategies might be employed, such as the use of community newspapers, newsletters, person-to-person solicitation, phone banks, and involvement of key opinion leaders (e.g., clergy, political figures, teachers, and health care professionals). Stratification of the population or setting may also be required to address different community characteristics. Environmental variables, such as rural and urban, presence of environmental hazards, or agricultural risk factors, present one type of stratification. Another type would reflect characteristics of the people, such as culture, ethnicity, values, and mores. Local history and geopolitical issues may present further indications for stratification. These strategies may represent a different path from traditional research approaches with individuals and small groups.

Analysis Issues

The methodological and analytical techniques used in community-level research are those used in any complex clinical study borrowing from epidemiology, health services, and nursing research. The field of health services research, grounded in public health science and statistics, has been concerned with discovering explanations for and resolution of variations in practice, cost, and quality differences (Sechrest, Perrin, & Bunker, 1990). Use of a health services research (HSR) approach may assist in the development of community-focused research strategies. Health services research methods texts provide discussion of methods to explicate causality in aggregated data of a nonexperimental nature (DeFriese, Ricketts, & Stein, 1989). A discussion of these strategies is beyond the scope of this chapter.

Some techniques useful in studies with individuals may be adapted for community-focused research. Multiple regression has been used in program evaluation to address specific methodological problems. For example, in the channeling studies of community-based long-term care as a substitute for institutionalization (R. S. Brown, 1988), regression techniques were employed when different data collection procedures were used, high attrition rates occurred, different individuals were surveyed (caregivers vs. patients), or proxies were used to provide information. Multiple regression analysis provided a means by which the impact of the interventions and effects of methodological differences or problems could be measured and explained.

Analysis of qualitative data on a communitywide scale also presents problems for investigators. Barton and colleagues (1993) identified a number of data analysis issues that arose during a series of community analysis studies conducted by faculty and students at the University of Colorado Health Sciences Center School of Nursing. These issues related to coordinating large volumes of data, large numbers of interviews, and a large number of interviewers; disagreements with interpretations of data among community members representing different stakeholder groups; disagreements between the researchers and community regarding what constitutes a community health problem; and difficulty in correlating the secondary data analysis with primary data analysis when the analyses conflict with one another.

In conclusion, although a number of pertinent issues related to the conduct and evaluation of community-focused practice and research have been discussed, a myriad of issues remain. We have discussed several issues from a scientific framework and provided evidence that many of the problems can be resolved. Conducting community-focused research requires attention to the delicate balance of competing demands of scientific and community interests. Why would individual or collaborating researchers choose to conduct this type of research in light of the multiplicity of issues discussed? Community-focused research is critically needed as the public becomes more aware of the relationship between community, environment, and personal health. Grassroots efforts toward health care reform indicate the impatience of the public to "get on with" the process of developing accessible and affordable health care services within their communities and their demands to be partners in this effort. The responsibility of nurse scientists and our colleagues is to design research that supports and evaluates the process and outcomes of community-level interventions.

State of the Science: Community-Focused Interventions and Outcomes

Research on the community level of client is in an early phase of development, yet a number of intervention studies have been conducted. In this section, we have selected several exemplars of community-focused interventions and outcomes research to demonstrate the state of the science in this area. Most of the studies have been conducted by nurse scientists, but some researchers outside the discipline have been included to expand the possibilities for future research.

Healthy Cities/ Communities Programs

The Healthy Cities/Communities programs currently being implemented in over 150 communities in 25 states and more than 1,500 communities worldwide are an outstanding example of a community-focused intervention following the principles of primary health care and related to the WHO movement of health for all by the year 2000 (Zagoras & Norris, 1994). Beginning in Toronto, Canada and spreading globally, the U.S. Healthy Communities initiative was stimulated by the National Civic League and the U.S. Department of Health and Human Services, Office of Health Promotion and Disease Prevention. A parallel program working with the WHO Healthy Cities Collaborating Center at Indiana University is under the direction of Dr. Beverly Flynn, a nurse scientist. The Healthy Cities/Communities programs work closely with other national and statewide organizations, such as the Healthcare Forum and the Colorado Trust (Flynn, Rider, & Bailey, 1992; Flynn, Rider, & Ray, 1991; Zagoras & Norris, 1994).

To form a foundation for Healthy Cities/Communities projects, the Healthcare Forum (1994) conducted a national telephone survey of 1,000 Americans to examine issues of community health, health care reform, quality of life, and community leadership. Respondents identified several determinants of a healthy community, including (in order of importance): low levels of crime and child abuse, public safety, good schools, strong family life, high environmental quality, healthy economy, excellent race relations, low teenage pregnancy, low homelessness, low infant mortality, and affordable housing. The terms "healthy community" and "community quality of life" were used interchangeably by respondents. A lack of trust in existing government and community leaders and desire for change in the health care system were identified. The researchers reported that the public is ready to participate proactively in the health of its communities; however, a need was indicated for education in community health problem solving and for a collaborative model of community leadership.

The Healthy Cities Indiana program is a community development collaborative effort of the Indiana University School of Nursing, the Indiana Public Health Association, and six Indiana cities. In this community-focused intervention, nurse scientists and their health professional colleagues are engaged in developing community leadership, assisting communities in program implementation and evaluation, and identifying outcomes indicators (Flynn, Rider, & Bailey, 1992). Long- and short-term indicators include changes in health status, community leadership development, and development of appropriate health policies. In addition, subjective methods (not described in detail in available literature) are used to observe process and the effects of the interventions. The program, now called Citynet Healthy Cities, supported in part by the W. K. Kellogg Foundation, is an excellent beginning toward development of community-focused interventions with full local participation and leadership (Rains & Wiles-Ray, 1995). A need is indicated for further development of research strategies to evaluate the process and outcomes of these efforts.

The Colorado Healthy Communities Initiative (CHCI), funded by the Colorado Trust, was established to develop local community-based programs for improvement of health and quality of life (Zagoras & Norris, 1992). Selected communities participate in a 1-year planning phase and a 2-year implementation phase, facilitated by the trust and the National Civic League. Competitive funding is then offered for implementation of health promotion projects related to Healthy People 2000 objectives. Noteworthy about the CHCI are the core premises: broadly defined health and community involvement, and the guiding principles, including shared values and vision, systems change, linkage of community initiatives, local definitions of community, measurement and benchmarking performance, building assets and capacities, and fostering collaborative leadership and decision making.

Each community first undertakes a community-specific assessment process, creating a localized Healthy Community Index. A manageable number of easily understood indicators are identified for the index, which is also used for future comparisons and benchmarking goals. Community strengths and weaknesses are identified and the community's civic infrastructure evaluated using the Civic Index (Zagoras & Norris, 1992). Following an action research process, the community stakeholders then identify key performance areas (KPAs) to prioritize action plans and strategies related to broadly defined

community health and quality of life. Examples of KPAs developed in the initial project cycle included strengthening families, building community leadership capacities, adolescent health, regional land use, and sustainable economic development. In the subsequent action phase, community stakeholders select and implement a few carefully selected initiatives, track progress, make changes as necessary, and evaluate their community development efforts. Evaluation efforts are ongoing, facilitated by periodic meetings of leaders in the selected communities to share experiences and ideas. Although the CHCI program is not being conducted by nurse scientists, in many communities public health nurses and other nurses are actively involved as stakeholders and leaders. Nurse scientists planning community-focused interventions and outcomes research would be well informed by the action research process developed in this program.

An example of community-focused nursing action research was reported by Rains and colleagues (1995). This participatory action research project was conducted in one of the Healthy Cities Indiana (Citynet Healthy Cities) communities (Flynn, Rider, & Ray, 1991). Working with the New Castle, Indiana Healthy Cities Committee, a multisectorial group of volunteers representing community segments such as health care, arts, business, education, labor, finance, and government, the nurse scientists assisted with community development, volunteer training, access and interpretation of Census data, survey research design, and data analysis. They viewed their role as developing community health leadership and community empowerment. Public health nursing professionals consider community empowerment essential for primary community health care; they emphasize a broad base of community leadership working closely with health professionals to develop a healthy, competent community (Eng, Salmon, & Mullan, 1992). Rains and colleagues (1995) assisted the community in interpretation of health statistics leading to the observation of higher-than-expected death rates, especially for heart disease and cancer. The community was also noted to have a high proportion of older adults. Following analysis of a community health survey examining health behaviors and lifestyle, a community action process was planned. Five viable projects were narrowed into one "winnable" issue: smoking policy and prevention. Multiple strategies in collaboration with numerous community groups are being implemented and will be evaluated over time. The authors recommend the participatory action research (PAR) process as a means of empowering local stakeholders and increasing community competence for health problem solving.

Community Analysis Research: Project GENESIS and Community Needs Assessments

Community analysis and needs assessments can be both assessment and intervention tools when used in partnership with communities to plan community-focused health care and community development activities. At the University of Colorado Health Sciences Center, a model of community analysis sometimes referred to as the GENESIS (general ethnographic nursing evaluation studies in the state) model has been implemented with graduate students and faculty since 1979 in over 25 communities (Barton, Smith, et al., 1993; Stoner et al., 1992). The model combines quantitative and qualitative research methods to assess health status and needs and recommend community interventions. The model is based on a recognition that community health is influenced by a variety of factors (e.g., physical, environmental, recreational, educational, political, social, and spiritual factors, as well as health care, social, and other community resources).

Methodologically, the model includes gathering and secondary analysis of existing epidemiological, census, historical, and other data about the community; conducting descriptive community surveys such as APEX; gathering of ethnographic data from key and primary informants or participants who describe the community and its health from their lived experience perspective; and ethnographic participant observation and interviews with persons living and working in the community. Secondary analysis of existing data, analysis of survey data, and ethnographic or thematic analysis of qualitatively generated data are synthesized in a full analysis and interpretation of themes; identification of community strengths, health problems, and concerns; and recommendations derived from the analysis (Barton, Smith, et al., 1993; Magilvy et al., 1987; Stoner et al., 1992).

The model can be used to analyze the health of an entire community, such as a rural town, Native American reservation, a small city, or a distinct neighborhood within a larger city. It can also be useful for analyzing the health needs of aggregates, groups, or organizations, such as adolescents in a high school, a church congregation, older adults served by a community center, or the area surrounding a primary care facility. When a GENE-

SIS-type community analysis study is conducted, the full participation and partnership with the designated community is essential. A variety of community participants is an integral part of study planning and implementation; for example, community leaders and residents, health and social service professionals, clergy, education and recreation leaders, youths, and older adults may be part of the process.

This model of community analysis and health needs assessment produces written and verbally presented reports to the community, incorporating community member feedback and, often, numerous photographs, as well as findings illustrated with rich quotations and descriptions. The reports are useful in the planning and implementation of primary, secondary, and tertiary prevention programs, community development, and grant-writing activities. At the University of Colorado Health Sciences Center, faculty and students have conducted several analyses across several community analysis study sites to identify specific problems such as the health needs of aging populations (Schultz & Magilvy, 1988) and racism (Supples & Smith, 1995). Several methodological issues common to this exploratory and evaluative type of research were discussed in the previous description of analysis issues. Other issues, such as novice researchers and their naive approach or fear of interviewing strangers, handling conflicting research findings, insider versus outsider views, and ways to facilitate study rigor, were identified. Overall, the model was found to be robust for identifying community health needs and educating nursing graduate students to take a leadership role in this area (Barton, Smith, et al., 1993). The model was later adapted for use in a major, federally funded assessment of a Superfund clean-up site, described in the next section.

Rocky Flats Community Needs Assessment

The Rocky Flats Community Needs Assessment was a study designed and implemented by faculty (Drs. Nancy Brown and Judith Barton) from the University of Colorado Health Sciences Center School of Nursing (UCHSC/SON) Division of Community, Health Systems and Policy, in partnership with the Division of Community Health Services of the Jefferson County Department of Health and Environment (JCDHE). An ad hoc task force of stakeholder groups, concerned individuals, and representatives of the State Department of Public Health and Environment, in addition to the university faculty and the local health department, petitioned the United States Department of Energy (DOE) to fund a community-based assessment of the communities adjacent to Rocky Flats. The goal of the study was to explore community members' health and safety concerns and needs during the clean-up of contamination at the Rocky Flats Environmental Technology Site (formerly the Rocky Flats Nuclear Weapons Plant) and to provide direction to the DOE as they designed and implemented health studies and programs during the clean-up.

The target community in this needs assessment was identified as the population living and working within a five-mile radius of the perimeter of Rocky Flats. A sample of 233 individuals from this population participated in either a key informant or a primary informant interview or focus group session and completed a demographic profile. A semistructured interview guide, developed by members of the ad hoc task force, was used for data collection. Data collection was carried out by community health nursing graduate students from the UCHSC/SON and by public health nurses from the JCDHE who were trained in data collection techniques by Drs. Brown and Barton. Information obtained and analyzed from these sources reflected community members' perceptions, attitudes, and beliefs regarding living or working in the shadow of Rocky Flats. In addition, historical data; media accounts of on-site activities; and mortality, morbidity, vital statistics, health status, and census data were collected on the target community.

To provide a framework for organizing the data collected in the needs assessment, an advanced triangle of epidemiology was used (Timmreck, 1994). This model recognizes the complexity of factors represented in the host, agent, and environment interaction and suggests that a change in any one of the components can alter an existing equilibrium to change the disease patterns. For purposes of this needs assessment, the host was defined as the community at risk for potential harm from the clean-up process at Rocky Flats. Agents of harm were defined as the perceived risks to the host. Environment was defined as factors, both positive and negative, that affect the interaction between the host and agents of harm.

Using data analysis worksheets prepared by Brown and Barton (N. J. Brown, Barton, & Bjork, 1996), each data collector coded his or her own recorded interview data, looking for noteworthy quotes, important ideas or themes, and inclusive "big ideas" (Kruger, 1994). Data collectors met as a total group for two 3-hour data analy-

sis sessions to review and compile the data. In the first session, convergent big ideas or themes were identified and categorized according to the framework of host, agent, and environment. During the second data analysis session, overall themes that were consistent across host, agents of harm, and environment, and across primary and secondary data sources, were identified. Outlier ideas were examined and included as appropriate in the final analysis.

The eight themes that emerged from the data were categorized as issues or problems related to (a) inaccessible, not understandable, and/or unreliable information and communication; (b) a lack of trust resulting from a lack of governmental and/or contractor accountability; (c) a lack of knowledge of an emergency plan and preparedness; (d) concerns about land development in neighborhoods around the site and on the site itself; (e) concerns about the impartiality and adequacy of environmental and health monitoring in the area; (f) fear of potential hazards related to the movement or storage of hazardous materials both on and off site; (g) feelings of social, emotional, financial, and physical vulnerability; and (h) perceptions of risk to personal health—in particular, cancer, birth defect, and general illness—related to living or working close to Rocky Flats.

A number of recommendations for action were developed and forwarded to the DOE, the site contractor, the Citizens Advisory Board, and other interested groups and individuals. They included (a) that the DOE fund a public information officer position, with a budget supporting outreach activities, to be jointly shared by and responsible to the Jefferson County Department of Health and Environment and Boulder County Health Department; (b) that the DOE continue (partial) funding of the cancer and birth defects registries and the Historical Public Exposure Studies at the Colorado Department of Public Health and Environment and expand these efforts to include support for epidemiological studies in the communities affected by Rocky Flats; (c) that a citizen oversight process be established to review the adequacy of environmental monitoring and to compare data from monitoring sources with disease rates in affected populations; (d) that there be a moritorium on building and other development in the area adjacent to the buffer zone until such time as the land is proven to be suitable for unrestricted use; and (e) that the DOE fund an ongoing community-based initiative to facilitate community input into the Rocky Flats clean-up process, continue the documentation of community members' concerns, solicit community member oral histories for archival records, and develop an outreach educational program that uses community members as the educators.

Most of the recommendations remain under review at this time; however, the Citizens Advisory Board has contracted with an outside, independent organization to review and assess the current environmental monitoring system at the site. Depending on the outcome of this review, a decision will be made regarding the establishment of an ongoing citizen oversight process. In addition, the DOE has contracted with Brown and Barton to formalize their needs assessment process in a guidebook to be used by other Superfund clean-up sites.

A Community-Focused Intervention Model: Parish Nursing

Consistent with a tradition of community and public health nursing's focus on healthier communities and environments and the provision of care to diverse populations in nontraditional settings, parish nursing is another emerging nursing practice model (Magilvy & Brown, 1997). Parish nursing is a community-based nursing practice set in communities of faith (i.e., churches, synagogues, temples, mosques, and other faith communities, referred to as "parishes" in the literature of this emerging area of practice). Founded on principles of primary health care, parish nursing facilitates community partnerships and is responsive to holistic health care needs of people of all ages who congregate in a specific self-defined intentional community, a place where they live, worship, and feel comfortable and safe in discussing health concerns (N. J. Brown, Congdon, & Magilvy, 1996).

Parish nursing practice involves health education, health assessment, counseling, referral, and support to members of a faith community congregation, and sometimes beyond to the community at large, promoting health and well-being, lifestyle change, improved access and use of health care services, increased involvement in and satisfaction with health care, and improved quality of life (McDermott & Burke, 1993). Part of the pastoral care team of the faith community, parish nurses provide care management and serve as a personal resource to families in crisis, as well as being a liaison between congregation and community (Magilvy & Brown, 1997). Parish nursing and other health ministry practices exist in thousands of faith communities in the United States and worldwide; still, research, especially outcomes studies, is limited. A need exists to identify appropriate com-

munity and/or population level, congregation level, and individual and family outcome measures to evaluate the effectiveness of parish nursing and compare it to community and national health standards (McDermott & Burke, 1993).

Other Studies of Culturally Diverse Populations

This chapter would not be complete without discussion of several excellent nursing research investigations of interventions and outcomes for specific, culturally diverse populations. Many of these studies are described in other chapters in this handbook, but Affonso, Jemmott, McFarlane, Harrell, and Lorig have produced exemplary investigations related to the community and population-focused emphasis of this chapter. The reader is referred to Affonso and colleagues (1992, 1993), who studied culturally sensitive prenatal care interventions in Hawaii; Jemmott and colleagues (Jemmott, 1993; Jemmott & Jemmott, 1991, 1992; O'Leary & Jemmott, 1995), who studied health risk behaviors and HIV/AIDS and STD prevention in community-dwelling low-income African-American teens and adults; McFarlane and colleagues (Mahon, McFarlane, & Golden, 1991; Rodriguez, McFarlane, Mahon, & Fehir, 1993) who conducted intervention and action research to improve prenatal care for women in one Hispanic neighborhood; Harrell and colleagues (Harrell & Frauman, 1994; Harrell et al., 1996), who studied use of knowledge and exercise interventions with rural and urban children in North Carolina to reduce cardiovascular risk factors; and Lorig and colleagues (Gonzalez, Stewart, Ritter, & Lorig, 1995; Lorig, 1996; Lorig & Holman, 1993; Lorig et al., 1996), whose program of research involved community-based interventions and outcomes for persons with multiple chronic conditions, emphasizing culturally sensitive measures and outcomes for Hispanic persons.

Advancing the Science: Recommendations for Further Research

Several recommendations arise from this examination of theories, methodological and practice issues, and state of the science in community-focused interventions and outcomes research. Recognizing the value and importance of this area of inquiry to nursing and health care practice, our primary recommendation is to continue and expand community-focused research. To accomplish this goal, nurse scientists must develop expertise to become increasingly involved in this complex and interdisciplinary research focus. The volume of research in this area must be expanded, and methodological studies will be an integral part of this process as well as investigations focused on a variety of populations and health concerns. To facilitate these efforts, we recommend that both private and public funding agencies expand their foci and acknowledge the importance of community-focused research when setting priorities for funding.

We call for additional interventions studies, methodological studies, and identification of appropriate, relevant, and culturally sensitive outcomes indicators and measures. We recognize that interventions research inclusive of multiple levels of analysis and environments, and participatory in nature, will be expensive in time, money, and other resources. This type of inquiry also requires expanded scientific and community expertise as well as development and nurturing of strong community partnerships. We need to increase the numbers of nurse scientists prepared to develop methodological expertise and conduct complex, multifaceted studies along with their colleagues in public health and epidemiology, health services research, and social, administrative, and policy sciences. We need to join with these disciplines as well as community partners to identify indicators and measures that are appropriate, relevant, and sensitive to the diverse populations comprising our global community.

Finally, we recommend that nursing faculty in doctoral education programs examine curricula to increase or develop content in epidemiology, health services re-

search, health care environments and contexts, and policy analysis and development. Preparing a cadre of nurse scientists skilled in community-focused inquiry should be a primary goal of nursing education for the future.

Conclusions

In this chapter, we have emphasized community-focused research as a valued and important role of nurse scientists congruent with the trend toward population and community-focused health care. We addressed the complex, interdisciplinary nature of community-focused research and offered three potential theoretical perspectives—primary health care, epidemiology, and action research—as guiding frameworks consistent with the principles of community-focused investigations. The complex, multifaceted nature of community health led to the identification of a number of issues in need of consideration in community-focused practice and research; several issues discussed were related to the culture, environment, and setting contexts of the project. Design and methodological issues were identified, and strategies were offered to improve the success and rigor of the studies. An overview of the state of the science in community-focused interventions and outcomes studies was presented, highlighting a number of excellent projects initiated or led by nurse scientists. Finally, several recommendations were offered for further research in this essential and emerging area of nursing science. We believe that the body of existing research, although a commendable initial effort, indicates the potential for further evolution of scientifically rigorous and collaborative community-focused inquiry.

References

Affonso, D. D., Mayberry, L. J., Graham, K., Shibuya, J., & Kunimoto, J. (1992). Adaptation themes for prenatal care delivered by public health nurses. *Public Health Nursing, 9*(3), 172-176.

Affonso, D. D., Mayberry, L. J., Graham, K., Shibuya, J., & Kunimoto, J. (1993). Prenatal and postpartum care in Hawaii: A community-based approach. *Journal of Obstetric, Gynecologic, and Neonatal Nursing, 22*(4), 320-325.

Anderson, R. M., & Davidson, P. L. (1996). Measuring access and trends. In R. M. Anderson, T. H. Rice, & G. F. Kominski (Eds.), *Changing the U.S. health care system: Key issues in health services, policy and management* (pp. 13-44). San Francisco, CA: Jossey-Bass.

Annese, M. (1995). Principles for creating "caring" community partnerships. In D. H. Bor, L. W. Chambers, T. S. Inui, & J. A. Showstack (Eds.), *Community health improvement through information and action.* San Francisco, CA: Health of the Public Program Office, University of California.

Barton, J. A., Brown, N. J., & Clark, L. (1997, November). *Establishing protocols for community needs assessments.* Paper presented at the 125th Annual Meeting of the American Public Health Association, Indianapolis, IN.

Barton, J., Smith, M. C., Brown, N., & Supples, J. (1993). Methodological issues in community analysis. *Nursing Outlook, 41*(4), 253-261.

Becker, D. M., Hill, D. R., Jackson, J. S., Levine, D. M., Stillman, F. A., & Weiss, S. M. (Eds.). (1992). *Health behavior research in minority populations: Access, design, and implementation* (NIH Pub. No. 92-2965). Washington, DC: U.S. Government Printing Office.

Bor, D. H., Chambers, L. W., Inui, T. S., & Showstack, J. A. (Eds.). (1995). *Community health improvement through information and action.* San Francisco, CA: Health of the Public Program Office, University of California.

Brown, L. (1995). Ten commandments of community-based research. In D. H. Bor, L. W. Chambers, T. S. Inui, & J. A. Showstack (Eds.), *Community health improvement through information and action.* San Francisco, CA: Health of the Public Program, University of California.

Brown, N. J., Barton, J. A., & Bjork, K. E. (1996). *Rocky Flats community needs assessment: Final report.* (Available from Rocky Flats Citizens Advisory Board, 9055 Wadsworth Parkway, Suite 2250, Westminster, CO 80021)

Brown, N. J., Barton, J. A., & Clark, L. (1997, November). *Needs assessment of a community in the shadow of a Superfund clean-up site.* Paper presented at the 125th Annual Meeting of the American Public Health Association, Indianapolis, IN.

Brown, N. J., Congdon, J. G., & Magilvy, J. K. (1996). An approach to care management for rural older adults: Parish nursing. *New Horizons, 5*(27), 7.

Brown, R. S. (1988). The evaluation of the national long term care demonstration: Estimation methodology. *Health Services Research, 23*(1), 23-50.

Courtney, R. (1995). Community partnership primary care: A new paradigm for primary care. *Public Health Nursing, 12*(6), 366-373.

Courtney, R., Ballard, E., Fauver, S., Gariota, M., & Holland, L. (1996). The partnership model: Working with individuals, families, and communities toward a new vision of health. *Public Health Nursing, 13*(3), 177-186.

DeFriese, G. H., Ricketts, T. C., & Stein, J. S. (1989). *Methodological advances in health services research.* Ann Arbor, MI: Health Administration Press.

Donabedian, A. (1980). *Explorations in quality assessment and monitoring* (Vol. 1). Ann Arbor, MI: Health Administration Press.

Donabedian, A. (1985). The quality of care: How can it be measured? *Journal of the American Medical Association, 260*(12), 1743-1748.

Eng, E., Salmon, M. E., & Mullan, F. (1992). Community empowerment: The critical base for primary health care. *Family and Community Health, 15*(1), 1-12.

Flynn, B. C. (1984). An action research framework for primary health care: A conceptual approach to the study of primary health care in communities. *Nursing Outlook, 32*(6), 316-318.

Flynn, B. C. (1997). Partnerships in health cities and communities: A social commitment for advanced practice nurses. *Advanced Practice Nursing, 2*(4), 1-6.

Flynn, B. C., Rider, M. S., & Bailey, W. W. (1992). Developing community leadership in healthy cities: The Indiana model. *Nursing Outlook, 40*(3), 121-126.

Flynn, B. C., Rider, M. S., & Ray, D. W. (1991). Healthy cities: The Indiana model of community development in public health. *Health Education Quarterly, 18*(3), 331-347.

Freire, P. (1970). *Pedagogy of the oppressed.* New York: Continuum.

Gonzalez, V. M., Stewart, A., Ritter, P. L., & Lorig, K. (1995). Translation and validation of arthritis outcome measures into Spanish. *Arthritis and Rheumatism, 38*(10), 1429-1446.

Green, L. W., Kreuter, M. W., Deeds, S. G., & Partridge, K. B. (1980). *Health education planning: A diagnostic approach.* Palo Alto, CA: Mayfield.

Gruenewald, P. J., Treno, A. J., Taff, G., & Klitzner, M. (1997). *Measuring community indicators: A systems approach to drug and alcohol problems.* Thousand Oaks, CA: Sage.

Habermas, J. (1971). *Knowledge and human interests.* Boston: Beacon.

Harrell, J. S., & Frauman, A. C. (1994). Cardiovascular health promotion in children: Program and policy implications. *Public Health Nursing, 11*(4), 236-241.

Harrell, J. S., McMurray, R. G., Bangdiwala, S. I., Frauman, A. C., Gansky, S. A., & Bradley, C. B. (1996). Effects of a school-based intervention to reduce cardiovascular disease risk factors in elementary-school children: The Cardiovascular Health in Children (CHIC) study. *Journal of Pediatrics, 128*(6), 797-805.

Healthcare Forum. (1994). *What creates health? Individuals and communities respond.* San Francisco, CA: Author.

Hegevary, S. T. (1991). Issues in outcomes research. *Journal of Nursing Quality Assurance, 5*(2), 1-6.

Institute of Medicine, Committee on Monitoring Access to Personal Health Services. (1993). *Access to health care in America.* Washington, DC: National Academy Press.

Jemmott, L. S. (1993). AIDS risk among Black male adolescents: Implications for nursing interventions. *Journal of Pediatric Health Care, 7*(1), 3-11.

Jemmott, L. S., & Jemmott, J. B. (1991). Applying the theory of reasoned action to AIDS risk behavior: Condom use among Black women. *Nursing Research, 40,* 228-234.

Jemmott, L. S., & Jemmott, J. B. (1992). Increasing condom-use intentions among sexually active Black adolescent women. *Nursing Research, 41,* 273-279.

Jones, K. R., Jennings, B. M., Moritz, P., & Moss, M. T. (1997). Policy issues associated with analyzing outcomes of care. *Image: The Journal of Nursing Scholarship, 29*(3), 261-267.

Kruger, R. A. (1994). *Focus groups: A practical guide for applied research* (2nd ed.). Thousand Oaks, CA: Sage.

Leavell, H. R., & Clark, E. G. (1965). *Preventive medicine for the doctor in his community.* New York: McGraw-Hill.

Lincoln, Y. S., & Guba, E. G. (1985). *Naturalistic inquiry.* Beverly Hills, CA: Sage.

Lorig, K., & Associates. (1996). *Patient education: A practical approach* (2nd ed.). Thousand Oaks, CA: Sage.

Lorig, K., & Holman, H. (1993). Arthritis self-management studies: A twelve-year review. *Health Education Quarterly, 20*(1), 17-28.

Lorig, K., Stewart, A., Ritter, P., Gonzalez, V., Laurent, D., & Lynch, J. (1996). *Outcomes measures for health education and other health care interventions.* Thousand Oaks, CA: Sage.

Magilvy, J. K., & Brown, N. J. (1997). Parish nursing: Advanced practice nursing model for healthier communities. *Advanced Practice Nursing Quarterly, 2*(4), 67-72.

Magilvy, J. K., McMahon, M., Bachman, M., Roark, S., & Evenson, C. (1987). The health of teenagers: A focused ethnographic study. *Public Health Nursing, 4*(1), 35-42.

Mahon, J., McFarlane, J., & Golden, K. (1991). *De madres a madres:* A community partnership for health. *Public Health Nursing, 8*(1), 15-19.

Martinez, R. J. (1995). *Close friends of God: An ethnography of health of older Hispanic people.* Unpublished doctoral dissertation, University of Colorado Health Sciences Center School of Nursing, Denver.

May, K. M., Mendelson, C., & Ferketich, S. (1995). Community empowerment in rural health care. *Public Health Nursing, 12*(1), 25-30.

McCarthy, P., Craig, C., Bergstrom, L., Whitley, E., Stoner, M. H., & Magilvy, J. K. (1991). Caring conceptualized for community nursing practice: Beyond caring for individuals. In M. J. Watson

& P. Chinn (Eds.), *Anthology on caring.* New York: National League for Nurses.

McDermott, M. A., & Burke, J. (1993). When the population is a congregation: The emerging role of the parish nurse. *Journal of Community Health Nursing, 10*(3), 179-190.

Milton, D. A., Verran, J. A., Gerber, R. M., & Fleury, J. (1995). Tools to evaluate reengineering progress. In *Reengineering nursing and health care* (pp. 195-202). Gathersburg, MD: Aspen.

Moritz, P. (1995). Outcomes research: Examining clinical effectiveness. *Communicating Nursing Research, 28,* 113-125.

National Association of County Health Officials. (1991). *Assessment protocol for excellence in public health.* Washington, DC: Author.

National Institute of Nursing Research. (1992). *Patient outcomes research: Examining the effectiveness of nursing practice* (NIH Pub. No. 93-3411). Bethesda, MD: U.S. Government Printing Office.

National Institute of Nursing Research. (1995). *Community-based health care: Nursing strategies* (NIH Pub. No. 95-3917). Bethesda, MD: U.S. Department of Health and Human Services.

Olds, D. (1992). Home visitation for pregnant women and parents of young children. *American Journal of Diseases of Children, 146,* 704-708.

Olds, D., & Kitzman, H. (1993). Review of research on home visiting. *Future of Children, 3*(4), 51-92.

O'Leary, A., & Jemmott, L. S. (1995). *Women at risk: Issues in the primary prevention of AIDS.* New York: Plenum.

O'Malley, J. (1997). Emergence of healthier communities. *Advanced Practice Nursing Quarterly, 2*(4), v-vi.

Porter-O'Grady, T. (1997). Building community health: The real work of advanced practice. *Advanced Practice Nursing Quarterly, 2*(4), 90-91.

Rains, J. W., & Wiles-Ray, D. W. (1995). Participatory action research for community health promotion. *Public Health Nursing, 12*(4), 256-261.

Rodriguez, R., McFarlane, J., Mahon, J., & Fehir, J. (1993). *De madres a madres:* A community partnership to increase access to prenatal care. *Bulletin of PAHO, 27*(4), 403-407.

Rogers, E. (1995). *Diffusion of innovations* (4th ed.). New York: Free Press.

Rohrer, J. E. (1996). *Planning for community-oriented health systems.* Baltimore, MD: American Public Health Association, United Book.

Schultz, P. R., & Magilvy, J. K. (1988). Assessing community health needs of elderly populations: Comparison of three strategies. *Journal of Advanced Nursing, 13,* 193-202.

Sechrest, L., Perrin, E., Bunker, J. (1990). *Research methodology: Strengthening causal interpretations of nonexperimental data* (DHHS Pub. No. 90-3454). Washington, DC: U.S. Department of Health and Human Services.

Stevens, P. E., & Hall, J. M. (1992). Applying critical theories to nursing in communities. *Public Health Nursing, 9*(1), 2-9.

Stoner, M. H., Magilvy, J. K., & Schultz, P. R. (1992). Community analysis in community health nursing practice: The GENESIS model. *Public Health Nursing, 9*(4), 223-227.

Stringer, E. T. (1996). *Action research: A handbook for practitioners.* Thousand Oaks, CA: Sage.

Supples, J. M., & Smith, M. C. (1995, August). East and west of Main Street: Racism in rural America. *Community Health Nursing, 12*(4), 235-241.

Timmreck, T. C. (1994). *An introduction to epidemiology.* Boston, MA: Jones and Bartlett.

Valanis, B. (1992). *Epidemiology in nursing and health care* (2nd ed.). Norwalk, CT: Appleton & Lange.

Verran, J. A., Gerber, R. M., & Milton, D. A. (1995). Data aggregation: Criteria for psychometric evaluation. *Research in Nursing and Health, 18,* 77-80.

Wilkin, D., Hallam, L., & Doggett, M. A. (1992). *Measures of need and outcome for primary health care.* New York: Oxford University Press.

World Health Organization. (1978). *Report of the International Conference on Primary Health Care.* Alma Ata, USSR.

Zagoras, M., & Norris, T. (1994). *Interim report: Colorado Health Communities Initiative.* Denver, CO: Colorado Trust and National Civic League.

Zambrana, R. E., Hernandez, M., Dunkel-Schetter, C., & Scrimshaw, S. (1991). Factors which influence use of prenatal care in low-income racial-ethnic women in Los Angeles County. *Journal of Community Health, 16*(5), 283-295.

PART
IIB

CLINICAL NURSING PRACTICE STRATEGIES AND NURSE SENSITIVE OUTCOMES

Joan L. F. Shaver

Of major relevance to the nursing profession and discipline is the ability to articulate the clinical nursing practice strategies that are sensitive and lead to outcomes that improve health status, either of individuals or groups. Increasing emphasis on "evidence-based" practice necessitates that we determine the "evidence" through nursing research. The three chapters in this section incorporate a suggested categorical schema and review of some key instruments for measuring outcomes sensitive to nursing practice in the chapter by Holzemer and Henry, and two chapters focus on considering individuals who are at high biological risk for an untoward health status trajectory. These include historical and emerging views on the nature of biological instability in individuals experiencing acute or critical illness episodes by Mitchell and a review of the nursing research applicable to preterm infants by Medoff-Cooper.

In the chapter "Therapeutic Outcomes Sensitive to Nursing Practice," Holzemer and Henry posit a conceptual model of quality of life with five broad categories of outcomes and review key instruments for measuring health status outcomes. The model includes, first, a biological and physiological component to refer to outcomes measured through physiochemical means; second, a symptom component to classify measures of self-report; third, a functional status component to refer to outcomes frequently falling in the realm of performance; fourth, a general health perceptions component to refer to global-level interpretations of health status; and last, an overall quality of life component to classify general satisfaction with life as a whole. Holzemer and Henry give examples of key instruments for the last four components in the model and examples of use in the nursing research literature. They also speak to six conceptual and methodological issues that are of importance to measuring outcomes sensitive to nursing practice. These include being able to assess a discipline-specific impact when care is interdisciplinary and concern for condition-specific versus generic instruments. Holzemer and Henry suggest paying attention to making risk adjustments in outcomes to account sufficiently for individual variations, as well as factoring in errors present in the context of giving care to groups of people. They point out the lack of normative data for many components against which to compare outcomes and the challenges of linking measured outcomes to specific interventions. Holzemer and Henry emphasize the importance of careful measurement of health status components, as it is critical to deriving therapeutic outcomes that reveal the positive impact of nursing interventions.

In the chapter titled "Promoting Physiological Stability," Mitchell discloses that "physiological stability" is a concept that is implicitly rather than explicitly used by nursing scientists, usually refers to physiological hemodynamics, and is defined by reference to population normative data. She discusses an emerging dialectic about the dynamics of physiological functions. The concept of "homeostasis" led to physiological stability, meaning predictable change in a narrow range as regulated through negative feedback systems. Similarly, the more recent idea of *allostasis* reinforces variation within a normal range that is relatively narrow. However, nonlinear dynamic analysis of some physiological phenomena reveals that narrow variability might indicate a less positive health dynamic, for instance in heart rate variability. Because few nursing researchers have focused their work on intervention studies to promote physiological stability, Mitchell delved into studies whereby the physiological responses to a variety of health problems or environmental stimuli were addressed. She found 10 papers in the nursing literature in which physiological stability as a goal of therapy was addressed. These were mainly reviews, clinical essays, or clinical guidelines. She asserts that definitions for physiological stability as human responses were most clear in studies of sleep, activity, or health status. The majority of physiological nursing research, according to Mitchell, could be classed as responses to biological or psychosocial stimuli. These include studies of cardiopulmonary or cerebrovascular responses to nursing care activities or interpersonal contacts. The majority of studies were descriptive, and few were based on a controlled design. Variability generally

was not used in analysis to examine issues of stability or explanatory contingencies for who was or was not responsive to stimuli or actions. Emerging assessment instruments for quantifying stability and instability are reviewed. Mitchell submits that we are in need of developing contingency models that predict physiological stability and instability and using nonlinear dynamic frameworks for characterizing physiological phenomena. As well, she urges that we embrace a conceptual shifting to consider how much stability in phenomena is optimal and in what contexts and that we consider environmental manipulations for their effects on facilitating optimum physiological stability or variability.

In the chapter "Therapeutic Actions and Outcomes for Preterm (Low Birth Weight) Infants," Medoff-Cooper and Holditch-Davis trace the beginnings of the study of high-risk preterm infants and understanding care for the effects of low birth weight on maturation or growth and development. Theory-driven work by nurse researchers began with infant stimulation research, based on the premise that neonatal nursery environments created deprivation. This transformed into a focus on infant organization and behavioral development, much of which has been centered on investigations into biological rhythms, especially sleep/wake. Similar to adults at risk for biological instability, the effects of handling and routine nursing procedures, painful procedures, and social interactions have been studied by nursing scientists. As feeding is logically related to growth promotion, this behavior also has received attention in the study of preterm infants. Over time, it is evident that early oral feeding is positive and breastfeeding is likely superior to bottle feeding for preterm infants, perhaps because of fewer negative effects on breathing patterns. Environmental challenges that have been studied for effects of nursing actions include body temperature maintenance, respiratory support, biological support during transport, and intravenous catheter maintenance. In infants, the effects of environment and modification of the environment have been studied for the effects on outcome indicators. The salient outcome indicators of maturation for this group of patients studied by nursing scientists are sleep/wake behaviors and sucking (both nutritive and non-nutritive) behaviors. Medoff-Cooper and Holditch-Davis review studies of lighting and noise modulation, temporal disruptions management, skin-to-skin care (kangaroo care), and stimulus modulation (e.g., waterbeds and massage). These authors assert that there is now a cadre of experienced researchers in this realm. Thematic work is being done around development during the preterm period, efficacy of care, environmental influences, and outcomes. Preterm development research with sucking (nutritive, non-nutritive) and sleep/wake behavior as the main indicators of maturation or behavioral organization is the most advanced. Physiological indicators of development deserve attention. Efficacy of care and environmental manipulation research has mainly revolved around pain management, the physical environment, and the use of massage and kangaroo care. The authors observe that the translation of results into practice is scant. Outcomes research needs better integration with the research on development and, overall, utilization projects are needed.

PROMOTING
PHYSIOLOGICAL STABILITY

Pamela H. Mitchell

We, as nurses, implicitly assume that promoting biologic stability in unstable clinical conditions is a goal of nursing interventions with acutely and critically ill people. We also assume this goal underlies both descriptive and intervention studies in these populations. Nursing and related science literatures were reviewed to ascertain whether these assumptions are supported in the clinical research literature and to ascertain the state of nursing science knowledge with respect to promoting physiological stability. An electronic literature search from 1966 to early 1997 used Medline, CINAHL, Current Contents, Expanded Academic Index, and PsycINFO with the following key words: "biologic(al) stability and nursing," "stability and nursing," "physiological stability and nursing," "physiological response and nursing," "physiological adaptation and nursing," "adaptive capacity and nursing," "physiological variability," and "nonlinear dynamics."

All key words except "biologic(al) stability and nursing" yielded some citations, but works known to be relevant were missing from the electronic searches. Therefore, the electronic search was supplemented with manual searches of references and the author's own knowledge of relevant work.

The majority of citations in the nursing literature was not research reports but conceptual or clinical essays, affirming the notion that outcome measures of physiologic stability have not been pursued extensively through research. A total of 86 citations were reviewed in detail for this chapter, distributed as follows: conceptual reviews (11), physiological stability as a goal of therapy (9), physiological stability and nursing (22), physiological responses and nursing (16), adaptive capacity and nursing (3), physiologic variability (11), and quantifying stability and variability (14). A working table and complete bibliography of these reports is available from the author.

AUTHOR'S NOTE: The author wishes to acknowledge the efforts of Susan Blackburn, Ph.D., R.N., Professor of Family and Child Nursing, University of Washington, in reviewing the material related to infants and children.

Points of View Found in the Literature

Biologic stability in basic science refers to the constancy or unchanged properties of cell membranes, chemical or biologic properties, and lack of degeneration of function and properties (see, for example, Leonard et al., 1993; Maysinger et al., 1996). The term *biologic stability* was never used in indexing nursing research, appearing only in reference to cell membrane properties and constancy of pharmaceutics. Without exception, *physiological stability* is the term used to refer to stability in adult care and in most of the literature regarding children and neonates. In clinical essays, maintaining patients' physiological stability or maintaining patients until stability occurs was frequently mentioned. Much of the extant research is centered on seeking to understand the conditions under which stability is threatened. Rarely is the goal of physiologic stability cited in intervention studies (see, for example, Crilly, Williams, Trenholm, & Hayes, 1989; Peters, 1992).

Physiological stability is often undefined but is assumed to be a reasonable goal in nursing texts, reviews of therapy, and the popular press (for example, see Bohachick, 1987, or Kelly-Rhyne, 1995). Operational definition is most commonly expressed by normal values of physiological hemodynamic variables, specifically mean arterial blood pressure. Similarly, the term *medical stability* is sometimes referred to as a goal or milestone and is defined as maintaining treatment-appropriate physiological measures within normal parameters. Examples include hematocrit in the case of splenic rupture (Lynch, Ford, Gardner, & Weiner, 1993), alveolar oxygenation in ventilator-dependent children (DeWitt, Jansen, Ward, & Keens, 1993), health status measures in frail elderly admitted to nursing homes (Engle & Graney, 1995), or not requiring frequent monitoring (Wright, Rao, Smith, & Harvey, 1996). The common denominator in these studies or reviews is a norm-referenced view of stability—specifically, *population normal* values define stability. In only two cases was the validity of norm referencing tested, when physiologic values or stability scoring system scores were correlated with indexes of metabolic demand beyond "normal" (Siegel et al., 1979; Steinhorn & Green, 1991).

The concept of *homeostasis* explicitly and implicitly has guided generations of physiological research and physiological nursing research. Within homeostasis as a concept, healthy function is characterized by the return of system parameters to set points or a regular and narrow range of fluctuation, mediated by system feedback loops. In the more recent concept of *allostasis,* fluctuations are regulated among multiple physiologic systems to maintain a range of variability (McEwen & Stellar, 1993; Shulkin, McEwen, & Gold, 1994). However, current concepts of *nonlinear dynamics* represent refutation that a narrow range of feedback or variability is the sine qua non of health. Rather, too little variability and predictable fluctuation may instead indicate loss of healthy adaptive responses (Lipsitz & Goldberger, 1992).

The ability to measure physiologic variables over time has clearly shown that nonregular oscillations and a dynamic state are the norm for living beings. More recently, nonlinear dynamics concepts have prompted some physiologists to coin a newer term: *homeokinesis* (Garfinkel, 1983; Yates, 1983). The general physiologic literature is moving to the use of analyses of physiological responsiveness and stability from a nonlinear perspective. The view of stability as the achievement of normal values and, therefore, as an optimal state is being challenged by recent work in understanding the nonlinear dynamics of physiological systems, sometimes known as *chaos* or *complexity* theory. Such work suggests that too much regularity characterizes diseased or disordered systems; a certain degree of irregularity is characteristic of more healthy neural and cardiac systems (Lipsitz & Goldberger, 1992). In fact, McKenna, McMullen and Shlesinger (1994) put forth the proposition that neural physiologic systems normally operate near instability, thereby allowing rapid and flexible responses.

Buchman (1996) builds on Siegel's concept of multiple physiological phase states in proposing interacting nonlinear mechanisms that promote stability in humans (Siegel et al., 1979). Whereas homeostatic concepts are based on each system using its own set of feedback loops and linear counterforces that return a "perturbed" system to a normal value, Buchman argues that systems are nested and respond to perturbations interactively. Thus, mechanisms returning any one component to the basal state may bring along the others as well (Buchman, 1996; Godin & Buchman, 1996). He provides several examples to argue that the irregularity in the signals from the various subsystems indicates their healthy connectedness, whereas increasing regularity among the system signals is found in clinical states of multisystem failure (Kim et al., 1995).

In proposing a nursing diagnosis, *decreased adaptive capacity,* I alluded to nonlinear dynamics but did not explicitly address these analyses in any of the subsequent published studies examining aspects of stability and instability in intracranial pressure (Mitchell, 1986a, 1986b; Mitchell, Habermann-Little, Johnson, VanInwegen-Scott, & Tyler, 1985). However, in our most recent work, we are finding that nonlinear waveform analysis techniques allow us to identify patients more at risk for instability, as manifested by multiple episodes of increased intracranial pressure (Mitchell, Kirkness, Burr, March, & Newell, 1998).

Only one nursing investigator has published research in normally accessible literature explicitly using nonlinear dynamic analyses. Mary Woo and colleagues used the concepts of nonlinear dynamics and the technique of phase space analysis in describing the heart rate variability parameters that differentiate normal people and those with congestive heart failure. In this work, heart rate variability was *more* stable and regular in patients with bigeminy (a form of cardiac arrhythmia) than in healthy controls, whose heart rate variability was characterized by a particular pattern seen in a variety of biological and nonbiologic examples of chaos (Woo, Stevenson & Moser, 1996; Woo, Stevenson, Moser, & Middlekauff, 1994; Woo, Stevenson, Moser, Trelease, & Harper, 1992; Woo, Woo, et al., 1992). Carlson-Sabelli and colleagues (1995) have published a research report in fugitive literature using the principles of nonlinear dynamics in linking psychosocial and physiologic responses, but they did not publish any of the mathematical models underlying the work that might allow one to evaluate the validity of the claims.

These contrasting views bring forth important questions for clinical research: Under what circumstances is stability a reasonable goal? Does the achievement of a single or an averaged normal value represent stability or appropriate variability? Over a decade ago, Barnard (1982) proposed that we did not have adequate theories to guide our interventions in promoting more healthy human responses. She proposed that the transitions between stable and unstable responses were the key areas for nursing therapeutics and proposed two hypotheses for nurse scientists to test. First, "in the presence of internal system instability the environment can provide regulators which assist the human system in reintegrating body processes" and, second, that "the organism benefits most from imposed external structuring when there is instability in the organism's functioning" (p. 7). Hall (1981, 1983), drawing examples from psychosocial behavior, proposed that stability, or persistence of behavior over time, rather than

growth and change, is the preferred state of human beings. We have not gotten far in testing these propositions in the ensuing years. Only one study was found that explicitly examined responses as a function or contingency of physiologic stability (Mitchell, Johnson, & Habermann-Little, 1985), although a few reported physiological responses to environmental stimuli as a function of infant behavioral state (Blackburn & Patteson, 1991; Osband, Blackburn, Casey, Zuill, & Mitchell, 1989; Stevens & Johnston, 1994; Taquino & Blackburn, 1994). Hall (1987) and Randall (1993) both provide qualitative data about organizational and maternal behaviors that support the persistence model in transitional states, but these studies are not generalizable to physiologic variables.

In the majority of nursing research involving description of or intervention in physiological responses, stability is represented by normal range values. However, it is entirely possible to have a mean arterial blood pressure that is normal but represents inadequate variability to accommodate the stress of changing position, for example. Similarly, it is possible to have a "normal" heart rate and yet manifest the reduced variability in heart rate that appears to be a key risk factor or predictor of sudden cardiac arrest and of death following myocardial infarction (Cowan, 1995).

The *American Heritage Dictionary* (1992) and *Taber's Cyclopedic Medical Dictionary* (1993) define stability as "without change" or "resistant to change, deterioration or displacement." Bingham (1994) uses the definition of "no net change" from physics to illustrate two very different versions of stability. For the first, picture a preterm infant resting in an indentation atop a parabola. Although there is fluctuation in the infant's physiological parameters, there is no net change, and it would take a large "push" to move the infant from this stable physiologic state to a deteriorating one. In contrast, picture the second infant as also "stable" in the sense of no net change in physiologic functions, but perched precariously on top of a steep physiologic slope, where a small perturbation could precipitate a serious deterioration. Both of these infants would be termed "stable" as defined by physiologic measurements within a defined range of "normal," but this static definition of stability without understanding of potential response to perturbation as defined by the slope on which measurement occurs does not provide an adequate picture of the infant's vulnerability to instability. Do our current research questions or designs about stability take into account dynamic features related to vulnerability to change, which, in Buchman's model, is predicated on multiple interacting physiological system phase states?

The State of the Science

Nursing research literature that incorporates descriptions of the parameters of stability and instability is relatively small. Had I confined the review to intervention studies where the intention was to promote physiologic stability, the literature would be very small indeed. Researchers examining physiological responses to a variety of health problems or environmental stimuli are more plentiful. This body of literature was examined when relevant to the larger issues of understanding the foundations for physiological stability. Despite the increasing interest among physiological scientists in complexity as a fundamental framework, the majority of the reviewed nursing research literature implicitly or explicitly stems from the school that views stability as homeostatic, within population or individually defined limits of "normal."

Physiologic Stability as a Goal

The 10 papers in the nursing literature that addressed physiological stability as a goal of therapy were primarily reviews of underlying physiology (Thomas, 1994), clinical care essays (for examples, see Bohachick, 1987; Brown, 1989; Buckley & Kudsk, 1994) or clinical guidelines (National Association of Neonatal Nurses, 1993). Unfortunately, no definition of stability was given in the clinical essays and guidelines reviewed here.

Barnard and Blackburn (1985) review their own and others' work explicitly within the concepts of stabilization of infant self-regulation. They described the ultradian rhythms of the human caregiving environment in a neonatal intensive care unit and the social entrainment of infant activity and biologic responses to it. Further, they demonstrated the caregiving social environment to be a modifiable component of the key factors in stabilizing 24-hour self-regulation in developing infants.

The only other nursing research in this category was a survey of nurses regarding their perceptions of patient hemodynamic instability while using closed tracheal suction (Crimlisk, Paris, McGonagle, Calcutt, & Farber, 1994). No definition of hemodynamic instability was provided, so it is likely that the survey responses reflected a variety of definitions regarding stability.

Surgical clinical investigators compared the use of cardiac output (CO) and hematocrit (Hct) to continuous venous oxygen saturation (SVO_2) for evaluating hemodynamic stability in a consecutive series of postoperative patients in a single institution (Cernaianu et al., 1992). Charted changes in CO and Hct or hemoglobin were used to validate the degree to which SVO_2 changes outside normal values indicated hemodynamic instability. The changes in the invasive measures of hemodynamic stability were reflected in the SVO_2 changes sufficiently enough for the authors to conclude that over 70% of the invasive determinations of CO and Hct were unnecessary to ascertain postoperative instability. This study exemplifies clinical research definitions of clinical instability as deviation outside "normal" values.

Physiologic Stability and Human Responses

Although relatively few research studies were retrieved from electronic searches using the terms *physiological* or *physiological stability,* a larger number could be classified in this category. Those with the most clear and reproducible working definitions of stability were in sleep, gerontology, and rehabilitation research describing the stability of sleep, activity, or health status in community or structured living settings. Only 7 of the 22 studies reviewed in this category were reported by nurse scientists (Carson & Drew, 1994; Lobo & Michel, 1995; Lynch et al., 1993; Meers et al., 1996; Mitchell, Johnson, et al., 1985; Shaver, Giblin, Lentz, & Lee, 1988; Taquino & Blackburn, 1994). Only two of these studies tested interventions to promote physiologic stability.

Meers et al. (1996) used a case control design to compare health-related quality of life and incidence of metabolic instability in dialysis patients, using a self-care versus full-service dialysis unit. Metabolic instability was found not to vary with the type of unit but was not sufficiently well-defined in the report to determine how it was ascertained. Taquino and Blackburn (1994) report a within-subject controlled design in preterm infants to evaluate physical containment of the infant as an intervention to reduce behavioral stress and physiologic instability during adverse procedures such as suctioning or blood drawing. They noted more rapid recovery of physiologic variables in the containment condition, but the abstract report does not contain sufficient data to evaluate either the definition of stability or the magnitude of difference between the two contained and uncontained conditions.

For the most part, the nursing and other disciplinary literatures on physiologic stability consist of descriptive typologies regarding the stability of various physiologic phenomena. Nursing investigators have described cardiopulmonary stability and disengagement cues during naturally occurring feeding in infants (Lobo & Michel, 1995), hematocrit stability as a criterion for discharge in children with splenic injury (Lynch et al., 1993), intracranial pressure stability as a predictor of intracranial pressure response to parental contact (Mitchell, Johnson, et al., 1985; Mitchell & Habermann, 1999), and a typology of sleep architecture stability in pre-, peri- and postmenopausal women (Shaver et al., 1988). The majority of these studies used population-based norms to differentiate stable from unstable patterns; however, our group constructed an intraindividual measure of resting variability against which to evaluate episodes of unstable intracranial pressure episodes (Mitchell, Johnson, et al., 1985; Mitchell & Habermann, 1999; Mitchell, Habermann-Little, Johnson, Tyler, Van Inwegen-Scott, Amos, et al., 1986).

More sophisticated analyses of stability occurred in the literature from other disciplines. For example, Hausdorff et al. (1996) described the stability of the stride interval in human gait over time. They used nonlinear dynamic analyses of power spectra and detrended fluctuation of the step-to-step fluctuations at usual, fast, and slow walking speeds. Stride fluctuations (irregular variability) were present at all speeds but were consistent among speeds (e.g., highly correlated or stable) and disappeared when a regular metronome pattern was superimposed on spontaneous walking. This study is notable for its use of nonlinear analyses and a clear operational definition of stability that is not synonymous with regularity. Similarly, the nursing study of sleep architecture in women and three studies regarding stability of sleep and activity in the elderly are notable for clear, standardized, and reproducible operational definitions of stability and variability within a time period and across time periods (Hoch, Reynolds, Kupfer, & Berman, 1988; Satlin, Volicer, Ross, Herz, & Campbell, 1992; Shaver et al., 1988; van Someren et al., 1996).

In several studies, investigators either used indexes of clinical stability as a condition for entry to the study (Meers et al., 1996), a predictor variable for discharge (Lynch et al., 1993), or readmission to an acute care facility (Wright et al., 1996). Definitions of clinical stability varied from precise operational definitions such as three consecutive hematocrit determinations with no change (Meers et al., 1996) to the rather vague "condition judged to require little or no monitoring" (Wright et al., 1996). Measurement issues were the focus of four studies, evaluating the repeatability over time of serum osmolality in nursing home residents (Weinberg, Pals, McGlinchey-Berroth, & Minaker, 1994), stride fluctuation (Hausdorff et al., 1996), health status measures (Engle & Graney, 1995), and temperature measurement in infants (Seguin & Vieth, 1996).

Only two of the studies correlated physiological stability with behavioral measures. Lobo and Michel (1995) examined changes in heart rate and respiratory rate in relation to behavioral disengagement cues during feeding of normal human infants and infants with congenital heart disease (CHD). The infants with CHD exhibited significantly more of the subtle disengagement cues, but magnitude of cardiopulmonary change was not related in any systematic way. In contrast, Sapolsky (1992) showed marked basal cortisol level changes in baboons when stability of the individual's social ranking was shifting, as indicated by the percentage of dominance behaviors. Individuals who were rising or falling in the social hierarchy had the most markedly elevated cortisol levels.

Physiological Responses

The majority of physiologic nursing research reports could be classified as examinations of physiological responses to biologic or psychosocial stimuli. In many cases, the studies are relevant to the work at hand, as a better understanding of the response patterns that underlie the goal of promoting stability is sought. Studies so classified were reviewed if explications in the findings included understanding mechanisms of stability or if there was a time series design that would allow interpretation of stability in relation to naturally occurring or controlled interventions.

The response studies largely addressed cardiopulmonary or cerebrovascular responses to a variety of stimuli generated by nursing care activities or interpersonal contacts and were conducted in both adults and infants. Cardiopulmonary responses typically included heart rate, direct or indirect measures of arterial blood pressure, and direct or indirect measures of oxygenation (Bjornson et al., 1992; Blackburn & Patteson, 1991; Doering, Dracup, Moser, Czer, & Peter, 1996; Peters, 1992; Stevens & Johnston, 1994; Stone, Bell, & Preusser, 1991; Stone, Talaganis, Preusser, & Gonyon, 1991; Summers, Dudgeon, Byram, & Zingsheim, 1990; Velasco-Whetsell, Evans, & Wang, 1992). Surface and core temperature were described in one study (Summers et al., 1990).

Cerebrovascular responses were either inferred from intracranial pressure or indirectly measured by cerebral blood flow velocity and cerebral perfusion pressure (a calculated variable derived from intracranial pressure and mean systemic arterial pressure) (Brucia & Rudy, 1996; Crosby & Parsons, 1992; Hepworth, Hendrickson, & Lopez, 1994; Johnson, Omery, & Nikas, 1989; March, Mitchell, Grady, & Winn, 1990; Osband et al., 1989; Peters, 1992; Prins, 1989; Rudy, Turner, Baun, Stone, & Brucia, 1991; Stevens & Johnston, 1994; Treloar, Nalli, Guin, & Gary, 1991). The stimuli were naturally occurring events such as family visits (Hepworth et al., 1994; Prins, 1989), painful stimuli (Stevens & Johnston, 1994), or routine nursing care (Osband et al., 1989; Peters, 1992), or controlled trials of nursing care interventions such as change in position (Doering et al., 1996; March et al., 1990), endotracheal suctioning (Brucia & Rudy, 1996; Crosby & Parsons, 1992; Rudy et al., 1991; Stone, Bell, et al., 1991; Stone, Talaganis, et al., 1991; Velasco-Whetsell et al., 1992), warming devices after surgery (Summers et al., 1990), and interpersonal conversation (Johnson et al., 1989; Treloar et al., 1991). Mitchell and colleagues (Mitchell, Kirkness, et al., 1998; Rauch, Mitchell, & Tyler, 1990) sought to identify clinically useful cerebrovascular waveform parameters that would be predictive of untoward, destabilizing responses to nursing care.

These studies were mainly descriptive and reports of changes in group means for physiological variables. However, a few incorporated a within-subject control, quasiexperimental design to control for intervening variables and from which one could infer stability or instability in response to various stimuli. Peters (1992), for example, used a single-case quasiexperimental design with replication to capture responses of individual infants to ongoing care activity in a neonatal intensive care unit. Data were analyzed with an implied framework of stability in that the units of interest were episodes of bradycardia, oxygen desaturation, hypoxia and hyperoxia, and increased intracranial pressure based on definitions established from each infant's undisturbed "normal" ranges. The study demonstrated substantial periods for each infant in which levels of intracranial pressure and oxygen saturation were unstable and at potentially harmful levels. Others compared within-subjects standardized conditions such as containment during infant suctioning (Velasco-Whetsell et al., 1992) or head of bed elevation (March et al., 1990).

Randomized controlled trials were used in very few of the studies. Summers et al. (1990) evaluated core and surface temperature stability with warmed blankets versus a commercial warming device after surgery but did not adequately control for operative time differences in the analysis to draw firm conclusions. In another set of studies, investigators evaluated responses to endotracheal suctioning in several patient populations, using a randomized order of conditions (Rudy et al., 1991; Stone, Bell, et al., 1991; Stone, Talaganis, et al., 1991). In both head-injured and cardiac surgery patients, successive suction catheter passes resulted in a cumulative increase in mean arterial pressure and in ICP in the head-injured patients. The study was not designed to ascertain if there were subsets of patients for whom this could be predicted. This same effect was demonstrated in a nonrandomized, within-subject controlled design (Crosby & Parsons, 1992). Further, these investigators identified patients with a higher mean ICP as being more adversely responsive to the suctioning protocol.

In nearly all studies of physiological responses, responses were analyzed comparing mean values for physiological variables before and after the natural or controlled interventions. Although graphs in several of the papers suggest considerable individual variability in physiologic measures within each of the pre and post time periods, this variability was not used in the analyses to examine issues of stability and contingencies that might have influenced those who were and were not responsive physiologically. Osband et al. (1989) and Blackburn and Patteson (1991) did response analyses with respect to infant behavioral state, as did Stevens and Johnston (1994). The latter investigators also analyzed variability of responses with respect to a scale of infant physiologic instability. Although behavioral state did interact with physiological response, an index representing overall physiologic instability did not (Stevens & Johnston, 1994).

Physiologic Variability

The literature regarding physiologic response is nearly devoid of attention to variability within individuals, but there is growing literature in both nursing science and general clinical science regarding physiologic variability phenomena—specifically, heart rate variability. Methodologies of calculating variability in the heart period (beat-to-beat or R-R interval) have been developed using the increased sophistication of computer modeling and bioengineering models for nonlinear and nonregular data. This variability reflects sympathetic and parasympathetic nervous system balance in regulating heart rate (see Cowan, 1995, and Woo, Stevenson, & Moser, 1996, for further discussion of heart rate variability and its measurement). Papers were selected for this review when the studies were conducted by nurse scientists, or when the review illuminated some relevant population or principle for further development of nursing science in understanding stability and variability. As with the physiological response literature, the majority of papers regarding heart rate variability are reviews of methods of analysis (Cowan, 1995; Woo, Stevenson, & Moser, 1996), reviews of descriptive studies (Lipsitz & Goldberger, 1992), or descriptive studies of preterm infants or adults in intensive care (Allen, Menke, & Hayes, 1995; Winchell & Hoyt, 1996), adult cardiac patients (Carlson-Sabelli et al., 1995; Woo, Stevenson, Moser, & Middlekauff, 1994; Woo, Stevenson, Moser, Trelease, et al., 1992), response to bedrest in healthy women (Goldberger, Mietus, Rigney, Wood, & Fortney, 1994), children with congenital central hypoventilation syndrome (Woo, Woo, et al., 1992), and healthy adults exposed to endotoxin (Godin et al., 1996).

Cowan and her group (Cowan, 1995; Cowan, Burr, et al., 1992; Cowan, Kogan, Burr, Hendershot, & Buchanan, 1990) have designed an intervention to increase heart rate variability in survivors of sudden cardiac arrest by respiratory rhythm training and self-management strategies designed to reduce sympathetic arousal. In a randomized controlled trial, they have demonstrated a significant reduction in recurrent sudden cardiac arrest through increasing heart rate variability (HRV) (Cowan, 1996). Training for increased HRV is an area ripe for nursing therapeutic studies.

Quantifying Stability: Physiologic Instability Scales

The search strategies located 15 methodological studies representative of those in which scales are being developed or used to quantify stability. Not all such scales or methods are related to physiological variables, but a few nonphysiological studies are included to illuminate the definitional issues in common with physiological studies. Three instruments appear frequently in the clinical research literature: a neonatal Neurological and Adaptive Capacity Score (NACS) (see, for example, Amiel-Tison et al., 1982; Eldredge & Salamy, 1988); the pediatric Physiologic Stability Index (PSI) (Georgieff, Mills, & Bhatt, 1989; Kissoon, Frewen, Block, Gayle, &

Stiller, 1989; Meert, Lieh-Lai, Sarnaik, & Sarnaik, 1991), which is a component of the Pediatric Risk of Mortality (PRISM) (Steinhorn & Green, 1991); and the Acute Physiology Score (APS) of the adult Acute Physiology and Chronic Illness Evaluation (APACHE II, APACHE III) (Knaus et al., 1991; Wagner, Knaus, & Draper, 1983), as well as similar adult severity scores (see Kollef & Schuster, 1994, for a comparative review).

Although the NACS is widely used to evaluate the effects on the newborn infant of drugs used in labor and delivery, it is more an evaluation of infant responsiveness and reflex activity than of stability or instability of the infant. It has been shown to be more effective in distinguishing infants at risk for delayed development from normal newborns than the neurophysiological measure of auditory brain stem response (Eldredge & Salamy, 1988).

The pediatric and adult scales used to quantify severity of physiologic abnormality in critical care are commonly referred to as "stability measures." Such scales provide weighted values for deviation from population norms for commonly measured variables in key organ systems affected by critical illness. The choice of clinically measured variables and weighting was initially based on the clinical judgment of experts. In the case of the APACHE tool, these have been modified based on empiric testing to predict mortality in a large national database (Knaus et al., 1991). Eldrege and Salamy (1988) validated the strong correlation of PSI scores with multiple biochemical and metabolic indicators in a pediatric sample. Empiric cutoff scores are sometimes used to classify patients who do and do not need intensive care monitoring, which, in turn, is sometimes used as a clinical criterion of stability (Knaus et al., 1991). These scores have also been found to be valid indexes of nursing resource use, particularly in pediatric populations (Georgieff et al., 1989; Kissoon et al., 1989; Meert et al., 1991; Steinhorn & Green, 1991).

This approach of quantifying stability according to "absence of deviation from norms" is quite consistent with the most common approaches in stability quantification in the social sciences—that is, stability as constancy, sameness, or regularity (Alleyne et al., 1996; Grant, 1996). Operationally, this view of stability is often defined by interclass correlations across time (see, for example, Kochersberger, McConnell, Kuchibhatla, & Pieper, 1996). Although many investigators use methods developed for instrument or interrater reliability, Mitchell and Woods (1996) took a different approach, using the method of Heise to differentiate instrument reliability from behavioral stability in behaviors that would be expected to change with intervention.

Summary and Recommendations for Future Research

Near the beginning of this chapter, I asked whether or not our current research questions or designs take into account dynamic features due to multiple interacting physiological states in relation to stability. The answer is clearly no. Current work is static with regard to both questions and measurements. At a minimum, contingency models are needed to judge under what circumstances stability is compromised or maintained and the linkages between stability and irregularity. Such models would better enable us to predict who is at risk for decompensatory responses, in whom therapies are warranted, and which therapies would be likely to be effective.

The growing work using nonlinear dynamic principles raises crucial questions such as, In which features that are necessary for life should stability be a clinical goal? When should stability be a goal? How far should one go to achieve stability? For example, in any given individual, are there some indicators of life function that require stability or constancy under any circumstances? What are the circumstances in which one might simultaneously have constancy in some functions and variability in others?

There is enormous potential for explicit use of nonlinear dynamic frameworks and techniques to characterize physiological variables or to shape interventions, but there is relatively little work using this framework in mainstream nursing research journals (Vicenzi, 1994). The majority of papers are in the journal *Complexity and Chaos in Nursing* (first issue called *Theoretic and Applied Chaos in Nursing*), an occasional, privately published journal with papers of varying accuracy and quality. In only one of the papers using chaos theory that were reviewed by Henderson, Hamilton, and Vicenzi (1995) were physiological variables examined, and in none were standard quantitative techniques found in the mainstream complexity literature used. Carlson-Sabelli et al. (1995) claim to have used time-series approaches to evaluate the complexity in the electrocardiogram and provide examples of phase-space diagrams, but these investigators

have not published their methods in accessible literature, nor have they described their interventions clearly in terms of mainstream science. No primary research by nurse investigators in nonlinear dynamical models was found in the mainstream literature except for that of Mary Woo and her colleagues (see Woo, Stevenson, & Moser, 1996; Woo, Stevenson, Moser, & Middlekauff, 1994; Woo, Stevenson, Moser, Trelease, et al., 1992). Relatively few medical investigators have reported descriptive or intervention studies using these models (Buchman, 1996; Lipsitz & Goldberger, 1992).

There is need for a conceptual shift to explore questions regarding *how much stability* is optimal and *under what conditions*. Barnard and Blackburn (1985) have outlined many of these questions for the preterm infant population, and we see glimmers of them reflected in analyses of responses under different behavioral states (under what conditions). Woo and colleagues (Woo, Stevenson, Moser, & Middlekauff, 1994) have ventured into the questions of how much stability (regularity) in examining the phase-space patterns of children with congenital cardiopulmonary disorders contrasted with normal children, but this work has not moved to intervention studies to discern under what conditions we should promote more or less physiological variability. Cowan and her group (Cowan, 1996) have pioneered the testing of a life-saving intervention to increase heart rate variability in sudden cardiac arrest survivors. However, no one has yet reported studies designed to test Buchman's (1996) proposals regarding nested, nonlinear models of multiple interacting physiologic phase states. His model supports Barnard's (1982) contention, for infants, that we should be examining transitions within the physiologic as well as the developmental phase shifts. The evidence that there are interacting and nested control systems mandates that we consider physiologic stability among systems, not based on single physiological variables measured at one point in time.

Last, Barnard's (1982) call to evaluate manipulation of environment as well as direct physiological treatments to facilitate optimal stability or variability has barely been heeded in the ensuing decade. A few investigators with preterm infants evaluated environmental support during noxious stimulation (containment methods), but none have used analytic methods for evaluating the variability as well as the average response. There is a paradigm shift under way in the understanding of stability and variability in biobehavioral phenomena. Because of our interest as nursing scientists in the combined person and environment factors influencing the health status of individuals, we are in a position to be in the forefront of the

science that will advance our understanding and shape physiological stability phenomena.

References

Allen, C. E., Menke, J. A., & Hayes, J. (1995). Nonlinearity of heart rate in the neonate. *American Journal of Perinatology, 12*(2), 116-121.

Alleyne, S., Reiss, D., Leonard, K. J., Turner-Musa, J., Wagner, B., Simmens, S., Holder, B., Kimmel, P. L., Kobrin, S., & Cruz, I. (1996). Staff security and work pressure: Contrasting patterns of stability and change across five dialysis units. *Social Science and Medicine, 43*(4), 525-535.

Amiel-Tison, C., Barrier, C., Shnider, S. M., Levinson, G., Hughes, S. C., & Stefani, S. J. (1982). A new neurologic and adaptive capacity scoring system for evaluating obstetric medications in full-term newborns. *Anesthesiology, 56*(5), 340-350.

Barnard, K. E. (1982). The research cycle: Nursing, the profession, the discipline. *Communicating Nursing Research, 15,* 1-12.

Barnard, K. E., & Blackburn, S. (1985). Making a case for studying the ecologic niche of the newborn. *Birth Defects Original Articles, 21*(3), 71-88.

Bingham, R. J. (1994). Stability. *Neonatal Network, 13*(8), 5-7.

Bjornson, K. F., Deitz, J. C., Blackburn, S., Billingsley, F., Garcia, J., & Hays, R. (1992). The effect of body position on the oxygen saturation of ventilated preterm infants. *Pediatric Physical Therapy, 4,* 109-115.

Blackburn, S., & Patteson, D. (1991). Effects of cycled light on activity state and cardiorespiratory function in preterm infants. *Journal of Perinatal and Neonatal Nursing, 4*(4), 47-54.

Bohachick, P. A. (1987). Pulmonary embolism in neurological and neurosurgical patients. *Journal of Neuroscience Nursing, 19,* 191-197.

Brown, M. E. (1989). Clinical management of the organ donor. *Dimensions of Critical Care Nursing, 8*(3), 134-141.

Brucia, J., & Rudy, E. (1996). The effect of suction catheter insertion and tracheal stimulation in adults with severe brain injury. *Heart and Lung, 25*(4), 295-303.

Buchman, T. G. (1996). Physiologic stability and physiologic state. *Journal of Trauma, 41,* 599-605.

Buckley, S., & Kudsk, K. A. (1994). Metabolic response to critical illness and injury. *AACN Clinical Issues in Critical Care Nursing, 5*(4), 443-449.

Carlson-Sabelli, L., Sabelli, H., Patel, M., Messer, J., Zbilut, J. P., Walthall, K., Sugerman, A., Tom, C., & Zdanics, O. (1995). Electropsychocardiography: Illustrating the application of process methods and chaos theory to the comprehensive evaluation of coronary patient. *Complexity and Chaos in Nursing, 2*(1), 16-24.

Carson, K. J., & Drew, B. J. (1994). Electrocardiographic changes in critically ill adults during intrahospital transport. *Progress in Cardiovascular Nursing, 9*(4), 4-12.

Cernaianu, A. C., Del Rossi, A. J., Boatman, G. A., Moore, M. W., Postner, M. A., Cilley, J. H. Jr., Baldino, W. A., & Santos, Z. L. (1992). Continuous venous oximetry for hemodynamic and oxygen transport stability post cardiac surgery. *Journal of Cardiovascular Surgery, 33*(1), 14-20.

Cowan, M. J. (1995). Measurement of heart rate variability. *Western Journal of Nursing Research, 17,* 32-48.

Cowan, M. J. (1996). Myocardial infarction and its impact from the cellular to the community level: Nineteen years of study. *Communicating Nursing Research, 29,* 97-107.

Cowan, M. J., Burr, R. L., Narayanan, S. B., Buzaitis, A., Strasser, M., & Busch, S. (1992). Comparison of autoregression and fast Fourier transform techniques for power spectral analysis of heart period variability of persons with sudden cardiac arrest before and after therapy to increase heart period variability. *Journal of Electrocardiology, 25*(Suppl.), 234-239.

Cowan, M. J., Kogan, H., Burr, R., Hendershot, S., & Buchanan, L. (1990). Power spectral analysis of heart rate variability after biofeedback training. *Journal of Electrocardiology, 23*(Suppl.), 85-94.

Crilly, R. G., Williams, D. A., Trenholm, K. J., & Hayes, K. C. (1989). Effects of exercise on postural sway in the elderly. *Gerontology, 35*(2-3), 137-143.

Crimlisk, J. T., Paris, R., McGonagle, E. G., Calcutt, J. A., & Farber, H. W. (1994). The closed tracheal suction system: Implications for critical care nursing. *Dimensions of Critical Care Nursing, 13*(6), 292-300.

Crosby, L. J., & Parsons, L. C. (1992). Cerebrovascular response of closed head-injured patients to a standardized endotracheal tube suctioning and manual hyperventilation procedure. *Journal of Neuroscience Nursing, 24*(1), 40-49.

DeWitt, P. K., Jansen, M. T., Ward, S. L., & Keens, T. G. (1993). Obstacles to discharge of ventilator-assisted children from the hospital to home. *Chest, 103,* 1560-1565.

Doering, L. V., Dracup, K., Moser, D. K., Czer, L.S.C., & Peter, C. T. (1996). Hemodynamic adaptation to orthostatic stress after orthotopic heart transplantation. *Heart & Lung, 25*(5), 339-351.

Eldredge, L., & Salamy, A. (1988). Neurobehavioral and neurophysiological assessment of health and "at-risk" full-term infants. *Child Development, 59,* 186-192.

Engle, V. F., & Graney, M. J. (1995). Black and White female nursing home residents: Does health status differ? *Journal of Gerontology, 50*(4, Series A, Biological Sciences and Medical Sciences), M190-M195.

Garfinkel, A. (1983). A mathematics for physiology. *American Journal of Physiology, 245*(Regulatory Integrative Comparative Physiology 14), R455-R466.

Georgieff, M. K., Mills, M. M., & Bhatt, P. (1989). Validation of two scoring systems which assess the degree of physiological instability in critically ill newborn infants. *Critical Care Medicine, 17*(1), 17-21.

Godin, P. J., & Buchman, T. G. (1996). Uncoupling of biological oscillators: A complementary hypothesis concerning the pathogenesis of multiple organ dysfunction syndrome. *Critical Care Medicine, 24*(7), 1107-1116.

Godin, P. J., Fleisher, L. A., Eidsath, A., Vandivier, R. W., Preas, H. L., Banks, S. M., Buchman, T. G., & Suffredini, A. F. (1996). Experimental human endotoxemia increases cardiac regularity: Results from a prospective, randomized, crossover trial. *Critical Care Medicine, 24*(7), 1117-1124.

Goldberger, A. L., Mietus, J. E., Rigney, D. R., Wood, M. L., & Fortney, S. M. (1994). Effects of head-down bed rest on complex heart rate variability: Response to LBNP testing. *Journal of Applied Physiology, 77*(6), 2863-2869.

Grant, L. A. (1996). Assessing environments in Alzheimer special care units. *Research on Aging, 18*(3), 275-291.

Hall, B. A. (1981). The change paradigm in nursing: Growth versus persistence. *Advances in Nursing Science, 3*(4), 1-6.

Hall, B. A. (1983). Toward an understanding of stability in nursing phenomena. *Advances in Nursing Science, 5*(3), 15-20.

Hall, B. A. (1987). Strategies of persistence in a professional bureaucracy: A field study of a psychiatric hospital. *Archives of Psychiatric Nursing, 1*(3), 183-193.

Hausdorff, J. M., Purdon, P. L., Peng, C. K., Ladin, Z., Wei, J. Y., & Goldberger, A. L. (1996). Fractal dynamics of human gait: Stability of long-range correlations in stride interval fluctuations. *Journal of Applied Physiology, 80*(5), 1448-1457.

Henderson, J. S., Hamilton, P., & Vicenzi, A. E. (1995). Chaos theory in nursing publications: Retrospective and prospective views. *Complexity and Chaos in Nursing, 2*(1), 36-40.

Hepworth, J. T., Hendrickson, S. G., & Lopez, J. (1994). Time series analysis of physiological response during ICU visitation. *Western Journal of Nursing Research, 16*(6), 704-717.

Hoch, C. C., Reynolds, C. F., Kupfer, D. J., & Berman, S. R. (1988). Stability of EEG sleep and sleep quality of healthy seniors. *Sleep, 11*(6), 521-527.

Johnson, S. M., Omery, A., & Nikas, D. (1989). Effects of conversation on intracranial pressure in comatose patients. *Heart & Lung, 18*(1), 56-63.

Kelly-Rhyne, C. (1995). Governmental affairs and political action: Dear Representative Brawley. *Tar Heel Nurse, 57*(6), 32.

Kim, R., Hsu, J., Kacin, M., Morgan, L., Szaflarski, N., & Seiver, A. (1995). Low-frequency, periodic fluctuation in physiologic variables of critically ill patients [Abstract]. *Critical Care Medicine, 23*(1 suppl.), A26.

Kissoon, N., Frewen, T. C., Block, M., Gayle, M., & Stiller, C. (1989). Pediatric organ donor maintenance: Pathophysiologic derangements and nursing requirements. *Pediatrics, 84,* 688-693.

Knaus, W. A., Wagner, D. P., Draper, E. A., Zimmerman, J. E., Bergner, M., Bastos, P. G., Sirio, C. A., Murphy, D. J., Lotring, T., Damiano, A., & Harrell, F. E. Jr. (1991). The APACHE III prognostic system: Risk prediction of hospital mortality for critically ill hospitalized adults. *Chest, 100*(6), 1619-1636.

Kochersberger, G., McConnell, E., Kuchibhatla, M. N., & Pieper, C. (1996). The reliability, valididty and stability of a measure of physical activity in the elderly. *Archives of Physical Medicine and Rehabilitation, 77,* 737-795.

Kollef, M. H., & Schuster, D. P. (1994). Predicting intensive care unit outcome with scoring systems: Underlying concepts and principles. *Critical Care Clinics, 10*(1), 1-18.

Leonard, S., Logel, J., Luthman, D., Casanova, M., Kirch, D., & Freedman, R. (1993). Biological stability of mRNA isolated from human postmortem brain collections. *Biological Psychiatry, 33*(6), 456-466.

Lipsitz, L. A., & Goldberger, A. L. (1992). Loss of "complexity" and aging: Potential applications of fractals and chaos theory to senescence. *Journal of the American Medical Association, 267,* 1806-1809.

Lobo, M. L., & Michel, Y. (1995). Behavioral and physiological response during feeding in infants with congenital heart diseases: A naturalistic study. *Progress in Cardiovascular Nursing, 10*(3), 26-34.

Lynch, J. M., Ford, H., Gardner, M. J., & Weiner, E. S. (1993). Is early discharge following isolated splenic injury in the hemodynamically stable child possible? *Journal of Pediatric Surgery, 28,* 1403-1406.

March, K., Mitchell, P. H., Grady, S., & Winn, R. (1990). Effects of backrest position on ICP and CPP. *Journal of Neuroscience Nursing, 22,* 375-381.

Maysinger, D., Krieglstein, K., Filipovic-Grcic, J., Sendtner, M., Unsicker, K., & Richardson, P. (1996). Microencapsulated ciliary neurotrophic factor: Physical properties and biological activities. *Experimental Neurology, 138*(2), 177-188.

McKenna, T. M., McMullen, T. A., & Shlesinger, M. F. (1994). The brain as a dynamical physical system. *Neuroscience, 60*(3), 587-605.

McEwen, B. S., & Stellar, E. (1993). Stress and the individual: Mechanisms leading to disease. *Archives of Internal Medicine, 153,* 2093-2101.

Meers, C., Singer, M. A., Toffelmire, E. B., Hopman, W., McMurray, M., Morton, A. R., & MacKenzie, T. A. (1996). Self-delivery of hemodialysis care: A therapy in itself. *American Journal of Kidney Diseases, 27*(6), 844-847.

Meert, K., Lieh-Lai, M., Sarnaik, I., & Sarnaik, A. (1991). The role of intensive care in managing childhood cancer. *American Journal of Clinical Oncology, 14,* 379-382.

Mitchell, E. S., & Woods, N. F. (1996). Symptom experience of midlife women: Observations from the Seattle midlife women's health study. *Maturitas: Journal of the Climacteric & Postmenopause, 25,* 1-10.

Mitchell, P. H. (1986a). Decreased adaptive capacity, intracranial: A proposal for a nursing diagnosis. *Journal of Neuroscience Nursing, 18*(4), 170-175.

Mitchell, P. H. (1986b). Intracranial hypertension: Influence of nursing care activities. *Nursing Clinics of North American, 21*(4), 563-576.

Mitchell, P. H., & Habermann, B. (1999). Rethinking stability: Touch and intracranial pressure. *Biology Research for Nursing, 1.*

Mitchell, P. H., Habermann-Little, B., Johnson, F. B., Tyler, D., Van Inwegen-Scott, D., Amos, D. E., & Astley, C. (1986). Nursing and ICP: Studies of two clinical problems. In J. D. Miller, G. M. Teasdale, J. O. Rowan, S. L. Galbraith, & A. D. Mendelow (Eds.), *Intracranial pressure VI* (pp. 701-704). Berlin: Springer-Verlag.

Mitchell, P. H., Habermann-Little, B., Johnson, F., VanInwegen-Scott, D., & Tyler, D. (1985). Critically ill children: The importance of touch in a high-technology environment. *Nursing Administration Quarterly, 9*(4), 38-46.

Mitchell, P. H., Johnson, F. B., & Haberman-Little, B. (1985). Promoting physiologic stability: Touch and ICP [Abstract]. *Communicating Nursing Research, 18,* 93.

Mitchell, P. H., Kirkness, C., Burr, R., March, K. S., & Newell, D. W. (1998). Waveform predictors of adverse response to nursing care [Abstract]. *Acta Neurochirugia, 71*(Suppl.), 420.

National Association of Neonatal Nurses. (1993). *Infant developmental care guidelines.* Petaluma, CA: Author.

Osband, B., Blackburn, S., Casey, L., Zuill, R., & Mitchell, P. H. (1989). Intracranial pressure in preterm infants: Effects of nursing care. In J. Hoff & A. L. Betz (Eds.), *Intracranial pressure VII* (pp. 511-513). Berlin: Springer-Verlag.

Peters, K. L. (1992). Does routine nursing care complicate the physiologic status of the premature neonate with respiratory distress syndrome? *Journal of Perinatal and Neonatal Nursing, 6*(2), 67-84.

Prins, M. M. (1989). The effect of family visits on intracranial pressure. *Western Journal of Nursing Research, 11*(3), 281-292.

Randall, B. P. (1993). Growth versus stability: Older primiparous women as a paradigmatic case for persistence. *Journal of Advanced Nursing, 18*(4), 518-525.

Rauch, M. E., Mitchell, P. H., & Tyler, M. L. (1990). Validation of risk factors for the nursing diagnosis decreased intracranial adaptive capacity. *Journal of Neuroscience Nursing, 22*(3), 173-178.

Rudy, E. B., Turner, B. S., Baun, M., Stone, K. S., & Brucia, J. (1991). Endotracheal suctioning in adults with head injury. *Heart & Lung, 20*(6), 667-674.

Sapolsky, R. M. (1992). Cortisol concentration and the social significance of rank instability among wild baboons. *Psychoneuroendocrinology, 17*(6), 701-709.

Satlin, A., Volicer, L., Ross, V., Herz, L., & Campbell, S. (1992). Bright light treatment of behavioral and sleep disturbances in patients with Alzheimer's disease. *American Journal of Psychiatry, 149*(8), 1028-1032.

Seguin, J. H., & Vieth, R. (1996). Thermal stability of premature infants during routine care under radiant warmers. *Archives of Disease in Childhood, 74,* F137-F138.

Shaver, J., Giblin, E., Lentz, M., & Lee, K. (1988). Sleep patterns and stability in perimenopausal women. *Sleep, 11*(6), 556-661.

Shulkin, J., McEwen, B. S., & Gold, P. W. (1994). Allostasis, amygdala and anticipatory angst. *Neuroscience and Behavioral Reviews, 18*(3), 385-396.

Siegel, J. H., Cerra, F. B., Coleman, B., Giovannini, I., Shetye, M., Border, J. R., & McMenamy, R. H. (1979). Physiological and metabolic correlations in human sepsis. *Surgery, 88,* 163-193.

Steinhorn, D. M., & Green, T. P. (1991). Severity of illness correlates with alterations in energy metabolism in the pediatric intensive care unit. *Critical Care Medicine, 19,* 1503-1509.

Stevens, B. J., & Johnston, C. C. (1994). Physiological responses of premature infants to a painful stimulus. *Nursing Research, 43*(4), 226-231.

Stone, K. S., Bell, S. D., & Preusser, B. A. (1991). The effect of repeated endotracheal suctioning on arterial blood pressure. *Applied Nursing Research, 4*(4), 152-158.

Stone, K. S., Talaganis, S. A., Preusser, B., & Gonyon, D. S. (1991). Effect of lung hyperinflation and endotracheal suctioning on heart rate and rhythm in patients after coronary artery bypass graft surgery. *Heart & Lung, 20*(5, Part 1), 443-450.

Summers, S., Dudgeon, N., Byram, K., & Zingsheim, K. (1990). The effects of two warming methods on core and surface temperature, hemoglobin oxygen saturation, blood pressure, and perceived comfort of hypothermic post-anesthesia patient. *Journal of Post Anesthesia Nursing, 5*(5), 354-364.

Taquino, L., & Blackburn, S. (1994). The effects of containment during suctioning and heelstick on physiological and behavioral responses of preterm infants. *Neonatal Network, 13*(7), 55.

Thomas, K. (1994). Thermoregulation in the neonate. *Neonatal Network, 13*(2), 15-22.

Treloar, D. M., Nalli, B. J., Guin, P., & Gary, R. (1991). The effect of familiar and unfamiliar voice treatments on intracranial pressure in head-injured patients. *Journal of Neuroscience Nursing, 23*(5), 295-299.

Van Someren, E.J.W., Hagebeuk, E.E.O., Lijzenga, C., Scheltens, P., de Rooij, S.E.J.A., Jonker, C., Pot, A.-M., Mirmiran, M., & Swaab, D. F. (1996). Circadian rest-activity rhythm disturbances in Alzheimer's disease. *Biological Psychiatry, 40,* 259-270.

Velasco-Whetsell, M., Evans, J. C., & Wang, M. S. (1992). Do post-suctioning transcutaneous PO_2 levels change when a neonate's movements are restrained? *Journal of Perinatology, 12*(7), 334-337.

Vicenzi, A. E. (1994). Chaos theory and some nursing considerations. *Nursing Science Quarterly, 7*(1), 36-42.

Wagner, D. P., Knaus, W. A., & Draper, E. A. (1983). Statistical validation of a severity of illness measure: Acute Physiology Score of APACHE. *American Journal of Public Health, 73*(8), 878-884.

Weinberg, A. D., Pals, J. K., McGlinchey-Berroth, R., & Minaker, K. L. (1994). Indices of dehydration among frail nursing home patients: Highly variable but stable over time. *Journal of the American Geriatric Society, 42*(10), 1070-1073.

Winchell, R. J., & Hoyt, D. B. (1996). Spectral analysis of heart rate variability in the ICU: A measure of autonomic function. *Journal of Surgical Research, 63,* 11-16.

Woo, M. A., Stevenson, W. G., & Moser, D. K. (1996). Comparison of four methods of assessing heart rate variability in patients with heart failure. *American Journal of Critical Care, 5*(1), 34-41.

Woo, M. A., Stevenson, W. G., Moser, D. K., & Middlekauff, H. R. (1994). Complex heart rate variability and serum norepinephine levels in patients with advanced heart failure. *Journal of the American College of Cardiology, 23*(3), 565-569.

Woo, M. A., Stevenson, W. G., Moser, D. K., Trelease, R. B., & Harper, R. M. (1992). Patterns of beat-to-beat heart rate variability in advanced heart failure. *American Heart Journal, 123*(3), 704-710.

Woo, M. S., Woo, M. A., Gozal, D., Jansen, M. T., Keens, T. G., & Harper, R. M. (1992). Heart rate variability in congenital central hypoventilation syndrome. *Pediatric Research, 31*(3), 291-296.

Wright, R. E., Rao, N., Smith, R. M., & Harvey, R. F. (1996). Risk factors for death and emergency transfer in acute and subacute inpatient rehabilitation. *Archives of Physical Medicine and Rehabilitation, 77,* 1049-1055.

Yates, F. E. (Ed.). (1983). *Self-organizing systems: The emergence of order.* New York: Plenum.

10

THERAPEUTIC ACTIONS AND OUTCOMES FOR PRETERM (LOW BIRTH WEIGHT) INFANTS

Barbara S. Medoff-Cooper
Diane Holditch-Davis

Although modern hospital care of preterm or low birth weight (LBW) infants has its origins in the development of incubators and gavage feeding techniques in the early decades of the 20th century, neonatal intensive care did not begin until 1965 with the first reported use of mechanical ventilation

161

to treat respiratory distress syndrome. Most of the initial medical and nursing care of LBW infants used trial and error, based on an understanding of the physiological bases of neonatal diseases. It is not surprising that the earliest nursing research on care of LBW infants was primarily atheroretical, although it was based in physiology and focused on testing the efficacy of nursing procedures. For example, Torrance (1968) showed that axillary thermometers needed to be held in place longer than rectal thermometers in preterm infants. Neal and Nauen (1968) found that challenging preterm infants with exposure to room temperature enabled more than half of them to transition to an open bed within 24 hours. Other nurse researchers examined the relationship between feeding regimens and growth in preterm infants (Hasselmeyer, de la Puente, Lundeen, & Morrison, 1963; Iffrig, 1956). Using a very small sample, Curran and Kachoyeanos (1979) compared the effectiveness of suctioning with and without chest physiotherapy. The combination of suctioning and chest physiotherapy with a vibrator was most effective in maintaining a high mean pO_2, although it resulted in the highest mean pCO_2 levels. Much of the early history of neonatal nursing research can be traced to these early studies, and an interest in providing high-risk infants with appropriate nursing care remains a major thrust of nursing research today. Moreover, the tradition of being part of an interdisciplinary area of research has also continued. Neonatal nursing researchers frequently have mentors and publish in other disciplines, and they almost always have interdisciplinary team members.

In this chapter, a brief overview of the history of neonatal nursing research is presented; however, the main focus of the discussion will be on modern investigators. Research in the infant organization tradition has concentrated as much on describing preterm or LBW infants and their hospital environment as it has on evaluating specific interventions. In addition, the tradition of atheoretical, physiologically focused studies for examining specific nursing interventions remains prominent in research literature on LBW infants. In this chapter, research on LBW infants is addressed from physiologic, behavioral, and theoretical perspectives.

Infant Stimulation

The infant stimulation research in the 1970s was the first time neonatal nurse researchers began to conduct

theoretically driven research. Studies grew out of the assumption present in psychology and nursing that the neonatal nursery was an environment lacking much of the stimulation that infants receive in the home and that this lack contributed to many of the developmental delays seen in older prematurely born children. In addition, stimulation was seen as one way to help preterm infants organize their immature behaviors and manage the environmental stress of the nursery. Therefore, researchers attempted to provide preterm infants with supplemental stimulation to compensate for these deficits. The flaw of these studies was the assumption that the preterm infant was in a stimulus-deprived environment. This was probably an accurate description of the nurseries for preterm infants in the 1950s, but it was not an accurate description of neonatal intensive care units in the 1970s. They had deficits of some types of stimulation, excesses of others, and inappropriate patterning of stimulation, as was pointed out by Cornell and Gottfried (1976). Most of the studies were experimental, with small samples and low power. Thus, none of these studies had lasting impact on neonatal nursing care.

Auditory stimulation was the primary type of stimulation used in the aforementioned studies. Neal (1979) found that preterm infants showed definite heart rate response to auditory stimuli, with younger infants showing deceleration and older infants acceleration followed by deceleration. Segall (1972) showed that the heart rates of preterm infants decelerated more to maternal voice than to an unfamiliar voice. Katz (1971) found short-term improvement in development indexes for preterm infants exposed to auditory stimuli. Chapman (1978, 1979) exposed preterm infants to their mother's voice, a lullaby, or ambient noise but found no group differences in gross motor activity. Likewise, the developmental status of the infants did not differ (Malloy, 1979).

In other studies, combinations of tactile and vestibular stimulation were tested. Neal concentrated her work on motion as she developed an incubator hammock to promote organization of infant behaviors ("Nurse Researchers Show," 1978). Unfortunately, she never published her findings, but she did produce a video that was widely distributed. Her work influenced a large number of the current researchers, and she was one of the first nurses to work with a biomedical engineer on instrumentation to improve both research and nursing care. Kramer and colleagues (Chamorro, Davis, Green, & Kramer, 1973; Kramer, Chamorro, Green, & Kundson, 1975) examined the effectiveness of providing extra tactile stimulation to preterm infants. Using a very small sample of

14 infants, they provided 48 minutes of stroking daily for at least 2 weeks. They did not find any differences in the social or physical development of the infants or in their plasma cortisol levels.

Behavioral Organization

The 1980s marked the era of modern neonatal nursing research, with many studies theoretically focused on infant organization. Probably the most common framework used by nurses studying behavioral organization is the Synactive Model of Behavioral Organization (Als, 1991). Als suggested that newborn behaviors are infants' primary expressions of brain function and the critical route of communication. Investigation of central mechanisms, which regulate the temporal organization of behavior, is essential to understanding the basic relationship between cerebral activity and behavior.

From this knowledge of central mechanisms underlying behaviors, the relations between abnormal brain functions and abnormal behaviors are understood by inference (Kephart, 1960; Prechtl & Stemmer, 1962). The behavior of preterm infants, both before and after term, and their developmental outcomes, differ markedly from those of healthy, full-term infants. These differences are probably the result of both specific neurological insults and atypical environment effects on the developing nervous system. Brain development in the fetal and neonatal periods is a process of "experience-expectant" development, through which normal species-typical experiences enable the brain to make the structural and functional changes necessary to progress to the next stages of development (Greenough, Black, & Wallace, 1987). This process is somewhat plastic; maintaining a balance between the needs of the present developmental stage and the anticipated needs of subsequent stages of maturation (Oppenheim, 1981). Thus, species-typical experiences are needed to provide adequate amounts and types of stimulation for appropriate adaptation. Although an individual may initially make a successful adaptation to an atypical environment, changes in the organism's developmental trajectory resulting from this adaptation may be maladaptive at older ages. In addition, these changes affect the future expression of genes (Gottlieb, 1996) and thus may lead to increasingly atypical development. Because the human brain normally develops in the uterine environment, preterm infants inevitably experience disturbed ad-

aptation as they mature in the neonatal intensive care unit environment. The effects of this developmental disturbance vary among individuals, depending on the timing and severity of environmental stresses, the interaction of prenatal history on individual genetic background, adaptations that may have been made to atypical uterine stresses (e.g., maternal chronic illness or placental insufficiency), and specific neurological insults resulting from neonatal illnesses.

Development of Behaviors in Preterm Infants

Nursing research on the behavioral development of preterm infants has been focused primarily on biological rhythms and sleep. The physiological systems of all organisms exhibit rhythms, many exhibiting approximately 24-hour periods, called *circadian*, or shorter periods, called *ultradian*. Nurse researchers have found that preterm infants exhibit both ultradian and circadian rhythms (Thomas, 1995), but because of their neurological immaturity, biological rhythms are inconsistent and may not be apparent until near to term (Thomas, 1991; Updike, Accurso, & Jones, 1985). Updike et al. (1985) found that healthy, near-term infants exhibited circadian rhythms in body temperature, oxygenation, and respiratory pauses. However, in studying younger preterm infants, Thomas (1991) found ultradian rhythms with periods of 2 to 6 hours in body temperature but in only three of five infants. Although these studies are intriguing, the research in this area is still too limited to draw conclusions for practice.

Sleeping and waking rhythms are present during the preterm period. Holditch-Davis and her colleagues (Holditch-Davis, 1990a; Holditch-Davis & Edwards, 1998) have conducted a detailed study of the development of waking and sleeping patterns of 71 preterm infants between the ages of 27 and 39 weeks gestation. Sleep-wake states were scored every 10 seconds for weekly 4-hour periods, using a behavioral state scoring system based on Thoman (1990). During the preterm as compared to the after-term period, infants were found to exhibit greater amounts of active sleep (as much as 60% to 70% of the day) and indeterminate states and lower amounts of waking states (Holditch-Davis, 1990a; Holditch-Davis & Edwards, 1998). The major developmental change during the preterm period was a decrease in the amount of active sleep and an increase in the organization of both sleep states, as measured by the percentages of the state with typical state criteria. In addition, quiet sleep and waking states, especially crying, increased. The mean duration and frequency of episodes of each state also changed over the preterm period: quiet waking, active waking, and sleep-wake transition episodes occurred more frequently, and active waking and quiet sleep bout length increased over age (Holditch-Davis & Edwards, in press).

The severity of illness that the infant experienced during the perinatal period was found to have immediate effects on sleeping and waking patterns, but these effects disappeared after the infant recovered, as long as there were no neurological complications (Holditch-Davis, 1990a, 1995; Holditch-Davis & Hudson, 1995; Holditch-Davis & Lee, 1993). Holditch-Davis and Hudson (1995) used changes in sleep-wake to identify a wide variety of acute medical complications in preterm infants, including hydrocephalus, sepsis, and cold stress. Yet the only difference in the development of sleeping and waking states in convalescent preterm infants was that more severely ill infants showed less fussing and somewhat poorer organization of quiet sleep (Holditch-Davis, 1990a). Holditch-Davis and Lee (1993) compared high-risk preterm infants with and without chronic lung disease from 32 to 36 weeks on sleep-wake states and sleep organization exhibited over 4-hour observations in the intermediate care unit. The only difference comparatively was that infants with chronic lung disease had more irregular respiration in quiet sleep. Infants with chronic lung disease exhibited more jitters and fewer smiles than other preterm infants (Holditch-Davis & Lee, 1993). There were also no differences in sleeping and waking when the infants with and without chronic lung disease were with caregivers (Holditch-Davis, 1995). Similarly, Medoff-Cooper (1988) found that during handling for a neurobehavioral assessment, infants with chronic lung disease exhibit more stress behaviors than other preterm infants, including more tachycardia, tachypnea, and bradycardia.

Sleep and wake states were also found to affect the frequency of central apnea in preterm infants. During sleep, brief apneic pauses of less than 20 seconds in length occurred more frequently in active sleep than quiet sleep in preterm infants, and the mean length of apneic pauses was longer in quiet sleep (Holditch-Davis, Edwards, & Wigger, 1994). However, sleep state did not affect the frequency of periodic respiration (cyclic breathing alternating with brief apneic pauses). To date, nursing re-searchers have not determined the extent to which these findings also apply to the longer pathologic apnea, as pathologic apnea is often too rare to permit statistical analyses comparing states (Holditch-Davis, Edwards, et al., 1994). There may be some association between active sleep and pathologic apnea, as theophylline, used to treat this condition, is known to increase the amount of wakefulness and decrease the amount of active sleep in addition to its direct effects on respiration (Thoman, Holditch-Davis, Raye, Philipps, Rowe, & Denenberg, 1985). However, in an experimental study by a different research team, oral-gustatory stimulation was shown to reduce the length of pathologic apnea without altering the infants' ongoing sleep state (Park, 1991).

Other studies have indicated that the sleeping and waking states of infants in the first month after reaching term differ dramatically from those of preterm infants, suggesting that the early extrauterine experience of preterm infants has a prolonged effect. During brief observations, preterm infants after reaching term have been found to be equally as alert and irritable as healthy full-term infants (Telzrow, Kang, Mitchell, Ashworth, & Barnard, 1982). However, over 7-hour observation periods in the home, preterm infants exhibited more alertness and nonalert waking activity and less drowsiness than full-term infants. The major developmental trends exhibited by preterm infants in the first month were a decrease in active sleep and an increase in the amount of alertness (Holditch-Davis & Thoman, 1987).

Effect of Neonatal Intensive Care Unit (NICU) Environmental Stimulation

Investigators from a variety of disciplines, including nursing, have suggested that the hospital provides stimulation that is inappropriate for the development of preterm infants (Graven et al., 1992). A number of nursing investigators have studied the NICU environment and its effects on infant physiology and behavior. The neonatal intensive care unit provides infants with an extremely bright and noisy environment with little diurnal variation and frequent interventions for technical procedures but little positive handling (Barnard & Blackburn, 1985; Blackburn & Barnard, 1985; Duxbury, Henly, Broz, Armstrong, & Wachdorf, 1984; Kitchin & Hutchinson,

1996; Philbin, Ballweg, & Gray, 1994; Pohlman & Beardslee, 1987; Thomas, 1989; Zahr & Balian, 1995). Preterm infants were handled by nurses and other health professionals about 14% to 25% of the day, mostly by nurses (Blackburn & Barnard, 1985; Evans, 1991; Pohlman & Beardslee, 1987; Werner & Conway, 1990). The sickest infants received the most handling (Duxbury et al., 1984; Pohlman & Beardslee, 1987; Zahr & Balian, 1995) even though they lacked the physiological reserves to cope with it. These infants became hypoxic in response to virtually any form of stimulation such as noise, technical procedures (Evans, 1991; Norris, Campbell, & Brenkert, 1981; Peters, 1992), and increases in lighting (Shogan & Schumann, 1993).

Routine nursing procedures are particularly likely to have negative physiological effects on preterm infants (Becker, Brazy, & Grunwald, in press). Norris et al. (1981) found that preterm infants on mechanical ventilation experienced significant decreases in oxygenation that lasted for several minutes after suctioning, repositioning, and heelsticks. Chest physiotherapy was associated with decreases in oxygenation and increases in blood pressure and intracranial pressure (Cheng & Williams, 1989; Evans, 1991; Peters, 1992). The sicker the infant was, as indicated by higher oxygen requirements, the greater the decreases it experienced (Cheng & Williams, 1989). During bathing, infants exhibited marked changes in heart rates and blood pressure, decreases in oxygenation, and increases in intracranial pressure (Peters, 1992, 1996). Other routine procedures, such as weighing, tape removal, and repositioning, had equally large negative impacts on infants (Evans, 1991; Peters, 1992). In addition, neonatal nurses and physicians have seldom considered infant sleep-wake states and other infant behaviors when choosing the time for routine interventions. Thus, nursing and medical interventions frequently result in state changes. The frequency of caregiver interventions in the NICU has been found to be as high as five times per hour (Duxbury et al., 1984). Preterm infants were found to change their sleep-wake states about six times per hour, and 78% of these changes are associated with either nursing interventions or NICU noise (Zahr & Balian, 1995). Nearly half of all rest periods between interventions were less than 10 minutes long (Evans, 1994). Preterm infants were rarely able to sustain quiet sleep during nursing interventions (Holditch-Davis, 1990b) and usually awakened with each intervention. Preterm infants normally spent only a small percentage of their time in waking states (Holditch-Davis, 1990a), but this percentage increased significantly when they were with nurses (Holditch-Davis, 1990b). Of note is that Becker et al. (in press) demonstrated that time spent in sleep and drowsy wakefulness was higher and time spent in alert, nonalert wakefulness and fussing or crying was lower with an individualized approach to nursing care designed to reduce stressors and support behavioral organization, as compared to routine caregiving.

Certain infants may be more vulnerable to the effects of environmental stimulation than others. Most studies have indicated that critically ill infants were particularly likely to have negative physiological responses to handling (Evans, 1991; Norris et al., 1981; Peters, 1992). In addition, preterm infants with chronic lung disease were vulnerable to stimulation effects. Although the sleep-wakes states of these infants were not altered by handling (Holditch-Davis, 1995), infants with chronic lung disease exhibited more negative physiological responses—tachycardia, tachypnea, and bradycardia—than other preterm infants (Medoff-Cooper, 1988). This increased sensitivity to handling might be due to delayed maturation of the central nervous system.

The care that infants have received previously affects vulnerability. The amount of time it takes infants to recover physiologically from handling ranged from 3 to 24 minutes (Evans, 1991; Norris et al., 1981), so infants who receive nursing interventions in quick succession are more likely to show negative responses. Preterm infants in the supine rather than prone position exhibit increased energy expenditures, decreased quiet sleep, and increased waking (Masterson, Zucker, & Schulze, 1987). Infants in open warmers experience more handling than infants in incubators (Pohlman & Beardslee, 1987).

Effect of Painful Procedures

Infants in intensive care inevitably experience painful procedures. Neonatal nursing researchers have conducted significant studies on the physiological and behavioral effects of pain and on interventions to minimize pain. Detailed reviews that synthesize the existing research for clinicians exist (D'Apolito, 1984; Shapiro, 1989; Stevens & Johnston, 1993). Primary nurse researchers in this area are Johnston and Stevens, whose findings have been verified by a variety of other researchers. For example, infants are more likely to be awake and less likely to be in quiet sleep during painful procedures compared to during routine nursing care

(Bozzette, 1993; Holditch-Davis & Calhoun, 1989; Van Cleve & Andrews, 1995; Van Cleve, Johnson, Andrews, Hawkins, & Newbold, 1995). All but the youngest and sickest preterm infants are likely to cry (Evans, Vogelpohl, Bourguignon, & Morcott, 1997; Stevens, Johnston, & Horton, 1993; Van Cleve et al., 1995). Infants in pain exhibited a number of negative facial expressions and behaviors, including mouth opening, brow furrowing, grimacing, muscle rigidity, moving away, and hand clenching (Bozzette, 1993; Stevens et al., 1993). In addition, their heart rates increase, oxygenation decreases, and intracranial pressure increases (Bozzette, 1993; Stevens & Johnston, 1994; Stevens et al., 1993; Van Cleve et al., 1995). Preterm infants tend to remain awake after a painful procedure, but this tendency is not any greater than the tendency to stay awake after routine handling (Holditch-Davis & Calhoun, 1989). Although these responses tend to become more pronounced the older the infant, infants who were born at younger gestational age and, thus, have more experience in the NICU environment, have less mature responses to pain than infants of similar postconceptional ages born at later gestational ages (Johnston & Stevens, 1996).

Isolated studies have been conducted on how nurses respond to preterm infant pain. Although these studies are not products of programs of research, they have had similar findings and they have built on each other. Nurses have been found to use changes in infant behaviors to identify pain and decide when to administer analgesia (Franck, 1987; Hultgren, 1990; Jones, 1989; Page & Halverson, 1991; Pigeon, McGrath, Lawrence, & MacMurray, 1989; Shapiro, 1993). Changes in infant behaviors are the bases for recently developed objective rating scales for infant pain (Lawrence et al., 1993). However, nurses use the vigor of behaviors as indicators of the severity of pain and thus are likely to rate preterm infants' pain as less severe than that of full-term infants (Shapiro, 1993).

Nursing comfort measures have the potential to minimize some of the effects of pain. Yet it is not clear how frequently practicing nurses actually use them; in one study, nurses were not found to use positive touches or talking any more frequently during painful procedures than during routine care (Holditch-Davis & Calhoun, 1989). Franck (1987) identified nine different comfort measures that nurses report using to soothe infants receiving painful procedures. To date, only a few of them have been studied. Tactile stimulation, music, and intrauterine sounds were found to be ineffective when given during a painful procedure for both preterm and full-term infants (Beaver, 1987; Marchette, Main, & Redick, 1989). However, pacifiers were found to reduce crying

and arousal in full-term infants when given during and after the procedure. Swaddling has also been shown to be effective with full-term infants, but less so than pacifiers, and infants were more likely to be alert if given pacifiers (Campos, 1989). Facilitated tucking, a form of swaddling, was effective in reducing the negative physiological effects of heelsticks in preterm infants (Corff, 1993). Thus, there is evidence that use of pacifiers or swaddling can help reduce the sleeping and waking changes caused by painful procedures. However, additional research is needed to determine the effects of other comfort measures and of combining different comfort measures.

Despite the large amount of nursing research on preterm infant pain, very little is known about severe pain, such as occurs after surgery. Virtually all the previously cited studies examined procedural pain, usually due to heelsticks. However, Norton (1988) conducted a chart review to compare infants sedated with fentanyl and those sedated with morphine. Half of the infants receiving morphine and 84% of the infants receiving fentanyl exhibited signs of withdrawal after discontinuation of the medication. The longer the infant had received the medication, the more likely they were to show signs of withdrawal. In addition, Holditch-Davis and Hudson (1995) described the responses of one infant who was two days past an inguinal hernia repair. Although the nurses had reported that this infant was very irritable on the two previous evenings, he exhibited a major decrease in arousal, and his amount of quiet sleep was increased, as compared to his other observations and to infants of the same age. These responses were interpreted as indicating mild postoperative pain because full-term infants experiencing stress are known to respond with increased amounts of quiet sleep (Brackbill, 1971), and, after circumcision, full-term infants exhibit increased amounts of quiet sleep (Emde, Harmon, Metcalf, Koenig, & Wagonfeld, 1971). Even in full-term infants, only one nursing study of postoperative pain has been conducted (Cote, Morse, & James, 1991). Yet for nurses, decision making about the need for pain medication or nonpharmacological interventions for infants is frequent. Thus, studies that examine preterm infants' responses to severe pain are greatly needed.

Social Interaction

Relatively little is known about the effect on LBW infants of social interactions. Mothers report being aware of the sleeping and waking behaviors of their preterm infants—especially eye movements, orientation, and body movements—when they attempt to interact. They report using specific infant responses as guides to increase or decrease their interactive activity (Oehler, Hannan, & Catlett, 1993). Waking, eye opening, increased body movements, positive facial expressions, and calming encouraged mothers to increase interaction. Body movements, negative facial expressions, and withdrawing discouraged maternal interaction. However, preterm infants exhibit the same positive interactive behaviors as full-term infants in smaller portions of the time with their mothers (Oehler, 1995). Moreover, Harrison has shown that social stimulation affects the physiological status of preterm infants (Harrison, Leeper, & Yoon, 1991). Infants were more aroused and awake at the beginning of touch, and those with younger gestational ages at birth showed greater variations in their oxygen saturations. Heart rate was not affected by touch, but birth weight and prior handling did affect heart rate (Harrison, Leeper, & Yoon, 1990). Parents used 14 different types of touches, with holding, stroking, and contact being most common. Mothers spent the most time touching the infant and fathers the least. Infants younger than 28 weeks experienced shorter durations of touch and fewer touch episodes than older infants (Harrison & Woods, 1991). Using a standardized protocol of social stimulation, Eckerman, Oehler, Medvin, and Hannan (1994) found that preterm infants of at least 33 weeks postconceptional age responded to talking by eye opening and arousal, but added touching led to increased periods of closed eyes and negative facial expressions. Infants with more neurological insults showed even greater negative responses to touching. This suggests that preterm infants are responsive to social stimulation of low intensity, but when intensity is increased, they cope less well. Medical complications further decrease infants' ability to cope with moderately intense social stimulation.

Very little is known about the type of stimulation provided by nurses and how infants respond to it. Nurses have been shown to be more concerned with routine procedures than with social interaction (Barnard & Blackburn, 1985; Blackburn & Barnard, 1985; Cusson, 1986). They were not sensitive to the preterm infant's behavior patterns, seldom responded to infant cues indicating readiness for interaction, and usually initiated interactions with the infant (Barnard & Blackburn, 1985; Pickler, 1993). However, during interactions, nurses were quite sensitive to infant behaviors indicating aversive responses (Pickler, 1993). The younger, smaller, or sicker the infant, the fewer the attempts to provide social stimu-

lation (Cusson, 1986). Preterm infants have also been found to respond differently to nurses and parents. Preterm infants spent more time in active sleep and less time in sleep-wake transition when with their parents than when with nurses (Miller & Holditch-Davis, 1992). Parents and nurses behaved differently toward infants, with nurses more likely to engage in routine nursing and medical procedures and parents more likely to hold infants and provide positive social stimulation. These findings suggest that preterm infants respond to less active, more social stimulation provided by parents at first by sleeping and then, as they mature, by awakening to engage in interaction. The early sleeping may serve to conserve energy consumption and promote growth.

Feeding and Sucking Behaviors

Factors affecting the growth of preterm infants have been examined only through chart reviews. Nelson and Heitman (1986) found that the combined effects of chronological age, amount of formula, birth weight, and 5-minute Apgar score accounted for 46% of the variance in growth rates while preterm infants were in the hospital. Smith, Kirchhoff, Chan, and Squire (1994) found that infants weighing less than 1,000 gm lost a greater proportion of their birth weight than infants weighing between 1,000 and 1,500 gm and took longer to reach their lowest weight. There were no significant differences between the groups in the time it took to regain birth weight. The only factor related to length of time to regain birth weight was the number of days on diuretics.

Several national surveys have been conducted of NICU enteral feeding techniques. The majority of NICUs reported using transpyloric feedings for less than 5% of their infants, primarily because of medical indications such as gastroesophageal reflux, feeding intolerance, and mechanical ventilation (Chan & Ferraro, 1991). There was little consensus about associated procedures, with hospitals differing on frequency of feedings, personnel appropriate to insert, and frequency of changing tubes. Shaio, Youngblut, Anderson, DiFiore, and Martin (1995) surveyed Level II and III nurseries about their gastric tube practices and found that the majority used both oro- and nasogastric tubes. There was great variability in whether tubes were indwelling or placed intermittently and how long indwelling tubes were left in place. In another survey, most NICU nurses reported no gastric residual refeeding prior to gavage, even though they knew this practice to be beneficial, because physicians did not order the practice (Hodges & Vincent, 1993).

One explanation for the diversity of practices is that there has been only limited study of gavage feeding practices to provide evidence-based practice. Symington, Ballantyne, Pinelli, and Stevens (1995) compared indwelling to intermittently placed nasogastric tubes. No differences in weight gain or episodes of apnea and bradycardia were found. The temperature of formula was found to affect the tolerance of gavage feedings; infants fed milk at body temperature had significantly smaller gastric residual volumes (Gonzales, Duryea, Vasquez, & Geraghty, 1995). Brennan-Behm, Carlson, Meier, and Engstrom (1994) examined the effect of infusing breast milk in different-sized gavage tubing. Standard-size tubing resulted in a loss of about 20% of the lipids, with a mean loss of 2.8 kcal/oz, whereas microbore tubing resulted in a loss of only 2.3 kcal/oz.

Both nutritive and non-nutritive sucking patterns have been studied extensively by nursing researchers. Sucking is a behavior that is initiated *in utero* and continues to develop in an organized pattern in the early weeks after birth. It involves the integration of multiple sensory and motor central nervous system functions. Nutritive sucking is organized as a continuous rhythmic pattern rather than alternations between unpredictable bursts of activity and rest periods (Wolff, 1968). Nutritive sucking provides reinforcement to an infant, thereby motivating a steady level of behavior that allows comparison of sucking records between two infants and with the same infant over time (Williams, Williams, & Dial, 1986). The first published studies of sucking behaviors appeared in the late 1800s by two physiologists, Basch (1893) and Von Pfaundler (1899). Today, nursing studies of sucking are being conducted to assess the neurobehavioral development of preterm infants (Medoff-Cooper & Gennaro, 1996), ability of LBW infants to nipple-feed (Mathew, Clark, Pronske, Luna-Solarzano, & Peterson, 1985; Medoff-Cooper, Weininger, et al., 1989), sucking patterns in breast-fed infants (DeMonterice, Meier, Engstrom, Crichton, & Mangurten, 1992), and the relationship of non-nutritive sucking to behavioral state and later feeding patterns (Gill, Behnke, Conlon, & Anderson, 1988; McCain, 1992).

Dr. Gene Cranston Anderson pioneered the research on feeding behaviors in preterm infants. Her earliest study (Adams Weaver & Cranston Anderson, 1988) of integrated sucking pressures and first bottle-feeding scores was noteworthy. It was the first nursing study to assess preterm infants' readiness to bottle-feed and the first to use a portable electronic measurement device. Thirty infants between 28 and 36 weeks' gestation at birth and who had not received their first bottle feeding were studied. No significant correlations were found between feeding ability, as measured by two feeding scales, and the four sucking parameters, but Dr. Anderson acknowledges that there were many intervening variables that may have influenced the outcome. The importance of this study is the establishment of simple, quantitative measures to assess the initiation of oral feedings in preterm infants.

Drs. Anderson and Vidyasagar (1979) continued to explore the development of sucking in preterm infants from the first to seventh day of life. Using a clinical scoring system, sucking responses were assessed for strength, duration, and rapidity of onset. In 10 preterm infants, the sucking scores did not correlate with gestational age at birth, but did increase with increasing gestational age. The exception to this linear relationship was the decrease in sucking performance on the third day, which was attributed to developing hyperbilirubinemia. Pilot findings from a more refined suckometer were also reported.

It was not until almost a decade later that interest in sucking patterns and sucking as an indicator of maturation re-emerged in the nursing literature. The sucking patterns of 42 full-term and 44 preterm infants with a mean gestational age at birth of 30.9 weeks were compared using an updated version of the suckometer described in the previous work (Medoff-Cooper, Weininger, et al., 1989). The measured pressures were used to calculate six characteristics of the sucking response. It was concluded that there were significantly different sucking profiles in healthy term infants as compared to healthy, stable preterm infants and, most important, that sucking profiles could be developed to become a clinically useful tool for nursing practice.

Further exploration of sucking patterns in preterm infants, across postconceptional age, revealed further support of the use of sucking as an index of maturation. Infants were able to generate more sucks, more sucks per burst, generate the bursts over a shorter period of time, and showed stronger sucking with increasing maturity. For example, when examining the sucking record of a preterm infant 3 weeks after a 30 weeks gestational birth, the infant demonstrated a beginning sucking rhythmicity of 18 bursts, each burst having an average of 8.16 sucks per burst. There were 158 sucks during the 5-minute sucking measurement, with an average maximum pressure of 123.5 mmHg. Two weeks later, this infant displayed a robust sucking pattern with 269 sucks, much longer bursts (a mean of 21.63 sucks per burst), and a mean maximum pressure of 205.72 mmHg (Medoff-Cooper, Verklan, & Carlson, 1993). When comparing sucking patterns in infants born at different gestational ages at birth with the same postconceptional age, there were significant differences in sucking patterns between infants of the same postconceptional age with different gestational ages at birth. At 34 and 35 weeks postconceptional age, infants born less than 32 weeks at gestation generated more bursts, sucks were longer in duration, and there were longer bursts than infants born at 34 or 35 weeks, gestation and measured during the first week of life. At 36 weeks, there were no differences between the infants born with a younger gestation and infants born at 36 weeks. This is an important clinical finding because we often do not take into consideration both gestational age and postconceptional age in making nursing care decisions. In this case, chronological age did make a difference in the infant's ability to organize its sucking behaviors (Medoff-Cooper, Verklan, et al., 1993).

The physiological cost of placing a nipple into the mouths of very young preterm infants has generated considerable interest. Medoff-Cooper, Verklan, et al. (1993) reported that preterm infants did not show an increase in physiological cost during sucking. Yet, data in the literature support the notion that sucking increases heart rate. However, the literature data is based on very small sample sizes and needs to be re-examined. When comparing pre- and full-term infants, very low birth weight (VLBW) infants of gestational ages less than 32 weeks at birth and with the most immature sucking patterns at 36 weeks postconceptional age had the highest heart rates (177-187 bpm), as compared to 150-160 bpm for the rest of the group. The high heart rates may indicate the infant's inability to maintain physiological stability during stimulation.

Heart rate alone does not appear to be the best predictor of physiological stability. Maturational differences of the autonomic nervous system in preterm and full-term infants using heart rate variability (HRV) measures have been investigated. When comparing responses to feeding between full- and preterm infants, HRV was significantly higher for term infants as compared to preterm infants. Moreover, for both age groups, HRV was substantially lower during the feeding period than at rest. The effects of feeding on HRV also last much longer for preterm babies than for full-term infants. Thus, feeding appears to have a greater impact on the autonomic nervous system

function in preterm infants than full-term infants, with a quicker recovery of HRV postfeeding for the full-term infant.

Non-nutritive sucking has long been thought of as a way to facilitate behavioral organization through decreasing restlessness and thereby decreasing the potential for depletion of energy reserves of the preterm infant. Results of one study indicated that non-nutritive sucking improved the oxygenation status of both ventilated and nonventilated infants, with lasting effects after the sucking opportunity (Burroughs, Asonye, Anderson, & Vidyasagar, 1978). Gill et al. (1988) reported that non-nutritive sucking assists infants in maintaining a level of behavioral organization. This is evident in several studies demonstrating that non-nutritive sucking increased transcutaneous oxygen in infants between 32 and 35 weeks postconceptional age. Using a randomized crossover design, Pickler, Frankel, Walsh, and Thompson (1996) reported a significant increase in pre- and postfeeding oxygen saturation when provided with a 2-minute period of non-nutritive sucking prior to a bottle feeding. Initiation of first nutritive suck was significantly sooner (5.57 seconds vs. 9.19 seconds) when the infants received a pacifier. In general, non-nutritive sucking has been heralded as a method of improving behavioral state and, ultimately, overall behavioral organization in preterm infants (Gill et al., 1988; McCain, 1992). Although there has been no literature to validate improvement of feeding patterns after periods of non-nutritive sucking, clinical impressions seem to support this notion. Further research in this area is needed.

Unlike the investigations of nutritive and non-nutritive sucking on physiological and behavioral variables, early oral feeding studies with preterm infants were primarily focused on safety issues, and even current research remains largely atheoretical, except for its having a strong physiological basis. For example, Shiao and her colleagues (Shaio, 1997; Shaio et al., 1995) have investigated the physiological effects of oral feedings. The presence of a nasal gastric (NG) tube was found to interfere with both breathing and sucking, resulting in lower tidal volumes, oxygenation saturations, less forceful sucking, and less intake of formula. Thus, the presence of an (NG) tube increases the probability that the nurses will need to supplement the oral feeding. The time of day at which oral feedings are given also affects the feeding of preterm infants (Shaio, 1997). In general, morning-fed infants were less effective feeders and had poorer coordination of sucking and swallowing. As well, when infants are continuously sucking, they consume more formula but also experience more breathing problems than when they have intermittent sucking (Shaio, 1997).

Feeding readiness and effectiveness of oral cues have been used to explore the issue of schedule versus demand feedings. In a group of 36 LBW infants (less than 2,500 grams), Collinge, Bradley, Perks, Rezny, and Topping (1982) demonstrated that demand-fed infants were bottle feeding well enough to be discharged earlier than scheduled-fed infants and needed fewer feedings per day and fewer total gavage feedings. When studying VLBW infants (less than 1,500 grams), partial demand versus scheduled feedings made no difference in weight gain or earlier discharge; however, infants were disturbed less frequently and had the opportunity to demonstrate hunger cues (Saunders, Friedman, & Stramoski, 1991).

Nurse researchers have investigated factors affecting the length of time it takes preterm infants to transition from the first oral feeding to complete oral feedings. Using a chart review, Mandich, Ritchie, and Mullett (1996) found that preterm infants with apnea, whether or not it was severe enough to treat with aminophylline, took longer from the first oral feeding to transition to complete oral feedings than preterm infants without apnea. Kennedy and Lipsitt (1993) found that preterm infants who began oral feedings within 3 days after birth reached total oral feedings in a third of the time that it took infants who waited longer than 7 days before beginning oral feedings. Infants in the two groups were selected so that they had similar birth weights and gestational ages at birth.

Efficacy of breast-feeding has been studied in VLBW infants to establish infant weight and maturation criteria for the initiation of breast feeding. Early on, mothers of preterm infants were not allowed to put infants to the breast until bottle feedings or a critical weight was achieved (Meier, 1988). This practice was based on the untested assumption that breast feeding was more physiologically stressful than bottle feeding. However, until the mid-1980s, little if any data existed to validate this assumption. Meier and Pugh (1985) were the first to conduct a longitudinal examination of feeding behaviors in three small preterm infants, who served as their own control for breast and bottle feeding. During breast feeding, infants were found to coordinate sucking and swallowing more efficiently. In general, breast feedings were longer than bottle feedings, which was attributed to infants being able to regulate the pace of the feeding. Meier (1988) then investigated the effects of bottle and breast feeding on transcutaneous oxygen pressure and

body temperature in small preterm infants. A typical pattern for the transcutaneous pO_2 was a decline during the periods of sucking for bottle feeding, with a return to or near baseline when sucking ceased. There was a period of plateau while the infant rested and a gradual decline between the end of the feeding and 10 minutes postfeeding. In contrast, during breast feeding, there was a cyclic pattern around the baseline during the sucking and rest periods. In addition, there was no period of decline postfeeding as was evident during bottle feeding. The results of this study were suggestive that ventilatory patterns are different for breast and bottle feeding, with less alteration during breast feeding. Although these findings were generated from a small sample, they made a significant contribution to our knowledge of the relationship between methods of feeding and physiological responses. For the first time in the nursing literature, evidence that breast feeding is not more stressful than bottle feeding pertained. On the contrary, bottle feeding appeared to precipitate more periods of sustained hypoxemia, especially in lower weight infants.

With the two early Meier studies, breast-feeding studies moved from the investigation of efficacy of breast feeding in VLBW infants to a more conceptual approach of alterations of physiological parameters. More recently, with infants serving as their own controls, patterns of sucking and breathing revealed that during bottle feeding, preterm infants do not breathe within sucking bursts at very early postconceptional age; instead, they alternate short bursts of sucking and breathing (Meier et al., 1993). This is in contrast to breast feeding sessions where the infants' breathing patterns were integrated within sucking bursts. Meier suggested that these data explain the previous finding that oxygenation remains more stable during breast feedings than bottle feedings for this populations of infants (Meier & Brown, 1996). Alterations in breathing patterns during feeding may be related to gestational age as well as the method of feeding. Medoff-Cooper and McGrath (1999) have inferred from their work with bottle feeding and breathing patterns that with maturation, there was a dramatic improvement of integration of breathing and sucking, which does not exist in the earliest feeding periods. Longitudinal investigations of both breast and bottle feeding would help clarify the controversies about breast versus bottle feeding for VLBW infants. It is not clear whether nursing research on bottle and breast feeding has had any impact on practice. In a survey of neonatal intensive caregivers regarding criteria used to determine readiness for oral feedings, a large variance was found, with only 50% of hospitals admitting to having a specific feeding policy (Siddell & Froman, 1994). Primary criteria were gestational age, weight, medical condition, and infant behaviors. In most hospitals, infants were started on bottle feedings prior to breast feedings.

Studies of Nursing Procedures for Preterm Infants

Nursing researchers have also examined nursing procedures for effectiveness and reducing harmful effects. Most studies are atheoretical and are limited in their contribution to the science base for understanding preterm infant health. Sustained work has been done in suctioning, wherein nurse researchers, using a combination of human and animal studies, are developing a core of knowledge about ventilation in these very vulnerable infants. Other nursing activities that have been studied include thermoregulation, respiratory support, intravenous catheter care, skin care, obtaining urine specimens, and stabilizing during transport.

Nurses have studied interventions to monitor and maintain the body temperature of preterm infants. Axillary temperatures were found to correlate closely with rectal temperatures and to be adequate for temperature monitoring even in preterm infants under radiant warmers (Haddock, Merrow, & Vincent, 1988; Moen, Chapman, Sheehan, & Carter, 1987). The accuracy of axillary temperatures was not affected by peripheral intravenous infusions in the arms (Abrams, Bucholz, McKenzie, & Merenstein, 1989) but was affected by length of time held in place, taking up to 11 minutes to stabilize versus 5 minutes for rectal temperatures (Haddock et al., 1988; Stephen & Sexton, 1987). However, the axillary temperature was within 0.20 degrees of the final temperature by 5 minutes (Stephen & Sexton, 1987). Electronic thermometers were found to obtain accurate axillary temperatures in preterm infants, although these axillary temperatures were somewhat lower than rectal temperatures (Weiss & Richards, 1994). Likewise, infrared thermometers, when used in the cal-surface mode, provided accurate estimates of rectal and axillary temperatures in preterm infants (Johnson, Bhatia, & Bell, 1991). Covering incubators, even when they were double walled, were found to have an insulating effect and to help to keep infants warm (Nelson, Thomas, & Stein, 1992). Medoff-Cooper (1994) demonstrated that preterm infants as small as 1,500 gm are able to be weaned from incubators to open cribs with appropriate insulation and that this weaning can be accomplished in less than 24 hours. However, despite strong support from the research, weaning practices have not significantly changed.

Nursing researchers have also examined a number of the procedures used to provide respiratory support during mechanical ventilation of preterm infants. Suctioning and chest physiotherapy have been found to be particularly stressful. A national survey of NICUs found that the majority of nurses hyperventilate infants prior to or during suctioning with levels of oxygen that vary according to the infants' needs (Tolles & Stone, 1990). Frequency of suctioning depended primarily on amount of the infant's secretions, and chest physiotherapy was usually done before suctioning only when ordered by a physician. Evans (1992) found that increasing the FIO_2 10% prior to suctioning and ventilating with 100% O_2 during suctioning eliminated apnea and bradycardia and reduced the incidence of hypoxic episodes in response to suctioning. Suctioning, however, was still stressful, with most infants displaying increased blood pressure during suctioning.

Using animal models to examine the physiological effects of suctioning, Gunderson, Stone, and Hamlin (1991) found that suctioning procedures resulted in decreased oxygenation due to the suctioning and also resulted in decreased heart rate due to vagal stimulation from passing the catheter. The effect on heart rate could be reduced by using body temperature saline rather than room temperature saline (Gunderson & Stoekle, 1995). The procedure of shallow suctioning caused less tracheal damage and decreased mucus production as compared to deep suctioning, but the majority of neonatalogists reported that their NICUs still use deep suctioning frequently or exclusively (Bailey, Kattwinkel, Teja, & Buckley, 1988). A few isolated nursing studies have been done on other aspects of respiratory care. Minimal differences were found in the effectiveness of nasopharyngeal catheters and nasal cannulas in delivering supplemental oxygen to preterm infants, and both types of equipment were found to be appropriate for this use (Wilson, Arnold, Connor, & Cusson, 1996). The accuracy with which pulse oximetry reflects arterial oxygen saturation was found to be affected by anemia, hyperbilirubinemia, vasopressor drugs, and lipid infusions (Gibson, 1996). Spontaneous extubation in preterm infants was primarily a function of longer periods of intubation (more than 5 days) in infants who were motorically active at the time of extubation (Kleiber & Hummel, 1989).

Most preterm infants receive intravenous infusion because gastrointestinal immaturity at birth precludes the exclusive use of oral feeding in the first few days of life and because many of them are critically ill. Tobin (1988) studied the use of teflon catheters for intravenous infusions and found a mean life of 30 hours, with about half of the catheters lasting less than 24 hours. A study of the placement of umbilical catheters found that low placement was associated with more cyanosis and blanching of the extremities and more hematuria than high placement (Scanlon, Grylack, & Borten, 1982). The addition of heparin to IV locks did not prolong the duration of patency or reduce complications over the use of saline without heparin (Kotter, 1996).

Only two nursing studies of skin care were found, both of which were atheoretical tests of procedures. Dollison and Beckstrand (1995) compared the taping of a nasogastric tube directly to the skin of the face to taping it to a pectin barrier placed on the face. Each infant experienced both conditions. Skin breakdown was apparent in the majority of instances with direct taping within 5 days, whereas in the majority of cases with the pectin barrier, the skin was still intact at 21 days. Gordon and Montgomery (1996) conducted a research utilization project to improve skin care of the small preterm infant (less than 100 gm) by reducing use of tape on these infants and increasing use of skin barrier products. They monitored compliance with the new procedures for 5 months and found over 90% compliance and decreased amount of skin breakdown.

Several nursing researchers have examined the accuracy of techniques for obtaining urine specimens from preterm infants. One study showed that urine-specific gravity could be reliably obtained from a diaper sample up to 4 hours after the infant voided (Lybrand, Medoff-Cooper, & Munro, 1990; Stebor, 1989). The accuracy of urine volume estimates from diapers depended on both the type of the diaper, with cloth diapers being least accurate, and the infant's environment, with radiant warmers leading to the greatest loss of fluid due to evaporation (Fox, 1991).

Preterm infants with critical illnesses are commonly transported from community hospitals to tertiary medical centers to receive specialized care. A few nurse researchers have examined the transport process. The oxygenation of infants during transport was found to be increased by

placing them in the prone position (Squire & Kirchhoff, 1992). Danzig (1984) conducted a survey of neonatal transport teams and found that half of the hospitals had nurse-led teams, and the longer the geographic distance traveled by the teams the more likely they were to be led by nurses. Sherwood, Donze, and Giebe (1994) found that the vibration levels varied in different locations of a transport vehicle. They were able to decrease the amount of vibration reaching the infant by using a gel-filled mattress and modifying the incubator tray to reduce vibration.

Neonatal Nurse Practitioners

Mitchell-DiCenso and colleagues (1996) compared the effectiveness and costs of having nurse practitioners manage the care of high-risk infants with that of traditional pediatric resident managed care. There were no differences between the groups in the health or developmental outcomes of the infants, parental satisfaction, or hospital costs.

Testing Interventions to Improve the Development of Preterm Infants

In view of the problems with routine NICU care for preterm infants, it is not surprising that several researchers have attempted to alter this environment to make it less stressful. Als, Lawhon, Brown, et al. (1986) and Als, Lawhon, Duffy, et al. (1994) developed a system of individualized interventions for preterm infants that included sensitivity to infant cues and careful avoidance of sleep disruptions. The experimental infants did not exhibit different state patterns but did have fewer medical complications, improved performance on the Asssessment of Preterm Infant Behavior (APIB), and earlier bottle feedings compared to control infants. As well, infants in the experimental group displayed reduced incidence of chronic lung disease, as indicated by fewer days on the ventilator, and fewer days of supplemental oxygen. Using a modification of Als's intervention system, Becker, Grunwald, Moorman, and Stuhr (1993) also found improvements in experimental infant morbidity but no differences in state behaviors on the Neonatal Behavioral Assessment Scales (NBAS) at the time of hospital discharge. Experimental infants showed higher oxygen saturations, fewer disorganized movements, and more alertness during nursing care than did controls (Becker, Grunwald, et al., 1993). Becker also found that infants receiving developmental handling slept more, had smaller decreases in oxygenation, less heart rate increase, less respiration rate decrease, and fewer disorganized movements than infants receiving traditional handling (Becker, 1995; Becker, Brazy, & Grunwald, in press).

Zahr and colleagues also used a modification of Als's (Als, Lawhon, Brown, et al., 1986) individualized care to provide developmental care and teach mothers about their preterms' behaviors (Parker, Zahr, Cole, & Brecht, 1992; Zahr, Parker, & Cole, 1992). Control infants received developmental care plans without maternal involvement. The experimental infants scored significantly higher on the Bayley Mental scale at 4 and 8 months and on the Bayley Motor scale at 4 months (Parker et al., 1992; Zahr et al., 1992). The home environment of the experimental group was also more positive at 4 months.

Premji and Chapman (1997) conducted a qualitative study of nurses' experiences in working with the Neonatal Individualized Development Care and Assessment Program (NIDCAP) in their nursery. Nurses described the basic process of developmental care as putting the baby first. This process involved three phases: learning, reacting, and advocating/nonadvocating. Each phase involved four aspects: encountering conflict with other nurses and health professionals, appraising their own abilities and the responses of the infants to developmental care, finding resources and individuals to support their efforts, and gaining sensitivity to the subtleties and outcomes of developmental care.

A number of researchers have tested the effects of altering environmental lighting or sounds. Ackerman, Sherwonit, and Williams (1989) found that placing a blanket over the incubators of preterm infants to shield them from light did not decrease the incidence of retinopathy of prematurity. Blackburn and Patteson (1991) compared preterm infants in a nursery with continuous lighting with one where the lighting was dimmed at night. Infants in cycled light exhibited less motor activity during the night and lower heart rates over the entire day than the control infants. When preterm infants in the intermediate care unit were given four 1½-hour nap periods a day during which their incubators were covered and they received no nursing or medical procedures, they exhibited less quiet waking and longer uninterrupted sleep bouts than preterm infants without naps (Holditch-Davis,

Barham, O'Hale, & Tucker, 1995). Furthermore, they experienced a more rapid decline in apneas and more rapid weight gain (Torres, Holditch-Davis, O'Hale, & D'Auria, in press). Strauch, Brandt, and Edwards-Beckett (1993) reduced noise levels for 1 hour on each nursing shift. As a result, the infants experienced more sleep and fewer state changes. Positioning interventions have also been examined. Short, Brooks-Brunn, Reeves, Yeager, and Thorpe (1996) swaddled preterm infants so that their upper and lower extremities were maintained in flexion. Swaddled infants exhibited better motor development at 34 weeks postconceptional age. Altogether, these findings suggest that neonatal nurses need to examine their routine practices to see if changes could be made to better promote stable sleeping and waking patterns in infants.

Kangaroo care, or skin-to-skin contact, has been tested for stabilizing effects on physiological and behavioral patterns for VLBW infants. Kangaroo care involves placing a diaper-clad infant upright between the maternal breast for skin-to-skin contact. The name is, obviously, derived from the similarities to marsupial care. In marsupial caregiving, the immature infant is maneuvered into the maternal pouch and is kept warm, contained, and in close proximity to the mother's breast (Ludington-Hoe, Thompson, Swinth, Hadeed, & Anderson, 1994). Kangaroo care was first tested and implemented as a standard of care in Bogota, Colombia by Drs. Rey and Martinez (1983). Anderson (1995) suggests that kangaroo care studies has been applied at four time periods determined by the health status of the infant. Late kangaroo care usually begins days or weeks postbirth, when the infant is stable. Intermediate kangaroo care generally begins about 1 week postbirth, with infants who might be unstable and ventilated. Early kangaroo care begins during the first hours or day of life for infants who might require oxygen or intravenous fluids. Very early kangaroo care begins in the delivery room approximately 30 to 40 minutes postbirth and is most often limited to more mature LBW infants.

The first nursing study for examining the relationships between oxygen saturation, thermoregulation and cardiorespiratory parameters, and kangaroo care during interfeeding intervals (Ludington-Hoe, Hadeed, & Anderson, 1991) was very favorable. Kangaroo care was deemed safe for the 12 stable preterm infants. Ludington-Hoe, Thompson, et al. (1994) continued exploring the effect of kangaroo care on physiological parameters in less stable preterm infants. These infants received intermediate kangaroo care on Days 1 and 5 and for at least 1 hour on Days 2, 3, and 4. The results were extremely encouraging in that these infants with a history of mild apneas and bradycardia had no incidence of apneas during kangaroo care. In addition, apnea density and duration were decreased from pretest to kangaroo care and increased from kangaroo care to post-test, compared to no differences in the control infants. It was concluded that kangaroo care appeared safe and effective in reducing the frequency and duration of apneas and thus contributed to the general level of behavioral organization in preterm infants. Dr. Ludington is continuing this work with small, medically stable, ventilated preterm infants. In all of these studies, kangaroo care has been compared to leaving the infant alone in the incubator rather than to other approaches for enhancing infant organization and parental involvement. Another research study of note was conducted in Sweden (Wahlberg, Affonso, & Peterson, 1992) using early and intermediate kangaroo care. Infants given kangaroo care were younger when weaned to an open crib, had shorter average hospital stays, and were more frequently breast-fed at discharge. Once again, there appeared to be evidence that kangaroo care was contributing to the overall level of behavioral and physiological stability. It should be noted, however, that the control group was retrospective.

Pilot randomized clinical trials (RCT) have supported the efficacy of kangaroo care for LBW infants. Eight infants were assigned at 1 hour postbirth to the kangaroo care group or the hospital routine care group. The kangaroo care infants rapidly thermoregulated and showed excellent levels of behavioral organization. The mothers rapidly developed a large milk volume, had no signs of engorgement, and had no complaints of breast or nipple pain. Once the mothers were discharged, the infants were cared for in the normal newborn nursery. In contrast, the control infants were discharged in 14.2 days, on average spending 3 days in the NICU and 5.8 in the step-down unit. At 1 year of age, infants in the control group had experienced higher levels of morbidity than the kangaroo care infants (Syfrett & Anderson, 1996). This pilot work led to an RCT now in progress with 100 mothers with infants of gestational ages between 32 and 35 weeks (Anderson, in press). In general, the seven RCTs with preterm infants have demonstrated greater physiological stability using commonly accepted measures such as body temperatures, crying time, heart rates, respiratory patterns with periodic breathing and apneas, time to establish circadian patterns, and periods of sleep in kangaroo care infants as compared to incubator regular care infants (Anderson, in press). Parental acceptance of

kangaroo care is also a potential problem, as not all parents are comfortable with skin-to-skin contact that requires partial undressing.

Other interventions that have been tested with LBW infants are designed to provide extra stimulation to compensate for stimulation missing in the NICU. A meta-analysis of stimulation studies from a variety of disciplines found that these interventions had physiological benefits for preterm infants with both large and small birth weights (Krywanio, 1994). Nurse researchers have tested several of these stimulation interventions. For example, water beds are used to provide compensatory vestibular-proprioceptive stimulation for preterm infants who are largely deprived of this form of stimulation in the NICU. Infants on water beds exhibit increased amounts of active and quiet sleep, less irritability, fewer state changes, and decreased crying with less energy expenditure as indicated by lower heart rates (Deiriggi, 1990). In addition, water beds and water-filled pillows have been suggested to reduce head molding in preterms, but findings are equivocal, with some studies showing reductions in molding (Schwirian, Eesley, & Cueller, 1986) and others no effects (Hemingway & Oliver, 1991). Likewise, a foam pressure-relief mattress did not affect head molding (Chan, Kelley, & Khan, 1993).

Infant massage is another common infant stimulation technique. It provides both tactile and kinesthetic stimulation; it is necessary to move the infant to provide tactile stimulation to different parts of the body. The purpose of this type of stimulation is primarily to promote growth and augment development. Jay (1982) studied the effect of providing mechanically ventilated preterm infants with 48 minutes of stroking per day for 10 days. There were no significant differences in the health outcomes of the experimental infants compared to a retrospective control group. More recently, White-Traut and Pate (1987) studied the Rice Infant Sensimotor Stimulation, a 10-minute structured massage of the infant's entire body. They found that during massage infants were more alert. However, this effect may have been due to taking the infants out of the incubator for the massage and, thus, changing the infants' thermal environment. As a result, infants exhibited minor temperature decreases and heart and respiratory rate increases that stabilized prior to the conclusion of the massage (White-Traut & Goldman, 1988). Although not statistically significant, there was a trend for the experimental infants to show more rapid weight gain and shorter hospitalizations (White-Traut & Tubezewski, 1986). In another study, the intervention protocol was altered to be more contingent to infant cues (Burns, Cunningham, White-Traut, Silvestri, & Nelson, 1994). The experimental infants showed increased alertness during the intervention that continued for 30 minutes afterwards (White-Traut, Nelson, Silvestri, Patel, & Kilgallon, 1993). In another study, mothers provided the massage stimulation (White-Traut & Nelson, 1988). These mothers exhibited more maternal positive behaviors on a standardized assessment than either mothers receiving an educational intervention or mothers taught to talk to their infants. Infant behaviors did not differ between groups. In a study of the effectiveness of stimulation protocols involving just auditory; just tactile; a combination of auditory, tactile, and visual; and a combination of auditory, tactile, visual, and vestibular stimulation, these were compared to control preterm infants not receiving stimulation (White-Traut, Nelson, Silvestri, Cunningham, & Patel, 1997). Infants receiving the tactile stimulation protocols showed higher arousal levels and higher heart and respiration rates during stimulation than the other infants. Tactile-only protocols resulted in the highest number of episodes of heart rate above 180, whereas the infants receiving the combination protocol that included vestibular stimulation showed increased arousal after the stimulation.

Other researchers combining tactile and kinesthetic stimulation have found similar effects for preterm infants. Rausch (1981) provided massage and rocking to preterm infants and found that treated infants had more stools and increased feeding intake. Barnard and Bee (1983) found that gentle, interactional touch decreased crying, increased weight gain, and improved developmental status at 1 year of age. Tactile stimulation combined with visual and auditory stimulation that were individualized to the responses of the preterm infant were found to be safe even for ventilated preterms and much less stressful than routine nursing care (Eylers et al., 1989). Placing growing preterm infants on artificial lambswool pads did not affect their growth rate (Nelson, Heitman, & Jennings, 1986).

Several studies have shown that intermittent patterned auditory stimulation, such as music, may lead to improved outcomes in preterm infants. Collins and Kuck (1991) found that exposing agitated preterm infants to a recording of female singing and intrauterine sounds led to lower arousal and lower heart rates. Standley and Moore (1995) compared music and maternal voice as stimulation for preterm infants. They found that infants listening to music initially had higher oxygen levels, and throughout the intervention they had fewer periods of hypoxia than infants listening to maternal voice.

Long-Term Developmental and Health Status of Preterm Infants

Most research on the developmental and health outcomes of preterm infants has been conducted by physicians and psychologists, probably because of their easy access to neonatal follow-up programs. Nevertheless, there is a small body of nursing research in this area that has both examined possible predictors of outcomes and described the outcomes.

A predictor of outcomes is the Neurobiologic Risk Score (NBRS), which measures the severity of specific neurological insults (Oehler, Goldstein, Catlett, Boshoff, & Brazy, 1993). In a group of high-risk preterm infants, the NBRS scores during hospitalization correlated at between $r = -.37$ and $r = -.65$, with Bayley Mental and Motor scores obtained from 6 to 24 months corrected age, and at $r = .60$, with neurological examinations at 6 and 15 months (Brazy, Eckerman, Oehler, Goldstein, & O'Rand, 1991; Brazy, Goldstein, Oehler, Gustafson, & Thompson, 1993). One component of the NBRS, metabolic acidosis, was significantly related to cognitive, motor, and neurological outcomes through the age of 2 years; respiratory acidosis was related to outcomes only at 6 months (Goldstein, Thompson, Oehler, & Brazy, 1995). NBRS scores showed stronger relationships with mental and physical development than did measures of the social environment before 2 years. At 2 years, socioeconomic status was a slightly stronger predictor of mental development than NBRS scores, but the NBRS was still the strongest predictor of physical development (Thompson et al., 1994).

Sucking behaviors are thought to be an excellent barometer of central nervous system organization, and sucking behaviors of preterm infants as related to outcomes have been examined by Medoff-Cooper. The idea of evaluating the vitality and central nervous system integrity of neonates by assessing sucking is not new. The patterns can be quantified in detailed analysis and are disturbed to various degrees by neurological problems. Wolff (1968) described the study of sucking rhythms to investigate serial order in behavior and development, which has remained among the most resistant to empirical investigation. Medoff-Cooper, Verklan, et al. (1993) have shown a strong correlation between more organized sucking patterns and increasing maturation. A follow-up question is whether sucking patterns are predictive of developmental outcomes for high-risk infants during the first year of life. In a small group of infants ($N = 19$), sucking patterns correctly predicted developmental outcomes, with 80% sensitivity and 85% specificity. Sucking pressure, burst length, time between bursts, and time between sucks were significantly correlated with psychomotor skills as measured on the Bayley Scales of Infant Development. Although the sample size was small, these findings provide support for the predictability of sucking patterns for later developmental outcomes (Medoff-Cooper & Gennaro, 1996).

Another promising predictor of outcomes is neonatal heart rate variability, a measure of central nervous system organization. DiPietro, Caughy, Cusson, and Fox (1994) found that heart rate variability showed acceptable test-retest reliability over a few days and over weeks. Infants with low variability required more respiratory support, had more perinatal complications, were more likely to be male, and had longer hospitalizations.

Medoff-Cooper and Schraeder (1982) found that 42% of 26 preterm infants between 4 and 14 months were at risk for developmental problems, but there was no correlation between developmental status and quality of the home environment at either this age or a year later (Schraeder & Medoff-Cooper, 1983). However, there were correlations between home environment and infant distractibility and mood. In other reports, the home environment was found to have greater effects. During the first year, quality of the home environment accounted for 67% of the variance in the mother's report of the child's developmental status, with health status variables having only a minor impact (Schraeder, 1986). At 36 months, the quality of the home environment, especially language stimulation and stimulation of academic behaviors, remained the most important predictor of the mother's report of development, followed by length of hospitalization and degree of intraventricular hemorrhage (Schraeder, Rappaport, & Courtwright, 1987). The quality of the home environment was equally predictive of 48-month learning abilities determined by an examiner and of academic achievement at 7 years (Schraeder, Heverly, O'Brien, & McEvoy-Shields, 1992; Schraeder, Heverly, & Rappaport, 1990b). At 5 years, children who were more immature and hyperactive had caretakers who experienced higher levels of daily stress and less positive home environments (Tobey & Schraeder, 1990).

Schraeder (1993) also compared the usefulness of three different preschool screening tests in identifying preterm children who would have school problems. An information-processing-based tool was most effective, but no tool was able to identify more than two thirds of the children who later had academic problems.

Other nurse researchers have had similar findings. Censullo (1994) found that 2-year-old children born preterm scored lower on the Bayley Mental Development Index (MDI) than did children born at term, but they did not differ on the Psychomotor Developmental Index. The quality of the home environment accounted for more of the variance in MDI scores than either infant characteristics or distal environmental factors (such as paternal employment and SES). Thompson et al. (1994) found that neonatal neurological insults and maternal stress were related to Bayley Mental scores at each age; whereas SES and race, more general measures of parenting risk, were only related at 24 months. Psychomotor scores were related to neonatal neurological insults, gender, maternal stress, and maternal education. Feingold (1994) also found that the quality of the home environment was the only variable correlated with the Bayley Mental Development Index (MDI) for prematurely born toddlers. Maternal education was positively correlated with the Home Observation for the Measurement of the Environment (HOME) score, and maternal depression scores and infant birth weight were negatively correlated with the HOME. In addition, the more choice mothers of preterm infants felt they had about employment the better the cognitive and motor outcomes of their infants (Youngblut, Loveland-Cherry, & Horan, 1993).

The presence of behavioral, learning, and temperament problems in preterm infants is also related to the home environment. Preterm infants had more difficult temperaments than full-term infants, and their temperaments were related to both the quality of their home environments and their illness severity (Medoff-Cooper, 1986). Preschoolers born preterm showed more behavioral problems than children born at term, and these behavioral problems were related to temperamental difficulties (Schraeder, Heverly, & Rappaport, 1990a). Brandt, Magyary, Hammond, and Barnard (1992) found that prematurely born children with learning problems displayed less positive behavior during a teaching situation at 8 months, had less positive home environments at 24 months, and lived in families with more stresses— particularly financial problems and maternal job loss— than did children without learning problems. Children with behavioral and emotional problems displayed less positive behavior during a teaching situation at 8 months and lived in families with more stress (Brandt et al., 1992).

Fischel and Imbruglio (1989) used the telephone for developmental screening in 60% of 2-year-old infants who had been lost to a developmental follow-up program. Three of the 30 contacted infants failed the telephone screening. Many of the parents expressed concern about their child's development with the callers. This study showed that telephone screening could be effectively used to supplement developmental follow-up.

Preterm infants are also at risk for health problems. About three fourths of preterm infants experienced acute care visits by 18 months, primarily for respiratory problems (Termini, Brooten, Brown, Gennaro, & York, 1990). In addition, a quarter of these infants were rehospitalized, with three quarters of these hospitalizations occurring in the first 6 months after discharge.

State of the Science on Care for Preterm (Low Birth Weight) Infants

Over the past 15 to 20 years, neonatal nursing research has progressed from a group of very young researchers to a strong cadre of experienced researchers. In the preceding review, we have identified at least 12 nurse investigators with established research programs, including Anderson on feeding and kangaroo care, Holditch-Davis on sleep-wake states, Medoff-Cooper on nutritive sucking and temperament, Meier on breastfeeding, Harrison on touch, and Johnston and Stevens on pain. In addition, several new investigators, such as Shaio and Peters, show promise of moving the science forward.

Substantively, several different research themes have emerged: development during the preterm period, efficacy of care, environmental influences, and outcomes. Of these themes, the preterm developmental studies have been the most theoretical and provide the basis for the other areas. Preterm developmental research has primarily focused on sucking, both nutritive and non-nutritive, and on sleeping and waking. The understanding gained about the maturational changes in these behaviors allows a better interpretation of the numerous nursing studies that use sucking and/or sleep/wake state as outcome measures for testing intervention effects. Interestingly, physiological measures of maturation have re-

ceived less attention, with only heart rate variability and thermoregulation receiving much attention by nursing scientists. Together, the behavioral and physiological modalities provide us with an index of maturation or behavioral organization. Behavioral and physiological indicators of maturation include increased alert state during non-nutritive sucking, changes in sucking patterns with increasing age, improved sleep/wake patterns, increased heart rate variability, and evident and stable circadian rhythms.

The efficacy of care and environment themes have been studied, but only in a few cases have the results been widely incorporated into practice. The three areas showing the greatest use in practice are the studies on neonatal pain, the NIDCAP program, and kangaroo care. However, the significant interest of clinicians in conducting neonatal research suggests that there is a potential for using clinicians to conduct the utilization studies, such as the weaning to open crib study that was organized by the Association for Women's Health, Obstetrical and Neonatal Nursing (AWHONN) (Medoff-Cooper, 1994).

Outcomes research is the least developed. There are a number of promising studies of the prediction of developmental outcomes that are strongly theoretically based. However, long-term outcome studies remain atheoretical. Nursing science would benefit from a concentration on outcomes as related to theory testing.

Recommendations for Future Research

Great progress has been made in understanding preterm infant behavior and care, yet much is left to be done. Continued efforts to examine maturation using more physiological parameters will greatly enhance the interpretations of future clinical investigators. More cognizance of the heterogeneity of the preterm population in nursing research is needed. Studies are needed to examine the effects of interventions on infants of varying gestational ages at birth and varying chronological ages. As even younger preterm infants survive, often with more serious health complications, there is an increasing need to know when it is appropriate to begin and end particular interventions. It has been the assumption of most researchers that gender and ethnicity have minimal effects on the behavioral and physiological responses of preterm infants. However, these notions must be empirically determined. With the increasing body of knowledge about the behavioral and physiological patterns in the preterm infant, it behooves nursing scientists to engage in a concerted effort to advance these findings and test nursing practices through research utilization projects.

References

Abrams, L., Bucholz, C., McKenzie, N. S., & Merenstein, G. B. (1989). Effect of peripheral IV infusion on neonatal axillary temperature measurement. *Pediatric Nursing, 15*(6), 630-632.

Ackerman, B., Sherwonit, E., & Williams, J. (1989). Reduced incidental light exposure: Effect on development of retinopathy of prematurity in low birth weight infants. *Pediatrics, 83*(6), 958-962.

Adams Weaver, K., & Cranston Anderson, G. (1988). Relationship between integrated sucking pressures and first bottle-feeding scores in premature infants. *Journal of Obstetric, Gynecologic, and Neonatal Nursing, 17*(2), 113-120.

Als, H. (1991). Neurobehavioral organization of the newborn: Opportunity for assessment and intervention. *NIDA Research Monographs, 114,* 106-116.

Als, H., Lawhon, G., Brown, E., Gibes, R., Duffy, F. H., McAnulty, G., & Blickman, J. G. (1986). Individualized behavioral and environmental care for the very low birth weight preterm infant at high risk for bronchopulmonary dysplasia: Neonatal intensive care unit and developmental outcome. *Pediatrics, 78,* 1123-1132.

Als, H., Lawhon, G., Duffy, F. H., McAnulty, G. B., Gibes-Grossman, R., & Blickman, J. G. (1994). Individualized developmental care for the very-low-birth-weight preterm infant: Medical and neurofunctional effects. *Journal of the American Medical Association, 272*(11), 853-858.

Anderson, G. C. (1995). Touch and the kangaroo method. In T. Field (Ed.), *Touch and infancy* (pp. 35-51). Hillsdale, NJ: Lawrence Erlbaum.

Anderson, G. C. (in press). Kangaroo care of the premature infant. In E. Goldson (Ed.), *Nurturing the premature infant: Developmental interventions in the neonatal intensive care nursery.* New York: Oxford University Press.

Anderson, G. C., & Vidyasagar, D. (1979). Development of evoking in premature infants from 1 to 7 days post birth. *Birth Defects: Original Article Series, 15*(7), 145-171.

Bailey, C., Kattwinkel, J., Teja, K., & Buckley, T. (1988). Shallow versus deep endotracheal suctioning in young rabbits: Pathologic effects on the tracheobronchial wall. *Pediatrics, 82*(5), 726-751.

Barnard, K. E., & Bee, H. L. (1983). The impact of temporally patterned stimulation on the development of preterm infants. *Child Development, 54,* 1156-1167.

Barnard, K. E., & Blackburn, S. (1985). Making a case for studying the ecological niche of the newborn. *NAACOG Invitational Research Conference. Birth Defects: Original Article Series, 21*(3), 71-88.

Basch, K. (1893). *Archiv Gynakologie, 44,* 15.

Beaver, P. K. (1987). Premature infants' response to touch and pain: Can nurses make a difference? *Neonatal Network, 5*(6), 13-17.

Becker, P. T. (1995). Studies of developmental nursing care for very low birth weight infants. In S. G. Funk, E. M. Tornquist, M. T. Champagne, & R. A. Wiese (Eds.), *Key aspects of caring for the acutely ill: Technological aspects, patient education and quality of life* (pp. 79-94). New York: Springer.

Becker, P. T., Brazy, J. E., & Grunwald, P. C. (in press). Behavioral state organization of very low birth weight infants: Effects of developmental handling during care giving. *Infant Behavior and Development.*

Becker, P. T., Grunwald, P. C., Moorman, J., & Stuhr, S. (1993). Effects of developmental care on behavioral organization in very-low-birth-weight infants. *Nursing Research, 42,* 214-220.

Blackburn, S. T., & Barnard, K. E. (1985). Analysis of caregiving events relating to preterm infants in the special care unit. In A. W. Gottfried & J. L. Gaiter (Eds.), *Infant stress under intensive care: Environmental neonatology* (pp. 113-129). Baltimore: University Park Press.

Blackburn, S., & Patteson, D. (1991). Effects of cycled light on activity state and cardiorespiratory function in preterm infants. *Journal of Perinatal and Neonatal Nursing, 4*(4), 47-54.

Bozzette, M. (1993). Observation of pain behavior in the NICU: An exploratory study. *Journal of Perinatal and Neonatal Nursing, 7*(1), 76-87.

Brackbill, Y. (1971). Cumulative effects of continuous stimulation on arousal level in infants. *Child Development, 42,* 17-26.

Brandt, P., Magyary, D., Hammond, M., & Barnard, K. (1992). Learning and behavioral-emotional problems of children born preterm at second grade. *Journal of Pediatric Psychology, 17,* 291-311.

Brazy, J., Eckerman, C., Oehler, J., Goldstein, R., & O'Rand, A. (1991). Nursery Neurobiologic Risk Score: Important factors in predicting outcome in very low birthweight infants. *Journal of Pediatrics, 118,* 783-792.

Brazy, J., Goldstein, R., Oehler, J. M., Gustafson, K. E., & Thompson, R. J. Jr. (1993). Nursery Neurobiologic Risk Score: Levels of risk and relationships with nonmedical factors. *Journal of Developmental and Behavioral Pediatrics, 14,* 375-380.

Brennan-Behm, M., Carlson, G. E., Meier, P., & Engstrom, J. (1994). Caloric loss from expressed mother's milk during continuous gavage infusion. *Neonatal Network, 13*(2), 27-32.

Burns, K., Cunningham, N., White-Traut, R., Silvestri, J., & Nelson, M. N. (1994). Infant stimulation: Modification of an intervention based on physiologic and behavioral cues. *Journal of Obstetric, Gynecologic and Neonatal Nursing, 23*(7), 581-589.

Burroughs, A., Asonye, U., Anderson, G., & Vidyasagar, D. (1978). The effect of nonnutritive sucking on transcutaneous oxygen tension in noncrying, preterm neonates. *Research in Nursing and Health, 1,* 69-75.

Campos, R. G. (1989). Soothing pain-elicited distress in infants with swaddling and pacifiers. *Child Development, 60,* 781-792.

Censullo, M. (1994). Developmental delay in healthy premature infants at age two years: Implications for early development. *Journal of Developmental and Behavioral Pediatrics, 15*(2), 99-104.

Chamorro, I. L., Davis, M. L., Green, D., & Kramer, M. (1973). Development of an instrument to measure premature infant behavior and caretaker activities: Time sampling methodology. *Nursing Research, 22,* 300-309.

Chan, J., & Ferraro, A. R. (1991). The use of transploric feedings in the NICU: A national survey. *Neonatal Network, 10*(3), 37-42.

Chan, J.S.L., Kelley, M. L., & Khan, J. (1993). The effects of a pressure relief mattress on postnatal head molding in very low birth weight infants. *Neonatal Network, 12*(5), 19-22.

Chapman, J. S. (1978). The relationship between auditory stimulation and gross motor activity of short-gestation infants. *Research in Nursing and Health, 1*(1), 29-36.

Chapman, J. S. (1979). Influence of varied stimuli on development of motor patterns in the premature infant. *Birth Defects: Original Article Series, 15*(7), 1-80.

Cheng, M., & Williams, P. D. (1989). Oxygenation during chest physiotherapy of very-low-birth-weight infants: Relations among fraction of inspired oxygen levels, number of hand ventilation, and transcutaneous oxygen pressure. *Journal of Pediatric Nursing, 49*(6), 411-418.

Collinge, J.M., Bradley, K., Perks, C., Rezny, A., & Topping, P. (1982). Demand vs. scheduled feedings for premature infants. *Journal of Obstetric, Gynecologic, and Neonatal Nursing, 11*, 581-589.

Collins, S. K., & Kuck, K. (1991). Music therapy in the neonatal intensive care unit. *Neonatal Network, 9*(6), 19-24.

Corff, K. E. (1993). An effective comfort measure for minor pain and stress in preterm infants: Facilitated tucking [Abstract]. *Neonatal Network, 12*(8), 74.

Cornell, E. H., & Gottfried, A. W. (1976). Intervention with premature human infants. *Child Development, 47*, 32-39.

Cote, J., Morse, J. M., & James, S. G. (1991). The pain experience of the post-operative newborn. *Journal of Advanced Nursing, 16*, 378-387.

Curran, C. L., & Kachoyeanos, M. K. (1979). The effects on neonates of two methods of chest physical therapy. *MCN: The American Journal of Maternal-Child Nursing, 4*(5), 309-313.

Cusson, R. (1986, April). *Nurses' interactions with preterm infants.* Poster presented at the biennial International Conference on Infant Studies, Los Angeles. (Abstract published in *Infant Behavior and Development, 9*[Special ICIS Edition], 92)

Danzig, D. (1984). Neonatal transport teams: A survey of functions and roles. *Neonatal Network, 3*(5), 41-56.

D'Apolito, K. (1984). The neonate's response to pain. *MCN: The American Journal of Maternal-Child Nursing, 9*, 256-258.

Deiriggi, P. M. (1990). Effects of waterbed flotation on indicators of energy expenditure in preterm infants. *Nursing Research, 39*, 140-146.

DeMonterice, D., Meier, P., Engstrom, J., Crichton, C., & Mangurten, H. (1992). Concurrent validity off a new instrument for measuring nutritive sucking in preterm infants. *Nursing Research, 41*, 342-346.

DiPietro, J. A., Caughy, M. O., Cusson, R., & Fox, N. A. (1994). Cardiorespiratory functioning of preterm infants: Stability and risk associations for measures of heart rate variability and oxygen saturation. *Developmental Psychobiology, 27*(3), 137-152.

Dollison, E. J., & Beckstrand, J. (1995). Adhesive tape vs. pectin-based barrier use in term infants. *Neonatal Network, 14*(4), 35-39.

Duxbury, M. L., Henly, S. J., Broz, L. J., Armstrong, G. D., & Wachdorf, C. M. (1984). Care giver disruptions and sleep of high-risk infants. *Heart and Lung, 13*, 141-147.

Eckerman, C. O., Oehler, J, M., Medvin, M. B., & Hannan, T. E. (1994). Premature newborns as social partners before term age. *Infant Behavior and Development, 17*, 55-70.

Emde, R. N., Harmon, R. J., Metcalf, D., Koenig, K. L., & Wagonfeld, S. (1971). Stress and neonatal sleep. *Psychosomatic Medicine, 33*, 491-496.

Evans, J. C. (1991). Incidence of hypoxemia associated with care giving in premature infants. *Neonatal Network, 10*(2), 17-24.

Evans, J. (1992). Reducing the hypoxemia, bradycardia, and apnea associated with suctioning in low birth weight infants. *Journal of Perinatology, 12*(2), 137-142.

Evans, J. C. (1994). Comparison of two NICU patterns of care giving over 24 hours for preterm infants [Abstract]. *Neonatal Network, 13*(5), 87.

Evans, J. C., Vogelpohl, D. G., Bourguignon, C. M., & Morcott, C. S. (1997). Pain behaviors in LBW infants accompany some "non-painful" caregiving procedures. *Neonatal Network, 16*(3), 33-40.

Eyler, F. D., Courtway-Meyers, C., Edens, M. J., Hellrung, D. J., Nelson, R. M., Eitzman, D. V., & Resnick, M. B. (1989). Effects of developmental intervention on heart rate and transcutaneous oxygen levels in low-birth-weight infants. *Neonatal Network, 8*(3), 17-23.

Feingold, C. (1994). Correlates of cognitive development in low-birth-weight infants from low-income families. *Journal of Pediatric Nursing, 9*(2), 91-97.

Fischel, J. E., & Imbruglio, L. R. (1989). Developmental evaluation of the newborn intensive care graduate: The lost-to-follow-up problem. *Neonatal Network, 8*(1), 23-27.

Fox, M. (1991). Urine measurement: diaper weight accuracy [Abstract]. *Neonatal Network, 9*(8), 73.

Franck, L. S. (1987). A national survey of the assessment and treatment of pain and agitation in the neonatal intensive care unit. *Journal of Obstetric, Gynecologic and Neonatal Nursing, 16*, 387-393.

Gibson, L. Y. (1996). Pulse oximeter in neonatal ICU: A correlational analysis. *Pediatric Nursing, 22*(6), 511-515.

Gill, N., Behnke, M., Conlon, M., & Anderson, G. (1988). Non-nutritive sucking: Effect on behavioral state in preterm infants prefeeding. *Nursing Research, 37*, 347-350.

Goldstein, R. F., Thompson, R. J. Jr., Oehler, J. M., & Brazy, J. E. (1995). Influence of acidosis, hypoxemia, and hypotension on neurodevelopmental outcome in very low birth weight infants. *Pediatrics, 95*(2), 238-243.

Gonzales, I., Duryea, E. J., Vazquez, E., & Geraghty, N. (1995). Effect of enteral feeding temperature on feeding tolerance in preterm infants. *Neonatal Network, 14*(3), 39-43.

Gordon, M., & Montgomery, L. A. (1996). Minimizing epidermal stripping in the very low birth weight infant: Integrating research and practice to affect infant outcome. *Neonatal Network, 15*(1), 37-44.

Gottlieb, G. (1996). A systems view of psychobiological development. In D. Magnusson (Ed.), *Individual development over the lifespan: Biological and psychosocial perspectives* (pp. 76-103). Cambridge, England: Cambridge University Press.

Graven, S. N., Bowen, F. W. Jr., Brooten, D., Eaton, A., Graven, M. N., Hack, M., Hall, L. A., Hansen, N., Hurt, H., Kavalhuna, R., Little, G. A., Mahan, C., Morrow, G. III, Oehler, J. M., Poland, R., Ram, B., Sauve, R., Taylor, P. M., Ward, S. E., & Sommers, J. G. (1992). The high-risk infant environment: Part 1. The role of the neonatal intensive care unit in the outcome of high-risk infants. *Journal of Perinatology, 12*(2), 164-172.

Greenough, W. T., Black, J. E., & Wallace, C. S. (1987). Experience and brain development. *Child Development, 58*, 539-559.

Gunderson, L. P., & Stoekle, M. L. (1995). Endotracheal suctioning of the newborn piglet. *Western Journal of Nursing Research, 7*(1), 20-31.

Gunderson, L. P., Stone, K. S., & Hamlin, R. L. (1991). Endotracheal suctioning-induced heart rate alterations. *Nursing Research, 40*(3), 139-143.

Haddock, B. J., Merrow, D. L., & Vincent, P. A. (1988). Comparisons of axillary and rectal temperatures in the preterm infant. *Neonatal Network, 7*(2), 67-71.

Harrison, L. L., Leeper, J. D., & Yoon, M. (1990). Effects of early parental touch on preterm infants' heart rates and arterial oxygen saturation levels. *Journal of Advanced Nursing, 15*, 877-885.

Harrison, L. L., Leeper, J., & Yoon, M. (1991). Preterm infants' physiologic responses to early parent touch. *Western Journal of Nursing Research, 13*, 698-713.

Harrison, L. L., & Woods, S. (1991). Early parental touch and preterm infants. *Journal of Obstetric, Gynecologic and Neonatal Nursing, 20*(4), 299-306.

Hasselmeyer, E. G., de la Puente, J., Lundeen, E. C., & Morrison, M. (1963). A weight chart for preterm infants. *Nursing Research, 12,* 222-231.

Hemingway, M. M., & Oliver, S. K. (1991). Water bed therapy and cranial molding of the sick preterm infant. *Neonatal Network, 10*(3), 53-56.

Hodges, C., & Vincent, P. A. (1993). Why do NICU nurses not refeed gastric residuals prior to feeding by gavage? *Neonatal Network, 12*(8), 37-40.

Holditch-Davis, D. (1990a). The development of sleeping and waking states in high-risk preterm infants. *Infant Behavior and Development, 13,* 513-531.

Holditch-Davis, D. (1990b). The effect of hospital care giving on preterm infants' sleeping and waking states. In S. G. Funk, E. M. Tornquist, M. T. Champagne, L. A. Copp, & R. A. Wiese (Eds.), *Key aspects of recovery: Improving nutrition, rest, and mobility* (pp. 110-122). New York: Springer.

Holditch-Davis, D. (1995). Behaviors of preterm infants with and without chronic lung disease when alone and when with nurses. *Neonatal Network, 14*(7), 51-57.

Holditch-Davis, D., Barham, L., O'Hale, A., & Tucker, E. (1995). The effect of standardized rest periods on convalescent preterm infants. *Journal of Obstetric, Gynecologic and Neonatal Nursing, 24,* 424-432.

Holditch-Davis, D., & Calhoun, M. (1989). Do preterm infants show behavioral responses to painful procedures? In S. G. Funk, E. M. Tornquist, M. T. Champagne, L. A. Copp, & R. A. Wiese (Eds.), *Key aspects of comfort: Management of pain, fatigue, and nausea* (pp. 35-43). New York: Springer.

Holditch-Davis, D., & Edwards, L. (1998). Modeling development of sleep-wake behaviors. II. Results of two cohorts of preterms. *Physiology and Behavior, 63*(1), 319-328.

Holditch-Davis, D., & Edwards, L. (in press). Temporal organization of sleep-wake states in preterm infants. *Developmental Psychobiology.*

Holditch-Davis, D., Edwards, L. J., & Wigger, M. C. (1994). Pathologic apnea and brief respiratory pauses in preterm infants: Relation to sleep state. *Nursing Research, 43*(5), 293-300.

Holditch-Davis, D., & Hudson, D. C. (1995). Using preterm infant behaviors to identify acute medical complications. In S. G. Funk, E. M. Tornquist, M. T. Champagne, & R. A. Wiese (Eds.), *Key aspects of caring for the acutely ill: Technological aspects, patient education, and quality of life* (pp. 95-120). New York: Springer.

Holditch-Davis, D., & Lee, D. A. (1993). The behaviors and nursing care of preterm infants with chronic lung disease. In S. G. Funk, E. M. Tornquist, M. Champagne, & R. A. Wiese (Eds.), *Key aspects of caring for the chronically ill: Hospital and home* (pp. 250-270). New York: Springer.

Holditch-Davis, D., & Thoman, E. B. (1987). Behavioral states of premature infants: Implications for neural and behavioral development. *Developmental Psychobiology, 20,* 25-38.

Hultgren, M. S. (1990). Assessment of post-operative pain in critically ill infants. *Progress in Cardiovascular Nursing, 5*(3), 104-112.

Iffrig, M. C. Sr. (1956). Nursing observations of one hundred premature infants and their feeding programs. *Nursing Research, 5*(2), 71-81.

Jay, S. S. (1982). The effects of gentle human touch on mechanically ventilated very-short-term-gestation infants. *Maternal-Child Nursing Journal, 11*(4), 199-257.

Johnson, K. J., Bhatia, P., & Bell, E. F. (1991). Infrared thermometry of newborn infants. *Pediatrics, 87*(1), 34-38.

Johnston, C. C., & Stevens, B. J. (1996). Experience in a neonatal intensive care unit affects pain response. *Pediatrics, 98,* 925-930.

Jones, M. A. (1989). Identifying signs that nurses interpret as indicating pain in newborns. *Pediatric Nursing, 15*(1), 76-79.

Katz, V. (1971). Auditory stimulation and developmental behavior of the premature infant. *Nursing Research, 20,* 196-201.

Kennedy, C., & Lipsitt, L. P. (1993). Temporal characteristics of nonoral feedings and chronic feeding problems in premature infants. *Journal of Perinatal and Neonatal Nursing, 7*(3), 77-89.

Kephart, N. (1960). *The slow learner in the classroom.* Cincinnati, OH: Merrill Boslow.

Kitchin, L. W., & Hutchinson, S. (1996). Touch during preterm infants resuscitation. *Neonatal Network, 15*(7), 45-51.

Kleiber, C., & Hummel, P. A. (1989). Factors related to spontaneous endotracheal extubation in the neonate. *Pediatric Nursing, 15*(4), 347-351.

Kotter, R. W. (1996). Heparin vs saline for intermittent intravenous device maintenance in neonates. *Neonatal Network, 15*(6), 43-47.

Kramer, M., Chamorro, I., Green, D., & Kundson, P. (1975). Extra tactile stimulation of the premature infant. *Nursing Research, 24,* 324-333.

Krywanio, M. L. (1994). Meta-analysis of physiological outcomes of hospital-based infant intervention programs. *Nursing Research, 43*(3), 133-137.

Lawrence, J., Alcock, D., McGrath, P., Kay, J., MacMurray, S. B., & Dulberg, C. (1993). The development of a tool to assess neonatal pain. *Neonatal Network, 12*(6), 59-66.

Ludington-Hoe, S. M., Hadeed, A., & Anderson, G. C. (1991). Physiologic responses to skin-to-skin contact in hospitalized premature infants. *Journal of Perinatology, 4,* 19-24.

Ludington-Hoe, S. M., Thompson, C., Swinth, J., Hadeed, A., & Anderson, G. C. (1994). Kangaroo care: Research results, and practice implications and guidelines. *Neonatal Network, 13,* 19-26.

Lybrand, M., Medoff-Cooper, B., & Munro, B. H. (1990). Periodic comparisons of specific gravity using urine from a diaper and collecting bag. *MCN: The American Journal of Maternal-Child Nursing, 15,* 238-239.

Malloy, G. B. (1979). The relationship between maternal and musical auditory stimulation and the developmental behavior of premature infants. *Birth Defects: Original Article Series, 15*(7), 81-98.

Mandich, M. B., Ritchie, S. K., & Mullett, M. (1996). Transition times to oral feeding in premature infants with and without apnea. *Journal of Obstetric, Gynecologic and Neonatal Nursing, 25,* 771-776.

Marchette, L., Main, R., & Redick, E. (1989). Pain reduction during neonatal circumcision. *Pediatric Nursing, 15,* 207-210.

Masterson, J., Zucker, C., & Schulze, K. (1987). Prone and supine positioning effects on energy expenditure and behavior of low birth weight neonates. *Pediatrics, 80*(5), 689-692.

Mathew, O., Clark, M., Pronske, M., Luna-Solarzano, H., & Peterson, M. (1985). Breathing pattern and ventilation during oral feeding in term newborn infants. *Journal of Pediatrics, 106,* 810-813.

McCain, G. C. (1992). Facilitating inactive awake states in preterm infants: A study of three interventions. *Nursing Research, 41*(3), 157-160.

Medoff-Cooper, B. (1986). Temperament in very low birth weight infants. *Nursing Research, 35*(3), 139-143.

Medoff-Cooper, B. (1988). The effects of handling on preterm infants with bronchopulmonary dysplasia. *Image: The Journal of Nursing Scholarship, 20*(3), 132-134.

Medoff-Cooper, B. (1994). Transitition of the preterm infant to the open crib. *Journal of Obstetric, Gynecologic, and Neonatal Nursing, 23*(4), 329-335.

Medoff-Cooper, B., & Gennaro, S. (1996). The correlation of sucking behaviors and Bayley Scales of Infant Development at six months of age in VLBW infants. *Nursing Research, 45,* 291-296.

Medoff-Cooper, B., & McGrath, J. (1998). *Nutritive sucking and neurobehavioral development in VLBW infants from 34 weeks PCA to term.* Unpublished manuscript, University of Pennsylvania.

Medoff-Cooper, B., & Schraeder, B. D. (1982). Developmental trends and behavioral styles in very low birth weight infants. *Nursing Research, 31,* 68-72.

Medoff-Cooper, B., Verklan, T., & Carlson, S. (1993). The development of sucking patterns and physiologic correlates in very low birth weight infants. *Nursing Research, 42,* 100-105.

Medoff-Cooper, B., Weininger, S., & Zukowsky, K. (1989). Neonatal sucking as a clinical assessment tool: Preliminary findings. *Nursing Research, 38,* 162-165.

Meier, P. (1988). Bottle and breast feeding: Effects on transcutaneous oxygen pressure and temperature in preterm infants. *Nursing Research, 37*(1), 36-41.

Meier, P. P., & Brown, L. P. (1996). State of the science: Breast feeding for mothers and low birth weight infants. *Maternal Fetal Nursing, 31*(2), 351-365.

Meier, P. P., Engstron, L. L., Mangurten, H. H., Estrada, E., Zimmerman, B., & Kopparthi, R. (1993). A model to provide breast feeding support services in the NICU. *Journal of Obstetric, Gynecologic and Neonatal Nursing, 22,* 338-347.

Meier, P., & Pugh, E. (1985). Breastfeeding behavior of small preterm infants. *MCN: The American Journal of Maternal-Child Nursing, 10,* 396-401.

Miller, D. B., & Holditch-Davis, D. (1992). Interactions of parents and nurses with high-risk preterm infants. *Research in Nursing and Health, 15*(3), 187-197.

Mitchell-DiCenso, A., Guyatt, G., Marrin, M., Goeree, R., Willan, A., Southwell, D., Hewson, S., Paes, B., Rosenbaum, P., Hunsberger, M., & Bauman, A. (1996). A controlled trial of nurse practitioners in neonatal intensive care. *Pediatrics, 98,* 1143-1148.

Moen, J. E., Chapman, S., Sheehan, A., & Carter, P. (1987). Axillary versus rectal temperatures in preterm infants under radiant warmers. *Journal of Obstetric, Gynecologic and Neonatal Nursing, 17*(5), 348-351.

Neal, M. V. (1979). Organizational behavior of the premature infant. *Birth Defects: Original Article Series, 15*(7), 43-60.

Neal, M. V., & Nauen, C. M. (1968). Ability of premature infant to maintain his own body temperature. *Nursing Research, 17*(5), 396-402.

Nelson, D., & Heitman, R. (1986). Factors influencing weight change in preterm infants. *Pediatric Nursing, 12*(6), 425-428.

Nelson, D., Heitman, R., & Jennings, C. (1986). Effects of tactile stimulation on premature infant weight gain. *Journal of Obstetric, Gynecologic and Neonatal Nursing, 15*(3), 262-267.

Nelson, H., Thomas, K., & Stein, M. (1992). Thermal effects of hooding incubators. *Journal of Obstetric, Gynecologic, and Neonatal Nursing, 21,* 377- 381.

Norris, S., Campbell, L., & Brenkert, S. (1981). Nursing procedures and alterations in transcutaneous oxygen tension in premature infants. *Nursing Research, 31,* 330-336.

Norton, S. J. (1988). Aftereffects of morphine and fentanyl analgesia: A retrospective study. *Neonatal Network, 7*(3), 25-28.

Nurse researchers show stimulation speeds development in prematures. (1978). *American Journal of Nursing, 78,* 968-1090.

Oehler, J. M. (1995). Development of mother-child interaction in very low birth weight infants. In S. G. Funk, E. M. Tornquist, M. T. Champagne, & R. A. Wiese (Eds.), *Key aspects of caring for the acutely ill: Technological aspects, patient education, and quality of life* (pp. 120-133). New York: Springer.

Oehler, J. M., Goldstein, R. F., Catlett, A., Boshoff, M., & Brazy, J. E. (1993). How to target infants at highest risk for developmental delay. *MCN: The American Journal of Maternal-Child Nursing, 18,* 20-23.

Oehler, J. M., Hannan, T., & Catlett, A. (1993). Maternal views of preterm infants' responsiveness to social interaction. *Neonatal Network, 12*(6), 67-74.

Oppenheim, R. W. (1981). Ontogenetic adaptations and retrogressive processes in the development of the nervous system and behavior. In K. Connolly & H. Prechtl (Eds.), *Maturation and behavior development* (pp. 73-109). London: Spastic Society.

Page, G. G., & Halverson, M. (1991). Pediatric nurses: The assessment and control of pain in preverbal infants. *Journal of Pediatric Nursing, 6,* 99-106.

Park, A. (1991). Preterm infants' respiratory responses to oral/gustatory and tactile stimulation during an apneic episode [Abstract]. *Neonatal Network, 10*(5), 79.

Parker, S. J., Zahr, L. K., Cole, J. G., & Brecht, M. L. (1992). Outcome after developmental intervention in the neonatal intensive care unit for mothers of preterm infants with low socioeconomic status. *Journal of Pediatrics, 120,* 780-785.

Peters, K. L. (1992). Does routine nursing care complicate the physiologic status of the premature neonate with respiratory distress syndrome? *Journal of Perinatal and Neonatal Nursing, 6*(2), 67-84.

Peters, K. L. (1996). Dinosaurs in the bath. *Neonatal Network, 15*(1), 71-73.

Philbin, M. K., Ballweg, D. D., & Gray, L. (1994). The effect of an intensive care unit sound environment on the development of habituation in healthy avian neonates. *Developmental Psychobiology, 27*(1), 11-21.

Pickler, R. H. (1993). Premature infant-nurse care giver interaction. *Western Journal of Nursing Research, 15*(5), 548-567.

Pickler, R. H., Frankel, H. B., Walsh, K. M., & Thompson, N. H. (1996). Effects of non-nutritive sucking on behavioral organization and feeding performance in preterm infants. *Nursing Research, 45*(3), 132-135.

Pigeon, H. M., McGrath, P. J., Lawrence, J., & MacMurray, S. B. (1989). Nurses' perceptions of pain in the neonatal intensive care unit. *Journal of Pain and Symptom Management, 4,* 179-183.

Pohlman, S., & Beardslee, C. (1987). Contacts experienced by neonates in intensive care environments. *Maternal-Child Nursing Journal, 16*(3), 207-226.

Prechtl, H., & Stemmer, C. (1962). The choreiform syndrome in children. *Developmental Medicine and Child Neurology, 4,* 119-123.

Premji, S.S.J.E., & Chapman, J. S. (1997). Nurses' experience with implementing developmental care in NICUs. *Western Journal of Nursing Research, 19,* 97-109.

Rausch, P. B. (1981). Effects of tactile and kinesthetic stimulation on premature infants. *Journal of Obstetric, Gynecologic and Neonatal Nursing, 10*(1), 34-37.

Rey, E. S., & Martinez, H. B. (1983, March 17-18). *Manjeo rational de niño prematuro.* Paper presented at the conferences curso de Medicinia Fetal y Neonatal, Bogota, Colombia.

Saunders, R. B., Friedman, C. B., & Stramoski, P. R. (1991). Feeding preterm infants: Schedule or demand? *Journal of Obstetric, Gynecologic and Neonatal Nursing, 20,* 212-218.

Scanlon, K. B., Grylack, L. J., & Borten, M. (1982). Placement of umbilical artery catheters: High vs. low. *Journal of Obstetric, Gynecologic and Neonatal Nursing, 11*(6), 355-358.

Schraeder, B. D. (1986). Developmental progress in very low birth weight infants during the first year of life. *Nursing Research, 35*(4), 237-242.

Schraeder, B. D. (1993). Assessment of measures to detect preschool academic risk in very-low-birth-weight children. *Nursing Research, 42*(1), 17-21.

Schraeder, B. D., Heverly, M. A., O'Brien, C., & McEvoy-Shields, K. (1992). Finishing first grade: A study of school achievement in very-low-birth-weight children. *Nursing Research, 41*(6), 354-361.

Schraeder, B. D., Heverly, M. A., & Rappaport, J. (1990a). Temperament, behavior problems, and learning skills in very low birth weight preschoolers. *Research in Nursing and Health, 13,* 17-34.

Schraeder, B. D., Heverly, M. A., & Rappaport, J. (1990b). The value of early home assessment in identifying risk in children who were very low birth weight. *Pediatric Nursing, 16*(3), 268-272.

Schraeder, B. D., & Medoff-Cooper, B. (1983). Development and temperament in very low birth weight infants: The second year. *Nursing Research, 32*(6), 331-335.

Schraeder, B. D., Rappaport, J., & Courtwright, L. (1987). Preschool development of very low birth weight infants. *Image: The Journal of Nursing Scholarship, 19*(4), 174-178.

Schwirian, P. M., Eesley, T., & Cueller, L. (1986). Use of water pillows in reducing head shape distortion in preterm infants. *Research in Nursing and Health, 9,* 203-207.

Segall, M. E. (1972). Cardiac responsivity to auditory stimulation in premature infants. *Nursing Research, 21,* 947-101.

Shaio, S.-Y.P.K. (1997). Comparison of continuous versus intermittent sucking in very-low-birth-weight infants. *Journal of Obstertric, Gynecologic and Neonatal Nursing, 26,* 313-319.

Shaio, S.-Y.P.K., Youngblut, J. M., Anderson, G. C., DiFiore, J. M., & Martin, R. J. (1995). Nasogastric tube placement: Effects on breathing and sucking in very low birth weight infants. *Nursing Research, 44*(2), 82-87.

Shapiro, C. (1989). Pain in the neonate: Assessment and intervention. *Neonatal Network, 8,* 7-21.

Shapiro, C. R. (1993). Nurses' judgements of pain in term and preterm neonates. *Journal of Obstetric, Gynecologic, and Neonatal Nursing, 22*(1), 41-47.

Sherwood, B., Donze, A., & Giebe, J. (1994). Mechanical vibration in ambulance transport. *Journal of Obstetric, Gynecologic and Neonatal Nursing, 23*(6), 457-463.

Shogan, M. G., & Schumann, L. L. (1993). The effect of environmental lighting on the oxygen saturation of preterm infants in the NICU. *Neonatal Network, 12*(5), 7-13.

Short, M. A., Brooks-Brunn, J. A., Reeves, D. S., Yeager, J., & Thorpe, J. A. (1996). The effects of swaddling versus standard positioning on neuromuscular development in very low birth weight infants. *Neonatal Network, 15*(4), 25-31.

Siddell, E. P., & Froman, R. D. (1994). A national survey of neonatal intensive care units: Criteria used to determine readiness for oral feedings. *Journal of Obstetric, Gynecologic and Neonatal Nursing, 19,* 209-220.

Smith, S. L., Kirchhoff, K. T., Chan, G. M., & Squire, S. J. (1994). Patterns of postnatal weight changes in infants with very low and extremely low birth weights. *Heart & Lung, 23,* 439-445.

Squire, S. J., & Kirchhoff, K. T. (1992). Positional oxygenation changes in air-transported neonates. *Heart & Lung, 21*(3), 255-259.

Standley, J. M., & Moore, R. S. (1995). Therapeutic effects of music and mother's voice on premature infants. *Pediatric Nursing, 21*(6), 509-512, 574.

Stebor, A. D. (1989). Posturination time and specific gravity in infants' diapers. *Nursing Research, 38*(4), 244-245.

Stephen, S. B., & Sexton, P. R. (1987). Neonatal axillary temperatures: Increases in readings over time. *Neonatal Network, 6*(4), 25-28.

Stevens, B. J., & Johnston, C. C. (1993). Pain in the infant: Theoretical and conceptual issues. *Maternal-Child Nursing Journal, 21*(1), 3-14.

Stevens, B. J., & Johnston, C. C. (1994). Physiological responses of premature infants to a painful stimuli. *Nursing Research, 43*(4), 226-231.

Stevens, B. J., Johnston, C. C., & Horton, L. (1993). Multidimensional pain assessment in premature neonates: A pilot study. *Journal of Obstetric, Gynecologic, and Neonatal Nursing, 22*(6), 531-541.

Strauch, C., Brandt, S., & Edwards-Beckett, J. (1993). Implementation of a quiet hour: Effect on noise levels and infant sleep states. *Neonatal Network, 12*(2), 31-35.

Syfrett, E. B., & Anderson, G. C. (1996, October 23-26). *Very early kangaroo care beginning at birth for 34-36 week infants: Effect on outcome.* Paper presented at the Meeting on Kangaroo Mother Care, Bureau of International Health, World Health Organization, Trieste, Italy.

Symington, A., Ballantyne, M., Pinelli, J., & Stevens, B. (1995). Indwelling versus intermittent feeding tube in premature neonates. *Journal of Obstetric, Gynecologic, and Neonatal Nursing, 24,* 321-326.

Telzrow, R. W., Kang, R. R., Mitchell, S. K., Ashworth, C. D., & Barnard, K. E. (1982). An assessment of the behavior of the preterm infant at 40 weeks conceptional age. In L. P. Lipsitt & T. M. Field (Eds.), *Infant behavior and development: Perinatal risk and newborn behavior* (pp. 85-96). Norwood, NJ: Ablex.

Termini, L., Brooten, D., Brown, L., Gennaro, S., & York, R. (1990). Reasons for acute car visits and rehospitalizations in very low-birth weight infants. *Neonatal Network, 8*(5), 23-26.

Thoman, E. B. (1990). Sleeping and waking states in infancy: A functional perspective. *Neuroscience and Biobehavioral Reviews, 14,* 93-107.

Thoman, E. B., Holditch-Davis, D., Raye, J. R., Philipps, A. F., Rowe, J. C., & Denenberg, V. H. (1985). Theophylline affects sleep-wake state development in premature infants. Neuropediatrics, 16, 13-18.

Thomas, K. A. (1989). How the NICU environment sounds to a preterm infant. *MCN: The American Journal of Maternal-Child Nursing, 14,* 249-251.

Thomas, K. A. (1991). The emergence of body temperature biorhythm in preterm infants. *Nursing Research, 40*(2), 98-102.

Thomas, K. A. (1995). Biorhythms in infants and the role of the care environment. *Journal of Perinatal and Neonatal Nursing, 9*(2), 61-75.

Thompson, R. J. Jr., Goldstein, R. F., Oehler, J. M., Gustafson, K. E., Catlett, A. T., & Brazy, J. E. (1994). Developmental outcome of very low birthweight infants as function of biological risk and psychosocial risk. *Journal of Developmental and Behavioral Pediatrics, 15*(4), 232-238.

Tobey, G. Y., & Schraeder, B. D. (1990). Impact of caretaker stress on behavioral adjustment of very low birthweight infants. *Nursing Research, 39,* 84-89.

Tobin, C. R. (1988). The teflon intravenous catheter: Incidence of phlebitis and duration of catheter life in the neonatal patient. *Journal of Obstetric, Gynecologic and Neonatal Nursing, 17*(1), 35-42.

Tolles, C. L., & Stone, K. S. (1990). National survey of neonatal endotracheal suctioning practices. *Neonatal Network, 9*(2), 7-14.

Torrance, J. T. (1968). Temperature readings of premature infants. *Nursing Research, 17*(4), 312-320.

Torres, C., Holditch-Davis, D., O'Hale, A., & D'Auria, J. (in press). Effect of standardized rest periods on apnea and weight gain of convalescent preterm infants. *Journal of Obstetric, Gynecologic and Neonatal Nursing.*

Updike, P. A., Accurso, F. J., & Jones, R. H. (1985). Physiologic circadian rhythmicity in preterm infants. *Nursing Research, 34,* 160-166.

Van Cleve, L., & Andrews, S. (1995). Pain responses of hospitalized neonates to venipuncture activities. *MCN: The American Journal of Maternal-Child Nursing, 20*(3), 148-152.

Van Cleve, L., Johnson, L., Andrews, S., Hawkins, S., & Newbold, J. (1995). Pain responses of hospitalized neonates to venipuncture. *Neonatal Network, 14*(6), 31-36.

Von Pfaundler, M. (1899). *Sommerfelds Handbuck der Michkunde.* Weisbaden, Germany.

Wahlberg, V., Affonso, D., & Peterson, B. (1992). A retrospective comparative study using the kangaroo method as a complement to standard incubator care. *European Journal of Public Health, 2*(1), 34-37.

Weiss, M. E., & Richards, M. T. (1994). Accuracy of electronic axillary temperature measurement in term and preterm neonates. *Neonatal Network, 13*(8), 35-40.

Werner, N. P., & Conway, A. E. (1990). Caregiver contacts experienced by premature infants in the neonatal intensive care unit. *Maternal-Child Nursing Journal, 19*(1), 21-43.

White-Traut, R. C., & Goldman, M.B.C. (1988). Premature infant massage: Is it safe? *Pediatric Nursing, 14*(4), 285-289.

White-Traut, R. C., & Nelson, M. N. (1988). Maternally administered tactile, auditory, visual, and vestibular stimulation: Relationship to later interactions between mothers and premature infants. *Research in Nursing and Health, 11,* 31-39.

White-Traut, R. C., Nelson, M., Silvestri, J. M., Cunningham, N., & Patel, M. (1997). Responses of preterm infants to unimodal and multimodal sensory intervention. *Pediatric Nursing, 23,* 169-175, 193.

White-Traut, R. C., Nelson, M. N., Silvestri, J. M., Patel, M. K., & Kilgallon, D. (1993). Patterns of physiologic and behavioral response of intermediate care preterm infants to intervention. *Pediatric Nursing, 19*(6), 625-629.

White-Traut, R. C., & Pate, C.M.H. (1987). Modulating infant state in premature infants. *Journal of Pediatric Nursing, 1*(2), 90-95.

White-Traut, R. C., & Tubezewski, K. A. (1986). Multimodal stimulation of the premature infant. *Journal of Pediatric Nursing, 1*(2), 90-95.

Williams, P., Williams, A., & Dial, M. (1986). Children at risk: Perinatal events, developmental delays and the effects of a developmental stimulation program. *Journal of Nursing Studies, 23,* 21-38.

Wilson, J., Arnold, C., Connor, R., & Cusson, R. (1996). Evaluation of oxygen delivery with the use of nasopharyngeal catheters and nasal cannulas. *Neonatal Network, 15*(4), 15-22.

Wolff, P. (1968). The serial organization of sucking in the young infant. *Pediatrics, 42,* 943-956.

Youngblut, J. M., Loveland-Cherry, C. J., & Horan, M. (1993). Maternal employment, family functioning, and preterm infant development at 9 and 12 months. *Research in Nursing and Health, 16,* 33-43.

Zahr, L. K., & Balian, S. (1995). Responses of premature infants to routine nursing interventions and noise in the NICU. *Nursing Research, 44*(3), 179-185.

Zahr, L. K., Parker, S., & Cole, J. (1992). Comparing the effects of neonatal intensive care unit intervention on premature infants at different weights. *Journal of Developmental and Behavioral Pediatrics, 13*(3), 165-172.

11

THERAPEUTIC OUTCOMES SENSITIVE TO NURSING

William L. Holzemer
Suzanne Bakken Henry

Nursing professionals are increasingly called upon to demonstrate the contributions of nursing practice to patient outcomes (American Nurses Association, 1995; Clark & Lang, 1992; Lange & Marek, 1992). Valid and reliable instruments that can be used in clinical settings and are sensitive to the impact of nursing interventions are essential to meeting this challenge (Crawford, Taylor, Seipert, & Lush, 1996; Jennings, 1991; Johnson & Maas, 1995; Martin, Scheet, & Stegman, 1993). In this chapter, we examine the state of the science related to the measurement of therapeutic outcomes sensitive to nursing care. The scope of the review excludes outcomes that are covered in detail elsewhere in this volume (e.g., biological stabilization, cognitive-behavioral) and is limited to those outcomes in which a patient is the unit of analysis. First, a conceptual model for patient outcomes that links clinical variables with health status measures (Wilson & Cleary, 1995) is reviewed and subsequently used as an organizing framework for a review

of measurement instruments. Second, 16 instruments are classified according to the model and critically analyzed. Third, the conceptual and methodological issues related to the measurement of therapeutic outcomes sensitive to nursing care are reviewed.

Conceptual Model

A conceptual model of health-related quality of life outlined in terms of patient outcomes (Figure 11.1), proposed by Wilson and Cleary (1995), links traditional clinical variables with health status. (The terms "health-related quality of life" and "health status" are used interchangeably by us.) Within the five component scheme—biological and physiological variables, symptom status, functional status, general health perceptions, and overall quality of life—health status is conceptualized as exist-

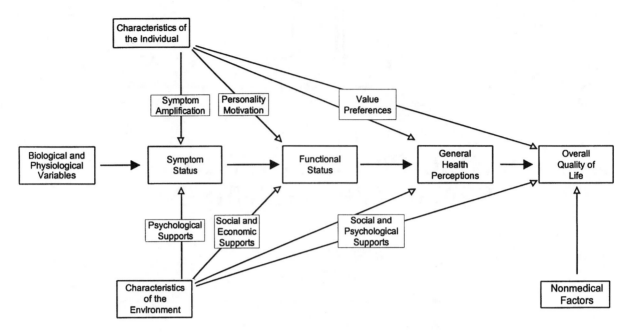

Figure 11.1 Conceptual Model of Health-Related Quality of Life in Terms of Patient Outcomes

ing on a continuum of increasing biological, social, and psychological complexity. Subsequently, the five components represent increasing measurement difficulty and number of intervening variables not outside the control of health care providers. The model also explicates specific causal linkages between the components but has yet to undergo empirical testing.

The model was selected as a heuristic for discussing therapeutic outcomes sensitive to nursing care for several reasons. First, the components of the model have served to define outcome variables in nursing studies; second, these components reflect human responses to illness that are the focus of nursing interventions. In the following paragraphs, therapeutic outcomes as categorical components of the model are defined.

Biological and Physiological Component

This category includes medical diagnoses, laboratory values, physical examination findings, and other measures of physiological functioning such as pulmonary, cardiovascular, or renal function tests. Although interventions related to many of these factors are within the purview of nursing, related measures are discussed elsewhere in this volume and not in this chapter.

Symptom Status Component

A symptom is defined as "a patient's perception of an abnormal physical, emotional, or cognitive state" (Wilson & Cleary, 1995, p. 61). Instruments exist that measure single symptoms such as pain (e.g., McGill Pain Questionnaire; Melzack, 1975) or fatigue (e.g., Visual Analogue Scale for Fatigue; Lee, Hicks, & Nino-Murcia, 1991); others include multiple symptoms (e.g., Symptom Distress Scale; McCorkle & Young, 1978). In her comprehensive review of patient care outcomes related to symptoms, Hegyvary (1993) emphasized that research into management of symptoms and symptom outcomes is an essential adjunct to research about disease and treatment.

Functional Status Component

Functional status is defined as "the ability of the individual to perform particular defined tasks" (Wilson & Cleary, 1995, p. 61; see Chapter 19 this volume, for further discussion of this variable). Four commonly identified domains of interest to patients, clinicians, and researchers are physical, social role, and psychological functions, often separated into emotional and cognitive. Instruments such as the Medical Outcome Study Short Form 36 (Ware & Sherbourne, 1992) and the Sickness

Impact Profile (Bergner, Bobbitt, Carter, & Gilson, 1981) are designed to measure a full range of functional status domains; others, including the Karnofsky Performance Status (Karnofsky, Abelmann, Craver, & Burchenal, 1948) and the Quality Audit Marker (Holzemer, Henry, Stewart, & Janson-Bjerklie, 1993), are focused on physical status. In her critical analysis of the literature, Leidy (1994) acknowledged the importance of functional status as a nursing-sensitive outcome measure and also highlighted the conceptual confusion related to its measurement. She proposes four dimensions of functional status—functional capacity, performance, reserve, and capacity utilization—but the majority of existing instruments measure only performance.

General Health Perceptions Component

Rather than being explicitly defined in the Wilson and Cleary model, general health perceptions are characterized as an integration of the previous concepts in the model: that is, biophysical variables, symptom status, and functional status, plus mental health. Involving a subjective rating, large variations in responses occur across the range of illness severity. General health perceptions are frequently measured by a single item, and a limited number of instruments exist that measure this component (e.g., the Medical Outcome Study Short Form 36) (Ware & Sherbourne, 1992).

Overall Quality of Life Component

Overall quality of life is defined as a general measure of happiness or satisfaction with life as a whole. It represents a synthesis of a wide range of experiences and feelings. As examples, the Quality of Life Index (Ferrans & Powers, 1985) measures both satisfaction with and importance of various domains of life using multiple items; the Medical Outcome Study Short Form 36 (Ware & Sherbourne, 1992) uses a single item to provide an overall rating.

Critical Analysis of Selected Instruments

Instruments chosen for inclusion in this review met three criteria: (a) they measured a component of the Wilson and Cleary model, (b) they had published evidence for reliability and validity, and (c) they had been used in at least one nursing research study. The intent of this selection process was to provide illustrative examples, not an exhaustive review.

Patient outcomes measured by each instrument are indicated in Table 11.1, and examples of nursing studies are shown in Table 11.2, both according to the components of the model. In the following paragraphs, instruments are described and the quality of the evidence for reliability and validity analyzed. Examples of each instrument's use in nursing studies are also provided.

Six instruments could be classified as measures of mainly symptom status and follow in alphabetical order.

Adolescent Pediatric Pain Tool (APPT)

Description. Modeled after the McGill Pain Questionnaire (Melzack, 1975), the APPT (Savedra, Tesler, Holzemer, Wilkie, & Ward, 1990) contains three parts: (a) a body outline to measure pain location; (b) a one-item, 10-cm word graphic rating scale to measure pain intensity; and (c) a word list of 43 pain descriptors to assess three dimensions of pain quality (sensory, affective, and evaluative) (Savedra, Holzemer, Tesler, & Wilkie, 1993). The APPT requires approximately 5 minutes to complete.

Reliability and validity. The APPT has been subjected to extensive validation to remove potential gender, ethnic, and developmental biases (Wilkie, Holzemer, et al., 1990). Strong evidence supports the content validity of the APPT and the test-retest reliability when administered within a short time frame (Tesler, Wilkie, Holzemer, & Savedra, 1994). The APPT has been demonstrated to provide valid and reliable estimates of adolescents' and children's self-reports of the location, intensity, and quality of pain.

Examples in nursing research. The APPT was used to measure change in pain intensity over time postsurgery in a sample of 131 children and adolescents (Tesler et al., 1994). The findings documented the undermedication of the children and the moderately severe pain the children were experiencing.

TABLE 11.1 Scale Dimensions, Classified by Wilson and Cleary (1995) Model

Instrument	Symptom Status			Functional Status				Role	Health Perceptions	Overall Quality of Life
	Physical	Cognitive	Emotional	Physical	Cognitive	Emotional	Social			
ADL				x						
APPT	x									
DVAS	x									
INV-2	x									
KPS				x						
MPQ	x									
MOS-SF36	x			x	x	x	x	x	x	x
MMSE					x					
PFSDQ	x			x			x	x		
POMS						x				
QAM			x	x						
QLI-Ferrans & Powers										x
QLI-Padilla & Grant	x			x		x				
SIP				x	x	x	x	x		
SDS	x	x	x							
VAS-F	x									

Dyspnea Visual Analogue Scale (DVAS)

Description. The DVAS (Janson-Bjerklie, Carrieri, & Hudes, 1986) is used to determine the amount of usual and worst dyspnea experienced. A 100-mm line is anchored at either end with the words "not breathless at all" and "extremely breathless." One line is marked to represent "usual dyspnea" and one line is marked to represent "worst dyspnea."

Reliability and validity. Evidence for concurrent validity of the DVAS has been demonstrated in a number of patient populations, including asthma (Gift, 1989; Janson-Bjerklie et al., 1986) and respiratory failure (Knebel, Janson-Bjerklie, Malley, Wilson, & Marini, 1994).

Examples in nursing research. Knebel et al. (1994) used the DVAS in a study of 21 patients ventilated for 3 days or more, comparing breathing comfort during weaning with similar levels of partial support provided by two types of ventilation modes. The DVAS was used as one measure of breathing comfort.

McGill Pain Questionnaire (MPQ)

Description. The MPQ (Melzack, 1975) has been widely used in pain research to assess adult self-reports of pain location, intensity, and quality. Unfortunately, since the early work of Melzack (1975) there has been very little clarity or consistency in the use of the various forms of the MPQ. Wilkie, Savedra, Holzemer, Tesler, and Paul (1990) provided a landmark meta-analysis of the MPQ and demonstrated how the scale has evolved into at least five different versions and how most investigators who use the MPQ fail to identify which version they are actually using. There is no standardized information regarding the scoring of the instrument.

Reliability and validity. Wilkie, Holzemer, et al. (1990) provided a synthesis of the literature on validity, reliability, and scoring of the MPQ. They also described normative data for pain intensity across seven different painful conditions. In general, the MPQ is thought to be a valid and reliable pain assessment tool for adults. However, little research has been conducted to explore potential gender, ethnic, or developmental biases.

Examples in nursing research. Wilkie, Savedra, et al. (1990) conducted a meta-analysis of 51 studies done to assess pain quality and pain intensity as measured by the

TABLE 11.2 Examples of Nursing Studies Using the Categories of Patient Outcomes

Authors	Instrument	Clinical Population
Symptom status		
Coward (1991)	SDS	Breast cancer
Lee et al. (1991)	VAS-F	Sleep disorders
Knebel et al. (1994)	DVAS	Respiratory failure
Lareau et al. (1994)	PFSDQ	COPD
Simms et al. (1993)	INV-2	Oncology
Slack and Faut-Callahan (1991)	MPQ	Critical care
Tesler et al. (1994)	APPT	Postoperative children and adolescents
Functional status		
Janson-Bjerklie et al. (1992)	QAM	AIDS
Ragsdale and Morrow (1990)	SIP	HIV disease
Rankin (1990)	POMS	Cardiac surgery
Sarna (1993)	KPS	Lung cancer
Stewart et al. (1995)	ADL	Elderly discharged from home health care agencies
Souren et al. (1995)	MMSE	Alzheimer's disease
General health perceptions		
Kantz et al. (1992)	MOS-SF36	Total knee replacement
Quality of life		
Daumer and Miller (1992)	QLI (Ferrans & Powers)	Coronary artery disease
Youngblood et al. (1994)	QLI (Padilla & Grant)	Oncology

MPQ in 3,624 subjects with seven painful conditions. McGuire et al. (1993) used the MPQ to describe pain in 47 patients undergoing bone marrow transplants. Giuffre, Asci, Armstein, and Wilkinson (1991) used the MPQ to assess postoperative pain following total hip or knee replacement surgery in a sample of 29 subjects.

Rhodes Index of Nausea and Vomiting-Form 2 (INV-2)

Description. The INV-2 (Rhodes, Watson, & Johnson, 1984; Rhodes, Watson, Johnson, Madsen, & Beck, 1987; Simms, Rhodes, & Madsen, 1993) is an 8-item self-report instrument that measures patients' perceived nausea duration, nausea frequency, nausea distress, vomiting amount, vomiting frequency, vomiting distress, dry heaves frequency, and dry heaves distress. A 5-point Likert-type scale is used to evaluate each of the items,

where 0 = no symptom experience. Total scores range from 0 to 32.

Reliability and validity. Concurrent and construct validity (Rhodes, Watson, Johnson, Madsen, et al., 1987) and internal consistency reliability (Troesch, Rodehaver, Delaney, & Yanes, 1993) have been established for the INV-2.

Examples in nursing research. The INV-2 has been used as an outcome measure in a number of nursing studies, including Troesch et al. (1993), which evaluated the impact of guided imagery on chemotherapy-related nausea and vomiting, and Simms et al. (1993), who compared two antiemetic regimens.

Symptom Distress Scale (SDS)

Description. There are at least two versions of the SDS currently reported in the literature. The original 10-item scale reported by McCorkle and Young (1978) includes the symptoms of nausea, mood, appetite, insomnia, pain, mobility, fatigue, bowel pattern, concentration, and appearance. A revised 13-item scale (McCorkle & Benoliel, 1983) appears to be the most commonly used version, and it includes the symptoms of frequency of nausea, intensity of nausea, appetite, insomnia, frequency of pain, intensity of pain, fatigue, bowel pattern, concentration, appearance, breathing, outlook, and cough. Holmes (1991) reports on an 11-item version of the SDS. Items are rated on a 5-point Likert-type scale where 1 = low/none and 5 = extreme/worst.

Reliability and validity. There is evidence for the content and concurrent validity of the SDS as well as internal consistency reliability; Cronbach's alpha has been reported in the range of 0.82 to 0.90.

Examples in nursing research. The SDS has been widely used in a number of clinical populations, including HIV disease (Lovejoy et al., 1991), bone marrow transplant (Larson, Viele, Coleman, Dibble, & Cebulski, 1993), and cancer (Coward, 1991; Munkres, Oberst, & Hughes, 1992).

Visual Analogue Scale-Fatigue (VAS-F)

Description. The VAS-F (Lee et al., 1991) is an 18-item scale that takes less than 2 minutes to complete. Each VAS has a bipolar anchor—for example, "not at all tired" to "extremely tired." The time frame for responding to the instrument is the respondent's perception of the energy and fatigue in the evening when going to bed and in the morning upon rising. There are four scores for the VAS-F, including energy morning, energy evening, fatigue morning, and fatigue evening. Subjects respond by placing a vertical mark somewhere along a 100-mm (10-cm) line. Scores are derived by measuring the actual number of millimeters from 0 to the vertical mark.

Reliability and validity. Support for the concurrent validity of the scale was demonstrated by high correlations with related scales on the Stanford Sleepiness Scale (Hoddes, Zarcone, Smythe, Phillips, & Dement, 1973) and the Profile of Mood States (POMS) (McNair, Lorr, & Droppleman, 1984). Cronbach's alpha for the subscales ranged from 0.94 to 0.96 in a sample of 75 healthy subjects and 57 subjects being evaluated for a sleep disorder.

Examples in nursing research. Lee, Hicks, and Nino-Murcia (1991) used the VAS-F to measure fatigue severity in a sample of 75 healthy individuals and 57 patients undergoing medical evaluation for sleep disorders.

Five instruments could be classed as measures of mainly *functional status,* be it physical or cognitive/emotional, as follows.

Activities of Daily Living (ADL)

Description. Initially titled the "Index of Independence in Activities of Daily Living" (ADL) (Katz, Ford, Moskowitz, Jackson, & Jaffe, 1963), the 6-item ADL is completed by a health care provider or investigator who rates the degree of independence observed related to bathing, dressing, toileting, transferring, continence, and feeding. Originally, the individual was scored on a 7-point scale, but later, a 3-level, Likert-type scale was applied to rate the degree of dependence for each of the 6 items. Therefore, scores range from 6 (total independence) to 18 (total dependence).

Reliability and validity. The ADL has been validated primarily on samples of frail elderly. Although there is excellent evidence of the validity of the scale, little work appears to have been focused on intrarater or interrater reliability.

Examples in nursing research. Hughes, Conrad, Manheim, and Edelman (1988) used the ADL to compare the severity of illness between convenience experimental and control groups at baseline in a four year follow-up study of home care clients. Stewart, Blaha, Weisfeld, and Yuan (1995) used the ADL as an outcome measure in an exploratory study of 57 elderly discharged from home care services.

Karnofsky Performance Status Scale (KPS)

Description. The KPS (Karnofsky et al., 1948) is a simple measure of physical performance and level of assistance needed. First used with lung cancer patients to assess the impact of palliative treatments (Karnofsky et al., 1948), the KPS is a scale from 0 to 100 with 11 stages of functioning. A score of 100 indicates absence of disease, normal independent functioning, and the ability to work (Bowling, 1991). It has been used primarily as a global assessment of patient function by professionals providing direct care.

Reliability and validity. Interrater reliability and validity have been established in a number of clinical populations. More recently, researchers have used the KPS scale as an outcome measure in HIV+ individuals treated with Zidovudine versus a placebo (Fischl, Richman, Grieco, et al., 1987; Fischl, Richman, Hansen, et al., 1990; Wu et al., 1990).

Examples in nursing research. Sarna (1993) used the KPS to measure physical activities (functional status) over a 1-month period with 24 patients with non-small-cell lung cancer.

Mini-Mental State Exam (MMSE)

Description. The MMSE (Folstein, Folstein, & McHugh, 1975) is an 11 item provider-administered questionnaire that is used to screen for cognitive impairment. Scores range from 0 to 30; total scores less than 23 or 24 have been reported to indicate disturbance of cognition.

Reliability and validity. Validity and reliability of the MMSE have been established and normative data reported for those above age 40. Test-retest reliabilities have ranged from 0.56 to 0.98. Interrater reliability has been consistently reported above 0.82. There is some evidence of false positives being assessed with subjects who have low levels of education (Anthony, LeResche, Niaz, Von Korff, & Folstein, 1982).

Examples in nursing research. A recent study by Souren, Franssen, and Reisberg (1995) examined the associations between contractures and cognitive and functional decline in Alzheimer's disease in a sample of 161 subjects. The MMSE was used to measure cognitive decline.

Profile of Mood States (POMS)

Description. The POMS (McNair, Lorr, & Droppleman, 1984, 1992) is a 65-item scale that measures six affective states or moods (tension-anxiety, depression-rejection, anger-hostility, vigor-activity, fatigue-inertia, and confusion-bewilderment). Subjects rate each of the six dimensions on a 5-point Likert-type scale where 0 = *not at all* and 4 = *extremely*. The POMS takes 3 to 7 minutes to complete. The scores are summed to also create a Total Mood Disturbance (TMD) score. Higher scores suggest increases in disturbance of mood.

Reliability and validity. Extensive reliability and validity testing have been reported.

Examples in nursing research. In a study of appraisal of illness, symptom distress, self-care burden, and mood states in 60 patients receiving chemotherapy, Munkres et al. (1992) did not find anticipated mood differences between two groups of cancer patients (initial and recurrent). However, symptom distress was a significant predictor of both affective mood and somatic mood as measured by the POMS.

Sickness Impact Profile (SIP)

Description. There have been several versions of the SIP (Bergner et al., 1981; Gilson, Gilson, et al., 1975), but the most commonly used version today consists of 136 items and is scored in 12 categories (sleep and rest, eating, work, home management, recreation and pastime, ambulation, mobility, body care and movement, social interaction, alertness behavior, emotional behavior, and communication) (de Bruin, de Witte, Stevens, & Diederiks, 1992). In addition to the 12 categories plus total score, there are two additional factor scores that can be reported: physical (ambulation, mobility, body care & movement) and psychosocial (social interaction, alertness behavior, emotional behavior, and communication). It takes approximately 20 to 30 minutes to complete the instrument, either in a self-report or interview format. Respondents are asked to mark only those items that are related to their health and that describe them on a given day. It is conceptualized as a behaviorally based measure of the impact of sickness.

Reliability and validity. Extensive literature exists supporting the validity and reliability of the SIP. A Chicano version of the SIP has also been validated (Gilson, Erickson, Chavez, Bobbitt, Bergner, & Carter, 1980).

Examples in nursing research. The SIP has been used extensively in oncology (Frederickson, Jackson, Strauman, & Strauman, 1991), COPD (Leidy, 1995), and HIV disease (Ragsdale & Morrow, 1990) populations.

No selected instruments represent a pure measure of *general health perceptions,* and one represents a measure of mainly *overall quality of life,* as follows.

Quality of Life Index (QLI-Ferrans & Powers)

Description. The QLI-Ferrans & Powers (Ferrans & Powers, 1985) is a 64-item scale based upon 18 life domains (health care, physical health and functioning, marriage, family, friends, stress, standard of living, occupation, education, leisure, future retirement, peace of mind, personal faith, life goals, personal appearance, self-acceptance, general happiness, and general satisfaction). Respondents rate the items on 6-point Likert-type scales in two parts: 32 items focus upon satisfaction (*very satisfied* to *very dissatisfied*) and 32 items assess importance (*very important* to *very unimportant*) of the domains. An adjusted item level score is calculated for the responses to the matched items by adjusting the satisfaction score with the importance score, resulting in one score for each of the 32 items.

Reliability and validity. Evidence for the content and construct validity, as well as the internal consistency reliability, has been published by a number of authors. Ferrans and Powers (1992) conducted a factor analysis in a sample of 349 dialysis patients, resulting in a four-factor solution (health and functioning, socioeconomic, psychological/spiritual, and family). The Cronbach alphas ranged from 0.77 to 0.90 for the scales. Similar evidence for reliability and validity has been reported for patient samples (Belec, 1992; Daumer & Miller, 1992).

Examples in nursing research. Belec (1992) used the QLI-Ferrans & Powers to measure quality of life in a sample of 24 adults receiving bone marrow transplantation. Daumer and Miller (1992) used it to measure quality of life in a study of the effects of cardiac rehabilitation on psychosocial functioning and life satisfaction in a sample of 47 patients with coronary artery disease.

Pulmonary Functional Status and Dyspnea Questionnaire (PSFDQ)

Description. The PSFDQ (Lareau, Carrieri-Kohlman, Janson-Bjerklie, & Ross, 1994) is a 164-item self-administered questionnaire that measures two constructs (dyspnea and functional abilities). For the dyspnea component, respondents rate, on a 10-point Likert-type scale, the general dyspnea experience and the usual intensity of dyspnea associated with 79 activities comprising six scales (self-care, mobility, eating, home management, social, and recreational).

Reliability and validity. In a sample of 131 adult males with chronic obstructive pulmonary disease, the scale demonstrated adequate validity and reliability (Lareau et al., 1994).

Examples in nursing research. The only study located that has used the PSFDQ is that by Lareau et al. (1994).

The remaining four instruments represent measures of a mixture of the model components, including three that combine symptom and functional status measurement and one that combines those two components plus general health perceptions and overall quality of life, as follows.

Quality Audit Marker (QAM)

Description. The QAM was designed to measure changes in the status of hospitalized AIDS patients (Holzemer et al., 1993). The 10-item QAM includes three scales: Self-Care (6 items), Ambulation (2 items), and Psychological Distress (2 items). Four- and 5-point Likert-type scales are used. A high score on the QAM indicates high functional status and low patient symptoms (Janson-Bjerklie, Holzemer, & Henry, 1992). The QAM is completed by a trained observer according to the observer's judgment about the patient's status based on multiple data sources (e.g., observation, interview, chart). Estimated time to complete this instrument is less than 2 minutes.

Reliability and validity. The internal consistencies of the three scales of the QAM were high in a study of 201 hospitalized AIDS patients with *Pneumocystis carinii* pneumonia. Cronbach's alphas for the self-care, ambulation, and psychological distress scales were 0.89, 0.88, and 0.84, respectively. Adequate content, construct, concurrent, and predictive validity for patient mortality at 3 and 6 months were reported in the same sample (Holzemer et al., 1993). Adequate reliability and validity have also been demonstrated for samples of homeward bound elderly (Brown, 1992) and total joint replacement patients (Ireson, 1993).

Examples in nursing research. Kataoka-Yahiro, Portillo, Henry, and Holzemer (1996) used the self-care score from the QAM in a study of the physical and social correlates of perceived psychological support among 168 hospitalized AIDS patients.

Quality of Life Index (QLI-Padilla & Grant)

Description. The initial QLI-Padilla & Grant consisted of 14 linear analogue scale items (100-mm visual analogue scale) measuring general physical condition, normal activities, and personal attitudes. The factor analysis, using data from a cancer sample, resulted in four factors (psychological well-being [5 items], physical well-being [5 items], symptom control [3 items] and financial protection [1 item] (Padilla, Presant, Grant, Metter, Lipsett, & Heide, 1983). The fourth factor was subsequently dropped. The scale was expanded for use with a sample of colostomy patients into a 23-item scale (Padilla & Grant, 1985) comprising six factors: psychological well-being, physical well-being, body image, diagnosis/treatment (surgical) response, diagnosis/treatment (nutritional) response, and social concerns. In a discussion of a synthesis of the different versions of the QLI, Padilla and Grant suggest that there are four factors to the scale: psychological well-being, physical well-being, symptom/side effects, and nutrition. An overall summative quality of life score can also be obtained.

Reliability and validity. Padilla et al. (1983) reported relatively poor test-retest scores and modest evidence of concurrent validity. In a subsequent study with a sample of colostomy patients, internal consistencies of the factor scales ranged from 0.48 to 0.90. Additional support for the construct validity of the scale was demonstrated in a sample of patients undergoing outpatient cancer treatment (Youngblood, Williams, Eyles, Waring, & Runyon, 1994), with a significant inverse correlation between self-reported toxic symptoms of therapy and QLI-Padilla & Grant scores.

Examples in nursing research. Sherman and Johnson (1991) used the QLI-Padilla & Grant as an outcome measure in a study of the effectiveness of case management on a 36-bed study unit. Ferrell et al. (1992) used it to study the meaning of quality of life for 119 bone marrow transplant survivors.

Medical Outcomes Study Short-Form General Health Survey (MOS-SF36)

Description. The MOS-SF36 is used to measure a mixture of symptom status, functional status, and general health perceptions. Based upon the extensive work of the Medical Outcomes Study, the MOS-SF36 (Ware & Sherbourne, 1992) is a short form of the larger research instrument and contains 36 items. It measures the following concepts: physical functioning (10 items), role limitations due to physical problems (4 items), social functioning (2 items), bodily pain (2 items), general mental health (5 items), role limitations due to emotional problems (3 items), vitality (4 items), and general health perceptions (5 items). The history of the instruments, as well as a copy of the scale and the varied response format, is presented by Ware and Sherbourne (1992). It has been reported that the scale takes between 5 and 20 minutes to complete, depending upon the age and severity of illness of the sample.

Reliability and validity. The evidence for the validity of the MOS-SF36 is reviewed by McHorney, Ware, and Raczek (1993) and the reliability testing by McHorney, Ware, Lu, and Sherbourne (1994). The reliability coefficients for the subscales ranged from a low of 0.65 to a high of 0.94 (median = 0.85).

Examples in nursing research. Overall, the MOS-SF36 has quickly become the standard scale for clinical practice, research, health policy evaluations, and general population surveys related to health concepts. To date, there has been limited use of the MOS-SF36 in nursing research. For a nursing research example, see Kantz, Harris, Levitsky, Ware, and Davies (1992).

The 16 instruments in this analysis varied in methods of administration, time for completion, and scope.

Twelve instruments were designed to be completed by the patient. Four measures reflect the provider's judgment rather than the patient's self-report (i.e., the ADL, KPS, MMSE, and QAM). Some instruments require only a few minutes for completion (e.g., the QAM); others can take as long as 30 minutes (e.g., the SIP). The measures vary in scope across the categories of the Wilson and Cleary (1995) model, with most focused on a single symptom or specific area of functional status, and three including multiple categories. There was also a range in the patient populations in which the instruments had been validated, with some (e.g., the QLI-Padilla & Grant) being used primary in the oncology population and others across multiple patient groups (e.g., the MOS-SF36). The critical review of these 16 instruments provided a sample of reliable and valid measures appropriate for use in nursing intervention studies. However, a number of conceptual and methodological issues warrant further discussion.

Conceptual and Methodological Issues

Six conceptual and methodological issues are of prime importance when measuring nursing-sensitive patient outcomes. These are (a) difficulty of assessing the impact of a single discipline on patient outcomes in a multidisciplinary, patient-focused care environment; (b) advantages of condition- or problem-specific versus generic outcome measures; (c) role of patient preferences in outcomes measurement; (d) need for appropriate risk-adjustment strategies; (e) lack of normative data; and (f) linkage of interventions and outcomes.

Assessing the Impact of a Single Discipline on Patient Outcomes

Efforts such as the Nursing Minimum Data Set (Werley, Lang, & Westlake, 1986), the Unified Nursing Language System (McCormick & Zielstorff, 1995), the International Classification of Nursing Practice (Clark & Lang, 1992), and the Nursing-Sensitive Outcomes Classification (NOC) (Johnson & Maas, 1995) are aimed at increasing the visibility of the influence of nursing practice on patient outcomes. Interpretation of the term *nursing-sensitive patient outcome* is difficult. For example, does it mean that nursing care influences the outcome or that the outcome can be attributed exclusively to nursing practices? One approach to addressing this question is illustrated in a recent study by Lush, Jones, and the Outcomes Taskforce (1995) who surveyed a random sample of nurses ($N = 538$) within an HMO, asking them to rate how much independent nursing assessment and intervention affected patient outcomes in three areas of care. The sample believed their interventions had a moderate effect on functional status, in contrast to a large effect on engagement in health care and mental and social well-being.

Hegyvary (1991) cautioned nurses to avoid failing to account for the multiple contributions to patient outcomes, stating that "future studies using a multivariate analytical approach will enable us to determine the levels of variance explained by nursing, medicine, organizational, demographic, environmental, and numerous other variables" (p. 5). Clearly, the approach to measuring the contribution of nursing therapeutics to patient outcomes must include both a focus on the disciplinary perspective (Lange & Marek, 1992) and an acknowledgment of the multiple disciplinary contributions to patient outcomes.

Condition-Specific Versus Generic Outcome Measures

Outcome measures can be viewed according to two broad perspectives: condition specific and generic. Traditional hospitalization outcome measures such as length of stay, mortality, and readmission rate, as well as the majority of the measures reviewed earlier in this chapter, are considered generic outcome measures applicable across a broad range of clinical populations. Another example of a generic outcome indicator is patient adherence to a discharge plan, which is under consideration for inclusion in the "Nursing Care Report Card for Acute Care" (American Nurses Association, 1995). In contrast, two standardized classification schemes for nursing include outcome measures related to specific problems. In the Omaha Community Health System (Martin et al., 1993), problem status, patient knowledge, and patient behavior are rated and examined for changes over time. The Georgetown Home Health Care Classification System (Saba, 1992) offers a unidimensional rating (improved, deteriorated, or unchanged) of problem status over time. In another approach, Crawford et al. (1996) recently described the development of a generic outcomes infrastructure for measuring nursing-sensitive patient outcomes in three categories (functional status, psychological status, and health care engagement) across the continuum of care. Only a few studies (Kantz et al., 1992) have compared the utility of condition-specific (e.g., joint mobility after total joint replacement) and generic outcome measures.

Congruent with the Wilson and Cleary model, it is likely that outcomes studies of most value will include both condition-specific and generic outcome measures as complementary dimensions (Bombardier et al., 1995).

Patient Preferences

The influence of patient preference for a specific outcome on the selection of therapeutic strategies and achievement of the outcome cannot be underestimated. Lohr (1988) states that

> the desirability of one outcome rather than another in any given clinical situation (e.g., palliation rather than extension of life in the terminally ill patient) may differ markedly according to the values and preferences of patients, factors that to date are rarely taken explicitly into account in outcome studies. (p. 38)

Longo (1993) proposed a new model for examination of practice variation that includes patient practice style variation. The Wilson and Cleary (1995) model specifies the influence of individual characteristics such as values and preferences, but little research has been done to examine this influence on model components, with the exception of quality of life.

The application of normative decision theoretic techniques, such as classical decision analysis or multiple criteria models, is a strategy for incorporating patient preferences in treatment planning, monitoring, and outcome evaluation that has been underused in nursing (Brennan, 1995; Goldstein et al., 1994). Other efforts are focused on eliciting patient preferences as part of a decision-making process shared by patients and professionals (Kasper, Mulley, & Wennberg, 1992).

Risk Adjustment for Outcomes

Comparative report cards are being published by national organizations, professional associations such as the American Nurses Association (1995), consumer groups, and government agencies, among others. However, if the outcomes reported do not take into account patient characteristics that can be considered dimensions of risk, there is the possibility that erroneous conclusions will be drawn about the quality of the care provided. Factors affecting the use of specific outcome measures in comparing the quality of care among providers can be illustrated using the following equation (McAuliffe, cited in Thomas, Hollaway, & Guire, 1993):

$$Var (O) = Var (V) + Var (SE) + Var (RE).$$

Var (O) is the observed variability in patient outcomes across providers, Var (V) is the part of Var (O) "validly" attributable to quality of care differences among providers, Var (SE) is the systematic error related to differences in patient-specific characteristics among providers, and Var (RE) is the random error related to residual variability caused by unknown or unmeasured factors.

Iezzoni (1994) identified 11 patient characteristics or sources of systematic error that may be related to the risk of variation in patient outcomes: age; gender; acute clinical stability; principal diagnosis or case mix; severity of principal diagnosis; extent and severity of comorbidities; physical functional status; psychological, cognitive, and psychosocial functioning; cultural, ethnic, and socioeconomic attributes and behaviors; health status and quality of life; and patient attitudes and preferences for outcomes. Many of these risk factors are identified in the Wilson and Cleary (1995) model, either as outcome categories or as individual or environmental characteristics.

Patient characteristics are controlled for by the use of risk-adjustment models (Blumberg, 1986; DesHarnais, Chesney, Wroblewski, Flemming, & McMahon, 1988). The aim of risk adjustment, according to Wu (1995), is "to find a parsimonious representation of those patient characteristics which have a strong relation to mortality and that could, without proper attention, confound the results of a particular analysis" (p. 149). Although there is extensive research focused on risk adjustment of outcomes such as mortality (Green, Wintfeld, Sharkey, & Passman, 1990; Krakauer et al., 1992) and hospital length of stay (Horn et al., 1991; Knaus, Wagner, Zimmerman, & Draper, 1993), little is known about how to risk adjust for outcomes such as symptom status, functional status, and quality of life.

Lack of Normative Data

Normative data exist for clinical variables such as laboratory values or pulmonary function tests; however, there is a dearth of normative data about health-related quality of life (Greenfield & Nelson, 1992). This lack of normative data makes it difficult for providers to interpret the levels of a particular outcomes score and to understand the meaning of a unit of change. Efforts are under way to gather normative data for widely used instruments such as those from the Medical Outcomes Study. However, Greenfield and Nelson (1992) caution that "the ref-

erence values are instrument-dependent and contingent on controlling for many sources of variability, as is done with laboratory tests" (p. MS35).

Linking Interventions and Outcomes

In the absence of carefully controlled randomized clinical trials, the attribution of outcomes to specific interventions is complex. A particular complication is choosing the time for outcome measurement, as little is known for most interventions about dose response or peak and sustained effects (Greenfield & Nelson, 1992). For example, changes in functional status may not be apparent until several weeks after a particular intervention. However, the longer the period of observation, the more likely that extraneous variables (including the patient practice variation mentioned earlier) will intervene on the linkages between interventions and outcomes (Lohr, 1988). Wilson and Cleary (1995) point out that, in addition to health care interventions, individual and environmental characteristics and other nonmedical factors affect patient outcomes.

The complexity of these issues highlights the need for information systems and informatics techniques to assist in outcomes measurement (Henry, 1995). For example, the vision of the computer-based patient record described by the authors of the Institute of Medicine report (Dick & Steen, 1991) includes the collection of health status data across the life span and the continuum of care. Integrated information systems provide the capacity to link a broad variety of data from different types of computer systems thus facilitating appropriate risk-adjustment of outcomes based on individual characteristics of patients. Another important approach is the use of computer-based multimedia to facilitate a shared decision making process between patients and providers.

Conclusion

The Wilson and Cleary (1995) model provided a framework for reviewing instruments for and issues in measuring therapeutic outcomes that may perhaps be sensitive to nursing care. The review demonstrated that reliable and valid instruments exist for measuring the categories of the model and that these instruments have been applied in nursing research studies. The instruments vary according to respondent reporting (patient versus provider), length of time for completion, scope of model components tested, and clinical populations in which the instruments have been used. The unresolved conceptual and methodological issues provide direction for future research related to the measurement of therapeutic outcomes sensitive to nursing care.

The rapidly changing health care environment has generated a mandate for all health care professionals to document their contributions to patient outcomes. The profession of nursing must meet this challenge by providing evidence of the impact of nursing care on health status. In doing this, it is important to heed the warning of Ware (1992), who cautions against the premature

adoption of "brief or completely transparent" systems. He notes that

anything worth measuring is worth measuring well. Before clinicians decide whether it is possible to settle for less, they need to gain experience with the use of health status data from the best possible measures. The time and burden involved in completing a standardized health survey are important considerations, but they do not preclude precise measurements. I suspect that most patients spend more time in elevators and lounges waiting for laboratory tests than it takes to fill out the entire Sickness Impact Profile. (p. MS209)

References

American Nurses Association. (1995). *Nursing care report card for acute care.* Washington, DC: American Nurses Publishing.

Anthony, J. C., LeResche, L., Niaz, U., Von Korff, M. R., & Folstein, M. F. (1982). Limits of the "Mini-Mental State" as screening test for dementia and delirium among hospital patients. *Psychological Medicine, 12,* 397-408.

Belec, R. H. (1992). Quality of life: Perceptions of long-term survivors of bone marrow transplantation. *Oncology Nursing Forum, 19,* 31-37.

Bergner, M., Bobbitt, R. A., Carter, W. B., & Gilson, B. S. (1981). The Sickness Impact Profile: Development and final revision of a health status measure. *Medical Care, 19,* 787-805.

Blumberg, M. (1986). Risk adjusting health care outcomes: A methodologic review. *Medical Care Review, 43*(2), 351-393.

Bombardier, C., Melfi, C. A., Paul, J., Green, R., Hawker, G., Wright, J., & Coyte, P. (1995). Comparison of a generic and a disease-specific measure of pain and physical function after knee replacement surgery. *Medical Care, 33,* AS131-AS144.

Bowling, A. (1991). *Measuring health: A review of quality of life measurement scales.* Philadelphia: Open University Press.

Brennan, P. F. (1995). Patient satisfaction and normative decision theory. *Journal of the American Medical Informatics Association, 2,* 250-259.

Brown, D. S. (1992). *Hospital discharge preparation for homeward bound elderly.* Unpublished dissertation, University of California, San Francisco.

Clark, J., & Lang, N. M. (1992). Nursing's next advance: An international classification for nursing practice. *International Nursing Review, 39,* 109-112.

Coward, D. D. (1991). Self-transcendence and emotional well-being in women with advanced breast cancer. *Oncology Nursing Forum, 18,* 857-863.

Crawford, B. L., Taylor, L. S., Seipert, B. S., & Lush, M. (1996). The imperative of outcomes analysis: An integration of traditional and nontraditional outcome measures. *Journal of Nursing Care Quality, 10*(2), 33-40.

Daumer, R., & Miller, P. (1992). Effects of cardiac rehabilitation on psychosocial functioning and life satisfaction of coronary artery disease clients. *Rehabilitation Nursing, 17*(2), 69-86.

de Bruin, A. F., de Witte, L. P., Stevens, F., & Diederiks, J.P.M. (1992). Sickness Impact Profile: The state of the art of a generic func-

tional status measure. *Social Science and Medicine, 35,* 1003-1014.

DesHarnais, S. I., Chesney, J. D., Wroblewski, R. T., Flemming, S. T., & McMahon, L. F. (1988). The risk-adjusted mortality index: A new measure of hospital performance. *Medical Care, 26*(12), 1129-1148.

Dick, R. S., & Steen, E. B. (1991). *The computer-based patient record.* Washington, DC: National Academy Press.

Ferrans, C. E., & Powers, M. J. (1985). Quality of Life Index: Development and psychometric properties. *Advances in Nursing Science, 8*(1), 15-24.

Ferrans, C. E., & Powers, M. J. (1992). Psychometric assessment of the Quality of Life Index. *Research in Nursing and Health, 15,* 29-38.

Ferrell, B., Schmidt, G. M., Grant, M., Rhiner, M., Whitehead, C., Fonbuena, P., & Forman, S. J. (1992). The meaning of quality of life for bone marrow transplant survivors. *Cancer Nursing, 15,* 153-160.

Fischl, M. A., Richman, D. D., Grieco, M. H., Gottlieb, M. S., Volberding, P. A., Lasking, O. L., Leedom, J. M., Groopman, J. E., Mildvan, D., Schooley, R. T., Jackson, G. G., Durack, D. T., King, D., & the AZT Collaborative Working Group. (1987). The efficacy of azidothymidine (AZT) in the treatment of patients with AIDS and AIDS-related complex: A double-blind, placebo controlled trial. *New England Journal of Medicine, 317,* 185-191.

Fischl, M. A., Richman, D. D., Hansen, N., Collier, A. C., Carey, J. T., Para, M. F., Hardy, W. D., Dolin, R., Powderly, W. G., Allan, J. D., Wong, B., Mertgan, T. C., McAuliffe, V. J., Hyslop, N. E., Rhame, F. S., Balfour, H. H., Spector, S. A., Volberding, P., Pettinelli, C., Anderson, A., & the AIDS Clinical Trials Group. (1990). The safety and efficacy of Zidovudine (AZT) in the treatment of subjects with mildly symptomatic immunodeficiency virus type 1 (HIV) infection: A double-blind, placebo-controlled trial. *Annals of Internal Medicine, 112,* 727-737.

Folstein, M. F., Folstein, S. E., & McHugh, P. R. (1975). Mini-Mental State: A practical method for grading the cognitive state of patients for the clinician. *Journal of Psychiatric Research, 12,* 189-198.

Frederickson, K., Jackson, B. S., Strauman, T., & Strauman, J. (1991). Testing hypotheses derived from the Roy adaptation model. *Nursing Science Quarterly, 4*(4), 168-174.

Gift, A. G. (1989). Validation of a vertical visual analogue scale as a measure of clinical dyspnea. *Rehabilitation Nursing, 14,* 323-325.

Gilson, B. S., Erickson, D., Chavez, C. T., Bobbitt, R. A., Bergner, M., & Carter, W. B. (1980). A Chicano version of the Sickness Impact Profile (SIP). *Culture, Medicine and Psychiatry, 4*(2), 137-150.

Gilson, B. S., Gilson, J. S., Bergner, M., Bobbitt, R. A., Kressel, S., Pollard, W. E., & Vesselago, M. (1975). The Sickness Impact Profile: Development of an outcome measure of health care. *American Journal of Public Health, 65,* 1304-1310.

Giuffre, M., Asci, J., Arnstein, P., & Wilkinson, C. (1991) Postoperative joint replacement pain: Description and opioid requirement. *Journal of Post Anesthesia Nursing, 6,* 239-245.

Goldstein, M. K., Clarke, A. E., Michelson, D., Garber, A. M., Bergen, M. A., & Lenert, L. A. (1994). Developing and testing a multimedia presentation of a health state. *Medical Decision Making, 14,* 336-344.

Green, J., Wintfeld, N., Sharkey, P., & Passman, L. J. (1990). The importance of severity of illness in assessing hospital mortality. *Journal of the American Medical Association, 263*(2), 241-246.

Greenfield, S., & Nelson, E. (1992). Recent developments and future issues in the use of health status assessment measures in clinical setting. *Medical Care, 30,* MS23-MS41.

Hegyvary, S. T. (1991). Issues in outcomes research. *Journal of Nursing Quality Assurance, 5*(2), 1-6.

Hegyvary, S. T. (1993). Patient care outcomes related to management of symptoms. In J. Fitzpatrick & J. S. Stevenson (Eds.), *Annual review of nursing research* (pp. 145-168). New York: Springer.

Henry, S. B. (1995). Informatics: Essential infrastructure for quality assessment and improvement in nursing. *Journal of the American Medical Informatics Association, 2,* 169-182.

Hoddes, E., Zarcone, V., Smythe, H., Phillips, R., & Dement, W. C. (1973). Quantification of sleepiness: A new approach. *Psychophysiology, 10,* 431-436.

Holmes, S. (1991). Preliminary investigations of symptom distress in two cancer patient populations: Evaluation of a measurement instrument. *Journal of Advanced Nursing, 16,* 439-446.

Holzemer, W. L., Henry, S. B., Stewart, A., & Janson-Bjerklie, S. (1993). The HIV Quality Audit Maker (HIV-QAM): An outcome measure for hospitalized AIDS patients. *Quality of Life Research, 2,* 99-107.

Horn, S. D., Sharkey, P. D., Buckle, J. M., Backofen, J. E., Averill, R. F., & Horn, R. A. (1991). The relationship between length of stay and mortality. *Medical Care, 29*(4), 305-317.

Hughes, S., Conrad, K. J., Manheim, L. M., & Edelman, P. L. (1988). Impact of long-term home care on mortality, functional status, and unmet needs. *Health Services Research, 23*(2), 269-294.

Iezzoni, L. I. (1994). Dimensions of risk. In L. I. Iezzoni (Ed.), *Risk adjustment for measuring health care outcomes* (pp. 29-118). Ann Arbor, MI: Health Administration Press.

Ireson, C. L. (1993). *Psychometric analysis of the Quality Audit Marker in patients undergoing total joint replacements.* Unpublished manuscript, University of Kentucky.

Janson-Bjerklie, S., Carrieri, V. K., & Hudes, M. (1986). The sensations of pulmonary dyspnea. *Nursing Research, 35,* 155-159.

Janson-Bjerklie, S., Holzemer, W. L., & Henry, S. B. (1992). Patient's perceptions of problems and nursing intervention during hospitalization for *Pneumocystis carinii* pneumonia. *American Journal of Critical Care, 1,* 114-121.

Jennings, B. M. (1991). Patient outcomes research: Seizing the opportunity. *Advances in Nursing Science, 14,* 59-72.

Johnson, M., & Maas, M. (1995). Classification of nursing-sensitive patient outcomes. In N. M. Lang (Ed.), *Nursing data systems: The emerging framework.* Washington, DC: American Nurses Publishing.

Kantz, M. E., Harris, W. J., Levitsky, K., Ware, J. E., & Davies, A. R. (1992). Methods for assessing condition-specific and generic functional status outcomes after total knee replacement. *Medical Care, 30,* MS240-MS252.

Karnofsky, D. A., Abelmann, W. H., Craver, L. F., & Burchenal, J. H. (1948). The use of nitrogen mustards in the palliative treatment of carcinoma with particular reference to bronchogenic carcinoma. *Cancer, 1,* 634-656.

Kasper, J. F., Mulley, A. G. Jr., & Wennberg, J. E. (1992). Developing shared decision-making programs to improve quality of health care. *Quality Review Bulletin, 18,* 183-190.

Kataoka-Yahiro, M. R., Portillo, C. J., Henry, S., & Holzemer, W. L. (1996). Physical and social correlates of perceived psychological support among hospitalized AIDS patients. *Journal of Advanced Nursing, 24,* 167-173.

Katz, S., Ford, A. B., Moskowitz, R. W., Jackson, B. A., & Jaffe, M. W. (1963). Studies of illness in the aged: The Index of ADL: A standardized measure of biological and psychosocial function. *Journal of the American Medical Association, 185,* 914-919.

Knaus, W. A., Wagner, D. P., Zimmerman, J. E., & Draper, E. A. (1993). Variations in mortality and length of stay in intensive care units. *Annals of Internal Medicine, 118*(10), 753-761.

Knebel, A. R., Janson-Bjerklie, S. L., Malley, J. D., Wilson, A. G., & Marini, J. J. (1994). Comparison of breathing comfort during weaning with two ventilatory modes. *American Journal of Respiratory and Critical Care Medicine, 149,* 14-18.

Krakauer, H., Bailey, R. C., Skellan, K. J., Stewart, J. D., Harta, A. J., Kuhn, E. M., & Rimm, A. (1992). Evaluation of the HCFA model for the analysis of mortality following hospitalization. *Health Services Research, 27*(3), 317-335.

Lange, N. M., & Marek, K. D. (1992). Outcomes that reflect clinical practice. In *Patient outcomes research: Examining the effectiveness of nursing practice* (NIH Pub. No. 93-3411, pp. 27-38). Washington, DC: U.S. Department of Health and Human Services.

Lareau, S. C., Carrieri-Kohlman, V., Janson-Bjerklie, S., & Roos, P. J. (1994). Development and testing of the Pulmonary Functional Status and Dyspnea Questionnaire (PFSDQ). *Heart & Lung, 23,* 242-250.

Larson, P. J., Viele, C. S., Coleman, S., Dibble, S. L., & Cebulski, C. (1993). Comparison of perceived symptoms of patients undergoing bone marrow transplant and the nurses caring for them. *Oncology Nursing Forum, 20,* 81-88.

Lee, K. A., Hicks, G., & Nino-Murcia, G. (1991). Validity and reliability of a scale to assess fatigue. *Psychiatry Research, 36,* 291-298.

Leidy, N. K. (1994). Functional status and the forward progress of merry-go-rounds: Toward a coherent analytical framework. *Nursing Research, 43,* 196-202.

Leidy, N. K. (1995). Functional performance in people with chronic obstructive pulmonary disease. *Image: The Journal of Nursing Scholarship, 27*(1), 23-24.

Lohr, K. N. (1988). Outcome measurement: Concepts and questions. *Inquiry, 25,* 37-50.

Longo, D. R. (1993). Patient practice variation: A call for research. *Medical Care, 31,* YS81-YS85.

Lovejoy, N. C., Paul, S., Freeman, E., & Christianson, B. (1991). Potential correlates of self-care and symptom distress in homosexual/bisexual men who are HIV seropositive. *Oncology Nursing Forum, 18,* 1175-1185.

Lush, M. T., Jones, D. L., & the Outcomes Taskforce. (1995). Developing an outcomes infrastructure for nursing. In R. M. Gardner (Ed.), *Proceedings of the Nineteenth Annual Symposium on Computer Applications in Medical Care* (pp. 625-629). Philadelphia: Hanley & Belfus.

Martin, K. S., Scheet, N. J., & Stegman, M. R. (1993). Home health clients: Characteristics, outcomes of care, and nursing interventions. *American Journal of Public Health, 83,* 1730-1734.

McCorkle, R., & Benoliel, J. Q. (1983). Symptom distress: Current concerns and mood disturbance after diagnosis of life threatening disease. *Social Science and Medicine, 17,* 431-438.

McCorkle, R., & Young, K. (1978). Development of a symptom distress scale. *Cancer Nursing, 5,* 373-378.

McCormick, K. A., & Zielstorff, R. (1995). Building a Unified Nursing Language System (UNLS). In N. M. Lang (Ed.), *Nursing data systems: The emerging framework.* Washington, DC: American Nurses Publishing.

McGuire, D. B., Altomonte, V., Peterson, D. E., Wingard, J. R., Jones, R. J., & Grochow, L. B. (1993). Patterns of mucositis and pain in patients receiving preparative chemotherapy and bone marrow transplantation. *Oncology Nursing Forum, 20,* 1493-1502.

McHorney, C. A., Ware, J. E., Lu, J.F.R., & Sherbourne, C. D. (1994). The MOS 36-item Short-Form Health Survey (SF-36): III. Test of data quality, scaling assumptions, and reliability across diverse patient groups. *Medical Care, 32,* 40-66.

McHorney, C. A., Ware, J. E., & Raczek, A. E. (1993). The MOS 36-item Short-Form Health Survey (SF-36): II. Psychometric and clinical tests of validity in measuring physical and mental health constructs. *Medical Care, 31,* 247-263.

McNair, D. M., Lorr, M., & Droppleman, L. (1984). *Profile of Mood States.* San Diego, CA: Educational and Industrial Testing Service.

McNair, D. M., Lorr, M., & Droppleman, L. F. (1992). *Edits manual for the Profile of Mood States.* San Diego, CA: Educational and Industrial Testing Service.

Melzack, R. (1975). The McGill Pain Questionnaire: Major properties and scoring methods. *Pain, 1,* 277-299.

Munkres, A., Oberst, M. T., & Hughes, S. H. (1992). Appraisal of illness, symptom distress, self-care burden, and mood states in patients receiving chemotherapy for initial and recurrent cancer. *Oncology Nursing Forum, 19,* 1201-1209.

Padilla, G. V., & Grant, M. M. (1985). Quality of life as a cancer nursing outcome variable. *Advances in Nursing Science, 8*(1), 45-60.

Padilla, G. V., Presant, C., Grant, M. M., Metter, G., Lipsett, J., & Heide, F. (1983). Quality of Life Index for patients with cancer. *Research in Nursing and Health, 6,* 117-126.

Ragsdale, D., & Morrow, J. R. (1990). Quality of life as a function of HIV classification. *Nursing Research, 39,* 355-359.

Rankin, S. H. (1990). Differences in recovery from cardiac surgery: A profile of male and female patients. *Heart & Lung, 19,* 481-485.

Rhodes, V. A., Watson, P. M., & Johnson, M. H. (1984). Development of reliable and valid measures of nausea and vomiting. *Cancer Nursing, 7,* 33-41.

Rhodes, V. A., Watson, P. M., Johnson, M. H., Madsen, R. W., & Beck, N. C. (1987). Patterns of nausea, vomiting, and distress in patients receiving antineoplastic drug protocols. *Oncology Nursing Forum, 14,* 35-44.

Saba, V. K. (1992). Home health care classification. *Caring Magazine, 11,* 58-60.

Sarna, L. (1993). Fluctuations in physical function: Adults with non-small cell lung cancer. *Journal of Advanced Nursing, 18,* 714-724.

Savedra, M. C., Tesler, M. D., Holzemer, W. L., Wilkie, D. J., & Ward, J. A. (1990). Testing a tool to assess postoperative pediatric and adolescent pain. *Advances in Pain Research Therapy, 15,* 85-93.

Savedra, M. C., Holzemer, W. L., Tesler, M. D., & Wilkie, D. J. (1993). Assessment of postoperation pain in children and adoles-

cents using the adolescent pediatric pain tool. *Nursing Research, 42*(1), 5-9.

Sherman, J. J., & Johnson, P. K. (1991). Nursing case management. *American College of Medical Quality, 6,* 142-145.

Simms, S. G., Rhodes, V. A., & Madsen, R. W. (1993). Comparison of prochlolorperazine and lorazepam antiemetic regimens in the control of postchemotherapy symptoms. *Nursing Research, 42,* 235-239.

Slack, J. F., & Faut-Callahan, M. (1991). Efficacy of epidural analgesia for pain management of critically ill patients and the implications for nursing care. *AACN Clinical Issues, 2,* 729-740.

Souren, L.E.M., Franssen, E. H., & Reisberg, B. (1995). Contractures and loss of function in patients with Alzheimer's disease. *Journal of the American Geriatrics Society, 43,* 650-655.

Stewart, C. J., Blaha, A. J., Weisfeld, L., & Yuan, W. (1995). Discharge planning from home health care and patient status post-discharge. *Public Health Nursing, 12,* 90-98.

Tesler, M. D., Wilkie, D. J., Holzemer, W. L., & Savedra, M. C. (1994). Postoperative analgesics for children and adolescents: Prescription and administration. *Journal of Pain and Symptom Management, 9,* 85-95.

Thomas, J. W., Holloway, J. J., & Guire, K. E. (1993). Validating risk-adjusted mortality as an indicator for quality of care. *Inquiry, 30,* 6-22.

Troesch, L. M., Rodehaver, C. B., Delaney, E. A., & Yanes, B. (1993). The influence of guided imagery on chemotherapy-related nausea and vomiting. *Oncology Nursing Forum, 20,* 1179-1185.

Ware, J. E. (1992). Comments on the use of health status assessment in clinical settings. *Medical Care, 30,* MS205-MS209.

Ware, J. E., & Sherbourne, C. D. (1992). The MOS 36-item Short-Form Health Survey (SF-36): I. Conceptual framework and item selection. *Medical Care, 30,* 473-483.

Werley, H. H., Lang, N. M., & Westlake, S. K. (1986). Brief summary of the Nursing Minimum Data Set Conference. *Nursing Management, 17*(7), 42-45.

Wilkie, D. J., Holzemer, W. L., Tesler, M. D., Ward, J. A., Paul, S. M., & Savedra, M. C. (1990). Measuring pain quality: Validity and reliability of children's and adolescents' pain language. *Pain, 41,* 151-159.

Wilkie, D. J., Savedra, M. C., Holzemer, W. L., Tesler, M. D., & Paul, S. M. (1990). Use of the McGill Pain Questionnaire to measure pain: A meta-analysis. *Nursing Research, 39*(1), 36-41.

Wilson, I. B., & Cleary, P. D. (1995). Linking clinical variables with health-related quality of life: A conceptual model of patient outcomes. *Journal of the American Medical Association, 273,* 59-65.

Wu, A. W. (1995). The measure and mismeasure of hospital quality: Appropriate risk-adjustment methods in comparing hospitals. *Annals of Internal Medicine, 122,* 149-150.

Wu, A. W., Mathews, W. C., Brysk, L. T., Atkinson, J. H., Grant, I., Abramson, I., Kennedy, C. J., McCutchan, J. A., Spector, S. A., & Richman, D. D. (1990). Quality of life in a placebo-controlled trial of Zidovudine in patients with AIDS and AIDS-related complex. *Journal of Acquired Immune Deficiency Syndromes, 3,* 683-690.

Youngblood, M., Williams, P. D., Eyles, H., Waring, J., & Runyon, S. (1994). A comparison of two methods of assessing cancer therapy-related symptoms. *Cancer Nursing, 17,* 37-44.

PART IIC

FAMILIES IN HEALTH, ILLNESS, AND LIFE TRANSITIONS

Suzanne L. Feetham

This section examines the state of the science of nursing research of families from three perspectives: research in normative family transitions, non-normative family transitions, and the correspondence of nursing research of families with policy. The chapter authors provide specific recommendations for advancing the science and improving the correspondence among research, practice, and policy. Common themes are identified in the analysis conducted for each chapter. These themes relate to the need for family theory development in nursing research, increased progress in intervention research, and increased integration of research and practice.

All authors reported evidence of progress in the scientific merit of the research. They also found increasing numbers of studies addressing specific problems and developing substantive theoretical frameworks. Feetham and Meister documented examples of deliberate theory development and testing in four programs of research by using multiple methods of inquiry. Gilliss and Knafl make a unique contribution to the science as they provide

a synthesis across the many integrated reviews conducted on nursing research of families. They note that advances in the science are limited because of the failure to build on the conclusions of such reviews in subsequent research or practice. Although the use of multiple methods to address complex research questions is becoming normative in nursing research of families, Gilliss and Knafl conclude that qualitative researchers often fail to clarify the philosophical or methodological underpinnings of their work. Increasingly, family studies incorporate multiple methods in a single study and give voice to multiple family members.

The ability to identify the science of research of families is becoming more difficult, as it does not belong solely to nursing, and nurses and non-nurses publish much of the relevant work outside of the nursing literature. This diversity in the dissemination of our science has two sides. One is an increase in the difficulty of identifying and evaluating nursing science; the other side is the opportunity to inform other scientists through dissemination of nursing research across disciplines. All the authors in this section stress the significance of interdisciplinary research and the dissemination of the nursing research of families beyond nursing.

The transfer of knowledge between research and practice is a continuing challenge across nursing and the family sciences. Gilliss, Knafl, and McCubbin note that not only is the translation from research to practice lacking, we also lack methods of ensuring the translation of practice knowledge to research. Gilliss and Knafl recommend a systematic analysis of the clinical literature to identify the themes and patterns that contribute to our knowledge of families. Clinical knowledge can also be used to advance the science of intervention research by assisting in defining the components of interventions and the outcomes (Feetham, 1993; Levenstein, 1996). McCubbin identifies other processes critical to increasing the translation between practice and research. These include having a strong theoretical base to clinical research and asking the tangible outcome question of how will the research make a difference with families? Feetham and Meister state that the correspondence between research and practice and research and policy are not separate issues. They urge that increasing the correspondence with policy, and nursing research of families will build on and contribute to the correspondence between research and practice.

All the authors speak to the interdependence among nursing of families, research, and policy. Feetham and Meister assess the state of the correspondence of nursing research of families with policy and present frameworks to guide our efforts to improve the correspondence. These frameworks define the components of policy development, identify domains of policies that affect the health and well-being of families, and clarify the steps by which successful interventions are gradually transformed into programs, which in turn are then sustained by policies. These frameworks guide the selection of the design, methods, measures, and data interpretation, resulting in research with a greater correspondence with policy deci-

sions. The research provides data for the issues facing policy makers to use to inform their decisions. It can also unite practice and policy by helping to transform successful interventions into the centerpiece of programs and policies.

Feetham and Meister also discuss the emergence of science policy that currently guides the nature of nursing research of families and the preparation of researchers. Changes in science policy are proposed as a strategy to increase the correspondence with policy and to promote the further development of a cadre of researchers who are capable of transforming interventions into service programs by policy.

All the authors provide recommendations to advance the science in nursing and other disciplines. Readers are challenged to attend to the complex and continuing pressures on families as they respond to the issues of changes in health systems and financing, the aging population, the imbalance in the distribution of resources, and the burgeoning technologies in every aspect of their lives. Scholars in nursing research of families have led the science in moving away from deficit models or frameworks to those identifying and building on family strengths. Nurse scientists often seek to examine the strengths, strategies, and predictors that enable families to successfully manage family challenges or stresses such as chronic illness, risk behaviors in family members, and caregiving responsibilities. Identifying these factors positions researchers to develop interventions that enhance these characteristics and, in some families, enable them to develop protective factors that can prevent adverse threats to the family.

A family nursing agenda for increasing the correspondence among practice, education, research, and policy is necessary and will make an important contribution to the health and well-being of families for the next millenium. The authors make it clear that this correspondence is not easy to accomplish. Progress to improve correspondence must be done in a programmatic way and by extending the contexts of our current research.

References

Feetham, S. (1993). Family outcomes: Conceptual and methodological issues. In P. Moritz (Ed.), *Patient outcomes research: Examining the effectiveness of nursing practice.* Bethesda, MD: National Center for Nursing Research, NIH.

Levenstein, C. (1996). Policy implications of intervention research: Research on the social context for intervention. *American Journal of Industrial Medicine, 29,* 358-361.

12

NORMATIVE FAMILY TRANSITIONS AND HEALTH OUTCOMES

Marilyn McCubbin

Historically, normative family transitions have been a focus of nursing practice in addition to care for individuals and families during times of illness. Normative transitions have health consequences that require nursing assessment and intervention at all levels of prevention—primary, secondary, and tertiary. Nurses intervene to promote optimal functioning at times of family transition, recognize and intervene if early signs of malfunctioning appear, and provide active support and referral in cases of severe dysfunction and deterioration.

In this chapter, the nursing research on normative family transitions and health outcomes is reviewed. First, the concept of transition is defined as an integral part of nursing practice; theoretical perspectives for examining normative family transitions are reviewed; the existing body of nursing research on normative family transitions is examined, using a family life cycle stage trajectory; and, finally, conclusions and recommendations for advancing the nursing science on normative family transitions are discussed. The review builds on prior reviews

of family nursing research (Feetham, 1984; Ganong, 1995; Whall & Loveland-Cherry, 1993).

Concept of Transition

Transition has been defined as the "passage or movement from one life phase, condition, status, or place to another" (Chick & Meleis, 1986, p. 239). Psychosocial transitions have been defined as "major changes in life space which are lasting in their effects, which take place over a relatively short period of time, and which affect large areas of the assumptive world" (Parkes, 1971, p. 103). A strong argument has been made that transition is a central concept in nursing (Chick & Meleis, 1986; Meleis & Trangenstein, 1994; Schumacher & Meleis, 1994). Five types of transitions pertinent for nursing (Meleis & Trangenstein, 1994) have been identified: (a) individual developmental (e.g., adolescence, midlife), (b) family developmental (e.g., childbearing, child rearing), (c) situational (e.g., immigration, unemployment), (d) health/illness (e.g., hospitalization, diagnosis of chronic or life-threatening illness), and (e) organizational (e.g., managed health care, changes in advanced nursing practice roles). In this chapter, the emphasis is on the nursing research related to family developmental transitions or those transitions that are normative and expected as part of the family life cycle. Because of the interdependence and mutual influence of individual and family developmental transitions (Benson & Deal, 1995), however, both individual and family normative transitions are represented in the research review.

Several characteristics of transitions deserve attention when examining this body of research. Transition is a process (Chick & Meleis, 1986) involving change (Schumacher & Meleis, 1994) over time. There is a beginning or onset of the transition, a period of disorganization as the individual and family attempt to respond and adapt to the transition, and a new level of functioning or performance as a result of the transition. The disorganization in the transition process is accompanied by feelings of disconnectedness (Chick & Meleis, 1986). There is a loss of the old and familiar as new roles, relationships, and identities for both the individual and the family unit must be forged. Because transitions are disruptive, resolution of the uncertainty in this situation (Selder, 1989) may require the acquisition of new knowledge and skills (Schumacher & Meleis, 1994).

Transitions can also be viewed as opportunities for growth, with gains for both the individual and family (Chick & Meleis, 1986). For example, the transition to parenthood, although stressful, can bring much joy and pleasure for new parents as they nurture and interact with their infant. Transitions can bring satisfaction and a sense of achievement and mastery. In their nursing model of transition, Schumacher and Meleis (1994) depict subjective well-being, mastery, and well-being of relationships as indicators of healthy transition.

The meaning or perception of the transition is vitally important and can vary considerably from individual to individual and family to family, however. This variability in perception influences both the patterns of response and transition outcomes (Chick & Meleis, 1986). Expectations also play a role in this process and may be unrealistic or unclear (e.g., what it is like to have a new baby in the family). Here again, providing information and assisting with skill acquisition may help in clarifying expectations and restructuring reality (Selder, 1989). The

level of planning and problem solving ability; environmental supports such as social support, "family friendly" policies, and community resources; and individual physical and emotional health are also important factors that have an influence on transitional outcomes (Schumacher & Meleis, 1994).

Transition may be conceptualized as either an independent or a dependent variable in the research design (Chick & Meleis, 1986). As an independent variable, transitions have three potential outcomes relevant to nursing research: changes in health status, changes in health seeking behaviors, and/or changes in health care utilization (Chick & Meleis, 1986). Transition, as a dependent variable, could be viewed as an outcome due to changes in health status (the independent variable) (Chick & Meleis, 1986). Changes in health status due to Alzheimer's disease in a husband, for example, may eventually necessitate institutionalization, with this change in living arrangements representing a transition for the couple.

Family Science Theories and Normative Family Transitions

Theories from family science have been used to guide some of the nursing research on normative family transitions. Family development theory has been the family theory most closely linked with normative family transitions and developmental change in families over time (Aldous, 1996). In this theory, the family unit is viewed as progressing through a series of stages beginning with the formation of the couple relationship (traditionally viewed as marriage rather than cohabitation) and ending with the family in later life and the death of both spouses. The first or oldest child is the marker for entering a new child-rearing stage—family with infants and toddlers, preschool children, school-aged children, adolescents, launching stage of children leaving home as young adults, followed by the middle years of empty nest through retirement, and family in retirement years and old age (Duvall, 1977, and Duvall & Miller, 1985, as adapted in Friedman, 1992). At each stage, families complete certain developmental tasks or growth responsibilities to meet biological and cultural requirements and the family's own goals and aspirations (Duvall, 1977). Specific health concerns have also been described for each stage (Friedman, 1998). Nurses have found this developmental task framework helpful with assessment, anticipatory guidance, and direction for interventions with families.

Later reformulations of family development theory (Aldous, 1996; Rodgers & White, 1993) have specifically addressed the concept of transition. Family transitions encompass the concepts of stage, event, and time (Rodgers & White, 1993). A transition occurs "when the family moves from one qualitatively distinct stage to another stage" (Rodgers & White, 1993, p. 238). A specific event (e.g., birth of a child) signifies the move into a new stage that is very different from the previous stage. This new stage involves changes in roles or role transitions (Aldous, 1996). The transition to a new stage is viewed as a period of disorganization and disequilibrium for the family unit, but the time within a stage is viewed as being relatively stable.

Time refers to both event and stage sequencing and stage duration. An event can be "on time or off time." Age is one indicator of time; too-early childbearing (when the woman is an adolescent) and delayed childbearing (when the woman is in her 40s) can be considered "off time" events due to age. Event and stage sequencing is the expected order and progression of stages—specifically, marriage, then birth of first child. The family sequence of birth, marriage, divorce is quite different. The duration of a stage also influences the course of family development. For example, the longer a couple stays childless, the less apt they are to have a child. A long cohabitation or engagement may preclude the couple's marrying. Cross-institutional norms also affect the family's developmental course. Educational and occupational career norms, such as completing education before marriage or meeting career goals before starting a family, may be in conflict with the family's timing and goals.

The major criticism of family development theory has been the difficulty of application to non-nuclear and non-Caucasian families. Societal changes such as increasing divorce rates and changing roles for men and women have made it increasingly difficult to determine what a normal family life cycle is (McGoldrick, Heiman, & Carter, 1993). Research concerns have centered on the theory's failure to demonstrate predictive and explanatory power (Rodgers & White, 1993).

Family stress theory addresses the concept of family adaptational change. In this theory, families are seen as adapting to stressor events, including family developmental transitions, that are occurring either within the family, within the family's interactions with the outside environment, or both at the same time. Life transitions highlight the role of individual and family adaptation. To navigate developmental transitions, a restructuring of the psychological sense of self and a reorganization of interpersonal relationships must take place (Cowan, 1991). From this perspective, the concepts of risk and vulnerability, protective factors, and resiliency factors are appropriate to consider when analyzing family responses to transitional events (Cowan, 1991). Recent developments in family stress theory (McCubbin & McCubbin, 1993, 1996), guided by the concept of resiliency, have emphasized the importance of changing patterns of family functioning, appraisal processes, resources, and coping in the family's adaptation to normative family transitions and have focused on the ability of families to endure, recover, and grow from these life experiences.

The most recent family stress model, the Resiliency Model of Family Stress, Adjustment, and Adaptation (McCubbin & McCubbin, 1993, 1996), depicts family response to stressor events as occurring in two phases: adjustment and adaptation. Adjustment is seen as the process families go through as a response to more minor events that do not require major changes in family functioning. In most developmental transitions, however, family system changes and modified patterns of functioning are necessary and expected. A family "crisis" occurs, calling for these changes.

This crisis, or state of family disorganization, is the start of the adaptation phase in the Resiliency Model. The level of family adaptation is influenced by the family's vulnerability, depicted as the accumulation of stressors, strains, and transitions happening to the family. Resiliency factors of newly established patterns of family functioning encompassing modifications in roles, boundaries, and rules (e.g., sharing child care responsibilities and decline in social behaviors are predictable changes in couple behaviors in reponse to the addition of a first child); resources of informal and formal social support; family appraisal processes; and problem-solving and coping strategies assist the family in this adaptation process. The positive outcome is *bonadaptation,* or restoration of harmony and balance in the functioning of individual family members, the family unit, and the relationships of the family to the broader community. Adaptation is a cyclical process, not a linear one. Families try out new strategies for family functioning, resource use, and coping; if unsuccessful, *maladaptation* occurs, putting the family back into crisis, with the process of finding new ways to manage the situation beginning all over again.

In this theory, normative family transitions would be viewed as requiring adaptation rather than adjustment because major changes in family functioning need to be made. The idea of using both family development theory and family stress theory to analyze family response to transitional events has already been advanced (Mederer & Hill, 1983). Families experience a series of critical transitions over the life cycle (family development theory) that require the family to reorganize and establish new patterns of functioning to adapt (family stress theory). Thus, although family development emphasizes the discrete stages and the developmental tasks to be accomplished within those stages, family stress theory can aid in analyzing the critical variables involved in the *process* by which families reorganize in the face of developmental change and also how families transition from one stage to another.

Family scientists (Rodgers & White, 1993; White, 1991) have argued that it is important to distinguish between developmental, maturational, and adaptational change. They contend that maturational change occurs at the individual level and is not applicable to the family unit, but adaptational change encompasses a family's efforts to align itself with the environment. Although these conceptual differences are important, one can argue that families undergo maturational change too; as the adolescent matures, for example, parental roles and relationhips must be re-examined. In this sense, the parents "mature" and learn to "let go" to allow the adolescent increased autonomy and independence in preparation for adulthood. This "maturation" does not occur in a vacuum; individual family members and the family unit are engaged in a continual process of seeking a "fit" with the environment so that both the adolescent, the parents, and the family unit are meeting the norms set by the culture and other societal institutions.

Family systems theory has also been used as a framework for normative family transitions. This theory emphasizes the mutual interdependence and interaction of family members and transactions within the family and between the family and the larger environment (Whitchurch & Constantine, 1993). Subsystems within the family are the adult couple, the parent-child, and the sibling subsystems. Much of the nursing research on normative family transitions has focused on a subsystem (couple, parent-child) rather than on the entire family unit.

In this theory, families that are open systems readily receive information and support from the outside environment and seek new resources with which to manage family transitions. Families negotiate their boundaries to either encourage or limit input and to determine the degree of separation between the family and the environment. Input is processed by the family using rules of transformation. These rules encompass the various ways in which families manage input; families who have a variety of ways to do this possess the systems property of *equifinality,* or the ability to use many routes to achieve their goals (Whitchurch & Constantine, 1993). Feedback loops provide the family with information about how it is doing in this regard. Negative feedback indicates that the family should maintain its present state and promote stability (morphostasis); positive feedback indicates the need for change, or morphogenesis (Broderick & Smith, 1979). Normative family transitions would be viewed as creating the need for morphogenesis.

A key concept in family systems theory is nonsummativity, or the premise that the family unit is different than just the sum of its individual members. Another key assumption is that what affects one family member affects all members and the family unit. Thus, normative transition for one family member (e.g., retirement) will affect all family members—the spouse or partner, any children, and the functioning of the family group.

Family systems theory concepts are abstract and can be difficult to operationalize for research purposes (Whitchurch & Constantine, 1993). Strategies of measurement to capture the nonsummativity property of families, for example, have generated considerable debate in family research and the "proper" use of individual- and family-level scores (Ransom, Fisher, Phillips, Kokes, & Weiss, 1990).

Symbolic interactionism depicts human interaction as being based on symbols that have meanings that are derived from living in the environment. The behavior of the individual and family is influenced by the meanings that are attached to these symbols. For example, in Hawaiian American families, food is a symbol that carries a meaning of respect. Traditionally, Hawaiians had great regard for the food they grew, harvested, and ate. Children are still taught to eat some of everything they are served. The wisdom of the elders states that "you never belittle the food you eat, for some day you will starve" (McCubbin & McCubbin, 1997). For the individual, a sense of self develops from these symbols and their meanings. Family behaviors are influenced by the meanings that develop over time around shared events, experiences, and cultural beliefs.

During normative family transitions, the meaning of the transition would be emphasized in this theory. How family roles are constructed, developed, negotiated, carried out, and changed over time is the focus of role theory, which has been linked to the interactionist perspective (Burr, Leigh, Day, & Constantine, 1979). Role taking, or taking on the role behaviors of others in a similar role, and role making, or creating and modifying a role to better fit an individual's situation, are both part of the socialization process and are used in family role transitions such as becoming a spouse, parent, or sibling.

Exchange theory has been used infrequently in nursing research on normative family transitions but more often in long-term family caregiving in chronic illness and disability. When applied to the family, this theory focuses on how relationships are developed, experienced, and maintained through patterns of fairness, equity, reciprocity, decision making, dominance, control, and power (Sabatelli & Shehan, 1993). The overall assumption is that individuals seek to maximize their rewards and minimize their costs in a relationship with the standards used for evaluating this ratio changing over time. In general, a comparison level is used for evaluation that addresses whether the individual is getting what is realistic, attainable, and satisfying, as well as reflective of what others are getting in similar situations. The exchange process is mediated by resources, dependencies, and alternatives to the present situation. If the ratio of rewards to costs is positive, the relationship is maintained; if it is negative and better alternatives exist, the relationship changes and may end (Sabatelli & Shehan, 1993).

Nursing theories have not been used as often as a theoretical perspective for research on normative family transitions. Orem's self-care deficit theory was used to examine women's pregnancy outcomes (Hart, 1995). Roger's Life Process Model formed part of the framework for Fawcett's studies of body image and symptoms in expectant couples (Fawcett, 1989). The Roy Adaptation Model served as the framework for the intervention study on preparation for cesarean childbirth by Fawcett, Pollio, et al. (1993).

These family science and nursing theories, even though the latter are less well developed for family research, provide important frameworks for nursing research on family transitions. Each theory uses a slightly different set of lenses with which to measure and analyze both the process and outcomes of family transitions. These theories can provide critical guidance as to specific factors that might be most amenable to interventions to reduce risk and promote health in normative family transitions (Muehrer & Koretz, 1992).

Criteria and Process for Research Review

▬ *Definition of Family*

A clear definition of the family has been noted as a criteria for evaluating research of families (Feetham, 1990). Among family scholars, there is no agreed-upon definition of the family (Levin & Trost, 1992), and there is great diversity in families in today's society. In this review, the definition of the family was based on dyadic units, as recommended by Trost (1988), to include a variety of family forms. Any nursing research study on normative family transitions using a dyadic unit as the stated or implied definition of family was included in this review.

▬ *Study Inclusion Criteria and Retrieval Process*

Study selection was also limited to family-related or family research (Feetham, 1990). Family-related research "refers to research that focuses on relationships between family members, using data derived from individuals" (Feetham, 1990, p. 35). Family research focuses on "the family unit as a whole" (Feetham, 1990, p. 35). Research that focused solely on individual-level variables in normative family transitions was excluded. Studies on a situational transition accompanying a normative transition (e.g., birth of a child with a disability) were excluded. Other family transitions that are increasing in society today and are still considered non-normative, such as adolescent pregnancy and parenthood, were also excluded. In summary, this research review defined family as at least one dyadic unit, included studies with dyadic and/or family variables and measures, and represents both family-related and family research on normative family transitions over the family life cycle.

The retrieval process for studies included both computerized and manual searching methods. Key words such as *family, transition, life cycle stage, family development, transition to parenthood, aging family,* and so on were used to retrieve pertinent published nursing research studies in computerized databases in nursing and other disciplines (psychology, family studies, sociology).

In addition, a manual search of nursing journal indexes was conducted using the past 10 years of nursing research journals (1986 to early 1996) and the past 5 years of clinical nursing journals (1990 to early 1996). A published directory of U.S. nursing journals was used to guide this search process (Swanson, McCloskey, & Bodensteiner, 1991).

Overall, the research questions addressed by the nursing research on normative family transitions have included:

a. What are the risk factors that increase the probability of family dysfunction and ill health for family members during normative family transitions?

b. What are the protective factors that help family members and family units manage normative transitions more successfully?

c. What is the process that family members and the family unit go through when experiencing a normative family transition?

d. What nursing interventions can provide support for families experiencing normative transitions over the family life cycle?

Nursing Research on Normative Family Transitions

No published nursing research was found that focused on the transition to marriage. Therefore, this review begins with the second life cycle stage, divided into research on pregnancy and the transition to parenthood.

Pregnancy as a Family Transition

The nursing research on pregnancy would support this family event as a transition because the evidence indicates that the family moves from one qualitatively distinct stage to another. Nursing research on the family transition of pregnancy has included similarities and differences in spouses' experiences during pregnancy and postpartum; the marital relationship during pregnancy; maternal and paternal fetal attachment, dimensions of expectant fatherhood; mother-daughter relationships during pregnancy; diverse families and pregnancy; and factors predicting family functioning during pregnancy.

Couple Relationships During Pregnancy

Using the theoretical framework of the family as a "living, open system" (Fawcett, 1975) drawn from Martha Rogers' Life Process Model, Fawcett and colleagues (Drake, Verhulst, Fawcett, & Barger, 1988; Fawcett, 1989; Fawcett, Bliss-Holtz, Haas, Leventhal, & Rubin, 1986; Fawcett & York, 1986) examined similarities and differences in spouses' perceptions of body image changes and reports of physical and psychological symptoms during pregnancy and postpartum. Based on couple mutual influence and interdependence, it was hypothesized that husbands and wives would experience similarities in pregancy and postpartum experiences and that these similarities would be positively related to the strength of their identification.

Perceived body space, one component of body image, was similar between spouses in an initial study of 40 couples (Fawcett, 1978), but this finding was not replicated in subsequent studies of 54 U.S. couples (Fawcett, 1987; Fawcett, Bliss-Holst, et al., 1986) and 20 Canadian couples (Drake, Verhulst, Fawcett, & Barger, 1988). Spouses did report some similar physical and psychological symptoms in the Canadian sample (Drake, Verhulst, & Fawcett, 1988) and another sample of 70 U.S. couples (Fawcett & York, 1986, 1987). However, the relationships between body image and symptoms and the couples' strength of identification were not supported in any of the studies. Given these results, the credibility of this theoretical perspective of the family system and the view of pregnancy as a family experience was questioned (Fawcett, 1989). The need for other measures of couple mutual interaction, such as the quality of the marital relationship and different definitions and measures of the husband's experience and involvement during pregnancy, were indicated (Fawcett, 1989).

Pregnancy as a couple experience has been supported in more recent research for couples with a history of infertility. Systems theory, with a focus on the interdependency and mutuality in the spousal subsystem, was the theoretical framework for a study of fertility status and physical and affective symptoms in 58 expectant Caucasian couples (Holditch-Davis, Black, Sandelowski, Harris, & Belyea, 1995). Expectant couples with a history of infertility ($N = 37$) were found to experience the unique phenomenon of symptom attunement, as they reported similar amounts of general types of symptoms and were also experiencing symptoms in a more globally consistent manner. The investigators concluded that this reflected attempts to restore equilibrium to the spousal subsystem after the strain and estrangement of infertility treatment (Holditch-Davis et al., 1995).

In cross-sectional studies, Brown developed an instrument to measure supportive behaviors by partners and others during pregnancy (1986a); described and compared the physical and psychological symptoms of expectant mothers and fathers (1988); and examined relationships between stress, social support, and expectant parents' health (1986b) in a sample of 313 mostly Caucasian couples. Time of data collection ranged from 21 to 42 weeks of the pregnancy. Factor analysis of her instrument, the Supportive Behaviors Inventory, based on House's (1981) categories of emotional, material, information, and appraisal support, indicated a unidimensional construct of perceived degree of experienced support during pregnancy (Brown, 1986a). The subsequent report (Brown, 1986b), however, used the two subscales of the instrument—Satisfaction with Partner's Support and Other People's Support. Stress and partner support, but not support from others, were significant predictors of both parents' health, with women's health also being influenced by a history of chronic illness.

In a more recent cross-sectional study, Brown (1994) added an additional independent variable of marital discord to explore the relationships between stress, social support, and health in a sample of 431 expectant couples during the 15 to 42 weeks of pregnancy. Only partner support was used for the analysis. One yes or no item was used to measure occurrence of marital discord during pregnancy. Patterns of couple responses were used to configure four groups: both spouses reporting discord (both yes), husband yes and wife no, husband no and wife yes, and both spouses no for comparison. Expectant parents who both reported marital discord reported higher stress, lower partner support, and poorer health. Strengths of Brown's studies included large sample sizes using responses of both expectant mothers and fathers and the use of pattern scores (Ransom et al., 1990). Instruments to measure stress, support, and health, however, were all in the early stages of psychometric development by the author. Application of well-tested instruments used in family science could have been used for concurrent validity. Replication of the study in other samples using a well-validated measure of marital discord would be an important area of future inquiry.

Expectations for mutual support after childbirth in expectant couples was examined by Coffman, Levitt, and Brown (1994), who tested Levitt's (1991) support expectations model in 99 men and 105 women in childbirth education classes. This nursing-psychology research team also tested an experimental intervention based on this model, which states that both close support and confirmation of that support contribute to satisfaction in close relationships. Relationship satisfaction was viewed as a mediator leading to higher individual emotional well-being and more positive parenting attitudes. Results supported the model, as parents with greater confirmation of their support expectations had more positive relationship satisfaction, emotional affect, and attitudes towards the baby. Gender differences were found, however, with confirmation of support being more important for women and actual level of received support being more important for men. For the experimental intervention, a couple and group discussion focusing on the expectant couple clarifying their expectations for support after childbirth was carried out, using an index of 14 support functions. Control group participants completed a sex role behavior index, also using both couple and group discussion. Outcome data, collected 3 months after delivery, indicated that the experimental intervention was not related to confirmation of support expectations nor to relationship satisfaction, emotional affect, and attitude towards the baby. The one-time intervention may not have been "strong" enough to produce lasting changes in the relationship once the baby arrived.

Prenatal Attachment

Nurse investigators have directed much attention to studying prenatal attachment, based on the belief that prenatal attachment has a strong influence on future parent-child relationships and the child's development. Previous review articles (Gaffney, 1988; Muller, 1992) have documented the progress and directions for future research in this area; therefore this review will build on those reviews and examine only the prenatal attachment studies published since 1992. Muller (1992) notes that five research questions have been addressed: (a) How do pregnant women experience prenatal attachment? (b) Can prenatal attachment be measured? (c) What factors have relationships with prenatal attachment? (d) Will interventions influence attachment? (e) Does prenatal attachment predict postnatal attachment? The dominant theoretical perspective has been attachment theory, drawing on the work of Bowlby (1979, 1988). Concerns about nursing prenatal attachment research have focused on the measurement of prenatal attachment. Most nurse investigators have used Cranley's Maternal Fetal Attachment Scale (MFAS). Paternal fetal attachment also has been measured using this instrument but less frequently (Mercer, Ferketich, May, DeJoseph, & Sollid, 1988). As Muller (1992) notes, this does allow comparison across study findings, but serious questions about the validity of the MFAS instrument (Mercer, Ferketich, May, et al., 1988; Muller & Ferketich, 1992, 1993) have been raised, namely the inability of factor analyses to produce the conceptual dimensions of the instrument.

Two more recent studies (Hart, 1995; Zachariah, 1994a), however, also used the MFAS. Using Orem's nursing theory of self-care, Hart (1995) combined the MFAS measure of prenatal attachment with a measure of the readiness to assume the maternal role to represent the foundations for dependent-care agency in Orem's theory. Foundations for dependent care agency had a direct effect on the infant's birth weight and were positively related to basic prenatal care actions (prenatal health activities such as nutrition, activity and rest, etc.). Zachariah (1994a) also used the MFAS to examine the influence of both mother-daughter and husband-wife relationships on maternal fetal attachment (MFA). Although both of these relationships were correlated with each other, neither predicted maternal fetal attachment. The investigator raised questions about the adequacy of MFA measurement.

The epistemology of expectant parenthood was examined by Sandelowski and Black (1994) via a secondary analysis of 288 interviews with 62 childbearing couples. They concluded that much of pregnancy work is directed at getting to know the fetus, with both fetal attachment and fetal acquaintance as two distinct components of this process. However, there is a lack of clarity between these two components.

The complexity of prenatal attachment and acquaintance with the fetus as one of the primary processes for couples during pregnancy has been highlighted by this body of research. A revision of the MFAS or new measures of prenatal attachment and acquaintanceship, as well as postnatal attachment, are critically needed. Development of the Prenatal Attachment Inventory (Muller, 1993), with initial evidence of reliability and validity, is a step in this direction. More information is also needed about the process of getting to know the fetus for the father. Is it similar to the mother's process? How does the mother influence the father in this process, and vice versa? Although interventions for promoting fetal attachment have been undertaken (Gaffney, 1988; Muller, 1992), it would seem necessary to address measurement issues first before undertaking further intervention studies.

Expectant Fatherhood

Increased societal expectations for father participation in pregnancy and childbirth have generated a small body of research on this transition for fathers. Grounded theory has been used to describe the experience of fathers at this family life cycle stage. Donovan's (1995) extensive interviews with six expectant fathers during the second trimester of pregnancy uncovered five theoretical constructs: (a) fathers' ambivalence in the early stages of pregnancy; (b) perception of the relationship with the baby as not real; (c) questioning, How should I be as a father? (d) coping with changing roles and lifestyles; and (e) disequilibrium in relationship with female partner. Fathers' emotional distress and anxiety influenced the differing expectations of the couple about becoming parents. In a grounded theory study of 56 expectant and new fathers, Jordan (1990) found an overall theme of "laboring for relevance," which involved (a) grappling with the reality of the pregnancy and child; (b) struggling for recognition from others—partner, the infant, other family members, coworkers, friends, and society; and (c) plugging away at role making of involved fatherhood. Findings supported the importance of maternal support in promoting paternal behavior, couple communication, and emotional sharing of the childbearing experience. In a grounded theory study of 20 couples, using postbirth interviews and birth observations, Chapman (1991) found that fathers who were present during labor and birth were "searching for their place." This process involved "identifying a new role, engaging in it, testing it out, and gauging the effectiveness of the role" (Chapman, 1991, p. 27). Fathers' roles during labor of coach, teammate, and witness were influenced by labor guides—the laboring mother first and then health care providers who performed gatekeeping, directive, and informational functions. Different levels of physical and mental engagement were found in each role, with both types of engagement present in the coach role.

Expectant fathers' (*N* = 108) stressors centered around the health and birth condition of the baby, childbirth pain for the partner, and unexpected events during childbirth (Glazer, 1989). High anxiety levels were not found in these expectant fathers; however, higher stress levels were associated with higher anxiety. Fathers who were young, less educated, and had lower incomes had higher stress and anxiety.

Themes of paternal uncertainty and role ambiguity, anxiety about the mother during the birth experience and about the baby's health, and both tensions and support in the couple relationship have been documented as part of fathers' experience during the family transition of pregnancy and birth. Conclusions in these studies indicated that fathers desired pregnancy and birth participation but felt they lacked the knowledge and skills to participate (Jordan, 1990), current childbirth preparation classes were not meeting fathers' needs (Donovan, 1995), and fathers should not automatically be assigned the role of coach during labor but be given options for a role that is congruent and comfortable for them (Chapman, 1991).

Mother-Daughter Relationships During Pregnancy

Earlier research had noted the importance of both the spousal and mother-daughter relationships on the mother's physical and emotional health during pregnancy (Lederman, 1984). Although Zachariah (1994a) did not find a relationship between mother-daughter relationship and fetal attachment, both mother-daughter and husband-wife attachment, as well as the woman's age, were significant predictors of psychological well-being in 115 Canadian Caucasian pregnant women (Zachariah, 1994b). A qualitative study using content analysis examined the mother-daughter relationship in pregnancy in 64 daughters (99% Caucasian) and 60 mothers (Martell, 1990). Themes encompassed (a) changes in the mother-daughter relationship, such as desire for more frequent contact and need to resolve past conflicts; (b) help exchanged between mothers and daughters, mostly in the form of emotional and psychological support; and (c) the impact of others, especially the daughter's husband, on the relationship that generated both support and conflict (e.g., who would be present at the birth). Intergenerational relationships during pregnancy in more diverse samples have not been reported.

Family Diversity and the Pregnancy Transition

The vast majority of studies on the pregnancy transition for families have used middle-class Caucasian samples, frequently drawn from expectant parents attending childbirth education classes (Brown, 1986a, 1986b, 1988, 1994; Coffman, Levitt, & Brown, 1994; Zachariah, 1994a, 1994b). Two groups of nursing researchers have examined pregnancy transitions in more diverse populations. Norbeck and Anderson (1989a) examined life stress, social support, and anxiety in mid- and late-pregnancy in 190 low-income women equally di-

vided among African American, Hispanic, and White groups. All study variables showed stability over time. Controlling for race and marital status, social support was a significant buffer between stress and anxiety, with partner support the critical source at both time points. Support from the woman's mother was also significant at midpregnancy. Highest anxiety was associated with high life stress and low partner support. Lower social support from the woman's partner or mother was also a predictor for higher labor and delivery and gestation complications in African-American women, but not in Hispanic women (Norbeck & Anderson, 1989b). Hispanic women, however, had very low rates of complications and low life stress and substance use. For Whites, support had a negative influence, suggesting that this support might encourage unhealthful practices during pregnancy, such as smoking and drug use.

Affonso et al. (1993) used a focus group methodology to describe themes of stressors for pregnant Filipino, Japanese, and Hawaiian women living in Hawaii. Five groups of 7 to 10 women each were convened—one for each ethnic group, one for health care providers, and one for local neighborhood women who were community leaders representing all three ethnic groups. The family focus was addressed by asking "What kinds of events, feelings, or concerns happen within a family that are hard for a pregnant woman to deal with?" (Alfonso et al., 1993, p. 12). For Hawaiian women, stress, conflict, and control issues with the spouse or partner and overprotectiveness of the pregnant woman by the family were concerns. For Filipino women, difficulties fulfilling familial and social roles and obligations due to fatigue and symptoms of pregnancy were noted, with social ostracism resulting if the woman did not fulfill expected roles. For Japanese women, who were better educated and more affluent than the other two groups, family concerns centered on the stress of multiple work and family roles and being burdened by intergenerational differences of pregnancy and life philosophies. This created much tension for the women.

Only one nursing study was found on pregnancy that compared family coping and anticipated problems in 40 traditional nuclear families and 40 stepfamilies (Dietz-Omar, 1991). The nuclear families were expecting a subsequent child; stepfamilies were expecting their first child together. Unexpectedly, nuclear family wives anticipated the most problems. The stepcouple looked forward to having their first child together. Stepfamily wives used more internal family coping strategies (using resources within the family) than nuclear family wives.

Both nuclear family husbands and stepfamily wives used more external family coping (resources outside the family) than stepfamily husbands.

Family Functioning During Pregnancy

Only two groups of nursing researchers have examined family system functioning during pregnancy. Tomlinson, White, and Wilson (1990) used the Family Dynamics Measure (FDM), developed by a group of nurse researchers (Lasky et al., 1985) to assess family functioning and determine relationships between family functioning and sociodemograhic variables in a U.S. sample of 160 women and 65 of their partners during the third trimester of pregnancy. Couples who were married and had a higher social status had higher family functioning, which was thought to be due to better resources. Race, parity, and maternal age were not related to family functioning. The FDM has also been used to measure family functioning during pregnancy in Nordic countries (Hakulinen, Paunonen, & Turunen, 1993; Hall, Wulff, White, & Wilson, 1994).

The largest and most comprehensive nursing study of family transition during pregnancy, postpartum, and early infancy to date has been the longitudinal research carried out by Mercer and colleagues (Mercer & Ferketich, 1990, 1994a, 1994b, 1995; Mercer, Ferketich, DeJoseph, et al., 1988; Mercer, Ferketich, May, et al., 1988; Mercer, May, Ferketich, & DeJoseph, 1986), who tested a multivariate model, based on family development theory (Mercer, May, et al., 1986), to determine the effect of antepartum stress on the family in four groups: 218 low-risk pregnant women and 147 partners and 153 high-risk pregnant women and 75 partners, during the 24th through 34th weeks of pregnancy. Follow-up data were obtained at four time points: during early postpartum and 1, 4, and 8 months after the infant's birth. High-risk women were hospitalized during the pregnancy (these data were collected in the early 1980s) and had a higher rate of infant health complications. Individual, dyadic, family system, and intergenerational variables were included in the model. Outcomes included family functioning (Mercer & Ferketich, 1990; Mercer, Ferketich, DeJoseph, et al., 1988), partner relationships (Mercer, Ferketich, & DeJoseph, 1993), health status of the men (Ferketich & Mercer, 1989) and women (Mercer & Ferketich, 1995), and maternal and paternal role transition (Ferketich & Mercer, 1994, 1995b; Mercer & Ferketich, 1994a, 1995).

Family functioning was measured by the Feetham Family Functioning Survey (Roberts & Feetham, 1982;

Sawin & Harrigan, 1995). Comparisons of family functioning were carried out between risk groups and between partners within risk groups. As expected, during pregnancy, high-risk women and men reported lower family functioning than low-risk women and men. High-risk women and men reported similar family functioning; low-risk men reported more optimal family functioning than low-risk women. For low-risk women, depression was the major predictor of family functioning, followed by perceived support. Sense of mastery, stress (negative life events), and health perception affected family functioning indirectly through depression. Self-esteem, pregnancy risk, stress, and health perception explained significant variance in mastery. Negative life events had indirect effects on family functioning through sense of mastery, self-esteem, depression, health perception, and perceived support. For low-risk men, more optimal health status, less stress, more frequent present contact with their fathers, and greater perceived support were linked to more optimal family functioning.

For high-risk women, sense of mastery, trait anxiety, and relationship as a child with father were direct predictors of family functioning, with stress and self-esteem having indirect effects through sense of mastery. Perceived support, relationship with their mother as a teen, and negative life events (stress) were the direct predictors of family functioning for high-risk men, explaining 48% of the variance, with no indirect effects found. The model for high-risk men was the simplest model of the four and explained the most variance (Mercer, Ferketich, DeJoseph, et al., 1988). In these models, perceived support for men was more critical than for women. This finding, along with the findings from the qualitative studies on expectant fatherhood noted earlier, indicate that the support men receive during pregnancy appears to be critical in managing the role ambiguity and uncertainty they experience as expectant parents. Women, on the other hand, were more affected by the stress during pregnancy, and the authors concluded that this made support also important for women during pregnancy (Mercer, Ferketich, DeJoseph, et al., 1988). The importance of parent personality and psychological variables also cannot be overlooked during pregnancy.

Family development, family systems, role theory, and family stress theory all have provided guidance for nursing research on pregnancy as a family transition. It appears that concepts of transition are quite relevant at this stage—a major change in life space (Parkes, 1971) is taking place, with disruption, uncertainty, and the need to acquire new knowledge and skills becoming evident to make the transition to parenthood. One pregnancy intervention study was reported on preparing pregnant women for the possibility of cesarean birth (Fawcett, Pollio, et al., 1993). No differences on perception of birth experience, physical distress, self-esteem, mothers' functional status, feelings about the baby, or marital relationship quality were found between the women who received extensive information about cesarean birth ($n = 74$) and those who received only limited information ($n = 48$). The provision of no information about cesarean birth to the control group was not possible due to ethical concerns; this may also have influenced study results (Fawcett, Pollio, et al., 1993). Here again, the information may not have been "strong" enough to produce a lasting effect, and the authors acknowledge it may not have been realistic to expect an intervention given several weeks before delivery to have an impact after delivery, given the major disruption taking place at this time. Perhaps larger samples, especially in the control group, would have brought about different results. The measures used to detect changes also may have lacked specificity and sensitivity.

Transition to Parenthood

Early family science research on the couple's initial transition to parenthood focused on a debate about the amount of crisis associated with this transition. Study limitations were related to how crisis was defined and retrospective data collection (Hobbs, 1965; Hobbs & Cole, 1977; LeMasters, 1957). Later research (Belsky & Rovine, 1990; Belsky, Spanier, & Rovine, 1983; Cowan & Cowan, 1992) was guided by five domains: (a) quality of relationships in the new parents' family of origin, (b) quality of new parents' couple relationship, (c) quality of mother-infant and father-infant relationship, (d) stress and social support in this expanding family, and (e) health or distress of individual parents and child (Cowan & Cowan, 1995). These domains have all been addressed in the nursing research, although most of the emphasis has been on the last four.

Couple relationship. Family scientists have reported a decline in marital satisfaction over the transition to parenthood (Belsky & Rovine, 1990; White & Booth, 1985), and this has been supported in nursing research (Dalgas-Pelish, 1993; Tomlinson, 1987). Both new mothers and fathers reported a decline in marital satisfaction from the last trimester of pregnancy to 3 months postbirth, but not to dysfunctional levels (Tomlinson, 1987). However, new parents' levels of marital satisfaction were higher than

nonparents both before and after birth, so it was concluded that this transition did not represent a crisis (Tomlinson, 1996). New mothers reported the greatest decline in marital satisfaction (Tomlinson, 1996).

The reason for this decline may lie in concepts from exchange and role theory. Equity in the marital relationship was a predictor for both women's and men's marital satisfaction postbirth, with a traditional sex role orientation also a negative contributor for women but not for men (Tomlinson, 1987). Difficulty reaching agreement with the spouse on tasks, activities, goals, and values contributed to the decline in marital satisfaction for new mothers (Tomlinson, 1996). Using grounded theory, Hall (1992) found that redefining roles was the core process in dual-earner families following the birth of the first child (Hall, 1992). New mothers took on multiple roles, experienced more role strain than fathers, and then reduced role strain. New fathers monitored role strain that arose from unmet needs and then limited role strain by taking on more family responsibilities (Hall, 1991, 1992). Mothers, however, whether employed or not, were found to continue to do the majority of the infant's care over the first year in 351 families of healthy infants. Fathers' proportion of infant care did increase as hours of maternal employment increased but was not more than mothers in any realm of infant care (Jones & Heermann, 1992). Rustia and Abbott (1990) found that it took 2 years for the 53 couples in their sample to agree on suitable patterns of child-care roles. Over time, fathers' willingness and actual participation in child care increased although not as much as these fathers originally expected to do. Fathers' care also lagged behind mothers' expectations, but by 2 years, fathers increased their participation and mothers lowered their expectations so the two merged into a more functional pattern. Mercer (1990) notes in her commentary on this study that the intense mother-infant relationship in early infancy may force the father out of the picture, with his role resurfacing again at the time of maternal individuation when the infant is around 8 months to 1 year old. Maternal preoccupation with the infant was thought to explain why mothers who reported less spousal interaction and care participation had higher sensitivity to the infant (Broom, 1994).

In Mercer and Ferketich's longitudinal study (1990) of high- and low-risk pregnant women and their partners, declines in family functioning at 8 months after birth, as measured by the Feetham Family Functioning Scale (Roberts & Feetham, 1982; Sawin & Harrigan, 1995), were found for both low-risk women and men, with low-risk women reporting lower levels than their partners.

This suggests that disorganization and change is still going on within the family system 8 months after birth, even for low-risk parents. For high- and low-risk women, depression had a direct effect on family functioning. Lower depression, greater perceived support, and lower life stress were the shared variables associated with more optimal family functioning for both high- and low-risk women. Whether a family member's depression causes lower family functioning or whether lower family functioning results in depression has been debated, however (Keitner & Miller, 1990). Family functioning had a direct effect on low-risk women's health status but only indirect effects on high-risk women's health status 8 months after birth (Ferketich & Mercer, 1990). For high-risk men, state anxiety at 4 months and the mate's pregnancy risk were significant predictors, explaining 50% of the variance in family functioning at 8 months. For low-risk men, perceived support 1 month after birth, medical treatment for health problems during pregnancy, and relationship with their father as a child were significant predictors, explaining 33% of the variance in family functioning at 8 months. No indirect effects were found in men's models (Mercer & Ferketich, 1990).

The transition to parenthood for older (over 30) mothers as a unique group of new parents has also been examined, reflecting the societal trend for delayed childbearing. Women in these samples were typical of the later childbearer—well educated, in professional careers, with a possible history of fertility problems. Older mothers had lower responses to the positive aspects of parenting and also tolerated the negative aspects of parenting better in a cross-sectional study of 68 women over the age of 29 during their first year of parenting (Meisenhelder & Meservey, 1987). In a longitudinal correlational study of 82 first-time mothers over age 35, high levels of stress 1 year after birth were associated with being employed and having poorer maternal health. Stress was inversely related to positive partner or spousal relationships, partner involvement with the infant, support for parenting from family and friends, and having the women's parents in close proximity. Women who were in longer lasting relationships had lowered confidence in parenting, suggesting that this transition may be more difficult in long-established couple relationships (Reece, 1995). In Mercer's (1986) subsample of 90 older mothers ages 30 to 42, slightly over half (51.8%) experienced decreased personality integration and two thirds (67.8%) reported decreased self-concept 8 months after the infant's birth. Mercer concluded that older mothers "warrant greater attention to prepare [them] for the realities of mother-

hood" (p. 32) and that older mothers may have unrealistically high expectations for themselves and their infants.

The influence of past and present relationships with the family of origin at this stage of transition to parenthood has not been a major focus in nursing research. In a grounded theory study, 13 of 14 Canadian fathers of 2-month-old infants indicated that they wanted to have a more nurturing, emotionally connected relationship with their child, as opposed to the relationship with their own father, whom they saw as a distant, emotionally detached figure serving only in an instrumental role (Anderson, 1996). Intergenerational family processes among parents, grandparents, and first-born infants in three families have been examined during the transition to parenthood, also using grounded theory (Bright, 1992). *Making place* was a family process that began before birth and encompassed both physical and social aspects, with reorganized interpersonal patterns and expanded boundaries across the generations.

Transition to the maternal role. Maternal and, to a lesser degree, paternal role attainment has been another focus of nursing research, as this is felt to be a strong influence on the well-being of both the parent and the infant and can be a focus of nursing intervention. The nursing studies on maternal role are family related (Feetham, 1990) where this role is examined from an individual and dyadic (mother-child) perspective but not in the context of the broader family system and family functioning. Maternal role attainment (MFA) has been described as both an interactional and a developmental process encompassing infant attachment, caretaking skills, and pleasure and gratification in the maternal role (Mercer, 1985). Koniak-Griffin (1993), in a state of the science review on MFA, has noted that maternal characteristics of age, parity, marital status, perceptions of the birth experience, personality, and psychological health of the mother; role conflict and role strain; infant characteristics of temperament; health status; environmental stress; and social support have all been found to influence maternal role attainment. The research has been limited by lack of a clear operationalization of MFA and incongruity between measures (Koniak-Griffin, 1993).

Most research on MFA has compared primiparas with multiparas without regard to specific parity. Grace (1993) examined role attainment in women having their first, second, or third child and found that women having a third child were highest on their evaluations of their performance as a mother and knowledge of the child and had the lowest life-change scores. These results may reflect self-selection, however, as women who enjoy parenting and the maternal role may tend to have subsequent children (Grace, 1993).

Self-esteem and mastery predicted maternal role competence in both low- and high-risk women; no differences in role competence were found between the two groups. Role competence increased at 4 and 8 months postpartum (Mercer & Ferketich, 1994a). Maternal role competence was also similar in experienced and inexperienced mothers over the first 8 months of parenthood, with inexperienced mothers' role competence increasing when the infant was 4 and 8 months old. Maternal self-esteem was the consistent predictor for both experienced and inexperienced mothers (Mercer & Ferketich, 1995). At 4 months, the partner relationship was a significant predictor for experienced mothers' role competence, suggesting that the partner's assistance at this time in larger families may help the mother's functioning (Mercer & Ferketich, 1995).

Using transition theory (Chick & Meleis, 1986), Pridham and Chang (1992) examined a model of transition for being a new mother of an infant during the first 3 months, focusing on maternal problem-solving tasks and self-appraisals of problem-solving competence and parenting. Mothers kept daily logs of both infant knowledge and caretaking issues they encountered. Mothers who had higher everyday supports identified higher numbers of both types of issues; younger mothers who identified higher numbers of caretaking issues were more likely to use lay problem-solving help; the number of caretaking issues a mother identified was positively related to use of clinician help. As previous mothering experience contributed very little to the model, this suggested that each infant presents a unique situation with new challenges the mother must manage (Pridham & Chang, 1992).

Transition to paternal role. Beliefs about father-infant bonding across the first transition to parenthood decreased after birth for both mothers and fathers in a sample of 35 Caucasian, well-educated, mostly dual-earning couples expecting their first child (Palkovitz, 1992). Fathers' beliefs about bonding were enhanced by longer initial father-infant contact with the mother present, extended contact beyond the delivery setting, and a number of supportive staff present. Drawing on data from a sample of 114 fathers, Jones and Lenz (1986) concluded that encouraging new fathers to stay with their partners and hold their infants was related to father's perceived competence in the early newborn period. Preg-

nancy risk and previous fathering experience were not influences on paternal role competence (Ferketich & Mercer, 1994, 1995b) but the father's psychological health appears to be a critical factor in transition to the paternal role. Anxiety was the major predictor of paternal role competence in partners of high-risk women; a sense of mastery and depression were major predictors of paternal role competence for partners of low-risk women (Ferketich & Mercer, 1994). Depression was also a major predictor for role competence in experienced fathers at 1, 4, and 8 months, with partner relationships as an additional predictor at 1 and 4 months. For inexperienced fathers, sense of mastery and family functioning were consistent predictors across time, with inexperienced fathers reporting greater anxiety and depression at 4 and 8 months after birth (Ferketich & Mercer, 1995a).

Sibling relationships. Facilitating and hindering conditions for sibling mutuality between a school-aged child and an infant sibling using multiple sources of longitudinal data (videotapes, interviews, children's drawings) were identified in a grounded theory study of nine families by Murphy (1990). The child's interest in the infant; high-quality parental relationship with the older child; and parents providing opportunities for uncensored, uninterrupted interaction with the infant and inclusion in the infant's care promoted sensitive, caring sibling interactions. Parents hindered sibling mutuality by interrupting or correcting sibling-infant interaction, limiting opportunities for contact, and discrepant treatment of the older child and newborn (Murphy, 1990, 1993). Distress and autonomy in 80 firstborn preschool children during the mothers' second pregnancy was examined by Gottlieb and Bailles (1995). Although distress varied by age, gender, and the time of the pregnancy, with girls being the most stressed group during late pregnancy, this nurse/psychologist research team concluded that the mother's pregnancy was not particularly stressful for these children but did require new ways of coping for them.

Families of Infants, Toddlers, and Preschool Children

The major focus of the nursing research at this life cycle stage of early child rearing has been on parent-infant (young child) relationships and parenting behaviors. Infant, parent, and, to a lesser extent, family environmental characteristics (marital relationship, family functioning) have been examined for their influence on the parent-infant relationship.

Parent-infant relationships. The underlying assumption behind the studies on parental role attainment and competence was that positive parental role competence and role attainment would be associated with more positive parent-infant relationships. A positive relationship was found between paternal role competence and paternal attachment, using self-report measures (Ferketich & Mercer, 1995a). Using a behavioral measure of mother-infant interaction, a relationship between maternal role attainment and mother's parenting behaviors was supported for primiparas but not multiparas in the early postpartum period (Walker, Crain, & Thompson, 1986a; 1986b). Because of differences in measurement of parental role compentence and attainment, the parent-infant relationship, and the time of data collection, it is difficult to draw conclusions. Many studies on parental role attainment did not examine the parent-child relationship as an outcome but focused instead on parents' confidence in the role or on maternal identity.

Support from other persons, recognizing and prioritizing the infant's needs, and mutual influence of the mother's and infant's emotional state were major influences on maternal responsiveness to infants in 30 healthy middle-class mothers (Blank, Schroeder, & Flynn, 1995). Mother's perception of the infant's temperament was related to maternal appraisals of parenting and problem-solving competence, controlling for infant gender, maternal attributes (education and parity), and parental context (life change and infant centrality) in a sample of 117 mothers. Infant temperament had more influence at 1 month than at 3 months. The role of the couple relationship or father's support was not explored in this study (Pridham, Chang, & Chiu, 1994).

Marital quality was found to have a direct influence on mother's infant sensitivity, but for fathers, the effect of marital quality was indirect through psychological well-being in a sample of 71 married couples with healthy 3-month-old infants. However, only a small amount (6%) of variance was explained for fathers (Broom, 1994). Parent attachment to the infant over the first 8 months did not differ between inexperienced (first child) and experienced (subsequent child) mothers and fathers (Ferketich & Mercer, 1995a; Mercer & Ferketich, 1994b). Support in the partner relationship during the first month was critical for experienced mothers, with a sense of mastery being important for inexperienced mothers (Mercer & Ferketich, 1994b). Men's attachment was independent of

environmental factors but more dependent on fetal attachment, with negative effects of depression noted in both inexperienced and experienced fathers at varying times during the early infancy period (Ferketich & Mercer, 1995a, 1995b). Measurement of parent-infant attachment by various self-report measures has been a concern in this body of research.

Videotapes of father-infant interaction in 114 father-newborn pairs indicated that new fathers began early to learn to read and respond to the infant's cues (Jones & Lenz, 1986; Jones & Thomas, 1989), with the infant's state (awake, asleep, crying) influencing fathers' interactional behavior. Infant crying predicted affective and comforting behavior by fathers (Jones & Lenz, 1986) but was also stressful for fathers and was related to elevations in systolic blood pressure (Jones & Thomas, 1989). An unexpected finding in Harrison's (1990) study of parental interactions with preterm ($n = 28$) and term ($n = 31$) infants was a positive correlation between the mother's satisfaction with the father's participation in child care and fathers' responsive, sensitive paternal behavior in both preterm and term infant groups. The conclusion was that positive feedback from the mother about the father's child-care assistance may help the father be more responsive to the infant (Harrison, 1990).

Although not specifically identified as linked to family stress theory, stress models of the early child-rearing stage of the family life cycle have been tested, using data primarily from mothers. A causal model of parenting stress tested in a sample of 101 mothers of 6-week-old infants showed that pregnancy stress, but not labor and delivery stress, was positively related to parenting stress. Social support and prior experience with childbearing had direct negative effects on pregnancy stress; personality strength had direct negative effects on parenting stress (Younger, 1991). In 173 mothers of 2- to 13-month-old infants (mean = 6.8 months), the effects of stressors (being employed and infant difficultness) on maternal identity were negatively mediated by the mothers' global perception of stress, with a health-promoting lifestyle having a direct and positive relationship to maternal identity (Walker, 1989a). In the follow-up study of 119 mothers (69% sample retention) when the mean infant age was 13.3 months, the model was replicated except that the stress effects of early infant difficultness on maternal identity had diminished (Walker, 1989b). In a longitudinal study of 193 families who were followed from pregnancy to 48 months after birth, maternal life change in the first year of the child's life was negatively correlated with the child's IQ and language development at 4 years of age. Mothers who had both low personal coping resources (as indicated by low education) and low social support were at higher risk for having children with lower IQ and language development (Bee, Hammond, Eyres, Barnard, & Snyder, 1986). Prior maternal illness and life change were significant predictors of subsequent maternal illness in 155 mothers of 6-month-old infants. A buffering effect of support was not found; the size of the support network was the only characteristic of support that was negatively related to illness (Lenz, Parks, Jenkins, & Jarrett, 1986).

Ventura (1986), in a replication of an earlier study, examined relationships between both parents' coping, their psychological health, and the infants' temperament in 47 mother-father pairs of 2- to 3-month-old infants. Mothers and fathers with higher depression perceived their infants as having a more difficult temperament (Ventura & Stevenson, 1986). Paternal depression was related to limited use of social support and perceptions of the infant as fearful and distressed. Mothers perceived their infants as more soothable and approachable than fathers. Mothers who viewed their infant as optimal in temperament sought social support, maintained family integrity, and said they were religious, thankful, and content. Unexpectedly, families who had higher socioeconomic status had higher parental depression and reported more difficult infant temperament (Ventura & Stevenson, 1986).

Capacity for empathy was found to be the best predictor of parent sensitivity for both mothers and fathers of 32 first-born infants in an unvideotaped observational study. Attitudes toward infant care also predicted mothers' sensitivity but not fathers' (Graham, 1993).

The majority of nursing studies on parent-infant attachment have examined the parent's attachment to the infant (Coffman, 1992). Factors influencing the infant's attachment to the mother were examined by Kemp (1987) and Coffman, Levitt, and Guacci-Franco (1995), using Ainsworth's Strange Situation procedure. Infant temperament predicted infant attachment group (Kemp, 1987) and was more strongly related to infant attachment than maternal responsiveness (Coffman, Levitt, & Guacci-Franco, 1995).

The above studies used samples that were predominantly White and middle class. There have been far fewer studies on early parenting in economically and socially at-risk families. In 88 low-income minority women, early contact with the infant helped develop maternal attachment; however, it was concluded that this need not take place right after delivery (Troy, 1993).

Depressive symptoms were found in 59.6% of a sample of 225 low-income single mothers who had at least one child between 1 and 4 years old; poorer family functioning, less tangible support, higher everyday stressors, and greater use of avoidance coping predicted higher depressive symptoms. Neither social resources nor coping strategies buffered the stress-depression relationship. Higher depressive symptoms and poorer quality of the primary intimate relationship predicted parenting attitudes. Parenting attitudes were the strongest predictor of child behavior problems; the quality of the intimate relationship did not affect child behavior (Hall, Gurley, Sachs, & Kryscio, 1991). A high rate (74%) of depressive symptoms was also found in a sample of 19 socially high-risk (single, poor, low education, higher history of child protection involvement) mothers of 6- to 9-month-old infants (Karl, 1995). Maternal depression was associated with less responsiveness to infants' cues and frequent physical unavailability of the mother to the infant (Karl, 1995).

Maternal and paternal parenting of toddlers, based on Bandura's self-efficacy theory, has been the focus of nursing research by Gross and colleagues (Gross, Conrad, Fogg, & Wothke, 1994; Gross, Fogg, & Tucker, 1995; Gross, Rocissano, & Roncoli, 1989; Gross & Tucker, 1994). Mothers of both preterm-born ($n = 62$) and full-term-born ($n = 70$) toddlers were quite confident in their parenting, with the mother's pre-childbearing child-care experience an important predictor (Gross, Rocissano, et al., 1989). A longitudinal model of maternal toddler parenting using data from 272 mothers of 1- and 2-year-olds indicated that the more depressed a mother feels, the more likely she is to rate the child's temperament as difficult; a perception of difficult child temperament leads to lower perceptions of maternal self-efficacy (confidence in parenting); the lower maternal self-efficacy, the greater the depression, with depression at an earlier time predicting depression 6 months later (Gross, Conrad, et al., 1994). In contrast, fathers' ($N = 46$) depression had no relationship to paternal confidence; the intensity of the toddler's behavior was the only variable influencing fathers' confidence (Gross & Tucker, 1994). This finding is in sharp contrast to Ferketich and Mercer's results (1994, 1995b) showing that fathers' depression was a predictor of paternal role competence in infancy.

An experimental study of a 10-week intervention program designed to teach mothers and fathers how to interact effectively with their toddlers found that experimental group mothers ($n = 10$) had increased self-efficacy, decreased stress, and improvement in mother-toddler interactions, but no effects were found for fathers ($n = 10$). The latter results were thought to be due to limited or no attendance by fathers at the intervention sessions (Gross, Fogg, et al., 1995).

Using a risk-and-resilience framework, these studies indicate that life change, parenting stress, difficult infant temperament, and parents' depression constitute risk factors for parenting in the early child-rearing years. Economic and social risk places mothers at higher risk for depression, which then has an influence on mother-child relationships and parenting. Although the results are mixed for the buffering benefits of social support, in general, partner support, father participation in child care, parent personality strengths (self-esteem, sense of mastery), and a health-promoting lifestyle have been found to promote resiliency at this stage of the family life cycle. Gross, Fogg, et al. (1995) conducted the only intervention study at this life cycle stage. Although the sample was small ($N = 23$ families), experimental group mothers ($n = 10$) did show improvement in parenting toddlers, as recorded by videotaped interactions. Despite increased societal interest in parenting by fathers, fathers' lack of participation in this study's intervention sessions was disappointing. This may be unique to this sample, but it could reflect the view that mothers still bear the primary responsibility for early child rearing.

These nursing studies on families with infants and toddlers have not explored family system functioning at this stage. The research has focused on individual variables such as the psychological state and health of the parents, child characteristics and behaviors, the dyadic relationship between parent and child, life stress, and the role of social support. Thus the contribution of family functioning as either an independent or a dependent variable is lacking in the nursing research on this family life cycle stage.

Families and School-Age Children

Nursing research on families with school-age children is sparse, with the main focus on the mother-child dyad and the influence of maternal psychological and role variables on the child's development and behavior.

Maternal role indicators assessed during early postpartum were not found to be strong predictors of the school-age child's socioemotional development 9 years later (Walker & Montgomery, 1994). In the 77 women (63%) who were retained out of the original sample of 124, only maternal identity as an affective response to the baby was a significant predictor, explaining 7% to 20%

of the variance, depending on parity and SES. Perceived and demonstrated role attainment were not predictors. Use of maternal role indicators at later stages in the infant's first year may have produced different results (Walker & Montgomery, 1994). A causal model of maladjustment in school-age children indicated the importance of family interpersonal relationships (McClowry et al., 1994). Mothers who reported their child's temperament as high in negative reactivity and who responded intensely to daily hassles perceived their child as more maladjusted. Maternal psychiatric symptoms, major life events, and maternal temperament intensity explained 54% of the variance in maternal hassles. Both the child's temperament and the mother's response to daily hassles influenced the child's behavior. Both of these studies used predominantly Caucasian samples.

Hall, Schaefer, and Greenberg (1987) and Hall and Farel (1988) have studied families of school-age children in samples that were 76% and 73% African American, respectively. In 214 mostly low-income mothers with an average of two to three children who were followed up from an earlier study of maternal attachment, associations between quality and quantity of social support and maternal psychosomatic symptoms (defined as subjectively expressed bodily feelings indicative of depression and anxiety) were examined using logistic regression. Interestingly, the quality of the relationship, if the woman's primary intimate was a husband or boyfriend, was not a predictor of psychosomatic symptoms. Significant predictors were the quantity of social ties (this was true for all women regardless of the primary intimate), relationship quality modified by the type of primary or intimate, and the baseline level of psychosomatic symptoms measured 5 years earlier.

In a sample of 115 low-income mothers of 5- and 6-year-old children, maternal everyday stressors plus life events were predictive of child behavior problems; maternal depressive symptoms were associated with everyday stressors but did not mediate the relationship between stressors and child behavior. Mothers who perceived their everyday lives as stressful may also perceive their child's behavior as more difficult (Hall & Farel, 1988).

Using a family stress framework, Murata (1994, 1995) studied 23 African-American inner-city single-mother-headed families of school-age sons between 8 and 12 years old who had exhibited disruptive behavior in school. These families were found to have high stress, particularly in the area of family relationship strains, and lower social support, with mothers reporting more depression and using more verbal aggression and less reasoning in interactions with their children. Sample data were compared to study instrument norms. Sons were found to have low social competence and little participation in social groups. The author recommended interventions targeted at reducing intrafamily stress and increasing social support to these families (Murata, 1995).

From these studies focusing on mother-child relationships at this stage, it can be seen that event stress, daily hassles, and intrafamily strains, as well as the mother's psychological status and maternal and child temperament, contributed to the school-age child's development and behavior. Social support appears to play a protective role for mother's well-being, with family support being more important than partner support in one study. All studies used mother's self-reports of child temperament or behavior that were not substantiated by other raters, so personal bias may have influenced the results.

One study was found that addressed family functioning during the school-age and adolescent years (Richards, 1989). Three levels of functioning (individual, dyadic, and family) were measured in 60 volunteers, predominantly well-educated professional couples. As expected, subjects who perceived themselves to be more emotionally mature and perceived their marriages to be more compatible, reported more cohesive family functioning (Richards, 1989).

Families With Adolescents

The adolescent or launching stage of the family life cycle has been noted to be the most stressful stage (Olson, McCubbin, et al., 1983). Developmental tasks of adolescence, coupled with developmental tasks of middle adulthood of the parents, are "ripe for conflict" (Riesch & Forsyth, 1992, p. 34). Young adolescents are very self-conscious, have easily bruised egos, are undergoing physical changes, attach increasing significance to peer relationships, and challenge authority, especially that of parents. Middle-aged parents of these adolescents are often at the peak of their careers and earning power, may be concerned about their own parents' health and living situation, and are aware of the reported difficulties of parenting a teen and anxious about entering this life cycle stage (Riesch & Forsyth, 1992).

Maternal role satisfaction in parenting a teen, however, was found to be high in a sample of 102 well-educated, mostly married, employed mothers (Ohashi, 1992). These mothers reported high satisfaction with their own adult development as well. Expectations for the role were less important than value attainment (role per-

formance was congruent with own values for the role) in predicting role satisfaction. Experiencing at least one positive surprise in parenting a teen, obtained from qualitative data, was an additional factor in role satisfaction (Ohashi, 1992). These results may have been influenced by the sample characteristics and the use of the investigator's newly developed instruments to measure expectations and satisfaction specific to the mother role. However, this study was unique in that the focus was on one parent's satisfaction at this life cycle stage rather than the predominant focus being on the stress and problems associated with rearing adolescents.

Despite the increased emphasis on peer relationships during adolescence, the stress and support in family relationships have been shown to have a significant influence on the lives of adolescents in the nursing research literature. Difficult life events identified by 847 young adolescents ages 11 to 14 years reflected distinct family concerns: (a) losses of significant persons due to death, divorce, relocation, or siblings leaving the family; (b) threats towards family integrity or relationships, personal or family health, personal family safety, and family violence; (c) feelings of being hassled by parents' limits and expectations and sibling disagreements and conflicts; and (d) testing limits and their own maturity (Riesch, Jacobson, & Tosi, 1994).

Parents were the most frequently reported stressful relationship in a sample of 130 adolescent boys 15 to 19 years of age, with girlfriends being the second most stressful relationship (Barron & Yoest, 1994). Using an individual stress and coping framework, the researchers found that the boys used more problem-oriented than emotion-oriented coping, with emotion-focused coping being associated with emotional distress (Barron & Yoest, 1994). Situational variables of perceived maternal and paternal expressiveness, close friend solidarity, and perceived social support were negative predictors of loneliness in 212 adolescent, 15- to 21-year-olds. With increase in adolescent age, the influence of close friend support increased and the role of parent expressiveness decreased. Personality characteristics were slightly stronger predictors than situational variables for 113 younger adolescents 11 to 14 years old (Mahon & Yarcheski, 1992).

The adolescent's perception of a poor-quality parental relationship, and not whether the parents were married or separated/divorced, was associated with poor life satisfaction, low sense of future, and higher anxiety in 244 adolescents (mean age = 16.6 years) in a largely female (68%), middle-class Canadian sample (Grossman &

Rowat, 1995). Coping strategies and received support did not mediate the relationship between the parental relationship and adolescent well-being in either married or divorced households. For adolescents with married parents, use of emotion-focused coping was found to be associated with a poor parental relationship. Study findings may have been influenced by the mean time of 6 years since the divorce for adolescents from divorced family households (Grossman & Rowat, 1995). Other research has shown that most adolescents have adjusted to parental divorce after 2 or more years (Hetherington & Anderson, 1987; Wallerstein, 1985).

One family-level study based on the Circumplex Model of Marital and Family Systems (Olson, Sprenkle, & Russell, 1979) was designed to test an intervention to improve communication skills between parents and young adolescents with 258 parent-adolescent pairs (Riesch, Tosi, et al., 1993). Mothers, but not fathers, perceived their communication with their young adolescents as more open, as did the young adolescent with the mother. There was no change in father-adolescent communication by self-report, but observations of fathers and young adolescents in the experimental group showed decreased antisocial content in their interactions; control group adolescents became more negative in their communication (Riesch, Tosi, et al., 1993). A limitation of the study design was nonrandom assignment, as families who were willing to take the training sessions were assigned to the experimental group; thus this group may have been more motivated to improve communication.

Divorce and Remarriage

Divorce and remarriage, although not considered normative in traditional views of the family life cycle, have become an increasingly common transition for many families. Although the divorce rate in the 1990s declined somewhat from the 1980s, it was estimated that divorce will affect over a million children each year (Behrman & Quinn, 1994). The few nursing research studies on this transition have focused on the effects of divorce on women and children.

Self-esteem and emotional distress in 36 recently divorced women were predicted only for women who perceived themselves as unable to prevent the divorce; causes of the divorce were attributed more to the spouse than to themselves (Barron, 1987). The personal goals of 250 recently divorced women included independence and economic self-reliance, employment and education,

parenting skills, environmental goals (better housing, neighborhood, schools), and mental health. Older women were more likely to report employment and environmental goals than younger women (Duffy, 1990). Women did experience a decrease in support network size and received support in the 2 years following divorce, but the sources of support—friends and family—remained stable (Duffy, 1993). Family support was more common in women with younger children who received more direct assistance, often in the form of child care (Duffy, 1989). Older women used nonkin as primary support (Duffy, 1989). Qualities of the primary support relationship were continuity, availability, and understanding (Duffy, 1989). Unmet needs of these women centered on emotional support, financial help, need for a "significant other" relationship, time for self, and child care (Duffy, 1993).

A pilot intervention study with 21 mothers and their 3- to 6-year-old children following a recent marital separation employed a two-group experimental design using "two doses" of a COPE (Creating Opportunities for Parent Empowerment) intervention program of audiotaped information and parent-child activities for enhancing parenting and children's coping. The control group received information about preschool children's normal growth and development. Short-term outcomes after 3½ months were positive, with experimental group mothers showing decreased anxiety and negative mood. Scores on the HOME inventory and the NCAST teaching scales also improved. Teachers reported an increase in problem behaviors for control-group children and a decrease in internalizing behaviors for experimental-group children (Melnyk & Alpert-Gillis, 1996). The authors report that a larger study is planned.

One study by a nurse investigator, reported in the family science literature, examined the impact of late-life divorce on family rituals (Pett, Lang, & Gander, 1992). Almost three fourths (71.3%) of 73 female and 42 male adult children reported negative changes in family relationships since the divorce of their middle-aged parents after at least 15 years of marriage. Loss of family unity, difficulty in arranging and restructuring family gatherings, problems with seeing both parents separately, parents' hostility towards one another creating tensions within the parent-child relationship, loss of their children's relationship with grandparents, and not feeling a part of the parent's remarried family were common stressors. It was felt that this transition required years of continued negotiation and restructuring (Pett et al., 1992).

Health effects on either adult child or parent were not examined in this study.

The effects of remarriage on health have been studied by two family scientists who reported their findings in the nursing literature (Ganong & Coleman, 1991). No health differences between the remarried 105 women and 100 men were found; however, women had more health complaints after remarriage. Higher marital satisfaction was associated with better health for both men and women. More family decision-making power was associated with better health for men. Women with fewer children, less family decision-making power, and where the household children were all hers reported better health. Thus women living in stepfather families had better health than those women in complex and stepmother families (Ganong & Coleman, 1991).

Later Life Families

The predominant focus of nursing research on later life families has been on family caregiving for chronically ill or mentally impaired members, with much less attention to normative transitions at this stage. Creation of a marital enhancement program at retirement was the purpose of a research study by Johnston (1990). This purposive sample of 10 couples who had retired within the previous 6 to 18 months reported the significant stressors as changes in identity and roles. They talked more about thoughts than feelings; regarded children as important topics of conversation and sources of pride and thought; showed increasing awareness of partner's faults, with men being more satisfied with retirement; and noted that hobbies and time spent together or with children did not increase. Adult children were frequently unaware of parents' struggles and changes with retirement. Nineteen recommendations for a couples' post-retirement enhancement program were generated (Johnston, 1990).

The health-protective function of marriage in older individuals has been examined in three studies. In an investigation based on Roy's Adaptation Model, older married women had higher stress and poorer health in a random sample of 900 older adults over 65 in the northeastern United States (Preston & Dellasega, 1990). However, how high and low categories were derived for the subjective measures of stress and health was not indicated in this report. A strong level of attachment, primarily to a spouse (67%), in 100 community-dwelling older men was a significant predictor of quality of life (Rickelman, Gallman, & Papra, 1994). Exchange and equity theory, conjugal support, family coping behaviors, and partners' psychological well-being (life satisfaction) were examined over a 2-year period in a sample of 135 over-65 Canadian couples (Ducharme, 1995). Conjugal support, reciprocity, and cognitive coping strategies (reframing and active appraisal) were associated with higher life satisfaction for both older men and women. Husbands had more positive perceptions of conjugal support and used more spiritual support over time; wives reported more use of informal supports over time (Ducharme, 1995).

Health-promoting behaviors in later life couples were also examined in one study. Older spouses ($N = 104$, or 52 couples) had similar health-promotion behaviors related to exercise, stress management, self-actualization, health responsibility, and interpersonal support, as reported by both Pender's Health Promoting Lifestyle instrument and open-ended questions (Conn & Armer, 1995). Older wives reported more nutrition-related behaviors (e.g., eating low-fat foods and vegetables, limiting salt, and drinking adequate fluids) than husbands. Correlations between the spouses' health-promotion behaviors were small to moderate ($r = .24-.58$), indicating some variability, with the highest similarity in nutrition, exercise, and positive attitude behaviors. Patterns of health promotion influence between older spouses remain to be investigated (Conn & Armer, 1995).

Finally, the only other nursing study addressing the later life cycle stage compared the developmental trajectories of 80 women, ages 60 to 95 years, divided into older mother ($n = 50$) and nonmother ($n = 30$) groups. The trajectories were similar, but mothers reported more transitional events, such as those related to children and grandchildren's transitions, than nonmothers (Mercer, Nichols, & Doyle, 1988).

Transition to Widowhood

This last transition in the family life cycle has been studied by nurse researchers using both qualitative (Porter, 1994a, 1994b), quantitative (Gass, 1987; Gass & Chang, 1989; Kirschling & McBride, 1989), and a combination of both methods (Anderson & Dimond, 1995), but with a focus on the individual. The absence of a family orientation (e.g., changes in relationships, roles, boundaries) is evident in the nursing research on this transition; Gass-Sternas (1995) has documented the lack of research on single-parent widows in particular.

Stress and coping has been the dominant framework (Gass, 1987; Gass & Chang, 1989; Kirschling & McBride, 1989) for quantitative work with descriptions of distressful feelings, physical symptoms, special hardships of loneliness, ways of coping and self-sustenance, reducing risks of living alone, and negotiating reliance and support emerging from the qualitative data (Anderson & Dimond, 1995; Porter, 1994a, 1994b). Younger widows who experienced the sudden death of a spouse experienced more stress and difficulties coping (Anderson & Dimond, 1995; Kirschling & McBride, 1989). Social support, strong religious beliefs, practice of rituals, belief in control over bereavement, greater number of resources, lower threat appraisal, use of more problem-focused and less emotion-focused coping, and good previous mental health were related to less physical and/or psychosocial dysfunction in 100 older widows and 59 widowers who had experienced the loss of a spouse during the previous year (Gass, 1987; Gass & Chang, 1989).

Conclusions and Recommendations

This section summarizes the existing state of knowledge on normative family transitions from the nursing research to date and how this body of nursing research relates to the family science research on family transitions. The theoretical and methodological issues in this body of work will also be addressed.

The predominant focus of nursing research on normative family transitions has been focused on the family life cycle stages of childbearing and early child rearing, as noted in other reviews (Ganong, 1995). No research was found on the transition to marriage or becoming a couple, only on the first stage of the family life cycle. Given the empirical evidence of the importance of the couple relationship in the initial transition to parenthood and the increased attention to preconceptual health at an individual level, research is needed to guide nursing assessment and intervention to sustain and increase couple relationship strengths in preconceptual couples.

For nurse practitioners in primary care settings, evaluation of the use of a brief screening tool such as the Family APGAR (Adaptation, Partnership, Growth, Affection, Resolve) (Smilkstein, 1978) may provide evidence as to the utility of this approach to address any concerns an individual might have about his or her couple or family functioning and relationships. The unique contribution of nursing research at this stage can be focused on the influence of the couple relationship on health promotion practices because both of these have been shown to have an impact on subsequent normative transitions. In the family science literature, improvement of couple communication and relationship satisfaction, as well as lower divorce rates, has been found for couples participating in the Prevention and Relationship Enhancement Program (PREP) developed by Markman and colleagues (Markman, 1981; Markman, Floyd, Stanley, & Storasli, 1988; Markman, Renick, Floyd, Stanley, & Clements, 1993). These U.S. samples included couples with and without children; however, in both these and a Dutch sample (Van Widenfelt, Hosman, Schapp, & van der Staak, 1996), couples who had been together a shorter period of time tended to decline study participation.

Research on other inventories such as PREPARE (Premarital Personal and Relationship Evaluation) and ENRICH (Enriching and Nurturing Relationship Issues, Communication and Happiness) (Olson, Fournier, & Druckman, 1986) for premarital and married couples, respectively, has documented the utility of these reliable and valid instruments for assessment, intervention, and prediction of divorce in couple relationships (Olson, 1993; Olson, McCubbin, et al. 1986). These instruments may provide a sound measurement base for examining couple relationships and how they relate to health promotion behaviors for use in nursing research.

There has been considerable attention by nurse researchers to the transitions associated with pregnancy and parenthood. Negative life event stress, pregnancy risk, marital discord, individual psychological health (depression, anxiety) and conflict in intergenerational relationships have been found to be risk factors during pregnancy for both men and women. Support from partner, overall greater perceived support, and individual personality characteristics (self-esteem, sense of mastery) have been shown to be protective factors. The contribution of prenatal attachment to pregnancy and parenthood outcomes remains unclear because of measurement concerns.

Nursing research evidence supports the decline in marital satisfaction during the transition to parenthood found in the family science literature. Marital satisfaction has been used both as a dependent variable (Tomlinson, 1987, 1996) and as an independent variable influencing sensitivity to the infant (Broom, 1994). Traditional prenatal classes have been structured around preparation for labor and delivery and care of the infant. Little research attention has been paid to the effects of education about changes in couple and family relationships following the infant's birth. Because nurses have had a strong role in childbirth preparation, intervention studies are needed of prenatal education classes that include anticipated changes in the couple relationship (Tomlinson, 1987, 1996), the mother's preoccupation with the infant up to 8 months or longer (Broom, 1994; Mercer & Ferketich, 1990), sexual relationship adjustments, discussion of division of labor and support expectations postchildbirth (Coffman, Levitt, & Brown, 1994), influence of parental moods (anxiety, depression) on couple and family functioning (Mercer & Ferketich, 1990), intergenerational influences on parenting (Anderson, 1996), and negotiating new relationships and roles with extended family (Bright, 1992). An intervention prebirth may not have lasting influence postbirth due to considerable family reorganization (Coffman, Levitt, & Brown, 1994; Tomlinson, 1996), so additional "booster" doses of the couple- and family-relationship-focused interventions would be indicated and followed with longitudinal data collection over the first year. In addition, "single-agent" interventions may not be adequate to produce effects at this stage, given the multiple changes occurring at this time (Coie et al., 1993).

The grounded theory studies on expectant fatherhood (Chapman, 1991; Donovan, 1995; Jordan, 1990) have highlighted the uncertainty and ambiguity of this family transition for men. Increased personal and societal expectations for more father involvement in pregnancy and parenting have put pressures on men to be active participants at this stage. Interventions designed specifically to assist in role taking and role making for fathers during this transition are needed. Couple communication, maternal and extended family support, mutual discussion of father's role during labor and delivery, as well as postbirth, are areas that have been identified as needed for fathers in their transition to parenthood.

Mercer and colleagues' longitudinal study on pregnancy and early postpartum and parenthood remains the most comprehensive nursing research on this transition (Mercer, May, et al., 1986). Replication of this investigation would be indicated; since these data were collected, changes in the health care system due to managed care and shorter maternity hospitalizations have had an impact on this family transition. A multisite study to better detect regional differences and use of both self-report and observational measures with families during pregnancy and at least the first year of the infant's life would be ideal. Mercer and colleagues have acknowledged the limitations of sample attrition in their publications of study findings. Obtaining multiple types of data from at least two

family members at this time of family disorganization and upheaval remains a challenge.

The research on the transition to parent roles indicates that pregnancy risk and previous parenting experience may not influence this process as originally hypothesized (Mercer & Ferketich, 1994a, 1994b, 1995). Replication of these findings is needed. Self-report measures were used to measure role competence, and questions about adequacy of measurement have been raised (Ferketich & Mercer, 1994). Videotapes (Jones & Lenz, 1986) and observations (Broom, 1994) of parent-infant interaction have addressed issues of parent sensitivity and responsivity to the infant's cues.

One of the findings in the body of nursing research on pregnancy and preadolescent parenthood has been the prevalence of depression in the parents, especially the high rates found in low-income minority women (Hall & Farel, 1988; Hall, Schaefer, & Greenberg, 1987). Almost all of these studies used the Center for Epidemiological Studies (CES-D) depression scale to subjectively measure depression. This is not a clinical diagnosis, but it does raise concerns about the psychological health of parents at these stages. A meta-analysis of these studies would be warranted to synthesize these findings and provide direction for future research and intervention.

As the family life cycle advances, the nursing research becomes more sparse. There have been few studies on families with school-age children and adolescents, despite evidence from family science that the adolescent or launching stage is the most stressful stage of the family life cycle. No nursing research was located on families at the launching and empty-nest stages of the middle years. With the Baby Boomer cohort now reaching this stage and much media attention on menopause for both women and men, the family and health implications for this stage remain to be investigated by nurses. Nursing research could address the influence and impact of family system functioning and relationships on the physiological changes occurring for both men and women at this stage, as well as on health decision making. Is there mutuality and similarity or difference in "change of life" symptoms at this stage between men and women in couple relationships (as examined in the earlier stage of pregnancy in the nursing research)? Is women's use of hormonal replacement therapy based only on physiological criteria, individual personality, and psychological variables, or does the family system play a role as well?

The later life family has been viewed through the lens of family caregiving by nurse researchers. Although this work has made a significant contribution to the field, normative transitions at this stage involving retirement, family influences on maintaining physical and psychological health, and a healthy lifestyle have received far less attention. With the aging of the population, the family transitions at this stage need to be examined from a health-promotion perspective (e.g., Antonovsky's salutogenic model) as well as examining the impact of physical and mental decline. Connections between later life family strengths and positive health outcomes need to be made.

For the existing body of nursing research on normative family transitions, theoretical and methodological issues have also been raised.

Theoretical issues. Is the concept of transition central to nursing? The nursing literature on family normative transitions would indicate that it is. Certainly there is evidence that these family transitions occur over time, produce change in the family unit, and have health consequences (Brown, 1986b; Fawcett & York, 1986; Ferketich & Mercer, 1990; Grossman & Rowat, 1995; Norbeck & Anderson, 1989a; Walker & Montgomery, 1994). Disorganization and disconnectedness (Chick & Meleis, 1986) are evident, with disruptiveness and uncertainty also present. New knowledge and skills are needed, and the few intervention studies that have been carried out are targeted toward this goal. The meaning and perception of these transitions has been described using qualitative approaches, with the contributions of environmental or social support and individual physical and emotional health being documented in the quantitative studies.

Normative family transitions have usually been viewed as independent variables "causing" some outcome for the individual, dyadic subsystem, or family. To the three outcomes of changes in health status, health-seeking behaviors, and/or health care utilization posited by Chick and Meleis (1986), the evidence from this body of research would add changes in family roles, boundaries, and interactions as another outcome.

The importance of stage, event, and timing from family development theory has been evident. Societal changes such as delayed fertility and childbearing for women and an increase in dual-earner families have been addressed in the research questions and sampling. Transition events have been viewed as stressor events from family stress theory; consideration of the effects of both negative life events (Mercer, Ferketich, DeJoseph, et al., 1988a) and daily hassles (Hall, Gurley, et al., 1991) are evident. Support, especially from the spouse or partner (Coffman, Levitt, & Brown, 1994), with less emphasis

on coping, has been reported as a factor in managing stress during these transitions. Role strain, role competence and role attainment, particularly related to the transition to parenthood, have been addressed. Concepts of equity, fairness, and reciprocity from an exchange perspective have been used in the transition to parenthood (Tomlinson, 1987) and in older couples (Ducharme, 1995).

The use of an ecological framework (Bronfenbrenner, 1979) or feminist perspective (Cardwell, 1993; Thompson, 1992) has been lacking in this body of nursing research. Cardwell (1993) has noted the nursing research emphasis on women's reproductive and childrearing roles, and this chapter supports that observation. For example, women who have experienced success in other societal roles, such as the samples of "older" mothers, have been studied in terms of their adaptation to the maternal role. A broader environmental perspective and a view of the influence of societal patriarchal bias would provide additional insight into normative family transitions.

Much of the work on normative family transitions by nurses, however, has been atheoretical. Sometimes a framework, such as stress and coping, is implied but not explicitly stated. Stronger grounding of this research from a theoretical base is needed. Some researchers have argued that only nursing theories can be used to study phenomena of interest to nursing (Fawcett & Whall, 1990). However, to date, nursing theory development has focused more on the individual rather than the family. The source of theory for a given research study on normative family transitions, however, may not be as critical as the "fit" of a theory with the research purpose and the specific research questions being asked.

Future nursing theory development need not be viewed as addressing either just individuals or just families. Continuation of the dichotomy between nursing of individuals and of families may not be in nursing's best interest (Robinson, 1995). Bridging individual and family perspectives and integrating the mutual influence between the two would seem appropriate for nursing research as well as for research in child development and family science (Benson & Deal, 1995).

Methodological issues. Although many of the studies in this body of nursing research have been cross-sectional, an increase in longitudinal studies over the past 10 years was found. Because these family transitions take place over time, the longitudinal perspective is essential (Coie et al., 1993). Increased use of qualitative methods, mainly grounded theory, has shed light on individual and family meanings and processes related to fatherhood (Hall,

1991, 1994), expectant parenthood (Sandelowski & Black, 1994), transition to parenthood in dual-earner families (Hall, 1992), cross-cultural family influences on pregnancy (Affonso et al., 1993), and sibling relationships with a new baby (Murphy, 1990). Qualitative approaches have been sparse in the later stages of the family life cycle.

The results of the few intervention studies on family transitions have produced mixed results. Interventions on couple discussions of mutual support expectations after childbirth (Coffman, Levitt, & Brown, 1994) and provision of information on cesarean birth to expectant couples (Fawcett, Pollio, et al., 1993) did not produce differences between experimental and control groups. Fawcett's study pointed out the difficulty of incorporating a true control group when information about a given procedure is routinely given, and, ethically, one cannot withhold this type of care. Interventions by Gross, Fogg, et al. (1995) on parenting of toddlers and by Riesch, Tosi, et al. (1993) to improve parent-early adolescent communication were more effective for mothers than for fathers. Getting fathers to participate in these interventions was a challenge, and this situation is not unique to nursing (Dumka, Roosa, Michaels, & Suh, 1995).

Results of Melnyk and Alpert-Gillis's (1996) pilot study on enhancing mothers' and young children's coping following marital separation were encouraging. Their study points to some of the characteristics necessary for intervention studies: designing a reproducible type of intervention, random assignment of families if ethically possible, manipulation checks to be sure participants are absorbing and retaining information given, "booster" doses of the intervention, and sensitive outcome measures to detect differences between experimental and control groups. Because of multiple systems of influence on normative family transitions, a single type of intervention directed at one aspect of these systems may not be adequate to produce a difference (Coie et al., 1993).

Despite the challenges in designing, executing, and evaluating interventions directed at normative family transitions, one of the critical issues in today's changing health care environment is, How do nurses make a difference at these crucial times for families? A longitudinal randomized trial of nurse home visitation with socially disadvantaged women during pregnancy, postpartum, and up to 2 years after the child's birth has shown that nursing intervention resulted in greater use of community services and increased informal support during pregnancy and early postpartum, with improved pregnancy and birth outcomes for adolescents and smokers (Olds,

Henderson, & Kitzman, 1994; Olds, Henderson, Tatelbaum, & Chamberlin, 1986, 1988). Long-term effects from nurse home visitation were improved educational and employment outcomes for the poor White women in the sample, with fewer second pregnancies and postponement of a second pregnancy (Olds, Henderson, Tatelbaum, et al., 1988). Improved safety of the children, fewer behavioral and parental coping problems, and fewer emergency room visits were also found for the nurse-visited group (Olds, Henderson, & Kitzman, 1994). One nurse member (H. Kitzman) of the research team has been a coauthor of several study publications. Other research team members represent other disciplines. It is vital that nursing researchers play a visible role in the systematic examination of nursing interventions during family transitions, especially for those families at risk due to health or socioeconomic factors.

More sample diversity is needed in all of the research on normative family transitions. This is true in both nursing and other disciplines. Inclusion of single-parent families who are so by choice, separation, or divorce; stepfamilies; gay and lesbian families, low-income families; and non-Caucasian families is badly needed. This is an ongoing challenge; many of these families may not be able to access the health care system easily for assistance during times of transition and are not represented in childbirth education classes, clinics, or other sites traditionally used for sample recruitment.

A dyadic or family subsystem has been the predominant unit of interest, measurement, and analysis in the nursing research on normative family transitions. Family system functioning has rarely been a unit of interest or measurement in this body of research. Mercer, Ferketich, DeJoseph, et al.'s (1988) study on pregnancy and early infancy; Tomlinson et al.'s (1990) work on family dynamics during pregnancy; Riesch, Tosi, et al. (1993) and Richards's (1989) measurement of family functioning at the adolescent stage and examination of family system coping in nuclear/stepfamily expectant couples (Dietz-Omar, 1991) and later life couples (Ducharme, 1995) are the exceptions. Self-report measures—Feetham's Family Functioning Scale (Roberts & Feetham, 1982; Sawin & Harrigan, 1995), the Family Dynamics Measure (Lasky et al., 1985); Olson, Portner, and Lavee's (1985) FACES (Family Adaptability & Cohesion Evaluation Scale) instrument on cohesion and adaptability, and the F-COPES (Family Crisis Oriented Personal Scales) for family coping (McCubbin, Olson, & Larsen, 1996)—have been used to measure family functioning in these six studies. Overall, the nursing research on normative family transitions lacks information on family system functioning, with the few findings presenting an "insider's view" of family functioning.

A major limitation is the lack of a family *systemic* perspective in this body of research, which is one of the hallmarks of advanced practice in family nursing (Bell, 1996). Not only is there a lack of information on family system functioning, there is also a lack of information on the mutual influence and interdependency among family members at times of family transitions. Although data have often been collected from more than one family member (a definite improvement over earlier family research), this information has been analyzed comparing one family member group (i.e., mothers) with another family member group (i.e., fathers). Unequal sample sizes for men (smaller) and women (larger) also enter into the findings of some of the group comparisons (Mercer & Ferketich, 1990; Mercer, Ferketich, DeJoseph, May, et al., 1988). Using the subsample of *paired* high-risk couples (*n* = 73) from Mercer, Ferketich, DeJoseph, May, et al.'s study (1988) of expectant parenthood, Feetham, Perkins and Carroll (1993) used exploratory data analysis (scatter diagrams, box plots, and stem and leaf displays) to illustrate distributional differences between the men's and women's scores. These differences were also confirmed by plotting the scores on a graph but were not evident in the nonsignificant correlations and *t*-test comparisons between the two groups as an aggregate.

The conceptual or theoretical framework, research questions, measurement methods, and analysis strategies need to reflect a systemic perspective. Family science theories are in place to provide guidance and continued development of nursing theories to reflect that a family systems orientation is ongoing. Research questions such as, What is the influence of *mothers'* depression, anxiety, sense of mastery on *paternal* role competence? What is the influence of *fathers'* depression, anxiety, sense of mastery on *maternal* role competence? How does *mothers'* psychological health status influence *fathers'* perceptions of the marriage and family functioning and vice versa? reflect a systems orientation and could provide needed information about normative family transitions.

Debate continues about the desirability and appropriateness of strategies for taking data from individuals about their family and translating this family-related data into a "family" score (Feetham, 1990; Ransom et al., 1990; Sullivan & Fawcett, 1990; Uphold & Strickland, 1989). Almost all the data were family related in the nursing research on normative family transitions; self-report measures predominate. However, these measures have usually been psychometrically sound, with established reliability and validity.

Brown (1994) provided one example of how data on marital discord during pregnancy were examined using patterns of couple scores. Even though the measure of marital discord could have been stronger in this study, the findings do provide a more systemic view of how the couple's congruent (both spouses perceived high or low discord) or discrepant perspectives (husband high and wife low and vice versa) of marital discord influenced the individual's health. Larger samples are needed for adequate score distributions with this procedure. Cutting points using median values for high and low groups also blurs the placement of scores around the median. But despite these considerations and limitations, pattern scores are worth exploring (Ransom et al., 1990).

Correlations between spouses' pregnancy symptoms, based on fertility status (Holditch-Davis et al., 1995) and health-promoting lifestyle behaviors of older couples (Conn & Armer, 1995), have been reported to show differences and similarities in the couple subsystem. Pattern scores can also illuminate these findings and help point the way to couples who are functioning well and to those who may be at risk.

In summary, we have made continued progress in family research in nursing, but much remains to be done. Fawcett's (1989) summary of her program of research exhibits the strengths of nursing research on a specific normative family transition (pregnancy): (a) sound conceptual, theoretical, and empirical linkages; (b) longitudinal design; (c) use of valid and reliable instruments; (d) home data collection to ensure independent completion of study instruments; (e) multivariate analyses; (f) replication in U.S. and Canadian samples with adequate sample size; and (g) publication of study results, as well as a summary of all the findings from this program of research.

Although Ganong (1995) has indicated that nursing is about 10 years behind family disciplines in research sophistication, nursing has wrestled with many of the same issues as other disciplines studying families (e.g., theoretical, measurement, and analysis), and this is well documented in the nursing literature. Nursing has much to offer other disciplines in the areas of both normative and non-normative family transitions; the strong applied focus inherent in nursing research has the potential to make a critical difference for families in their daily lives, with the results not resting on the dusty shelves of academe. However, as Ganong (1995) has noted, nursing has exhibited a "relatively high degree of disciplinary isolation and segregation" (p. 192). A recent review of the transition to parenthood research (Cowan & Cowan, 1995) from the family science literature did not cite any research from nursing! Nurses must discard parochial blinders and disseminate findings from well-designed studies in other disciplinary journals and publications. Interdisciplinary research teams also can help in this effort. Three research teams of nursing and psychology collaboration (Coffman, Levitt, & Brown, 1994; Gottlieb & Baillies, 1995; Melnyk & Alpert-Gilliss, 1996) and one nursing-family studies team (Rustia & Abbott, 1990) are represented in this review. Certainly more interdisciplinary collaboration is indicated and is important to advance the field (Dumka et al., 1995), as well as publication of nursing research in the journals of other disciplines.

Nurses, too, need to tap into the existing body of knowledge in other disciplines on family normative transitions. In previous reviews of family research, Feetham (1984) incorporated findings from other disciplines; Whall and Loveland-Cherry (1993) did to some extent as well. In their critical review of fatherhood research, Tiedje and Darling-Fisher (1996) addressed the contribution of multiple disciplines in this body of research. Too rarely, however, only the nursing literature is cited in published reports in both nursing research and clinically oriented nursing articles.

Nurses must continue to assist families at times of normative transitions, based on a sound research knowledge base, and intervene to assist families at these times of disorganization and change for the family unit. As societal supports are reduced or withdrawn, the role of nurses remains critical to support positive outcomes for families at these expected junctures in the life cycle. The unique contribution of nursing research is to demonstrate how to optimize health outcomes during normative family transitions and how to promote health for both individual family members and the family unit at these times. Nursing can also make a unique contribution when normative family transitions are accompanied by situational events such as acute, chronic, or catastrophic life-threatening illness.

In general, nursing has focused on dysfunction and risk during normative family transitions, with less emphasis on what Antonovsky (1987) has called the salutogenic approach. Why families stay healthy during normative transitions and what patterns of functioning are found in families successfully negotiating transitions throughout the family life cycle has received less attention. Future research goals must include further explication of the processes of family transitions, test well-designed timely interventions to maximize health outcomes, and explore ways of increased interdisciplinary collaboration in these efforts.

References

Affonso, D., Mayberry, L., Shibuya, J., Kunimoto, J., Graham, K., & Sheptak, S. (1993). Themes of stressors for childbearing women on the island of Hawaii. *Family and Community Health, 16*(2), 9-19.

Aldous, J. (1996). *Family careers: Rethinking the developmental perspective.* Thousand Oaks, CA: Sage.

Anderson, A. (1996). Factors influencing the father-infant relationship. *Journal of Family Nursing, 2,* 306-324.

Anderson, K., & Dimond, M. (1995). The experience of bereavement in older adults. *Journal of Advanced Nursing, 22,* 308-315.

Antonovsky, A. (1987). *Unraveling the mystery of health.* San Francisco: Jossey-Bass.

Barron, C. (1987). Women's causal explanations of divorce: Relationships to self-esteem and emotional distress. *Research in Nursing and Health, 10,* 345-353.

Barron, C., & Yoest, P. (1994). Emotional distress and coping with a stressful relationship with adolescent boys. *Journal of Pediatric Nursing, 9*(1), 13-20.

Bee, H., Hammond, M., Eyres, S., Barnard, K., & Snyder, C. (1986). The impact of parental life change on the early development of children. *Research in Nursing and Health, 9,* 65-74.

Behrman, R., & Quinn, L. (1994). Children and divorce: Overview and analysis. *Future of Children, 4,* 4-14.

Bell, J. (1996). Advanced practice in family nursing: One view. *Journal of Family Nursing, 2*(3), 244-248.

Belsky, J., & Rovine, M. (1990). Patterns of marital change across the transition to parenthood. *Journal of Marriage and the Family, 52,* 109-123.

Belsky, J., Spanier, G., & Rovine, M. (1983). Stability and change in marriage across the transition to parenthood. *Journal of Marriage and the Family, 45,* 567-577.

Benson, M., & Deal, J. (1995). Bridging the individual and the family. *Journal of Marriage and the Family, 57,* 561-566.

Blank, D., Schroeder, M., & Flynn, J. (1995). Major influences on maternal responsiveness to infants. *Applied Nursing Research, 8*(1), 34-38.

Bowlby, J. (1979). *The making and breaking of affectional bonds.* London: Tavistock.

Bowlby, J. (1988). *A secure base: Parent-child attachment and healthy human development.* New York: Basic Books.

Bright, M. (1992). Making place: The first birth in an intergenerational family context. *Qualitative Health Research, 2,* 75-98.

Broderick, C., & Smith, J. (1979). The general systems approach to the family. In W. Burr, R. Hill, F. Nye, & I. Reiss (Eds.), *Contemporary theories about the family* (Vol. 2, pp. 112-129). New York: Free Press.

Bronfenbrenner, U. (1979). *The ecology of human development.* Cambridge, MA: Harvard University Press.

Broom, B. (1994). Impact of marital quality and psychological well-being on parental sensitivity. *Nursing Research, 43,* 138-143.

Brown, M. (1986a). Social support during pregnancy: A unidimensional or multidimensional construct? *Nursing Research, 35,* 4-9.

Brown, M. (1986b). Social support, stress, and health: A comparison of expectant mothers and fathers. *Nursing Research, 35,* 72-76.

Brown, M. (1988). A comparison of health responses in expectant mothers and fathers. *Western Journal of Nursing Research, 10,* 527-549.

Brown, M. (1994). Marital discord during pregnancy: A family systems approach. *Family Systems Medicine, 12,* 221-234.

Burr, W., Leigh, G., Day, R., & Constantine, J. (1979). Symbolic interaction and the family. In W. Burr, R. Hill, F. Nye, & I. Reiss (Eds.), *Contemporary theories about the family* (Vol. 2, pp. 42-111). New York: Free Press.

Cardwell, M. (1993). Family nursing research: A feminist critique. In S. Feetham, S. Meister, J. Bell, & C. Gilliss (Eds.), *The nursing of families: Theory, research, education, practice* (pp. 200-210). Newbury Park, CA: Sage.

Chapman, L. (1991). Searching: Expectant fathers' experiences during labor and birth. *Journal of Perinatal and Neonatal Nursing, 4*(4), 21-29.

Chick, N., & Meleis, A. (1986). Transitions: A nursing concern. In P. Chinn (Ed.), *Nursing research methodology: Issues and implementation* (pp. 237-257). Rockville, MD: Aspen.

Coffman, S. (1992). Parent and infant attachment: Review of nursing research 1981-1990. *Pediatric Nursing, 18,* 421-425.

Coffman, S., Levitt, M., & Brown, L. (1994). Effects of clarification of support expectations in prenatal couples. *Nursing Research, 43*(2), 111-116.

Coffman, S., Levitt, M., & Guacci-Franco, N. (1995). Infant-mother attachment: Relationships to maternal responsiveness and infant temperament. *Journal of Pediatric Nursing, 10*(1), 9-18.

Coie, J., Watt, N., West, S., Hawkins, J., Asarnow, J., Markman, H., Ramey, S., Shure, M., & Long, B. (1993). The science of prevention: A conceptual framework and some directions for a national research program. *American Psychologist, 48,* 1013-1022.

Conn, V., & Armer, J. (1995). Older spouses: Similarity of health promotion behaviors. *Journal of Family Nursing, 1,* 397-414.

Cowan, C., & Cowan, P. (1992). *When partners become parents: The big life change for couples.* New York: Basic Books.

Cowan, C., & Cowan, P. (1995). Interventions to ease the transition to parenthood: Why they are needed and what they can do. *Family Relations, 44,* 412-423.

Cowan, P. (1991). Individual and family life transitions: A proposal for a new definition. In P. Cowan & M. Hetherington (Eds.), *Family transitions* (pp. 3-30). Hillsdale, NJ: Lawrence Erlbaum.

Dalgas-Pelish, P. (1993). The impact of the first child on marital happiness. *Journal of Advanced Nursing, 18,* 437-441.

Dietz-Omar, M. (1991). Family coping: A comparison of stepfamilies and traditional nuclear families during pregnancy. *Applied Nursing Research, 4*(1), 31-33.

Donovan, J. (1995). The process of analysis during a grounded theory study of men during their partner's pregnancies. *Journal of Advanced Nursing, 21,* 708-715.

Drake, M., Verhulst, D., & Fawcett, J. (1988). Physical and psychological symptoms experienced by pregnant Canadian women and their husbands. *Journal of Advanced Nursing, 13,* 436-440.

Drake, M., Verhulst, D., Fawcett, J., & Barger, D. (1988). Spouses' body image changes during and after pregnancy: A replication in Canada. *Image: The Journal of Nursing Scholarship, 20,* 88-92.

Ducharme, F. (1995). Longitudinal change in conjugal support and coping behaviors of elderly marital partners. *Journal of Family Nursing, 1,* 281-302.

Duffy, M. (1989). The primary support received by recently divorced mothers. *Western Journal of Nursing Research, 11,* 676-693.

Duffy, M. (1990). Personal goals of recently divorced women. *Image: The Journal of Nursing Scholarship, 22,* 14-17.

Duffy, M. (1993). Social networks and social support of recently divorced women. *Public Health Nursing, 10,* 19-24.

Dumka, L., Roosa, M., Michaels, M., & Suh, K. (1995). Using research and theory to develop prevention programs for high risk families. *Family Relations, 44,* 78-86.

Duvall, E. (1977). *Family development* (5th ed.). Philadelphia: Lippincott.

Duvall, E., & Miller, B. (1985). *Marriage and family development* (6th ed.). New York: Harper & Row.

Fawcett, J. (1975). The family as a living open system: An emerging conceptual framework for nursing. *International Nursing Review, 22,* 113-166.

Fawcett, J. (1978). Body image and pregnant couple. *MCN: The American Journal of Maternal Child Nursing, 3,* 227-233.

Fawcett, J. (1987). Re: "Spouses' body image changes during and after pregnancy: A replication and extension" (Letter). *Nursing Research, 36,* 220-243.

Fawcett, J. (1989). Spouses' experiences during pregnancy and the postpartum: A program of research and theory development. *Image: The Journal of Nursing Scholarship, 21,* 149-152.

Fawcett, J., Bliss-Holtz, V., Haas, M., Leventhal, M., & Rubin, M. (1986). Spouses' body image changes during and after pregnancy: A replication and extension. *Nursing Research, 35,* 220-223.

Fawcett, J., Pollio, N., Tully, A., Baron, M., Henklein, J., & Jones, R. (1993). Effects of information on adaptation to cesarean birth. *Nursing Research, 42,* 49-53.

Fawcett, J., & Whall, A. (1990). Family theory development in nursing. In J. Bell, W. Watson, & L. Wright (Eds.), *The cutting edge of family nursing* (pp. 17-23). Calgary, Alberta: Family Nursing Unit Publications.

Fawcett, J., & York, R. (1986). Spouses' physical and psychological symptoms during pregnancy and postpartum. *Nursing Research, 35*(3), 144-148.

Fawcett, J., & York, R. (1987). Spouses' strength of identification and reports of symptoms during pregnancy and the postpartum. *Florida Nursing Review, 2*(2), 1-10.

Feetham, S. (1984). Family research, issues and directions for nursing. In H. Werley & J. Fitzpatrick (Eds.), *Annual review of nursing research* (pp. 3-16). New York: Springer.

Feetham, S. (1990). Conceptual and methodological issues in research of families. In J. Bell, W. Watson, & L. Wright (Eds.), *The cutting edge of family nursing* (pp. 35-49). Calgary, Alberta: Family Nursing Unit Publications.

Feetham, S., Perkins, M., & Carroll, R. (1993). Exploratory analysis: A technique for the analysis of dyadic data in research of families. In S. Feetham, S. Meister, J. Bell, & C. Gilliss (Eds.), *The nursing of families: Theory, research, education, practice* (pp. 99-107). Newbury Park, CA: Sage.

Ferketich, S., & Mercer, R. (1989). Men's health status during pregnancy and early fatherhood. *Research in Nursing and Health, 12,* 137-148.

Ferketich, S., & Mercer, R. (1990). Effects of antepartal stress on health status during motherhood. *Scholarly Inquiry for Nursing Practice, 4,* 127-149.

Ferketich, S., & Mercer, R. (1994). Predictors of paternal role competence by risk status. *Nursing Research, 43,* 80-85.

Ferketich, S., & Mercer, R. (1995a). Paternal-infant attachment of experienced and inexperienced fathers during pregnancy. *Nursing Research, 44,* 31-37.

Ferketich, S., & Mercer, R. (1995b). Predictors of role competence for experienced and inexperienced fathers. *Nursing Research, 44,* 89-95.

Friedman, M. (1998). *Family nursing: Research, theory and practice.* Stamford, CT: Appleton & Lange.

Gaffney, K. (1988). State of the science: Prenatal maternal attachment. *Image: The Journal of Nursing Scholarship, 20,* 106-109.

Ganong, L. (1995). Current trends and issues in family nursing research. *Journal of Family Nursing, 1,* 171-206.

Ganong, L., & Coleman, M. (1991). Remarriage and health. *Research in Nursing and Health, 14,* 205-211.

Gass, K. (1987). The health of conjugally bereaved older widows: The role of appraisal, coping and resources. *Research in Nursing and Health, 10,* 39-47.

Gass, K., & Chang, A. (1989). Appraisals, of bereavement, coping, resources, and psychosocial health dysfunction in widows and widowers. *Nursing Research, 38,* 31-38.

Gass-Sternas, K. (1995). Single parent widows: Stressors, appraisal, coping, resources, grieving responses and health. *Marriage and Family Review, 20*(3/4), 411-445.

Glazer, G. (1989). Anxiety and stressors of expectant fathers. *Western Journal of Nursing Research, 11,* 47-59.

Gottlieb, L., & Baillies, J. (1995). Firstborns' behaviors during a mother's second pregnancy. *Nursing Research, 44,* 356-362.

Grace, J. (1993). Mothers' self-reports of parenthood across the first 6 months postpartum. *Research in Nursing and Health, 16,* 431-439.

Graham, M. (1993). Parental sensitivity to infant cues: Similarities and differences between mothers and fathers. *Journal of Pediatric Nursing, 8,* 376-384.

Gross, D., Conrad, B., Fogg, L., & Wothke, W. (1994). A longitudinal model of maternal self-efficacy, depression, and difficult temperament during toddlerhood. *Research in Nursing and Health, 17,* 207-215.

Gross, D., Fogg, L., & Tucker, S. (1995). The efficacy of parent training for promoting positive parent-toddler relationships. *Research in Nursing and Health, 18,* 489-499.

Gross, D., Rocissano, L., & Roncoli, M. (1989). Maternal confidence during toddlerhood: Comparing preterm and fullterm groups. *Research in Nursing and Health, 12,* 1-9.

Gross, D., & Tucker, S. (1994). Parenting confidence during toddlerhood: A comparison of mothers and fathers. *Nurse Practitioner, 19*(10), 25-34.

Grossman, M., & Rowat, K. (1995). Parental relationships, coping strategies, received support, and well-being in adolescents of separated or divorced and married parents. *Research in Nursing and Health, 18,* 249-261.

Hakulinen, T., Paunonen, M., & Turunen, L. (1993). Family dynamics of mothers and fathers expecting their first or second child. *Hoitotiede Journal of Nursing Science, 5*(3), 120-127.

Hall, E., Wulff, T., White, M., & Wilson, M. (1994). Family dynamics during the third trimester of pregnancy in Denmark. *International Journal of Nursing Studies, 31,* 87-95.

Hall, L., & Farel, A. (1988). Maternal stress and depressive symptoms: Correlates of behavior problems in young children. *Nursing Research, 37,* 156-161.

Hall, L., Gurley, D., Sachs, B., & Kryscio, R. (1991). Psychosocial predictors of maternal depressive symptoms, parenting attitudes, and child behavior in single-parent families. *Nursing Research, 43,* 214-220.

Hall, L., Schaefer, E., & Greenberg, R. (1987). Quality and quantity of social support as correlates of psychosomatic symptoms in mothers with young children. *Research in Nursing and Health, 10,* 287-298.

Hall, W. (1991). The experience of fathers in dual-earner families following the births of their first infants. *Journal of Advanced Nursing, 16,* 423-430.

Hall, W. (1992). Comparison of the experience of women and men in dual-earner families following the birth of their first infant. *Image: The Journal of Nursing Scholarship, 24,* 33-38.

Hall, W. (1994). New fatherhood: Myths and realities. *Public Health Nursing, 11,* 219-228.

Harrison, M. (1990). A comparison of parental interactions with term and preterm infants. *Research in Nursing and Health, 13,* 173-179.

Hart, M. (1995). Orem's self care deficit theory: Research with pregnant women. *Nursing Science Quarterly, 8,* 120-126.

Hetherington, M., & Anderson, E. (1987). The effects of divorce and remarriage on early adolescents and their families. In M. Levine & E. McAnarney (Eds.), *Early adolescent transitions* (pp. 49-67). Lexington: D. C. Heath.

Hobbs, D. (1965). Parenthood as crisis: A third study. *Journal of Marriage and the Family, 27,* 367-372.

Hobbs, D., & Cole, S. (1977). Transition to parenthood: A decade replication. *Journal of Marriage and the Family, 38,* 723-731.

Holditch-Davis, D., Black, B., Sandelowski, M., Harris, B., & Belyea, M. (1995). Fertility status and symptoms in childbearing couples. *Research in Nursing and Health, 18,* 417-426.

House, J. (1981). *Work, stress, and social support.* Menlo Park, CA: Addison-Wesley.

Johnston, T. (1990). Retirement: What happens to the marriage. *Issues in Mental Health Nursing, 11,* 347-359.

Jones, L., & Heermann, J. (1992). Parental division of infant care: Contextual influences and infant characteristics. *Nursing Research, 41,* 228-234.

Jones, L., & Lenz, E. (1986). Father-newborn interaction: Effects of social competence and infant state. *Nursing Research, 35,* 149-153.

Jones, L., & Thomas, S. (1989). New fathers' blood pressure and heart rate: Relationships to interaction with their newborn infants. *Nursing Research, 38,* 237-241.

Jordan, P. (1990). Laboring for relevance: Expectant and new fatherhood. *Nursing Research, 39,* 11-16.

Karl, D. (1995). Maternal responsiveness of socially high-risk mothers to the elicitation cues of their 7 month old infants. *Journal of Pediatric Nursing, 10,* 254-263.

Keitner, G., & Miller, I. (1990). Family functioning and major depression: An overview. *American Journal of Psychiatry, 174,* 1128-1137.

Kemp, V. (1987). Mothers' perceptions of children's temperament and mother-child attachment. *Scholarly Inquiry for Nursing Practice, 1,* 51-68.

Kirschling, J., & McBride, A. (1989). Effects of age and sex on the experience of widowhood. *Western Journal of Nursing Research, 11,* 207-218.

Koniak-Griffin, D. (1993). State of the science: Maternal role attainment. *Image: The Journal of Nursing Scholarship, 25,* 257-262.

Lasky, P., Buckwalter, K., Whall, A., Lederman, R., Speer, J., McLane, A., King, J., & White, M. (1985). Developing an instrument for the assessment of family dynamics. *Western Journal of Nursing Research, 7,* 40-52.

Lederman, R. (1984). Anxiety and conflict in pregnancy: Relationship to maternal health status. *Annual Review of Nursing Research, 2,* 28-61.

LeMasters, E. (1957). Parenthood as crisis. *Marriage and Family Living, 19,* 352-355.

Lenz, E., Parks, P., Jenkins, L., & Jarrett, G. (1986). Life change and instrumental support as predictors of illness in mothers of 6-month olds. *Research in Nursing and Health, 9,* 17-24.

Levin, I., & Trost, J. (1992). Understanding the concept of family. *Family Relations, 41,* 348-351.

Levitt, M. (1991). Attachment and close relationships: A life span perspective. In J. Gewirtz & W. Kurtines (Eds.), *Intersections with attachment* (pp. 183-206). Hillsdale, NJ: Lawrence Erlbaum.

Mahon, N., & Yarcheski, A. (1992). Alternate explanations of loneliness in adolescents: A replication and extension study. *Nursing Research, 41*(3), 151-156.

Markman, H. (1981). Prediction of marital distress: A five-year follow up. *Journal of Consulting and Clinical Psychology, 49,* 760-762.

Markman, H., Floyd, F., Stanley, S., & Storasli, R. (1988). The prevention of marital distress: A longitudinal investigation. *Journal of Consulting and Clinical Psychology, 54,* 210-217.

Markman, H., Renick, M., Floyd, F., Stanley, S., & Clements, M. (1993). Preventing marital distress through communication and conflict management training: A 4-year and 5-year follow-up. *Journal of Consulting and Clinical Psychology, 61,* 70-77.

Martell, L. (1990). The mother-daughter relationship during daughter's first pregnancy: The transition experience. *Holistic Nursing Practice, 4*(3), 47-55.

McClowry, S., Giangrande, S., Tommasini, N., Clinton, W., Foreman, N., Lynch, K., & Ferketich, S. (1994). The effects of child temperament, maternal characteristics, and family circumstances on the maladjustment of school-age children. *Research in Nursing and Health, 17,* 25-35.

McCubbin, H., & McCubbin, L. (1997). Hawaiian American families. In M. DeGenova (Ed.), *Families in a cultural context.* Mountain View, CA: Mayfield.

McCubbin, H., Olson, D., & Larsen, A. (1996). Family Crisis Oriented Personal Scales (F-COPES). In H. McCubbin, A. Thompson, & M. McCubbin (Eds.), *Family assessment: Resiliency, coping and adaptation—Inventories for research and practice* (pp. 455-507). Madison: University of Wisconsin System.

McCubbin, M., & McCubbin, H. (1993). Family coping with illness: The Resiliency Model of Family Stress, Adjustment, and Adaptation. In C. Danielson, B. Hamel-Bissell, & P. Winstead-Fry (Eds.), *Families, health and illness: Perspectives on coping and intervention* (pp. 21-63). St. Louis, MO: Mosby.

McCubbin, M., & McCubbin, H. (1996). Resiliency in families: A conceptual model of family adjustment and adaptation in response to stress and crisis. In H. McCubbin, A. Thompson, & M. McCubbin (Eds.), *Family assessment: Resiliency, coping and adaptation—Inventories for research and practice* (pp. 1-64). Madison: University of Wisconsin System.

McGoldrick, M., Heiman, M., & Carter, B. (1993). The changing family life cycle: A perspective on normalcy. In F. Walsh (Ed.), *Normal family processes* (2nd ed., pp. 405-443). New York: Guilford.

Mederer, H., & Hill, R. (1983). Critical transitions over the family life span: Theory and research. *Marriage and Family Review, 6,* 39-60.

Meisenhelder, J., & Meservey, P. (1987). Childbearing over thirty: Description and satisfaction with mothering. *Western Journal of Nursing Research, 9,* 527-541.

Meleis, A., & Trangenstein, P. (1994). Facilitating transitions: Redefinition of the nursing mission. *Nursing Outlook, 42,* 255-259.

Melnyk, B., & Alpert-Gillis, L. (1996). Enhancing coping outcomes of mothers and young children following marital separation: A pilot study. *Journal of Family Nursing, 2,* 266-285.

Mercer, R. (1985). The process of maternal role attainment over the first year. *Nursing Research, 34,* 198-204.

Mercer, R. (1986). Predictors of maternal role attainment at one year postbirth. *Western Journal of Nursing Research, 8,* 9-32.

Mercer, R. (1990). Commentary. *Western Journal of Nursing Research, 12,* 156-158.

Mercer, R., & Ferketich, S. (1990). Predictors of family functioning eight months following birth. *Nursing Research, 39,* 76-82.

Mercer, R., & Ferketich, S. (1994a). Maternal-infant attachment of experienced and inexperienced mothers during pregnancy. *Nursing Research, 43,* 344-351.

Mercer, R., & Ferketich, S. (1994b). Predictors of maternal role competence by risk status. *Nursing Research, 43,* 38-43.

Mercer, R., & Ferketich, S. (1995). Experienced and inexperienced mothers' maternal competence during infancy. *Research in Nursing and Health, 18,* 333-343.

Mercer, R., Ferketich, S., & DeJoseph, J. (1993). Predictors of partner relationships during pregnancy and infancy. *Research in Nursing & Health, 16,* 45-56.

Mercer, R., Ferketich, S., DeJoseph, J., May, K., & Sollid, D. (1988). Effect of stress on family functioning during pregnancy. *Nursing Research, 37,* 268-275.

Mercer, R., Ferketich, S., May, K., DeJoseph, J., & Sollid, D. (1988). Further exploration of maternal and paternal fetal attachment. *Research in Nursing and Health, 11,* 83-95.

Mercer, R., May, K., Ferketich, S., & DeJoseph, J. (1986). Theoretical models for studying the effect of antepartum stress on the family. *Nursing Research, 35,* 339-346.

Mercer, R., Nichols, E., & Doyle, G. (1988). Transition over the life cycle: A comparison of mothers and nonmothers. *Nursing Research, 37,* 144-150.

Muehrer, P., & Koretz, D. (1992). Issues in preventive intervention research. *Current Directions in Psychological Science, American Psychological Society, 1*(3), 109-112.

Muller, M. (1992). A critical review of prenatal attachment research. *Scholarly Inquiry for Nursing Practice, 6,* 5-26.

Muller, M. (1993). Development of the Prenatal Attachment Inventory. *Western Journal of Nursing Research, 15,* 199-215.

Muller, M., & Ferketich, S. (1992). Assessing the validity of the dimensions of prenatal attachment. *Maternal-Child Nursing Journal, 20,* 1-10.

Muller, M., & Ferketich, S. (1993). Factor analysis of the Maternal Fetal Attachment Scale. *Nursing Research, 42,* 144-147.

Murata, J. (1994). Family stress, social support, violence, and sons' behavior. *Western Journal of Nursing Research, 16,* 154-168.

Murata, J. (1995). Family stress, mothers' social support, depression, and sons' behavior problems: Modeling nursing interventions for low-income inner-city families. *Journal of Family Nursing, 1,* 41-62.

Murphy, S. (1990). Using multiple forms of family data: Identifying pattern and meaning in sibling-infant relationships. In J. Gilgun, K. Daly, & G. Handel (Eds.), *Qualitative methods in family research* (pp. 146-171). Newbury Park, CA: Sage.

Murphy, S. (1993). Siblings and the new baby: Changing perspectives. *Journal of Pediatric Nursing, 8,* 277-288.

Norbeck, J., & Anderson, N. (1989a). Life stress, social support, and anxiety in mid- and late-pregnancy among low income women. *Research in Nursing and Health, 12,* 281-287.

Norbeck, J., & Anderson, N. (1989b). Psychosocial predictors of pregnancy outcomes in low income Black, Hispanic, and White women. *Nursing Research, 38,* 204-209.

Ohashi, J. (1992). Maternal role satisfaction: A new approach to assessing parenting. *Scholarly Inquiry for Nursing Practice, 6,* 135-150.

Olds, D., Henderson, C., & Kitzman, H. (1994). Does prenatal and infancy nurse home visitation have enduring effects on qualities of parental caregiving and child health at 25-50 months of life? *Pediatrics, 93,* 89-98.

Olds, D., Henderson, C., Tatelbaum, R., & Chamberlin, R. (1986). Improving the delivery of prenatal care and outcomes of pregnancy: A randomized trial of nurse home visitation. *Pediatrics, 77,* 16-28.

Olds, D., Henderson, C., Tatelbaum, R., & Chamberlin, R. (1988). Improving the life-course development of socially disadvantaged mothers: A randomized trial of nurse home visitation. *American Journal of Public Health, 78,* 1436-1445.

Olson, D. (1993). Circumplex model of marital and family systems: Assessing family functioning. In F. Walsh (Ed.), *Normal family processes* (2nd ed., pp. 104-137). New York: Guilford.

Olson, D., Fournier, D., & Druckman, J. (1986). *PREPARE and EN-RICH Inventories* (2nd ed.). Minneapolis, MN: PREPARE/EN-RICH, Inc.

Olson, D., McCubbin, H., Barnes, H., Larsen, A., Muxem, A., & Wilson, M. (1983). *Families: What makes them work.* Beverly Hills, CA: Sage.

Olson, D., McCubbin, H., Barnes, H., Larsen, A., Muxen, M., & Wilson, M. (1986). *Family inventories.* St. Paul: University of Minnesota Family Social Science.

Olson, D., Portner, J., & Lavee, Y. (1985). *FACES III.* St. Paul: Family Social Science, University of Minnesota.

Olson, D., Sprenkle, D., & Russell, C. (1979). Circumplex model of marital and family systems. I: Cohesion and adaptability dimensions, family types, and clinical applications. *Family Process, 18,* 3-28.

Palkovitz, R. (1992). Changes in father-infant bonding beliefs across couples: First transition to parenthood. *Maternal-Child Nursing Journal, 20,* 141-154.

Parkes, C. (1971). Psycho-social transitions: A field for study. *Social Science and Medicine, 5,* 101-115.

Pett, M., Lang, N., & Gander, A. (1992). Late-life divorce: Its impact on family rituals. *Journal of Family Issues, 13,* 526-552.

Porter, E. (1994a). Older widows' experience of living at home. *Image: The Journal of Nursing Scholarship, 26,* 19-24.

Porter, E. (1994b). "Reducing my risks": A phenomenon of older widows' lived experience. *Advances in Nursing Science, 17*(2), 54-65.

Preston, D., & Dellasega, C. (1990). Elderly women and stress: Does marriage make a difference? *Journal of Gerontological Nursing, 16*(4), 27-32.

Pridham, K., & Chang, A. (1992). Transition to being the mother of a new infant in the first 3 months: Maternal problem solving and self-appraisal. *Journal of Advanced Nursing, 17,* 204-216.

Pridham, K., Chang, A., & Chiu, Y. (1994). Mothers' parenting self-appraisals: The contribution of perceived infant temperament. *Research in Nursing and Health, 17,* 381-392.

Ransom, D., Fisher, L., Phillips, S., Kokes, R., & Weiss, R. (1990). The logic of measurement in family research. In T. Draper & A. Marcos (Eds.), *Family variables: Conceptualization, measurement, and use* (pp. 48-63). Newbury Park, CA: Sage.

Reece, S. (1995). Stress and maternal adaptation in first-time mothers more than 35 years old. *Applied Nursing Research, 8*(2), 61-66.

Richards, E. (1989). Self-reports of differentiation of self and marital compatibility as related to family functioning in the third and fourth stages of the family life cycle. *Scholarly Inquiry for Nursing Practice, 3,* 163-180.

Rickelman, B., Gallman, L., & Papra, H. (1994). Attachment and quality of life in older, community-residing men. *Nursing Research, 43,* 68-72.

Riesch, S., & Forsyth, D. (1992). Preparing to parent the adolescent: A theoretical overview. *Journal of Child and Parent Nursing, 5*(1), 32-40.

Riesch, S., Jacobson, G., & Tosi, C. (1994). Young adolescents' identification of difficult life events. *Clinical Nursing Research, 3,* 393-413.

Riesch, S., Tosi, C., Thurston, C., Forsyth, D., Kuenning, T., & Kestly, J. (1993). Effects of communication training on parents and young adolescents. *Nursing Research, 42,* 10-16.

Roberts, C., & Feetham, S. (1982). An instrument for assessing family functioning across three areas of relationships. *Nursing Research, 31,* 231-235.

Robinson, C. (1995). Beyond dichotomies in the nursing of persons and families. *Image: The Journal of Nursing Scholarship, 27,* 116-120.

Rodgers, R., & White, J. (1993). Family development theory. In P. Boss, W. Doherty, R. LaRossa, W. Schumm, & S. Steinmetz (Eds.), *Sourcebook of family theories and methods: A contextual approach* (pp. 225-254). New York: Plenum.

Rustia, J., & Abbott, D. (1990). Predicting paternal role enactment. *Western Journal of Nursing Research, 12,* 145-160.

Sabatelli, R., & Shehan, C. (1993). Exchange and resource theories. In P. Boss, W. Doherty, R. LaRossa, W. Schumm, & S. Steinmetz (Eds.), *Sourcebook of family theories and methods* (pp. 385-411). New York: Plenum.

Sandelowski, M., & Black, B. (1994). The epistemology of expectant parenthood. *Western Journal of Nursing Research, 16,* 601-622.

Sawin, K., & Harrigan, M. (1995). Well established self-report instruments: Feetham Family Functioning Survey. In P. Woog (Ed.), *Measures of family functioning for research and practice* (pp. 42-47). New York: Springer.

Schumacher, K., & Meleis, A. (1994). Transitions: A central concept in nursing. *Image: The Journal of Nursing Scholarship, 26,* 119-127.

Selder, F. (1989). Life transition theory: The resolution of uncertainty. *Nursing and Health Care, 10,* 437-440; 449-451.

Smilkstein, G. (1978). The family APGAR: A proposal for a family function test and its use by physicians. *Journal of Family Practice, 6,* 1231-1239.

Sullivan, J., & Fawcett, J. (1990). The measurement of family phenomena. In A. Whall & J. Fawcett (Eds.), *Family theory development in nursing* (pp. 69-84). Philadelphia: F. A. Davis.

Swanson, E., McCloskey, J., & Bodensteiner, A. (1991). Publishing opportunities for nurses: A comparison of 92 U.S. journals. *Image: The Journal of Nursing Scholarship, 23,* 33-38.

Thompson, L. (1992). Feminist methodology for family studies. *Journal of Marriage and the Family, 54,* 3-18.

Tiedje, L., & Darling-Fisher, C. (1996). Fatherhood reconsidered: A critical review. *Research in Nursing and Health, 19,* 471-484.

Tomlinson, B., White, M., & Wilson, M. (1990). Family dynamics during pregnancy. *Journal of Advanced Nursing, 15,* 683-688.

Tomlinson, P. (1987). Spousal differences in marital satisfaction during transition to parenthood. *Nursing Research, 36*(4), 239-243.

Tomlinson, P. (1996). Marital relationship change in the transition to parenthood: A reexamination as interpreted through transition theory. *Journal of Family Nursing, 2*(3), 286-305.

Trost, J. (1988). Conceptualizing the family. *International Sociology, 3,* 301-308.

Troy, N. (1993). Early contact and maternal attachment among women using public health care facilities. *Applied Nursing Research, 6,* 161-166.

Uphold, C., & Strickland, O. (1989). Issues related to the unit of analysis in family nursing research. *Western Journal of Nursing Research, 11*(4), 405-417.

Van Widenfelt, B., Hosman, C., Schaap, C., & van der Staak, C. (1996). The prevention of relationship distress for couples at risk:

A controlled evaluation with nine-month and two-year follows. *Family Relations, 45,* 156-165.

Ventura, J. (1986). Parent coping: A replication. *Nursing Research, 36,* 77-80.

Ventura, J., & Stevenson, M. (1986). Relations of mothers' and fathers' reports of infant temperament, parents' psychological functioning, and family characteristics. *Merrill-Palmer Quarterly, 32,* 275-289.

Walker, L. (1989a). A longitudinal analysis of stress process among mothers of infants. *Nursing Research, 38,* 339-343.

Walker, L. (1989b). Stress process among mothers of infants: Preliminary model testing. *Nursing Research, 38,* 10-16.

Walker, L., Crain, H., & Thompson, E. (1986a). Maternal role attainment and identity in the postpartum period: Stability and change. *Nursing Research, 35,* 68-71.

Walker, L., Crain, H., & Thompson, E. (1986b). Mothering behavior and maternal role attainment during the postpartum period. *Nursing Research, 35,* 352-355.

Walker, L., & Montgomery, E. (1994). Maternal identity and role attainment: Long-term relations to children's development. *Nursing Research, 43,* 105-110.

Wallerstein, J. (1985). Children of divorce: Preliminary report of a ten year follow up of older children and adolescents. *Journal of the American Academy of Child Psychiatry, 24,* 545-553.

Whall, A., & Loveland-Cherry, C. (1993). Family unit-focused research: 1987-1991. In J. Fitzpatrick, J. Stevenson, & A. Jacox (Eds.), *Annual review of nursing research* (pp. 227-247). New York: Springer.

Whitchurch, G., & Constantine, L. (1993). Systems theory. In P. Boss, W. Doherty, R. LaRossa, W. Schumm, & S. Steinmetz (Eds.), *Sourcebook of family theories and methods: A contextual approach* (pp. 325-352). New York: Plenum.

White, J. (1991). *Dynamics of family development: A theoretical perspective.* New York: Guilford.

White, L., & Booth, A. (1985). The transition to parenthood and marital quality. *Journal of Family Issues, 6,* 435-450.

Younger, J. (1991). A model of parenting stress. *Research in Nursing and Health, 14,* 197-204.

Zachariah, R. (1994a). Mother-daughter and husband-wife attachment as predictors of psychological well-being during pregnancy. *Clinical Nursing Research, 3,* 371-392.

Zachariah, R. (1994b). Maternal-fetal attachment: Influence of mother-daughter and husband-wife relationships. *Research in Nursing and Health, 17,* 37-44.

13

NURSING CARE OF FAMILIES IN NON-NORMATIVE TRANSITIONS

The State of Science and Practice

Catherine L. Gilliss
Kathleen A. Knafl

The effort people make to organize themselves in some semblance of family is one of the most imperishable habits of the human race. Over time and across cultures, people have arranged themselves in multiple family forms, and the family as a recognizable unit has endured as a fundamental social structure, a structure that is critical to both its individual members and the larger social order. Families have also been the focus of considerable scholarly attention, providing the grist for great literary works, ideological debates, and systematic inquiry. The health professions, such as nursing, medicine, social work, and clinical psychology, have also shown strong interest in the family, as there is evidence that illness can have a profound impact on family life and families can play a crucial role in individual adaptation to illness (Campbell, 1986; Litman,

1974; Patterson & Garwick, 1994; Schwenk & Hughes, 1983). As such, each of these fields has directed effort to developing a scholarly basis for its work with families.

Like the other helping professions, nursing's long-standing interest in the family is grounded in its practice imperative, with research concerns both evolving from and contributing to the practice base. Whall and Fawcett (1991) traced nursing's interest in family to the origins of the profession, noting,

> It is clear, then, that family phenomena were of interest from the beginning of modern nursing. Although formal middle-range family theory development efforts were not undertaken by Nightingale, she sensitized nurses to the view that family members were an important focus for nursing care. (p. 9)

231

These authors (Whall & Fawcett, 1991) also highlighted the upsurge in the amount and range of nursing scholarship related to family. Not only do both graduate and undergraduate clinical texts typically include sections on the family, there are a number of nursing texts devoted entirely to family. Typically, these texts reflect a combined focus on family theory, practice, and research (Bomar, 1989; Clements & Roberts, 1983; Friedman, 1986; Hanson & Boyd, 1996; Wegner & Alexander, 1993). In addition, considerable research is being reported in a variety of both research- and clinically focused journals, and in February 1996, the *Journal of Family Nursing* was launched, with Dr. Janice Bell as its editor. Moreover, the volume of family nursing research has been sufficient to generate multiple reviews, which have categorized the focus of this research, synthesized the results, and critiqued its methodological and conceptual underpinnings (Feetham, 1984; Gilliss, 1989; Hayes, 1993; Whall & Loveland-Cherry, 1993). Other reviews have focused on more circumscribed areas of family research, such as family adaptation to childhood chronic illness (Austin, 1991) and family violence (Campbell, Harris, & Lee, 1995). In addition, attention has been directed to specifying the defining characteristics of family nursing and to debating issues related to family nursing practice and family nursing research (Gilliss, 1991).

The purpose of this chapter is to examine the state of nursing science related to families facing non-normative, health-related challenges such as chronic illness, dementia, or organ transplantation, as well as the related practice developments. Our examination incorporates prior reviews of the state of the science, current research, and theoretical discussions about family nursing practice and research. The decision to include both empirical studies and position papers reflects our conviction that efforts in both these realms are making important contributions to the advancement of family nursing science. Further, in charting future directions for the field, it is useful to examine the extent and ways in which empirical and theoretical efforts inform one another. Because of our focus on the state of the science, we have not included clinical case studies or articles based on the authors' personal experiences. Although such articles also make important contributions to our understanding of families and family nursing, there are no clear guidelines for either evaluating or integrating these contributions into the scientific underpinnings of the profession, an issue we will return to in the discussion section of this chapter. This review also excludes articles focusing entirely on methodological issues or approaches because this topic has been the subject

TABLE 13.1.   Major Sources of Data for Review

Prior reviews of the literature

Comprehensive reviews
   Feetham, 1984
   Gilliss, 1989
   Whall and Loveland-Cherry, 1993
   Hayes, 1993
   Ganong, 1995

Focused reviews
   Snelling, 1990
   Austin, 1991
   Campbell, Harris, and Lee, 1995
   Loukissa, 1995
   Rennick, 1995
   Ford-Gilboe and Campbell, 1996

Position papers

Nature of family nursing research and theory
   Moriarity, 1990
   Wright and Leahey, 1990, 1994
   Gilliss, 1991
   Anderson and Tomlinson, 1992
   Lansberry and Richards, 1992
   Shaw and Halliday, 1992
   Woods and Lewis, 1992
   Wright and Levac, 1992
   Robinson, 1993
   Forchuk and Dorsay, 1995
   Lynn, 1995

Promising frameworks for advancing family nursing
   Beckingham and Baumann, 1990
   Bridges and Lyman, 1993

Current research, 1991-1996
   Research and clinical specialty journals

of several prior reviews (Feetham, 1991; Gilliss, 1983; Thomas, 1987).

Method

Table 13.1 summarizes the data sources used in this review. Relevant sources were identified through a combination of computer-based and hand searches of the published literature. Identification of prior reviews and position papers was based on searches of nursing journals and texts from 1980 to 1996. Current research was drawn from articles published between 1991 and 1996 in major nursing research and specialty journals.

The selection of current research for this chapter included both research that focused on the family unit and studies addressing family roles and relationships. The inclusion criteria, which were consistent with those used in prior reviews (Feetham, 1984; Gilliss, 1989; Hayes, 1993; Whall & Loveland-Cherry, 1993), included the requirements that reports (a) be theoretically grounded, (b) represent a contribution to knowledge about families, and (c) be relevant to nursing. The review was limited to published articles because this is the work that is currently shaping the field. Identification of articles entailed a two-step process. First, articles addressing any aspect of family (e.g., maternal coping, caregiver role) were identified through a combination of computer and hand searches, yielding over 300 articles. Each article was then reviewed, and only those that met the above criteria and were pertinent to the topic of this chapter (i.e., non-normative transitions) were retained ($N = 100$).

Theoretical discussions and position papers were identified primarily through hand searches. These articles included both general statements about the defining characteristics of family nursing; position papers and debates about the differences between family nursing, the nursing of families, and the nursing of the individual in the context of the family; and research and discussions of selected frameworks or approaches that were viewed as particularly relevant to family nursing. Our intent was to be as inclusive as possible with regard to representing the multiple viewpoints of nurses engaged in family research.

In the next section, we discuss prior efforts to evaluate the state of family nursing research, as well as efforts to define the unique characteristics of family nursing research and practice. This section draws on past reviews of the literature and theoretical papers related to family nursing. The subsequent section reviews current research, with an eye to identifying conceptual and methodological trends, as well as substantive contributions. In the final section, we draw conclusions regarding the extent to which current research is building on the lessons and recommendations revealed in past reviews, reflects theoretical positions about the nature of family nursing, and provides empirical grounding for practice.

Prior Reviews and Discussions

Comprehensive Reviews

Prior reviews of family nursing research set the stage for evaluating current (1991-1996) research efforts. Reviews by Feetham (1984), Gilliss (1989), Whall and Loveland-Cherry (1993), and Hayes (1993) were especially useful because of the authors' comprehensiveness and efforts to build on one another's work. Table 13.2

summarizes the major reviews with regard to their purpose, sampling criteria, conclusions, and recommendations regarding the state of family science in nursing.

Although each of the reviews focused on critically assessing the state of family nursing science and offered recommendations for future directions, the selection criteria for identifying relevant literature varied. Whall and Loveland-Cherry (1993) used the most restrictive sampling criteria and limited their review to studies that focused on the family, used family measures, and obtained data from multiple family members. In contrast, the other reviews included studies of family roles and relationships as well as the family unit and did not set limits on the types of measures or subjects used in the research. Feetham (1984), Gilliss (1989), and Hayes (1993) all specified that the article should be theoretically grounded and relevant to nursing to be included in the review, although many were not.

Later reviews explicitly took into account the selection criteria of the earlier reviews and presented well-articulated rationales for their sampling criteria and approach. Thus, Whall and Loveland-Cherry (1993) justified their decision to exclude topics that had been the focus of major prior reviews, Gilliss (1989) discussed her decision to adapt Feetham's selection criteria, and Hayes (1993) presented her rationale for expanding the sampling frame used by Gilliss. Feetham's (1984) original distinctions between family and family-related research and between full and partial theoretical models of family research guided subsequent reviewers' efforts to define and analyze family nursing research.

In spite of their somewhat differing purposes and approaches, the conclusions reached by the authors of these reviews were remarkably similar in their identification of major trends in the field, enduring challenges facing family nursing researchers, and recommendations for the future. There is evidence of enduring interest in family and family-related research in nursing. Feetham's review identified 30 articles meeting her criteria for family research in the 20-year time span between 1963 and 1983. She found that the number of family-related research articles had grown threefold during that period (S. Feetham, personal communication, April 15, 1997). Gilliss, who included both family and family-related research in her sample, identified 76 articles during the next 4 years. On the other hand, Hayes's (1993) more recent review, which encompassed a longer time span than that of Gilliss, identified fewer articles and concluded that the quantity, though not the quality, of family nursing research was decreasing. Across all reviews there is evi-

TABLE 13.2. Comparison of Major Prior Reviews

Review	Purpose	Sample	Conclusion	Recommendation
Feetham, 1984	Review and assess the development of family nursing research.	All studies through 1983 meeting criteria for family research: conceptualization of family, result in knowledge about family structure or function, operational definition of family, relevance to nursing, theoretical grounding. Final sample of 30 research reports.	Studies focused on families defined as abnormal, focused on internal family dynamics, relied on mother as primary data source, and reflected a lack of consensus about the family unit system and subsystem that should be measured.	Develop programs of research, establish interdisciplinary ties, ground research in full theoretical model of family, incorporate family strengths, define and predict family well-being.
Gilliss, 1989	Offer direction in family nursing research by reviewing types of research questions addressed and designs and methods used.	All studies between 1983 and 1986 in which one or more authors was a nurse, a theoretical framework was tested or developed, the family or family member was a focus, relevance to nursing was addressed. Limited to six nonspecialty nursing journals. Final sample of 76 articles.	Majority of research addressed maternal-child issues, focused on family roles rather than the family unit, failed to use a full theoretical model, was based on cross-sectional designs. Evidence of an increase in family research.	Situate all family research in a full theoretical model, focus more on nontraditional and culturally diverse families and on family ties to other systems, use a wider array of methods.
Whall and Loveland-Cherry, 1993	Answer the following questions: Is the term family defined? Is the study design appropriate? Are the various aspects of the study conceptually congruent? Are the findings consistent with the intent of the research?	All studies published between 1984 and 1991 in which the family unit was the focus, data on more than two family members were collected, family-focused instruments were used. Final sample of 51 articles.	Studies focused on family transitions and evolving structures, cross-cultural family research, and family needs. Few studies addressed how the family as a unit of analysis was defined. Evidence of development of middle-range theory related to family transitions and appreciation for family strength and health.	Focus more on cross-cultural research, increase methodological diversity, expand intervention research to include community settings.
Hayes, 1993	Examine the current state of the science related to family nursing.	Literature not sampled by Feetham or Gilliss that met inclusion criteria of one or more authors a nurse; clinically relevant; theoretically grounded; methodologically sound; addressed family roles, relationships, or relationship of family to external systems. Final sample of 54 articles.	Articles focused on conceptual issues or literature reviews, instrumentation, or research reports, with cross-sectional, observational designs being dominant. Family nursing research declining in quantity though not quality.	Pay greater attention to specifying the family as a unit of analysis and focus on theory development and testing. Direct more studies to nontraditional family types, families of the elderly, and well-functioning families.

dence that researchers have addressed both normative and non-normative transitions. However, studies in the non-normative domain, the focus of this chapter, have predominated. Studies addressing non-normative transitions focus on the impact of illness on families and family members and families' efforts to adapt to illness. In particular, nurse researchers have been interested in family caregiving for the elderly and in family coping with childhood chronic illness.

Conceptual, methodological, and design issues identified by Feetham (1984) in the first major review of the field were evident in subsequent reviews as well. As a group, the reviews found that family nursing studies have been characterized by their failure to specify the investigator's underlying assumptions or stance regarding the family-illness interface. Thus, Hayes (1993), in the most recent review, concluded, as did Feetham (1984) in the earliest review, that researchers needed to specify the nature of their family focus and clarify whether it was on the family unit or on family roles and relationships. In much of the early research, it was unclear whether the family was being conceptualized as (a) the context for understanding the individual's response to illness, (b) the system responding to an illness challenge, or (c) the etiology of the illness or adaption problems in the ill family member.

Moreover, early researchers rarely grounded their studies of family roles and relationships in a broader family theoretical perspective. In addition, the authors of these four comprehensive reviews admonished investigators to expand their samples to include more culturally diverse families and more non-traditional family forms and to address the links between the family and the external system or environment, as well as internal family dynamics.

In general, the authors of these major reviews did an excellent job of building on one another's efforts, and their efforts provide both a comprehensive assessment of the quality of family nursing research and a useful direction for future efforts, especially with regard to the design and conceptual underpinnings of family nursing research. On the other hand, because of their comprehensiveness, these reviews tended to focus on broad topical, methodological, and conceptual issues and trends. They were less successful in identifying the collective substantive contributions generated by the studies they reviewed. Broad areas of focus were identified, but a critical summary of the knowledge generated was not provided.

One final review of the family nursing research also merits discussion. In 1995, Ganong examined issues and trends in family nursing research. Basing his discussion on the reviews just described, he identified a number of major shortcomings of family nursing research in comparison to family research being conducted in other fields and concluded that "with the exception of the development of qualitative approaches, family nursing research conceptually and methodologically is about a decade behind family research in disciplines such as family studies, sociology, and psychology" (p. 192). Although his review offers some interesting challenges to family nursing researchers, it is impossible for the reader to evaluate the validity of Ganong's overall assessment of the state of family science in nursing, as no information is provided to support his interdisciplinary comparisons. Unfortu-

nately, his opinions were disconnected from clear examples and thus appeared to be conjectural.

Focused Reviews

Reviews have also been completed in more focused, substantive areas of family nursing. Austin (1991), Loukissa (1995), and Snelling (1990) each reviewed literature related to family and chronic illness, and Rennick (1995) explored the research on the family's experience of acute hospitalization. Austin's (1991) review of family adaptation to childhood chronic illness was the most rigorous of these, giving careful attention to definitional considerations in identifying relevant literature. She found that across the 39 articles she reviewed, stress and coping was the predominant conceptual framework, with approximately half the studies having no explicit theoretical grounding. Although Austin found that investigators in this area were generating knowledge in four domains (family adaptation processes, illness effect on family members, illness effect on mother-infant interactions, relationship between family and child characteristics), she concluded that "current research in nursing does not provide a consistent body of knowledge about family adaptation to chronic illness in a child to guide nursing practice" (pp. 114-115). Like Feetham, she concluded that research has focused too exclusively on internal family dynamics and has often failed to specify the investigator's conceptualization or underlying assumptions about family. She also found that researchers rarely took into account time since onset of illness when studying family adaptation, and she recommended that greater attention be paid to family adaptation over time. On the other hand, Austin (1991) also found that data were collected from multiple family members in over half the studies, suggesting that researchers in this area are responding to prior criticisms that family researchers have relied too heavily on the mother as the spokesperson for the family. The degree to which the data were analyzed to reflect individual or family reactions and processes was not discussed.

Loukissa (1995) took a chronological perspective in reviewing the research from 1960 to 1993 on family burden in chronic mental illness. She found that, over time, there has been a shift from studies that sought to document the existence of burden and explore the correlates of burden to research that explores interventions or supports that ameliorate family burden. Rennick's (1995) look at the research on the family experience of an acutely ill hospitalized child served to document the dearth of work being done in this area and concluded with a "call to action" for family nursing researchers to direct greater attention to the experiences and needs of these families.

Snelling's (1990) review of the role of the family in relation to chronic pain was the only one that focused on the contribution of the family to the etiology or maintenance of pathology. Her review suggests that chronic pain is an area strongly dominated by a "deficit view" of families. Unfortunately, her discussion fails to address the implications of such a view for working with families or possibilities for incorporating a more balanced perspective that takes family strengths as well as deficits into account. As such, it fails to incorporate the recommendations of earlier reviews (Feetham, 1984; Hayes, 1993) that pointed to the importance of understanding family strengths.

In contrast to the prior reviews, all of which were done from a nonideological position, Campbell, Harris, and Lee's (1995) and Ford-Gilboe and Campbell's (1996) work supports the insights that can be gained from a critical or ideologically based synthesis of the literature. In their review of the nursing research on family violence, Campbell, Harris, and Lee (1995) argue that nursing research on victimization, because of its advocacy orientation, has approximated a critical theoretical approach and avoided the victim-blaming and deficit orientation that has characterized the research in other disciplines. Similarly, Ford-Gilboe and Campbell's (1996) review of the 17 nursing journal articles on single-parent families found that there were few studies in this area being done from a feminist perspective. They concluded that the absence of a feminist perspective had resulted in the single-parent family typically being viewed as deviant and less functional than the traditional nuclear family, and they advocated the use of feminist approaches as a vehicle for supporting research that eliminates androcentric and ethnocentric biases and contributes to the development of research agendas *for* rather than *on* women.

▬ Defining Family Nursing Practice and Research

Family nursing scholars have also directed their efforts to conceptualizing the defining characteristics of family nursing practice and research. The work of Wright and Leahey (1990, 1994) and the Family Nursing Unit (FNU) of the University of Calgary has been especially influential in developing and articulating the nature of family nursing practice. Based on observations grounded

in their clinical practice, Wright and Leahey (1990) distinguished between family nursing and family systems nursing. Whereas family nursing views the individual in the context of the family or the family with the individual as context, family systems nursing maintains a simultaneous focus on both the individual and the family. As developed by Wright and Leahey, family systems nursing emphasizes the importance of the family's belief system in shaping its response to illness and the development of collaborative interaction between the nurse and the family in promoting both individual and family growth and healing in the context of illness. Other authors (Lansberry & Richards, 1992; Shaw & Halliday, 1992; Wright & Levac, 1992) continue to elaborate specific aspects of family systems nursing and discuss its relevance for nursing practice.

Forchuk and Dorsay (1995) argue in favor of combining family systems nursing, as conceptualized by Wright and Leahey, with Peplau's nursing theory. Pointing to the congruity between the two approaches, they conclude that combining the two has the advantage of adding a family perspective to Peplau and grounding Wright and Leahey in a nursing theory.

Robinson (1993), also, has been interested in defining the nature of family nursing. Her work expands Wright and Leahey's efforts to view the family and the individual simultaneously, although she argues against using the term *family systems nursing* and contends that it perpetuates false dichotomies between the family and the individual family member that limit nursing practice. She provides a schema of four different focuses on nursing practice with individuals and families: nursing the individual/family member; nursing the individual/family subgroup; nursing the family group; nursing the individual/family system. Robinson's (1993) schema was developed to take into account the person both as individual and family member, and it includes progressively more complex conceptualizations of the family unit. Although her framework provides a useful heuristic for viewing the various ways in which nurses focus on individuals and families, her critique of the concept of family nursing as leading to false dichotomies is unconvincing and fails to recognize that neither family nursing as conceptualized by Gilliss, Highley, Roberts, and Martinson (1989) or family systems nursing as conceptualized by Wright and Leahey (1984, 1994) precludes a simultaneous focus on both the family and the individual.

Arguing that "the absence of a critical dialogue regarding what constitutes family nursing prevents the further development of the specialty area of family nursing,"

Gilliss (1991, p. 19) identified nine challenges confronting family nursing. The challenges, which encompassed practice, research, and education, were based on the assumption that family nursing deliberately targets the family group as the unit of interest. Summarizing the challenges she identified as facing the field, Gilliss concluded,

> We must begin by clarifying the nature of the preparation for specialty practice in family nursing. Next, we must move beyond the declaration of our practice intentions to demonstrate family nursing practice and its *real* outcomes. Our theoretical explanations of family nursing need refinement; observing practice outcomes offers considerable promise for theory development. (p. 22)

The issues identified by Gilliss are a continuing focus of lively discussion and debate.

Other authors (Gilliss & Davis, 1992; Lynn, 1995; Moriarty, 1990; Woods & Lewis, 1992) have discussed the defining characteristics of family nursing research and have identified conceptual and methodological issues faced by investigators in this area. In many ways, their conclusions mirror those of the authors who completed comprehensive reviews of the literature (Feetham, 1984; Gilliss, 1989; Hayes, 1993; Whall & Loveland-Cherry, 1993). They point to the importance of studying the family as a unit and of focusing on family strengths and competencies as well as problematic areas of family life. Gilliss and Davis (1992), in particular, stress the importance of targeting research that develops and evaluates family care interventions. Anderson and Tomlinson (1992) speak to the importance of specifying and further developing the concept of family health and linking it to family structure and function. They propose that a nursing perspective on family health should incorporate interactive, developmental, coping, and integrity processes as well as those related to health. Developing these theoretical ideas in a theoretically rigorous fashion represents yet another challenge.

▬ *Promising Frameworks*

Finally, several authors have advocated the use of certain frameworks that to date have received little recognition by family nursing researchers. Bournaki and Germain (1993) discussed the usefulness of esthetics as a vehicle for drawing on the untapped experiential knowledge of the nurse as a basis for shaping nursing practice in the future. Bridges and Lynam (1993), on the other hand, argue that nursing as a profession needs to examine its practice from the perspective of broader social, political, and economic contexts and suggest that Marxist theory provides a useful framework for raising questions about the taken-for-granted aspects of nursing practice. Marxist theory is viewed as a mechanism for moving nursing practice from an individual and family focus to the social system and policy arena.

▬ *Summary*

Taken together, these prior reviews and position papers provide a useful backdrop for reviewing and assessing current research. They synthesize the knowledge from which contemporary investigators can build, identify critical methodological and conceptual issues, and offer insights into especially promising lines of inquiry.

Contemporary Research in Family Nursing

In an effort to more closely examine current research in the field of family nursing, we initiated a review of research reports authored by nurses that addressed family or family-related issues in non-normative health circumstances. As has been described, the review covered the period from 1991 to 1996 and included electronic strategies (keywords and personal authors) and hand searches of nursing journals that publish research reports. Parenthetically, the task was more difficult than ever before, suggesting that there are more papers appearing in more varied journals than previously. All articles identified were reviewed to determine (a) purpose, (b) source of information, (c) health or medical problem, (d) conceptual framework, (e) the family phenomenon addressed, and (f) the findings about the family. A summary document, which included the abstracts of each citation, served as a working document for organizing observations included in this analysis; the citations are listed in the reference list for this chapter.

▬ *Purpose*

The majority of the 100 research reports reviewed described the experiences of families and individuals in family relationships responding to some aspect of the illness experience. Many of these articles attempted to explain the experience in a meaningful and generalizable way. More reports focus on an adult member with a health problem than address the response of a family to a child member who was ill.

Of the papers included in this review, only two described traditional tests of nursing care (Archbold, Stewart, Miller, et al., 1995; Ferrell, Grant, Chan, Ahn, & Ferrell, 1995). That is, those reports described completed experiments of interventions that could be replicated by others. Although this suggests that the research-based knowledge of family nursing intervention is surprisingly limited, a second, important segment of intervention research literature is growing.

Although not traditional reports of the outcomes of care, the number of papers reviewed that described care outcomes in a manner not conforming to a traditional scientific "test" seems to be growing. Nine reports that describe the results of naturally occurring interventions and the experiences of patients, families, and nurses throughout interventions appeared in the identified literature. These papers present the descriptive results of the events that families experienced, or experienced in relation to family nursing care. Although these are not traditional research reports, they, also, can provide useful insights into effective nursing interventions and direction for future research projects. Eight of the nine papers addressed aspects of home management of care for elders or children and included successful approaches taken by families or nurses or both (Bull, 1993; Davis & Grant, 1994; Langner, 1993; Magilvy, Congdon, & Martinez, 1994; Patterson & Garwick, 1994; Reinhard, 1994; Rhiner, Ferrell, Shapiro, & Dierkes, 1994; Taylor, Ferrell, Grant, & Cheyney, 1993). The growth of this segment of the literature may suggest that traditional science, as evaluated with the randomized clinical trial, is more difficult and less useful in the study of *particular* families who are struggling with *particular* problems in *particular* ways.

Source of Information

Research reports about families have sometimes been described as "mother" or "wives" sociology, as the common strategy for accessing information about the "family" has been to interview the mother/wife (Safilios-Rothschild, 1969). This approach has been appropriately criticized, as it generalizes the individual mother's experience to other individual family members and does not always assess the relational and transactional aspects of family life (Fisher, Kokes, Ransom, Phillips, & Rudd, 1985). As summarized in Table 13.3, the majority of papers reviewed continue to seek data from one family member (most often a caregiver, the mother, or one "parent"), and a growing number of studies are seeking data from more than one family participant, as was noted in some of the prior reviews. Common informant combinations include mother and father or patient and family caregiver. Novel approaches to resourcing data have been reported using triadic or multiple combinations of perspectives, such as patient/partner/adult child (Snelling, 1994), patient/nurse/caregiver (Ferrell, Taylor, Grant, Fowler, & Corbisiero, 1993; Taylor et al., 1993), nurse/patient/physician/family member (Magilvy, Congdon, & Martinez, 1994), and patient/partner/child (Germino, Fife, & Funk, 1995; Germino & Funk, 1993).

Efforts at actually capturing a family-level experience remain limited and seem best assessed through qualitative methods (Chesla, 1991; Elfert, Anderson, & Lai, 1991; Gagliardi, 1991; Hough, Lewis, & Woods, 1991; Klein-Berndt, 1991; Knafl, Breitmayer, Gallo, & Zoeller, 1996; McCarthy & Gallo, 1992; Sharkey, 1995; Whyte, 1992).

The Health or Medical Problem

Table 13.4 provides an overview of the health problems that were studied in the research reviewed for this chapter. Although most women would indicate that family caregiving activities span the life cycle, the literature tends to focus on the discrete experiences of families in relationship to particular illness episodes or developmental periods. The experiences of families with ill children are reported less frequently than the experiences of families with ill adult members (45% versus 55%, respectively). However, far fewer children have serious illnesses than do adults, suggesting that the concerns and disruptions addressed in the literature about childhood illness are particularly significant (Feetham & Frink, 1998). Within the adult-focused reports, the literature addressing problems of frail and demented elders dominates. In addition, AIDS in children and adults, cancer in the young and old, and home-care experiences with children and elders are frequently covered topics. Research on the family participation in pain control is developing, as is the literature about the family experiences related to organ donation. Untimely death and the experiences of bereavement have been explored in a number of cultural groups (Martinson, Davis, et al., 1995; Martinson, McClowry, Davies, & Kuhlenkamp, 1994), adding to our understanding of the cultural meanings assigned to death and cancer. Chesla (1989) has investigated the family's

TABLE 13.3. Source of Information

Mothers
Andrews, Williams, and Neil, 1993
Cohen, Nehring, Malm, and Harris, 1995
Frye and D'Avanzo, 1994
Gallo, Breitmayer, Knafl, and Zoeller, 1993
Keltner, Keltner, and Farren, 1990
King, 1993
LoBiondo-Wood, Bernier-Henn, and Williams, 1992
McClowry, Giangrande, Tommasini, Clinton, Foreman, Lunch, and Ferketich, 1994
Saiki, Martinson, and Inano, 1994
Sawyer, 1992
Youngblut, Loveland-Cherry, and Horan, 1993

Elders and caregivers
Archbold, Stewart, Greenlick, and Harvath, 1990
Archbold, Stewart, Miller, Harvath, Greenlick, Van Buren, Kirschling, Valanis, Brody, Schook, and Hagan, 1995
Bull, 1992
Bull, 1993
Given, Stommel, Collins, King, and Given, 1990
Grafstrom, Norberg, and Hagberg, 1993
Langner, 1995
Langner, 1993
Lewis, Curtis, and Lundy, 1995
Magilvy, Congdon, and Martinez, 1994
Phillips, Morrison, Steffl, Young, Cromwell, and Russell, 1995
Wallhagen, 1992

Couples
Lewis and Deal, 1995
Powell-Cope, 1995

Caregiver, other pair
Atkinson, 1992
Ferrell, Johnson, Grant, Fowler, and Corbisiero, 1993
Given, Given, Stommel, Collins, King, and Franklin, 1992
Reinhard, 1994
Robinson, 1990
Stuifbergen, 1990

Parents
Chesla, 1991
Chesla, 1989
Cohen, 1995
Cohen and Martinson, 1988
Dashiff, 1993
Donnelly, 1994
Dragone, 1990
Hirose and Ueda, 1990
Hymovich, 1993
Jerrett, 1994
Kachoyeanos and Selder, 1993
Lemmer, 1991
Leonard, Brust, and Nelson, 1993
Miles, Funk, and Kasper, 1992
Najarian, 1995
Patterson, Jernell, Leonard, and Titus, 1994
Ray and Ritchie, 1993
Rhiner, Ferrell, Shapiro, and Dierkes, 1994
Van Riper, Ryff, and Pridham, 1992

Family
Brackley, 1994
Brown and Powell-Cope, 1993
Bull, 1990
Cohen, 1995
Cohen, 1993
Cornman, 1993
Cossette, Levesque, and Laurin, 1995
Davis and Grant, 1994
Dodd, Dibble, and Thomas, 1992
Elfert, Anderson, and Lai, 1991
Failla and Jones, 1991
Ferrell, Grant, Chan, Ahn, and Ferrell, 1995
Ferrell, Rhiner, Shapiro, and Dierkes, 1994
Fink, 1995
Fleming, Challela, Eland, Hornick, Johnson, Martinson, Nativio, Nokes, Nokes, Riddle, Steele, Sudele, Thomas, Turner, Wheele, and Young, 1994
Gagliardi, 1991

Family (*continued*)
Halm, Titler, Kleiber, Johnson, Montgomery, Craft, Buckwalter, Nicholson, and Megivern, 1993
Hartshorn and Byers, 1994
Hilton, 1994
Hilton and Starzomski, 1994
Hough, Lewis, and Woods, 1991
Klein-Berndt, 1991
Lingren, 1990
Mackenzie and Holroyd, 1995
McCarthy and Gallo, 1992
McShane, Bumbalo, and Patsdaughter, 1994
Norbeck, Chafetz, Wilson, and Weiss, 1991
Pelletier, 1993
Prudhoe and Peters, 1995
Sayles-Cross, 1993
Schumaker, Dodd, and Paul, 1993
Sharkey, 1995
Snelling, 1994
Snowdon, Cameron, and Dunham, 1994
Taylor, Ferrell, Grant, and Cheyney, 1993
Tomlinson, White, and Wilson, 1990
Tomlinson and Mitchell, 1992
Woods, Haberman, and Packard, 1993
Woods and Lewis, 1995
Whyte, 1992
Wuest, Ericson, and Stern, 1994
Youngblut, Brennan, and Swegart, 1994
Robinson, 1990
Germino, Fife, and Funk, 1995
Germino and Funk, 1993
Knafl, Breitmayer, Gallo, and Zoeller, 1996

Spouse
Artinian and Duggan, 1993
Bohachick and Anton, 1990
Hilbert, 1994

"explanatory model" of schizophrenia among Anglo and Filipino families and is now exploring how Anglo and Latino couples in which one person has non-insulin-dependent diabetes understand what causes and influences the diabetes (Fisher, Chesla, Bartz, Gilliss, & Kantor, NIH/NIDDK Grant No. 1 R01 DK49816, *NIDDM in Anglo and Hispanic Families*).

Conceptual Framework

Despite a long-standing call for the inclusion of theoretical or conceptual frameworks, descriptions of theory in the reviewed reports were surprisingly limited. The majority of reports described the use of qualitative

TABLE 13.4. Health Problems Under Study

AIDS
  Andrews, Williams, and Neil, 1993
  Brown and Powell-Cope, 1993
  Cohen, Nehring, Malm, and Harris, 1995
  McShane, Bumbalo, and Patsdaughter, 1994
  Powell-Cope, 1995

Asthma
  Donnelly, 1994

Broncho-pulmonary dysplasia and preterms
  Klein-Berndt, 1991
  Miles, Funk, and Kasper, 1992
  Youngblut, Loveland-Cherry, and Horan, 1993

Cancer, child and adult
  Cohen, 1995a
  Cohen, 1995b
  Cohen, 1993
  Cohen and Martinson, 1988
  Cornman, 1993
  Dodd, Dibble, and Thomas, 1992
  Ferrell, Rhiner, Shapiro, and Dierkes, 1994
  Ferrell, Grant, Chan, Ahn, and Ferrell, 1995
  Ferrell, Johnson, Grant, Fowler, and Corbisiero, 1993
  Hilton, 1994
  Hough, Lewis, and Woods, 1991
  Hymovich, 1993
  Martinson, Davis, Liu-Chiang, Yi-Hua, Qiao, and Gan, 1995
  Martinson, McClowry, Davies, and Kuhlenkamp, 1994
  Lewis and Deal, 1995
  Rhiner, Ferrell, Shapiro, and Dierkes, 1994
  Saiki, Martinson, and Inano, 1994
  Schumaker, Dodd, and Paul, 1993
  Taylor, Ferrell, Grant, and Cheyney, 1993

Cardiac
  Artinian and Duggan, 1993
  Bohachick and Anton, 1990
  Hilbert, 1994

Chronic illness
  Dragone, 1990
  Elfert, Anderson, and Lai, 1991
  Gallo, Breitmayer, Knafl, and Zoeller, 1993
  Jerrett, 1994
  McCarthy and Gallo, 1992
  Ray and Ritchie, 1993
  Sharkey, 1995
  Stuifbergen, 1990
  Woods and Lewis, 1995
  Whyte, 1992

Conduct disorders
  Keltner, Keltner, and Farren, 1990

Critical care
  Chesla, 1996
  Halm, Titler, Kleiber, Johnson, Montgomery, Craft, Buckwalter, Nicholson, and Megivern, 1993
  Klein-Berndt, 1991
  Prudhoe and Peters, 1995
  Tomlinson and Mitchell, 1992

Cystic fibrosis
  Sawyer, 1992

Death
  Kachoyeanos and Selder, 1993
  Lemmer, 1991

Diabetes
  Dashiff, 1993

Disabled dependents
  Atkinson, 1992
  Failla and Jones, 1991
  Snowdon, Cameron, and Dunham, 1994
  Van Riper, Ryff, and Pridham, 1992

Frail elders
  Archbold, Stewart, Greenlick, and Harvath, 1990
  Archbold, Stewart, Miller, Harvath, Greenlick, Van Buren, Kirschling, Valanis, Brody, Schook, and Hagen, 1995

Cerebral palsy
  Hirose and Ueda, 1990

Caregiving
  Brackley, 1994
  Bull, 1990
  Bull, 1992
  Bull, 1993
  Cossette, Levesque, and Laurin, 1995
  Davis and Grant, 1994
  Fink, 1995
  Given, Given, Stommel, Collins, King, and Franklin, 1992
  Given, Stommel, Collins, King, and Given, 1990
  Grafstrom, Norberg, and Hagberg, 1993
  King, 1993
  Langner, 1995
  Langner, 1993
  Lewis and Deal, 1995
  Lingren, 1990
  MacKenzie and Holroyd, 1995
  Magilvy, Congdon, and Martinez, 1994
  Phillips, Morrison, Steffl, Young, Cromwell, and Russell, 1995
  Robinson, 1990
  Sayles-Cross, 1993
  Wallhagen, 1992
  Wuest, Ericson, and Stern, 1994

Liver/pediatrics
  Simon and Smith, 1992

Medically fragile children
  Leonard, Brust, and Nelson, 1993
  Patterson, Jernell, Leonard, and Titus, 1994
  Youngblut, Brennan, and Swegart, 1994

Muscular distrophy
  Gagliardi, 1991

Organ donation
  Hilton and Starzomski, 1994
  LoBiondo-Wood, Bernier-Henn, and Williams, 1992
  Pelletier, 1993

Pain (see also Cancer)
  Snelling, 1994

Schizophrenia and mental health
  Chesla, 1991
  Najarian, 1995
  Norbeck, Chafetz, Wilson, and Weiss, 1991
  Reinhard, 1994

Seizure disorders
  Hartshorn and Byers, 1994

Technology dependents
  Fleming, Challela, Eland, Hornick, Johnson, Martinson, Nativio, Nokes, Riddle, Steele, Sudele, Thomas, Turner, Wheele, and Young, 1994

Temperament
  McClowery, Giangrande, Tommasini, Clinton, Foreman, Lynch, and Ferketich, 1994

Violence
  Frye and D'Avanzo, 1994

methods or listed no theoretical perspectives when using quantitative methods. Of the qualitative approaches employed, many authors did not identify a qualitative approach or a research stance or perspective.

Among the theories or frameworks employed, some well-known theories were identified, as were a promising number of new, substantive frameworks. The most often appearing grand or middle-range theories were those derived from symbolic interaction: stress and coping approaches and family stress (McCubbin, Patterson), role theory, or family adaptation and family hardiness (McCubbin). Systems theories were also evident, especially in the adult-focused literature. In keeping with the move toward substantive theory development, the focus of many of the reviewed reports was on the specific illness situation faced by families (e.g., pain control), rather than the broader and more illusive concepts of coping or adaptation. As such, these reports were contextualized in the most difficult and common health care problems of our times: cancer or chronic illness in children, medically fragile children cared for at home, HIV/AIDS-care in the home, and caregiving for the elderly.

Among those employing qualitative approaches for data collection and analysis, the most frequently cited method was grounded theory, followed by content analysis, ethnography, and phenomenology. Rigorous use of these methods appeared variable at best, and little attempt was made to address the issues of rigor in the majority of the reports. Generally, these reports sought to develop a concept or a beginning framework to explain a family's experience in managing an illness.

The development of substantive frameworks that relate to families and the health care issues they face is one important aspect of this review. Although the theories and frameworks address more specific areas of concern for families and nursing practice, few have attempted to identify approaches to nursing intervention. Since the mid-1980s, Knafl and Deatrick have been adding to our understanding of how the parents of ill children manage the child's illness (Deatrick & Knafl, 1988, 1990; Deatrick, Knafl, & Walsh, 1988; Knafl, 1985; Knafl & Deatrick, 1986, 1987). Their Family Management Style Model was developed through both careful concept analysis and data collection and analysis. Following a symbolic interaction tradition, the framework conceptualizes family response to childhood chronic illness as the interplay between how individual family members define and manage their situation. When dealing with a chronic condition, research based on the Family Management

Style Framework suggests that many families try to "normalize" the child's and the family's existence. This framework, developed over a decade and across a variety of samples, provides direction for further exploration of what matters to which families and how to be helpful to them.

Austin's program of research with children who have epilepsy has resulted in a Model of Family Adaptation to New-Onset Epilepsy (Austin, 1996). Building on the Double ABCX Model of McCubbin and Patterson (1983), Austin's model proposes that the characteristics at onset (family demands and resources, as well as the child's characteristics and illness features and functioning) influence an adaptation process (changes in the family demands, resources, and child seizure condition, as well as parent and child attitudes and coping responses) that can be influenced by psychosocial nursing care. Adaptation outcomes result for both the child and the family. Although nursing care is introduced into this model, the nature of that care is not specified, as "families need different types and levels of care based on the child's condition and the family characteristics" (p. 86). Clearly, the focus of the next stage of work with this framework will be to further develop the details of this soundly established framework.

LaMontagne has employed a stress and coping framework to develop a model of Parental Stress and Coping when children are patients in critical care (LaMontagne, Johnson, & Hepworth, 1995). This model also proposes that coping interventions can address the problem-focused issues or the emotion-focused issues faced by parents. However, the author notes, "Coping interventions will differ according to the person factors, such as the age of the child and age of the parent, and the situational factors, such as the type of support available during the experience" (p. 217). However, no approaches to intervention are proposed.

Ferrell's work appeared in the late 1980s and early 1990s. The Impact of Pain on the Dimensions of Quality of Life Model has resulted from the work of her team with families of persons with cancer who were trying to manage pain at home (Ferrell, Rhiner, Cohen, & Grant, 1991; Ferrell, Rhiner, Shapiro, & Dierkes, 1994; Ferrell & Schneider, 1988). The model depicts four domains of pain: physical well-being and symptoms; psychological well-being; social well-being; and spiritual well-being. Using this model, Ferrell and colleagues have evaluated the positive impact of pain education on the knowledge and attitudes of caregivers. As pain management is a significant problem for many caregivers and can contribute to their sense of caregiving burden, this model and the related intervention provide a specific example of how to be helpful in the family management of this specific problem.

Lewis and colleagues tested a multidimensional theoretical model to determine how the individual effects of a mother's illness would affect her children, the marriage, and the parent-child relationship (Lewis, Hammond, & Woods, 1993). This program of research serves as an example of a longitudinal, statistically sophisticated effort. The authors found that illness demands were predictive of depressed mood, which was significantly associated with poorer marital quality. Families in which the marital relationship was of poorer quality functioned less well, as reflected in problem solving and providing feedback to one another. Social supports reduced the likelihood of depression for mothers, and, surprisingly, higher levels of economic status predicted lower levels of marital adjustment. Although the authors suggest that this recursive approach to unidirectional causality probably oversimplifies the life of a family, the findings provide invaluable insights into individual and family response to illness. The model suggests that one useful intervention involves lowering the illness demands experienced by the family.

Gilliss and colleagues (Gilliss, Gortner, et al., 1993) tested an intervention with individuals recovering from cardiac bypass and valve surgery and their caregiving partner (usually spouse). Based on the Double ABCX Model, nurses provided advice and support to recovering couples by telephone for 3 months following hospital discharge. This intervention was conceptualized as an additional resource to families. Although patients reported improved exercise ability in early recovery, the experimental families did not demonstrate significance on any of the family measures through the first 6 months following discharge. This study employed a family theoretical approach and used a controlled clinical trial design to evaluate the effect of an intervention. A significant effect of the treatment was not detected for families. The fit between family and intervention, reported to be the reason that no intervention effect could be identified in the frameworks described earlier, could have been the missing piece in this effort. In other words, some efforts must be made to determine which intervention will be useful for which family, based on the family's situation and characteristics. A framework has not yet developed within nursing that acknowledges the importance of that fit. Additionally, Archbold and Stewart (1992) have noted that measures able to detect effects for families are not abundant.

▦ Family Phenomena

The specific aspect of family life addressed in the literature is presented in Table 13.5. The language with which the life of the family is described relies heavily on the language used to describe the individual family member. Thus, although relationships are often the focus of inquiry, most identified variables describe some aspect of one person's experience and not in relationship to another's. Common examples include stress, burden, caring, caregiving, appraisal, mood, resources, demands, symptoms, self-esteem, marital satisfaction, and parenting role. Given the prominence of symbolic interaction in the family science literature, the examination of individual variables in relationship to each other might be expected, but it is not evident.

Our review suggests that some findings might be grouped to address the family's, or some aspect of the family's, experience with illness. Several over-time processes common among families can be seen. Generally, families must formulate an initial response to illness, including defining the threat, impact, and experience and a beginning understanding of how to adapt family life, garner resources, and treat the illness. The initial response is followed by a period in which the family must continue to develop and refine its management of the illness but must also learn to manage the illness in light of other, ongoing aspects of life that are not illness specific (e.g., driving the car pool, supervising homework or playing). The balancing of life's demands with those of the illness has been referred to by some as "keeping the illness in its place" (Robinson, 1993; Wright, Watson, & Bell, 1996). Despite the fact that this phenomenon has been the subject of an increasing number of investigations, few theorists or reviews seem to document this trend. The net effect, of course, is that new studies do not build on this idea, which may limit the development of the science. In addition, the literature continues to feature papers on caregiving across the life cycle (e.g., parent-child, spouse caring for ill spouse, caregiving for the elderly), with a rapidly proliferating focus on caregiving for the elderly.

One growing area is the relationship between the family and the caregiving system (see also the special issue of *Journal of Family Nursing*, 2(2), 1996, Sandra Faux and Kathleen Knafl, editors, devoted to relationships between health care providers and families). This relationship, especially challenging to measure, is one of the foci of the work of Magilvy, Congdon, and Martinez (1994).

TABLE 13.5. Phenomena Under Study

Recovery and transition	Parental or familial distress	Parental or familial distress *(continued)*
Bull, 1993	Bohachick and Anton, 1990	McShane, Bumbalo, and Patsdaughter, 1994
Familial bonds	Cohen, Nehring, Malm, and Harris, 1995	Miles, Funk, and Kasper, 1992
Andrews, Neil, and Williams, 1993	Cohen, 1995	Najarian, 1995
	Cohen, 1993	Norbeck, Chafetz, Wilson, and Weiss, 1991
Caregiving	Cohen and Martinson, 1988	Pelletier, 1993
Archbold, Stewart, Greenlick, and Harvath, 1990	Cornman, 1993	Powell-Cope, 1995
Archbold, Stewart, Miller, Harvath, Greenlick, Van Buren, Krischling, Valanis, Brody, Schook, and Hagen, 1995	Dashiff, 1993	Prudhoe and Peters, 1995
	Dodd, Dibble, and Thomas, 1992	Ray and Ritchie, 1993
Artinian and Duggan, 1993	Donnelly, 1994	Rhiner, Ferrell, Shapiro, and Dierkes, 1994
Atkinson, 1992	Dragone, 1990	Saiki, Martinson, and Inano, 1994
Brackley, 1994	Elfert, Anderson, and Lai, 1991	Sawyer, 1992
Brown and Powell-Cope, 1993	Failla and Jones, 1991	Schumaker, Dodd, and Paul, 1993
Bull, 1990	Ferrell, Rhiner, Shapiro, and Dierkes, 1994	Sharkey, 1995
Bull, 1992	Fink, 1995	Simon and Smith, 1992
Chesla, 1989	Fleming, Challela, Eland, Hornick, Johnson, Martinson, Nativio, Nokes, Riddle, Steele, Sudele, Thomas, Turner, Wheele, and Young, 1994	Shelling, 1994
Chesla, 1991		Snowdon, Cameron, and Dunham, 1994
Cohen, 1995	Frye and d'Avanzo, 1994	Stuifbergen, 1990
Cossette, Levesque, and Laurin, 1995	Gagliardi, 1991	Taylor, Ferrell, Grant, and Cheyney, 1993
Davis and Grant, 1994	Gallo, Breitmayer, Knafl, and Zoeller, 1993	Tomlinson, White, and Wilson, 1990
Ferrell, Grant, Chan, Ahn, and Ferrell, 1995	Halm, Titler, Kleiber, Johnson, Montgomery, Craft, Buckwalter, Nicholson, and Megivern, 1993	Tomlinson and Mitchell, 1992
Ferrell, Johnson, Grant, Fowler, and Corbisiero, 1993		Van Riper, Ryff, and Pridham, 1992
Given, Given, Stommel, Collins, King, and Franklin, 1992	Hartshorn and Byers, 1994	Woods, Haberman, and Packard, 1993
Given, Stommel, Collins, King, and Given, 1990	Hilbert, 1994	Woods and Lewis, 1995
	Hilton, 1994	Wuest, Ericson, and Stern, 1994
Grafstrom, Norberg, and Hagberg, 1993	Hilton and Starzomski, 1994	Youngblut, Brennan, and Swegart, 1994
King, 1993	Hirose and Ueda, 1990	Youngblut, Loveland-Cherry, and Horan, 1993
Langner, 1995	Hough, Lewis, and Woods, 1991	Younger, 1991
Langner, 1993	Hymovich, 1993	
Lewis, Curtis, and Lundy, 1995	Jerrett, 1994	
Lingren, 1996	Kachoyeanos and Selder, 1993	
MacKenzie and Holroyd, 1995	Keltner, Keltner, and Farren, 1990	
Magilvy, Congdon, and Martinez, 1994	Klein-Berndt, 1991	
Patterson, Jernell, Leonard, and Titus, 1994	Lemmer, 1991	
Phillips, Morrrison, Steffl, Young, Cromwell, and Russell, 1995	Leonard, Brust, and Nelson, 1993	
	Lewis and Deal, 1995	
Reinhard, 1994	LoBiondo-Wood, Bernier-Helm, and Williams, 1992	
Robinson, 1990	McCarthy and Gallo, 1992	
Sayles-Cross, 1993	McClowery, Giangrande, Tommasini, Clinton, Foreman, Lynch, and Ferketich, 1994	
Wallhagen, 1992		
Whyte, 1992		

The relationship of families to their larger community context is of practical interest to nurses, but measurement and theoretical barriers have limited our understanding of the nature of these relationships.

▰ *What Do We Know About Families?*

In fact, based on our empirical scientific work, we may know less about families than we would wish to acknowledge. This chapter suggests that traditional scientific work in the nursing of families continues to be largely atheoretical, with few empirical findings leading to intervention studies that might ultimately guide nursing practice. Few programs of qualitative work have developed to a point where useful generalizations can be offered. For some qualitative programs, generalizations are not an expected outcome. For instance, Heideggerian phenomenology, as represented through interpretive phenomenology, seeks to understand rather than to generalize. In doing so, the nurse/scientist/clinician is changed and potentially open to new possibilities in future interactions. In the development of grounded theory, a framework for understanding is sought. This framework can serve as a way of organizing the empirical world.

With respect to midlife families and acute or chronic illness, many investigators have described the stress experienced by female spouses in caring for their male (patient) partners. More recently, the microdynamics possibly underlying that stress have been described (Coyne & Smith, 1991) as a process by which the wife ignores aspects of family life or illness management that she believes will result in conflict. Rather than engage in this distressing conflict, she silently endures the distress, often leading to increased depression, distress, or physical symptomology. Coyne and Smith have referred to this as "protective buffering." Learning how to manage conflict and personal responsibility for illness management may be helpful to these men and women; helping couples deal with new and frightening experiences may be the appropriate family intervention.

With aging families, the literature on caregiving has produced some reliable findings on who is burdened, by what, and if or when they will institutionalize the ill family member. Interventions have been aimed at key variables in this theoretical equation. Nonetheless, this literature has lacked precision, ignoring the effects of family role and gender on the caregiving relationship. The contribution of these two master variables has not been evaluated in nursing research.

Where Do We Go From Here?

A number of critical questions remain to be addressed as we advance our understanding of how to be caring and helpful to families experiencing non-normative health care transitions.

1. When should we intervene? The timing of interventions is important, as they will likely vary as to content and possibly according to the family's openness to change. Although some aspects of timing will be particular to each family, some issues in timing may relate to the illness process. During diagnosis, a focus on the meaning that the family attributes to the situation may be more relevant than a focus on the way in which it manages the

illness. Although some of the developing literature locates its theoretical explanations in the timing of the illness, much of it does not. It would be useful to have more studies of how nurses have worked with families early in the illness experience to shape the meaning (definition of the situation) in a way that facilitates coping, as described by Wright and colleagues (Wright, Watson, & Bell, 1996). These interventions are likely to be substantively different from interventions that help families to address ongoing problems. In fact, the question of when to intervene with families may be the wrong question; a particular intervention might be appropriate at any time. Perhaps the question should be, How should the intervention vary according to the stage of illness? as proposed by Rolland (1984).

2. Why do we still think that there is one "right" outcome for all families? The review suggests that researchers are still trying to attain one specific outcome, rather than a typology or range of outcomes, for families. As written, most contemporary theories continue to suggest that there is one "right" way for each family to behave, and only one correct end point (for example, for families to *discuss* problems or *reach agreement* on solutions). Given the inability of most analyses to account for more than 45% of the variance, this seems unwarranted and unfruitful. Perhaps families should be invited to define their own outcomes, as suggested by Wright, Watson, and Bell (1996)? If this were to be the case, how would nurses and families work together so that professional and practical expertise from both parties informs the desired outcome?

What do we know about how outcomes change over time? Endpoints are ever changing. The transitioning of responsibility for illness management from parent to child varies over time. First, the parent assumes most of the responsibility. Then the aging child takes on and masters the treatment regimen. Next the child begins learning how to adapt that treatment regimen in ways that balance issues of health with quality of life.

The fit of intervention to the family must also receive greater attention. Given the style and characteristics of a particular family, what intervention would they select? Which intervention would be effective for them?

3. What are the relationships among clinicians, theorists, and researchers? Is there interaction and collaboration? Family therapists, theorists, and researchers from other disciplines have long recognized that they use different theories to support their work and that researchers cannot always measure the effects of therapeutic intervention (Campbell & Patterson, 1995). Although we hope for more in nursing, the results appear similar to those in other fields and may suggest one reason why our theoretical models are not accounting for variance: The models are not based on a practical reality with corresponding empirical referents. As mentioned earlier, the traditional scientific approach to development and testing of interventions fails to consider the wide variation in circumstances of families, illness characteristics, developmental levels of people and families, and the social and community circumstances that influence family life. Perhaps, as suggested by Chesla (personal communication, February 12, 1997), it is time to thoughtfully observe and report on real practice to learn what works in family nursing.

Campbell and Patterson (1995) point out that we are just beginning to understand what family variables are important to physical health and how they exert their influences. They write that four types of family intervention are reported in the literature: family therapy, family psychoeducation, family information and support, and direct care. Different families may need different services at different times; different services may produce effects that are measurable, even though others do not. In an integrative review and meta-analysis of a collection of interdisciplinary studies reporting the results of family psychoeducation, information, and support, Gilliss and Davis (1993) found significant effects of these interventions. Thus, we conclude that, like other professional groups, we continue to struggle with difficult questions to find answers that we believe can be found. However, forging a closer link between those who care for families and those who study families is likely to bring us to better answers.

4. Is family nursing science building cumulatively? Why, despite all the periodic reviews of family research, is there not a better sense of the accumulation of our knowledge? According to Whall and Loveland-Cherry (1993), few programs of research have described family experience and gone on to demonstrate the effects of intervention. Perhaps, as noted above, this traditional pattern will not be observed in family nursing. Unlike Hayes's (1993) conclusion, our review suggests that interest in family nursing research and practice continues to grow. Further, it is increasingly difficult to locate this literature, as nurse authors increasingly publish with interdisciplinary teams in interdisciplinary journals. Unlike past reviews of the state of family nursing science,

where the papers were easily located in nursing journals, in this review it was discovered that contemporary papers appear in both nursing and interdisciplinary journals. The improved scientific rigor of nursing research may be responsible for this distribution, but cataloging the work has become more challenging.

Perhaps more attention needs to be given to the rigor with which critical reviews are conducted, both in summarizing the literature and in developing background knowledge sections for ongoing scientific work. Useful guidelines exist for conducting integrative reviews (Broome, 1993; Ganong, 1987) and these ensure that the review process is systematic and results in a critical synthesis of the literature. Moreover, these guidelines help clarify the purpose of the review (e.g., focus on method, substantive results). Dunkin (1996) provides an especially useful discussion of the errors that often occur in knowledge synthesis efforts—unexplained selectivity, lack of discrimination of research quality, erroneous detailing, double counting (different reports from the same study used as evidence for the same finding), nonrecognition of faulty author conclusions, unwarranted attributions, suppression of contrary findings, consequential errors, and failure to marshal all evidence relevant to a generalization. Guidelines such as these support the effective synthesis of the literature.

Conclusion

As we noted throughout our own work on this chapter, our contemporary understanding of the family is based on a blurring of disciplinary boundaries. No one discipline "owns" the family, and, as a result, the general literature is fragmented and presented from many disciplinary perspectives. To specifically identify what we know in nursing creates both an impossible task and an artificial boundary. Can we identify what we know about pain control that is solely a function of nursing science and theory, independent of basic science? Family nursing theory, research, and intervention is similarly integrated, making the specific identification of nursing knowledge difficult.

However, what does appear to be clear is that the current nursing literature does not provide significant empirical evidence for the effect of nursing interventions with families. Although many have called for revisions of scientific approach or technique to remedy this, we would also invite the reader to reconsider the literature that we are overlooking when we exclude reports of clinical work with families from our periodic reviews of nursing science. There may be invaluable insights in these reports.

Progress in this field is achieved through many approaches, including new theoretical paradigms, new treatments, and new approaches to the conduct of our research. One additional important activity is the periodic and self-conscious review of our developing literature. These analyses have the potential to stimulate midcourse corrections and identify new directions for our work. We have enjoyed the chance to work together to develop this review, and we hope that it will be useful to those who care about and for families.

References

Anderson, K. H., & Tomlinson, P. S. (1992). The family health system as an emerging paradigmatic view for nursing. *Image: The Journal of Nursing Scholarship, 24,* 57-63.

Andrews, S., Williams, A., & Neil, K. (1993). The mother-child relationship in the HIV-1 positive family. *Image: The Journal of Nursing Scholarship, 25,* 193-198.

Archbold, P. G., & Stewart, B. J. (1992). Nursing intervention studies require outcome measures that are sensitive to change: Part one. *Research in Nursing and Health, 5,* 477-481.

Archbold, P., Stewart, B., Greenlick, M., & Harvath, T. (1990). Mutuality and preparedness as predictors of care giver role strain. *Research in Nursing and Health, 13,* 375-384.

Archbold, P. G., Stewart, B. J., Miller, L. L., Harvath, T. A., Greenlick, M. R., Van Buren, L., Kirschling, J. M., Valanis, B. G., Brody, K. K., Schook, J. E., & Hagen, J. (1995). The PREP system of nursing interventions: A pilot test with families caring for older members. Preparedness (PR), enrichment (E) and predictability (P). *Research in Nursing and Health, 18,* 3-16.

Artinian, N., & Duggan, C. (1993). Patterns of demands experienced by spouses following coronary bypass surgery. *Clinical Nursing Research, 2,* 278-295.

Atkinson, I. (1992). Experiences of informal care givers providing nursing support for disabled dependants. *Journal of Advanced Nursing, 17,* 835-840.

Austin, J. (1991). Family adaptation to a child's chronic illness. *Annual Review of Nursing Research, 9,* 103-120.

Austin, J. (1996). Model of Family Adaptation to New-Onset Childhood Epilepsy. *Journal of Neuroscience Nursing, 28*(2), 82-92.

Bohachick, P., & Anton, B. (1990). Psychosocial adjustment of patients and spouses to severe cardiomyopathy. *Research in Nursing and Health, 13,* 385-392.

Bomar, P. (Ed.). (1989). *Nurses as family health promotion.* Baltimore: Williams & Wilkins.

Bournaki, M., & Germain, C. P. (1993). Esthetic knowledge in family-centered nursing care of hospitalized children. *Advances in Nursing Science, 16*(2), 81-89.

Brackley, M. (1994). The plight of American family care givers: Implications for nursing. *Perspectives in Psychiatric Care, 30*(4), 14-20.

Bridges, J. M., & Lynam, M. J. (1993). Informal care givers: A Marxist analysis of social, political, and economic forces underpinning the role. *Advances in Nursing Science, 15*(3), 33-48.

Broome, M. (1993). Integrative reviews in the development of concepts. In B. Rodgers & K. Knafl (Eds.), *Concept development in nursing.* Philadelphia: W. B. Saunders.

Brown, M., & Powell-Cope, G. (1993). Themes of loss and dying in caring for a family member with AIDS. *Research in Nursing and Health, 16,* 179-191.

Bull, M. J. (1990). Factors influencing family care giver burden and health. *Western Journal of Nursing Research, 12,* 758-776.

Bull, M. (1992). Managing the transition from hospital to home. *Qualitative Health Research, 2,* 27-41.

Bull, M. J. (1993). Use of formal community services by elders and their family care givers 2 weeks following hospital discharge. *Journal of Advanced Nursing, 19*(3), 503-508.

Campbell, J. C., Harris, M. J., & Lee, R. K. (1995). Violence research: An overview. *Scholarly Inquiry for Nursing Practice: An International Journal, 9*(2), 105-126.

Campbell, T., & Patterson, J. (1995). The effectiveness of family interventions in the treatment of physical illness. *Journal of Marital and Family Therapy, 21,* 545-583.

Campbell, T. L. (1986). Family's impact on health: A critical review and annotated bibliography. *Family Systems Medicine, 4,* 135-328.

Chesla, C. (1989). Parents' illness models of schizophrenia. *Archives of Psychiatric Nursing, 3,* 208-225.

Chesla, C. (1991). Parents' caring practices of their schizophrenic offspring. *Qualitative Health Research, 1,* 446-468.

Clements, I. W., & Roberts, F. B. (1983). *Family health: A theoretical approach to nursing care.* New York: John Wiley.

Cohen, F., Nehring, W., Malm, K., & Harris, D. (1995). Family experiences when a child is HIV-positive: Reports of natural and foster parents. *Pediatric Nursing, 21,* 248-254.

Cohen, M. (1993). The unknown and the unknowable: Managing sustained uncertainty. *Western Journal of Nursing Research, 15*(1), 77-96.

Cohen, M. (1995a). The stages of the prediagnostic period in chronic, life-threatening childhood illness: A process analysis. *Research in Nursing and Health, 18,* 39-48.

Cohen, M. (1995b). The triggers of heightened parental uncertainty in chronic, life-threatening childhood illness. *Qualitative Health Research, 5,* 63-77.

Cohen, M., & Martinson, I. (1988). Chronic uncertainty: Its effect on parental appraisal of a child's health. *Journal of Pediatric Nursing, 3,* 89-96.

Cornman, B. (1993). Childhood cancer: Differential effects on the family members. *Oncology Nursing Forum, 20,* 1559-1566.

Cossette, S., Levesque, L., & Laurin, L. (1995). Informal and formal support for care givers of a demented relative: Do gender and kinship make a difference? *Research in Nursing and Health, 18,* 437-451.

Coyne, J. C., & Smith, D. A. (1991). Couples coping with a myocardial infarction: A contextual perspective on wives' distress. *Journal of Personality and Social Psychology, 6,* 404-412.

Dashiff, C. (1993). Parent's perceptions of diabetes in adolescent daughters and its impact on the family. *Journal of Pediatric Nursing, 8,* 361-369.

Davis, L. L., & Grant, J. S. (1994). Constructing the reality of recovery: Family home care management strategies. *Advances in Nursing Science, 17*(2), 66-76.

Deatrick, J. A., & Knafl, K. A. (1988). Developing programs for hospitalized children: Clinical significance of qualitative research. *Journal of Pediatric Nursing, 3,* 123-126.

Deatrick, J. A., & Knafl, K. (1990). Family management behaviors: Concept synthesis. *Journal of Pediatric Nursing, 5,* 15-22.

Deatrick, J. A., Knafl, K. A., & Walsh, M. (1988). The process of parenting a child with a disability: Normalization through accommodations. *Journal of Advanced Nursing, 13,* 15-21.

Dodd, M., Dibble, S., & Thomas, M. (1992). Outpatient chemotherapy: Patients' and family members' concerns and coping strategies. *Public Health Nursing, 9,* 37-44.

Donnelly, E. (1994). Parents of children with asthma: An examination of family hardiness, family stressors and family functioning. *Journal of Pediatric Nursing, 9,* 398-408.

Dragone, M. (1990). Perspectives of chronically ill adolescents and parents on health care needs. *Pediatric Nursing, 16,* 45-50.

Dunkin, M. (1996). Types of errors in synthesizing research in education. *Review of Educational Research, 66*(2), 87-97.

Elfert, H., Anderson, J. M., & Lai, M. (1991). Parents' perceptions of children with chronic illness: A study of immigrant Chinese families. *Journal of Pediatric Nursing, 6,* 114-120.

Failla, S., & Jones, L. (1991). Families of children with developmental disabilities: An examination of family hardiness. *Research in Nursing and Health, 14,* 41-50.

Faux, S. A., & Knafl, K. A. (Eds.). (1996). Relationships between health care providers and families. *Journal of Family Nursing, 2*(2) [Special issue].

Feetham, S. (1984). Family research: Issues and directions in nursing. In H. Werley & J. Fitzpatrick (Eds.), *Annual review of nursing 2* (pp. 3-25). New York: Springer.

Feetham, S. (1991). Conceptual and methodological issues in research of families. In A. Whall & J. Fawcett (Eds.), *Family theory development in nursing: State of the science and art* (pp. 55-68). Philadelphia: F. A. Davis.

Feetham, S. L., & Frink, B. B. (1998). Issues in health services research: Children and families. In M. Broome, K. Pridham, K. Knafl, & S. Feetham (Eds.), *Handbook of children and families in health and illness* (pp. 280-297). Thousand Oaks, CA: Sage.

Ferrell, B., Rhiner, M., Cohen, M., & Grant, M. (1991). Family factors influencing cancer pain management. *Postgraduate Medicine, 67*(Suppl. 2), S64-S69.

Ferrell, B., & Schneider, C. (1988). Experience and management of cancer pain at home. *Cancer Nursing, 11,* 84-90.

Ferrell, B. R., Grant, M., Chan, J., Ahn, C., & Ferrell, B. A. (1995). The impact of cancer pain education on family care givers of elderly patients. *Oncology Nursing Forum, 22,* 1211-1218.

Ferrell, B. R., Rhiner, M., Shapiro, B., & Dierkes, M. (1994). The experience of pediatric cancer pain, Part I: Impact of pain on the family. *Journal of Pediatric Nursing, 9,* 368-379.

Ferrell, B. R., Taylor, E. J., Grant, M., Fowler, M., & Corbisiero, R. M. (1993). Pain management at home: Struggle, comfort, and mission. *Cancer Nursing, 16,* 169-178.

Fink, S. (1995). The influences of family resources and family demands on the strains and well-being of care giving families. *Nursing Research, 44,* 139-146.

Fisher, L., Kokes, R., Ransom, D., Phillips, S., & Rudd, P. (1985). Alternative strategies for creating relational family data. *Family Process, 24,* 213-224.

Fleming, J., Challela, M., Eland, J., Hornick, R., Johnson, P., Martinson, I., Nativio, D., Nokes, K., Riddle, I., Steele, N., Sudele, K., Thomas, R., Turner, Q., Wheele, B., & Young, A. (1994). Impact

on the family of children who are technology dependent and cared for in the home. *Pediatric Nursing, 20,* 379-388.

Forchuk, C., & Dorsay, J. P. (1995). Hildegard Peplau meets family systems nursing: Innovation in theory-based practice. *Journal of Advanced Nursing, 21,* 110-115.

Ford-Gilboe, M., & Campbell, J. (1996). The mother-headed single-parent family: A feminist critique of the nursing literature. *Nursing Outlook, 44,* 173-183.

Friedman, M. M. (1986). *Family nursing: Theory and assessment* (2nd ed.). Norwalk, CT: Appleton-Century-Crofts.

Frye, B., & D'Avanzo, C. (1994). Cultural themes in family stress and violence among Cambodian refugee women in the inner city. *Advances in Nursing Science, 16*(3), 64-77.

Gagliardi, B. A. (1991). The family's experience of living with a child with Duchenne muscular dystrophy. *Applied Nursing Research, 4*(4), 159-164.

Gallo, A., Breitmayer, B., Knafl, K., & Zoeller, L. (1993). Mother's perception of sibling adjustment and family life in childhood chronic illness. *Journal of Pediatric Nursing, 8,* 318-324.

Ganong, L. H. (1987). Integrative reviews in nursing research. *Research in Nursing and Health, 10,* 1-11.

Ganong, L. H. (1995). Current trends and issues in family nursing research. *Journal of Family Nursing, 1,* 171-206.

Germino, B. B., Fife, B. L., & Funk, S. G. (1995). Cancer and the partner relationship: What is its meaning? *Seminars in Oncology Nursing, 11*(1), 43-50.

Germino, B. B., & Funk, S. G. (1993). Impact of a parent's cancer on adult children: Role and relationship issues. *Seminars in Oncology Nursing, 9*(2), 101-106.

Gilliss, C. (1983). The family as a unit of analysis: Strategies for the nurse researchers. *Advances in Nursing Science, 5*(3), 50-59.

Gilliss, C. (1991). Family nursing research: Theory and practice. *Image: The Journal of Nursing Scholarship, 23,* 19-22.

Gilliss, C., & Davis, L. (1993). Does family intervention make a difference? An integrative review and meta-analysis. In S. Feetham, S. Meister, J. Bell, & C. Gilliss (Eds.), *The nursing of families* (pp. 259-265). Newbury Park, CA: Sage.

Gilliss, C., Gortner, S., Hauck, W., Shinn, J., Sparacino, P., & Tompkins, C. (1993). A randomized trial of nursing care for recovery from cardiac surgery. *Heart & Lung, 22*(2), 125-133.

Gilliss, C. L. (1989). Family research in nursing. In C. Gilliss, B. Highley, B. Roberts, & I. Martinson, *Toward a science of family nursing.* New York: Addison-Wesley.

Gilliss, C. L., & Davis, L. L. (1992). Family nursing research: Precepts from paragons and peccadilloes. *Journal of Advanced Nursing, 17,* 28-33.

Gilliss, C. L., Highley, B., Roberts, B., & Martinson, I. (1989). *Toward a science of family nursing.* New York: Addison-Wesley.

Given, B., Stommel, M., Collins, C., King, S., & Given, C. (1990). Responses of elderly spouse care givers. *Research in Nursing and Health, 13,* 77-85.

Given, C., Given, B., Stommel, M., Collins, C., King, S., & Franklin, S. (1992). The care giver reaction assessment (CRA) for care givers to persons with chronic physical and mental impairments. *Research in Nursing and Health, 15,* 271-283.

Grafstrom, M., Norberg, A., & Hagberg, B. (1993). Relationships between demented elderly people and the families: A follow-up study of care givers who had previously reported abuse when caring for their spouses and parents. *Journal of Advanced Nursing, 18,* 1747-1757.

Halm, M., Titler, M., Kleiber, C., Johnson, S., Montgomery, L., Craft, M., Buckwalter, K., Nicholson, A., & Megivern, K. (1993). Behavioral responses of family members during critical illness. *Clinical Nursing Research, 2,* 414-437.

Hanson, S.M.H., & Boyd, S. T. (1996). *Family health care nursing: Theory, practice and research.* Philadelphia: F. A. Davis.

Hartshorn, J., & Byers, V. (1994). Importance of health and family variables related to quality of life in individuals with uncontrolled seizures. *American Association of Neuroscience Nurses, 26,* 288-297.

Hayes, V. (1993). Nursing in family care. In S. Feetham, S. Meister, J. Bell, & C. Gilliss (Eds.), *The nursing of families* (pp. 18-29). Newbury Park, CA: Sage.

Hilbert, G. (1994). Cardiac patients and spouses. *Clinical Nursing Research, 3,* 243-252.

Hilton, B. (1994). Family communication patterns in coping with early breast cancer. *Western Journal of Nursing Research, 16,* 336-391.

Hilton, B., & Starzomski, R. (1994). Family decision making about living related kidney donation. *American Nephrology Nurses Association Journal, 21,* 346-355.

Hirose, T., & Ueda, R. (1990). Long-term follow-up of cerebral palsy and coping behaviour of parents. *Journal of Advanced Nursing, 15,* 762-770.

Hough, E. E., Lewis, F. M., & Woods, N. F. (1991). Family response to mother's chronic illness: Case studies of well- and poorly adjusted families. *Western Journal of Nursing Research, 13,* 568-596.

Hymovich, D. (1993). Child-rearing concerns of parents with cancer. *Oncology Nursing Forum, 20,* 1360-1993.

Jerrett, M. (1994). Parents' experience of coming to know the care of their chronically ill child. *Journal of Advanced Nursing, 19,* 1050-1056.

Kachoyeanos, M., & Selder, F. (1993). Life transitions of parents at the unexpected death of a school-aged and older child. *Journal of Pediatric Nursing, 8,* 41-49.

Keltner, B., Keltner, N., & Farren, E. (1990). Family routines and conduct disorders in adolescent girls. *Western Journal of Nursing Research, 12,* 161-174.

King, T. (1993). The experience of midlife daughters who are care givers for their mothers. *Health Care for Women International, 14,* 419-426.

Klein-Berndt, S. (1991). Bronchopulmonary dysplasia in the family: A longitudinal case study. *Pediatric Nursing, 17,* 607-611, 621.

Knafl, K. A. (1985). Living with chronic pain: The spouse's perspective. *Pain, 23,* 259-271.

Knafl, K. A., Breitmayer, B., Gallo, A., & Zoeller, L. (1996). Family response to childhood chronic illness: Description of management styles. *Journal of Pediatric Nursing, 11,* 315-326.

Knafl, K. A., & Deatrick, J. (1986). How families manage chronic conditions: An analysis of the concept of normalization. *Research in Nursing and Health, 9,* 215-222.

Knafl, K. A., & Deatrick, J. (1987). Conceptualizing family response to a child's chronic illness or disability. *Family Relations, 36,* 300-304.

LaMontagne, L. L., Johnson, B. D., & Hepworth, J. T. (1995). Evolution of parental stress and coping processes: A framework for critical care practice. *Journal of Pediatric Nursing, 10,* 212-218.

Langner, S. R. (1993). Ways of managing the experience of care giving to elderly relatives. *Western Journal of Nursing Research, 15,* 582-594.

Langner, S. (1995). Finding meaning in caring for elderly relatives: loss and personal growth. *Holistic Nursing Practice, 9*(3), 74-84.

Lansberry, C. R., & Richards, E. (1992). Family nursing practice paradigm perspectives and diagnostic approaches. *Advances in Nursing Science, 15*(2), 66-75.

Lemmer, C. (1991). Parental perceptions of caring following perinatal bereavement. *Western Journal of Nursing Research, 13,* 475-493.

Leonard, B., Brust, J., & Nelson, R. (1993). Parental distress: Caring for medically fragile children at home. *Journal of Pediatric Nursing, 8,* 22-30.

Lewis, F., & Deal, L. (1995). Balancing out lives: A study of the married couple's experience with breast cancer recurrence. *Oncology Nursing Forum, 22,* 943-953.

Lewis, F. M., Hammond, M. A., & Woods, N. F. (1993). The family's functioning with newly diagnosed breast cancer in the mother: The development of an explanatory model. *Journal of Behavioral Medicine, 16,* 351-370.

Lewis, M., Curtis, M., & Lundy, K. (1995). He calls me his angel of mercy: The experience of caring for elderly parents in the home. *Holistic Nursing Practice, 9*(4), 54-65.

Litman, T. J. (1974). The family as the basic unit in health and medical care: A social-behavioral overview. *Social Science and Medicine, 8,* 495-519.

LoBiondo-Wood, G., Bernier-Henn, M., & Williams, L. (1992). Impact of the child's liver transplant on the family: Maternal perception. *Pediatric Nursing, 18,* 461-466.

Loukissa, D. A. (1995). Family burden in chronic mental illness: A review of research studies. *Journal of Advanced Nursing, 21,* 248-255.

Lynn, M. R. (1995). Family research: Consideration of who to study. *Journal of Pediatric Nursing, 10,* 383-384.

Mackenzie, A., & Holroyd, E. (1995). An exploration of the perceptions of care giving responsibilities in Chinese families. *Journal of Clinical Nursing, 4,* 267-270.

Magilvy, J. K., Congdon, J. G., & Martinez, R. (1994). Circles of care: Home care and community support for rural older adults. *Advances in Nursing Science, 16*(3), 22-33.

Martinson, I. M., Davis, A. J., Liu-Chiang, C. Y., Yi-Hua, L., Qiao, J., & Gan, M. (1995). Chinese mothers' reactions to their child's chronic illness. *Health Care for Women International, 16,* 365-375.

Martinson, I. M., McClowry, S. G., Davies, B., & Kuhlenkamp, E. J. (1994). Changes over time: A study of family bereavement following childhood cancer. *Journal of Palliative Care, 10*(1), 19-25.

McCarthy, S. M., & Gallo, A. M. (1992). A case illustration of family management style. *Journal of Pediatric Nursing, 7,* 395-402.

McClowry, S., Giangrande, S., Tommasini, N., Clinton, W., Foreman, N., Lynch, K., & Ferketich, S. (1994). The effects of child temperament, maternal characteristics and family circumstances on the maladjustment of school-age children. *Research in Nursing and Health, 17,* 25-35.

McCubbin, H., & Patterson, J. (1983). The family stress process: The Double ABCX Model of Adjustment and Adaptation. *Marriage and Family Review, 6,* 7-37.

McShane, R., Bumbalo, J., & Patsdaughter, C. (1994). Psychological distress in family members living with HIV/AIDS. *Archives of Psychiatric Nursing, 8*(1), 53-61.

Miles, M., Funk, S., & Kasper, M. (1992). The stress response of mothers and fathers of preterm infants. *Research in Nursing and Health, 15,* 261-269.

Moriarty, H. J. (1990). Key issues in the family research process: Strategies for nurse researchers. *Advances in Nursing Science, 12*(3), 1-14.

Najarian, S. (1995). Family experience with positive client response to Clozapine. *Archives of Psychiatric Nursing, 9*(1), 11-21.

Norbeck, J., Chafetz, L., Wilson, H., & Weiss, S. (1991). Social support needs of family care givers of psychiatric patients from three age groups. *Nursing Research, 40,* 208-213.

Patterson, J. M., & Garwick, A. W. (1994). The impact of chronic illness on families: A family systems perspective. *Annals of Behavioral Medicine, 16*(2), 131-142.

Pelletier, M. (1993). Emotions experienced and coping strategies used by family members of organ donors. *Canadian Journal of Nursing Research, 25*(2), 63-73.

Phillips, L., Morrison, E., Steffl, B., Young, M., Cromwell, S., & Russell, C. (1995). Effect of situational context and interactional process on the quality of family care giving. *Research in Nursing and Health, 18,* 205-216.

Powell-Cope, G. (1995). The experience of gay couples affected by HIV infection. *Qualitative Health Research, 5,* 36-62.

Prudhoe, C., & Peters, D. (1995). Social support of parents and grandparents in the neonatal intensive care unit. *Pediatric Nursing, 21,* 140-146.

Ray, L., & Ritchie, J. (1993). Caring for chronically ill children at home: Factors that influence parents' coping. *Journal of Pediatric Nursing, 8,* 217-225.

Reinhard, S. C. (1994). Living with mental illness: Effects of professional support and personal control on care giver burden. *Research in Nursing and Health, 17,* 79-88.

Rennick, J. E. (1995). The changing profile of acute childhood illness: A need for the development of family nursing knowledge. *Journal of Advanced Nursing, 22,* 258-266.

Rhiner, M., Ferrell, B. R., Shapiro, B., & Dierkes, M. (1994). The experience of pediatric cancer pain, Part II: Management of pain. *Journal of Pediatric Nursing, 9,* 380-387.

Riesch, S., Tosi, C., Thurston, C., Forsyth, D., Kuenning, T., & Kestly, J. (1993). Effects of communication training on parents and young adolescents. *Nursing Research, 4,* 10-16.

Robinson, C. (1993). Managing life with a chronic condition: The story of normalization. *Qualitative Health Research, 3,* 6-28.

Robinson, K. (1990). The relationship between social skills, social support, self-esteem and burden in adult care givers. *Journal of Advanced Nursing, 15,* 788-795.

Rolland, J. (1984). Chronic illness and the family. *Family Systems Medicine, 2,* 245-262.

Safilios-Rothschild, C. (1969). Family sociology or wives' family sociology? A cross-cultural examination of decision making. *Journal of Marriage and the Family, 31,* 290-301.

Saiki, S., Martinson, I., & Inano, M. (1994). Japanese families who have lost children to cancer: A primary study. *Journal of Pediatric Nursing, 9,* 239-250.

Sayles-Cross, S. (1993). Perceptions of family care givers of elder adults. *Image: The Journal of Nursing Scholarship, 25,* 88-92.

Sawyer, E. (1992). Family functioning when children have cystic fibrosis. *Journal of Pediatric Nursing, 7,* 304-311.

Schumaker, K., Dodd, M., & Paul, S. (1993). The stress process in family care givers of persons receiving chemotherapy. *Research in Nursing and Health, 16,* 395-404.

Schwenk, T., & Hughes, C. (1983). The family as a patient in family medicine: Rhetoric or reality. *Social Science and Medicine, 17,* 1-16.

Sharkey, T. (1995). The effects of uncertainty in families with children who are chronically ill. *Home Healthcare Nurse, 13,* 37-42.

Shaw, M. C., & Halliday, P. H. (1992). The family, crisis and chronic illness: An evolutionary model. *Journal of Advanced Nursing, 17,* 537-543.

Simon, N., & Smith, D. (1992). Living with chronic pediatric liver disease: The parents' experience. *Journal of Pediatric Nursing, 18,* 453-458, 489.

Snelling, J. (1990). The role of the family in relation to chronic pain: Review of the literature. *Journal of Advanced Nursing, 15,* 771-776.

Snelling, J. (1994). The effect of chronic pain on the family unit. *Journal of Advanced Nursing, 19,* 543-551.

Snowdon, A., Cameron, S., & Dunham, K. (1994). Relationships between stress, coping resources, and satisfaction with family func-

tioning in families of children with disabilities. *Canadian Journal of Nursing Research, 26,* 63-76.

Stuifbergen, A. (1990). Patterns of functioning in families with a chronically ill parent: An exploratory study. *Research in Nursing and Health, 13,* 35-44.

Taylor, E. J., Ferrell, B. R., Grant, M., & Cheyney, L. (1993). Managing cancer pain at home: The decisions and ethical conflicts of patients, family care givers, and homecare nurses. *Oncology Nursing Forum, 20,* 919-927.

Thomas, R. (1987). Methodological issues and problems in family health care research. *Journal of Marriage and the Family, 49,* 65-70.

Tomlinson, P., & Mitchell, K. (1992). On the nature of social support for families of critically ill children. *Journal of Pediatric Nursing, 7,* 386-394.

Von Riper, M., Ryff, C., & Pridham, K. (1992). Parental and family well-being in families of children with Down syndrome: A comparative study. *Research in Nursing and Health, 15,* 227-235.

Wallhagen, M. (1992). Care giving demands: Their difficulty and effects on the well-being of elderly care givers. *Scholarly Inquiry for Nursing Practice, 6,* 111-127.

Wegner, G. D., & Alexander, R. J. (Eds.). (1993). *Readings in family nursing.* Philadelphia: Lippincott.

Whall, A. L., & Fawcett, J. (1991). The family as a focal phenomenon in nursing. In A. L. Whall & J. Fawcett (Eds.), *Family theory development in nursing* (pp. 7-29). Philadelphia: F. A. Davis.

Whall, A., & Loveland-Cherry, C. (1993). Family unit-focused research: 1984-1991. *Annual Review of Nursing Research, 11,* 227-247.

Whyte, D. A. (1992). A family nursing approach to the care of a child with a chronic illness. *Journal of Advanced Nursing, 17*(3), 317-327.

Woods, N., & Lewis, F. (1995). Women with chronic illness: Their views of their families' adaptation. *Health Care for Women International, 16,* 135-148.

Woods, N. F., & Lewis, F. M. (1992). Design and measurement challenges in family research. *Western Journal of Family Research, 14,* 397-403.

Wright, L., Watson, W., & Bell, J. (1996). *Beliefs: The heart of healing in families and illness.* New York: Basic Books.

Wright, L. M., & Leahey, M. (1984). *Nurses and families.* Philadelphia: F. A. Davis.

Wright, L. M., & Leahey, M. (1990). Trends in nursing of families. *Journal of Advanced Nursing, 15,* 148-154.

Wright, L. M., & Leahey, M. (1994). Calgary Family Intervention Model: One way to think about change. *Journal of Marital and Family Therapy, 20,* 381-395.

Wright, L. M., & Levac, A. M. (1992). The non-existence of noncompliant families: The influence of Humberto Maturana. *Journal of Advanced Nursing, 17,* 913-917.

Wuest, J., Ericson, P., & Stern, P. (1994). Becoming strangers: The changing family care giving relationship in Alzheimer's disease. *Journal of Advanced Nursing, 20,* 437-443.

Youngblut, J., Brennan, P., & Swegart, L. (1994). Families with medically fragile children: An exploratory study. *Pediatric Nursing, 20,* 463-468.

Youngblut, J., Loveland-Cherry, C., & Horan, M. (1993). Maternal employment, family functioning, and preterm infant development at 9 and 12 months. *Research in Nursing and Health, 16,* 33-43.

Younger, J. (1991). A model of parenting stress. *Research in Nursing and Health, 14,* 197-204.

14

NURSING RESEARCH OF FAMILIES

State of the Science and
Correspondence With Policy

Suzanne L. Feetham
Susan B. Meister

Introduction

In nursing research of families, we have always aimed to achieve a high degree of correspondence with practice. The two preceeding chapters focus on the state of the science in nursing research of families and the degree of correspondence between science and practice. Such correspondence is important because research that is closely tied to practice clarifies our understanding of the relative value of an intervention for specific groups of families. If the intervention has enough value, it should become the centerpiece of a well-designed service program, and the evaluation of that program should guide the development of policies to sustain the program.

However, what usually happens after research based in practice demonstrates the utility of an intervention?

Too often, too little. Our research rarely includes the information that enables us to preceed with designing programs and tailoring policies to support them.

In the interest of closing that gap, this chapter focuses on the state of science and the degree of correspondence between science and policy. The first sections present eight frameworks related to policy development, policy and families, and the steps in transforming interventions into programs and policies. We chose these eight frameworks because they will help researchers design and conduct studies that correspond with both practice and policy.

Here, we use the same frameworks to assess the state of the science. They structure our assessment of the correspondence between nursing research of families and policy. To provide some perspective, we also use the frameworks to assess the degree of correspondence between nursing research in general and policy.

Next, we bring correspondence with policy into focus by discussing four programs of nursing research of families. The programs were chosen because they demonstrate use of one or more of the eight frameworks.

As with the chapters about the state of the science in relation to practice, we close with strategies for improving the state of the science. But before turning to the strategies, we describe the evolution of the science policy that currently guides both nursing research of families and the preparation of researchers. Our strategies make use of that science policy. We propose changes that would, in our view, expand the aims of family studies beyond the correspondence between research and practice to include policy as well. The changes would have related effects on the preparation of scientists, to assure the development of a cadre of researchers who are capable of helping to transform successful interventions into service programs that are sustained by policy.

Frameworks

This section presents eight frameworks that clarify relationships between family interventions and policy. They offer a succint overview of the fields we want to bridge, they provide the structure for assessing the correspondence between science and policy, and inform the design and conduct of new projects.

Components of Policy Development

Health policy consists of a broad range of policies that, directly or indirectly, define a plan of action regarding the allocation of resources related to key determinants of health such as health care, education, and employment (Abdellah, 1991; Natapoff, 1990b). The plan may be adopted by a government, organization, or individual, and it will be affected by the public and private sectors (Jacox, 1998). Research contributes to the development of health policy because policies result from the interactions of knowledge base, social strategy, and political will.

Of the many models of health policy, we have used Richmond and Kotelchuck's (1983) because it is based on their extensive experience and scholarship in child health policy, including the development of Head Start and neighborhood health centers and Richmond's service as surgeon general. The model has guided 15 years of successful interdisciplinary work in child health policy at Harvard, demonstrating that the model can be applied to all levels of policy development (Meister, 1997). This is important to nursing because the discipline is concerned with a wide range and multiple levels of policies, including practice policies affecting patients, families, and communities; institutional policies shaping health care delivery; national health policy emanating from legislation and professional organizations; and international policies (Hinshaw, 1988, 1992). Finally, the model can accommodate a wide range of health issues and policy efforts. This is important to family research because families' dependencies on social and health policies are multiple and multivariate (Milio, 1984; Moynihan, 1986; Natapoff, 1990a).

The Richmond and Kotelchuck (1983) model defines *policy* as the outcome of changes in and interaction of three components: knowledge base, political will, and social strategies. The *knowledge base* includes the accrued knowledge for and about practice, as well as for and about research. *Political will* includes the hopes, concerns, willingness to act, and aspirations of many groups, including citizens, taxpayers, and community leaders, as well as policy makers. *Social strategies* include plans for improving health outcomes for an aggregate—such as programs of service delivery and the financial and organizational context for such programs. The best social strategies are often based on programs built around successful interventions (Feetham, 1997; Schorr, 1991, 1997).

Currently, the three components of policy development have triggered rapid, dramatic innovations and experiments by states, employers, and communities in their organization and financing of health and social welfare programs (Aiken, 1992; Akula, 1997; Blumenthal, 1995; Field & Shapiro, 1993; Perrin, Kahn, et al., 1994; Reforming States Group, 1997; Rosenbaum, Serrano, Magar, & Stern, 1997). State laws, regulations guiding the design and operation of programs, and institutional policies are in a similar state. In other words, there is a great deal of opportunity created by fluidity in many systems. Families could benefit if nursing research brought an understanding of successful interventions to these developments in programs and policies, but we are hampered by the limited correspondence between research and policy.

Domains of Policies Affecting Families

We define policies affecting families in relation to family outcomes. The outcomes are based on the findings of the National Forum on the Future of Children and Families of the Institute of Medicine and National Research Council (Both & Garduque, 1989). The Forum studied 22 recent reports on child health produced by national panels, commissions, and government agencies. They identified four outcomes for children: education for work, health and well-being, employment and income, and poverty and welfare (well-being).

Although they focused on the subset of families with children, the Forum's findings are important here because they demonstrate the correspondence of outcomes to specific sets of policies. Applying the Forum's findings to families in general allows us to recognize the broad range of pertinent policies. For example, we would include school district policies about graduation standards (education for work), municipal policies about the coordination of elder services (health and well-being), state initiatives to employ non-college-bound youths (employment and income), and welfare reform (poverty and welfare).

Steps in Transforming Successful Interventions Into Programs and Policies

Policy development hinges upon having both a successful intervention and the research to provide strong empirical support for the impact, applicability, feasibility, and effectiveness of the program that provides the intervention (Feetham, 1997; Newhouse, 1986, 1991; Perrin, Shayne, & Bloom, 1993; Rosenbaum & Johnson, 1986; Schorr, 1988, 1991, 1997). The research must have scientific credibility, must produce a body of knowledge that corresponds with family outcomes as well as with policy development, and must clarify ways of making wider use of effective interventions (Davis, 1986; Feetham, 1992, 1997; Hinshaw, 1992; Mechanic & Aiken, 1986; Meister, 1993; Schorr, 1997).

These empirical linkages do not come easily. Ginzberg (1991) and Shortell and Reinhardt (1992) surveyed the field of health services research and concluded that the usefulness of research is limited when it fails to anticipate the questions that concern decision makers or when it fails to translate what is already known about problems into simple and understandable lessons. Fur-

ther, they note that the gap between analytical research and policy prescriptions increases when there is a large difference between public needs and tax revenues. In most cases, clinical and health services research are part of the early stages of policy development. The research produces and tests ideas that are then incorporated into later stages of negotiating health policy.

Shortell and Rienhart's (1992) framework to guide clinical and health services research is intended to shape research for policy. The research should produce explicit consideration of interdependencies of policies, a better understanding of delivery systems from all three perspectives (patient, provider, and institution), and criteria for clinical and fiscal accountability. Ideally, interventions are tested in many contexts that influence the effectiveness of an intervention, such as the individual, family, health system, and community.

It is important to recognize the time lag between the research and the application of findings to policy. Nursing research of families needs to be conducted with attention to the current policy context, but investigators must also address the anticipated future policy context because the findings from current research may inform policy makers over the next decade. The time lag is accentuated with the current state of the science of nursing research of families because much of the research continues to focus on the description of family phenomena, with few intervention studies and limited attention to policies affecting families.

Recognizing the importance of using research to transform a successful intervention into a program sustained by policy, in the following sections we look more closely at the steps between those endpoints: converting interventions into programs, evaluating programs, addressing bureaucracies, and informing policy decisions.

Converting Interventions Into Service Programs

Palfrey (1994) provides an especially relevant analysis of moving successful interventions into service programs. Her analysis is grounded in extensive clinical practice and research and is enlightened by her recognition of the need to enlist the full complement of policies in support of effective programs. Based on analysis of years of efforts to build community child health, Palfrey sets forth an action plan that includes several key elements: choosing important and achievable goals, creating linkages among providers, developing community support (moral and fiscal), changing legislation and/or regulation, carrying out pilot programs with ample evaluation, and establishing larger programs.

Similarly, Rossi and Freeman (1993) point out that when successful interventions become programs, the distinctions between policy studies of interventions and technical-administrative studies are artificial. When programs are developed to make use of successful interventions, it is necessary to define the problem precisely, assess its extent, describe the elements of the intervention, and accurately define the target population (Rossi & Freeman, 1993).

The question for nurse researchers is, Do we keep these concepts in mind when we take on the business of conducting intervention research with families? If the current research is any kind of benchmark, usually not.

Evaluating Programs and Addressing Bureaucracy

A strong evaluation of a program should be designed to produce empirical findings that will guide policy development. The evaluation sciences have developed a range of methods and designs because evaluations generally require ongoing revision and modification. For any particular evaluation, the choice of methods, design, and revisions should be guided by a strong theoretical base, the nature of the context, the volatility of social programs, a balance between scientific and pragmatic postures, the use of multiple methods and perspectives, and the nature of the policies that can be affected (Rossi & Freeman, 1993; Schorr, 1997).

Many methodologies are relevant to the evaluation of programs. Meta-analyses are sometimes used instead of controlled experiments with service programs. Meta-analyses are less expensive but have the limitation of failing to predict the outcomes of actual trials 35% of the time (LeLorier, Gregoire, Benhaddad, Lapierre, & Derderian, 1997). Controlled experiments are the gold standard for evaluations. When they are done well and are focused on enduring questions, the benefits in the caliber of knowledge far outweigh the costs and the demands on the funding agency (Newhouse, 1991).

In light of our goal of improving the correspondence with policy development, it is important that program evaluations include three sets of measures. The evaluation should establish the extent and fidelity of the implementation of the program, it should isolate the effects of the intervention and estimate their magnitude, and it

should provide a frame of reference for relating costs to program results (Rossi & Freeman, 1993).

Schorr's (1988, 1991, 1997) policy analysis from the evaluation of child- and family-based programs is also useful here. She has developed the concept of "scaling up" to describe extending successful programs and policies. For example, Head Start has been "scaled up" from an original program in one community to many programs existing in communities across the country. The process of scaling up required that policies be created and developed to define and support the bureaucratic structures within which Head Start programs are housed. This process, although difficult and complex, forms a critical base to sustain programs. Schorr's work dovetails with the evaluation sciences and highlights the pivotal role of administrative and functional contexts in efforts to scale up successful programs (Rossi & Freeman, 1993; Stokey & Zeckhauser, 1978).

Based on a national study of successful programs, Schorr identified five impediments that are related to organization and financing policies and that, when unresolved, hamper the extension or "scaling up" of successful programs. They are relevant here because they illustrate the bureaucratic conflicts that must be addressed when converting interventions into sustained service programs. The impediments are (a) successful programs are comprehensive, but funding for programs is generally categorical; (b) successful programs emphasize flexibility and discretion for the front-line workers, but traditions in professional training and conventional management do not; (c) successful programs tailor the intensity and scope of services for the individual, but bureaucracy is pressured to ensure equity despite insufficient funds; (d) successful programs are oriented toward prevention, which is at odds with pressures for immediate payoffs; and (e) successful programs evolve over time, but funding is usually short-term and unpredictable (Schorr, 1988, 1991, 1997).

Virtually all of Schorr's studies demonstrate that although providers often understand the system changes that are needed for scaling up, they usually cannot implement those changes. Funders and policy decision makers, acting on an understanding that can be informed by research, are able to make those all-important changes. Nursing research must rise to this challenge.

Informing Policy Decisions

Research that includes evaluation as described above is well positioned to guide policy decisions. In

TABLE 14.1. Improving Correspondence Between Nursing Research and Policy

	Frameworks	Types of Research		
		All Research	Intervention Research	Program Research
Policy development	Relate to components of policy development: knowledge base, political will, social strategy (Richmond & Kotelchuck, 1983)	X	X	X
Policies affecting families	Relate to family interventions and outcomes: education for work, health, and well-being, employment/income/poverty/welfare (the Forum; see Both & Garduque, 1989)	X	X	X
Steps from interventions to programs and policy	Define the problem precisely, assess the extent of the problem, describe the elements of the intervention, define the target population accurately (Rossi & Freeman, 1993)		X	X
	Define important and achievable goals, create linkages between providers, develop community support, change legislation/regulation, pilot service program and evaluate, establish larger program (Palfrey, 1994)			X
	Evaluate program fidelity, impact, and efficiency (Rossi & Freeman, 1993)			X
	Address the system and the institution (Schorr, 1997)			X
	Address the balance of bureaucracy and clinical practice (Schorr, 1997)			X
	Address financing and organization issues: which services are covered, to what extent, how much cost sharing, mix of premiums and taxes, administration issues (Newhouse, 1991)			X

their classic primer of policy analysis, Stokey and Zeckhauser (1978) refer to this phase as "putting the analysis to work." Looking over their five steps, the potential contribution of nursing research of families—if it is shaped for policy as well as practice—is clear:

— establish the context (What is the problem? What are the objectives?)
— lay out the alternatives (which program design, which bureaucracies)
— predict the consequences of the alternatives
— value the outcomes (What is success? How should heterogeneous outcomes be compared?)
— make a choice for preferred course of action (Stokey & Zeckhauser, 1978).

Again, the research should go beyond describing the intervention. It should assess the fidelity, impact, and efficiency of the service program. As noted in Table 14.1, it should include findings that define the importance of the systems and institutional context and remove obstacles by creating a new balance between essential bureaucratic protections and the autonomy, flexibility, and variation needed by clinicians (Schorr, 1991). However, when the analysis extends beyond the intervention into

economic and political factors, it is imperative that the analysts include the health professions so that the focus remains on what will improve and restore health (Shine, 1998).

Research that supports the process will reflect a foundation in both practice and science. It will build upon nursing's unique knowledge base regarding the nature of families, the needs of families, and interventions that promote the well-being of families. Similarly, programs to prepare nurse researchers will incorporate the knowledge bases and experiences that are necessary to conduct work that makes use of these frameworks.

In Table 14.1, we summarize eight frameworks related to the components of policy development, domains of policies affecting families, and the steps in moving from interventions to programs and policies. Including these frameworks in the design of nursing research of families will increase the correspondence with policy. It is important to note, however, that certain frameworks relate best to specific types of research. Although the frameworks regarding components of policy development (Richmond & Kotelchuck, 1983) and policies domains affecting families (Both & Garduque, 1989) are applicable to any type of research, the other frameworks apply more to intervention research (Rossi & Freeman, 1993) or re-

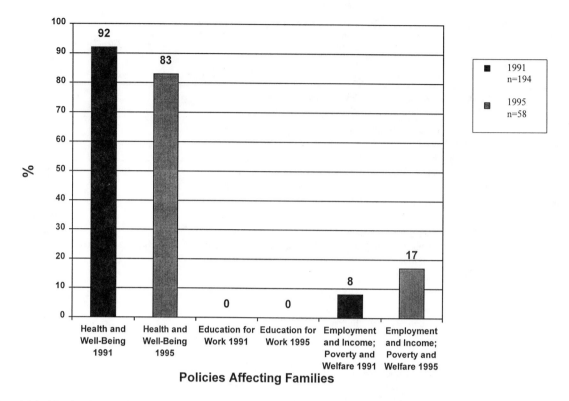

Figure 14.1. Nursing Research of Families: Correspondence With Policies Affecting Families
NOTE: For 1991, *n* = 194; for 1995, *n* = 58.

search on programs (Newhouse, 1991; Palfrey, 1994; Schorr, 1997).

These frameworks apply to nursing research in general, as long as the type of research is considered in selecting the frameworks that should be incorporated. In the following section, we discuss our assessment of the current degree of correspondence between nursing research of families and policy, including a review of four programs of nursing research of families that illustrate the application of some of these frameworks.

Assessment

Nursing research of families builds upon practice and thus has a vital and unique foundation for developing and testing interventions. McCubbin (Chapter 12), and Gilliss and Knafl (Chapter 13) found that nursing research of families rarely includes studies of interventions. What are the implications of that shortcoming in relation to policy? It prevents effective interventions from being understood as strategies—strategies capable of inspiring programs and policies. Thus nursing research

of families falls short in two senses. It does not test the effectiveness of interventions for individual families. Furthermore, it does not test the utility of those interventions when applied to specific aggregates of families, and thus it does not contribute to converting effective interventions into service programs.

We used two analyses to assess the current degree of correspondence between nursing research and policy. First, we analyzed reported research from 1991 and 1995. This analysis was designed to describe the distribution of nursing research in relation to three domains of policies affecting families and three components of policy development. The findings are summarized in Figures 14.1 and 14.2. The second analysis focused on four programs of nursing research of families. It was designed to identify how each program of research makes use of one or more of the frameworks listed in Table 14.1 to increase the correspondence with policy.

Current Degree of Correspondence With Policy

Three samples of nursing research reports were used in this analysis: family research reported in 1991, family

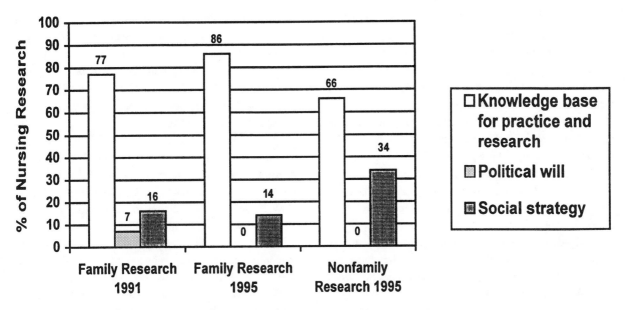

Figure 14.2. Nursing Research: Correspondence With Components of Policy Development
NOTE: Family research 1991, $N = 194$; family research 1995, $N = 58$; nonfamily research 1995, $N = 114$.

research reported in 1995, and nonfamily research reported in 1995. The 1991 sample of family research comprised the abstracts accepted for the 1991 Second International Conference on Family Nursing, held in Portland, Oregon. Their correspondence with policy has already been described (Meister, 1993). The 1995 samples of family research and nonfamily nursing research were composed of the research reports published during 1995 in *Nursing Research, Nursing Outlook, Image: The Journal of Family Nursing, Annual Review of Nursing Research,* and the *Reports of the Expert Panels of the American Academy of Nursing.* These publications were selected because together they are a current, comprehensive, and respected force within nursing research. The 1995 reports were sorted as "family" or "nonfamily." We defined family research quite broadly, accepting a study if there was evidence of using family variables, frameworks, or concepts, even if in a minor way. This process produced 194 family research reports in 1991, 58 family research reports in 1995, and 114 nonfamily research reports in 1995.

We pursued two questions about the correspondence between research and policy: How well does family research address the components of policy development and the domains of policies affecting families? and Does all nursing research address policy in the same way, or are there patterns that are specific to the nursing research of families? In other words, how well does family re-

search correspond to policies and policy development, and is that degree of correspondence related to *family* or to *nursing*?

First, we compared the correspondence between nursing research of families and three domains of policies affecting family outcomes (the Forum; see Both & Garduque, 1989) (see also Figure 14.1). When we applied the Forum's four domains of policies to quantify the correspondence between nursing research of families and policy, we collapsed the domains of employment income and poverty/welfare, resulting in three domains of policies. The distribution of nursing research lends some specificity to our thinking about which domains of policy are addressed, and the two samples of family research allowed us to examine trends within the field.

Looking first at the correspondence between nursing research of families and policies affecting family outcomes, it is not surprising that the data show that the studies emphasize health and well-being. No studies included issues related to education for work. The third category of outcomes (employment/income, poverty/welfare) was included in the lowest number of studies—but the percentage was twice as high in 1995 (17%) as in 1991 (8%).

Next, we examined the correspondence between each of the three research samples and the three components of policy development (Richmond & Kotelchuck, 1983). The analysis permits two comparisons: the distribution of nursing research of families in 1991 compared to the distribution of nursing research of families in 1995 and the distribution of those two samples compared to the distribution of nonfamily nursing research in 1995. This would enable us to see what, if anything, characterized family research in relation to policy.

In terms of family research, the correspondence with the components of policy development is dominated by studies contributing to the knowledge base. As seen in Figure 14.2, the percentage of studies contributing analyses of social strategies is steady at about 15%, but the small amount of interest seen in political will in 1991 (7%) is absent in 1995.

We noted above that both samples of family studies emphasized the knowledge base and that they have virtually identical, and modest, attention to interventions as strategies. This is seen again in Figure 14.2, but, more important, the modest attention to strategies is seen to be even more modest in contrast to nonfamily nursing research. In the nonfamily studies, 34% went beyond the knowledge base and included analyses of strategies—more than twice as many as seen in the two samples of family studies.

Overall, despite its limited correspondence with policy development and policies affecting family outcomes and its lack of attention to intervention strategies, nursing research of families has produced a body of knowledge that is based in the intersection of research and practice. On one hand, the interdependence of the family and its environment, the relationships between disciplinary research and policy, and the unique knowledge that emerges from the diversity of practice settings and broad scopes of practice have been described (Feetham, 1984; Feetham & Meister, 1994; Milio, 1984; Natapoff, 1990a). On the other hand, the work is generally descriptive in nature, emphasizing the childbearing and child-rearing stages of families (McCubbin, Chapter 12). Furthermore, a framework has not yet developed within nursing that acknowledges the importance of the fit between interventions, family situation, and family characteristics (Gilliss & Knafl, Chapter 13).

Nursing research of families can do better. Schorr (1991) lays out a pertinent agenda for nurse researchers to extend the influence of their research; that is, to conduct the work accurately and rapidly enough to shape resource allocation and other policy decisions in the near future. She emphasizes the importance of providing information to the general public that would inspire confidence in the efforts to transform successful interventions into programs and policy (Schorr, 1991).

The larger body of nursing research provides several lines of inquiry that can contribute as well. For example, a cluster of reviews of innovations in service delivery found progress in melding clinical, financial, and organizational data but also the need for advances in certain analytical skills and improvement in the coordination of nursing research with priorities in health care (Fralic, 1994; Sanders, 1994; Tierney, 1994; Verran, 1994). The issue of coordination has been discussed in greater specificity in relation to reconceptualizing health issues as health care financing issues (Feetham, 1992; McTeer, 1996; Meister, 1989, 1993), and in relation to politics (Cohen et al., 1996; Kalisch & Kalisch, 1982).

Nursing outcomes research is another relevant line of inquiry, and one that has a history of analysis (Strickland & Waltz, 1988, 1990; Waltz & Strickland, 1988, 1990). This body of work is consistent with the recommendations of Rossi and Freeman (1993), Palfrey (1994), and Schorr (1991, 1997) and includes a framework for advancing studies of the outcomes of successful nursing interventions. The framework directs scientists to use conceptual models of appropriate scope, to design clinical trials that are likely to identify changes, and to conduct interventions so that they can be replicated (Strickland, 1997).

Progress needs to be made in nursing research of families in a number of areas, including designing research so that it addresses the needs of society and is relevant to multiple levels of policy development; developing greater skill in analytical techniques that can address complex variables embedded in the context and target populations of interventions; and moving purposefully through series of empirical tests, including randomized trials of innovations (Abdellah & Levine, 1994; Cohen et al., 1996; Conn & Armer, 1996; Davis, 1986; Hinshaw, 1988; Newhouse, 1986, 1991; Rosenbaum et al., 1997; Schorr, 1988, 1991, 1997).

Examples: Four Programs of Nursing Research Demonstrating Use of the Frameworks

In this chapter, we have selected eight frameworks to define policy development, policies affecting families, and steps to transform interventions into programs and policies. Advancing the state of the science for nursing research of families requires overt attention to the frameworks. Four programs of nursing research of families are analyzed in this section to identify how each program of research demonstrates use of one or more of the frameworks listed in Table 14.1 to increase their correspondence with policy.

The four programs of research are Archbold and Stewart's studies of family caregivers (Archbold, 1980, 1981, 1982a, 1982b, 1983, 1992; Archbold, Stewart, Greenlick, & Harvath, 1990); Knafl and Deatrick's studies of family management styles and normalization in families of children with health problems (Deatrick & Knafl, 1988, 1990; Deatrick, Knafl, & Walsh, 1988; Knafl, 1985; Knafl & Deatrick, 1990; Knafl, Gallo, Zoeller, & Breitmayer, 1993); Loveland-Cherry's studies of family-based interventions to decrease substance misuse in adolescents (Dielman, Leech, & Loveland-Cherry, 1995; Loveland-Cherry, Leech, Laetz, & Dielman, 1996; Loveland-Cherry, Ross, & Kaufman, in press); and McCubbin and colleagues' studies of families responding to normative and non-normative transitions and other family stresses (McCubbin, 1989; McCubbin, McCubbin, & Thompson, 1986, 1988b; Svavarsdottir & McCubbin, 1996). These programs were selected because they span developmental ages and stages and because they address health promotion, disease prevention, and health and illness with culturally and racially diverse populations (McCubbin, Thompson, Thompson, McCubbin, & Kaston, 1993; Nkongho & Archbold, 1995, 1996; Ross, Loveland-Cherry, Leech, & Laetz, in press).

The primary criterion used to select these four programs was evidence that they applied one or more of the frameworks described above and listed in Table 14.1. These programs of research are also conducted by interdisciplinary teams and have sustained extramural funding. They couple scientific merit with clinical and policy relevance. The sources of data for the assessment of these four programs were publications, grants, personal communication, and unpublished summaries of their programs of research. In general, the four programs of research echo the findings in our analyses of nursing research of families and nonfamily nursing research. As in Figure 14.1, the four programs emphasize the knowledge base, with little attention to political will or social strategies. As in Figure 14.2, the four programs emphasize health and well-being, with little attention to the other domains of policies affecting families. However, the four programs stand out because they grapple with the frameworks that help to transform successful interventions into programs and policies. In Table 14.2 and later in this chapter, we discuss the details of how these programs have made use of the frameworks that guide our efforts to increase the correspondence with policy.

Components of Policy Development

As noted earlier in this chapter, Richmond and Kotelchuck (1983) define *policy* as the outcome of the interaction of *knowledge base, political will,* and *social strategies.*

The *knowledge base* includes the accrued knowledge for and about practice, as well as for and about research. The contributions to the knowledge base for nursing research and care with families are extensive in these four programs and demonstrate (a) deliberate application and testing of family theory or conceptual frameworks, (b) the development and testing or revision of family measures, (c) the use of multiple research methods, and (d) wide dissemination of knowledge in nursing and interdisciplinary journals (Knafl & Deatrick, 1986, 1987, 1993, in press; Knafl, Deatrick, & Kirby, in press). The evidence is in their numerous conceptual, methodological, and data-based publications. These scholars have led the science in moving away from deficit models or frameworks to those identifying and building on family strengths. A focus in each of these programs of research is to identify the characteristics or factors that enable some families and family members to manage illnesses and reduce high-risk behaviors that threaten health. These scientists seek to examine the strengths, strategies, and predictors that enable families to successfully manage family challenges or stresses such as chronic illness, risk behaviors in family members, and caregiving responsibilities. Identifying these factors positions these researchers to target interventions that enhance these characteristics, and in some families, it enables them to develop protective factors to prevent adverse threats to the family.

Another characteristic of these programs of research demonstrating use of one or more of the frameworks for increasing correspondence with policy is the attention to the concept of the complexity of context in relation to family processes and outcomes. Deatrick, Knafl, and Murphy-Moore (in press) state that the importance and complexity of context was reinforced in their reanalysis of the concept of normalization. The authors note that the family perspective needs to be synthesized within social, cultural, ethical, and moral perspectives. Archbold and Stewart (Archbold & Stewart, 1996a, 1996b; Archbold, Stewart, Miller, et al., 1995; MacVicar & Archbold, 1976) and Loveland-Cherry and colleagues (Loveland-Cherry, Leech, Laetz, & Dielman, 1996; Loveland-Cherry & Ross, in press) have developed multifaceted interventions in recognition of the complexity and criti-

TABLE 14.2. Four Programs of Nursing Research of Families: Correspondence With Policy

		Programs of Research			
	Frameworks	*Archbold and Stewart*	*Knafl and Deatrick*	*Loveland-Cherry*	*McCubbin*
Policy development	Relate to components of policy development:				
	knowledge base	x	x	x	x
	political will	x	x	x	x
	social strategy	x	o	x	o
	(Richmond & Kotelchuck, 1983)				
Policies affecting families	Relate to policies affecting families:				
	health and well-being	x	x	x	x
	education for work	o	x	x	o
	employment/income and poverty/welfare	o	o	o	o
	(Both & Garduque, 1989)				
Steps from interventions to programs and policy	Define the problem precisely	x	x	x	x
	Assess the extent of the problem	x	o	x	o
	Describe the elements of the intervention	x	x	x	o
	Define the target population accurately	x	x	x	x
	(Rossi & Freeman, 1993)				
	Define important and achievable goal	x	x	x	x
	Create linkages between providers	o	o	o	o
	Develop community support	x	o	x	o
	Change legislation/regulation	o	o	o	o
	Pilot service program and evaluate	x	o	o	o
	Establish larger program	o	o	o	o
	(Palfrey, 1994)				
	Evaluate program fidelity, impact, and efficiency	o	o	o	o
	(Rossi & Freeman, 1993)				
	Address the system and the institution	o	o	o	o
	(Schorr, 1997)				
	Address the balance of bureaucracy and clinical practice	o	o	o	o
	(Schorr, 1997)				
	Address financing issues	x	o	o	o
	Address organization issues	o	o	o	o
	Address administration issues	o	o	o	o
	(Newhouse, 1991)				

NOTE: x = demonstrated; O = not demonstrated.

cal nature of context for the family. This attention to family context and its complexity is consistent with the policy frameworks used in this chapter (Palfrey, 1994; Richmond & Kotelchuck, 1983; Rossi & Freeman; Schorr, 1991, 1997) and with Feetham's (1997) characteristics of successful family interventions.

The contributions to the knowledge base for practice and research from these four programs extend beyond data-based publications. Their contributions include publications on issues such as measurement (Stewart & Archbold, 1992, 1993, 1997) and research methods

(Archbold, 1986a, 1986b; Deatrick & Knafl, 1988; Hoeffer & Archbold, 1983; Knafl, 1990; Knafl & Breitmayer, 1989; Knafl & Deatrick, in press), interdisciplinary research (Archbold, 1991a, 1991b), and concept analyses (Deatrick & Knafl, 1990; Deatrick, Knafl, & Guyer, 1993; Deatrick, Knafl, & Murphy-Moore, in press; Deatrick, Knafl, & Walsh, 1988; Knafl, Gallo, Breitmayer, Zoeller, & Ayres, 1993). Knafl and Deatrick (1993) have affirmed the value of concept analysis and other integrative activities that lead to synthesis and furthering knowledge development. Loveland-Cherry's work is notable for her comprehensive evaluation of a common family measure (Loveland-Cherry, Youngblut, & Leidy, 1989). This publication is recognized in nursing and the family sciences as a model for the evaluation of the conceptual and analytical integrity of family measures. For McCubbin and colleagues, a strength of their multifaceted program of research is the reporting of their deliberate efforts of theory building and testing (Kosciulek, McCubbin, & McCubbin, 1993; McCubbin, McCubbin, & Thompson, 1998a). McCubbin coauthored the resiliency model of family stress, adjustment, and adaptation, used as the theoretical framework for research on normative and non-normative family transitions in the United States and internationally. For two decades, these investigators have challenged, reframed, and retested the theory (McCubbin, McCubbin, & Thompson, 1988a). Since 1983, the start of the Archbold and Stewart collaboration, studies were proposed with the goals of refining the conceptualization of caregiving, developing measures of caregiving concepts, conducting a longitudinal study of family caregiving, and developing family interventions focused on the doing of caregiving for families caring for frail elderly. The application of the conceptual basis for this program of research has focused on role and symbolic interaction theories and frameworks that have a strong history in the social sciences, particularly the family sciences (Klein & White, 1996).

McCubbin and colleagues have developed instruments to measure aspects of family functioning such as family hardiness, family problem solving, communication, and parental coping with children's chronic illness (McCubbin, 1988; McCubbin, McCubbin, & Thompson, 1986, 1988a, 1988c). In the seven studies conducted by Archbold and Stewart, the Family Care Inventory and other measures were tested (Archbold & Stewart, 1996b; Archbold, Stewart, Greenlick, et al., 1990; Archbold, Stewart, Miller, et al., 1995; Cartwright, Archbold, Stewart, & Limandri, 1994; Nkongho & Archbold, 1995, 1996; Schumacher, Stewart, & Archbold, 1998; Stewart, Archbold, Harvath, & Nkongho, 1993).

Political will, as an interactive component of policy development, includes the hopes, concerns, willingness to act, and aspirations of many groups such as citizens, taxpayers, community leaders, and politicians (Richmond & Kotelchuck, 1983). There is evidence in the four programs of research of some correspondence with this component of policy development. For example, the programs of research address issues recognized as public

health problems affecting significant numbers of the population. These are problems that are of high cost to health systems and families and have current social and health policies related to these issues. These policy issues are aging and family caregiving, substance misuse in adolescents, and living with chronic illness.

Loveland-Cherry's family-based program of research derives from her practice in public health and addresses substance use and misuse in adolescents, a serious health problem affecting individuals, families, and the public's health. Substance use and misuse in adolescents is on the rise, with children consuming alcohol and other drugs in larger quantities at earlier ages than in previous years (Bachman, Johnson, & O'Malley, 1998). Substance use and misuse is associated with negative consequences, including a variety of problem behaviors in adulthood (Andrews, Hops, Ary, Tildesley, & Harris, 1993; Miller, 1994). The family context is a known correlate to substance use in children (Ross & Hill, in press; Wills, Schreibman, Benson, & Vaccaro, 1992, 1994). Loveland-Cherry's work is consistent with the growing consensus on the importance of identifying both protective factors and risk factors in relation to adolescent substance use and misuse. These factors are interdependent and include family, peer, psychological, and behavioral characteristics. In addition to the health and well-being of families, this program of research also addresses the policies affecting family outcomes of education for work, employment, poverty, and welfare.

The Archbold and Stewart program of research is based on evidence that many families want to provide care for family members. Therefore their work has focused on (a) understanding family care, (b) improving skill in family care, and (c) improving access to services for and by family members. The societal context of this program of research is the importance of family care for frail elders and the need for research on family care interventions. In 1990, the percentage of the U.S. population over 65 years old was 12.5%. In 2030, it will be 20.1%. The percentage of the U.S. population over age 85 has more than quadrupled since 1970. Forty-nine percent of persons over 85 years old require assistance in activities of daily living (ADL). Public policy in the United States demonstrates several assumptions about family care. These assumptions are that (a) families should provide the care needed by ill or frail family members, (b) they have the knowledge and skill to provide that care, and (c) they know how to access the resources needed to provide the care. This program of research will continue to demonstrate clinical and policy relevance, as in the next 50 years there will be an unprecedented increase in the number of persons living to old age. Although our society increasingly relies on families to provide elder care, health care systems have not developed effective ways to support families in this role.

The programs of research of Knafl and Deatrick and McCubbin address a key policy concern of the distribution of health resources to children with chronic illness and their families. Several factors influence the distribution of health resources to children and their families. Although 10% of the children, those with disabilities and chronic illness, consume over 70% of the total health resources, the number of children experiencing illness is far less than the number of adults (Feetham & Frink, 1997). Conditions with a high incidence in children tend to have low severity (Homer et al., 1996), which results in less policy attention to children's health and family problems (Feeg, 1996). The focus of these programs—identifying predictors of family outcomes in caring for family members with chronic illness—can be used to inform policy analysts and decision makers.

Social strategies, as a component of policy development, include plans for improving health outcomes for an aggregate, such as programs of service delivery and the financial and organizational context for such programs (Richmond & Kotelchuck, 1983).

An underlying reason for the Archbold and Stewart program of research to test the Preparedness Enrichment Predictability (PREP) intervention is that current Medicare guidelines allow for only minimal support of families in their care of elders—specifically in consideration of the "skilled care" needs of the elder. Archbold states that provision of more low-intensity service (such as PREP) can avert higher intensity service use, such as hospitalizations. Currently, Medicare allows for interventions with the Medicare enrollee only (except for some teaching of caregivers in relation to skilled care). The premise of these scientists is that focusing on the entire family (including the health of caregivers) is necessary to promote optimum health of all family members. A goal is to affect Medicare regulations to allow for PREP or PREP-like services for frail elders and their families (P. Archbold, personal communication, July 1998).

Policies Affecting Families

All of these programs emphasize health and well-being. None of the programs directly address education for

work, although Loveland-Cherry's program affects the outcomes of the adolescents completing their high school education (Dielman et al., 1995; Loveland-Cherry & Ross, in press). All of the programs include high-risk, low-income families, and the outcomes of the two programs with interventions could affect the employment and, therefore, the income of the program participants. Direct measures of these outcomes would help to better position these programs to inform health and social policy. What is missing in these programs of research is evidence of deliberate application of the findings to inform policy analysis and decisions.

Steps From Interventions to Programs and Policy

Intervention research is a step in the process of developing service programs, so it is important to increase its correspondence with policy. The four programs of research demonstrate various ways to do so. Archbold and Stewart (Archbold & Stewart, 1996a, 1996b; Archbold, Stewart, Greenlick, et al., 1990; Archbold, Stewart, Miller, et al., 1995; Cartwright et al., 1994; Nkongho & Archbold, 1995, 1996; Schumacher et al., 1998; Stewart et al., 1993) and Loveland-Cherry and colleagues (Loveland-Cherry, Leech, Laetz, et al., 1996; Loveland-Cherry & Ross, in press) have published results from intervention studies. McCubbin and colleagues have not conducted intervention studies, but an intervention study with high-risk families is in process (M. McCubbin, personal communication, April 1998). The work of McCubbin and colleagues (McCubbin, 1993; McCubbin, McCubbin, et al., 1986; Svavarsdottir & McCubbin, 1996) and Deatrick, Knafl, and Murphy-Moore (in press) provide specific information to guide the development of interventions. These four programs of research focus on discovering and testing factors that explain why some families recover and manage the illness of a family member and others remain vulnerable and, in some cases, deteriorate in similar circumstances.

The research of Archbold and Stewart and Loveland-Cherry and colleagues has tested interventions with tangible outcomes that could be incorporated into existing or new service programs. The PREP intervention developed by Archbold and Stewart (Archbold & Stewart, 1996a, 1996b; Archbold, Stewart, Miller, et al., 1995; Harvath et al., 1994) meets Feetham's (1992, 1997) and Schorr's (1991, 1997) criteria for successful interventions. Loveland-Cherry's two programs, Adolescent Drug Abuse Prevention (ADAP) and Child and Parent

Relations (CAPR), also meet these criteria. These multi-faceted interventions include systematic assessments, a family focus, family and nursing collaboration, early identification of problematic transitions, and the inclusion of multiple individualized strategies.

The Archbold and Stewart program of research is directed to address some of the impediments described by Schorr (1997). Archbold and Stewart recognize that the recent transition to a more managed care approach to health care has been implemented by some profit-making health care organizations in ways that have off-loaded care previously provided by health care personnel onto families. In this process, families were not asked about this—and in some cases, policy makers may not be aware that it has happened, as it is "hidden" within the home, unless there is a severe untoward consequence. These researches perceive that PREP—with its ongoing monitoring and 24-hour call-in system—can provide a safety net for families in these situations (P. Archbold, personal communication, July 1998).

Researchers from health services, economics, and policy analysis are developing better models to examine costs and methods to address institutional and broad system issues (Newhouse, 1991; Rossi & Freeman, 1993). Stewart and Archbold (1992, 1993), in their discussion of measurement issues in intervention research, give directions for family researchers to better position themselves to address these issues. Archbold and Stewart have also examined costs to the individual family member, the family, and the health systems (Archbold & Hoeffer, 1981; Miller, Hornbrook, Archbold, & Stewart, 1996). Attention to the costs of the caregiver role have been addressed through the inclusion of economists on the research team. Cost differences were demonstrated, with their intervention group having total hospital costs of $34,716 and the control group $87,945, a savings per family of $3,800 in a 3-month period. This study also demonstrated that the strategies for collecting use and cost data were accurate, feasible for most participants, and not a burden to families (Miller et al., 1996). Although Archbold and Stewart have the cost data, none of the four programs have included analyses within the context of the components of policy development.

In future phases, for these programs of research to demonstrate improved correspondence with policy will require evidence of applying more of the frameworks for transforming interventions to programs and policy. These frameworks include creating links with the providers, developing community support, evaluating and monitoring larger programs, and addressing the bal-ance of bureaucracy and clinical practice (Table 14.1) (Newhouse, 1991; Palfrey, 1994; Rossi & Freeman, 1993; Schorr, 1997).

In summary, analysis of the correspondence with policy for these four programs of research is consistent with our findings for nursing research and nursing research of families (see Figures 14.1 and 14.2 and Table 14.2). Although the programs of research relate to policy development, the correspondence is limited primarily to the knowledge base component. Similarly, the research corresponds best with policies affecting families' health and well-being, leaving out the domains of education for work, employment, income, poverty, and welfare. All of the programs contribute to the knowledge base in multiple ways, but political will is addressed indirectly. Only in the Archbold and Stewart and the Loveland-Cherry programs of research are the interventions conceptualized as social strategies. None of the programs directly address education for work, although Loveland-Cherry's program does affect the outcomes of the adolescents for completing their high school education (Loveland-Cherry, Leech, Laetz, et al., 1996; Loveland-Cherry & Ross, in press). Also, in a secondary analysis of the Knafl data, Zoeller (1996) examined the relationships between children with chronic illnesses, their families, and the school system. All of the programs include diverse cultural and racial groups, high-risk and at-risk groups, and families in poverty. Although it is more overt in the Loveland-Cherry program, the outcomes of the two programs with interventions could affect the employment and therefore the income of the program participants. To better position these programs to inform health and social policy, direct measures of these outcomes are necessary. Some of the investigators have programs in mind that could serve as demonstration models to affect state and national policy (C. J. Loveland-Cherry, personal communication, April 1998; B. J. Stewart, personal communication, April 1998).

These programs of research serve as illustrations of the state of the science, but it is important to note that the evidence of correspondence was derived from multiple sources. Identifying the evidence required sources beyond traditional publications such as grant proposals, personal communication, presentations, and unpublished reports of the programs of research. To improve the correspondence with policy, this important evidence should be included as part of publications. The use of a variety of data sources reinforces the point that correspondence with policy is not easy to accomplish. It is also evident that to achieve correspondence, a deliberate, programmatic process is required to transform interventions to programs and to policy.

Strategies

Successful interventions are the heart of practice and, once validated by research, serve well as the centerpiece of programs and policy. However, broad analyses of family nursing and research consistently show that there is, at best, only partial empirical support for the effectiveness of interventions (Campbell & Patterson, 1995; Gilliss & Davis, 1993; Feetham, 1984, 1991, 1997; see also Chapters 12 and 13). And yet, in practice, nurses are reported to provide exemplary services to the full range of families, addressing a broad set of problems in virtually any context (Feetham & Meister, 1994). The discrepancies between practice, research, and policy are troubling and, we believe, unnecessary.

Reviews of nursing research of families coalesce around a cluster of unanswered questions about family interventions: Which outcomes are we able to influence? Which interventions are most effective for which types of families? Which interventions are most effective for which clinical problems? Which interventions are cost-effective and under what conditions? (Campbell & Patterson, 1995; Gilliss & Davis, 1993; Feetham, 1984, 1991, 1997; see also Chapters 12 and 13). Without answers to such basic questions, it is impossible to address the second-order questions related to policy decisions.

Policy demands a broader context and better answers. The context is broader because programs are designed, implemented, and funded at levels ranging from a home-care program in a community hospital to federal programs to support family caregivers. The answers must be better because the questions are complex. For example, policy decisions on health care financing take place along at least five dimensions: (a) What services should be covered? (b) How well should they be covered? (c) How much cost-sharing should there be? (d) How should care be financed (mix of taxes and premiums)? and (e) What are the administrative issues? (Newhouse, 1991).

How do we move forward? How can we improve the degree of correspondence between nursing research of families and policies? We recommend a strategy that makes use of another form of policy—science policy.

The Role of Science Policy

In general, science policy defines what is recognized as science, and, therefore, guides the development of research and education. It is a big umbrella for many types of issues. Examples of science policy include the recommendations made by the president's science policy advisor, the National Research Council's national science education standards, and the research methodology standards applied by the National Institutes of Health.

The importance of science itself is seen in its applications. Science is used to achieve a number of goals, including designing plans to build the knowledge base, creating the ability to make decisions, and preparing for expected or chosen applications (Pratt & Zeckhauser, 1985; Rossi & Freeman, 1993). Science policy is important because it is a determinant of science. For example, the new director general of the World Health Organization (WHO) plans to bring science, policy, and science policy to bear on efforts to improve world health. Science will be a strong underpinning to policy, and WHO calls for science policy makers in governments, agencies, foundations, and industry to underwrite the interdisciplinary research needed for such science (Brundtland, 1998).

Viewed through the lens of a discipline, science policy becomes a powerful mechanism for advancing a field. It establishes the standards for science and, thus, the standards for academic programs (distribution of credits, emphasis within coursework, levels of expertise to be achieved, kinds of research experience) and the standards for empiricism. Science policy consists of decisions that, formally or informally, shape the allocation of scarce resources to support the training of scientists and to support scientific work. Although those allocation decisions are commonly viewed as unrelated, we also need to view them as a whole. They define how nurse scientists are prepared and who they are prepared to work with as colleagues. Eventually, science policy is a strong factor in the nature of the work of nurse scientists and the field itself.

Science Policy and Nursing Research of Families

The concept of science policy is central to this discussion because we are relating research to a number of applications. Does nursing research of families meet the goal of expanding the science base for practice and education? Does it meet the goal of expanding the knowledge base for policy development? If we know where nursing research of families should go next, how can we shape our science policy accordingly, to bring our goal of correspondence into focus and allocate resources accordingly?

In 1984, Feetham analyzed the field of nursing research of families and identified criteria for family-related research and family research that also served as guidelines for the development and review of research of families—which is to say, a summary of the then-extant science policy. In 1991, Feetham's survey of conceptual and methodological issues in research of families produced a comprehensive summary of the purposes of the research and the criteria for evaluating the research. That survey also described an evolution in the science policy.

The criteria, as revised in 1991, were (a) there is a family conceptual or theoretical framework; (b) there is an explicit conceptualization of the family; (c) the definition of the family is consistent with the conceptualization, design, and methods; (d) the findings add to the knowledge of family functioning and family structure; (e) for family-related research, the responses of individual family members and/or concepts related to families or family members are examined; and (f) for family research, the conceptualization, measurement, and analysis reflect the family as the unit or system, and this adds to knowledge of the family system. Feetham also noted that in a practice discipline, research demonstrates practice relevance (Feetham, 1984, 1991).

Feetham (1991) also described five purposes for nursing research of families: (a) to examine the responses of families and family members to various states of health, (b) to examine responses of families and family members to expected and unexpected life transitions, (c) to test theories of the effect of nursing on family members and families, (d) to formulate theories of predictors of family outcomes, and (e) to identify factors most predictive of successful family outcomes.

Together, Feetham's criteria and purposes describe a science policy. Research of families should:

1. be conceptually and methodologically rigorous,
2. focus on circumstances in which families are likely to need help,
3. contribute to the development and testing of interventions, and

4. be conducted in the broadest context of relevance to the individual and family (community, health system, environment, social, and health policy).

This science policy is important because it shapes what we define as science in nursing research of families. It also defines, perhaps indirectly, what we establish as standards for the preparation of nurse researchers in this field. These two impacts are powerful determinants of the nature of nursing science about families. As stated earlier, the nature of that science is vital because policies will result from the interaction of knowledge base, social strategy, and political will (Richmond & Kotelchuck, 1983).

The assessment of the four programs of research in this chapter tracks with the evolution of the science policy in a number of ways. Students and other scientists have applied their conceptual and methodological publications. As noted by Deatrick, Knafl, and Murphy-Moore (in press), other scientists have applied their concept analysis to further the analyses of the concept of normalization. They have also affirmed the value of concept analysis and other integrative activities leading to synthesis and furthering knowledge development (Knafl & Deatrick, 1993). Archbold and Stewart and Loveland-Cherry have advanced the science for intervention research by identifying critical criteria for outcome measures and specifying processes for identifying the integrity of family measures. These scientists have also promoted the evolution of science policy through their roles on national and international research advisory committees and in research study sections in nursing and other disciplines (WHO Study Group, 1994).

⋙ Recommendations

First, we recommend that the standards for nursing research of families be recognized as a science policy. Those standards guide more than reviews of the literature; they also guide decisions about the content of academic programs that prepare nursing scientists, as well as decisions about the content of research programs conducted by nurse scientists.

Second, we propose revision to the science policy, to promote the kinds of education and scholarship that will increase both the correspondence between practice and research and the correspondence between research and public policy.

We recommend expanding the third standard, derived from Feetham's criteria and purposes, to make the importance of testing interventions and strategies explicit, and adding a standard addressing communication with policy analysts and decision makers at many levels. Thus research of families should:

1. be conceptually and methodologically rigorous;
2. focus on circumstances in which families are likely to need help;
3. contribute to the development and testing of interventions and assessment of strategies;
4. be conducted in the broadest context of relevance to the individual and family, such as in the community, health system, environment, and social and health policy; and
5. provide guidance to institutions and agencies.

In short, the research must (a) be based on valid conceptualizations of families, health services, practice, and policies, so that appropriate knowledge bases (i.e., clinical, bench, economic, organizational sciences) are aligned; (b) assess the impact and efficiency of interventions as a basis for service programs and evaluate their potential to serve as social strategies for policy development; (c) recognize, although not necessarily bow to, political will; and (d) apply methodologies that address the impediments to policies evolving around successful service programs. Research may focus on any level of policy development, from institution to community to municipal and beyond, but it should make use of the frameworks presented here.

It is imperative that research continue to develop so that it may guide practice, but it is also vital that research be conducted in such a way that the results can be translated to inform policies that affect families. It is time to commit to increasing the effectiveness of nursing research of families by strengthening the correspondence with policy in general, emphasizing in particular research to promote the development of interventions into social strategies for improving family health and well-being.

This will require research that is articulated with various levels of application, links the building blocks of science, builds upon the knowledge base of practice, includes variables related to changes in bureaucracy and systems, and makes use of the evaluation sciences. It also requires nurse scientists who have been prepared to participate in the challenges of interdisciplinary work as colleagues.

Designs of academic programs will, in large measure, define what the nurse researcher will be prepared to contribute, as well as how those contributions will be made. Science policy indirectly guides technical choices about graduate programs and research training (distribution of credits, emphasis in coursework, level of expertise to be achieved, kinds of research experience). Do the programs produce credible health scientists, capable of providing high-quality advice to policy deliberations?

For example, do the programs produce nurse researchers who understand the most common tools for carrying out the work of policy analysis and development? Understanding those tools is a prerequisite for communicating with the multidisciplinary cadre of policy analysts. Reviewing session topics for annual meetings of the Association for Health Services Research, tables of contents for survey texts on health policy, and the coursework of a leading doctoral program in health policy, core topics for health services researchers and policy analysts include: access, quality, and appropriateness of care; vulnerable populations; and the role of poverty. These and other researchers and analysts have been trained in analytic methods such as forecasting, legal studies, economic theory regarding competition, demand, geographic variations, decision analysis, cost-benefit analysis, technology assessment, financial and accounting methods, and meta-analysis. Although clinical nurse scholars have valuable knowledge about these topics, they must be able to communicate it to the public, health services researchers, and policy analysts.

Trends in nursing research itself are heartening. In 1997 and 1998, editorials in several of the journals that we used to develop our 1995 samples of family and nonfamily research discussed the increasing credibility of, interest in, and involvement with applications to policy (Bell, 1997; Dougherty, 1997, 1998; Downs, 1997; Henry, 1998). The president and the Expert Panels of the American Academy of Nursing reported successes in building organizational structures that can support policy-related initiatives (Fitzpatrick, 1997, 1998; *Expert Panels Report,* 1997). The academy has also worked with the Agency for Health Care Policy and Research, as well as the National Institute of Nursing Research, to create two senior scholars in residence positions. Both *Maternal-Child Nursing Journal* and *Nursing Outlook* added features focused on the future of health care and bridges between empiricism and practice (Patterson & Lipman, 1998; Pesut, 1997). *Image: the Journal of Nursing Schol-*

arship routinely includes features on health policy and research (Buerhaus, 1998; Henry, 1998; Hirschfeld, 1998; Holleran, 1998; Jones, Jennings, Moritz, & Moss, 1997). The *American Journal of Nursing* "Issues Updates" in 1998 included discussions of why nurses' commitment to health care compels our attention to welfare reform and how our front-line position translates into unique principles to guide the evolution of managed care (Keepnews, 1998; Trossman, 1998).

The social capital of nursing is, perhaps, the most encouraging factor. Nursing is viewed as an honest broker in health care—as a discipline that bases its efforts on the best interests of patients and their families and that can be looked to for committed service (McBride, 1997; Salmon, 1998; Sigma Theta Tau, 1996). Recently, the American people confirmed that view. In a national survey by Blendon and colleagues (1998), participants were asked who was doing "a good job" of providing services. With an approval rating of 83%, nurses stand head and shoulders above the others. Doctors were next (69%), but

hospitals were lower (61%), and insurance companies (44%) and managed care companies (34%) were very low. Blendon et al.'s (1998) report illustrates the strong, positive political will Americans have for nurses. This social capital can be used to articulate solutions to the public and to all levels of policy makers (Wakefield, 1998; *Woodhall Study,* 1998).

Professions advance through constant reassessment of their roles in society. In addition to such evolving reassessment, there are more defining moments which make us aware of a transformation in professional practice (Richmond, 1994). Our assessment of the state of nursing research of families demonstrates that the profession has made progress—uneven and limited, but progress even so—in a transformation to increase the correspondence between practice, research, and policy. There are frameworks and a science policy to support more progress. Families have much to gain if nursing research of families applies the frameworks to improve correspondence with policy. The gap is ours to close.

References

(NOTE: This list does not include references for the 366 research reports and abstracts that we classified into the matrix.)

Abdellah, F. G. (1991). *Nursing's role in the future: A case for health policy decision making.* Indianapolis: Center Nursing Press, Sigma Theta Tau International.

Abdellah, F. G., & Levine, E. (1994). *Preparing nursing research for the 21st century: Evolution, methodologies, challenges.* New York: Springer.

Aiken, L. H. (1992). Charting nursing's future. In L. H. Aiken & C. M. Fagin (Eds.), *Charting nursing's future: Agenda for the 1990s* (pp. 3-12). New York: J. B. Lippincott.

Akula, J. L. (1997). Insolvency risk in health carriers: Innovation, competition and public protection. *Health Affairs, 16,* 9-33.

Andrews, J. A., Hops, H., Ary, D. V., Tildesley, E., & Harris, J. (1993). Parental influence on early adolescent substance use: Specific and nonspecific effects. *Journal of Early Adolescence, 13*(3), 285-310.

Archbold, P. (1980). Impact of parent-caring on middle-aged offspring. *Journal of Gerontological Nursing, 6*(2), 78-85.

Archbold, P. (1981). Ethical issues in the selection of a theoretical framework for gerontological nursing research. *Journal of Gerontological Nursing, 7,* 408-411.

Archbold, P. (1982a). All-consuming activity: The family as caregiver. *Generations, 7*(2), 12-13.

Archbold, P. (1982b). An analysis of parent-caring by women. *Home Health Care Services Quarterly, 3*(2), 5-26.

Archbold, P. (1983). Impact of parent-caring on women. *Family Relations: Journal of Applied Family and Child Studies, 32*(1), 39-45.

Archbold, P. (1986a). Qualitative methods in caregiving support. *Japanese Journal of Nursing Research, 19*(1), 81-104.

Archbold, P. (1986b). The interaction between qualitative and quantitative methods in caregiving research. *Japanese Journal of Nursing Research, 19*(1), 105-116.

Archbold, P., & Hoeffer, B. (1981). Using debate to reframe the issue: Third-party reimbursement for nurses. *Nursing Outlook, 29*(7), 423-427.

Archbold, P. G. (1991a). An interdisciplinary approach to family caregiving research. *Communicating Nursing Research, 24,* 27-42.

Archbold, P. G. (1991b). Distinguished research lectureship: An interdisciplinary approach to family caregiving research. *Communicating Nursing Research, 24,* 27-42.

Archbold, P. G. (1992). Reflections on a program of caregiving research. In Western Institute of Nursing (Ed.), *The anniversary issue 1956-1992.* Boulder, CO: Western Institute of Nursing.

Archbold, P. G., & Stewart, B. J. (1996a). Thinking about intervention classification. *Image: The Journal of Nursing Scholarship, 28*(4), 290.

Archbold, P. G., & Stewart, B. J. (1996b). The nature of the family caregiving role and nursing interventions for caregiving families. In E. A. Swanson & T. Tripp-Reimer (Eds.), *Advances in gerontological nursing* (pp. 133-156). New York: Springer.

Archbold, P. G., Stewart, B. J., Greenlick, M. R., & Harvath, T. (1990). Mutuality and preparedness as predictors of caregiver role strain. *Research in Nursing and Health, 13*(6), 375-384.

Archbold, P. G., Stewart, B. J., Miller, L. L., Harvath, T. A., Greenlick, M. R., Van Buren, L., Kirschling, J. M., Valanis, B. G., Brody, K. K., Schook, J. E., & Hagan, J. M. (1995). The PREP system of nursing interventions: A pilot test with families caring for older members. *Research in Nursing and Health, 18*(1), 3-16.

Bachman, J. G., Johnson, L. D., & O'Malley, P. M. (1998). Explaining recent increases in students' marijuana use: Impacts of perceived risks and disapproval, 1976 through 1996. *American Journal of Public Health, 88*(6), 887-892.

Bell, J. M. (1997). Year 3: A state of the union address. *Journal of Family Nursing, 3,* 115-119.

Blendon, R. J., Brodie, M., Benson, J. M., Altman, D. E., Levitt, L., Hoff, T., & Hugick, L. (1998). Understanding the managed care backlash. *Health Affairs, 17,* 80-94.

Blumenthal, D. (1995). Health care reform—past and future. *New England Journal of Medicine, 332,* 465-468.

Both, D. R., & Garduque, L. (Eds.). (1989). *Social policy for children and families: Report of the Steering Group of the National Forum on the Future of Children and Families.* Washington, DC: National Academy Press.

Brundtland, G. H. (1998). Reaching out for world health [Editoral]. *Science, 280,* 2027.

Buerhaus, P. I. (1998). Financing, demographic, and political problems confronting medicare in the United States. *Image: The Journal of Nursing Scholarship, 30,* 117-123.

Campbell, T. L., & Patterson, J. M. (1995). The effectiveness of family interventions in the treatment of physical illness. *Journal of Marital and Family Therapy, 21,* 545-583.

Cartwright, J. C., Archbold, P. G., Stewart, B. J., & Limandri, B. (1994). Enrichment processes in family caregiving to frail elders. *Advances in Nursing Science, 17*(1), 31-43.

Cohen, S. S., Mason, D. J., Kovner, C., Leavitt, J. K., Pulcini, J., & Sochalski, J. (1996). Stages of nursing's political development: Where we've been and where we ought to go. *Nursing Outlook, 44,* 259-266.

Conn, V. S., & Armer, J. M. (1996). Meta-analysis and public policy: Opportunity for nursing impact. *Nursing Outlook, 44,* 267-271.

Davis, K. (1986). Research and policy formulation. In L. H. Aiken & D. Mechanic (Eds.), *Applications of social science to clinical medicine and health policy* (pp. 113-125). New Brunswick, NJ: Rutgers University Press.

Deatrick, J. A., & Knafl, K. A. (1988). Developing programs for hospitalized children: Clinical significance of qualitative research. *Journal of Pediatric Nursing, 3,* 123-126.

Deatrick, J., & Knafl, K. (1990). Family management behaviors: Concept synthesis. *Journal of Pediatric Nursing, 5,* 15-22.

Deatrick, J., Knafl, K., & Guyer, K. (1993). The meaning of caregiving behaviors: Inductive approaches to family theory development. In S. Feetham, J. Bell, S. Meister, & K. Gilliss (Eds.), *The nursing of families* (pp. 38-45). Newbury Park, CA: Sage.

Deatrick, J., Knafl, K., & Murphy-Moore, C. (in press). Clarifying the concept of normalization. *Image: The Journal of Nursing Scholarship.*

Deatrick, J. A., Knafl, K. A., & Walsh, M. (1988). The process of parenting a child with a disability: Normalization through accommodations. *Journal of Advanced Nursing, 13,* 15-21.

Dielman, T. E., Leech, S. L., & Loveland-Cherry, C. J. (1995). Parents' and children's reports of parenting practices, and parent and child alcohol use. *Drugs and Society: A Journal of Contemporary Issues, 8,* 3-4, 83-87.

Dougherty, M. (1997). Continuity and change. *Nursing Research, 46,* 187.

Dougherty, M. (1998). Changes. *Nursing Research, 47,* 1.

Downs, F. S. (1997). The completion of an evolutionary step. *Nursing Research, 46,* 65.

Expert panels report. (1997). Washington, DC: American Academy of Nursing.

Feeg, V. D. (1996). Now is the time for a kid version of Medicare [Editorial]. *Pediatric Nursing, 22,* 466, 499.

Feetham, S. L. (1984). Family research: Issues and directions for nursing. In H. H. Werley & J. J. Fitzpatrick (Eds.), *Annual review of nursing research* (pp. 3-26). New York: Springer.

Feetham, S. L. (1991). Conceptual and methodological issues in research of families. In A. L. Whall & J. Fawcett (Eds.), *Family theory development in nursing: State of the science and art* (pp. 55-68). Philadelphia: F. A. Davis.

Feetham, S. (1992). Family outcomes: Conceptual and methodological issues. In P. Moritz (Ed.), *Patient outcomes research: Examining the effectiveness of nursing practice* (pp. 103-111). Bethesda, MD: National Center for Nursing Research, NIH.

Feetham, S. L. (1997). Families and health in the urban environment. In O. Reyes, H. J. Wallberg, & R. P. Weissberg (Eds.), *Interdisciplinary perspectives in children and youth* (pp. 321-359). Thousand Oaks, CA: Sage.

Feetham, S. L., & Frink, B. B. (1997). Issues in health services research: Children and families. In M. Broome, K. Pridham, K. Knafl, & S. Feetham (Eds.), *Handbook of children and families in health and illness* (pp. 280-297). Thousand Oaks, CA: Sage.

Feetham, S. L., & Meister, S. B. (1994). Innovations in providing maternal and child health nursing services. In H. M. Wallace, R. P. Nelson, & P. J. Sweeney (Eds.), *Maternal and child health practices* (4th ed., pp. 149-159). Oakland, CA: Third Party.

Field, M. J., & Shapiro, H. T. (1993). *Employment and health benefits.* Washington, DC: National Academy Press.

Fitzpatrick, J. J. (1997). The president's message. *Nursing Outlook, 45,* 277-279.

Fitzpatrick, J. J. (1998). The president's message. *Nursing Outlook, 46,* 136-137.

Fralic, M. F. (1994). Comments on innovative practice and delivery systems research. In J. J. Fitzpatrick, J. S. Stevenson, & N. S. Polis (Eds.), *Nursing research and its utilization: International state of the science* (pp. 159-166). New York: Springer.

Gilliss, C. L., & Davis, L. L. (1993). Does family intervention make a difference? An integrative review and meta-analysis. In S. L. Feetham, S. B. Meister, J. M. Bell, & C. L. Gilliss (Eds.), *The nursing of families* (pp. 259-265). Newbury Park, CA: Sage.

Ginzberg, E. (1991). The challenges ahead. In E. Ginzberg (Ed.), *Health services research: Key to health policy* (pp. 315-332). Cambridge, MA: Harvard University Press.

Harvath, T. A., Archbold, P. G., Stewart, B. J., Gadow, S., Kirschling, J. M., Miller, L., Hagan, J., Brody, K., & Schook, J. (1994). Establishing partnerships with family caregivers: Local and cosmopolitan knowledge. *Journal of Gerontological Nursing, 20*(2), 29-35, 42-43.

Henry, B. (1998). To journal readers, report and requests. *Image: The Journal of Nursing Scholarship, 30,* 2.

Hinshaw, A. S. (1988). Using research to shape health policy. *Nursing Outlook, 36,* 21-24.

Hinshaw, A. S. (1992). The impact of nursing science on health policy. In *Communicating nursing research* (Vol. 25, pp. 15-26). Boulder, CO: Western Institute of Nursing.

Hirschfeld, M. J. (1998). WHO priorities for a common nursing research agenda. *Image: The Journal of Nursing Scholarship, 30,* 114.

Hoeffer, B., & Archbold, P. G. (1983). Problems in doing nursing research: Interfacing qualitative and quantitative methods. *Western Journal of Nursing Research, 5*(3), 254-257.

Holleran, C. (1998). New leader from Normandy for the World Health Organization. *Image: The Journal of Nursing Scholarship, 30,* 113.

Homer, C. J., Szilagyi, P., Rodewald, L., Bloom, S. R., Greenspan, P., Yazdgerdi, S., Leventhal, J. M., Finkelstein, D., & Perrin, J. M. (1996). Does quality of care affect rate of hospitalization for childhood asthma? *Pediatrics, 98,* 18-23.

Jacox, A. (1998). Health policy. In J. J. Fitzpatrick (Ed.), *Encyclopedia of nursing research* (pp. 234-235). New York: Springer.

Jones, K., Jennings, B. M., Moritz, P., & Moss, M. T. (1997). Policy issues associated with analyzing outcomes of care. *Image: The Journal of Nursing Scholarship, 29,* 261-268.

Kalisch, B. J., & Kalisch, P. A. (1982). *Politics of nursing.* Philadelphia: J. B. Lippincott.

Keepnews, D. (1998). Welfare reform and health care. *American Journal of Nursing, 98,* 55-56.

Klein, D. M., & White, J. M. (1996). *Family theories: An introduction.* Thousand Oaks, CA: Sage.

Knafl, K., & Deatrick, J. (1990). Family management style: Concept analysis and refinement. *Journal of Pediatric Nursing, 5,* 4-14.

Knafl, K., & Deatrick, J. A. (1993). Knowledge synthesis and concept development in nursing. In B. Rodgers & K. Knafl (Eds.), *Concept development in nursing: Foundations, techniques, and applications* (pp. 35-50). Philadelphia: Saunders.

Knafl, K., & Deatrick, J. (in press). Research careers and concept development: The case of normalization. In B. Rodgers & K. Knafl (Eds.), *Concept development in nursing* (2nd ed.). Philadelphia: Saunders.

Knafl, K., Deatrick, J., & Kirby, A. (in press). Normalization promotion. In M. Craft-Rosenberg & J. Dennehy (Eds.), *Nursing interventions for childbearing and childrearing families.* Thousand Oaks, CA: Sage.

Knafl, K., Gallo, A., Breitmayer, B., Zoeller, L., & Ayres, L. (1993). One approach to conceptualizing family response to illness. In S. Feetham, J. Bell, S. Meister, & K. Gilliss (Eds.), *The nursing of families* (pp. 70-78). Newbury Park, CA: Sage.

Knafl, K., Gallo, A., Zoeller, L., & Breitmayer, B. (1993). Family response to a child's chronic illness: A description of major defining themes. In S. Funk & E. Tomquist (Eds.), *Key aspects of caring for the chronically ill: Home and hospital* (pp. 290-303). New York: Springer.

Knafl, K. A. (1985). How families manage a pediatric hospitalization. *Western Journal of Nursing Research, 7,* 151-168.

Knafl, K. A. (1990). Concept development. In *Monograph of the Invitational Conference on Research Methods for Validating Nursing Diagnosis* (pp. 37-63). St. Louis, MO: North American Nursing Diagnosis Association.

Knafl, K. A., & Breitmayer, B. (1989). Triangulation in qualitative research: Issues of conceptual clarity and purpose. In J. Morse (Ed.), *Qualitative nursing research: A contemporary dialogue* (pp. 209-220). Rockville, MD: Aspen.

Knafl, K. A., & Deatrick, J. (1986). How families manage chronic conditions: An analysis of the concept of normalization. *Research in Nursing and Health, 9,* 215-222.

Knafl, K. A., & Deatrick, J. A. (1987). Conceptualizing family response to a child's chronic illness or disability. *Family Relations, 36,* 300-304.

Kosciulek, J. F., McCubbin, M. A., & McCubbin, H. I. (1993). A theoretical framework for family adaptation to head injury. *Journal of Rehabilitation, 59*(3), 40-45.

LeLorier, J., Gregoire, G., Benhaddad, A., Lapierrre, J., & Derderian, F. (1997). Discrepancies between meta-analysis and subsequent large randomized controlled trials. *New England Journal of Medicine, 337,* 536-542.

Loveland-Cherry, C. J., Leech, S., Laetz, V. B., & Dielman, T. E. (1996). Correlates of alcohol use and misuse in fourth-grade children: Psychosocial, peer, parental, and family factors. *Health Education Quarterly, 23*(4), 497-511.

Loveland-Cherry, C. J., & Ross, L. T. (in press). Effects of a family intervention to decrease adolescent alcohol use and misuse. *Journal of Studies in Alcoholism.*

Loveland-Cherry, C. J., Ross, L. T., & Kaufman, S. R. (in press). Effects of a family intervention to decrease adolescent alcohol use and misuse. *Journal of Studies in Alcoholism.*

Loveland-Cherry, C. J., Youngblut, J. M., & Leidy, N. W. (1989). A psychometric analysis of the Family Environment Scale. *Nursing Research, 38*(5), 262-266.

MacVicar, M., & Archbold, P. (1976). A framework for family assessment in chronic illness. *Nursing Forum, 15*(2), 180-184.

McBride, A. B. (1997). Nursing and the women's movement: The legacy of the 1960s. *Reflections, 23,* 38-41.

McCubbin, M. A. (1988). Response to "Measures of stress and related constructs." *Scholarly Inquiry for Nursing Practice, 2*(1), 71-75.

McCubbin, M. A. (1989). Family stress and family strengths: A comparison of single- and two-parent families with handicapped children. *Research in Nursing and Health, 12*(2), 101-110.

McCubbin, M. A. (1993). Family stress theory and the development of nursing knowledge about family adaptation. In S. L. Feetham, S. B. Meister, J. M. Bell, & C. L. Gilliss (Eds.), *The nursing of families* (pp. 46-58). Newbury Park, CA: Sage.

McCubbin, M. A., McCubbin, H. I., & Thompson, A. I. (1986). Family Hardiness Index. In H. I. McCubbin (Ed.), *Family stress, coping and health project, School of Human Ecology* (pp. 237-303). Madison: University of Wisconsin System.

McCubbin, M. A., McCubbin, H., & Thompson, A. (1988a). *Family assessment: Resiliency, coping and adaptation—Inventories for research* Madison: University of Wisconsin System.

McCubbin, M. A., McCubbin, H., & Thompson, A. (1988b). Resiliency in families: A conceptual model of family adjustment and adaptation in response to stress and crises. In M. A. McCubbin, H. McCubbin, & A. Thompson (Eds.), *Family assessment: Resiliency, coping and adaptation—Inventories for research* (pp. 1-61). Madison: University of Wisconsin System.

McCubbin, M. A., McCubbin, H., & Thompson, A. (1988c). Family problem solving communication. In H. I. McCubbin, A. I. Thompson, & M. A. McCubbin (Eds.), *Family assessment: Resiliency, coping and adaptation—Inventories for research* (pp. 639-686). Madison: University of Wisconsin System.

McCubbin, H. I., Thompson, E. A., Thompson, A. I., McCubbin, M. A., & Kaston, A. J. (1993). Culture, ethnicity, and the family: Critical factors in childhood chronic illnesses and disabilities. *Pediatrics, 91*(Suppl. 5, part 2), 1063-1070.

McTeer, M. A. (1996). Social security and welfare reform: Their impact on families. *Journal of Family Nursing, 2,* 3-9.

Mechanic, D., & Aiken, L. H. (1986). Social science, medicine and health policy. In L. H. Aiken & D. Mechanic (Eds.), *Applications of social science to clinical medicine and health policy* (pp. 1-9). New Brunswick, NJ: Rutgers University Press.

Meister, S. B. (1989). Health care financing, policy, and family nursing practice: New opportunities. In C. L. Gilliss, B. H. Highley, B. M. Roberts, & I. M. Martinson (Eds.), *Toward a science of family nursing* (pp. 146-155). New York: Addison-Wesley.

Meister, S. B. (1993). The family's agents: Nursing and policy. In S. L. Feetham, S. B. Meister, J. M. Bell, & C. L. Gilliss (Eds.), *The nursing of families: Theory, research, education, practice* (pp. 3-10). Newbury Park, CA: Sage.

Meister, S. B. (1997). *Policy for children's health: Scholarship, practice and principles: Harvard's Working Group on Early Life and*

Adolescent Health Policy. Boston: Harvard Center for Children's Health.

Milio, N. (1984). Nursing research and the study of health policy. In H. H. Werley & J. J. Fitzpatrick (Eds.), *Annual review of nursing research* (pp. 291-306). New York: Springer.

Miller, L. L., Hornbrook, M. C., Archbold, P. G., & Stewart, B. J. (1996). Development of use and cost measures in a nursing intervention for family caregivers and frail elderly patients. *Research in Nursing and Health, 19*(4), 273-285.

Miller, T. Q. (1994). A test of alternative explanations for the stage-like progression of adolescent substance use in four national samples. *Addictive Behaviors, 19*(3), 287-293.

Moynihan, D. P. (1986). *Family and nation.* San Diego, CA: Harcourt, Brace, Jovanovich.

Natapoff, J. N. (1990a). Conclusions and recommendations: A policy agenda. In J. N. Natapoff & R. R. Wieczorek (Eds.), *Maternal-child health policy: A nursing perspective* (pp. 323-329). New York: Springer.

Natapoff, J. N. (1990b). Introduction. In J. N. Natapoff & R. R. Wieczorek (Eds.), *Maternal-child health policy: A nursing perspective* (pp. 1-16). New York: Springer.

Newhouse, J. P. (1986). Social experiments in health. In L. H. Aiken & D. Mechanic (Eds.), *Application of social science to clinical medicine and health policy* (pp. 229-250). New Brunswick, NJ: Rutgers University Press.

Newhouse, J. P. (1991). Controlled experimentation as research policy. In E. Ginzberg (Ed.), *Health services research: Key to health policy* (pp. 161-194). Cambridge, MA: Harvard University Press.

Nkongho, N. O., & Archbold, P. G. (1995). Reasons for caregiving in African American families. *Journal of Cultural Diversity, 2*(4), 116-123.

Nkongho, N. O., & Archbold, P. G. (1996). Working-out caregiving systems in African American families. *Applied Nursing Research, 9*(3), 108-114.

Palfrey, J. S. (1994). *Community child health: An action plan for today.* Westport, CT: Praeger.

Patterson, E. T., & Lipman, T. H. (1998). Toward evidenced-based practice. *Maternal Care Nursing, 23,* 166-167.

Perrin, J. M., Kahn, R., Bloom, S., Davidson, S., Guyer, B., Hollingshead, W., Richmond, J., Walker, D. K., & Wise, P. (1994). Health care reform and the special needs of children. *Pediatrics, 3,* 504-506.

Perrin, J. M., Shayne, M. W., & Bloom, S. R. (1993). *Home and community care for chronically ill children.* New York: Oxford University Press.

Pesut, D. J. (1997). Future think. *Nursing Outlook, 45,* 107.

Pratt, J. W., & Zeckhauser, R. J. (1985). Principals and agents: An overview. In J. W. Pratt & R. J. Zeckhauser (Eds.), *Principals and agents: The structure of business* (pp. 1-35). Boston: Harvard Business School Press.

Reforming States Group and the Milbank Memorial Fund. (1997). *State oversight of integrated health systems.* New York: Milbank Memorial Fund.

Richmond, J. B. (1994). Introduction. In J. S. Palfrey (Ed.), *Community child health: An action plan for today* (pp. 8-9). Westport, CT: Praeger.

Richmond, J. B., & Kotelchuck, M. L. (1983). Political influences: Rethinking national health policy. In C. H. McGuire, R. P. Foley, A. Gorr, R. W. Richards, & Associates (Eds.), *Handbook on health professions education* (pp. 386-404). San Francisco: Jossey-Bass.

Rosenbaum, S., & Johnson, K. (1986). Providing health care for low-income children: Reconciling health goals with child health financing realities. *Milbank Quarterly, 64,* 442-478.

Rosenbaum, S., Serrano, R., Magar, M., & Stern, G. (1997). Civil rights in a changing health care system. *Health Affairs, 16,* 90-115.

Ross, L. T., & Hill, E. M. (in press). Drinking and parental unpredictability among adult children of alcoholics. *International Journal of the Addictions.*

Ross, L. T., Loveland-Cherry, C. J., Leech, S. L., & Laetz, V. (in press). Parental, peer and personal correlates of adolescent substance use and misuse: Race and gender comparisons. *Journal of Research and Adolescence.*

Rossi, P. H., & Freeman, H. E. (1993). *Evaluation: A systematic approach* (5th ed.). Newbury Park, CA: Sage.

Salmon, M. E. (1998). Nursing, equity and social justice. *Reflections, 24,* 8-11.

Sanders, N. F. (1994). Measuring the effectiveness of innovative patient care delivery systems: A multivariate model. In J. J. Fitzpatrick, J. S. Stevenson, & N. S. Polis (Eds.), *Nursing research and its utilization: International state of the science* (pp. 119-128). New York: Springer.

Schumacher, K. L., Stewart, B. J., & Archbold, P. G. (1998). Conceptualization and measurement of doing family caregiving well. *Journal of Nursing Scholarship, 30*(1), 63-69.

Schorr, L. B. (1988). *Within our reach: Breaking the cycle of disadvantage.* New York: Doubleday.

Schorr, L. B. (1991). *Successful programs and the bureaucratic dilemma: Current deliberations.* New York: National Center for Children in Poverty.

Schorr, L. B. (1997). *Common purpose: Strengthening families and neighborhoods to rebuild America.* New York: Doubleday.

Shine, K. I. (1998). The health sciences, health services research and the role of the health professions. *Health Service Research, 33,* 439-445.

Shortell, S. M., & Reinhardt, U. E. (1992). Creating and executing health policy in the 1990's. In S. M. Shortell & V. E. Reinhardt (Eds.), *Improving health policy and management* (pp. 3-36). Ann Harbor, MI: Health Administration Press.

Sigma Theta Tau. (1996). *Nursing leadership in the 21st century.* Indianapolis, IN: Center Nursing Press, Sigma Theta Tau International.

Stewart, B. J., & Archbold, P. G. (1992). Nursing intervention studies require outcome measures that are sensitive to change: Part one. *Research in Nursing and Health, 15*(6), 477-481.

Stewart, B. J., & Archbold, P. G. (1993). Nursing intervention studies require outcome measures that are sensitive to change: Part two. *Research in Nursing and Health, 16*(1), 77-81.

Stewart, B. J., & Archbold, P. G. (1997). Guest editorial. A new look for measurement validity. *Journal of Nursing Education, 36*(3), 99-101.

Stewart, B. J., Archbold, P. G., Harvath, T. A., & Nkongho, N. O. (1993). Role acquisition in family caregivers for older people who have been discharged from the hospital. In B. J. Stewart, P. G. Archbold, T. A. Harvath, & N. O. Nkongho (Eds.), *Key aspects of caring for the chronically ill: Hospital and home* (pp. 219-231). New York: Springer.

Stokey, E., & Zeckhauser, R. J. (1978). *A primer for policy analysis.* New York: W. W. Norton.

Strickland, O. L. (1997). Are we rigorous enough? *Reflections, 23,* 8-10.

Strickland, O. L., & Waltz, C. F. (1988). *Measurement of nursing outcomes: Measuring nursing performance* (Vol. 2). New York: Springer.

Strickland, O. L., & Waltz, C. F. (1990). *Measurement of nursing outcomes: Measuring client self-care and coping skills* (Vol. 4). New York: Springer.

Svavarsdottir, E. K., & McCubbin, M. (1996). Parenthood transition for parents of an infant diagnosed with a congenital heart condition. *Journal of Pediatric Nursing, 11*(4), 207-216.

Tierney, A. (1994). Innovative practice and delivery systems research: A perspective from the United Kingdom. In J. J. Fitzpatrick, J. S. Stevenson, & N. S. Polis (Eds.), *Nursing research and its utilization: International state of the science* (pp. 135-140). New York: Springer.

Trossman, S. (1998). Quality managed care: A nursing perspective. *American Journal of Nursing, 98*(6), 56-58.

Verran, J. A. (1994). The effects of practice model implementation. In J. J. Fitzpatrick, J. S. Stevenson, & N. S. Polis (Eds.), *Nursing research and its utilization: International state of the science* (pp. 129-134). New York: Springer.

Wakefield, M. (1998). Capitalizing on our currency. *Nursing Outlook, 46,* 89-90.

Waltz, C. F., & Strickland, O. L. (1988). *Measurement of nursing outcomes: Measuring client outcomes* (Vol. 1). New York: Springer.

Waltz, C. F., & Strickland, O. L. (1990). *Measurement of nursing outcomes: Measuring clinical skills and professional development in education and practice* (Vol. 3). New York: Springer.

Wills, T. A., Schreibman, D., Benson, G., & Vaccaro, D. (1992). The role of life events, family support, and competence in adulthood substance use: A test of vulnerability and protective factors. *American Journal of Community Psychology, 20,* 349-374.

Wills, T. A., Schreibman, D., Benson, G., & Vaccaro, D. (1994). Impact of parental substance use on adolescents: A test of mediational model. *Journal of Pediatric Psychology, 19*(5), 537-555.

WHO Study Group. (1994). *Nursing beyond the year 2000: Report of a WHO study group.* Geneva, Switzerland: World Health Organization.

Woodhall study on nursing and the media. (1998). Indianapolis, IN: Center Nursing Press, Sigma Theta Tau.

Zoeller, L. H. (1996). *The school experience of families with chronically ill children: Conceptualization and correlates.* Unpublished dissertation, University of Illinois at Chicago.

PART
IID

HEALTH PROMOTION
AND RISK REDUCTION

Nola J. Pender

Health promotion and risk reduction services are becoming a vital part of comprehensive health care for persons of all ages. The science that provides the base for health promotion and risk reduction is expanding rapidly, but we have much more to learn. However, we already know a great deal about what behavioral and environmental changes are needed to promote health. We know less about how to bring about positive changes. Nurse scientists are in an ideal position to help build the sciences of health promotion and risk reduction. Their holistic orientation to health care is ideally suited to designing and testing the multidimensional approaches that are needed to create health-strengthening environments and positive health behavior norms. Most health promotion and disease prevention research to date has been descriptive and correlational in nature. Few prospective studies have explored causal relationships among variables that are theoretically proposed as influencing health behavior outcomes. Even fewer longitudinal studies have been conducted to track the developmental trajectory of healthy behaviors and risky behaviors over time.

The ultimate goal of scientists in health promotion is to design and test theoretically based and culturally appropriate interventions that will inform nurses and other health professionals about which interventions work to create healthy environments and positive health behavior patterns in varying populations and which interventions are ineffective. Conduct of intervention research is the most efficient way to identify strategic health promotion and disease prevention services that should be integrated into primary care and into health promotion programs offered in schools and at worksites.

Research to determine the efficacy and acceptability of interventions must be conducted in multiple ethnic and racial populations. Further, to ensure culturally relevant health promotion services for diverse populations, collaborative research and service partnerships need to be developed with communities. As scientists and communities work together, critical problems can be identified, appropriate measurement tools developed, and tailored interventions designed that will be more likely to fit the life context and life ways of people who are intended to benefit from newly created programs. Community partnerships to develop and test health promotion interventions can narrow the current gap between expectations of health care recipients and responsiveness of providers, as well as improving the quality of care provided by nurses and other health professionals to target populations.

Lifestyles and social and physical environments, interacting with genetics, contribute to health. Thus, we must discover how biology, behavior, and environment either promote or impair health. We need to understand when an ecological or population-based approach versus an individually or behaviorally based approach is likely to be most effective. Often, both environmental and behavioral changes that are enduring must occur simultaneously to improve the health of populations, especially those most vulnerable due to genetic makeup, age, socioeconomic status, or other life circumstances.

New communication technologies will also play a role in the future character of health promotion and prevention services. Worldwide information systems will provide access to a range of health information that will empower individuals and families to act on their own behalf to protect and enhance health. Nurses will play an important role in structuring the assessment tools and information available and in testing the effectiveness of tailoring information to meet the unique needs of persons at different points in the lifespan and with different genetic profiles, behavioral patterns, and environments. Some of the studies reported in this chapter incorporate the latest information technology in nursing intervention research. Designing and testing information and communication systems of care that provide the appropriate balance between face-to-face contact with health care providers and interactive, distance communication is an important frontier for scientific advances in health promotion intervention research.

The chapters in this section have been prepared by outstanding nurse researchers actively involved in investigating health promotion and disease prevention processes and related interventions. The chapter authors provide an in-depth discussion of the state of the science of health promotion and risk reduction in the areas of preventing and treating hypertension in Black Americans, lowering risk for cardiovascular disease in children and adolescents, promoting health in adolescents, and promoting health and preventing disease in worksite populations. The reader will find a wealth of information about strengths and gaps in nursing science relevant to health promotion and risk reduction, extant conceptual and theoretical perspectives, important clinical issues and questions in the field, and recommendations for advancing nursing science relevant to health promotion and risk reduction. A critical analysis of these chapters will enrich the work of nurse scientists and contribute to improving the quality of clinical and counseling services provided by nurses in primary care as well as in other health care settings.

15

INTERVENTIONS FOR PROMOTING HEALTH IN ADOLESCENTS

Carol J. Loveland-Cherry

Overview

Adolescence is a tremendously important transition period. It is marked by complex biological, physical, behavioral, and social transformations. According to the report of the Carnegie Council on Adolescent Development (1995), "The events of this crucially formative phase can shape an individual's life course and thus the future of the whole society" (p. 19). Adolescence is a period of experimentation and learning; behaviors that have significant implications for immediate and long-term health are tried out and adopted, especially during early adolescence. Clearly, adolescence is a critical period for implementing interventions to promote the health of an important segment of the population.

Nursing has intervened with adolescents in a variety of settings and around many health issues. Although the preponderance of nursing care to adolescents has occurred in the context of illness, growing numbers of nursing interventions are focused on health promotion with adolescents. Nurses in schools, clinics, health centers, public health agencies, communities, and other traditional and nontraditional settings are well positioned to develop, implement, and evaluate health promotion interventions with adolescents. Unfortunately, relatively few of these nursing interventions have been subjected to empirical verification of their effectiveness within a systematic research context. As research with adolescents becomes more interdisciplinary, it is often difficult to identify nursing research. Consequently, a computer literature search using Medline was initially run using the keywords of *intervention, health promotion, adolescents,* and *risk reduction.* All identified references were scanned to determine if the article was a research report and if a nurse was an author. If there was any difficulty in deciding either of these two issues, a copy of the article was obtained and examined. Hand searches of major relevant interdisciplinary journals (e.g., *Journal of Health Promotion*) were completed to identify articles that might have been missed in a computer search.

In this chapter, the state of the science for promoting health for adolescents is evaluated and recommendations made for advancing the science in this field of study. Two major areas of review and critique are undertaken: a description of the conceptual and theoretical perspectives used to develop interventions with adolescents and an evaluation of the current scientific basis for intervening with adolescents.

Introduction

If primarily physical parameters are considered, adolescents have been thought to be one of the healthiest segments of the population. However, if other dimensions of health (i.e., psychological, social, environmental) are considered, multiple unmet needs are evident (Millstein, Petersen, & Nightingale, 1993). In fact, adolescents have been one of the most neglected groups in terms of health promotion (Shalala, 1995). Recent work has highlighted the needs of this segment of the population. Much of the growing concern arises from recent data on the health and well-being of adolescents. The Year 2000 Objectives for the Nation (U.S. Department of Health and Human Services [USDHHS], 1990) identified two major categories of preventable health concerns for adolescents and young adults: "injuries and violence that kill or disable and developing lifestyle behaviors" (p. 571). Within the Year 2000 Objectives for the Nation, adolescence is one of the phases of the lifespan for which age-specific objectives were formulated. The areas of intervention needed to promote the health of adolescents are clear.

The overall objective is to reduce the death rate for adolescents and young adults by 15% to no more than 85 per 100,000. Specific objectives for this segment of the population target nutrition, physical activity and fitness, sexual activity and the associated risks of unwanted pregnancy and sexually transmitted diseases (including

HIV/AIDS), suicide, homicide, unintentional injury, and substance use (alcohol, tobacco, marijuana, and other drugs—ATOD). The foci of these objectives provide the structure for the review of the science. Efforts to reduce overweight (including physical activity and nutrition) are often associated with reducing cardiovascular risk. Because interventions for reducing hypertension in African Americans and for reducing cardiovascular risk in children are addressed in Chapters 16 and 17, efforts to reduce overweight in adolescents are not addressed in this chapter. Specific attention is paid to efforts to (a) promote positive parenting in adolescent parents; (b) to delay or postpone early sexual behavior; (c) to reduce homicide and suicide; and (d) to reduce alcohol, tobacco, and other drug use. These areas are also consistent with those targeted in the final report of the Carnegie Council on Adolescent Development: promoting the delay or postponement of early sexual behavior, preparing for healthy parenthood, and preventing drug abuse.

In this chapter, adolescence is defined as the period from 10 to 19 years old. Three distinct phases of adolescence have been identified in the literature: early (10-12), middle (13-15), and late (16-19). Each phase is marked by a critical school transition that is accompanied by important social, cognitive, and environmental transitions. Early adolescence is the phase when the important transition from elementary to middle or junior high school occurs. During middle adolescence, adolescents move from middle or junior high school to high school. Late adolescence is the time when many adolescents leave the family home for college, other training, or work. Although there are commonalties across the three phases, there are also differences among the three that are reflected in health outcomes. For example, the leading cause of death for all adolescents, at all ages, is motor vehicle accidents. However, homicide is the next leading cause of death for adolescents age 15 to 19 years, in contrast to unintentional injury for the younger group (Carnegie Council on Adolescent Development, 1995). It is not clear that stage of adolescence has been acknowledged in interventions with this population. Consequently, one of the criteria that will be used in critiquing the literature is whether attention is given to the stage of adolescence.

The Priority Expert Panel F: Health Promotion for Older Children and Adolescents, one of a series of expert panels convened by the then National Institute of Nursing Research, recommended priorities for research with this population (USDHHS, 1993). The three broad priority recommendations for 1992 to 1997 were:

1. Examine the interactive effects of behavioral and biological processes, including the timing of developmental and social transitions, on health actions and outcomes.

2. Investigate family, school, and community strategies for adopting and maintaining health-promoting behaviors among youth in rural and urban settings. Special attention should be given to highly vulnerable youth who are economically disadvantaged, homeless, school dropouts, members of racial or ethnic minority groups, immigrants, gay or lesbian, alienated or chronically ill or disabled.

3. Develop and test culturally appropriate, innovative health promotion interventions that incorporate both educational and contextual components in outreach settings and focus on the collaboration of nurses with other health professionals. (USDHHS, 1993, p. 10).

The current literature of nursing interventions to promote the health of adolescents is evaluated within the context of these three recommendations.

As part of the evaluation of the status of nursing interventions to promote health in adolescents, the various conceptual and theoretical perspectives and schools of thought are summarized and examined in terms of similarities and diversity of views. In the context of this background, clinical issues and questions regarding health promotion in adolescents are identified.

The nursing literature and relevant literature from other disciplines, with emphasis on the former, are synthesized. This process focuses on identifying what is known, what needs to be known, strengths and weaknesses in this area of science, and an evaluation of the state of the science.

In the final section of this chapter, recommendations for advancing nursing science related to health in adolescents are presented.

Perspectives in Interventions to Promote Health in Adolescents

Conceptual and Theoretical Perspectives

Several issues are evident, related to conceptual or theoretical perspectives relevant to interventions to promote health in adolescents. The lack of an identified theoretical approach to structure interventions has been con-

sistently identified as a problem in the intervention research literature. This atheoretical state is characteristic of early nursing research, as well as that in other disciplines, and is evident in reports of nursing interventions. As a consequence, it was often difficult to determine why an intervention worked or didn't work and to know if the intervention could be generalized to other settings or groups. A major emphasis in graduate education programs in nursing has been to stress the need for theory-based intervention; thus one would expect to see a shift to the use of theoretical perspectives for development of nursing interventions.

Principles of what should be included in the development and implementation of interventions are presented in the literature. For example, Hamburg, Millstein, Mortimer, Nightingale, and Petersen (1993) identify characteristics of successful programs as follows: (a) programs "must be acceptable to the relevant individuals, cultural groups and communities"; (b) programs must "incorporate basic knowledge about adolescent development into their design, acknowledging the capabilities and needs of adolescents at different ages"; (c) programs should foster health-enhancing environments that are "supportive in the long term and direct adolescents toward autonomy"; (d) programs should promote the development and practice of skills (interpersonal and communications skills, cognitive skills, employability skills, coping skills, functional skills), and program messages and goals need to be "consistent with the cultural milieu of the adolescent"; (e) programs need to "link adolescents to social institutions that support their healthy development"; (f) programs "must be explicit and realistic about the goals they aim to reach"; (g) special attention needs to be given to health promotion of poor adolescents; and (h) programs for minority youth should recognize their uniqueness and simultaneously enhance "successful negotiation within the dominant group and societal institutions" (pp. 379-383). Finally, a need for theory-based interventions is consistently identified in the literature.

Indeed, reports of interventions to promote health in adolescents that are externally funded (i.e., by foundations or the National Institutes of Health [NIH]) are very likely, but not always, to be developed from an identified theoretical perspective. For example, the work of Jemmott, Jemmott, and colleagues (Jemmott & Jemmott, 1991, 1992a, 1992b, 1993, 1994; Jemmott, Jemmott, & Fong, 1992; Jemmott, Jemmott, & Hacker, 1992; Jemmott, Jemmott, Spears, Hewitt, & Cruz-Collins, 1992) is developed within the context of Social Learning Theory

(Bandura, 1986) and the Theory of Planned Behavior (Ajzen, 1985, 1991). Eggert and colleagues have framed their work within a conceptualization that integrates empirically supported work from social learning, social control, strain theories and nursing theories of therapeutic use of self, brief counseling theory, and motivational interviewing (Eggert, Seyl, & Nicholas, 1990; Eggert, Thompson, Herting, & Nicholas, 1994; Eggert, Thompson, Herting, Nicholas, & Dicker, 1994). In fact, the studies reviewed were more likely than not to include a conceptual or theoretical framework.

The variety of theoretical approaches that underlie health promotion interventions for adolescents reflects the broad range of health issues (e.g., adolescent parenting, HIV/AIDS, substance use, suicide) that are targeted and the focus of the intervention (e.g., family, individual, community). A number of individually focused theories, including Social Learning Theory (Bandura, 1986), the Health Promotion Model (Pender, 1996), and Problem Behavior Theory (Jessor & Jessor, 1980), were evident in structuring interventions related to reducing risk behaviors such as substance use (Dielman, Laetz, Leech, & Loveland-Cherry, 1994; Eggert, Thompson, Herting, & Nicholas, 1994; Loveland-Cherry, Ross, & Laetz, 1996), early sexual behavior, and risky sexual behavior (Guthrie, Wallace, et al., 1996; Jemmott & Jemmott, 1991, 1992a, 1992b, 1993). Measures to promote positive parenting in adolescents were likely to be approached from role-related theories, such as a role supplementation model (Clarke & Strauss, 1992), Orem's Self-Care Theory (Buckley, 1990), or maternal role theory (Koniak-Griffin & Verzemnieks, 1991). Conceptual constructs missing in all of the studies that were reviewed were development and gender. Theoretical, clinical, and empirical literature emphasize the importance of understanding and considering developmental aspects as well as more commonly included factors such as attitudes, knowledge, and values. Although it is generally agreed that there are at least three distinct phases of adolescence, little attention has been paid to acknowledging the potential differences among phases of adolescence. Adolescence is a time of change, and understanding the transitions inherent in this developmental period is proposed to facilitate the design of appropriate interventions for adolescents (USDHHS, 1993).

▬ Level of Intervention

There is a growing consensus that effective approaches to adolescent health promotion need to address not only individual factors but also important environmental factors, such as family, school, and community (Eccles et al., 1993; Eggert, Thompson, Herting, & Nicholas, 1994; Guthrie, Loveland-Cherry, Frey, & Dielman, 1994; USDHHS, 1993). Although the majority of the nursing interventions that were reviewed were focused on the individual adolescent, several acknowledged and incorporated the need to move to more comprehensive, ecological approaches (Bearinger & Gephart, 1987; Eggert, Thompson, Herting, & Nicholas, 1994; Guthrie, Wallace, et al., 1996). Environmental targets for intervention were most often the family (Loveland-Cherry, Ross, et al., 1996), the school (Eggert, Thompson, Herting, & Nicholas, 1994), and peer groups (Guthrie, Wallace, et al., 1996).

▬ Approach to Intervention: Risk Reduction Versus Protection

A second area of growing consensus is the advocation of a strength- or skill-enhancing empowerment approach to health promotion in adolescents (Hawkins, Catalano, & Miller, 1992; Igoe, 1991; Kumpfer, 1990; Schinke, Botvin, & Orlandi, 1991; USDHHS, 1993). This represents a shift from an emphasis solely on a threat-avoidance approach to one that includes competence building and an acknowledgment that interventions must go beyond information transmission to effect changes in behavior. Bogenschneider (1996) succinctly summarizes the strengths and limitations of the two approaches in understanding factors that contribute to healthy adolescent development. The epidemiological risk-focused approach was adapted from the medical field and emphasizes the identification and reduction of the multiple risks that adolescents encounter. In contrast, the protective-factor etiological perspective focuses on "enhancing youngsters' ability to resist stressful life events and promote adaptation and competence" (p. 129).

Bogenschneider (1996) argues effectively for an approach that integrates the two approaches (the Ecological Risk/Protective Theoretical Model) and asserts that they are complementary to each other rather than contradictory. Both approaches offer multiple opportunities for intervention; an integrative approach, therefore, provides a framework that may be even more effective for addressing the complexity of adolescent health promotion. Bogenschneider proposes that the protective model is "especially appropriate when targeted toward high-risk youth, whereas the risk model potentially benefits all youth" (p. 130). The integrated model is an intriguing challenge to the development of nursing interventions for adolescent health promotion. The use of such an integrated approach is evident in several nursing intervention programs (Eggert, Thompson, Herting, & Nicholas, 1994; Guthrie, Wallace, et al., 1996; Jemmott & Jemmott, 1991, 1992, 1994; Loveland-Cherry, Ross, et al., 1996).

Outcome of Intervention: Abstinence Versus Responsible Behavior

Adolescence has been described as being "in between" childhood and adulthood. Although adolescence is, indeed, a distinct developmental phase, this description reflects the dilemma of determining realistic and appropriate behavioral goals for interventions with this population. On the one hand, abstinence is the most appropriate behavioral outcome, especially when considering substance use, sexual behavior, and suicide. On the other hand, arguments have been made that with certain behaviors, specifically alcohol use and sexual activity, it may be more realistic and beneficial in the long run to focus on developing responsible behavior while not actually promoting initiation of behavior. Many adolescents experiment with alcohol use and do not develop alcohol misuse problems. In fact, large numbers of adolescents report limited alcohol use in supervised situations, such as religious, family, and holiday celebrations. However, selling or serving alcohol to minors (under age 21 in most states) is illegal. The dilemma is whether there is a social responsibility to prepare individuals to responsibly consume alcoholic beverages. A similar dilemma exists around sexual activity. The argument is made that because a high percentage of adolescents report being sexually active, preparing them to do so responsibly is a viable goal. In both instances, but more so with sexual activity, there is a tension between abstinence and responsible behavior as a behavior goal for intervention. The counterargument is that sex- and HIV-intervention programs may encourage the onset of sexual activity. A national evaluation of 25 such programs (Kirby et al., 1994) found that this was not the case and, in fact, results of six of the studies indicated a delay in onset of sexual intercourse.

Demonstrating Effectiveness of Interventions

Demonstrating the effectiveness of health promotion interventions is difficult and can be costly. Studies have been more successful in demonstrating short-term effectiveness than long-term outcomes. A related issue is that of costs and benefits. Few studies evaluate the cost of interventions or the feasibility of implementing the interventions outside of the context of a research project.

The notion that it is more effective to target interventions to specific at-risk groups has received increased support. Prevention interventions can be directed towards the general population (primary prevention and health promotion) or targeted to specific groups: toward subgroups who are identified as being at high risk and in the early stages of problem behaviors (secondary prevention, early intervention) or toward specific groups or individuals who display problem behaviors (tertiary prevention or treatment, rehabilitation). Debate continues on where the emphasis for interventions is most effective in this continuum. On the one hand, an argument can be made for the effectiveness and efficiency of a focus on groups identified as high risk. A counterargument is that all adolescents are at risk for the major factors that potentially affect their health and that intervening at this level is most cost effective. The evidence for the level of choice for intervention is not yet available and will require multiple controlled studies to adequately determine which approach is most effective.

Multidisciplinary Collaboration

The health issues of adolescents are complex, and it is unlikely that any one discipline alone can adequately address them. A broad range of disciplines (including, for example, social science, health disciplines, economics, education) is involved in health promotion efforts for adolescents. Interdisciplinary, collaborative interventions are needed to effectively address the health promotion needs of adolescents (National Institute of Nursing Research [NINR], 1993). An interdisciplinary approach requires integration of conceptual approaches and philosophical perspectives. Some disciplines (e.g., psychology) work within paradigms that are largely derived from a personal, individual health view. Other disciplines, such as sociology and public health, come from more ecological traditions. Nursing encompasses elements of both perspectives. Implementation of the holistic perspective advocated more recently in nursing fits well with the need for an integrated approach. As such, nursing brings unique skills and perspectives to collaborative interventions.

Ethnic and Cultural Relevance

The ethnic and cultural diversity of the U.S. population necessitates the evaluation of ethnic and cultural relevance in health promotion interventions. What are the commonalties across ethnic and cultural groups? What are the differences? Interventions are often developed and, if systematically evaluated, their effectiveness is determined for specific populations of adolescents. The generalizability of conclusions about appropriateness and effectiveness are often assumed and not systematically evaluated. Determination of the need for ethnically specific versus general interventions is a priority for health promotion interventions with adolescents. Guidelines for addressing ethnic dimensions in research are evolving (Porter & Villarruel, 1993). Researchers have employed a variety of techniques for structuring culturally relevant interventions, including the use of interviews and focus groups with adolescents from the population of interest.

Summary

The challenges inherent in health promotion intervention with adolescents are complex. The limited number of intervention studies, both in nursing and in other disciplines, is not surprising. In fact, it is encouraging to see that nursing has responded to the health promotion needs of this population to the extent that it has.

Synthesis of the State of the Science

The diversity of the areas for nursing interventions to promote health in adolescents makes it difficult to evaluate the literature as a whole. A more pragmatic approach is taken. The nursing research on interventions in each of the four areas (responsible sexual behavior; positive parenting; homicide and suicide; alcohol, tobacco, and other drug use) is synthesized and evaluated. Conclusions regarding health promotion interventions *across* the four areas are presented in a summary section.

Responsible Sexual Behavior

Early sexual activity and prevention of potential consequences (adolescent pregnancy and repeat pregnancy, sexually transmitted disease [STD], HIV/AIDS) have long been foci of both nursing clinical intervention and research. Of the 12 studies that address sexual behavior, there are six related to interventions to prevent HIV/AIDS (Guthrie et al., 1996; Jemmott & Jemmott, 1992a, 1992b; Jemmott et al., 1993; Naughton, Edwards, & Reed, 1991; Yturri-Byrd, Glazer-Waldman, Hedl, Bernardez, & Grover, 1992), one on prenatal education for fathers (Westney, Cole, & Munford, 1988), one on encouraging pregnant teens and teen parents to complete their high school education (Palmore & Millar, 1996), one on reducing low birth weight in high-risk adolescent pregnancies (Piechnik & Corbett, 1985), and one to reduce rapid repeat pregnancy (Covington et al., 1991).

The six interventions to prevent HIV/AIDS all focused on groups of adolescents; parents were not included. All were community based and located in a school-based clinic, an outpatient clinic, and other community sites such as school buildings. Regardless of which of a variety of approaches was used, including interactive games, peer counseling, brochures, and use of videos, results across the studies indicated the ability to increase knowledge about HIV/AIDS, promote more positive attitudes toward use of condoms, increase self-efficacy to avoid risky sexual behavior, increase intention to practice safe sex behavior, and reduce participation in risky sexual behaviors at a 3-month follow-up in Black males. Two teams of researchers (Jemmott and Jemmott, Guthrie and colleagues) report the use of interviews and focus groups prior to development of strategies to enhance the relevance of the interventions. However, no evaluation of the effectiveness of these approaches was evident. The results of work by Jemmott and colleagues provide preliminary evidence that social-cognitive approaches are more effective in changing behavioral intentions and behavior than are either an information-alone intervention or a general health promotion intervention (Jemmott & Jemmott, 1994). All of the samples consisted of urban adolescents and included both European-American and African-American adolescents. The existence of a large body of work, both theoretical and empirical, in reducing a variety of adolescent risk behaviors provides a strong basis for intervention research in the area of HIV/AIDS, especially with nurse researchers as integral members of interdisciplinary teams.

The number of studies of interventions designed to effect positive outcomes in adolescent pregnancy is limited. Further, the variety among the target outcomes and structure of the interventions across studies makes it difficult to come to any valid conclusions, despite the initial positive outcomes for a number of the studies. For example, although one study of the effects of prenatal education on adolescent fathers' knowledge and supportive behavior (Westney et al., 1988) indicates positive outcomes, additional studies are required to substantiate the findings. Interestingly, the knowledge-only intervention increased not only the fathers' knowledge but also their reports of supportive behavior. An interdisciplinary program designed to improve current pregnancy outcomes, improve parenting skills, and decrease rapid repeat pregnancy (Covington et al., 1991) uses a variety of media and experiential techniques similar to those described in the HIV/AIDS programs and encourages participation of significant others. Evaluation outcomes were not yet available at the time of the 1991 publication. Two reports support the effectiveness of interventions that are managed by nurse-midwives and use an interdisciplinary team approach in terms of labor and delivery outcomes for adolescents and their infants (Piechnik & Corbett, 1985; Smoke & Grace, 1988). No theoretical framework for any of the studies is explicated, but physiological and social-cognitive underpinnings are implied. Consequently, this is a general area that warrants further development of basic models to understand the dynamics of apparently effective nursing interventions.

Promoting Positive Parenting

Four studies that report interventions to promote effective parenting among adolescents were found (Buckley, 1990; Clarke & Strauss, 1992; Koniak-Griffin & Verzemnieks, 1991; O'Sullivan & Jacobsen, 1992). Promoting positive outcomes for adolescent parents and their infants is an area of nursing research that is characterized by a sound theoretical foundation. Earlier work of scholars in nursing (for example, Barnard, 1980; Meleis, 1975; Mercer, 1981, 1985, 1986) and other disciplines provides the basis for the development of nursing interventions with adolescent parents. The theoretical rationale derives from the general work on role theory, specifically on the constructs of maternal role attainment and role supplementation. One study (Buckley, 1990) was based on Orem's Self-Care Theory, which has a number of commonalties with role theory. Of the four reports of interventions, two (Clarke & Strauss, 1992; O'Sullivan & Jacobsen, 1992) are extensions of earlier projects. Results of the earlier projects by O'Sullivan and Jacobsen provide evidence of the effectiveness of these approaches to improving outcomes for adolescent parents and their

infants. Three of the four studies (Buckley, 1990; Clarke & Strauss, 1992; Koniak-Griffin & Verzemnieks, 1991) in this group enrolled participants prenatally, and the fourth study (O'Sullivan & Jacobsen, 1992) enrolled them during the immediate postpartum period. No rationale is given for the timing of enrollment; evaluation of the relative benefits of each could provide important information for implementation decisions. Although the Koniak-Griffin and Verzemnieks (1991) study demonstrated intervention effects in enhancing maternal-fetal attachment, analogous effects were not apparent in actual mothering behaviors. The sample for this study was small ($N = 20$), and there is the possibility that there was not adequate power to detect differences. A methodological concern with this population of high-risk adolescent mothers is the large attrition rate for both the experimental (60%) and control (82%) groups reported by O'Sullivan and Jacobsen (1992).

Promoting Adolescent Health: Reducing Risk of Suicide and Substance Use

There is clear consensus in the literature that problem behaviors (substance use, delinquency, school dropout, depression, potential for suicide) tend to occur in clusters among adolescents (Botvin, Baker, Dusenburg, & Botvin, 1990; Eggert, Thompson, Herting, & Nicholas, 1994; Jessor, 1993; Jessor & Jessor, 1980). The obvious implication is that interventions that target one of these behaviors could also affect other cluster behaviors. This perspective is consistent with the holistic approach to health that is advocated in the nursing literature. Of the nine articles in the nursing literature that included the word *intervention* related to preventing suicide, substance use, depression, or school problems, four were not reports of research studies (Ladely & Puskar, 1994; Long, 1986; Roberts & Quillian, 1992; Valente, 1989) and are not addressed here.

Two major programs of research, one focused on suicide prevention (Eggert, Seyl, et al., 1990; Eggert, Thompson, Herting, & Nicholas, 1994, 1995) and one focused on prevention of substance abuse (Dielman, Laetz, et al., 1994; Loveland-Cherry, Leech, Laetz, & Dielman, 1996; Loveland-Cherry, Ross, et al., 1996), and a third study that was a dissertation (Walsh, 1993) constitute the remaining nursing research in this area. The two programs of research illustrate the two sides of the debate regarding universal prevention intervention versus targeted prevention intervention (Peters & McMahon, 1996). Eggert, Thompson, Herting, and Nicholas (1994) have implemented an interdisciplinary program of research that targets high-risk students (potential high-school dropouts) for intervention to decrease school deviance, drug involvement, and suicide potential. In contrast, Loveland-Cherry and colleagues have established an interdisciplinary program of research that focuses on the general population of adolescents through universal interventions. Both programs of research are based within conceptual and theoretical frameworks that acknowledge the importance of critical environments for understanding and affecting adolescent risk behaviors. The conceptual frameworks for both programs of research integrate social learning theory with other theoretical perspectives and are complemented with the use of appropriate theoretical perspectives from nursing (e.g., therapeutic use of self). The common conceptual elements result in the examination of a number of similar constructs (including risk factors, protective factors, and intervention strategies). Both interventions focus on enhancing environments and building skills.

There are also differences in the two programs. Eggert and colleagues (Eggert, Thompson, Herting, & Nicholas, 1994, 1995; Eggert, Thompson, Herting, Nicholas, & Dicker, 1994) have structured a school-based intervention that is operational as an elective class (Personal Growth Class [PGC]) in the regular high school curriculum. Both proximal (school deviance, drug involvement, and depression) and distal (suicide behaviors) outcomes are specified. Loveland-Cherry and colleagues (Dielman, Leech, & Loveland-Cherry, 1995; Loveland-Cherry, Leech, et al., 1996; Loveland-Cherry, Ross, et al., 1996) have designed both a family-focused intervention and a school-based intervention for two studies (Adolescent Drug Abuse Prevention [ADAP] and Child and Parent Relations [CAPR]). In the ADAP project, the impact of both a family intervention and a school intervention on delaying the initiation and decreasing the use of alcohol, tobacco, marijuana, and inhalants are the target behaviors. The school intervention is a five-session program that is presented as a module during classroom time. In the CAPR project, the impact of a family intervention on delaying the initiation and decreasing the use of alcohol is evaluated.

Results of the evaluation study of the PGC intervention indicate that proposed differences among the three study groups (assessment and one semester of PGC, assessment and two semesters of PGC, and assessment only) were evident in some instances (anger, perceived

personal control) but not in others (e.g., suicide risk behaviors, depression, hopelessness, stress, self-esteem, social network support). No gender differences were found. Preliminary results for the CAPR program indicate support for the proposed effects on enhancing parenting skills and for slowing the increase in reported quantity and frequency of adolescent use and misuse of alcohol. The effects for alcohol use are as proposed for males but not for females; there are no gender differences for the impact on misuse. In both instances, the increase that would be anticipated as adolescents transition from elementary to middle school is less for those in the intervention group. Data on the post intervention measures for the ADAP study are not yet available for analysis. Both short-term and long-term outcomes are being evaluated in the CAPR project, with posttests into high school (a total of 5 to 6 years). These two programs of research demonstrate similarities and differences in health promotion intervention research with adolescents.

The only other nursing intervention study identified for review took a very different approach to intervention with suicidal adolescents. The effectiveness of a creative art future-image intervention (AFI) was evaluated. Although not statistically significant, the AFI group showed greater positive changes than the attention placebo group. Interestingly, the AFI was revised and used to help develop a positive identity and enhance self-efficacy to assist a group of adolescents deal with the stress following Hurricane Hugo (Walsh & Hardin, 1994). An integrated conceptual framework that draws from work on self-esteem, self-efficacy, behavioral and cognitive work, future-time perspective theory, and goal attainment aspects of King's (1992) theory and group work serves as the basis for the intervention. The purpose of AFI is "for teenagers to develop enhanced identity and increased self-efficacy" through the creation of "a caricature poster that shows their projected, idealized image of themselves in the future, both physically and vocationally" (Walsh & Hardin, 1994, p. 26). The AFI was implemented in 2-hour-long sessions at the end of the school day. At posttest (spring 1991, pretest fall 1990), self-efficacy scores for both intervention and control adolescents had declined; however, the decrease was less for those students in the intervention group. Walsh and Hardin suggest that effect of the intervention may be delayed and/or that the results may have been affected by involvement of significant persons for the study students in the Persian Gulf War, which occurred at the time of the study.

The duration of interventions and the evaluation of both short-term and long-term outcomes are important considerations for research examining health promotion interventions in adolescents (Weissberg & Elias, 1993).

▬ *General Health Promotion*

A final group of studies evaluated nursing interventions to promote more general health dimensions in adolescents. A self-help nursing intervention to build psychosocial competence was evaluated in a community sample of adolescents (N = 34) (Walker, Sandor, & Sands, 1994). The intervention was developed within the context of the importance of personal problem solving from a stress-coping perspective. Although short-term effects of the workbook intervention indicated positive effects in several areas, the longer term evaluation indicated that the only significant difference among the three groups (intervention, delayed intervention, and control) was for scholastic competence. Following an unanticipated suicide of one of the study participants, psychosocial competence was evaluated in the peer suicide survivors following a supportive community intervention (Sandor, Walker, & Sands, 1994). The results indicated a decay in effects of the intervention over time, similar to that seen in the larger study. That is, initial gains in problem-solving appraisal and global self-worth declined 2 months after the intervention. One intervention to evaluate a health education program (HEP) to promote general health behaviors in inner city adolescents was found (Fowler, 1991). The intervention was developed within Festinger's (1957) cognitive dissonance framework. The results indicated improvement in some of the health behaviors (e.g., nutrition, sleep/rest, self-belt or safety helmet use), but they were not statistically significant.

Summary

Taken as a whole, the nursing literature on health promotion interventions for adolescents is encouraging. The behaviors targeted for intervention reflect the foci identified in the Year 2000 Objectives for the Nation and the associated expertise of nurse researchers. The greatest number of studies examined the promotion of responsible sexual behavior (12), followed by approximately equal emphasis on prevention of suicide and substance use (7) and promoting positive parent behaviors among adolescents (5). A final, eclectic group of studies (3) addressed more general health promotion concerns. Although nursing research on interventions to promote

adolescent health is limited, several encouraging patterns are emerging.

If the National Institute of Nursing Research (NINR) Priority Expert Panel's recommendations (NINR, 1993) are used to evaluate the current science in health promotion among adolescents, it is evident that considerable progress has been made in several areas but not in others. Few studies examined the interactive effects of behavioral and biological processes on adolescent health behaviors and outcomes. Indeed, more attention was given to behavioral processes than to biological ones. Transitions such as movement to parenthood or movement from one level of school to another are used as opportune times to intervene, but less attention is given to examining the influences of developmental and social transitions on health behaviors and outcomes. Longitudinal designs are used, but, with few exceptions (e.g., Loveland-Cherry, Ross, et al., 1996), follow-up is limited to 3 months to 1 year following the intervention. This pattern is consistent with studies by other disciplines and is supported by other reviews of prevention interventions (see, for example, Janz et al., 1996; Kirby et al., 1994). Considerably more work needs to be done to meet this recommendation.

There has been progress toward meeting the objectives inherent in the second recommendation regarding investigating family, school, and community strategies for adolescent health promotion, especially with highly vulnerable youth. Although the majority of the studies reviewed described programs that focused on adolescents as the target of the intervention, several used theoretical frameworks that acknowledge the importance of critical environments. Interventions were delivered in clinics, schools, community facilities, and in the home. Interventions were both universal and targeted and included diverse groups of adolescents. Sexually active adolescents and those who have been identified as having school or emotional difficulties have been targeted for interventions. Urban youth, European-American, African-American, and, less frequently, Latino youth were represented in the samples for intervention. In at least four instances (e.g., Guthrie, Wallace, et al., 1996; Jemmott & Jemmott, 1991, 1993; Jemmott, Jemmott, & Fong, 1992), specific efforts were made to develop ethnically and culturally relevant interventions via the use of such techniques as focus groups. Increased attention and effort needs to be given to evaluating which interventions are most relevant and effective with diverse groups.

Interventions incorporated a variety of techniques and components. Nearly every intervention had a component that focused on increasing adolescents' knowledge regarding the behavior of interest. Other components were dependent either on the theoretical approach used or on techniques that were found to be effective in the literature. In studies that used an identified theoretical framework, the framework was used to structure the intervention and to evaluate outcomes. Several investigators used theoretical frameworks that integrated concepts and relationships from multiple theoretical perspectives and that had been derived and tested in earlier work. Because of the variety of theoretical frameworks used, it is difficult to identify common elements across the studies. These integrated frameworks commonly included components of social cognitive theory, especially the notions of role models, behavioral rehearsal, and self-efficacy. A variety of strategies were used in the interventions: for example, small group sessions, one-to-one counseling, videos, games, and role play. The one study (Yturri-Byrd et al., 1992) that evaluated the effectiveness of three different techniques found positive intervention effects for knowledge and attitudes about self-protection strategies but no significant differences in outcomes among the three types of interventions. There is limited evidence regarding which strategies are most effective with different developmental and ethnic groups.

There is recognition of the importance of interdisciplinary, collaborative teams in addressing adolescent health promotion needs, both in research and intervention. The programs of research that are becoming evident in adolescent health promotion are often interdisciplinary (e.g., Eggert, Thompson, Herting, & Nicholas, 1994, 1995; Eggert, Thompson, Herting, Nicholas, & Dicker, 1994; Jemmott & Jemmott). Likewise, interventions initiated by clinicians include other disciplines, such as social work and nutrition. However, there is a clear lack of collaboration with colleagues who could assist with strengthening the interactive effects of behavioral and biological processes.

The costs of interventions were seldom addressed. Only two studies (Eggert, Seyl, et al., 1990; O'Sullivan & Jacobsen, 1992) addressed the issue of costs. O'Sullivan and Jacobsen noted that although the actual costs of the intervention with first-time adolescents and their infants was less than that for usual care, this was an artificial difference because of personnel used in the program. The conclusion was reached that costs for the experimental program were probably comparable to those of usual care. Eggert, Seyl, et al. estimated a cost of $634 per student for a school-based prevention program for poten-

tial dropouts and drug abusers. They point out a favorable comparison with the costs of either outpatient or inpatient treatment.

Recommendations for Advancing the Science

In spite of some demonstrated success in developing interventions for adolescent health promotion, there is limited evidence of long-term effects on behavioral change or health outcomes. Multi-site field trials with diverse populations of the most promising interventions would provide the discipline with opportunity to more efficiently determine long-term outcomes. Further, this approach would provide additional information on the effectiveness of tailoring interventions for specific groups of adolescents.

The growing consensus that problem behaviors tend to occur in clusters points out the need to evaluate the effects of interventions on multiple behaviors. Certainly, there is compelling evidence that enhancing self-efficacy, life skills, decision-making skills, and perceptions of norms for specific behaviors can result in positive outcomes in other behaviors.

Although considerable progress has been made in moving to theoretical approaches that acknowledge the multiple environments that affect adolescent health and related behaviors (e.g., Bogenschneider, 1996; Weissberg & Elias, 1993), additional efforts are needed to operationalize these approaches in interventions. To accomplish this, the many individuals and institutions that influence adolescents' lives need to be incorporated into intervention strategies. Important environments, such as schools, need to be considered as partners in planning and implementing intervention programs. Most important, adolescents themselves need to be involved in the planning and implementation of programs.

To understand why some interventions are effective and others are not, it is important to continue to examine the dynamics of the interventions. This requires continued evaluation of the theoretical underpinnings, especially in the effects of mediating and moderating factors. At the same time, the impact of different modalities and technologies in delivery of theoretically based interventions needs to be considered. Perhaps one of the most needed pieces of knowledge is if and how the phase of adolescence affects the development, delivery, and effects of interventions. In other words, can the same intervention be used for early, middle, and late adolescents? Increased emphasis also needs to be placed on the development and evaluation of ethnically and culturally relevant interventions, with a focus on the relative effects of doing so. There are examples in nursing (e.g., Guthrie, Wallace, et al., 1996; Jemmott & Jemmott, 1992) and in other disciplines (e.g., Szapocznik, Kurtines, Santisteban, & Rio, 1990) that provide direction for the types of efforts that enhance the design of culturally sensitive interventions with adolescents.

An aspect of adolescent health promotion and risk reduction research that was not evident in the studies evaluated for the current review is that of genetic implications. Further, the role that genetics play in health needs to be considered within the context of environmental influences. This is a relatively new area for nursing and one that warrants additional attention. For example, how might interventions focused on promoting physical health in adolescents be structured for groups with varying genetic risk and different environmental risks?

Unfortunately, even interventions that have demonstrated effectiveness often are not able to be sustained after funding for a project ends. It is important, therefore, that costs of interventions be documented and efforts made to structure interventions that can be incorporated into currently existing delivery systems. To sustain successful interventions, nursing will need to become more involved in strategies to inform and influence health policy (NINR, 1993).

In summary, considerable progress has been made in nursing to intervene to promote health in adolescents. The broad range of behaviors and the variety of settings in which nursing is involved with adolescents have resulted in interventions that focus both on individuals in clinical settings and community-based populations. Nursing's extensive clinical experiences with health promotion among adolescents provides a strong basis from which to develop programs of intervention research. This strong clinical base is complemented by the discipline's commitment to building partnerships with clients, including communities, and to a theoretical perspective that encompasses the importance of context. As a result, nursing is quickly assuming a position of leadership in intervention research for adolescent health promotion, including the use of innovative approaches and the development of appropriate measures and designs.

Nursing has clearly recognized the need for interdisciplinary, collaborative approaches to address the complex issues of adolescent health promotion. If these initial efforts are to be expanded and sustained, the discipline needs to commit to a priority for health promotion for this important segment of the population.

References

Ajzen, I. (1985). From intentions to actions: A theory of planned behavior. In J. Kuhl & J. Beckman (Eds.), *Action control: From cognition to behavior* (chap. 2). New York: Springer-Verlag.

Ajzen, I. (1991). The theory of planned behavior. *Organizational Behavior and Human Decision Processes, 50,* 179-211.

Bandura, A. (1986). The explanatory and predictive scope of self-efficacy theory. *Journal of Social and Clinical Psychology, 4*(3), 359-373.

Barnard, K. E. (1980). Knowledge for practice: Directions for the future. *Nursing Research, 29,* 208-212.

Bearinger, L. H., & Gephart, J. (1987). Priorities for adolescent health: Recommendations of a national conference. *Mucinous Cystic Neoplasms, 12,* 161-164.

Bogenschneider, K. (1996). Family related prevention programs: An ecological risk/protective theory for building prevention programs, policies, and community capacity to support youth. *Family Relations, 45,* 127-138.

Botvin, G. J., Baker, E., Dusenbury, L., & Botvin, E. M. (1990). Preventing adolescent drug abuse through a multimodel cognitive-behavioral approach: Results of a 3-year study. *Journal of Consulting and Clinical Psychology, 58,* 437-446.

Buckley, H. B. (1990). Nurse practitioner intervention to improve postpartum appointment keeping in an outpatient family planning clinic. *Journal of the American Academy of Nurse Practitioners, 2*(1), 29-32.

Carnegie Council on Adolescent Development. (1995). *Great transitions: Preparing adolescents for a new century.* New York: Carnegie Corporation of New York.

Clarke, B. A., & Strauss, S. S. (1992). Nursing role supplementation for adolescent parents: Prescriptive nursing practice. *Journal of Pediatric Nursing, 7*(5), 312-318.

Covington, D. L., Churchill, P., Wright, B. D., Plummer, J., Cushing, D., & McCorkle, B. J. (1991). Adolescent rapid repeat pregnancy: Problem and intervention in a North Carolina hospital. *Health Values 15*(5), 43-48.

Dielman, T. E., Laetz, V., Leech, S., & Loveland-Cherry, C. J. (1994, June). *The effectiveness of a home-based parenting skills intervention.* Research presented at the Research Society on Alcoholics (RSA) Annual Scientific Meeting, Maui, Hawaii.

Dielman, T. E., Leech, S. L., & Loveland-Cherry, C. J. (1995). Parents' and children's reports of parenting practices, and parent and child alcohol use. *Drugs and Society: A Journal of Contemporary Issues, 8*(3/4), 83-87.

Eccles, J. S., Midgley, C., Wigfield, A., Buchanan, C. M., Reuman, D., Flanagan, C., & MacIver, D. (1993). Development during adolescence: The impact of stage-environment fit on young adolescents' experiences in schools and in families. *American Psychologist, 48*(2), 90-101.

Eggert, L. L., Seyl, C. D., & Nicholas, L. J. (1990). Effects of a school-based prevention program for potential high school dropouts and drug abusers. *International Journal of the Addictions, 25*(7), 773-801.

Eggert, L. L., Thompson, E. A., Herting, J. R., & Nicholas, L. J. (1994). Prevention research program: Reconnecting at-risk youth. *Issues in Mental Health Nursing, 15,* 107-135.

Eggert, L. L., Thompson, E. A., Herting, J. R., & Nicholas, L. J. (1995). Reducing suicide potential among high-risk youth: Tests of a school-based prevention program. *Suicide and Life-Threatening Behavior, 25*(2), 276-296.

Eggert, L. L., Thompson, E. A., Herting, J. R., Nicholas, L. J., & Dicker, B. G. (1994). Preventing adolescent drug abuse and high school dropout through an intensive school-based social network development program. *American Journal of Health Promotion, 8*(3), 202-215.

Festinger, L. A. (1957). *A theory of cognitive dissonance.* Stanford, CA: Stanford University Press.

Fowler, B. (1991). A health education program for inner city high school youths: Promoting positive health behaviors through intervention. *ABNF Journal, 2*(3), 53-58.

Guthrie, B. J., Loveland-Cherry, C. J., Frey, M. A., & Dielman, T. E. (1994). A theoretical approach to studying health behaviors in adolescents: An at-risk population. *Journal of Family and Community Health, 17*(3), 35-48.

Guthrie, B. J., Wallace, J., Doerr, K., Janz, N., Schottenfeld, D., & Selig, S. (1996). Girl talk: Development of an intervention for prevention of HIV/AIDS and other sexually transmitted diseases in adolescent females. *Public Health Nursing, 13*(5), 318-330.

Hamburg, D. A., Millstein, S. G., Mortimer, A. M., Nightingale, E. O., & Petersen, A. C. (1993). Adolescent health promotion in the twenty-first century: Current frontiers and future directions. In S. G. Millstein, A. C. Petersen, & E. O. Nightingale (Eds.), *Promoting the health of adolescents: New directions for the twenty-first century* (pp. 375-388). New York: Oxford University Press.

Hawkins, J. D., Catalano, R. F., & Miller, J. Y. (1992). Risk and protective factors for alcohol and other drug problems in adolescence and early adulthood: Implications for substance abuse prevention. *Psychological Bulletin, 112,* 64-105.

Igoe, J. B. (1991). Empowerment of children and youth for consumer self-care. *American Journal of Health Promotion, 6,* 55-65.

Janz, N. K., Zimmerman, M. A., Wren, P. A., Israel, B. A., Freudenberg, N., & Carter, R. J. (1996). Evaluation of 37 AIDS prevention projects: Successful approaches and barriers to program effectiveness. *Health Education Quarterly, 23*(1), 80-97.

Jemmott, J. B. III, & Jemmott, L. S. (1993). Alcohol and drug use during sexual activity: Predicting the HIV-risk-related behaviors of inner-city black male adolescents. *Journal of Adolescent Research, 8*(1), 41-57.

Jemmott, J. B. III, & Jemmott, L. S. (1994). Interventions for adolescents in community settings. In R. J. DiClemente & J. L. Peterson (Eds.), *Preventing AIDS: Theories and methods of behavioral interventions* (pp. 141-174). New York: Plenum.

Jemmott, J. B. III, Jemmott, L. S., & Fong, G. T. (1992). Reductions in HIV risk-associated sexual behaviors among Black male adolescents: Effects of an AIDS prevention intervention. *American Journal of Public Health, 82*(3), 372-377.

Jemmott, J. B. III, Jemmott, L. S., & Hacker, C. (1992). Predicting intentions to use condoms among African-American adolescents: The theory of planned behavior as a model of HIV risk-associated behavior. *Ethnicity and Disease, 2,* 371-380.

Jemmott, J. B. III, Jemmott, L. S., Spears, H., Hewitt, N., & Cruz-Collins, M. (1992). Self-efficacy, hedonistic expectancies, and condom-use intentions among inner-city black adolescent women: A social cognitive approach to AIDS risk behavior. *Journal of Adolescent Health, 13*(6), 512-519.

Jemmott, L. S., & Jemmott, J. B. III. (1991). Applying the theory of reasoned action to AIDS risk behavior: Condom use among Black women. *Nursing Research, 40*(4), 228-234.

Jemmott, L. S., & Jemmott, J. B. III. (1992b). Family structure, parental strictness, and sexual behavior among inner-city Black male adolescents. *Journal of Adolescent Research, 7*(2), 192-207.

Jemmott, L. S., & Jemmott, J. B. III (1992a). Increasing condom-use intentions among sexually active Black adolescent women. *Nursing Research, 41*(5), 273-278.

Jessor, R. (1993, February). Successful adolescent development among youth in high-risk settings. *American Psychologist, 48*(2), 117-126.

Jessor, R., & Jessor, S. (1980). A social-psychological framework for studying drug use. *National Institute on Drug Abuse Research Monograph, 30,* 102-109.

King, I. M. (1992). King's theory of goal attainment. *Nursing Science Quarterly, 5*(1), 19-26.

Kirby, D., Short, L., Collins, J., Rugg, D., Kolbe, L., Howard, M., Miller, B., Sonenstein, F., & Zabin, L. S. (1994). School-based programs to reduce sexaul risk behaviors: A review of effectiveness. *Public Health Reports, 109*(3), 339-360.

Koniak-Griffin, D., & Verzemnieks, I. (1991). Effects of nursing intervention on adolescents' maternal role attainment. *Issues in Comprehensive Pediatric Nursing, 14*(2), 121-138.

Kumpfer, K. L. (1990). Environmental and family-focused prevention: The Cinderellas of prevention want to go to the ball, too. In K. H. Rey, C. L. Faegre, & P. Lowry (Eds.), *Prevention research finding: 1988* (Office for Substance Abuse Prevention [OSAP] Prevention Monograph 3, DHHS Pub. No. ADM-89-1615, pp. 194-222). Washington, DC: Government Printing Office.

Ladely, S. J., & Puskar, K. R. (1994). Adolescent suicide: Behaviors, risk factors, and psychiatric nursing interventions. *Issues in Mental Health Nursing, 15,* 497-504.

Long, K. A. (1986). Suicide intervention and prevention with Indian adolescent populations. *Issues in Mental Health Nursing, 8,* 247-253.

Loveland-Cherry, C. J., Leech, S., Laetz, V. B., & Dielman, T. E. (1996). Correlates of alcohol use and misuse in 4th grade children: Psychosocial, peer, parental and family factors. *Health Education Quarterly, 23*(4), 497-511.

Loveland-Cherry, C. J., Ross, L. T., & Laetz, V. B. (1996, June). *Effects of a family intervention on adolescent alcohol misuse.* Poster presented at the Joint Scientific Meeting of the Research Society on Alcoholism and the International Society for Biomedical Research on Alcoholism, Washington DC.

Meleis, A. I. (1975). Role insufficiency and role supplementation: A conceptual framework. *Nursing Research, 24,* 264-271.

Mercer, R. T. (1981). A theoretical framework for studying the factors that impact on the maternal role. *Nursing Research, 30*(2), 73-77.

Mercer, R. T. (1985). The process of maternal role attainment over the first year. *Nursing Research, 34*(4), 198-204.

Mercer, R. T. (1986). *First-time motherhood: Experiences from teens to forties.* New York: Springer.

Millstein, S. G., Petersen, A. C., & Nightingale, E. O. (Eds.). (1993). *Promoting the health of adolescents: New directions for the twenty-first century.* New York: Oxford University Press.

National Institute of Nursing Research. (1993). *Health promotion for older children and adolescents: A report of the NINR priority ex-*

pert panel on health promotion. Bethesda, MD: U.S. Department of Health and Human Services.

Naughton, S. S., Edwards, L. E., & Reed, N. (1991). AIDS/HIV risk assessment and risk reduction counseling in a school-based clinic. *Journal of School Health, 61*(10), 443-445.

O'Sullivan, A. L., & Jacobsen, B. S. (1992). A randomized trial of a health care program for first-time adolescent mothers and their infants. *Nursing Research, 41*(4), 210-215.

Palmore, S., & Millar, K. (1996). Some common characteristics of pregnant teens who choose childbirth. *Journal of School Nursing, 12*(3), 19-22.

Pender, N. J. (1996). *Health promotion in nursing practice* (3rd ed.). Stamford, CT: Appleton & Lang.

Peters, D. R., & McMahon, R. J. (Eds.). (1996). *Preventing childhood disorders, substance abuse, and delinquency.* Thousand Oaks, CA: Sage.

Piechnik, S. L., & Corbett, M. A. (1985). Reducing low birth weight among socioeconomically high-risk adolescent pregnancies: Successful intervention with certified nurse-midwife-managed care and a multidisciplinary team. *Journal of Nurse-Midwifery, 30*(2), 88-98.

Porter, C. P., & Villarruel, A. M. (1993). Nursing research with African American and Hispanic people: Guidelines for action. *Nursing Outlook, 41*(2), 59-67.

Roberts, C., & Quillian, J. (1992). Preventing violence through primary care intervention. *Nurse Practitioner, 17*(8), 62-70.

Sandor, M. K., Walker, L. O., & Sands, D. (1994). Competence-building in adolescents, part II: Community intervention for survivors of peer suicide. *Issues in Comprehensive Pediatric Nursing, 17,* 197-209.

Schinke, S. P., Botvin, G. J., & Orlandi, M. A. (1991). *Substance abuse in children and adolescents: Evaluation and intervention.* Newbury Park, CA: Sage.

Shalala, D. E. (1995, October). *New visions for adolescent health issues.* Paper presented at American Public Health Association 123rd Annual Meeting and Exhibition, "A Decision Making in Public Health: Priorities, Power, and Ethics," San Diego, CA.

Smoke, J., & Grace, M. C. (1988). Effectiveness of prenatal care and education for pregnant adolescents: Nurse-midwifery intervention and team approach. *Journal of Nurse-Midwifery, 33*(4), 178-184.

Szapocznik, J., Kurtines, W., Santisteban, D. A., & Rio, A. T. (1990). Interplay of advances between theory, research, and application in treatment interventions aimed at behavior problem children and adolescents. *Journal of Consulting and Clinical Psychology, 58*(6), 696-703.

U.S. Department of Health and Human Services. (1990). *Healthy people 2000: National health promotion and disease prevention objectives* (DHHS Publication No. [PHS] 91-50212). Washington, DC: USDHHS, Public Health Service.

Valente, S. M. (1989). Adolescent suicide: Assessment and intervention. *Journal of Child and Adolescent Psychiatric and Mental Health Nursing, 2*(1), 34-39.

Walker, L. O., Sandor, M. K., & Sands, D. (1994). Competence-building in adolescents, part I: A self-help nursing intervention. *Issues in Comprehensive Pediatric Nursing, 17,* 179-195.

Walsh, S. M. (1993). Future images: An art intervention with suicidal adolescents. *Applied Nursing Research, 6*(3), 111-118.

Walsh, S. M., & Hardin, S. B. (1994). An art future image intervention to enhance identity and self-efficacy in adolescents. *Journal of Child and Adolescent Psychiatric Nursing, 7*(3), 24-34.

Weissberg, R. P., & Elias, M. J. (1993). Enhancing young people's social competence and health behavior: An important challenge for educators, scientists, policymakers, and funders. *Applied and Preventive Psychology, 2,* 179-190.

Westney, O. E., Cole, O. J., & Munford, T. L. (1988). The effects of prenatal education intervention on unwed prospective adolescent fathers. *Journal of Adolescent Health Care, 9,* 214-218.

Yturri-Byrd, K., Glazer-Waldman, H., Hedl, J. J., Bernardez, S., & Grover, R. (1992). Teaching teenagers about AIDS. *Journal of the American Academy of Physician Assistants, 5,* 432-437.

16

PREVENTION AND TREATMENT
OF HYPERTENSION
IN BLACK AMERICANS

Martha N. Hill

Overview

Hypertension, or high blood pressure (HBP), is the most common chronic disease in the Black American population. Recently published data from the 1989-1991 National Health and Nutrition Examination Survey (NHANES III) indicate that the prevalence of high blood pressure in the U.S. population is greater for both male and female non-Hispanic Blacks of all ages than for non-Hispanic Whites and Mexican Americans (Burt, Cutler, et al., 1995; Burt, Whelton, et al., 1995). Although age-specific prevalence rates have decreased for every age-sex-race subgroup except Black men 50 years old and older, the prevalence of hypertension is estimated to be 30% higher in urban Black Americans than in Caucasians (38% vs. 29%). Approximately 5,672,000 non-Hispanic Black U.S. adults are affected. Black Americans of all ages, especially men, bear a disproportionate burden from high blood pressure. At severely elevated levels (DBP ≥ 115 mm Hg), hypertension prevalence is four times greater in Black American men than in White men (Sempos, Cooper, Kovar, & McMillian, 1988). Non-Hispanic Black women bear the highest rates for all female age groups, and Non-Hispanic Black men bear the highest rates among men, except in the age group of 80 years or older, when rates are highest in Mexican-

American men. The higher prevalence of hypertension persists when controlled for age, adiposity, and socioeconomic status.

Although mortality rates from heart disease and stroke have decreased dramatically in the past two decades, coronary artery disease and other cardiovascular diseases remain the most frequent cause of death for the total population, and stroke remains the third leading cause (American Heart Association, 1997). Together, they are responsible for more deaths than all other causes combined. Mortality rates attributable to hypertension increase with age and peak earlier in Black Americans, who, in general, have shorter life spans (Heckler, 1985; Keil & Saunders, 1991). Complications of uncontrolled hypertension, especially cerebral vascular accidents, left ventricular hypertrophy, congestive heart failure, acute myocardial infarction, and end-stage renal disease (ESRD), are more common in Black Americans than in White Americans. Most people with hypertension know that they have the condition and that improvements in lifestyle and pharmacologic treatment are effective in controlling blood pressure (Joint National Committee, 1993). Of all people in the United States with hypertension, only 29% now have blood pressures controlled to below 140/90 mm Hg (Burt, Cutler, et al., 1995). Fewer than 50% of those treated for hypertension were controlled (below 140/90 mm Hg) in each of the six age, sex, and race groups analyzed. In the editorial accompanying the release of the NHANES III prevalence data, *Hypertension* Editor-in-Chief E. D. Froelich (1995) writes, "This is a totally unacceptable [situation]. . . . We can still do better in hypertension control" (p. 303).

The prevention and treatment of hypertension in Black Americans is targeted in many of the Year 2000 objectives. Two of the major goals for the nation, increase the span of healthy life for Americans and reduce health disparities among Americans, directly relate to the adverse impact of hypertension on morbidity and mortality. In the Index of *Healthy People 2000,* two strategies are listed under high blood pressure control: educational programs at the worksite and screenings (U.S. Department of Health and Human Services, 1990). Section 15, "Heart Disease and Stroke," contains several health status and risk reduction objectives (15.1, 15.2, 15.3, 15.4, and 15.5) that specifically address the hypertension problem (see Table 16.1). Three risk reduction objectives in the same section (15.9, reduce dietary fat intake; 15.10, reduce overweight; and 15.11, increase regular physical activity) are related to achieving blood pressure control through lifestyle modification. Additional objectives for

TABLE 16.1. Hypertension Health Status, Risk Reduction Objectives, and Lifestyle Modification Objectives for Blood Pressure Control

Hypertension health status and risk reduction objectives

15.1 Reduce coronary heart disease deaths to no more than 100 per 100,000 people

15.2 Reduce stroke deaths to no more than 20 per 100,000 people

15.3 Reverse the increase in end-stage renal disease (requiring maintenance dialysis or transportation) to attain an incidence of no more than 13 per 100,000

15.4 Increase to at least 50% the proportion of people with high blood pressure whose blood pressure is under control

15.5 Increase to at least 90% the proportion of people with high blood pressure who are taking action to help control their blood pressure

Lifestyle modification

15.9 Reduce dietary fat intake to an average of 30% of calories or less and average saturated fat intake to less than 10% of calories among people 2 years old and older

15.10 Reduce overweight to a prevalence of no more than 20% among people 20 years old and older and no more than 15% among adolescents 12 through 19 years old

15.11 Increase to at least 30% the proportion of people 6 years old and older who engage regularly, preferably daily, in light to moderate physical activity for at least 30 minutes per day

SOURCE: USDHHS (1990).

"Alcohol and Other Drugs" and "Educational and Community Based Programs" are also pertinent. All of these objectives connect nursing practice and research to blood pressure control in multicultural populations, particularly in Black Americans.

This chapter presents a synopsis and critique of the major areas of research that can guide future directions in nursing science and nursing practice in the prevention and treatment of hypertension in Black Americans. An in-depth synthesis of the science, illustrated in a case study, is accompanied by clinical interpretation. Gaps in information for nursing practice and directions for future clinical practice and research are identified. Emphasis is placed on ecological and multidisciplinary approaches to advancing the field of nursing science and practice.

Background Literature

The literature on prevention and treatment of hypertension in Black Americans relating to nursing research and practice is enormous. The majority of the clinical research literature is reports of epidemiologic surveys and clinical trials evaluating new treatments. Because the implications of this literature for nursing practice and research are extensive, this literature is included in this chapter. A major difficulty in synthesizing the state of the science in nursing research is the inability to clearly identify nursing research within the hypertension literature.

Factors Associated With Hypertension

Biological, genetic, demographic, behavioral, and psychosocial factors have all been associated with the development of hypertension (Blaustein & Grim, 1991; Hildreth & Saunders, 1991; Joint National Committee, 1993; Kaplan, 1994). Although the mechanisms are not thoroughly understood, age, race, sex, socioeconomic status, alcohol intake, family history of HBP, obesity, salt intake, and degree of physical activity contribute to the development and/or control of high blood pressure. Additional possible important independent risk factors include potassium intake, calcium intake, and fasting insulin level (Working Group on Primary Prevention of Hypertension, 1993). Environmental factors, especially low income and educational level, have been shown to be important correlates of hypertension, as has dark skin, especially in Black Americans with lower levels of education (Heckler, 1985; Klag, Whelton, Coresh, Grim, & Kuller, 1991; Murray, 1991). Low-income Black Americans have reported more psychological distress, influenced by the combined burden of poverty and racism, than lower and high-income Whites or than high-income Black Americans. Stressful residential environments, characterized by poverty, crowding, and crime, are related to anxiety, depression, somatic conditions, lower levels of perceived control, and enhanced sympathetic nervous system activity (James & Kleinbaum, 1976). "John Henryism," a behavioral pattern of hard work and determination against overwhelming odds, has also been associated with HBP among Black Americans, particularly those with low socioeconomic status (James, Hartnett, & Kalsbeck, 1983).

Factors Associated With Hypertension Prevention

The primary prevention of hypertension has begun to receive research and policy attention as a complementary approach to the detection and treatment efforts to control hypertension. Recent clinical trials in humans have produced evidence of the importance of lifestyle modification or nonpharmacologic approaches to preventing, delaying, or minimizing the progressive increase in blood pressure seen with age and other socioeconomic factors. The "National High Blood Pressure Education Program Working Group Report on Primary Prevention of Hypertension" (Working Group on Primary Prevention of Hypertension, 1993) presents the rationale and strategies for primary prevention. The Primary Prevention of Hypertension Trial, the Hypertension Prevention Trial, and the Trials of Hypertension Prevention (TOHP) Phase I are reviewed. Black Americans comprised 13% to 23% of the participants in different arms of these studies. In general, results tend to be similar in Black Americans and Caucasians.

The efficacy of 11 interventions to prevent hypertension, the feasibility of implementation, and policy recommendations are described in the primary prevention report. The intervention evidence is strongest for weight loss, reduced sodium intake, aerobic exercise, and reduced alcohol consumption as means to prevent hypertension. Evidence supporting stress management; potassium, fish oil, calcium, magnesium, or fiber supplementation; and micronutrient alteration (fat, fatty acids, carbohydrate, and protein) is more limited. The degree of high blood pressure reduction is related to the extent of weight loss, although even modest decrements in weight can produce a favorable impact on blood pressure. Interventions in clinical and community settings demonstrate that the behavior changes needed to achieve blood pressure reductions are feasible. Sustainability of these interventions, however, has been elusive.

Recently, the second Trial of Prevention of Hypertension (TOPH II) examined the separate and combined effect of decreased sodium and weight loss intake in 2,382 overweight participants, 17.7% of whom were Black Americans (Trials of Hypertension Prevention Cooperative Research Group, 1996). The goal was to decrease blood pressure by 2 mm Hg, which would be equivalent to a population benefit expected from the detection and treatment of all patients with diastolic blood pressures greater than 90 mm Hg; that is, a 6% decrease in coronary heart disease and a 13% to 16% decrease in stroke rates. The effects of the separate and combined interventions were equal. At the 3-year follow-up, 45% of the usual care group had developed incident (new) hypertension (≥ 140/90 mm Hg). Although the actual outcome in mm Hg was half of what was expected, risk was reduced 15% at 36 months. Differences in the reduction in blood pressure were greatest 6 months after the trial began and decreased over time, perhaps due to varied and diminishing compliance, particularly with sodium restriction. The Trial of Nonpharmacologic Interventions in the Elderly (TONE) study was designed to examine the benefit of weight reduction and sodium restriction (alone or combined) in controlling blood pressure of individuals 60 to 80 years of age who were withdrawn from antihypertensive medication (Whelton et al., 1998). The intensive intervention delivered by nutritionists and behavioral psychologists focused on adoption and maintenance of eating patterns and enhanced physical activity. Of the 975 participants, 23.5% were Black Americans, representing 28% of the obese and 17% of the nonobese members of the study population. Blacks and Whites achieved and sustained a 7- to 10-pound weight loss over a follow-up period of 1.5 to 3 years. The investigative teams for TOPH and TONE were composed of hypertension specialists with expertise in epidemiology, nutritionists, and behavioral scientists. A nurse investigator (Martha Hill), conducted an ancillary study at one TOPH II center and is currently examining predictors of enrollment, compliance, and outcomes.

Factors Associated With Hypertension Control

Control of hypertension is dependent upon appropriate detection, treatment, and patient adherence or compliance to treatment recommendations. By the end of the 1980s, 73% of the U.S. adult population with hypertension were aware of their hypertension (Burt, Cutler, et al., 1995; Burt, Whelton, et al., 1995). A more recent report indicates that 96% of hypertensive Black American adults in an underserved inner-city neighborhood knew they had hypertension (Hill, Bone, Barker, et al., 1995). Progress has been made in the control of hypertension nationally, but only 29% of individuals with this problem have adequately controlled blood pressure (< 140/90 mm Hg) (Burt, Cutler, et al., 1995; Burt, Whelton, et al., 1995). This problem is particularly noteworthy in urban populations with high unemployment, lower educational attainment, lower income, and psychosocial stressors in an unsafe environment, as well as among Black men.

The individual, the provider, and the health care system, as well as sociocultural factors, are associated with high blood pressure control. Response to treatment and high blood pressure control differences in Black Americans and Whites have been associated with physiological, sociocultural, economic, psychological, behavioral, and/or programmatic factors, including delayed entry and remaining in care (Bone, Hill, & Levine, 1994). Available studies indicate that the specific attitudes, beliefs, and concerns of Black Americans influence control rates. Important beliefs about causes and prevention of cardiovascular disease and perceptions about HBP care and treatment have been reported by Black Americans (Heurtin-Roberts, 1990; Livingston, Levine, & Moore, 1990). Behavioral factors are major impediments to HBP control in low-socioeconomic-status Black Americans. For example, eating patterns in many Black Americans resulting in excess weight gain, such as eating foods high in total saturated fat, cholesterol, and sodium, are associated with excess high blood pressure and cardiovascular risk factors such as obesity and diabetes (Kumanyika, 1990). Additionally, sedentary lifestyle is common among Black Americans, and achievement of recommended physical activity is low (Kumanyika & Adams-Campbell, 1991).

Lack of social support in Black Americans is another major factor associated with low rates of follow-up and adherence to treatment recommendations and the disproportionate burden of hypertension in Black Americans. In a study of predominantly female Black Americans with HBP, educational-behavioral interventions including individualized participant counseling sessions after the physician visit, a home visit to the family member or friend identified by the participant as the major source of social support, and group discussions were significantly associated with the following outcomes: improved follow-up, appointment keeping, compliance with medicine taking, weight loss, BP control, and less HBP-related morbidity, 5-year HBP related mortality, and 5-year all-cause mortality (Levine, Green, et al., 1979; Morisky et al., 1983). Social integration, social support, and material resources, all measures of social ties, have been associated with more positive health status and better control of HBP (Strogatz & James, 1986). Livingston and colleagues (1990) evaluated the role of social integration (defined in terms of employment, marriage, church affiliation, group affiliation, and having someone to talk to when needed) in explaining variation in BP in a sample of 1,420 Black American Maryland residents. They noted that only church affiliation was inversely associated with BP when adjusting for covariates, including age, education, body mass index, physical exercise, use of antihypertensive medications, and cigarette smoking.

Individual behavior, especially infrequent health-care seeking and low adherence to treatment recommendations, is a major impediment to blood pressure control in low-socioeconomic-status Black Americans (Heckler, 1985; Shea, Misra, & Francis, 1992). Adherence to treatment is associated with simplifying the regimen, involving the patient in decision making about the regimen, and addressing the aforementioned patient-related and system or provider factors (Bone, Levine, Parry, Morisky, & Green, 1984; Dunbar, 1990; Dunbar-Jacob, Dwyer, & Dunning, 1991; Working Group on Health Education and High Blood Pressure Control, 1987). In addition, drug treatment specific issues, including complexity of the regimen, cost, and side effects, are well-documented factors associated with adherence. Moreover, lifestyles of subgroups of Black Americans, for example those with high rates of unemployment and/or alcohol consumption, and concerns of daily life present barriers to seeking care and following treatment recommendations (Branche, Batts, Dowdy, Field, & Francis, 1991; Clark, 1991; Francis, 1991; Shea, Misra, Ehrlich, Field, & Francis, 1992a, 1992b). Thus, human resource needs are as important, if not more salient, than the perceived need for medical care and treatment for HBP. Compelling evidence exists that hypertensive patients improve their adherence to therapeutic regimens and their continuity of care when practitioners provide care in a multidisciplinary approach and identify patients' specific needs for information and supports, address the patients' specific concerns, and reinforce their progress at every visit (Hill & Houston-Miller, 1996; Roter & Hall, 1991).

Provider inadequacy in involving the patient in decisions regarding the regimen, including assessing the readiness of the participant to engage in treatment and eliciting the participant's concerns, has been identified as a major contributing factor to noncompliance (Working Group on Health Education and High Blood Pressure Control, 1987). Further, the patient's perception that the physician is too busy contributes to the lack of an effective patient-provider relationship, a critical component of the care process (Bone, Levine, et al., 1984; German, 1988; Roter & Hall, 1991). Thus, provider failure to assess the readiness of the patient to engage in treatment, elicit patients' concerns, and involve the patient in decisions regarding the regimen has been identified as a contributing factor to noncompliance.

Long-recognized physical, logistical, structural, and economic problems, such as no health insurance, no follow-up appointments, lack of continuity of providers, ab-sence of and inconvenient transportation, lengthy waiting times, and inconvenient locations and appointment times, are associated with low rates of entry into and remaining in care and achieving adequate HBP control (Bone, Levine, et al., 1984; Bone, Mamon, et al., 1989; Finnerty, Mattie, & Finnerty, 1973; Finnerty & Shaw, 1973a, 1973b; Shea et al., 1992b; Smith, Curb, Hardy, Hawkins, & Tyroler, 1982). The two most important factors correlated with nonadherence to hypertension treatment in an inner city minority population in a recent examination by Shea and colleagues (1992b) were having their BP checked in an emergency room and lack of a primary care physician.

In the past few decades, emergency departments (EDs) in hospitals have increasingly had to provide nonurgent services, as EDs are the usual source of primary care for those without health insurance, especially young unemployed men (Bone, Mamon, et al., 1989; Heckler, 1985; Pane, Farner, & Kym, 1991). Thus, as the hospital's most accessible entry point, they have had to become responsive to the needs of the surrounding communities and interested in minority health care. In one urban ED, an HBP demonstration program increased the follow-up appointment-keeping rate threefold after a follow-up clinic was established next to the ED (Anwar, Roberts, & Wagner, 1977). Several other studies have documented the beneficial contribution of paraprofessionals with specified responsibilities to the ED's effectiveness as a site of HBP detection, referral, and short-term follow-up (Bone, Mamon, et al., 1989; Fletcher, Appel, & Bourgeons, 1975).

The cultural insensitivity of many traditional HBP control methods to Black American populations and communities is an additional important factor associated with HBP control. Research in general, and ours in Baltimore specifically, suggests that HBP control interventions for Black Americans will be most effective if the interventions are culturally specific and relevant, if the indigenous population is involved in their development, and if they are community based and owned. The efficacy of planned health education programs, built on appropriate behavioral theory and principles, enhances the control of hypertension and decreases related morbidity and mortality (Levine, Green, et al., 1979; Levine & Bone, 1990; Morisky et al., 1983). Nurse-trained and -supervised community health workers (CHWs) capable of providing culturally sensitive care have been shown to be effective in supplementing providers' detection, treatment, and follow-up of hypertensive Black Americans

(Hill & Becker, 1995; Hill, Bone, & Butz, 1996). A recent Pew Health Professions Commission report (1994a) refers to the CHW as an "integral yet often overlooked member of the health care work force." In our East Baltimore experience, community health workers were successful in improving entry into care and appointment keeping in 66% of the population (Bone, Mamon, et al., 1989) and were a central part of a community intervention that resulted in significantly increasing BP control from 12% to 40% (Levine & Bone, 1990). The literature identifies the importance of having nurses actively involved in the use of community health workers, to define these workers' tasks and relationship with health care providers; to plan and implement programs; and to provide training, support, and supervision of the community health workers to increase the likelihood of program sustainability (Hill, Bone, & Butz, 1996; Walt, 1988).

Since 1972, the Coordinating Committee of the National Heart, Lung and Blood Institute's National High Blood Pressure Education Program has spearheaded extensive professional education activities and mass media campaigns about high blood pressure awareness, diagnosis, and control. Over 40 member organizations participate in the program. The American Nurses Association was an early member. As worksite programs gained prominence in the late 1970s, the American Association of Occupational Health Nurses joined. In the early 1980s, the National Black Nurses Association joined, when efforts to address hypertension in Black Americans became a program priority. The National High Blood Pressure Education Program produced a series of influential consensus reports from the Joint National Committee on Detection, Evaluation, and Treatment of High Blood Pressure (Joint National Committee, 1993) and other groups (Working Group on Health Education and High Blood Pressure Control, 1987; Working Group on Management of Patients with Hypertension and High Blood Cholesterol, 1991; Working Group on Primary Prevention of Hypertension, 1993; Working Group to Define Critical Behaviors in High Blood Pressure Control, 1979). The High Blood Pressure Education Program, the American Heart Association, the American Society of Hypertension, the International Society of Hypertension, and the International Society for Hypertension in Blacks have all focused extensive research and educational efforts on increasing understanding of basic, clinical, and population sciences related to the prevention and treatment of hypertension. The needs of Black Americans are well recognized and frequently focused upon.

Description and Comparison Across Various Perspectives

Despite widespread recognition of the prevalence of HBP and the cost of diagnosis, evaluation, and treatment, as well as the benefits of treatment, especially among Black Americans, the reasons why there has not been more improvement in control rates are not clearly understood. Potential explanations influencing nursing research and practice may be found in the following comparison of differing approaches. Controversial issues and contrasting theoretical perspectives dominate discussions about how to prevent and treat high blood pressure. These differing views will be presented prior to reviewing and evaluating what is known scientifically.

Individual Versus Population Approach

The National High Blood Pressure Education Program has pursued the dual strategy of professional and public education. Membership on the Program's Coordinating Committee is predominantly filled by cardiology and hypertension professional organizations and societies. This is explained in large part by early and ongoing recognition that practicing physicians were not detecting, diagnosing, or effectively treating hypertension. Improving detection of hypertension in all settings, as well as physicians' care of individual patients and control of hypertension in their offices, has been this national program's focus to reduce hypertension-related morbidity and mortality. Simultaneously, population-based approaches, primarily through mass media campaigns, greatly increased the public's awareness of the importance of high blood pressure and knowledge of blood pressure levels.

Medical Versus Multidisciplinary Models of Care

With physicians as the primary professional target audience for continuing education, the traditional medical model emphasized diagnosis and treatment of disease. The pathophysiology of elevated blood pressure and the associated target organ damage and physician-ordered pharmacologic treatment to lower blood pressure to minimize or prevent complications were of primary interest. The Stepped Care approach to sequential prescribing of single or combination drugs (which has always stressed individualized care, despite what its critics argue) is one strategy to synthesize a huge body of literature and to make practical practice guidelines (Joint National Committee, 1993). The emphasis on pharmacologic treatment in medical continuing education programs has contributed, in part, to the pharmaceutical industry's generous support and advertising of these programs. The critics of the medical model approach to hypertension prevention and treatment make two major points. First, within medical care settings, hypertension care is best delivered by multidisciplinary teams that include nursing, pharmacy, and nutrition as a basis. Second, blood pressure is influenced by environmental, psychological, behavioral, and socioeconomic factors that are not within the traditional purview of medicine. Yet, the multidisciplinary team approach demonstrated in clinical trials to reduce risk has been insufficiently incorporated into standard clinical practice, and the national program and most hypertension-focused medical continuing education programs stress physician care and control by pharmacological methods. The recently reported low national control rates for hypertension control are a clear reminder that the predominant strategies are entirely insufficient (Burt, Cutler, et al., 1995; Burt, Whelton, et al., 1995). To control hypertension effectively, multidisciplinary strategies, offering supportive care in culturally relevant approaches, are needed to improve intervention effectiveness and sustainability.

Goal-Directed Versus Nontargeted Treatment

For more than 20 years, U.S. policy and most research has been based on consensus agreement that a blood pressure level of equal to or greater than 140/90 mm Hg was the established dichotomous definition of high blood pressure. Initially, equal to or greater than 160/95 mm Hg was the definition for hypertension. It still is in much of the rest of the world. Scientists and some health professionals appreciate that these cut offs are arbitrary and that blood pressure risk is continuously and positively associated with the level of the pressure. Recently, sophisticated computer-assisted analysis of epidemiologic and clinical trial data has increased awareness of the positive health benefits of lower blood pressure levels, particularly for subgroups such as individuals with diabetes and/or decreased renal function. This has brought increasing attention internationally to the value

of risk stratification and differing goals for subgroups as well as lower level criteria for "normal" blood pressure (Alderman, Cushman, Hill, Krakoff, & Pecker, 1993). In 1993, the Fifth Joint National Committee on the Detection, Evaluation and Treatment of Hypertension issued a new classification schema of blood pressure that includes systolic as well as diastolic levels, the new class of "high normal" blood pressure (130-139/85-89 mm Hg) and four stages of high blood pressure, numbered 1 to 4, rather than using the misleading terms *mild, moderate,* and *severe* for the previous three levels (Joint National Committee, 1993) (see Table 16.2). The increasing emphasis on lower blood pressure in the United States, with a desirable goal of less than 130/85 mm Hg, is controversial internationally as well as within the United States. A criterion and goal of less than 140/90 mm Hg is considered by some to be too low, necessitating too-aggressive therapy at unfavorable risk and cost/benefit ratios. This is one reason why the blood pressure performance measure to be adopted by the National Committee on Quality Assurance (NCQA) is undergoing further evaluation and testing prior to inclusion in the Health Plan Employer Data and Information Set (HEDIS) 3.0.

Categorical Versus Multiple Risk Factor Approach

The federal government's approach to cardiovascular risk factors evolved historically, with resources devoted to individual risk factors or category of risk factor, as information became available from epidemiologic and clinical trial data. The National High Blood Pressure Education Program established in 1972 preceded the National Cholesterol Education Program (established in 1985) and the Obesity Initiative (established in 1991). Considerable overlap exists in the membership of the programs' coordinating committees, their professional as well as their patient and public target audiences, and content of their educational messages. The need for integrated multiple risk factor intervention approaches has been recognized; however, historic and political considerations seem to promote continuing the categorical approach at the federal level. Opponents of the categorical approach argue that many patients at risk for coronary heart disease have, or are at risk for, more than one risk factor. To be effective, primary prevention interventions for the person predisposed to or with multiple risk factors must be integrated. This is particularly true because of the importance of common physiological pathways such

TABLE 16.2.   Preventing, Monitoring, and Addressing Problems of Adherence

Educate about conditions and treatment

- Assess patient's understanding and acceptance of the diagnosis and expectations of being in care.
- Discuss patient's concerns and clarify misunderstandings.
- Inform patient of blood pressure level.
- Agree with patient on a goal blood pressure.
- Inform patient about recommended treatment and provide specific written information.
- Elicit concerns and questions and provide opportunities for patient to state specific behaviors to carry out treatment recommendations.
- Emphasize need to continue treatment, that patient cannot tell if blood pressure is elevated, and that control does not mean cure.

Individualize the regimen

- Include patient in decision making.
- Simplify the regimen.
- Incorporate treatment into patient's daily lifestyle.
- Set, with the patient, realistic short-term objectives for specific components of the treatment plan.
- Encourage discussion of side effects and concerns.
- Encourage self-monitoring.
- Minimize cost of therapy.
- Indicate you will ask about adherence at next visit.
- When weight loss is established as a treatment goal, discourage quick weight loss regimens, fasting, or unscientific methods, since these are associated with weight cycling, which may increase cardiovascular morbidity and mortality.

Provide reinforcement

- Provide feedback regarding blood pressure level.
- Ask about behaviors to achieve blood pressure control.
- Give positive feedback for behavioral and blood pressure improvement.
- Hold exit interviews to clarify regimen.
- Make appointment for next visit before patient leaves office.
- Use appointment reminders and contact patients to confirm appointments.
- Schedule more frequent visits to counsel nonadherent patients.
- Contact and follow up patients who missed appointments.
- Consider clinician-patient contracts.

Promote social support

- Educate family members to be part of the blood pressure control process and provide daily reinforcement.
- Suggest small group activities to enhance mutual support and motivation.

Collaborate with other professionals

- Draw upon complementary skills and knowledge of nurses, pharmacists, dieticians, optometrists, dentists, and physician assistants.
- Refer patients for more intensive counseling.

SOURCE: Joint National Committee (1993).

as obesity and diabetes and behavioral strategies such as appointment keeping and physical activity and eating patterns; all of these require integrated approaches. Furthermore, quality of life, economic, and safety concerns mandate an integrated approach.

Treatment Versus Prevention Emphasis

As described above, community-based efforts to increase public awareness and knowledge of blood pressure levels and physician office-based treatment of individuals with hypertension have been emphasized. Critics of this treatment-focused approach cite the variable success achieved thus far in controlling blood pressure and argue for targeting the population broadly through public health and regulatory approaches to healthier lifestyles. They point out that application of lifestyle interventions in the general population to achieve a downward shift in the distribution of blood pressure is also necessary if the hypertension epidemic is to be brought under control. The well-established interventions to lower blood pressure, even if only several mm Hg, subsequently lower the

risk of the complications. Interest from a public health standpoint has therefore begun to focus on prevention of the risk factor itself. This approach calls for lifestyle changes at the family, community, or population levels and targets adverse lifestyle factors, including a high sodium intake, an excessive consumption of calories, physical inactivity, excessive alcohol consumption, and a low intake of potassium (Joint National Committee, 1993; Working Group on Primary Prevention of Hypertension, 1993). The recent Surgeon General's report, *Physical Activity and Health* (U.S. Department of Health and Human Services, 1996), emphasizes the importance of physical activity in promoting health as a primary prevention strategy and as a vehicle to promote weight control within secondary prevention.

Theoretical Versus Applied Research

Controversy surrounds the balance in funding both investigator-initiated basic research and applied clinical or programmatic research. In a time of scarce resources, especially at the National Institutes of Health (NIH), the debate has become more intense. One issue in the debate is the expense of large multisite clinical trials in diverse populations, compared to the much larger number of laboratory-based studies that could be supported for the same amount of money. The need for basic research continues because the fundamental mechanisms underlying hypertension are not fully explicated. New basic science discoveries may influence the development of increasingly effective and well-tolerated therapies. Although the value of basic research is appreciated by clinical and epidemiologic investigators, they argue that effective interventions are needed now to blunt the costly hypertension epidemic. The role of theory-guided research, as opposed to pragmatic program-guided research, in addressing prevalent public health problems is controversial as well. Some have criticized nursing and health education for striving to be accepted as disciplines by imitating the social and biomedical sciences, which develop theory and test hypotheses. Others argue that developing theory is a luxury that does not address the need to find effective solutions to pressing health problems and that resources should be devoted to testing practical solutions. Moreover, some of these critics argue that to develop effective interventions it is necessary for investigators to understand that major public health problems are socially produced and maintained and that they are not randomly distributed. Many interventions known to be effective have been tested primarily at one level—the individual, the social network, or the organizational structure—with inconsistent sustained application of beneficial findings. An interesting example of these controversies within nursing research can be found in the debate about qualitative methodology to develop theoretical understanding and measurement capability versus quantitative methodology to determine intervention outcomes. These arguments, basic science versus clinical research, theory-driven versus practical intervention, and quantitative versus qualitative methodology, are something of a "red herring." All approaches are needed and are complementary.

Black Versus White Hypertension Myths

As the type and amount of research on ethnicity and hypertension improves, widely held beliefs about racial differences in hypertension are being dispelled (Flack, 1993). One myth is that there is a fundamental ethnic difference in the relationship between high blood pressure and cardiovascular disease. Although Black Americans may have higher absolute level of risk at a given level of blood pressure, the shape of the relationship and the predominant associated factors are the same: The higher the blood pressure, the higher the risk; the higher the income, the lower the blood pressure; and although people may be in care and on medication, the high blood pressure is not necessarily controlled. The belief that diastolic blood pressure is more important than systolic blood pressure is not supported by data. Increases in systolic blood pressure are important with or without increases in diastolic pressure. Another myth that is not supported by data is the belief that the elderly do not benefit from treatment and that the risk-benefit ratio of treatment is unfavorable for the elderly with hypertension.

Synthesis of the State of Nursing Science and Practice

It is not always possible to separate nursing science from nursing practice when reviewing nursing research because much of the research literature examines nursing practice interventions. There is a paucity of nursing research (in which the principal or other identifiable investigators are nurses) in hypertension prevention and control in general and in Black Americans in particular. For example, the internationally recognized work of L. Bone, M.P.H., R.N., and colleagues, particularly D. Levine, M.D., to improve hypertension detection, care, and control in inner-city Black Americans is published in the public health, health education, and medical literature (Bone, Hill, & Levine, 1994; Bone, Mamon, et al., 1989). This literature would not be identified through searching the nursing literature, nor would an author search identify Bone as a nurse. She is an example of nurse investigators who are in schools of public health or medicine, not nursing, and whose nursing focus is conceptualized within a discipline other than nursing. Importantly, the public health nursing perspective that Bone, who also is a health educator, brings to the research team with which she works enhances its multidisciplinary approach to research, which includes behavioral science, medicine, nursing, health education, and health services research. With the addition of a doctorally prepared NIH-funded principal investigator (M. Hill), who is primarily based in a school of nursing, the nursing research visibility and impact of this team's work is increasing. Additionally, the work by Hill, Bone,

Levine, and colleagues is the only program of research identified that specifically focuses on urban, underserved, hypertensive Black men, the least studied age/sex/race group with the lowest hypertension detection, treatment, and control rates.

If one's definition of nursing research includes investigation of nursing practice (i.e., what nurses do and what difference it makes for patients), regardless of the discipline of the principal and other investigators, then the nursing research and practice literature about the treatment of hypertension, although not necessarily in Black Americans, is considerably larger.

Nursing Research

In the 1970s and early 1980s, several nurse scientists published reports of their investigations. The most notable of these, perhaps, is the work of Swain and Steckle (1981), who tested the effectiveness of contingency contracting in comparison to routine clinic care or patient education on improving adherence with treatment recommendations in 115 patients randomized to one of the three groups. Nurses and patients negotiated certain behaviors to lower blood pressure that the patient would carry out, specific goals, and the incentive or reward the patient would receive at the next visit if the goal was met. Written contracts were signed. The strategies of establishing partnership, goal setting, negotiation, motivation, problem solving, feedback, and rewards are featured in this behavioral approach. Patient education produced an untoward effect of increasing a dropout rate higher than usual care. Contingency contracting significantly improved patient knowledge, adherence to requests for regular medical care, and decreased diastolic blood pressure. Hill and Reichgott (1979) reported quality of care outcomes in a hypertension clinic in which nurse practitioners and/or physicians cared for patients who were not randomized to provider type. These retrospective analyses documented the facts that nurses and physicians saw similar patient groups and did not differ in process documentation or outcome results (proportion of patients with controlled blood pressure). Moreover, nurses were managing patients as complex as those seen only by physicians, identifying important problems, and referring patients appropriately (Reichgott, Pearson, & Hill, 1983). Other reports of nurse-run screening and management clinics support effective nursing practice in the care of hypertensive patients (Jewell & Hope, 1988; Pheley et al., 1995). Spratlen (1982) described a school-based hypertension screening, education, and follow-up program

for adolescents with blood pressures at or above the 95th percentile. By oversampling Black students, Spratlen was able to accrue a sample in which Blacks comprised 37.6% of the adolescents screened in three Seattle schools. Approximately 4.1% of the males and 3.8% of the females had elevated systolic blood pressures, and 3.0% of males and 3.3% of females had elevated diastolic pressures. Black males and females had higher pressures than Whites except for the systolic pressures of the Black males. None of these studies were conducted in exclusively Black American samples, and, other than Spratlen's, they were not designed to examine racial differences.

The identifiable research published by nurse investigators about hypertension predominantly addresses these three areas: methodological issues, such as instrument development and accurate measurement of blood pressure; description of patient populations and factors associated with blood pressure control; and nursing interventions. For example, nurse investigators currently active in the hypertension field include G. Hamilton, who developed the Hamilton Health Belief Scale, which measures hypertension-related beliefs delineated by the Health Belief Model. Within an ongoing study (RO1 NR 03317), she is assessing the impact and cost-effectiveness of interventions aimed at improving adherence within an oral potassium supplementation to antihypertensive therapy. Thomas and Leihr have published several well-designed studies illustrating the effect of talking and listening on blood pressure levels and describing cardiovascular reactivity as an emerging risk factor (Leihr, 1992; Thomas & Friedman, 1994; Thomas & Leihr, 1995). The lifestyle profiles of 364 treated hypertensive patients, described by MacDonald and colleagues, illustrate the importance of dietary intake, perceived stress, and obesity, which vary by case and sex groupings (MacDonald, Sawatzky, Wilson, & Laing, 1991). In a multiple risk factor program staffed by a multidisciplinary team, a largely White sample of 135 patients completed 11 two-hour group sessions over 6 months. Significant decreases in both clinical and home recruitments of systolic and diastolic blood pressure occurred after intervention (Stuart et al., 1987). Although examining racial differences was not an aim of these studies, they are representative in that typically little or no information is provided about racial composition of the samples.

A review, "Nursing Blood Pressure Research, 1980-1990: A Bio-Psycho-Social Perspective" (Thomas, Leiher, Dekeyser, & Friedman, 1993), reports on 50 studies from three journals and notes that race was reported in

18 (30%) of the studies. Several nursing studies in Black Americans have been reported. In a sample of 160 subjects, 72% of whom were Black and 70% of whom were women, Powers and Woolridge (1982) used a factorial design to examine factors influencing knowledge, attitudes, and compliance of hypertensive patients. Despite significant decreases in blood pressure for patients in the educational program, variations in the approval had little or no effect on the actual blood pressure reduction. E. Smith and J. Charleston have conducted church-based programs. Smith evaluated the efficacy of an intervention in hypertensive subjects from Chicago Black churches. In a pilot study with 63 participants, 33 from a church that had a hypertension screening project and 30 from a church that did not, no relationship was found between support and compliance and blood pressure control (Smith, 1989). In the second study, there was a statistically significant increase in knowledge of the 32 participants, although no changes were noted in blood pressure or sodium intake 3 months after the educational intervention (Smith, 1992). In a larger study in Baltimore, 184 Black and 3 White women participated in a behaviorally oriented weight control program consisting of eight weekly 2-hour counseling and exercise sessions. The percent decrease in weight was significantly associated with decreases in systolic and diastolic blood pressure. Weight lost during the program was maintained or exceeded by 65% of the women (Kumanyika & Charleston, 1992). Hill, Bone, and colleagues have developed interventions with nurse-trained and -supervised community health workers to increase hypertension care and control in inner-city Black American populations (Hill, Bone, Barker, et al., 1995; Hill, Bone, & Butz, 1996; Hill, Bone, Stewart, et al., 1996a, 1996b). (Their ongoing NIH-funded studies are further described on pages 303-305.) Harrell and colleagues evaluated cardiovascular risk factors in textile workers (Harrell, Cometto, & Stutts, 1992). In this study, 40.6% of the 1,360 workers were not White, and all but four of them were Black Americans. Racial differences in risk factor prevalence were examined, and improvements were found in a subset of the workers after a 6-month nurse-administered educational intervention at the worksite. Approximately a third of the early-school-age participants studied by Grossman and colleagues to assess blood pressure rhythms were African Americans. There were no relationships found between race and the occurrence of significant blood pressure rhythms (Grossman, Parda, & Farr, 1994).

Much research has been reported that tested educational, behavioral, and treatment interventions delivered by nurses to effectively control blood pressure. In the large national multisite clinical trials upon which national consensus guidelines for treatment of hypertension are based, such as the Hypertension Detection and Follow-up Program (Hypertension Detection and Follow-up Program Cooperative Group, 1979), nurses were involved in a variety of roles: recruitment coordinators, data collectors, and interventionists (Cowley, Somelofski, Hill, Smith, & Buchwald, 1988). Nurses were not involved as investigators in any of these trials, with the exception of a nurse at the Yale site in the Systolic Hypertension in the Elderly Program (SHEP) Trial (SHEP Cooperative Research Group, 1991). Surveys of nurse coordinators' job satisfaction in these trials have been conducted by nurses; however, they are unpublished, with one exception (Kellen, Schron, McBride, Hale, & Campion, 1994). Thus, nursing research in large multisite hypertension clinical trials is scant. Black Americans were recruited into these multisite trials, with the proportion varying among the trials and among the sites within trials. In general, as in the primary prevention trials, Black Americans benefited from participation in the intervention studies (Saunders, 1991).

In nurse-run clinics, the effective advanced practice nursing role includes diagnosis and management of hypertension and other cardiovascular risk factors and prescribing therapies within the legal guidelines and policies of states and institutions (Hill & Becker, 1995). Results of numerous observational and uncontrolled intervention studies, as well as prospective clinical trials over a 30-year period, consistently show that nurses with specialty training can provide safe and efficacious care, achieving high rates of patient satisfaction, resulting in physician acceptance and cooperation and in treatment outcomes, including BP control, that are not significantly different from outcomes achieved by physicians (Hill & Reichgott, 1979; Jewell & Hope, 1988; Jones, Jones, & Katz, 1987; Perry et al., 1992; Pheley et al., 1995; Reichgott et al., 1983; Runyon, 1975; Schoenbaum & Alderman, 1976). In the large multisite clinical trials of hypertension control such as the Multiple Risk Factor Intervention Trial (MRFIT) (Multiple Risk Factor Intervention Trial Research Group, 1982), Hypertension Detection and Follow-up Program (HDFP) (Hypertension Detection and Follow-up Program Cooperative Group, 1979), and SHEP (SHEP Cooperative Research Group, 1991), nurses were actively involved in delivering multidisciplinary educational and behavioral interventions to improve hypertension control. More recently, large multisite prevention clinical trials such as Trials of Hypertension Prevention (TOHP I) used similar lifestyle modification strategies to prevent hypertension in individuals with high normal blood pressures (Trials of Hypertension Prevention Collaborative Research Group, 1992).

Nurses have also effectively managed other cardiovascular risk factors in a variety of settings. Using nurse practitioner and case management models in collaborative practice arrangements for consultation and referral, nurses working with physicians, pharmacists, and dietitians have effectively improved hypertension-related outcomes for patients with hypercholesterolemia (Blair, Bryant, & Bocuzzi, 1988), diabetes (Peters, Davidson, & Ossorio, 1995), smoking (Taylor, Miller, Killen, & DeBusk, 1990), and congestive heart failure (Rich et al., 1995). Nursing strategies integrated simultaneously in a case management system have been shown to improve outcomes for patients post-acute myocardial infarction (DeBusk et al., 1994). Using this case management system, known as MULTIFIT, specially trained nurses significantly improved smoking cessation, exercise training, diet-drug management of hyperlipidemia, and control of other risk factors in a 12-month randomized clinical trial conducted through a health maintenance organization. Mail and telephone contact decreased the number of physician or nurse office visits, and a computerized algorithm facilitated monitoring progress toward treatment goals and adjustments in recommendations. This and similar studies have nurse researchers as senior members of the investigative team and nationally visible proponents of advanced nursing practice (Rich et al., 1995). Black Americans were enrolled in these studies and benefited from the interventions, but none of the studies were designed to primarily address treatment of hypertension in Black individuals.

Identifiable hypertension research conceptualized, planned, and conducted by nurse investigators, whether principal investigator or not, remains scant. Dissertation titles indicate that some research has been done; however, subsequent articles in the literature are not always found. Further evidence for scarcity of nursing research in the prevention and treatment of hypertension can be found in the National Institute for Nursing Research portfolio. In 1994, within 338 titles of funded research, only three had hypertension or high blood pressure in the title: one title of a basic science study and two titles of clinical studies. Twelve additional titles indicated that other cardiovascular risk factors are being studied. In the 1996 portfolio, 13 hypertension-related grants were funded. Two of those specified Black American samples in their titles: R01 NR04119-01 (M. Hill, principal investigator),

"Comprehensive HBP Care for Young Urban Black Men," and R01 NR04290-01 (S. Picot, principal investigator), "Cardiovascular Responses in Black Female Care Givers." Although anecdotal examples are known of increasing numbers of studies in which nurse scientists are participating as members of multidisciplinary teams, it is difficult to identify these through the usual methods. This inability to identify nurse investigators may be a trade-off for the scientific gains derived from multidisciplinary work regardless of the discipline of the principal investigator, journal, or funding agency.

Nursing Practice

The literature contains numerous articles by nurses that focus on new knowledge about hypertension and its treatment, case studies, and approaches to patient care, including protocols and care plans. This literature and the previously mentioned literature by nurse investigators provide a firm base for nursing practice in high blood pressure control. In much of this literature, however, little or no mention is made specifically of the prevention and treatment of hypertension in Black Americans.

Nursing has contributed to improvements in hypertension detection and control through direct care, case management, supervision of allied personnel, and expertise in training for accurate measurement of blood pressure (Hill & Grim, 1991). Nursing's diverse and effective direct care role in hypertension control includes case finding, referral, patient education, follow-up, monitoring response to therapy, and improving adherence and treatment outcomes (Grim & Grim, 1981; Hill & Becker, 1995). Detection, education, referral, and follow-up have been conducted in nonclinic settings, including neighborhood clinics (Runyon, 1975), emergency departments (Bone, Mamon, et al., 1989), worksites (Schoenbaum & Alderman, 1976), churches (Kumanyika & Charleston, 1992; Smith, 1992) and schools (Spratlen, 1982). Community and public health nurses not only provide care to individuals and families in the community but also create linkages between traditional institutions and agencies and new and nontraditional partners. These nurses provide expertise in coordinating resources and managing programs encouraging sustainability by educating and mentoring community residents to maximize the likelihood of long-term success.

Nursing's roles, including advanced practice roles, have been recognized as an important part of primary care, as well as interdisciplinary education and teamwork in practice (Baldwin, 1994; Hill & Houston-Miller, 1996;

O'Neil, 1993; Pew Health Professions Commission, 1994b; Safriet, 1992). Nursing's contribution to high blood pressure control in a variety of settings, including care of people living in medically undeserved urban areas (Branche, Batts, Dowdy, Field, & Francis, 1991; Perry et al., 1992) and worksite programs, particularly those with union-supported worksite health programs (Schoenbaum & Alderman, 1976), is acknowledged in the literature. Care provided by family nurse practitioners in a rural clinic in which hypertension was the most common chronic condition in adults was associated with high rates of patient satisfaction (Ramsey, Edwards, Lenz, Odom, & Brown, 1993). This literature, which defines practice settings and roles as well as effectiveness of practice in some instances, does not describe or focus upon the racial composition of the patient population.

Patient education is a central role of the nurse in promoting cardiovascular health. Regardless of level of educational preparation and practice setting, nurses are prepared to help patients acquire skills, integrate treatment behaviors into daily life, make informed decisions, monitor progress, and resolve barriers to adherence with prescribed therapy. The focus of patient education is to bring about voluntary behavior change. Patient education strategies to promote adherence and desired treatment outcomes include (a) identify knowledge, attitudes, beliefs, and experience; (b) educate about condition; (c) tailor regimen to the patient; (d) provide reinforcement; (e) promote social support; and (f) collaborate with other professionals (Hill, 1989).

Areas of Substantiation and Gaps

The literature reviewed above converges to strongly support the role of nursing science and nursing practice in the prevention and treatment of hypertension in Black Americans. Yet, the aforementioned controversies clearly indicate that there are many research questions that need to be addressed and that would be enhanced by nursing's perspective. Important issues must be better understood if we are to improve hypertension prevention and treatment for Black Americans and expand nursing's contribution to this improvement.

What Is Known

The preceding description of the science documents evidence supporting the following areas of substantiated knowledge.

1. Hypertension is an important independent risk factor for coronary artery disease and stroke, the first and third causes of overall mortality in the United States.
2. Rich information is available about the prevalence of hypertension in Black Americans and factors associated with varying awareness, treatment, and control rates within age/race/gender subgroups, including geographic and socioeconomic differences.
3. A great deal is known about pharmacologic therapies and their beneficial effects on blood pressure, target organs, and health status. Knowledge about effective lifestyle interventions is increasing. Nursing research with varying research designs and educational-behavioral interventions has substantiated these findings.
4. The value of the multidisciplinary team approach and the contribution of the nurse are particularly well documented for eliciting increased compliance and blood pressure control with subsequent improved health outcomes.
5. Control rates for hypertension have improved, yet the national control rate is suboptimal (29%), and, among patients receiving treatment, only 55% are controlled to nonhypertensive levels. Among Blacks receiving antihypertensive treatment, 47% of men and 49% of women had controlled blood pressures.
6. The long-term sustainability of lifestyle changes such as weight control, restriction of sodium intake, and moderation of alcohol intake presents research and practice opportunities and challenges for nurses and other professionals.
7. Improved control rates and associated patient health status will require changes in behavior by patients, providers, and health care systems.

Gaps in Translating Knowledge Into Practice

Despite this knowledge, and improvements in the prevention and treatment of hypertension, uncontrolled high blood pressure remains a major health challenge in the United States. Several critical gaps reveal weaknesses in the clinical and public health application of knowledge.

1. Insufficient attention in research and practice is focused on the major health problem of hypertension, especially as it affects minority groups.

Overemphasis on office-based physician care and cutbacks in public health and community-based clinics may well be contributing to the unacceptable national control rates, particularly among underserved minority populations. For those individuals not in care or who are uninsured, individual physician office-based approaches offer little. Medical and behavioral approaches to hypertension prevention and management are inadequately integrated. They need to be addressed in research, education (journals and continuing education), and practice. The situation is aptly described in the following quote from the *Handbook of Black American Health*'s chapter "Hypertension: A Community Perspective" (Bone, Hill, & Levine, 1994):

> The gap between the development of research findings and policy recommendations about the detection, evaluation, and treatment of hypertension and effective application of this information at the individual and community levels are the basis of the current hypertension control problem. To narrow this gap, efforts need to be focused not only at the individual and community levels but also at the interface between them. The solution to decreasing hypertension can be found in applying scientific knowledge about behavior, pathophysiology, and therapeutics to individuals and communities. (p. 46)

2. There is little formal recognition about the importance and benefits of the multidisciplinary team approach and the contribution of the nurse in the delivery of care.

This gap between what we know works and what we are doing continues after 30 years. One explanation for the lack of recognition of the importance of the team approach may be that nurse-delivered interventions known for 30 years to be efficacious are not widely incorporated into practice. The reasons for this are complex and involve organizational, political, and financial factors. Moreover, little new information has been learned in educational and behavioral areas of provider and patient behavior. Early studies on provider behavior and interaction with patients have received scant attention in nursing and medical school curricula or in the continuing education for providers. Recent reviews, including one by Dunbar-Jacob and colleagues, indicate that no advances have been made in the compliance field since work done in 1970s and early 1980s, with the exception of computerized medication monitoring (Dunbar-Jacob et al., 1991; Rand, 1990).

Strategies to enhance the roles of nurses, pharmacists, dietitians, and health educators, as well as paraprofessionals such as community health workers, are needed. Moreover, if we are to make progress in the prevention and control of hypertension, additional disciplines will need to be brought onto the team. Behavioral psychologists are needed to further address the role of psychological and behavioral factors in "white coat" hypertension and the preventive and therapeutic contributions of biofeedback and relaxation. Anthropologists bring a helpful perspective in addressing persistent folk beliefs about hypertension (Heurtin-Roberts, 1990). Various disciplines outside the traditional medical model are needed to conceptualize how to demonstrate beneficial interventions and whether to incorporate them into medical care or have them remain outside accepted medical care. Finally, the health care system will need to place value on primary and secondary prevention and ways to implement strategies to achieve them. Because care improves and costs are less, "in many health care settings, the team approach will be the preferred technique for optimizing risk reduction" (Hill & Houston-Miller, 1996, p. 4). This will require organizational commitment, including new methods of reimbursement or coverage for services.

3. A discrepancy exists within the health care system between what the system expects of patients and what patients expect from the system.

The problems patients experience in accessing care and continuing with care providers, as well as in communicating with physicians and other providers, need to be examined more than before as managed care changes many policies and expectations. The national program and organizations concerned with prevention, detection, evaluation, and treatment need to de-emphasize the medical model and develop guidelines based on a more eclectic approach, giving increased attention to the community and worksite, other providers, and to strategies to promote adherence, self-monitoring, and self-care.

This gap between patient and system expectations can be expected to widen as our health care system continues to change. New creative, cost-effective, user-friendly approaches are needed as we manage multiple risk factors in individuals at varying stages of knowledge, readiness to change, and readiness to maintain behavior. Creative approaches will be needed to meet the needs of patients with differing values, beliefs, and available resources. Incorporating state-of-the-art behavioral science and health education into care of all Black Americans in effective ways remains an unmet patient need, as well as a provider and system challenge.

More needs to be learned about

- the risk/benefit ratio of prevention or treatment for any individual with a given blood pressure;
- efficient identification of those at highest or absolute risk or who will benefit the most from among at-risk populations;
- culturally relevant assessment tools and intervention strategies for heterogeneous subgroups;
- comprehensive interventions targeting environmental and psychosocial factors as well as medical outcomes;
- the effects of dietary patterns on blood pressure and the individual and the combined effects of potassium, magnesium, and fiber as strategies for primary and secondary prevention;
- self-monitoring and titrating medication, including step-down periods off medication;
- how to rigorously measure adherence and its effects on other outcomes; and
- cost/benefit ratio of different interventions.

Need for Ecological Approach

Further improvement in the nation's health, according to Pender and colleagues (Pender, Barkauskas, Hayman, Rice, & Anderson, 1992), will require (a) developing the self-care and health promotion potential of individuals, families, and communities; (b) creating healthier environments for all citizens; and (c) restructuring the present health care delivery system to include health promotion and prevention as reimbursable services. Critical review of multidimensional preventive and treatment approaches and the development and testing of health-related social-behavioral interventions are urgently needed (Robertson & Minkler, 1994). As Clark and McLeroy (1995a) noted, research is needed to improve the capacity of people, individually and collectively, to promote and maintain their health. Strategies that target individual behavior, as well as community and policy-level interventions, simultaneously offer enormous potential in improving health (Clark & McLeroy, 1995b). The impact of media tools, such as mass communication, and regulatory methods to restrict exposure to unhealthy substances are particularly effective.

The need for comprehensive approaches to hypertension prevention and management is evident. Even with social regulation such as smoking bans, mandatory food labeling, and walking and jogging trails, lifestyle

modification is difficult. The need to firmly address the social, cultural, and psychosocial factors affecting hypertension and its management in multidisciplinary and comprehensive ways is yet to be fully acknowledged in policy arenas. The most recent Joint National Committee consensus guidelines, published in 1993, continue to emphasize primarily the pharmacologic treatment of hypertension within the context of the physician-patient relationship.

The prevention and treatment of hypertension in Black Americans is an ideal area for nursing research within a broad multidisciplinary approach. With colleagues from nursing, medicine, and public health, we are conducting two studies to improve hypertension care and control in underserved inner-city Black Americans. Our work targeting young inner-city Black American men is the only research currently funded by the National Institutes of Nursing Research (NINR) (RO1 NR/HL 04 119) that tests nursing interventions in a Black American hypertensive population. We are one of five teams funded by the National Heart, Lung, and Blood Institute (NHLBI) to conduct hypertension control investigations in minority communities (HL-93-03 R18). Both of these areas of investigation are guided by the PRECEDE-PROCEDE framework (Green & Kreuter, 1991) (see Figure 16.1) and use nurse-trained and -supervised Black American community outreach workers as cointerventionists to help participants acquire skills, integrate treatment behaviors into daily life, make informed decisions, monitor progress, and resolve barriers (Hill, Bone, & Butz, 1996; Working Group to Define Critical Patient Behaviors in High Blood Pressure Control, 1979). Both investigations are also developed and conducted in partnership with community leaders and health and human services care providers, using state-of-the-art health education strategies. These more culturally appropriate approaches to closing the health status gap for Black Americans are used to increase long-term sustainability of effective programs, which has been a continuing, major problem. Moreover, both studies are designed to test the same general major hypothesis that more intensive intervention will result in significantly higher levels of (a) adherence to recommendations to enter or reenter care, remain in care, modify lifestyle, and take HBP medication and (b) lowering of blood pressure among hypertensive Black Americans.

The primary objective of the NINR-funded ongoing randomized clinic- and community-based clinical trial is to compare the differential reduction in BP in 250 inner

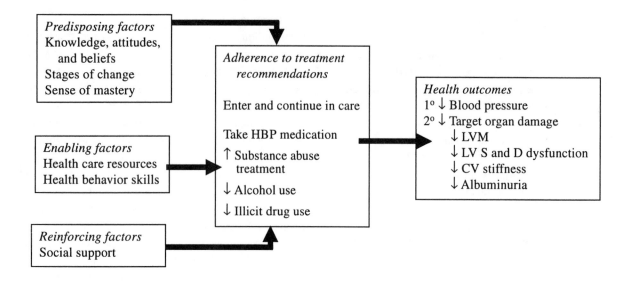

Figure 16.1. Conceptual Framework of Comprehensive High Blood Pressure Care for Young Urban Black Men
SOURCE: Green and Kreuter (1991).
NOTE: HBP = high blood pressure; LVM = left ventricular mass; LV S and D = left ventricular systolic and diastolic function; CV = cardiovascular.

city underserved hypertensive Black American men 18 to 49 years old. The study is designed to test the effectiveness of a comprehensive, educational-behavioral and treatment HBP control program provided by a nurse practitioner-community health worker team, compared to usual medical care available in the East Baltimore community. The intervention program addresses barriers to care and treatment and social support, as well as health care skills and use of health care and human services resources, with the goal of increasing entry into care, retention in care, and adherence to therapy. The intervention includes state-of-the-art clinical care, telephone contact, and home visits to the person to whom the participant turns for social support with his or her health matters. Participants in both groups will be evaluated at baseline and at 12 and 24 months by trained staff in the clinical research center who have been blinded to group assignment.

The aim of the ongoing NHLBI-funded population-based trial is to compare both the relative program effectiveness and the efficacy of educational-behavioral interventions to control high blood pressure delivered in the home by nurse-supervised community health workers on lowering blood pressure. Program effectiveness refers to the BP change in all hypertensive adults living on neighborhood blocks that have been randomized to an intervention, whether or not they actually participate in the intervention. Intervention efficacy refers to blood pressure

change in all hypertensive adults participating in either of the intervention groups, regardless of their level of adherence to recommendations. Residents of the local community are trained as nurse-supervised community health workers, to function as primary interventionists integrated into health and human service activities. They address barriers to treatment, health care resources, health-behavior-related skills, and social support. These factors are expected to affect adherence to four high blood pressure treatment recommendations, which are conceptualized as intervening variables: (a) enter or reenter care, (b) remain in care, (c) modify lifestyle, and (d) take HBP medication. Both intervention groups will receive usual medical care (including referral to care, if needed), community high blood pressure education, and HBP patient education materials. In addition, the more intensive intervention group will receive individualized education and counseling, outreach, and follow-up, including monitoring, and social support mobilization through family and peer reinforcement.

The long-term aims of both of these studies are to continue to build a multidisciplinary program of research to improve the health of underserved urban Black Americans and to improve the long-term sustainability of high blood pressure control programs. Toward this end, and building upon prior work, we have arranged to incorporate programmatic, managerial, and financial partnerships as critical parts of this work. The programmatic reliance on community health workers increases not only the acceptability of the interventions but provides employment and career opportunities for community residents. These studies are also planned and carried out in a manner that makes it possible to integrate them fully with other community services. Community leaders actively participate through scientific and/or community advisory committees. Community leaders in the social, human services, and economic development of the community who are already collaborating with both the public and private sectors serve as liaisons. Financial partnerships address sustainability through collaborative efforts with the public and private sectors to maximize (a) third-party reimbursement for health education and promotion, such as current efforts to reimburse community health workers through state funding; (b) additional federal and private funding to develop and empower the communities; and (c) employment and career opportunities for residents. Thus, our work extends from the academic and clinical settings into the community, acknowledging the multidimensionality and challenges in health promotion.

Recommendations for Advancing the Field of Nursing Science and Practice

The prevalence of hypertension and the benefits associated with its control demand our attention and action. Given the need to more effectively prevent and treat hypertension in Black Americans, we need to enhance nursing practice and develop the science upon which nursing practice is based. It is important for nurses to recognize the benefits of detecting those at risk, especially those at greatest absolute risk, and intervening accordingly. Much government, professional, and public attention has turned to other epidemic conditions, such as HIV/AIDS and tuberculosis, but detection of uncontrolled hypertension and improved management of hypertension are also necessary. The following recommendations are proposed to advance the field of nursing science.

Increase Focus on Behavioral Strategies

The importance of appropriately training and maintaining the skills of everyone who measures blood pressure—nurses, physicians, ancillary personnel, patients,

and families—cannot be overemphasized. Valid and reliable measurement, including home monitoring and appropriate use of 24-hour ambulatory monitoring, is necessary to prevent overdiagnosis and treatment and to assure accurate detection and appropriate treatment. It is well established that patient knowledge is necessary but insufficient for successful behavior change and sustainability of healthy behaviors. Moreover, knowledge and motivation are not necessarily associated with healthy behavior. We need to better understand how to predict and intervene to support positive behavior change and minimize relapse.

Screening programs to detect new cases of hypertension are no longer recommended (Joint National Committee, 1993). As part of public health programs, screening data can be helpful to determine prevalence; monitor awareness, treatment, and control rates; and evaluate program effectiveness, as well as educate and refer individuals with elevated levels of blood pressure. Care delivered in clinical settings can be supplemented by community-based intervention and follow-up programs. There is a clear need to evaluate the benefit and cost-effectiveness of nursing interventions in the community as well as in clinical settings. We need to know which individuals within a certain age/race/gender group and with a given level of blood pressure are at greatest risk for complications. This information will indicate more precisely which groups to target. We also need to develop and test effective, affordable outreach programs that extend nursing practice in culturally relevant ways (Hill, Bone, & Butz, 1996).

Primary prevention in adults and children through lifestyle modifications is an area that is ideally suited to nursing research and nursing practice. For example, the roles of obesity, sedentary lifestyle, hypertension, and cigarette smoking are important to understand within the context of culture and environment. The combination of nursing, public health, and health policy interventions offers an approach that complements and expands the more traditional one-on-one medical approach to the adult patient with diagnosed hypertension, with or without associated target organ damage. However, studies of primary and secondary prevention need to be relevant to cultural norms so that relevance, effectiveness, and sustainability are increased.

Attention must also be paid to proven strategies to lower high blood pressure, in addition to pharmacologic therapy. Lifestyle modification, especially weight control, and strategies to promote adherence and avoid relapse are effective fundamental components of blood pressure control practice. Multidisciplinary teams providing preappointment reminders, simple affordable regimens, goal setting, frequent monitoring, feedback, and reinforcement, as well as strategies to enhance social support, have all been shown to contribute to high rates of blood pressure control. Home visits and telephone contact are valuable strategies.

Design and Evaluate Culturally Relevant Programs

In the tradition of public health nursing, if the contextual issues in the environment in which the patient lives such as poverty and high stress are not addressed, we may see little advancement in the health of poor communities. The very nature of hypertension requires that we approach and work with individuals where they are—with their families and within their communities, not only in the doctor's office. To increase our understanding of patients' worldviews (Kauffman, 1994), it is necessary to consider the intrapersonal, interpersonal, organizational, community, cultural, and policy factors that affect their health and health care (Kaplan & Keil, 1993; McLeroy et al., 1993). Thus, simultaneous, feasible, patient-centered interventions, focused on multiple levels, are indicated if treatment leading to the reaching of a blood pressure goal is to be successful (McLeroy et al., 1993; Miller, Hill, Kottke, & Okene, 1997).

The main reasons for low hypertension control rates are inadequate entrance into and remaining in care, inadequately tailored treatment recommendations, and poor patient adherence to long-term treatment recommendations. Greater understanding of social, cultural, and psychosocial characteristics is needed if hypertension prevention and management are to improve. Studies of psychosocial determinants and integrated multidisciplinary and multilevel interventions are required to improve hypertension-related health status.

These studies are needed to increase understanding of ethnic and gender differences, recognizing that even within subgroups there is considerable heterogeneity. Including cultural and medical anthropologists as well as sociologists and behavioral scientists on research teams will bring their perspective to the development of more salient and effective community- and office-based interventions, such as new technologies to improve home monitoring and telecommunication of patient-collected data. At the same time, we need to understand much more about the cultural perspective of subgroups of our population. We therefore need medical anthropologists and sociologists involved in our research to increase the likelihood that community-based efforts will detect, refer, track, follow up, and intervene, especially in underserved populations. It will be necessary to include qualitative work and formative evaluation in major as well as pilot studies so that valid and reliable instruments and effective interventions can be tailored to different age, gender, and ethnic groups.

This recommendation is supported by concern about the cost and quality of health care. The current interest in documenting improved patient outcomes and outcomes research is great. What are the most prevalent, costly, and preventable conditions? What are we trying to accomplish in the provision of care? Are we succeeding? Which of our strategies is contributing to sustained behavior change and improved outcomes in a cost-effective manner? New models of delivering preventive and treatment services are needed. Reimbursement for alternative methods of delivering care will be dependent upon demonstrated cost benefit. The development, testing, and widespread application of strategies to improve adherence is urgently needed. Such strategies might include creative approaches to helping people incorporate lifestyle changes into daily life in their environment. Several recent multisite national studies to test educational and behavioral strategies to prevent hypertension have focused on nutritionists, physical activity specialists, and behavioral psychologists as the interventionists. Yet, the generalizability of these strategies, particularly in managed care settings, is questionable, and the role, if any, for nurses in delivering these interventions is unclear.

Implement Comprehensive Multidisciplinary Approaches

We cannot ignore coexisting social, psychological, physical, and economic issues or the presence of other cardiovascular risk factors such as diabetes, obesity, poverty, alcoholism, and substance abuse. To address these factors, we must understand and accept the variability of human behavior. The behavioral sciences are therefore an essential basis for further progress in hypertension prevention and control. Integration of biobehavioral approaches will help U.S. health personnel better understand casual and consequential pathophysiological factors and select the most appropriate treatment based on the risk profile of the individual patient.

Investigators concerned with the definition and measurement of interventions are encouraged to remember that patients do not live, and nurses do not practice, in isolation. Because it is impossible and impractical to isolate the nurse from all other providers and to isolate the patient from all other providers, it is extremely difficult to define and measure outcomes that are specifically nursing sensitive. Nurse investigators do need to be able to define and measure their interventions and the effect of their interventions with precision. The use of factorial designs, including an attention-only group, is one approach to consider. Additionally, to maximize their contribution by assessing the economic aspects of their interventions, nurse scientists should include an economist as coinvestigator.

In the recent decade, many of the barriers to interdisciplinary collaboration seem to be less obstructive as other professionals' awareness of nursing's competencies has increased. The larger number of doctorally prepared and funded nurse scientists and credentialed advanced practice nurses has increased successful collaborative activities in many settings. Exciting, cost-effective opportunities exist for nurse investigators to conduct ancillary, data-based, and substudies within clinical trials conducted by other investigators (Hill & Schron, 1992). Enhancing awareness of successful collaborations and attending to sensitive but timely issues such as protection of turf, legal constraints, economic disincentives, and organization of services are important to consider and address in practice as well as in research if nurses are to fulfill their potential in improving the health status of Black Americans.

▨ Collaborate to Advance Biobehavioral Science

New discoveries in understanding physiologic and genetic mechanisms promise to revolutionize our approaches to preventing and treating hypertension. New knowledge will greatly assist U.S. researchers in the identification of subtypes of hypertension and more precisely defined high-risk groups. The presence of coronary artery disease, diabetes mellitus, heart failure, asthma, chronic obstructive pulmonary disease, and depression has important implications for the selection of preventive and therapeutic antihypertensive therapy. The development of new classes of pharmacologic agents—for example, converging enzyme antagonists and angiotensin receptor blockers—are leading to new treatment com-

binations. Nurse researchers have unlimited opportunity and much to contribute by collaborating with investigators in other disciplines to creatively conceptualize how to maximize the scientific yield from laboratory and clinical studies in biomedical as well as biobehavioral research (Sigmon, Amende, & Grady, 1996).

The clinical association of hypertension, obesity, non-insulin-dependent diabetes mellitus, and other cardiovascular risk factors is well recognized. The role of insulin in mediating the association of insulin resistance with hyperinsulinemia, for example, needs to be delineated by in vivo studies of the role of hyperglycemia and may well contribute to our understanding of the increased risk of hypertension, particularly in the presence of diabetes. The roles of insulin and proinsulin in nondiabetic individuals and in the presence of other cardiovascular risk factors is a related area ripe for investigation. Blood pressure reduction is a proven surrogate for reduced cardiovascular risk. It may very well reverse important adverse effects of hypertension on left ventricular hypertrophy, obesity, mild hyperlipidemia, and insulin resistance. Additionally, as Anderson, McNeilly, and Myers (1991) stated, new models are needed to examine the interaction of psychological and physiological factors, such as autonomic reactivity and hypertension, in Blacks.

The advances in genetics may result in gene therapy as well as genetic interventions to prevent the development of hypertension. The polygenic nature of hypertension complicates advancing understanding of the genetic development of hypertension and the associated target organ damage. Nonetheless, the clinical importance of such advances is clear when one considers the disproportionate burden of end-stage renal disease in Black Americans, particularly among those with diabetes. The ethical issues surrounding the burgeoning field of genetics, especially regarding genetic conditions disproportionately found in minority groups, are of concern and merit careful consideration. The interactions among physiological phenomena within the blood vessel, such as turbulence and sheer stress, for example, with the role of growth factors on endothelium and plaque growth, promise exciting developments in the prevention of complications of atherosclerosis.

Primary prevention is a third area of biobehavioral science ideally suited to collaborative multidisciplinary research. The role of dietary interventions such as sodium, calcium, and potassium intake, and the contribution of homocystine and elevated fibrinogen levels even within normal range, need to be better understood as independent cardiovascular risk factors. Trials are needed to evaluate interventions to reduce excessive incidence of cardiovascular events. We are in need of information about racial subgroup differences, not only among Black Americans but among Hispanic subgroups. Nurses have opportunities to examine interactions among biological factors, behaviors, and health status—for example, sodium sensitivity, sodium intake, self-monitoring, and blood pressure.

Influence Policy Setting

To advance the field of nursing science and practice, nurses must influence both the research agenda and funding priorities, as well as practice standards and federal regulations. Nurses need to become involved in leadership positions not only in nursing associations but in multidisciplinary and disease-specific organizations as well. In these positions, they can participate in agenda setting and policy development. In public policy, nurses can participate in efforts to promote weight loss and control, foods that are lower in sodium and calorie content or higher in potassium content, physical activity, and moderation of alcohol consumption. Nurses can also influence legislative efforts through advocacy efforts. Members of the American Heart Association Council on Cardiovascular Nursing lobby annually on Capitol Hill with members of the other scientific councils. This activity is recognized as positively influencing increases in the NIH biomedical research budget. At the local level, nurses can act officially or through voluntary activities to create and increase community capacity at individual, family, and community levels. By influencing policy setting on multiple levels at once, nurses can contribute to these efforts, which are very powerful because of the potential to influence large numbers of people.

In practice and research, as well as in policy setting, nurses can emphasize the importance of sound evaluation and evidence-based recommendations. They can separate fact from opinion by taking the time to read primary references and data-based papers. They can document what they are doing and evaluate their effectiveness. It is hard to imagine having too much sound data to demonstrate the cost-effectiveness of nursing interventions in improving patient outcomes. As the proportion of care that is delivered in managed care settings increases, it is imperative that nurses be prepared to negotiate their roles with sound data that supports nursing practice.

There is a strong theoretical and empirical basis for hypothesizing that patients of nurse practitioners will benefit from improved access to care, continuity of care, and interpersonal treatment. The nurse practitioner maximizes the care process by using a comprehensive approach to identifying patients' needs and problems and referring or seeking consultation when indicated. Nurses with doctoral preparation can design conduct research studies as leaders or members of multidisciplinary teams. Nurses with exceptional expertise develop programs in communities and participate in government and organizational groups by setting policy and developing consensus guidelines for practice. To assure the effectiveness of these important roles, nurses must be actively involved in setting national and local policy.

Conclusion

Fundamental issues continue to challenge hypertension clinical research and practice. Exciting opportunities exist for nurses to design and test interventions to improve biobehavioral outcomes. The earlier recommendations to engage in theory-then-research to build the science base for nursing practice have been followed (Keller, 1990). Now, as cardiovascular nursing research matures, the proportion of theory and clinical studies is changing as behavior change and treatment efficacy trials increase. Nurse investigators realize that a balance continuously needs to be found so that qualitative and quantitative methods contribute to our increased knowledge. Much work needs to be done on a wide range of issues, including validity of self-report, technology transfer to improve patient self-monitoring and communication with providers, and valid biological markers of early target organ damage.

This is an exciting time for nursing to further develop its clinical expertise and take a leadership role in improving the health care of Black Americans. Optimists will appreciate the words on a much-photocopied sign seen on the bulletin board in someone's office: "There are no problems. There are only opportunities." The prevention and treatment of hypertension in Black Americans offers nurses unlimited research and practice opportunities and challenges to contribute to improving the health of the nation.

References

Alderman, M. H., Cushman, W. C., Hill, M. N., Krakoff, L. R., & Pecker, M. S. (1993). Report of international round table discussion of national guidelines for the detection, evaluation, and treatment of hypertension. *American Journal of Hypertension, 6,* 974-981.

American Heart Association. (1997). *1997 statistical update: Heart and stroke* (report). Dallas: Author.

Anderson, N. B., McNeilly, M., & Myers, H. (1991). Autonomic reactivity and hypertension in Blacks: A review and proposed model. *Ethnicity and Disease, 1,* 154-170.

Anwar, R.A.H., Roberts, J. R., & Wagner, D. K. (1977). The continuing emergency care clinic: Improving patient compliance with follow-up care. *Journal of the American College of Emergency Physicians, 6,* 251-253.

Baldwin, D. C. (1994). *The role of interdisciplinary education and teamwork in primary care and health care reform.* Washington, DC: U.S. Department of Health and Human Services.

Blair, T. P., Bryant, J., & Bocuzzi, S. (1988). Treatment of hypercholesterolemia by a clinical nurse using a stepped-care protocol in a non volunteer population. *Archives of Internal Medicine, 148,* 1046-1048.

Blaustein, M. P., & Grim, C. E. (1991). The pathogenesis of hypertension: Black-White differences. In E. Saunders (Ed.), *Cardiovascular disease in Blacks* (pp. 97-114). Philadelphia: Doris.

Bone, L. R., Hill, M. N., & Levine, D. M. (1994). Hypertension: A community perspective. In I. L. Livingston (Ed.), *Handbook of Black American health: The mosaic of conditions, issues, policies, and prospects* (pp. 46-58). Westport, CT: Green Wood.

Bone, L. R., Levine, D. M., Parry, R. E., Morisky, D. E., & Green, L. W. (1984). Update on the factors associated with high blood pressure compliance. *Maryland State Medical Journal, 33,* 201-104.

Bone, L. R., Mamon, J., Levine, D. M., Walrath, J. M., Nanda, J., Gurley, H. T., Noji, E. K., & Ward, E. (1989). Emergency department detection and follow-up of high blood pressure: Use and effectiveness of community health workers. *American Journal of Emergency Medicine, 7,* 16-20.

Branche, G. C. Jr., Batts, J. M., Dowdy, V. M., Field, L. S., & Francis, C. K. (1991). Improving compliance in an inner-city hypertensive patient population. *American Journal of Medicine, 91*(1A), 37S-41S.

Burt, V. L., Cutler, J. A., Higgins, M., Horan, M., Labarthe, D., Whelton, P. K., Brown, C., & Rocella, E. J. (1995). Trends in prevalence, awareness, treatment and control of hypertension in the adult U.S. population: Data from the health examination surveys 1960-1991. *Hypertension, 26,* 60-69.

Burt, V. L., Whelton, P. K., Rocella, E. J., Brown, C., Cutler, J. A., Higgins, M., Horan, M., & Labarthe, D. (1995). Prevalence of hypertension in the U.S. adult population: Results from the third national health and nutrition examination surveys, 1988-1991. *Hypertension, 25,* 305-313.

Clark, L. T. (1991). Improving compliance and increasing control of hypertension: Needs of special hypertensive populations. *American Heart Journal, 121,* 664-669.

Clark, N. M., & McLeroy, K. R. (1995a). Creating capacity through health education: What we know and what we don't. *Health Education Quarterly, 22*(3), 273-289.

Clark, N. M., & McLeroy, K. R. (1995b). Creating capacity: Establishing a health education research agenda [Editorial]. *Health Education Quarterly, 22*(3), 270-272.

Cowley, S. M., Somelofski, C., Hill, M. N., Smith, J., & Buchwald, H. (1988). Nursing and cardiovascular clinical trial research: Collaborating for successful outcomes. *Cardiovascular Nursing, 24,* 25-30.

DeBusk, R. F., Miller, N. H., Superko, R., Dennis, C. A., Thomas, R. J., Lew, H. T., Berger, W. E. III, Heller, R. S., Rompf, J., Gee, D., Kraemer, H. C., Bandura, A., Ghandour, G., Clark, M., Shah, R. V., Fisher, L., & Taylor, C. B. (1994). A case-management system for coronary risk factor modification after acute myocardial infarction. *Annals of Internal Medicine, 120,* 721-729.

Dunbar, J. (1990). Predictors of patient adherence: Patient characteristics. In S. Shumaker, E. B. Schron, & J. K. Okene (Eds.), *The handbook of health behavior change.* New York: Springer.

Dunbar-Jacob, J., Dwyer, K., & Dunning, E. J. (1991). Compliance with antihypertensive regimen: A review of the research in the 1980's. *Annals of Behavioral Medicine, 13,* 31-39.

Finnerty, F. A. Jr., Mattie, E. C., & Finnerty, F. A. III. (1973). Hypertension in the inner city, I: Analysis of clinic dropouts. *Circulation, 47,* 73-75.

Finnerty, F. A. Jr., & Shaw, L. W. (1973a). Hypertension in the inner city, I: Analysis of clinic dropouts. *Circulation, 47,* 73-75.

Finnerty, F. A. Jr. & Shaw, L. W. (1973b). Hypertension in the inner city, II: Detection and follow-up. *Circulation, 47,*76-78.

Flack, J. M. (1992). Lowering blood pressure yields benefits in young and old, Black and White. In National Heart, Lung and Blood Institute (Ed.), *The 4th National Forum on Cardiovascular Health, Pulmonary Disorders, and Blood Resources* (pp. 25-26). Washington, DC: National Heart, Lung and Blood Institute.

Fletcher, S. W., Appel, F. A., & Bourgeons, M. A. (1975). Management of hypertension: Effect of improving patient compliance for follow-up care. *Journal of the American Medical Association, 233,* 243-244.

Francis, C. K. (1991). Hypertension, cardiac disease, and compliance in minority patients. *American Journal of Medicine, 91,* 295-365.

Froelich, E. D. (1995). There's good news and not so good news [Editorial]. *Hypertension, 25,* 303-304.

German, P. S. (1988). Compliance and chronic disease. *Hypertension, 11,* 61-64.

Green, L. W., & Krueter, M. W. (1991). *Health promotion planning: An educational and environmental approach* (2nd ed.). Mountainview, CA: Mayfield.

Grim, C. M., & Grim, C. E. (1981). The nurse's role in hypertension control. *Family and Community Health, 4,* 29-40.

Harrell, J. S., Cornetto, A. D., & Stutts, W. C. (1992). Cardiovascular risk factors in textile workers. *American Association of Occupational Health Nurses Journal, 40,* 581-58.

Heckler, M. M. (1985). *Report of the secretary's task force on Black and minority health. Volume IV: Cardiovascular disease and cerebrovascular disease (Parts 1 and 2).* Washington, DC: U.S. Department of Health and Human Services.

Heurtin-Roberts, S. (1990). Health beliefs and compliance with prescribed medication among Black women—New Orleans, 1985-86. *Morbidity and Mortality Weekly Report, 39,* 701-707.

Hildreth, C., & Saunders, E. (1991). Hypertension in Blacks: Clinical overview. In E. Saunders (Ed.), *Cardiovascular disease in Blacks* (pp. 83-96). Philadelphia: Doris.

Hill, M. N. (1989). Strategies for patient education. *Clinical and Experimental Hypertension, A11,* 1187-1201.

Hill, M. N., & Becker, D. M. (1995). Role of nurses and health workers in cardiovascular health promotion. *American Journal of the Medical Sciences, 310,* S123-S126.

Hill, M. N., Bone, L. R., Barker, A. V., Baylor, I., Harris, C., Gelber, A. C., & Levine, D. M. (1995). Baseline household survey from urban minority community-based HBP trial [Abstract]. *Circulation, 92,* I-519.

Hill, M. N., Bone, L. R., & Butz, A. M. (1996). Enhancing the role of community health workers in research. *Image: The Journal of Nursing Scholarship, 25,* 221-226.

Hill, M. N., Bone, L. R., Stewart, M. C., Hilton, S. C., Kelen, G., & Levine, D. M. (1996a). A clinical trial to improve HBP care in young urban African American men. [Abstract]. *American Journal of Hypertension, 9,* 172A.

Hill, M. N., Bone, L. R., Stewart, M. C., Hilton, S. C., Kelen, G., & Levine, D. M. (1996b). Recruitment experience in a clinical trial to improve HBP care in young urban African American men [Abstract]. *American Journal of Hypertension, 9,* 1A-2A.

Hill, M. N., & Grim, C. M. (1991). How to take a precise blood pressure. *American Journal of Nursing, 91,* 38-42.

Hill, M. N., & Houston-Miller, N. (1996). Compliance enhancement: A call for multidisciplinary team approaches [Editorial]. *Circulation, 93,* 4-6.

Hill, M. N., & Reichgott, M. J. (1979). Achievement of standards for quality care of hypertension by physicians and nurses. *Clinical and Experimental Hypertension, 1,* 665-684.

Hill, M. N., & Schron, E. B. (1992). Opportunities for nurse researchers in clinical trials. *Nursing Research, 41,* 114-116.

Hypertension Detection and Follow-up Program Cooperative Group. (1979). Five-year findings of the Hypertension Detection and Follow-up Program I: Reduction in mortality of persons with high blood pressure, including mild hypertension. *Journal of the American Medical Association, 242,* 2562-2571.

James, S. A., & Kleinbaum, D. G. (1976). Socioecological stress and hypertension related mortality rates in North Carolina. *American Journal of Public Health, 66,* 354-358.

James, S. A., Hartnett, S. A., & Kalsbeck, W. D. (1983). John Henryism and blood pressure differences among Black men. *Journal of Behavioral Medicine, 6,* 259-278.

Jewell, D., & Hope, J. (1988). Evaluation of nurse-run hypertension clinic in general practice. *Practitioner, 232,* 484-487.

Joint National Committee. (1993). The fifth report of the Joint National Committee on the Detection, Evaluation and Treatment of High Blood Pressure (JNC V). *Archives of Internal Medicine, 153,* 154-183.

Joint National Committee. (1997). The sixth report of the Joint National Committee on Prevention, Detection, Evaluation and Treatment of High Blood Pressure. *Archives of Internal Medicine, 157,* 2413-2446.

Jones, P. K., Jones, S. L., & Katz, J. (1987). Improving follow-up among hypertensive patients using a health belief model intervention. *Archives of Internal Medicine, 147,* 1557-1560.

Kaplan, G. A., & Keil, J. E. (1993). Socioeconomic factors in cardiovascular disease. *Circulation, 88,* 1973-1998.

Kaplan, N. M. (1994). *Clinical hypertension.* Baltimore: Williams and Wilkins.

Kauffman, K. S. (1994). The insider/outsider dilemma: Field experience of a White researcher "setting in" a poor Black community. *Nursing Research, 43,* 179-183.

Keil, J. E., & Saunders, E. (1991). Urban and rural differences in cardiovascular disease in Blacks. In E. Saunders (Ed.), *Cardiovascular disease in Blacks* (pp. 17-28). Philadelphia: Doris.

Kellen, J. C., Schron, E. B., McBride, R., Hale, C., & Campion, J. (1994). A survey of clinical trial coordinators: Factors influencing job satisfaction and turnover. *Cardiovascular Nursing, 30,* 25-31.

Keller, C. (1990). Cardiovascular nursing research review: 1969-1988. *Progress in Cardiovascular Nursing, 5,* 26-33.

Klag, M. J., Whelton, P. K., Coresh, J., Grim, C. E., & Kuller, L. H. (1991). The association of skin color with blood pressure in U.S. Blacks with low socioeconomic status. *Journal of the American Medical Association, 265,* 599-602.

Kumanyika, S. (1990). Diet and chronic disease issues for minority populations. *Journal of Nutrition Education, 22,* 89.

Kumanyika, S., & Adams-Campbell, L. L. (1991). Obesity, diet, and psychological factors contributing to cardiovascular disease in Blacks. In E. Saunders (Ed.), *Cardiovascular diseases in Blacks* (pp. 85-94). Philadelphia: F. A. Davis.

Kumaniyka, S. K., & Charleston, J. B. (1992). Lose weight and win: A church-based weight loss program for blood pressure control among Black women. *Patient Education and Counseling, 19,* 19-32.

Leihr, P. (1992). Uncovering a hidden language: The effects of listening and talking on blood pressure and heart rate. *Archives of Psychological Nursing, 6,* 306-311.

Levine, D. M., & Bone, L. R. (1990). The impact of a planned health education approach on the control of hypertension in a high risk population. *Journal of Human Hypertension, 4,* 317-321.

Levine, D. M., Green, L. W., Deeds, S. G., Chwlow, J., Russell, P., & Finlay, J. (1979). Health education for hypertensive patients. *Journal of the American Medical Association, 241,* 1700-1703.

Livingston, I. L., Levine, D. M., & Moore, R. D. (1990). Social integration and Black interracial variation in blood pressure. *Ethnicity and Disease, 1,* 135-149.

MacDonald, M. B., Sawatzky, J. E., Wilson, T. W., & Laing, G. P. (1991). Lifestyle profiles of hypertensives. *Canadian Journal of Cardiovascular Nursing, 2,* 3-8.

McLeroy, K. P., Steckler, A. B., Simons-Morton, B., Goodman, R. M., Gottlieb, N., & Bordine, J. N. (1993). Social science theory in health education: Time for a new model? [Editorial]. *Health Education Research: Theory and Practice, 8,* 305-312.

Miller, N. H., Hill, M. N., Kottke, T., & Okene, I. S. (1997). The multilevel compliance challenge: Recommendations for a call to action. *Circulation, 95,* 1085-1090.

Morisky, D. E., Levine, D. M., Green, L. W., Shapiro, S., Russell, R. P., & Smith, C. R. (1983). Five-year blood pressure control and mortality following health education for hypertensive patients. *American Journal of Public Health, 73,* 153-162.

Multiple Risk Factor Intervention Trial Research Group. (1982). Multiple risk factor intervention trial: Risk factor changes and mortality results. *Journal of the American Medical Association, 248,* 1465-1477.

Murray, R. F. Jr. (1991). Skin color and blood pressure: Genetics or environment? *Journal of the American Medical Association, 265,* 639-640.

O'Neil, E. H. (1993). *Health professions education for the future: Schools in service to the nation.* San Francisco: Pew Health Professions Commission.

Pane, A. G., Farner, M. C., & Kym, S. A. (1991). Health care access problems of medically indigent emergency department walk-in patients. *Annals of Emergency Medicine, 20,* 730-733.

Pender, N. J., Barkauskas, V. H., Hayman, L., Rice, V. H., & Anderson, E. T. (1992). Health promotion and disease prevention: Toward excellence in nursing practice and education. *Nursing Outlook, 40,* 106-112.

Perry, H. M., Sambhi, M. P., Cushman, W. C., Frieds, E. D., Rutan, G., Bingham, S. F., Carmody, S., & Meyer, G. (1992, November). The VA hypertension screening and treatment program. *VA Practitioner,* pp. 54-60.

Peters, A. L., Davidson, M. B., & Ossorio, C. R. (1995). Management of patients with diabetes by nurses with support of subspecialists. *HMO Practice, 9,* 8-12.

Pew Health Professions Commission. (1994a). *Community health workers: Integral yet often overlooked members of the health care work force.* San Francisco: UCSF Center for the Health Professions.

Pew Health Professions Commission. (1994b). *Nurse practitioners: Doubling the graduates by the year 2000.* San Francisco: UCSF Center for the Health Professions.

Pheley, A. M., Terry, P., Pietz, L., Fowles, J., McCoy, C. E., & Smith, H. (1995). Evaluation of a nurse-based hypertension management program: Screening, management, and outcomes. *Journal of Cardiovascular Nursing, 9,* 54-61.

Powers, M. J., & Wooldridge, P. J. (1982). Factors influencing knowledge, attitudes, and compliance of hypertensive patients. *Research in Nursing and Health, 5,* 171-182.

Ramsey, P., Edwards, J., Lenz, C., Odom, J. E., & Brown, B. (1993). Types of health problems and satisfaction with services in a rural nurse-managed clinic. *Journal of Community Health Nursing, 10,* 161-170.

Rand, C. S. (1990). Issue in the measurement of adherence. In S. A. Shumaker, E. B. Schron, & J. K. Okene (Eds.), *The handbook of health behavior change.* New York: Spring.

Reichgott, M. J., Pearson, S., & Hill, M. N. (1983). The nurse practitioner's role in complex patient management: Hypertension. *Journal of the National Medical Association, 75,* 1197-1204.

Rich, M. W., Beckman, V., Wittenberg, C., Leven, C. L., Freedland, K. E., & Carney, R. M. (1995). A multidisciplinary intervention to prevent the readmission of elderly patients with congestive heart failure. *New England Journal of Medicine, 33,* 1190-1195.

Robertson, A., & Minkler, M. (1994). New health promotion movement: A critical examination. *Health Education Quarterly, 21,* 295-312.

Roter, D., & Hall, J. (1991). *Doctors talking with patients/patients talking to doctors: Improving communication in medical visits.* Westport, CT: Auburn.

Runyon, J. W. Jr. (1975). The Memphis chronic disease program: Comparison in outcome and the nurse's extended role. *Journal of the American Medical Association, 231,* 264-267.

Safreit, B. J. (1992). Health care dollars and regulatory sense: The role of advanced practice nursing. *Yale Journal on Regulation, 9,* 417-487.

Saunders, E. (Ed.). (1991). *Cardiovascular diseases in Blacks.* Philadelphia: F. A. Davis.

Schoenbaum, E. E., & Alderman, M. H. (1976). Organization for long-term management of hypertension: The recruitment, training, and responsibilities of the health team. *Bulletin of the New York Academy of Medicine, 52,* 699-708.

Sempos, C. T., Cooper, R., Kovar, M. G., & McMillian, M. (1988). Divergence of the recent trends in coronary mortality in the four major race-sex groups in the United States. *American Journal of Public Health, 78,* 1422-1427.

Shea, S., Misra, D., Ehrlich, M. H., Field, L., & Francis, C. K. (1992a). Correlates of nonadherence to hypertension treatment in an inner-city minority population. *American Journal of Public Health, 82,* 1607-1612.

Shea, S., Misra, D., Ehrlich, M. H., Field, L., & Francis, C. K. (1992b). Predisposing factors for severe, uncontrolled hypertension in an inner-city minority population. *New England Journal of Medicine, 82,* 776-781.

Sigmon, H. D., Amende, L. M., & Grady, P. A. (1996). Development of biological studies to support biobehavioral research at the National Institute of Nursing Research. *Image: The Journal of Nursing Scholarship, 28,* 88.

Smith, E. D. (1989). The role of Black churches in supporting compliance with antihypertension regimens. *Public Health Nursing, 6,* 212-217.

Smith, E. D. (1992). Hypertension management with church-based education: A pilot study. *Journal of Black Nurses Association, 6,* 19-28.

Smith, E. D., Curb, J. D., Hardy, R. J., Hawkins, C. M., & Tyroler, H. A. (1982). Clinic attendance in the hypertension detection and follow-up program. *Hypertension, 4,* 710-715.

Spratlen, L. P. (1982). Nurse-role dimensions of a school-based hypertension screening, education, and follow-up program. *Journal of School Health, 52,* 174-178.

Strogatz, D. S., & James, S. A. (1986). Social support and hypertension among Blacks and Whites in a rural, southern community. *American Journal of Epidemiology, 124,* 949-956.

Stuart, E. M., Caudill, M., Leserman, J., Dorrington, C., Friedman, R., & Benson, H. (1987). Nonpharmacologic treatment of hypertension: A multiple-risk-factor approach. *Cardiovascular Nursing, 1,* 1-14.

Swain, M. A., & Steckel, S. B. (1981). Influencing adherence among hypertensives. *Research in Nursing and Health, 4,* 213-222.

Systolic Hypertension in the Elderly Program Cooperative Research Group. (1991). Prevention of stroke by antihypertensive drug treatment in older persons with isolated systolic hypertension. *Journal of the American Medical Association, 265,* 3255-3264.

Taylor, C. B., Miller, N. H., Killen, J. C. & DeBusk, R. (1990). Smoking cessation after acute myocardial infarction: Effects of a nurse-managed intervention. *Annals of Internal Medicine, 113,* 118-123.

Thomas, S. A., & Friedman, E. (1994). Cardiovascular responses during verbal communication: Effect of rate of verbalization on blood pressure and heart rate. *Journal of Cardiovascular Nursing, 9,* 16-26.

Thomas, S. A., & Leihr, P. (1995). Cardiovascular reactivity during verbal communication: An emerging risk factor. *Journal of Cardiovascular Nursing, 9,* 1-11.

Thomas, S. A., Leihr, P., Dekeyser, F., & Friedman, E. (1993). Nursing blood pressure research 1980-1990: A bio-psycho-social perspective. *Image: The Journal of Nursing Scholarship, 25,* 157-164.

Trials of Hypertension Prevention Collaborative Research Group. (1992). The effects of nonpharmacological interventions on blood pressure of persons with high normal levels: Results of the Trials of Hypertension Prevention, Phase I. *Journal of the American Medical Association, 267,* 1213-1220.

Trials of Hypertension Prevention Cooperative Research Group. (1996). Effects of weight loss and sodium reduction on blood pressure and hypertension incidence in overweight nonhypertensive persons. *Journal of Hypertension, 14,* 15B.2.

U.S. Department of Health and Human Services. (1990). *Healthy people 2000: Full report, with commentary.* Boston: Jones and Bartlett.

U.S. Department of Health and Human Services. (1996). *Physical activity and health: A report of the surgeon general.* Atlanta, GA:

U.S. Department of Health and Human Services, Centers for Disease Control and Prevention, National Center for Chronic Disease Prevention and Health Promotion.

Walt, G. (1988). Community health workers: Are national programs in crisis? *Health Policy and Planning, 3,* 1-21.

Whelton, P. K., Appel, L. J., Espeland, M. A., Applegate, W. B., Ettinger, W. H. Jr., Kostis, J. B., Kumanyika, S., Lacy, C. R., Johnson, K. C., Folmar, S., & Cutler, J. A. (1998, March 18). Sodium reduction and weight loss in the treatment of hypertension in older persons: A randomized controlled Trial of Nonpharmacologic Interventions in the Elderly (TONE). *Journal of the American Medical Association, 279*(11), 839-846.

Working Group on Health Education and High Blood Pressure Control. (1987). *Improving adherence among hypertensive patients: The physician's guide.* Bethesda, MD: U.S. Department of Health and Human Services, Public Health Service, National Institutes of Health.

Working Group on Management of Patients with Hypertension and High Blood Cholesterol. (1991). National Education Programs working group on the management of patients with hypertension and high blood cholesterol. *Annals of Internal Medicine, 114,* 224-237.

Working Group on Primary Prevention of Hypertension. (1993). National High Blood Pressure Education Program Working Group Report on primary prevention of hypertension. *Archives of Internal Medicine, 153,* 186-208.

Working Group to Define Critical Behaviors in High Blood Pressure Control. (1979). Patient behavior for blood pressure control: Guidelines for professionals. *Journal of the American Medical Association, 241,* 2534-2537.

17

LOWERING RISK FOR CARDIOVASCULAR DISEASE IN CHILDREN AND ADOLESCENTS

Joanne S. Harrell
Barbara J. Speck

Introduction

Although many nurses are involved in the care of children and in promoting health across the life span, very little nursing research has focused on how to lower children's risk for future heart disease. Pediatric nurses generally focus on the care of sick children or on preventing common childhood diseases. Also, because cardiovascular disease (CVD) does not usually manifest itself until middle or late adulthood, nurses who study cardiovascular diseases have studied adults with heart disease (secondary prevention) or have focused their primary prevention efforts on adults. Only recently have nurse researchers and clinicians recognized the importance of intervening with children to prevent a disease that may not actually be evident for 30 or more years.

There is growing recognition that the atherosclerotic processes that cause most types of CVD actually begin in childhood (Kwiterovich, 1993; Williams, 1994). McGill (1984), in his landmark summary of the pathogenesis of atherosclerosis, notes that the earliest signs of atherosclerosis are fatty streaks, seen by age 10 years in the aorta and later in the coronary and cerebral arteries. These are followed by fibrous plaques with necrotic, lipid-rich cores that are surrounded by smooth muscle and connective tissue (third decade). Autopsy evidence demonstrates that adult fibrocalcific plaques can originate during the first two decades of life (Newman, Freedman, et al., 1986). Fatty streaks and atherosclerotic lesions have been found postmortem in the aorta and coronary vessels of 6- to 30-year-olds; these were related to antemortem CVD risk factors such as cholesterol and ponderal index in male subjects (Berenson, Wattigney, Tracy, et al., 1992). The Pathobiological Determinants of Atherosclerosis in Youth (PDAY) research group found that all subjects 15 to 34 years old had fatty streak lesions of the aorta on autopsy, with fibrous plaque lesions of the right coronary artery found in 11% to 15% of males and in 8% to 10% of females (PDAY, 1993). Coronary artery lesions were strongly related to serum cholesterol and smoking (PDAY, 1990). Autopsy studies of young soldiers who died in battle also confirm that the atherosclerotic process begins in youth. Coronary and aortic athero-sclerotic lesions were found in 77.3% of soldiers killed in Korea and 45% of those who died in Vietnam (Enos, Beyer, & Holmes, 1955; McNamara, Molot, & Stremple, 1971).

Two large interdisciplinary studies, the Muscatine Study (Mahoney, Lauer, Lee, & Clarke, 1991) and the Bogalusa Heart Study (Webber, Srinivasan, Wattigney, & Berenson, 1991), demonstrated that risk factors for future heart disease were present in school-age children and that these risk factors persist and even track over time. *Tracking* refers to the tendency for a child to remain in the same quintile (the same 20%) of risk within his or her age group over many years. Children who are in the top quintiles of weight (adjusted for height), blood pressure, and cholesterol are much more likely to be in the top two quintiles (top 40%) as adults (Lauer, Clarke, & Beaglehole, 1984; Mahoney et al., 1991; Webber et al., 1991).

A challenge in this field of research is that multiple risk factors for cardiovascular disease are recognized, and each has its own body of knowledge. The major risk factors now recognized by the American Heart Association (AHA) are hypertension, hypercholesterolemia, smoking, and physical inactivity, all of which are modifiable, as well as male sex and increased age (Fletcher et al., 1992). Although the AHA does not list obesity as a major risk factor in adults, it is related to hypertension, hyperlipidemia, and physical inactivity (Hensrud, Weinsier, Darnell, & Hunter, 1995; Katzel et al., 1995). Research indicates that obesity may be a more important risk factor in women than in men (Manson et al., 1990; Willett et al., 1995).

Nurses are in an excellent position to develop and implement theoretically sound, empirically based interventions to promote adoption of healthy lifestyles in children and youth. With a greater emphasis on intervening to lower CVD risk factors in youth, nurses could make significant contributions to improving the health of Americans. Potential collaborators with nurses in the area of cardiovascular risk reduction in children include cardiovascular epidemiologists, lipidologists, molecular biologists, endocrinologists, behaviorists, public health physicians, exercise physiologists, health educators, and psychologists.

A study of causes of death in the United States in 1990 showed that over half of all deaths could be attributed to lifestyles, particularly to tobacco use, diet, and activity patterns (McGinnis & Foege, 1993). Although the major causes of death in children are unintentional injuries, *Healthy Children 2000* (U.S. Department of Health and Human Services, 1992) devotes three of its 22 chapters to CVD risk factors (physical activity and fitness, nutrition, and tobacco) and one to heart disease and stroke. The transitional time between childhood and adulthood is a time when many physical changes are occurring and also when a sense of self and increased emotional independence is emerging (Willard & Schoenborn, 1995). Thus, the period of childhood through middle to late adolescence (elementary through high school years) is crucial in developing health behaviors that carry over into adulthood.

Much of the literature covering children or adolescents and CVD risk factors is in non-nursing journals. Thus, for the sake of completeness, selected major studies in other disciplines are discussed. However, as the intent of this chapter is to focus on nursing research, extensive efforts were made to find all relevant nursing literature. We first conducted a literature search that began with computerized searches in the Cumulative Index of Nursing and Allied Health Literature (CINAHL) and Medline (limited to nursing journals) for the years 1982 through 1996. The key words in all searches included "child or adolescent" and every combination of the risk factors discussed in this chapter. In addition, we hand searched 10 nursing journals for any relevant nursing articles using the above key words or phrases.

This chapter has three main sections. In the first section, we summarize and discuss relevant general research and all nursing research on each risk factor and summarize the nursing studies in a series of tables. We conclude the discussion of each risk factor with a summary of (a) conceptual perspectives used, (b) diverse views or controversies, and (c) clinical issues and questions. The second section presents a synthesis of the state of the science regarding CVD risk factors in children and youth; the third gives recommendations for advancing this field.

What Has Been Studied?

Cholesterol and Lipids

Normal total serum cholesterol values in children aged 2 to 19 are less than 170 mg/dl; values of 170 to 199 mg/dl are *borderline*, and values of 200 mg/dl or higher are termed *elevated* (National Cholesterol Education Program [NCEP], 1991). Mean cholesterol of children aged 5 to 14 years is about 160 mg/dl (Kwiterovich, 1991). Total cholesterol levels drop around puberty and then rise again at the end of pubertal development (Berenson, Srinivasan, Cresanta, Foster, & Webber, 1981). The mean levels of high-density lipoprotein (HDL), the "good" cholesterol, are about 52 to 56 mg/dl in those 5 to 14 years old; the levels of low-density lipoprotein (LDL), the "bad" cholesterol, average about 93 to 100 mg/dl (Kwiterovich, 1991). A small medical and epidemiological study measured total and HDL cholesterol on three successive weeks in 24 children, aged 6 to 9 years. This study verified those ranges but demonstrated a wide interperson variation in results; the average of the three readings was considered the best way to assign children to one of the three categories of total cholesterol risk (normal, borderline, or elevated) (Gillman, Cupples, Moore, & Ellison, 1992). Cholesterol levels track from childhood into adulthood (Lauer & Clark, 1990).

Lipids vary by race and sex in youth (Belcher et al., 1993; Srinivasan, Freedman, Webber, & Berenson, 1987). Webber, Harsha, et al. (1991) examined lipids in a large, ethnically mixed group of children (401 Hispanic, 1,207 African American, and 2,072 Caucasian), aged 5 to 17 years. Both total serum cholesterol and HDL cholesterol were higher in African-American than in Caucasian children. There were no significant differences by race in LDL cholesterol. The drop in total cholesterol during puberty was seen in all subjects but was most pronounced in Caucasian boys. A drop in HDL cholesterol was seen in all groups, beginning at about age 10. Triglyceride levels were 5 to 10 mg/dl lower for African-American children at almost all ages.

Nursing Research on Cholesterol and Lipids

Davidson, Bradley, Landry, Iftner, and Bramblett (1989) measured total cholesterol in 420 eighth-grade children, including girls (48.8%) and boys (51.2%). Subjects with levels over 200 mg/dl were tested 1 month later. The first test was done with the Kodak DT-60, the second with the Reflotron[7] (Boehinger Mannheim). The mean cholesterol of the children was 167 ± 29.4 mg/dl. Of the children with cholesterol values above 200 mg/dl at the initial testing, 83% had values above 185 mg/dl at the second testing. Counseling of parents and siblings was initiated for those who had elevated cholesterol levels at both testings. The procedure was well accepted by children, parents, and staff, was not time consuming, and the cost was small. The authors do not discuss a potential area of controversy: that associated with using two different instruments to measure cholesterol. Further, there was no control group.

Most of the nursing studies examining cholesterol also looked at other risk factors. Those studies are discussed at the end of this section (under "Multiple Risk Factors").

Conceptual/theoretical approaches. The only conceptual frameworks that can be inferred from the studies examining cholesterol are physiological. That is, there is often a search for the "biological plausibility" to explain why specific factors are associated with elevated serum lipids. In addition, the concept of heredity is inherent in much of the work. Although no studies have specifically mentioned it, a developmental approach could inform the study of cholesterol and lipids because the mean values change significantly with age in youth. Interventions to lower cholesterol in children and adolescents must be appropriate for their stage of development.

Controversies in the field. There is a considerable controversy concerning the importance, or even relevance, of routine cholesterol screening of children. The NCEP (1991) recommends that only children at risk be screened for cholesterol. Children considered at risk include those with a family history of premature coronary heart disease (CHD), myocardial infarction or sudden cardiac death in a parent or grandparent, or cholesterol of ≥ 240 mg/dl in at least one parent. In addition to those major criteria, a child should be screened if the family history is unknown or the child has other risk factors for CVD, including cigarette use, obesity, diabetes, hypertension, a diet high in fat and cholesterol, or is on lipid-raising medications such as corticosteroids. Although the American Academy of Pediatrics (1992) recommends that children with a family history of CVD receive cholesterol screening, studies indicate that such testing is often omitted, even in children with positive family histories of premature CVD (Arneson, Luepker, Pirie, & Sinaiko, 1992; Jessup & Harrell, 1996; Kluger, Morrison, & Daniels, 1991).

Those who recommend cholesterol screening for children include Buser, Riesen, and Mordasini (1990), Garcia and Moodie (1989), and Davidson et al. (1989). Buser et al. (1990) also recommend concomitant screening of parents. Garcia and Moodie (1989) studied 6,500 White children (mean age 6.4 years) during well-child visits; 19.3% had a level exceeding 185 mg/dl (90th percentile). As this is almost twice the expected yield, the authors suggest that routine cholesterol testing of all children is appropriate.

On the other hand, Newman, Browner, and Hulley (1990) reviewed the literature and concluded that there is no evidence that lowering cholesterol in childhood will have an effect on future CVD mortality. They also stated that children may be inappropriately placed on medications for many years, which would be expensive and could have serious long-term adverse effects. Further, they stated that the safety of low-fat, low-cholesterol diets on growing children had not been demonstrated. However, the Dietary Intervention Study in Children (DISC) (Dietary Intervention Study in Children Collaborative Research Group, 1995) in an intensive, 3-year study of children, ages 8 to 10 years old, demonstrated the safety of a diet containing only 28% of calories from fat and less than 150 mg of cholesterol per day. The diet sustained growth and iron stores in the children and produced a modest lowering of LDL cholesterol.

Lauer and Clarke (1990) report the results of longitudinal testing of 2,367 children (initially aged 8 to 18 years) who were followed to ages 20 to 30 years. Of that cohort, 249 (17%) were labeled positive for high cholesterol as children. When retested as young adults, 47% of the 17% who were positive as children had normal cholesterol levels (<200 mg/dl for adults), 36% had borderline (200 to 239 mg/dl), and 17% had high cholesterol (≥ 240 mg/dl). Only 2% of those who were negative as children had high cholesterol as adults. The authors concluded that, although universal screening of cholesterol

in all children is not warranted, there is a need to lower cholesterol in all children through proper diet.

Clinical issues and questions. Many questions must be answered about measuring cholesterol and other lipids. First, will a finger stick or a venous sample be used? There are pros and cons for each, as described by Smith (1989). In either method, a system of internal and external quality control must be in place to assure reasonable precision and lack of bias in measurement. Second, will blood be drawn when children are fasting? If not, then only total cholesterol and HDL cholesterol should be reported because triglyceride (and therefore LDL cholesterol) is affected by recent food intake. Third, has provision been made to give appropriate feedback to parents?

The most important clinical issues for nurses are how to motivate all children and adolescents to adopt a lifestyle of eating and activity patterns that will prevent them from developing dyslipidemias and how to treat those who have been diagnosed as dyslipidemic. We must discover new and effective ways to motivate children and adolescents to initiate healthy eating habits (lower fat content, increased fiber) and do this so they learn to enjoy healthy foods, which will encourage them to incorporate such habits into their permanent lifestyles. The entire family should be involved in incorporating these new healthier habits.

The issue of norms for lipids should also be addressed. The normative data presented by the NCEP panel were based on the Muscatine, Iowa data set and are thus more appropriate to Caucasians than to minorities. Clinicians and researchers should keep these differences in mind when analyzing lipid results.

Hypertension

Researchers have demonstrated that essential hypertension may begin in childhood (Berenson, Wattigney, Bao, et al., 1994; Lauer & Clarke, 1989). Studies have shown that adolescents and young adults can have the anatomical cardiovascular-renal changes typically found in those with essential hypertension. Thus, high blood pressure (HBP) in children and adolescents should not be ignored. Several studies have demonstrated that BP can track, but the level of tracking is lower than for other risk factors (Berenson, Wattigney, Bao, et al., 1994; Lauer et al., 1984). The degree of tracking varies among studies,

TABLE 17.1. Nursing Research on Hypertension

Authors and Publication Date	Theory Base	N	Gender (%)	Race (%)	Grades or Age	Design
Marsh et al., 1983	*	332	F = 50.3, M = 49.7	C = 79.2, non-C = 20.7	ninth	descriptive, prevalence
Thomas and Groer, 1986	*	323	F = 53.4, M = 46.6	C = 94, O = 7	ninth	descriptive
Grossman, 1991	*	40	*	*	8-10 years	descriptive
Grossman et al., 1994	*	60	F = 55, M = 45	C = 41.7, AA = 36.7, H = 13.3, O = 8.3	7-9 years	descriptive, replication
Bradley et al., 1997	*	2,207	F = 50.6, M = 49.4	C = 76.3, non-C = 23.7	third and fourth	descriptive

NOTE: * = not identified, M = male, F = female, C = Caucasian, AA = African American, H = Hispanic, O = other.

which may be due to the methods used for measuring BP and the great intraperson variability of BP.

Webber, Harsha, et al. (1991) examined the blood pressure of Hispanic, African-American, and Caucasian boys and girls aged 5 to 17 years. Systolic BP was remarkably similar in all boys across ages, but the systolic BP of African-American girls was about 3 to 4 mm Hg higher than Caucasian girls. Diastolic BP was slightly higher in Hispanic boys than in African-American or Caucasian boys; few consistent differences were seen in girls. The CHIC study of children in North Crolina found that systolic BP and diastolic BP were both about 2 mmHg higher in African-American than in Caucasian youth (Bradley et al., 1997).

The levels of BP that are considered abnormal in children are much lower than the adult criteria for clinical diagnosis of hypertension. All researchers studying BP in children and adolescents should be familiar with the new AHA-approved BP ranges presented by the National High Blood Pressure Education Program Working Group on Hypertension Control in Children and Adolescents (Falkner et al., 1996). There were two major changes from the previous recommendations of Horan et al. (1987). The first is that the use of K4 is no longer recommended for children; K5 can now be used. The second change is that the new blood pressure tables are adjusted for height, recognizing the importance of considering the size of the youth when evaluating BP. The cut-off points for elevated blood pressure and hypertension vary by age, gender, and height. Pressure at the 90th to below the 95th percentile is considered high-normal BP; "hypertension is an average systolic or diastolic greater than or equal to the 95th percentile for age or sex, measured on at least three sepa-

rate occasions" (Falkner et al., 1996, p. 650). Berenson, Wattigney, Bao, et al. (1994) found that BP in children and adolescents is more closely related to height and weight than to age and suggested that standard references for BP levels in growing children should be height, not age. The AHA now recommends age-, gender-, and height-referenced standards. Because BP varies directly with growth, it increases over time; also, large changes in BP occur in youth during activity, while at rest, and during sleep (Berenson, Wattigney, Bao, et al., 1994).

Intervention studies to prevent or reduce hypertension in youth usually involve older children or adolescents. An extensive diet intervention with boarding school students found that a diet that modified the fatty acid content of foods had no effect on BP (Goldberg et al., 1992). Howe, Cobiac, and Smith (1991) found that lowering the sodium content of food had no effect on BP of children aged 11 to 14 years. Others found that a low-sodium diet could reduce BP in girls but not in boys (Sinaiko, Gomez-Marin, & Prineas, 1993). A controlled study of hypertensive and normotensive children found that a physical activity training program reduced systolic and diastolic BP in both groups of children (Hansen, Froberg, Hyldebrandt, & Nielsen, 1991).

Nursing Research on Hypertension (see Table 17.1)

Marsh, Dubes, and Boosinger (1983) conducted a large hypertension screening program for 332 ninth graders. Hypertension (systolic BP ≥ 130 mm Hg and/or diastolic BP ≥ 85 mm Hg) was found in 10.5% of those assessed; overweight and increased triceps skinfold thickness were associated with diastolic but not systolic hypertension. Thomas and Groer (1986) examined the relationship of demographic, lifestyle, and stress variables to BP in 323 ninth graders. Significant predictors of higher systolic BP were age, gender, body mass index (BMI), and urban residence, and predictors of higher diastolic BP were BMI, smoking, and lack of regular exercise. They also found that males and females had different dietary and exercise patterns; males exercised more but had less healthy eating habits.

Two nursing studies compared BP rhythms of children of normotensive and hypertensive parents (Grossman, 1991; Grossman, Jorda, & Farr, 1994). Sixty children were studied; the 37 who showed significant rhythmic patterns in systolic BP weighed significantly more than the 23 other children. No relationship was found between blood pressure rhythms and parental hypertension (Grossman et al., 1994). These findings supported Grossman's earlier study of 40 children (1991).

Conceptual and theoretical perspectives. Few specific conceptual approaches could be found. The only attempt to add a conceptual approach was Grossman's work on circadian rhythms; although the results were not significant, they recognized the variability of BP and incorporated it into the research design.

Diversity of view or schools of thought. There is some difference of opinion as to the degree to which BP tracks from childhood through adolescence. Some studies support tracking; others, usually older studies, do not. Important questions are when and how to intervene to prevent hypertension in children and whether or not to target specific groups. Several of the studies suggest that interventions might need to be different for boys and girls; other studies recommend population-based interventions for primary prevention of hypertension.

Clinical issues and questions. A major clinical issue is the recognition that hypertension can begin in childhood. An additional problem is the increased difficulty of measuring BP in children due to the great variability in their arm circumference. Although a variety of pediatric cuffs are available, most clinical settings and even some research studies will only have one or two "pediatric" cuffs. A common mistake is to use a cuff that is too small. The new report gives standards on cuff size in children and adolescents and recommends a cuff bladder that will cover 80% to 100% of the circumference of the arm (Falkner et al., 1996).

An additional problem complicating diagnosis is the large variability of BP in children throughout the day, which makes it important to use multiple measures of BP over time to diagnose hypertension. Finally, the change in the AHA guidelines, eliminating K4, should make it easier to take BP but could cause some confusion if the implementation of the new standards is inconsistent.

▬ Smoking and the Use of Smokeless Tobacco

In the 1995 National Health Interview Survey of Youth Risk Behavior (NHIS-YRBS), 11.4% of eighth to twelfth graders used smokeless tobacco and 34.8% were current smokers (had smoked at least one day in the preceeding 30 days); however, only 16.1% smoked frequently (on at least 20 of the preceeding 30 days). Only 28.7% had never smoked (Kann et al., 1996). An excellent review article summarizes recent statistics on tobacco use in all ages (Giovino, Henningfield, Tomar, Escobedo, & Slade, 1995). Figure 17.1 shows that most smokers begin smoking in childhood or adolescence. National surveys of adolescents usually describe those who smoked at least once in the past 30 days as current smokers and define daily smokers as adolescents who averaged at least one cigarette daily in the previous 30 days. Smoking initiation increased markedly for adolescent girls around 1967. In the 1980s, prevalence for smoking was higher for girls than for boys, but in 1994, prevalence was 20% for both male and female high school seniors. As shown in Figure 17.2, the prevalence of cigarette smoking among Black adolescents has dropped sharply since the 1970s (Giovino et al., 1995). These figures emphasize the need to incorporate age, race, and gender when collecting data on tobacco use and demonstrate the need for studies to determine why the prevalence of smoking varies so markedly by race. Other demographic variables that should be included in studies are region of the country and urban or rural residence.

A recent federal publication reports that, if current patterns of smoking behavior persist, an estimated 5 million U.S. residents who were 0 to 17 years old in 1995 could die prematurely from smoking-related illnesses ("Projected Smoking-Related," 1996). Those patterns of smoking and smoking-related deaths could result in over $200 billion in health care costs in the future, or $12,000 per smoker, and approximately 64 million years of potential life lost, which is 12 to 21 years per smoking-related death ("Projected Smoking-Related," 1996).

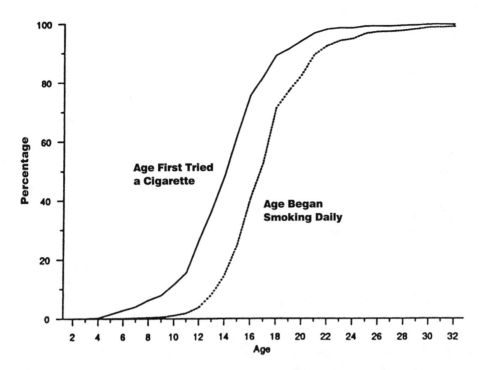

Figure 17.1 Cumulative age of initiation of cigarette smoking among persons aged 30-39 years who have smoked daily—United States, 1919.

SOURCE: National Household Survey on Drug Use (Giovino et al., *Epidemiology Reviews,* 1995, 17(1), 48-65.)

Nursing Research on Tobacco Use (see Table 17.2)

Blackford, Bailey, and Coutu-Wakulczyk (1994), in a cross-sectional telephone survey of tobacco use by 79 Canadian teenagers, found that cigarette smoking was fairly high (34.6%), but relatively few used smokeless tobacco (5.6%). Of the smokers, 25.8% had begun to smoke between the ages of 5 and 10 years, and 64.5% had started between the ages of 11 and 14 years. Common reasons for smoking were curiosity (45.2%) and peer pressure (35.5%). Curiosity and parental use were common reasons for using smokeless tobacco (SLT).

Murphy and Price (1988) examined the influence of self-esteem, parental smoking, and living in a tobacco-producing region on adolescent smoking behaviors. Many (55.3%) of the 1,513 subjects had at least one parent who smoked. Only 48.6% of the adolescents never smoked; 36.2% had tried smoking, and 15.2% were current smokers. About four times as many Caucasians (20.4%) as African Americans (5.8%) were current smokers. There was no significant difference between males and females in current smoking. Self-esteem was significantly related to smoking behavior; the lower the self-esteem the higher

the frequency of ever smoking. Adolescent smoking was positively associated with parental smoking. Harrell, Bangdiwala, Deng, Webb, and Bradley (1998) examined smoking initiation in children in the third through eighth grades. The mean age of initiation was 12.3 years, and smoking was more common in White children of parents with less education and in those with advanced pubertal development.

Several studies have examined SLT use in tobacco-growing states. Hill, Harrell, and McCormick (1992) determined the prevalence of SLT use by 2,020 North Carolina adolescents, as well as peer and parental influences on that use. Nearly 34% of boys and 12% of girls had used SLT at least once, and 8% of boys and 1% of girls were current users. Adolescents were 13.6 times more likely to use SLT if their peers were users, 6.0 times more likely if they were males, 2.8 times more likely if they were Caucasian, 8.0 times more likely if their mothers used SLT, and 2.8 times more likely to use SLT if their fathers used it. Scott (1989) examined the relationship of knowledge and health locus of control on use of SLT in 71 boys in western Kentucky. Those who had ever used smokeless tobacco had less knowledge about tobacco and were influenced by powerful others but not by chance. Scott also used gaming as a strategy to dissemi-

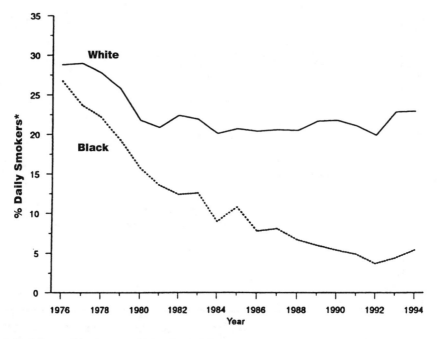

Figure 17.2 Trends in daily smoking* among high school seniors by race—United States, 1976-1994.
SOURCE: Institute for Social Research, University of Michigan (unpublished data). (Giovino et al., *Epidemiology Reviews,* 1995, 17(1), 46-65).
NOTE: *Smoking one or more cigarettes per day during the previous 30 days.

nate knowledge about smokeless tobacco; this significantly increased the knowledge of the subjects, but change in tobacco use was not studied.

Conceptual and theoretical perspectives. Several of the studies used Bandura's (1986) social learning (social cognitive) theory. One dissertation used Bandura's theory and Orem's Self Care Model. Some studies empha-

sized self-esteem but did not identify a corresponding conceptual framework.

Diversity of view and schools of thought. There was very little controversy about tobacco use by children. Researchers agree that smoking and use of SLT by youth must be prevented, as the majority of tobacco users start the habit well before adulthood. However, there is no

TABLE 17.2.   Nursing Research on Tobacco Use

Authors and Publication Date	Theory Base	N	Gender (%)	Race (%)	Grade	Design
Murphy and Price, 1988	*	1,513	F = 49, M = 51	C = 63.5, A = 34.4, O = 2.0	eighth	descriptive
Scott, 1989	Self-care, Social Learning Theory	71	M = 100	*	eighth	descriptive
Hill et al., 1992	Social Learning Theory	2,020	F = 48.8, M = 51.2	C = 74.8, AA = 21.3, H = 0.2, O = 3.7	sixth and seventh	descriptive, correlational
Blackford et al., 1994	*	179	F = 54.2, M = 45.8	*	fourth through college	cross sectional
Harrell, Gansky, McMurray, et al., 1998	*	1,970	*	C = 79.8, AA = 20.2	third through ninth	descriptive

NOTE: * = not identified, M = male, F = female, C = Caucasian, AA = African American, H = Hispanic, O = other.

consensus about the need to use physical measures such as metabolites of nicotine in body fluids or the amount of carbon monoxide in exhaled air to determine the accuracy of self-report of tobacco use. Although the age of the subjects, the type of study, and availability of funding are relevant, researchers should consider employing such validation techniques, at least on a randomly selected subsample.

Clinical issues and questions. An important issue is how to prevent children from initiating tobacco use. Several studies have tried to increase resistance to peer influence, others have attempted to increase the self-esteem of youths in an attempt to increase resistance to pressure to smoke or use SLT, and some have emphasized increasing knowledge about the dangers of smoking. But very little work has been done to provide insight into the best ways to help adolescents stop smoking, and few have actually examined the effect of the intervention on the actual behavior, that is, use of cigarettes or SLT. In addition, the importance of cessation of parental smoking must be addressed, as many studies have shown that parental role modeling is a very important factor in the use of tobacco, especially for children and younger adolescents.

A question that has not been addressed is the developmental trajectory of the initiation of tobacco use. Because most of the large epidemiological studies of smoking in youths are cross-sectional, we do not have good information as to the times during childhood when students are most vulnerable to the multiple pressures to smoke.

▬ *Physical Inactivity*

Studies of American youths partially verify the common belief that our children are relatively inactive. Researchers observed 24 third to sixth graders for 48 days and found no examples of aerobic activity (Baranowski, Hooks, Tsong, Cieslik, & Nader, 1987). In the 1995 Youth Risk Behavior Survey (YRBS) (Kann et al., 1996), of 10,904 youths from 110 high schools across the United States, 36.3% reported that they did *not* engage in vigorous activity at least three times a week. By gender, 25.6% of males and 47.9% of females did not meet this criteria for activity. The current Centers for Disease Control (CDC) recommendations for activity stress moderate activity, to be done on most days of the week (Pate et al., 1995). Very few (21.6%) engaged in moderate activity, such as walking or bicycling, at least five times a week (Kann et al., 1996). This tendency toward inactivity in-

creases as children get older and is more pronounced in girls than boys (Aaron et al., 1993; Rekers, Sanders, Rasbury, Strauss, & Morley, 1989; Sallis, 1993). Further, low fitness levels as children predict low physical activity as adults (Dennison, Straus, Mellits, & Charney, 1988).

Nursing Research on Physical Inactivity (see Table 17.3)

Several papers present results from the Cardiovascular Health in Children Study (CHIC). The conceptual framework for these studies is the Bruhn and Parcel (1982) Model of Heath Promotion in Children. McMurray, Harrell, and Bangdiwala (1994) describe the baseline aerobic power (cardiovascular fitness) and physical activity of 2,201 third and fourth graders; results are presented by age, sex, and race. The children were studied in 18 elementary schools across the state of North Carolina; half of the schools were in rural and half in urban areas. Aerobic power was higher in boys than in girls and higher in urban than in rural children; there were no racial differences in aerobic power. Although boys were more active than girls, the results indicated that both boys and girls have relatively low physical activity and low aerobic power. Harrell, Gansky, Bradley, and McMurray (1996) reported on the prevalence of common activities in third and fourth graders. McMurray, Bradley, et al. (1993) also examined parental influences on childhood fitness and physical activity. The physical activity scores of the children were not significantly correlated with their parents' attitudes or exercise habits, suggesting that other factors influence the activity habits of these children, or that the instruments used to measure activity need refinement. McMurray, Harrell, Bangdiwala, and Gansky (1995) examined the relative influence of biological versus environmental factors on predicted aerobic power of these same CHIC subjects at baseline. The biological factors of skinfolds and physical activity accounted for 44% of the variance in aerobic power for girls and 42% for boys; the environmental measure (rural vs. urban region) was a minor but significant predictor for boys and girls. Race was not a significant factor for boys or girls.

Trost et al. (1996) examined gender differences in physical inactivity in 365 fifth graders. Boys reported more vigorous and moderate-to-vigorous activities than girls, and there was a strong inverse association between physical activity and television watching. This study, which used Bandura's Social Cognitive Theory, found that boys scored higher than girls in perceived self-efficacy for overcoming barriers to physical activity.

TABLE 17.3.   Nursing Research on Physical Inactivity

Authors and Publication Date	Theory Base	N	Gender (%)	Race (%)	Grade	Design
McMurray, Bradley, et al., 1993	*	1,253 children, 1,253 parents	Children: F = 53, M = 47; Parents: F = 70, M = 21[a]	Children*; Parents: C = 82, AA = 13.8, O = 4	third and fourth	randomized, controlled, longitudinal
McMurray, Harrell, and Bangdiwala, 1994	*	2,201	F = 50.7, M = 49.3	C = 76.3, AA = 19.4, O = 4.3	third and fourth	randomized, controlled, longitudinal
Trost et al., 1995	Social Cognitive Theory	365	F = 51, M = 49	C = 25.5, AA = 72.9, O = 1.6	fifth	cross-sectional
Garcia, Broda, et al., 1995	Health Promotion Model	399	F = 51.7, M = 48.3	C = 62.6, AA = 30.4, O = 7.0	fifth, sixth, and eighth	descriptive, correlational
McMurray, Harrell, Bangdiwala, and Gansky, 1995	*	2,207	F = 50.6, M = 49.4	C = 76.3, AA = 19.4, O = 4.2	third and fourth	randomized, controlled, longitudinal
Harrell, Gansky, Bradley, et al., 1997	*	2,200	F = 50.7, M = 49.3	C = 76.3, AA = 19.4, O = 4.3	third and fourth	descriptive

NOTE: * = not identified, M = male, F = female, C = Caucasian, AA = African American, H = Hispanic, O = other.
a. Nine percent did not report gender.

Garcia et al. (1995) used a modification of the Health Promotion Model (Pender, Walker, Frank-Stromberg, & Sechrist, 1990) as the basis for the model of exercise prediction that was tested on 399 children in this study. Of the 14 model variables tested, only three (gender, benefits/barriers, and access to exercise facilities) were directly related to exercise behavior; six were indirectly related. The authors concluded that the model of exercise prediction needs further refinement. Boys were more active than girls, and African-American youth reported greater access to exercise facilities than White youth.

Conceptual and theoretical perspectives. The few studies that identified a conceptual framework had a nurse scientist on the team. Theories used were Bandura's Social Cognitive Theory, Pender's Health Promotion Model, and Bruhn and Parcel's conceptual framework on the development of health behaviors in children.

Diversity of view and schools of thought. There are several schools of thought as to the best way to facilitate the development of more active lifestyles in our children and adolescents. Some support the public health approach and advocate increasing physical activity at the school or community level. Others, who also believe in

the public health approach, suggest that the family be the focus of intervention efforts. However, there are some who believe that maximum efforts to increase physical activity should be focused on those who need it the most, that is, those who are at risk.

Several perspectives in this field should be clarified. Researchers must be clear as to whether they are studying exercise, an exercise regime, or habitual physical activity. Indeed, if the focus is habitual or regular physical activity, will that include only leisure-time activity, or will activity at school and work after school also be included? Researchers must be more careful to define their specific focus of study and find better ways to measure exercise and physical activity.

The focus of researchers is greatly influenced by their scientific discipline. Exercise physiologists are often more interested in the measurement of the five components of fitness that are seen as proximal outcomes of exercise programs. Fitness outcomes include (a) cardiovascular fitness (also called aerobic power, or VO_2), (b) body composition (including weight, BMI, percent body fat, and fat distribution), (c) muscular strength, (d) muscular endurance, and (e) flexibility (Kenney, 1995). Nurses and psychologists are generally more interested in activity behaviors and only one or two fitness outcomes. Physicians and nurses are also interested in the long-range impact of activity behaviors on obesity, lipids, and cardiovascular morbidity and mortality. There is a need for studies that incorporate physiological, psychological, and sociological variables in the study of the complex area of physical activity.

Clinical issues and questions. Now that the importance of physical activity at all ages is recognized, many other issues have arisen. What types of activities are most beneficial for heart health? Until very recently, we taught that, to be useful, the activity must be aerobic, of vigorous or high intensity, should last for at least 30 minutes at a time, and should be done at least three times a week. However, recently, Pate et al. (1995) concluded that less intensive, moderate activities can be beneficial and recommended that all children, adolescents, and adults engage in moderate activities for at least 30 minutes on most days of the week. Further, this activity can be accumulated throughout the day. More specific guidelines for adolescents were presented in a consensus conference (Sallis & Patrick, 1994). Two general population guidelines were stated:

> 1. All adolescents should be physically active daily, or nearly every day, as part of play, games, sports, work, transportation, recreation, physical education or planned exercise, in the context of family, school and community activities. . . . 2. Adolescents should engage in three or more sessions per week of activities that last 20 minutes or more at a time and that require moderate to vigorous levels of exertion. (Sallis & Patrick, 1994, pp. 307-308)

The first guideline is for general health, and the second is to develop fitness.

Another important issue is to identify activities that youth can enjoy and incorporate into their lifestyle as they mature. The key research questions here are not just the short- and long-term effects of specific exercise programs, although those should be studied. Even more important is to learn how nurses can provide and/or promote programs that will encourage youth to become active now and help them maintain a physically active lifestyle throughout their lives.

▧ *Obesity*

Obesity can be seen as a national epidemic in the United States. In the National Health and Nutrition Ex-

amination Surveys (NHANES), 1988 to 1991, the prevalence estimates for overweight in children and adolescents were either 22% (using the 85th percentile of BMI) or 10.9% (using the 95th percentile of BMI) (Troiano, Flegal, Kuczmarski, Campbell, & Johnson, 1995). That paper also showed that among boys 6 to 11 years old, obesity was most common in Hispanics, but in boys aged 12 to 17 years, there was little difference in obesity except that non-Hispanic Black males were least prone to obesity. The opposite was true for girls: obesity was more common in non-Hispanic Black females at ages 6 to 17 years. The National Heart, Lung and Blood Institute (NHLBI) Growth and Health Study (NHLBI Growth and Health Study Research Group, 1992) examined 2,379 girls aged 9 to 10 years at entry. African-American girls were taller and heavier and had a higher body mass index (17.5 vs. 18.4) than the Caucasian girls. Adeyanju, Creswell, Stone, and Macrina (1987) followed 356 matched cases (obese and nonobese) for 3 years and found a sharp increase in weight in African-American girls over time. They also found that the early onset of obesity was an indicator of obesity in the future, as students classified as obese as freshmen were more likely to be obese as seniors. Differences in health status seen by race may be confounded by other variables, such as income and educational status, both of which are commonly used as indicators of socioeconomic status (Balcazar & Cobas, 1993). In a study comparing Hispanic and Caucasian children aged 2 to 17 years, differences in height were small at early ages but greater in adolescence and were related to poverty (Martorell, Mendoza, & Castillo, 1989).

Most obesity intervention studies were designed for children who were already obese and involved small numbers of subjects. Many studies had poor outcomes; those that were successful typically included both diet and exercise (Epstein, Wing, Penner, & Kress, 1985; Hoerr, Nelson, & Essex-Sorlie, 1988). Typically, programs that are conducted for the family and continued over time tend to be more successful than short programs focusing just on the obese child (Nader et al., 1992). One study to reduce obesity in 36 Black adolescent girls (mean age 14.0 years) found that the type of intervention was not as important as mothers' attendance at the sessions. Weight reduction was associated with improvements in body composition, total serum cholesterol, and physiological status (Wadden et al., 1990). Review articles by leading researchers provide important insights into obesity in youth (Epstein, Coleman, & Meyers, 1996; Haddock, Shadish, Klesges, & Stein, 1994).

Nursing Research on Obesity

Sherman, Alexander, Gomez, Kim, and Marole (1992) present the results of an intervention given to 10 obese boys and 16 obese girls. The 9-week program addressed self-esteem, food choices and nutrition, physical activities, and fitness. The study compared pre- and posttest results on self-esteem, nutritional knowledge, exercise, body mass index, and skinfold thickness; there was no control group. The only variable that increased significantly was self-esteem ($p < .001$).

James (1991) used Orem's Self Care Model in her study of factors that influence the health behaviors of 100 obese adolescents. She found that mildly obese adolescents engaged in more self-care practices than those who were severely obese. In addition, those with higher perceived self-efficacy were more effective self-care agents.

Conceptual and theoretical perspectives. Two nurse researchers used Social Learning Theory. One of those also used Orem's Self Care Model.

Diversity of view and schools of thought. A few researchers address primary prevention of obesity through a public health approach using schools, communities, and families as sources of intervention. However, most of the intervention research has consisted of small clinical studies testing treatments for markedly obese children or adolescents. A major problem in this area is inconsistency in defining obesity. Some researchers use only weight, others use weight-for-height (BMI), some use skinfold measures at a variety of sites, and others use a combination of the above. Even among the researchers that select the same variable—that is, BMI—different standards are chosen. Criteria for obesity could be a BMI at or above the 85th, 90th, or 95th percentile according to national standards, which are old (National Center for Health Statistics, 1987). Finally, few researchers discuss the possibility that a subject may be heavy, even overweight, without having excess adipose tissue (i.e., may be overweight but not overfat).

Clinical issues and questions. Important clinical issues are how to get children to select healthy foods (low in fat, high in carbohydrates, fruits, and vegetables) and balance their food intake with expenditure of energy—that is, physical activity. In addition, as children and adolescents are at a stage in life with accelerated growth, it is vital that any recommended diet provide sufficient essential nutrients, especially proteins, vitamins, and minerals.

Family History

Family history of CVD has been shown to be an independent predictor of CVD risk factors (Grech, Ramsdale, Bray, & Faragher, 1992). Lee, Lauer, and Clarke (1986) found that 51% of the offspring of fathers with CHD had abnormal lipid profiles. The mean total cholesterol of pubertal children of patients with coronary heart disease (CHD) was significantly higher (195.1 mg/dl) than that of control subjects (176.6 mg/dl). The presence of a positive family history is particularly important, as current national guidelines for cholesterol screening recommend screening only children (up to 19 years old) who are at highest risk for CVD; that is, those with a parental history of coronary artery disease (CAD) or hypercholesterolemia (NCEP, 1991).

Children with a parental history of heart disease already show adverse risk factors, starting in childhood. Bao, Srinivasan, Wattigney, and Berenson (1995) studied 8,276 children and young adults. As compared with children of those who did not have CVD, the offspring of parents who had a myocardial infarction became significantly more overweight after puberty. In addition, they had significant increases in total and LDL cholesterol after age 18. Regardless of age, the offspring of hypertensive parents were more overweight and had higher blood pressure and higher serum triglycerides levels. Overweight was most pronounced in Black females with hypertensive parents. The impact of family history on the risk factors of children and youth was even more important if the CVD was premature; that is, beginning at less than 55 years (NCEP, 1991).

Nursing Research on Family History

Only one nursing study has focused primarily on family history. Jessup and Harrell (1996) sent questionnaires examining cardiovascular (CV) health promotion practices to all family nurse practitioners and a randomly selected sample of family physicians in North Carolina; 27% responded, yielding a sample of 94. Fewer than a quarter of the respondents reported that they always assessed family history of premature CVD. Although nurses reported more CV health promotion activities than physicians, those activities were similar for children with and without a positive family history of early CVD.

Conceptual and theoretical perspectives. No specific conceptual approaches could be found.

Clinical issues and questions. The literature is inconsistent as to what age should be used to determine "premature heart disease." The NCEP (1991) has stated that if the disease occurs before age 55 years it is considered premature. However, some studies use a different age criteria for men and women because the disease develops later in women. Whatever age is used for premature heart disease, the research reinforces the importance of taking a careful family history when clinically evaluating children or adolescents and when doing research about CVD. The family history should be obtained from a parent, not from the child.

Multiple Risk Factors for Cardiovascular Disease

A growing body of research examines clustering of risk factors for CVD. The national Class of 1989 study examined patterns of smoking, eating, and activity using serial cross-sectional samples of sixth through twelfth graders (Lytle, Kelder, Perry, & Klepp, 1995). Associations exist between smoking, unhealthy eating habits, and low levels of activity, and those associations are stronger in older children. The authors recommended comprehensive school-based health education as a way to develop a healthy lifestyle across multiple behaviors. Adeyanju and Creswell (1987) reported the clustering of smoking, poor diet, alcohol use, and stress in adolescents.

Other studies have examined the relationship of obesity with other risk factors such as cholesterol and blood pressure. Williams et al. (1992) found that high blood pressure and elevated total serum cholesterol in subjects 5 to 18 years of age were somewhat more common in the fattest males (body fat over 25%) and females (body fat over 30%).

Nursing Research on Multiple Risk Factors (see Table 17.4)

Purath, Lasinger, and Ragheb (1995) examined CVD risk factors in 357 elementary school children. Mean cholesterol of the children was 144.2 mg/dl; mean systolic BP was 108.5 and mean diastolic was 61.9 mmHg. More than 74% of the students did not meet the standards for excellence in fitness as measured by a one-mile walk-run. Although the students exercised about four times a week, they averaged 1.17 hours per day of TV viewing. Almost half (45.1%) lived with at least one smoker. There was no significant relationship between obesity and cholesterol in the children. There were sig-

nificant positive relationships between mother and child exercise patterns, and between cholesterol levels and the number of times the student ate in a restaurant per week. The amount of student exercise was inversely related to weekly restaurant visits.

Lipp and Trimble (1993) examined cardiovascular risk factors of 82 boys in a private high school; half of the subjects were on the school football team. Blood pressure, total cholesterol, BMI, percent body fat, eating habits, activity and tobacco use of the two groups were compared. The only significant differences were in BMI and body fat: Football players had a higher percent body fat and higher BMI than nonplayers. Although not statistically significant, smokeless tobacco was used by 9 of the 41 football players (22%) but by none of the nonplayers.

Hayman's research team examined CVD risk factors in twin children, comparing Type A behavior with the more traditional risk factors. This body of research is remarkable for its intensive measurement of lipids. Hayman, Meininger, Stashinko, Gallagher, and Coates (1988) measured blood pressure, obesity, lipids, and lipoproteins in 224 twin children ages 6 to 11 years and asked the children's teachers to rate the behavior of the children as Type A or B. The lipid profiles of Type A and Type B children were similar and were normal for children that age. However, the mean levels of total cholesterol, LDL cholesterol and Apo-B, were higher in Type B children. Meininger, Hayman, Coates, and Gallagher (1988) examined 71 monozygotic and 34 same-sex, dizygotic twin pairs to distinguish CVD risk factors with a large environmental component from those with a strong genetic basis. They found high heritability estimates for Type A behavior. For the physiological measures, heritability was higher for triglycerides and lower for LDL cholesterol and diastolic BP than what has been reported for other studies. The authors recommend that nursing interventions focus on improving weight, lipid profiles, and blood pressure, as those factors appear to have "substantial environmental as well as genetic origins" (Meininger et al., 1988, p. 345).

Hayman, Meininger, Coates, and Gallagher (1995) did a follow-up study of the 1988 work using matched-pair analyses of 105 sets of twins to look at nongenetic influences of obesity on the lipid profile and diastolic BP of children at two phases of development, school-age years and adolescence. In adolescence, obesity was associated with HDL cholesterol and total triglyceride. A change in obesity from school age to adolescence was directly related to a change in total triglyceride.

TABLE 17.4. Nursing Research on Multiple Cardiovascular Disease Risk Factors

Authors and Publication Date	Theory Base	N	Gender (%)	Race (%)	Grades or Age	Design
Hayman, Meininger, Stashinko, et al., 1988	*	224 (twins)	F = 57.7, M = 47.3	C = 100	6 to 11 years	descriptive, correlational
Meininger et al., 1988	*	210 (twins)	F = 53, M = 47	C = 100	6 to 11 years	descriptive, comparative
Cowell et al., 1989	*	2,120	*	*	sixth through eighth	program evaluation
Berg et al., 1992	*	452	F = 48, M = 52	C = 92, O = 7	tenth	descriptive
Cowell et al., 1992	*	195	F = 44.1, M = 55.9	*	ninth through eleventh	descriptive, longitudinal
Lipp and Trimble, 1993	*	82	M = 100	C = 100	14 to 18 years	descriptive
Harrell and Frauman, 1994	*	2,209	F = 50.6, M = 49.4	C = 74.6, AA = 19.4, O = 4.2	third and fourth	randomized, controlled, longitudinal
McMurray, Harrell, Levine, et al., 1995	*	1,092	F = 47.6, M = 52.4	C = 77.0, AA = 19.4, O = 3.6	third and fourth	randomized, controlled, longitudinal
Hayman, Meininger, Coates, et al., 1995	*	105 (twin pairs)	F = 55.4, M = 44.6	C = 100	9 to 17 years	descriptive, longitudinal
Purath et al., 1995	*	357	F = 51.8, M = 48	C = 90.1, AA = 4.3, H = 3.4, O = 2.2	first through fifth	descriptive, correlational
Stewart, Brown, et al., 1995	*	53	F = 51, M = 49	C = 98	fourth	9 to 11 years
Stewart, Lipis, et al., 1995	*	900	F = 50, M = 50	C = 92, AA = 7, O = 1	third	one group pretest, posttest; longitudinal
Harrell, McMurray, et al., 1996	Bruhn and Parcel	1,274	F = 51.6, M = 48.4	C = 74.3, AA = 20.4, O = 5.3	third and fourth	randomized, controlled, field trial
Felton et al., 1998	Jessor's adolescent risk behavior	352	F = 54, M = 46	C = 28, AA = 72	sixth	descriptive
Harrell, Gansky, McMurray, et al., 1998	Bruhn and Parcel	422	F = 52, M = 48	C = 72.5, AA = 22, O = 5.5	third and fourth	randomized, controlled, field trial

NOTE: * = not identified, M = male, F = female, C = Caucasian, AA = African American, H = Hispanic, O = other.

McMurrray, Harrell, Levine, and Gansky (1995) compared BP and total serum cholesterol of obese children with a sample of nonobese third- and fourth-grade children matched to be similar to the obese children in gender, race, age, and height. Obese children had higher systolic and diastolic BP and higher cholesterol levels than the nonobese children.

Stewart, Brown, et al. (1995) examined 900 fourth graders taking part in Food Re-education for Elementary School Health (FRESH), a school-based heart health program. Physical fitness and activity were higher in boys; fatness and serum triglycerides were higher in girls. Systolic BP was positively correlated with measures of fatness in girls ($r = 0.39 - 0.57$). Fitness was the primary correlate of total and LDL cholesterol, but it correlated positively in girls (not favorable) and negatively in boys (favorable).

Felton et al. (1998) examined health risk behaviors, defined as obesity, physical inactivity, smoking, and use of alcohol, in 352 sixth graders. Subjects were boys and girls from rural South Carolina; 72.5% were African American. Subjects were considered obese if they were at or above the 85th percentile (by age and sex) of the first National Health and Nutrition Survey (NHANES) in either body mass index or sum of skin folds. Only 32% of the youth had no health risk behaviors; 44% had one, and 24% had two or more. There was a clear linkage between inactivity and obesity only in girls; boys reported far more smoking than girls. Overall, 49% were obese, 33% were inactive, and 7% smoked.

Cowell, Montgomery, and Talashek (1989) present the results of an 8-year CVD screening program in Chicago. The program was large, involving four middle schools, but neither the subjects nor schools were randomly selected. Between 116 and 389 children were examined at each school every year from 1978 to 1986. The most prevalent risk factor was high total cholesterol: 25% of the total sample had cholesterol ≥ 180 mg/dl. The proportion of those at risk each year varied from 10.8% in 1979 to 35.9% in 1986. Unfortunately, the authors do not give mean values for cholesterol for any year. Over the years, 14.2% had average BP readings at or above the 90th percentile for gender and age. Obesity was present in 12.8% of the sample, but only 2.1% of the sample had low aerobic fitness. It is likely that the method of determining aerobic fitness was not sufficiently stringent. The authors note that, although a school-based health-education program had been in use for 8 years, CVD risk factors in the youth had not improved during that time. This descriptive, observational study included no control or comparison schools. Later, Cowell, Montgomery, and Talashek (1992) examined high school students who had participated in the risk reduction program 3 to 6 years earlier. The subjects' risks for obesity and high cholesterol were moderately stable: 58.3% of those who were obese in grade school were also obese in high school, and 39.6% of those with earlier high cholesterol still had high cholesterol. The tracking for BP was very low; only 16.2% had high BP both times. In general, the risk factor profile of the youth improved. Again, these data are difficult to interpret because no mean values are presented for cholesterol, BP, or BMI.

Berg, Swanson, and Juhl (1992) examined health records of 452 tenth graders from two high schools to determine their total serum cholesterol and other risk factors. Mean cholesterol for the total sample was 150.6 (+34.6) mg/dl, but the girls' mean (160.1 + 36.4) was higher than that of the boys (141.9 + 28.3). An additional analysis showed that the mean cholesterol of the 10 girls using oral contraceptives was 188.2 (+36.7) but that it was only 158.8 (+36.0) for the 206 girls who were not using them.

Harrell and Frauman (1994) used baseline data from the CHIC study as well as national data on CVD risk factors in children to discuss the policy implications of such research for health interventions and for local and state laws focused on protecting CV health. This was the only nursing paper found that discussed policies related to CV health in children.

Conceptual perspectives. Only one study that looked at multiple risk factors reported a conceptual framework. That was the Bruhn and Parcel (1982) conceptual framework used by Harrell and Frauman (1994). The lack of an organizing conceptual framework is a consistent limitation of these studies. Descriptive studies by other disciplines may or may not include a conceptual framework; this seems to be discipline specific. Epidemiological and medical studies seldom include a conceptual framework, but studies by health educators, psychologists, or sociologists may use one.

Diversity of view and schools of thought. The differences in viewpoint discussed with each of the individual risk factors apply to research with multiple risk factors. However, when doing research with multiple risk factors, it is especially important either to include nurses with expertise in each area or to assemble an interdisciplinary team of experts. The differing schools of thought thus represented can be stimulating and enhance the team approach or can result in blocks to conceptualization, design, and implementation. Conceptual definitions and operational definitions have to be developed that capture the health problem, measurement issues have to be addressed, and appropriate instruments must be carefully selected for each variable. A long measurement tool can negatively affect the quality of the data collected, as children have limited attention spans and may not have well-developed reading skills.

Because puberty can have an effect on many of the physical variables of interest, including cholesterol, body fat, weight, and height, it is critical to be able to measure stages of puberty. Many clinical studies use Tanner (1986) staging, but that requires the subjects to undress so the observer can directly assess the groin and breast areas. Such an invasive measure would not be feasible in school-based studies. Several paper-pencil methods are available that can allow subjects to provide information that can be related to Tanner stages, such as the Pubertal Development Scale (Petersen, Crockett, Richards, & Boxer, 1988; Petersen, Tobin-Richards, & Boxer, 1983). Another instrument uses pictures of the groin (and breasts for girls) and asks the child to select which is most like himself or herself (Brooks-Gunn, Warren, Rosso, & Gargiulo, 1987). Both instruments would benefit from further validation. In studies that examine lipids in adolescent girls, it is important to determine if the girls have entered menarche, if they use birth control pills, and to identify the stage of the menstrual cycle during data collection.

Clinical issues and questions. A study that examines many risk factors will usually require more time and resources than a study focusing on only one dependent variable. However, it is more efficient in the long run, as information obtained at one time may have several uses. Longitudinal studies are particularly needed to answer questions about the developmental trajectories of health behaviors and CVD physical outcomes such as lipids, blood pressure, and obesity. In the absence of such longitudinal studies, the smaller studies should compare their results to those of national studies whenever possible. Such comparisons can be facilitated by including questions or variables from the national databases when the smaller study is being designed.

▓ *Instrument Development and Measurement Issues: Nursing Studies*

Gilmer, Speck, Bradley, Harrell, and Belyea (1996) present the psychometric properties of the Youth Health Survey (YHS), an instrument developed for the CHIC study to assess CV health habits in adolescents. The eight subscales of the YHS assess eating, activity, and smoking habits of youth; their attitudes toward exercise (self and others); self-esteem; and the perceived health behaviors of the peers and parents. Test-retest reliability for six of the eight subscales ranged from .67 to .89. Internal consistency was determined with coefficient alpha (.74 to .89 for seven subscales); construct validity was assessed through factor analysis and found to be acceptable to excellent on 4 of 6 subscales. Thus, most of these scales could be used in other studies with adolescents.

Smith (1989) summarized clinical methods used to measure CV risk factors in children. She discusses issues in measuring BP, cholesterol, smoking behavior, physical fitness, and body composition, with emphasis on the need for careful training of testers. This important paper should be reviewed by nurses who intend to measure any of these variables in children.

The development of a board game to be used in interventions to improve health in schools is described by Bartfay and Bartfay (1994). This game could be used for a variety of health education themes, including heart health. In this pilot study, a pretest-posttest control group design was used to evaluate the effectiveness of the game. The experimental group increased significantly more in knowledge (+14.5) than the controls (+4.0).

A dissertation by Arvidson (1990) presented the development of the Children's Cardiovascular Health Promotion Attitude Scale, which was based on social learning theory and psychometric theory. The instrument, initially a 42-item four-point forced-choice Likert-type scale, was shortened to include 16 items covering these subscales: Physical Activity, Nutrition, Smoking, and Stress Control (confirmed with factor analysis). Coefficient alpha for the entire instrument was 0.799, with subscale values between 0.762 and 0.634. This would appear to be a very promising tool; unfortunately, we were not able to find any further publications by the author.

These few studies indicate a void in the literature. Additional instruments to measure cardiovascular health behaviors, attitudes, and knowledge in children need to be developed, and those that have been developed should be more widely tested. In addition, we need more studies testing the reliability and validity of instruments to measure physical variables in youth.

▓ *Intervention Studies*

There are a few large-scale, randomized, controlled studies of school-based programs to improve CVD risk in children. The Heart Smart Program modified school lunches, the physical education program, school health services, and extracurricular activities. Children in intervention schools showed some improvement in knowledge and a trend toward more healthful food choices; there was improvement in HDL cholesterol in one of the two intervention schools (Arbeit at al., 1992). Resnicow, Cross, LaCosse, and Nichols (1993) showed that a school-based screening program for children in eight Michigan elementary schools had positive effects on the attitude, knowledge, and behaviors of children with regard to CVD. Although they measured the BP, total serum cholesterol, and heart rate response to a step test, those results were used only to assess the children's risk factors; no intervention effects on those physical measures were reported.

Four research centers participated in the National Institute of Health (NIH) and NHLBI-funded Child and Adolescent Trial for Cardiovascular Health (CATCH) (Luepker et al., 1996). In CATCH, school-based, public-health-type intervention programs were provided to 5,106 children (initially in the third grade). There were 56 intervention and 40 control schools. In 28 schools, there was a classroom health curricula, enhanced physical activity, and modification of the food served at school. A family component was added to those measures in 28 other schools. After 3 years of intervention, the self-reported fat intake of the intervention children was reduced from 32.7% to 30.3% but was essentially unchanged in control children (32.6% to 32.2%). The intervention children also reported more minutes per day in vigorous exercise (58.6) as compared to the controls (46.5). There were no significant differences between intervention and control children in any of the physical measures (blood pressure, aerobic fitness, lipids, or skinfold thickness). The lack of physiological results suggests that the intervention may not have been sufficiently strong or that the postassessments were not made at times at which it was likely to capture relevant changes.

Nursing Intervention Studies

Stewart, Lipis, et al. (1995) reported results of a 3-year education program for children in the third through fifth grades; 92% of the subjects were Caucasian. The classroom intervention consisted of four 1-hour lessons taught by a health educator or dietitian, presented annually for 3 years. After 3 years, heart knowledge increased 30%, self-reported use of high-fat foods fell by 14%, and use of high-sodium foods fell by 16%. Although cholesterol was lower after 1 year, by the end of 3 years it was higher than baseline. No significant changes were seen in blood pressure, BMI, or body fat. The lack of either a control or comparison group makes it difficult to analyze these results, as some of the risk factors, particularly cholesterol, BP, and body fat, change naturally with growth in youth.

Harrell, McMurray, et al. (1996) presented the short-term results of a longitudinal, school-based intervention to improve CVD risk factors in 1,274 elementary school children. This federally funded study was a randomized, controlled field trial done at 12 elementary schools in North Carolina. One group of schools received a classroom-based intervention in which all children in the third and fourth grades received the 8-week intervention taught by their regular classroom teachers, using the American Heart Association School Site Kits, and by specially trained physical education teachers. A second group of schools served as the control (no intervention). Outcomes were measured within 2 weeks after the intervention or 9 to 10 weeks after the pretest for the control schools. As compared to the control subjects, children in the intervention group significantly increased their aerobic power and heart health knowledge and lowered their serum cholesterol and body fat.

Conceptual perspectives. The CATCH study used Bandura's social cognitive theory to guide its intervention (Bandura, 1986). The CHIC study used the Bruhn and Parcel (1982) Model of Health Promotion in children to select variables for study, but it did not inform the intervention.

Diversity of view and schools of thought. There is considerable debate as to the relative merits of a population-based, public health approach versus a risk-based approach, which would only provide interventions to youth who have been identified as having one or more risk factors. Many researchers recommend a population approach to improving CV health behaviors in children and adolescents (Harrell, McMurray, et al., 1996; Killen et al., 1988; Lawrence, Arbeit, Johnson, & Berenson, 1991; Newman, Freedman, et al., 1986; Perry, Klepp, & Shultz, 1988; Resnicow et al., 1993; Strong et al., 1992). This can be done through teaching and other interventions provided to all children in a variety of settings, such as schools and other community locations. The settings used by researchers often reflect their approach. Those who use the population approach usually study children at schools or community sites (Harrell, McMurray, et al., 1996; Perry et al., 1988; Resnicow et al., 1993); those who espouse the risk-based approach often collect data in clinics (Benuck, Gidding, & Donovan, 1995; Klein, Portilla, Goldstein, & Leininger, 1995).

An important concern is the lack of randomized, controlled intervention studies. Although this is true for nursing research, it is also true in general in this area of research. Randomized, controlled studies are particularly important with this age group, as most of the physical, behavioral, and even psychological variables would be expected to change over time as a consequence of normal growth. Without a control group, it is impossible to differentiate intervention from developmental effects.

Clinical issues and questions. The practical implications of the intervention for the anticipated setting must be considered. If designed for a school setting, is the intervention economical and practical? Does it meet state guidelines for educational curricula? If a community-based program, would it require more personnel and financial support than is practical in most communities? The researchers must consider whether the requirements of the individual program are too restrictive to be effectively maintained as lifetime behavior changes. Interventions that show significant results but cannot be implemented in practice will not be useful in reducing cardiovascular risk factors.

Synthesis of the State of the Science

The approaches to research in the field vary from intensive studies of subfractions of serum lipids (Hayman, Meininger, Stashinko, et al., 1988; Kwiterovich, 1991; Meininger et al., 1988) through targeted studies that focus on children who are obese (Epstein, Coleman, et al., 1996) to school-based interventions (Harrell et al., 1998; Luepker et al., 1996) and communitywide studies to improve CV health in youth (Kelder, Perry, & Klepp, 1993). There are many studies of the prevalence of risk factors in children but relatively few intervention studies. The large intervention studies are almost always multidisciplinary, making it more difficult to determine if a nurse was a member of the research team because "R.N." is seldom included as part of the author's title in nonnursing journals.

Most nursing studies described the prevalence of various risk factors, but they seldom included a large, representative sample. The subjects were usually samples of convenience and were seldom representative of the ethnic mix of the United States or even of the region in which the research was conducted.

Particularly scanty in nursing research are intervention studies. The few interventions tested often focus on "teaching" or "explaining" the importance of diet, with emphasis on understanding the scope of the problem rather than on facilitating the desired behaviors. Although several studies present uncontrolled intervention programs and discuss their effects, they do not incorporate formal program evaluation techniques. Only one nursing study testing an intervention used a control group and incorporated large numbers of subjects (Harrell et al., 1996).

There is a lack of consensus in defining some of the health behaviors in children. Although smoking habits in children are now defined fairly consistently, obesity and physical inactivity are still defined by researchers in multiple ways. Finding measurement tools for children and adolescents is complicated by the need to have tools that are developmentally appropriate and that also allow researchers to capture the behaviors across time.

There was a total absence of any qualitative studies of behaviors in children that would be related to future heart disease. Such studies would be an excellent way to design instruments to measure the health behaviors of children and could provide insights about possible interventions.

A few studies incorporate physiological measures with behaviors. Because nursing as a profession takes a holistic approach to clients, nurses are in an ideal position to include a wide variety of variables in their studies. Some relevant physical measures such as height, weight, and blood pressure are quite familiar to nurses and could fairly easily be incorporated into research studies. Others, such as skinfold thickness, aerobic power, and lipid subfractions, may require collaboration with researchers from other disciplines. Indeed, interdisciplinary research is most likely to be successful in developing clinically relevant knowledge for health promotion in general.

Conceptual frameworks or models are seldom reported. A conceptual framework may have been an integral part of the study design but not have been reported in the published papers. For example, the conceptual framework for Harrell's study team was Bruhn and Parcel's (1982) Model of Health Promotion in Children, but it is not identified in most of Harrell et al.'s published papers. It is possible that this is the case for other studies. This raises a philosophical question: Is reporting the conceptual framework (or lack of one) essential to scholarly publication? Other disciplines often do not report a conceptual framework. Yet a clearly stated conceptual framework is an excellent way to help readers understand the interrelationships of the study variables. For the researchers, such a framework provides a way of ensuring that constructs relevant to the research plan have been included as variables. For intervention studies, the conceptual framework needs to be included to avoid the un-scientific "black box" intervention approach (Lipsey, 1990); that is, concentrating on the input into and output or outcome from an intervention, with very little or no emphasis on a complete understanding of all the components of the intervention.

Little controversy was noted in the nursing research, most likely because so few studies have been done by nurses relating to cardiovascular health in children and adolescents. As the nursing knowledge develops in this field, controversies will inevitably surface. Potential controversies are optimal sites for interventions (home, school, community, or clinic), strengths and weaknesses of a public health approach targeting all subjects, or a risk-based approach targeting youth who already have one or more risk factors for future CVD.

Although interdisciplinary research has shown that CVD risk factors and mortality from CVD differ by race, few nursing studies have included samples that are representative of minorities. On the other hand, some studies include only minorities. Studies of minority groups are needed, but they only provide a partial picture of the problem. Studies should include samples that are representative of the entire target population. Recent work has made it apparent that some of the conclusions about ethnic variation in prevalence of CVD and risk factors is confounded by socioeconomic status (SES) (Link & Phelan, 1996; Rogers, 1992; Smith, Wentworth, Neaton, Stamler, & Stamler, 1996). Thus it is important to include a measure of SES in this research. The use of samples with representative numbers of both genders, major races, and a full range of SES is highly recommended.

Recommendations for Advancement of Nursing Science

This review emphasizes the need for nursing intervention studies to reduce cardiovascular risk in children. Table 17.5 summarizes what we have learned from research and areas that need further study. Recommendations for improving children's heart health are concisely presented in a report of a recent AHA conference (Gidding, Deckelbaum, Strong, & Moller, 1995). Other disciplines have firmly established the logical link between cardiovascular risk factors and cardiovascular disease: There is evidence that cardiovascular risk factors are present in children and adolescents and that many risk fac-

tors track from childhood to adulthood. This body of knowledge provides a critical basis for the advancement of nursing knowledge in the field of cardiovascular risk reduction in children and adolescents. The research of several nurses has made substantial contributions to the general knowledge. Hayman et al.'s work (Hayman, Meininger, Coates, et al., 1995; Hayman, Meininger, Stashinko, et al., 1988) has increased our understanding of the genetic and environmental aspects of risk factor development in youth, and the work of Harrell et al. (Harrell & Frauman, 1994; Harrell et al., 1996) has demonstrated the usefulness of school-based interventions to improve heart health in youth.

Additional epidemiological and prevalence studies by nurses to establish the extent of the knowledge in the nursing literature are unnecessary, but studies examining the prevalence of risk in certain vulnerable groups such as minorities, the poor, and those living in rural areas or inner cities would be useful. To be of real value, these studies should have samples that are truly representative of their populations, and at least some should be longitudinal. Longitudinal studies allow researchers to examine tracking of risk factors and the developmental trajectory of those factors through childhood and adolescence. In addition, researchers must account for normal growth and development, such as the impact of puberty on risk factors, particularly on obesity and cholesterol. Analyses should specifically examine for differences by sex and by race, controlling for SES and for pubertal level.

Intervention studies must be well designed and must be controlled because most of the outcome variables change naturally over time. Interventions should be focused on helping children develop healthy eating and activity habits that will last throughout their life. Interventions for smoking should be broadened to include any type of tobacco use and should focus not only on preventing use of tobacco products but also on helping young smokers quit the habit. Interventions that target parents and peers are particularly encouraged, although other, less comprehensive programs such as clinic-based programs for tobacco users are also needed. Instruments used to collect data from children must have been demonstrated to be reliable, valid, and feasible when used with the age group being studied. The issue of culturally sensitive instruments has not yet been addressed in children and should be included as new instruments are tested. These studies should incorporate state-of-the-art measures of relevant biological variables such as lipids, obesity, blood pressure, and cardiovascular fitness and provide evidence that these instruments have been used

TABLE 17.5.   Research Directing Practice

Risk Factor	What Research Has Shown	Areas Needing Further Research

Cholesterol	Normal values for children and youth:
	    variation by race and sex
	    drop in TC during puberty
	    values increased by birth control pills
	Levels track from childhood to adulthood
	Careful quality control needed in measurement
		Normal values for minorities
		Screening procedure:
		    importance of screening
		    who to screen

Hypertension	May begin in childhood
	Normal ranges (lower than adults)
	Significant relationship with other risk factors
	Measurement issues:
	    correct cuff size and technique
	    multiple measures needed for diagnosis
		Degree of tracking
		When and how to prevent
		Are different interventions needed for:
		    girls and boys?
		    different minority groups?

Tobacco use	Most begins in childhood or adolescence
	Positive relationship with peer use
	Positive relationship with parental use
	SLT : most common in Caucasian boys
	Smoking: less common in African Americans
		Developmental history of smoking and SLT use
		Verification by physiological measures
		Development and testing of interventions to:
		    prevent smoking and SLT use
		    help youth stop using tobacco

Physical inactivity	Inactivity increases with age
	
	Girls less active than boys
	
	Inactivity is related to:
	    obesity
	    higher blood pressure
		Best methods to measure activity in childhood
		
		Best approach to increase physical activity (public health versus at-risk)
		
		How to maintain lifelong regular physical activity
		Relation between physical fitness and activity in children not clear

Obesity	Prevalence of obesity is increasing Interventions with activity are most effective Obesity increases in puberty in girls, especially African-American girls	Clearer definitions of obesity Effective prevention methods How to build habits of eating healthy foods

Multiple risk factors	Smoking, inactivity, and poor eating habits are
	    associated, especially in older children
	Some school-based interventions have shown
	    these short-term effects:
	        improved eating habits
	        lowered cholesterol
	        lowered body fat
	Puberty has a major effect on cholesterol and
	    body fat
		Need controlled, longitudinal interventions to test
		    long-term effects
		Add physiological outcomes to behaviors and
		    attitudes
		Longitudinal studies to describe developmental
		    trajectories of risk factors
		
		Which sites are most effective for interventions with
		    children?
		Public health versus risk-based approach to improving
		    CV health
		Must clarify confounding effects of SES, race, and
		    ethnicity

NOTE: C = cholesterol, CV = cardiovascular, SLT = smokeless tobacco, TC = total cholesterol.

appropriately. The outcome measures for these intervention studies should encompass physical health outcomes and health behaviors, as well as health knowledge and other psychosocial variables from the conceptual framework guiding the study.

Research that is collaborative within the discipline—that is, nurse researchers working with nurse clinicians—is particularly needed. Nurse researchers can design and implement nursing intervention studies; nurse clinicians have a wealth of knowledge about children and have access to large populations of children through their practices. School nurses are in an ideal position to be collaborators with nurse researchers through school-based cardiovascular risk reduction programs. Community health and public health nurses also have in their practice large numbers of well children and are in a position to collaborate on community-based interventions. Nurse practitioners care for well children and families as well as children at high risk for cardiovascular disease due to family history and can be integral parts of individual or family-based intervention studies. All of these practicing nurses could be valuable members of research teams that can, through intervention studies, have the dual objectives of improving the cardiovascular health of children and families while adding to the scientific knowledge of nursing.

Another way to advance nursing knowledge in the field of cardiovascular risk reduction in children is for more nurse researchers to focus on development of programs of research in this field. For knowledge to be advanced, there is a need for nurse researchers to follow a consistent path of testing and retesting interventions, further developing the ones that are most successful in reducing cardiovascular risk factors in children. Many nurses have published one or two research articles related to this topic. Unrelated research requires replication and extension by other researchers and is difficult to connect to the larger body of knowledge already generated. As the area is so broad, there is room for many programs of research in cardiovascular risk reduction. Some researchers may choose to study specific risk factors extensively; others may be more interested in developing interventions for multiple risk factor reduction. Others may focus on the most appropriate sites and methods to deliver interventions to children and families. This approach (using similar outcome variables with a variety of differing samples and testing and retesting the interventions) does not place constraints on investigators but encourages development of a consistent and methodical program of research that also incorporates single studies from other nurse researchers. Such a process should expand the body of knowledge and advance the state of the science in nursing.

Another way to develop programs of research is through mentoring new researchers. As the number of new doctorally prepared nurses increases, there is great opportunity for them to begin a program of research. Nurses who have been successful researchers for a number of years have a responsibility to the profession to help doctoral students and recently prepared doctoral faculty achieve their research goals. In addition, clinicians and new researchers can initiate the mentoring process with senior investigators.

Large interdisciplinary research teams are currently studying cardiovascular risk reduction in children and contributing to the body of knowledge in this area. The specific knowledge of professionals such as exercise physiologists, nutritionists, educators, and cardiovascular and pediatric professionals is critical to the study of this complex problem. Some of these large studies include at least one nurse researcher. Whether these studies advance the state of the science in nursing is dependent upon the contribution of the nurse researcher to the development of the research questions or hypotheses. If interdisciplinary studies are to advance the nursing science related to promoting cardiovascular health in children and youth, they should include nurses in a leadership position, as principal investigator (PI) or co-PI, so the nurse can participate in the development of the research to address specific nursing questions in the context of the overall study.

Nursing has a unique perspective in that nurses use physiological as well as psychosocial knowledge of individuals, families, and communities in their practice. Further, doctorally prepared nurses usually have more extensive education in research methods and statistics than physicians, as well as a stronger clinical base than nonphysician researchers such as psychologists and sociologists. As nurses gain more experience and become senior researchers, nurses have the opportunity to be the leaders of research teams or significant contributors to the perspective of the study.

An exciting new area for nursing research will soon be opening as more advances are made in molecular biology. This genetic work, which is being spearheaded by the Human Genome Project, can lead to new treatments for cardiac disease and to improved identification of those at risk for diseases. The tissue plasminogen activator (t-PA) was the first commercial product of genetic engineering (Haber, 1995). Another area of progress is in gene transfer therapy; animal data indicate that liver-directed gene expression can modulate lipoprotein function to prevent the progression or even cause regression of atherosclerosis (Rader & Wilson, 1995). DNA probes will soon be available to provide tests to determine the risk of developing hypertension or coronary artery disease (Haber, 1995). New discoveries from genetic research may be of benefit to children as knowledge about the genetic causes of CV disease increases and new methods of diagnosis, such as presymptomatic diagnoses and carrier diagnoses, begin to be used. However, Williams and Lessick (1996) point out that these discoveries create ethical, social, and legal dilemmas regarding the health of children. Nurses specializing in genetics and ethics must be ready to conduct studies that examine the implications of genetic information, including the emotional implications of testing and the potential for denial of insurance. Research is needed to describe the problems that may arise with the application of more genetic testing, and then appropriate interventions can be developed and tested.

In conclusion, cardiovascular risk reduction in children and adolescents is a well-recognized and complex problem. Nurse researchers and nurse-directed research teams have a unique opportunity to expand and increase the body of knowledge in cardiovascular risk reduction in children. Focusing research to controlled intervention studies, particularly longitudinal studies, and developing programs of research, as well as nursing research in the newer area of genetic information, will advance this field of nursing science.

References

Aaron, D. J., Kriska, A. M., Dearwater, S. R., Anderson, R. L., Olsen, T. L., Cauley, J. A., & Laporte, R. E. (1993). The epidemiology of leisure physical activity in an adolescent population. *Medicine, Science, Sports and Exercise, 25*(7), 847-853.

Adeyanju, M., & Creswell, W. H. Jr. (1987). The relationship among attitudes, behaviors, and biomedical measures of adolescents "at risk" for cardiovascular disease. *Journal of School Health, 57*(8), 326-331.

Adeyanju, M., Creswell, W. H., Stone, D. B. & Macrina, D. M. (1987). A three-year study of obesity and its relationship to high blood pressure in adolescents. *Journal of School Health, 57*(3), 109-113.

American Academy of Pediatrics. (1992). Statement on cholesterol. *Pediatrics, 90,* 469-473.

Arbeit, M. L., Johnson, C. C., Mott, D. S., Harsha, D. W., Nicklas, T. A., Webber, L. S., & Berenson, G. S. (1992). The Heart Smart cardiovascular school health promotion: Behavior correlates of risk factor change. *Preventive Medicine, 21,* 18-32.

Arneson, T., Luepker, R., Pirie, P., & Sinaiko, A. (1992). Cholesterol screening by primary care pediatricians: A study of attitudes and practices in the Minneapolis-St. Paul area. *Pediatrics, 89,* 502-505.

Arvidson, C. R. (1990). *Children's cardiovascular health promotion attitude scale: An instrument development.* Unpublished doctoral dissertation, Texas Women's University, Denton.

Balcazar, H., & Cobas, J. A. (1993). Overweight among Mexican Americans and its relationship to life style behavioral risk factors. *Journal of Community Health, 18*(1), 55-67.

Bao, W., Srinivasan, S. R., Wattigney, W. A., & Berenson, G. S. (1995). The relation of parental cardiovascular disease risk factors in children and young adults: The Bogalusa Heart Study. *Circulation, 91*(2), 365-370.

Bandura, A. (1986). *Social learning theory.* Englewood Cliffs, NJ: Prentice Hall.

Baranowski, T., Hooks, P., Tsong, Y., Cieslik, C., & Nader, P. R. (1987). Aerobic physical activity among third to sixth-grade children. *Journal of Development and Behavioral Pediatrics, 8,* 203-206.

Bartfay, W. J., & Bartfay, E. (1994). Promoting health in schools through board games. *Western Journal of Nursing Research, 16,* 438-446.

Belcher, J. D., Ellison, R. C., Shepard, W. E., Bigelow, C., Webber, L. S., Wilmore, J. H., Parcer, G. S., Zucker, D. M., & Luepker, R. V. (1993). Lipid and lipoprotein distributions in children by ethnic group, gender, and geographic location: Preliminary findings of the child and adolescent trial for cardiovascular health (CATCH). *Preventive Medicine, 22,* 143-153.

Benuck, I., Gidding, S. S., & Donovan, M. (1995). Year-to-year variability of cholesterol levels in a pediatric practice. *Archives of Pediatrics & Adolescent Medicine, 149,* 292-296.

Berenson, G. S., Srinivasan, S. R., Cresanta, J. L., Foster, T. A., & Webber, L. A. (1981). Dynamic changes of serum lipoproteins in children during adolescence and sexual maturation. *American Journal of Epidemiology, 113,* 157-170.

Berenson, G. S., Wattigney, W. A., Bao, W., Nicklas, T. A., Jiang, X., & Rush, J. A. (1994). Epidemiology of early primary hypertension and implications for prevention: The Bogalusa heart study. *Journal of Human Hypertension, 8,* 303-311.

Berenson, G. S., Wattigney, W. A., Tracy, R. E., Newman, W. P., Srinivasan, S. R., Webber, L. S., Dalferes, E. R., & Strong, J. P. (1992). Atherosclerosis of the aorta and coronary arteries and cardiovascular risk factors in persons aged 6 to 30 years and studied at necropsy (the Bogalusa Heart Study). *American Journal of Cardiology, 70,* 851-858.

Berg, C. L., Swanson, D. J., & Juhl, N. (1992). Total blood cholesterol and contributory risk factors in an adolescent population. *Journal of School Health, 62,* 64-66.

Blackford, K. A., Bailey, P. H., & Coutu-Wakulczyk, G. M. (1994). Tobacco use in northeastern Ontario teenagers: Prevalence of use and associated factors. *Canadian Journal of Public Health, 85,* 89-92.

Bradley, C. B., Harrell, J. S., McMurray, R. G., Bangdiwala, S. I., Frauman, A. C., & Webb, J. P. (1997). Prevalence of high cholesterol, high blood pressure, and smoking among elementary schoolchildren in North Carolina. *North Carolina Medical Journal, 58*(5), 362-367.

Bruhn, J. G., & Parcel, G. S. (1982). Current knowledge about the health behavior of young children: A conference summary. *Health Education Quarterly, 9*(2&3), 142/228-166/262.

Brooks-Gunn, J., Warren, M. P., Rosso, J., & Gargiulo, J. (1987). Validity of self-report measures of girls' pubertal status. *Child Development, 58,* 829-841.

Buser, F., Riesen, W. F., & Mordasini, R. (1990). Lipid screening in pediatrics for early detection of cardiovascular risks. *Journal of Clinical Chemistry and Clinical Biochemistry, 28*(2), 107-111.

Cowell, J. M., Montgomery, A. C., & Talashek, M. L. (1989). Cardiovascular risk assessment in school-age children: A school and community partnership in health promotion. *Public Health Nursing, 6,* 67-73.

Cowell, J. M., Montgomery, A. C., & Talashek, M. L. (1992). Cardiovascular risk stability: From grade school to high school. *Journal of Pediatric Health Care, 6,* 349-354.

Davidson, D. M., Bradley, B. J., Landry, S. M., Iftner, C., & Bramblett, S. (1989). School-based blood cholesterol screening. *Journal of Pediatric Health Care, 3,* 3-8.

Dennison, B. A., Straus, J. H., Mellits, E. D., & Charney, E. (1988). Childhood physical fitness tests: Predictor of adult physical activity levels? *Pediatrics, 82*(3), 324-330.

Dietary Intervention Study in Children Collaborative Research Group. (1995). Efficacy and safety of lowering dietary intake of fat and cholesterol in children with elevated low-density lipoprotein cholesterol. *Journal of the American Medical Association, 273*, 1429-1462.

Enos, W. F., Beyer, J. C., & Holmes, R. H. (1955). Pathogenesis of coronary disease in American soldiers killed in Korea. *Journal of the American Medical Association, 152*, 1090-1093.

Epstein, L. H., Coleman, K. J., & Meyers, M. D. (1996). Exercise in treating obesity in children and adolescents. *Medicine and Science in Sports and Exercise, 28*, 428-435.

Epstein, L. H., Wing, R. R., Penner, B. C., & Kress, M. J. (1985). Effect of diet and controlled exercise on weight loss in obese children. *Journal of Pediatrics, 107*, 358-361.

Falkner, B., Daniels, S. R., Loggie, J.M.H., Horan, M. J., Prineas, R. J., Rosner, B., & Sinaiko, A. R. (1996). Update on the 1987 task force report on high blood pressure in children and adolescents: A working group report from the National High Blood Pressure Education Program. *Pediatrics, 98*, 649-658.

Felton, G. M., Pate, R. R., Parsons, M. A., Ward, D. S., Saunders, R. P., Trost, S., & Dowda, M. (1998). Health risk behaviors of rural sixth graders. *Research in Nursing and Health, 21*, 475-485.

Fletcher, G. F., Blair, S. N., Blumental, J., Caspersen, C., Chaitman, B., Epstein, S., Falls, H., Froelicher, E.S.S., Froelicher, V. F., & Pina, I. L. (1992). AHA statement on exercise. *Circulation, 86*, 340-344.

Garcia, A. W., Broda, M. A., Frenn, M., Coviak, C., Pender, N. J., & Ronis, D. L. (1995). Gender and developmental differences in exercise beliefs among youth and prediction of their exercise behavior. *Journal of School Health, 65*(6), 213-219.

Garcia, R. E., & Moodie, D. S. (1989). Routine cholesterol surveillance in childhood. *Pediatrics, 84*(5), 751-755.

Gidding, S. S., Deckelbaum, R. J., Strong, W., & Moller, J. H. (1995). Improving children's heart health: A report from the American Heart Association's children's heart health conference. *Journal of School Health, 65*, 129-132.

Gillman, M. W., Cupples, A., Moore, L. L. & Ellison, R. C. (1992). Impact of within-person variability on identifying children with hypercholesterolemia: Framingham Children's Study. *Journal of Pediatrics, 121*, 342-347.

Gilmer, M. J., Speck, B. J., Bradley, C. B., Harrell, J. S., & Belyea, M. (1996). The Youth Health Survey: Reliability and validity of an instrument for assessing cardiovascular health habits in adolescents. *Journal of School Health, 66*, 106-111.

Giovino, G. A., Henningfield, J. E., Tomar, S. L., Escobedo, L. G., & Slade, J. (1995). Epidemiology of tobacco use and dependence. *Epidemiologic Reviews, 17*, 48-65.

Goldberg, R. J., Ellison, R. C., Hosmer, D. W., Capper, A. L., Puleo, E., Gamble, W. J., & Witschi, J. (1992). Effects of alterations in fatty acid intake on the blood pressure of adolescents: The Exeter-Andover project. *American Journal of Clinical Nutrition, 56*, 71-76.

Grech, E. C., Ramsdale, D. R., Bray, C. L., & Faragher, E. B. (1992). Family history as an independent risk factor of coronary artery disease. *European Heart Journal, 13*, 1311-1315.

Grossman, D.G.S. (1991). Circadian rhythms in blood pressure in school-age children of normotensive and hypertensive parents. *Nursing Research, 40*, 28-34.

Grossman, D.G.S., Jorda, M. L., & Farr, L. A. (1994). Blood pressure rhythms in early school-age children of normotensive and hypertensive parents: A replication study. *Nursing Research, 43*, 232-237.

Haber, E. (1995). The impact of molecular biology on cardiovascular medicine. In E. Haber (Ed.), *Molecular cardiovascular medicine* (pp. 1-10). New York: Scientific American.

Haddock, C. K., Shadish, W. R., Klesges, R. C., & Stein, R. J. (1994). Treatments for childhood and adolescent obesity. *Annals of Behavioral Medicine, 16*, 235-244.

Hansen, H. S., Froberg, K., Hyldebrandt, N., & Nielsen, J. R. (1991). A controlled study of eight months of physical training and reduction of blood pressure in children: The Odense schoolchild study. *British Medical Journal, 303*, 682-685.

Harrell, J. S., Bangdiwala, S. I., Deng, S., Webb, J. P., & Bradley, C. (1998). Smoking initiation in youth: The roles of gender, race, socioeconomics, and developmental status. *Journal of Adolescent Health, 23*, 271-279.

Harrell, J. S., & Frauman, A. C. (1994). Cardiovascular health promotion in children: Program and policy implications. *Public Health Nursing, 11*, 236-241.

Harrell, J. S., Gansky, S. A., Bradley, C. B., & McMurray, R. G. (1997). Activities of elementary school children: The Cardiovascular Health in Children Study. *Nursing Research, 46*(5), 246-253.

Harrell, J. S., Gansky, S. A., McMurray, R. G., Bangdiwala, S. I., Frauman, A. C., & Bradley, C. B. (1998). School-based interventions improve heart health in children with multiple cardiovascular disease risk factors. *Pediatrics, 102*(2), 371-380.

Harrell, J. S., McMurray, R. G., Bangdiwala, S. I., Frauman, A. C., Gansky, S. A., & Bradley, C. B. (1996). The effects of a school-based intervention to reduce cardiovascular disease risk factors in elementary school children: The Cardiovascular Health in Children (CHIC) Study. *The Journal of Pediatrics, 128*, 797-805.

Hayman, L. L., Meininger, J. C., Coates, P. M., & Gallagher, P. R. (1995). Nongenetic influences of obesity on risk factors for cardiovascular disease during two phases of development. *Nursing Research, 44*, 277-283.

Hayman, L. L., Meininger, J. C., Stashinko, E. E., Gallagher, P. R., & Coates, P. M. (1988). Type A behavior and physiological cardiovascular risk factors in school-age twin children. *Nursing Research, 37*, 290-296.

Hensrud, D. D., Weinsier, R. L., Darnell, B. E., & Hunter, G. R. (1995). Relationship of co-morbidities of obesity to weight loss and four-year weight maintenance/rebound. *Obesity Research, 2*(3 Supplement), 217s-222s.

Hill, M. E., Harrell, J. S., & McCormick, L. K. (1992). Predictors of smokeless tobacco use by adolescents. *Research in Nursing and Health, 15*, 359-368.

Hoerr, S.L.M., Nelson, R. A., & Essex-Sorlie, D. (1988). Treatment and follow-up of obesity in adolescent girls. *Journal of Adolescent Health Care, 9*, 28-37.

Horan, M. J., Falkner, B., Kimm, S.Y.S., Loggie, J.M.H., Prineas, R. J., Rosner, B., Hutchinson, J., Lauer, R., Mueller, S., Riopel, D. A., Sinaiko, A., & Weidman, W. H. (1987). Report of the second task force on blood pressure control in children—1987. *Pediatrics, 79*, 1-25.

Howe, P.R.C., Cobiac, L., & Smith, R. M. (1991). Lack of effect of short-term changes in sodium intake on blood pressure in adolescent schoolchildren. *Journal of Hypertension, 9*, 181-186.

James, K. S. (1991). *Factors related to self-care agency and self-care practices of obese adolescents*. Unpublished dissertation, University of San Diego, San Diego, CA.

Jessup, A. N., & Harrell, J. S. (1996). Promotion of cardiovascular health in children by nurse practitioners and physicians in family practice. *Journal of American Academy of Nurse Practitioners, 8*, 467-475.

Kann, L., Warren, C. W., Harris, W. A., Collins, J. L., Williams, B. I., Ross, J. G., & Kolbe, L. J. (1996). Youth risk behavior surveillance—United States, 1995. *Morbidity and Mortality Weekly Report, 45*(SS-4), 1-83.

Katzel, L. I., Bleecker, E. R., Colman, E. G., Rogus, E. M., Sorkin, J. D., & Goldberg, A. P. (1995). Effects of weight loss versus aerobic exercise training on risk factors for coronary disease in healthy, obese, middle-aged, and older men: A randomized controlled trial. *Journal of the American Medical Association, 274,* 1915-1921.

Kelder, S. H., Perry, C. L., & Klepp, K. (1993). Community-wide youth exercise promotion: Long-term outcomes of the Minnesota Heart Health Program and the Class of 1989 study. *Journal of School Health, 63,* 218-223.

Kenney, W. L. (Ed.). (1995). *ACSM's guidelines for exercise testing and perscription* (5th ed.). Baltimore: Williams and Wilkins.

Killen, J. D., Telch, M. J., Robinson, T. N., Maccoby, N., Taylor, C. B., & Farquhar, J. W. (1988). Cardiovascular disease risk reduction for tenth graders: A multiple-factor school-based approach. *Journal of the American Medical Association, 260,* 1728-1733.

Klein, J. D., Portilla, M., Goldstein, A., & Leininger, L. (1995). Training pediatric residents to prevent tobacco use. *Pediatrics, 96,* 326-330.

Kluger, C. Z., Morrison, J. A., & Daniels, S. R. (1991). Preventive practices for adult cardiovascular disease in children. *Journal of Family Practice, 33,* 65-72.

Kwiterovich, P. O. (1991). Plasma lipid and lipoprotein levels in childhood. *Annals of New York Academy of Science, 623,* 90-107.

Kwiterovich, P. O. (1993). Prevention of coronary disease starting in childhood: What factors should be identified? *Coronary Artery Disease, 4,* 611-630.

Lauer, R. M., & Clarke, W. R. (1989). Childhood risk factors for high adult blood pressure: The Muscatine study. *Pediatrics, 84,* 633-641.

Lauer, R. M., & Clarke, W. R. (1990). Use of cholesterol measurement in childhood for the prediction of adult hypercholesterolemia: The Muscatine study. *Journal of the American Medical Association, 264*(23), 3034-3038.

Lauer, R. M., Clarke, W. R., & Beaglehole, R. (1984). Level, trend, and variability of blood pressure during childhood: The Muscatine study. *Circulation, 69,* 242-249.

Lawrence, M., Arbeit, M., Johnson, C. C., & Berenson, G. S. (1991). Prevention of adult heart disease beginning in childhood: Intervention programs. *Cardiovascular Clinics, 21,* 249-262.

Lee, J., Lauer, R. M., & Clarke, W. R. (1986). Lipoproteins in the progeny of young men with coronary artery disease: Children with increased risk. *Pediatrics, 78,* 330-337.

Link, B. G., & Phelan, J. C. (1996). Editorial: Understanding sociodemographic differences in health—The role of fundamental social causes. *American Journal of Public Health, 86,* 471-473.

Lipp, E. J., & Trimble, N. (1993). Health behaviors of adolescent male football athletes. *Pediatric Nursing, 19,* 395-399.

Lipsey, M. W. (1990). *Design sensitivity: Statistical power for experimental research.* Newbury Park, CA: Sage.

Luepker, R. V., Perry, C. L., McKinlay, S. M., Nader, P. R., Parcel, G. S., Stone, E. J., Webber, L. S., Elder, J. P., Feldman, H. A., Johnson, C. C., Delder, S. H., & Wu, M. (1996). Outcomes of a field trial to improve children's dietary patterns and physical activity: The Child and Adolescent Trial for Cardiovascular Health (CATCH). *Journal of the American Medical Association, 27*(10), 768-776.

Lytle, L. A., Kelder, S. H., Perry, C. L., & Klepp, K. (1995). Covariance of adolescent health behaviors: The Class of 1989 study. *Health Education Research, 10*(2), 133-146.

Mahoney, L. T., Lauer, R. M., Lee, J., & Clarke, W. R. (1991). Factors affecting tracking of coronary heart disease risk factors in children: The Muscatine Study. *Annals of the New York Academy of Science, 623,* 120-132.

Manson, J. E., Colditz, G. G., Stampfer, M. J., Willett, W. C., Rosner, B., Monson, R. R., Speizer, F. E., & Hennekens, C. H. (1990). A prospective study of obesity and risk of coronary heart disease in women. *New England Journal of Medicine, 322,* 882-889.

Marsh, B., Dubes, M., & Boosinger, J. K. (1983). Adolescent hypertension and significant variables: Weight, height, and skinfold thickness. *Pediatric Nursing, 9,* 287-289.

Martorell, R., Mendoza, F. S., & Castillo, R. O. (1989). Genetic and environmental determinants of growth in Mexican-Americans. *Pediatrics, 84,* 864-871.

McGill, H. C. (1984). Persistent problems in the pathogenesis of atherosclerosis. *Arteriosclerosis, 4*(5), 443-451.

McGinnis, J. M., & Foege, W. H. (1993). Actual causes of death in the United States. *Journal of the American Medical Association, 270,* 2207-2212.

McMurray, R. G., Bradley, C. B., Harrell, J. S., Bernthal, P. R., Frauman, A. C., & Bangdiwala, S. I. (1993). Parental influences on childhood fitness and activity patterns. *Research Quarterly for Exercise and Sport, 64,* 249-255.

McMurray, R. G., Harrell, J. S., & Bangdiwala, S. I. (1994). Aerobic power and physical activity of North Carolina elementary school children. *North Carolina Journal, 30*(2), 5-11.

McMurray, R. G., Harrell, J. S., Bangdiwala, S. I., & Gansky, S. A. (1995). Biologic and environmental factors influencing aerobic power in children. *Medicine, Exercise, Nutrition, and Health, 4,* 243-250.

McMurray, R. G., Harrell, J. S., Levine, A. A., & Gansky, S. A. (1995). Childhood obesity elevates blood pressure and total cholesterol independent of physical activity. *International Journal of Obesity, 19,* 881-886.

McNamara, J. J., Molot, M. A., & Stremple, J. F. (1971). Coronary artery disease in combat casualties in Vietnam. *Journal of the American Medical Association, 216,* 1185-1187.

Meininger, J. C., Hayman, L. L., Coates, P. M., & Gallagher, P. (1988). Genetics or environment? Type A behavior and cardiovascular risk factors in twin children. *Nursing Research, 37,* 341-346.

Murphy, N. T., & Price, C. J. (1988). The influence of self-esteem, parental smoking, and living in a tobacco production region on adolescent smoking behaviors. *Journal of School Health, 58,* 401-405.

Nader, P. R., Sallis, J. F., Abramson, I. S., Broyles, S. L., Patterson, T. L., Senn, K., Rupp, J. W., & Nelson, J. A. (1992). Family-based cardiovascular risk reduction education among Mexican- and Anglo-Americans. *Family and Community Health, 15,* 57-74.

National Center for Health Statistics. (1987). *Anthropometric reference data and prevalence of overweight: United States, 1976-80* (Report No. (PHS) 87-1688). Hyattsville, MD: Public Health Service. *Vital Health Statistics, 11,* 238.

National Cholesterol Education Program. (1991, September). *Report of the Expert Panel on Blood Cholesterol Levels in Children and Adolescents* (National Institutes of Health Pub. No. 91-2732). Bethesda, MD: National Heart, Lung, and Blood Institute.

National Heart, Lung and Blood Institute Growth and Health Study Research Group. (1992). Obesity and cardiovascular disease risk factors in Black and White girls: The NHLBI Growth and Health Study. *American Journal of Public Health, 82*(12), 1613-1620.

Newman, T. B., Browner, W. S., & Hulley, S. B. (1990). The case against childhood cholesterol screening. *Journal of the American Medical Association, 264*(23), 3039-3043.

Newman, W. P., Freedman, D. S., Voors, A. W., Gard, P. D., Srinivasan, S. R., Cresanta, J. L., Williamson, G. D., Webber, L. S., & Berenson, G. S. (1986). Relation of serum lipoprotein levels and systolic blood pressure to early atherosclerosis: The Bogalusa study. *New England Journal of Medicine, 314,* 138-144.

Pate, R. R., Pratt, M., Blair, S. N., Haskell, W. L., Macera, C. A., Bouchard, C., Buchner, D., Ettinger, W., Heath, G. W., King, A. C., Kriska, A., Leon, A. S., Marcus, B. H., Morris, J., Paffenbarger, R. S., Patrick, K., Pollock, M. L., Rippe, J. M., Sallis, J.,

& Wilmore, J. H. (1995). Physical activity and public health: A recommendation from the Centers for Disease Control and Prevention and the American College of Sports Medicine. *Journal of the American Medical Association, 273*(5), 402-407.

Pathobiological Determinants of Atherosclerosis in Youth. (1990). Relationship of atherosclerosis in young men to serum lipoprotein cholesterol concentration and smoking. *Journal of the American Medical Association, 264,* 3018-3024.

Pathobiological Determinants of Atherosclerosis in Youth. (1993). Natural history of aortic and coronary atherosclerotic lesions in youth. *Arteriosclerosis and Thrombosis, 13,* 1291-1298.

Pender, N. J., Walker, S. N., Frank-Stromberg, M., & Sechrist, K. R. (1990). *The health promotion model: Refinement and validation—Final report.* Bethesda, MD: National Center for Nursing Research.

Perry, C. L., Klepp, K., & Shultz, J. M. (1988). Primary prevention of cardiovascular disease: Community-wide strategies for youth. *Journal of Consulting and Clinical Psychology, 56,* 358-364.

Petersen, A. C., Crockett, L., Richards, M., & Boxer, A. (1988). A self-report measure of pubertal status: Reliability, validity, and initial norms. *Journal of Youth and Adolescence, 17,* 117-133.

Petersen, A. C., Tobin-Richards, M., & Boxer, A. (1983). Puberty: Its measurement and its meaning. *Journal of Early Adolescence, 3,* 47-62.

Projected smoking-related deaths among youth—United States. (1996). *Morbidity and Mortality Weekly Report, 45,* 971-974.

Purath, J., Lansinger, T., & Ragheb, C. (1995). Cardiac risk evaluation for elementary school children. *Public Health Nursing, 12,* 189-195.

Rader, K. J., & Wilson, J. M. (1995). Gene therapy for lipid disorders. In E. Haber (Ed.), *Molecular cardiovascular medicine* (pp. 97-114). New York: Scientific American.

Rekers, G. A., Sanders, J. A., Rasbury, W. C., Strauss, C. C., & Morley, S. M. (1989). Differentiation of adolescent activity participation. *Journal of Genetic Psychology, 150,* 323-335.

Resnicow, K., Cross, D., LaCosse, J., & Nichols, P. (1993). Evaluation of a school-site cardiovascular risk factor screening intervention. *Preventive Medicine, 22,* 838-856.

Rogers, R. G. (1992). Living and dying in the USA: Sociodemographic determinants of death among Blacks and Whites. *Demography, 29,* 287-303.

Sallis, J. F. (1993). Epidemiology of physical activity, fitness and health in children and adolescents. *Critical Reviews of Feed Science and Nutrition, 33*(4-5), 403-408.

Sallis, J. F., & Patrick, K. (1994). Physical activity guidelines for adolescents: Consensus statement. *Pediatric Exercise Science, 6,* 302-314.

Scott, D. L. (1989). *The relationship of knowledge and health locus-of-control of early adolescent males to the use of smokeless tobacco.* Unpublished doctoral dissertation, University of Alabama at Birmingham, Birmingham.

Sherman, J. B., Alexander, M. A., Gomez, D., Kim, M., & Marole, P. (1992). Intervention program for obese school children. *Journal of Community Health Nursing, 9,* 183-190.

Sinaiko, A. R., Gomez-Marin, O., & Prineas, R. J. (1993). Effect of low sodium diet or potassium supplementation on adolescent blood pressure. *Hypertension, 21,* 989-994.

Smith, B. A. (1989). Measurement of selected cardiovascular risk factors in children. *Applied Nursing Research, 2,* 143-146.

Smith, G. D., Wentworth, D., Neaton, J. D., Stamler, R., & Stamler, J. (1996). Socioeconomic differentials in mortality risk among men screened for the multiple risk factor intervention trial: II. Black men. *American Journal of Public Health, 86,* 497-504.

Srinivasan, S. R., Freedman, D. S., Webber, L. S., & Berenson, G. S. (1987). Black-white differences in cholesterol levels of serum high-density lipoproteins subclasses among children: The Bogalusa heart study. *Circulation, 76,* 272-279.

Stewart, K. J., Brown, C. S., Hickey, C. M., McFarland, L. D., Weinhofer, J. J., & Gottlieb, S. H. (1995). Physical fitness, physical activity, and fatness in relation to blood pressure and lipids in preadolescent children: Results from the FRESH study. *Journal of Cardiopulmonary Rehabilitation, 15,* 122-129.

Stewart, K. J., Lipis, P. H., Seemans, C. M., McFarland, L. D., Weinhofer, J. J., & Brown, C. S. (1995). Heart healthy knowledge, food patterns, fatness, and cardiac risk factors in children receiving nutrition education. *Journal of Health Education, 26,* 381-387.

Strong, W. B., Deckelbaum, R. J., Gidding, S. S., Kavey, R. E., Washington, R., Wilmore, J. H., & Perry, C. L. (1992). Integrated cardiovascular health promotion in childhood: A statement for health professionals from the Subcommittee on Atherosclerosis and Hypertension in Childhood of the Council on Cardiovascular Disease in the Young, American Heart Association [Special report]. *Circulation, 85,* 1638-1650.

Tanner, J. M. (1986). Normal growth and techniques of growth assessment. *Clinics in Endocrinology and Metabolism, 15,* 411-451.

Thomas, S. P., & Groer, M. W. (1986). Relationship of demographic, life-style, and stress variables to blood pressure in adolescents. *Nursing Research, 35,* 169-172.

Troiano, R. P., Flegal, K. M., Kuczmarski, R. J., Campbell, S. M., & Johnson, C. L. (1995). Overweight prevalence and trends for children and adolescents: The National Health and Nurtrition Examination Surveys, 1963 to 1991. *Archives of Pediatric and Adolescent Medicine, 149,* 1085-1091.

Trost, S. G., Pate, R. R., Dowda, M., Saunders, R., Ward, D. S., & Felton, G. (1996). Gender differences in physical activity and determinants of physical activity in rural fifth grade children. *Journal of School Health, 66*(4), 145-150.

U.S. Department of Health and Human Services. (1992). *Healthy children 2000.* Boston: Jones and Bartlett.

Wadden, T. A., Stunkard, A. J., Rich, L., Rubin, C. J., Sweidel, G., & McKinney, S. (1990). Obesity in Black adolescent girls: A controlled clinical trial of treatment by diet, behavior modification, and parental support. *Pediatrics, 85,* 345-352.

Webber, L. S., Harsha, D. W., Phillips, G. T., Srinivasan, S. R., Simpson, J. W., & Berenson, G. S. (1991). Cardiovascular risk factors in Hispanic, White, and Black children: The Brooks County and Bogalusa heart studies. *American Journal of Epidemiology, 133,* 704-714.

Webber, L. S., Srinivasan, S. R., Wattigney, W. A., & Berenson, G. S. (1991). Tracking of serum lipids and lipoproteins from childhood to adulthood. *American Journal of Epidemiology, 133,* 884-899.

Willard, J. C., & Schoenborn, C. A. (1995). Relationship between cigarette smoking and other unhealthy behaviors among our nation's youth: United States, 1992. *Advance Data, 263,* 1-11.

Willett, W. C., Manson, J. E, Stampfer, M. J., Conditz, G. A., Rosner, B., Sapeiver, F. E., & Hennikens, C. H. (1995). Weight, weight change, and coronary heart disease in women: Risk within the "normal" weight range. *Journal of the American Medical Association, 273*(6), 461-465.

Williams, C. L. (1994). Coronary heart disease prevention in childhood. Part I: Background and rationale. *Medicine, Exercise, Nutrition and Health, 3,* 194-205.

Williams, D. P., Going, S. B., Lohman, T. G., Harsh, D. W., Srinivasan, S. R., Webber, L. S., & Berenson, G. S. (1992). Body fatness and risk for elevated blood pressure, total cholesterol, and serum lipoprotein ratios in children and adolescents. *American Journal of Public Health, 82,* 358-363.

Williams, J. K., & Lessick, M. (1996). Genome research: Implications for children. *Pediatric Nursing, 22*(1), 40-46.

18

HEALTH PROMOTION AND DISEASE PREVENTION INTERVENTION IN WORKSITES

Sally Lechlitner Lusk

Overview

Occupational health nursing, with its goal to prevent worker illness and injury and to maintain worker health, is the smallest specialty in nursing. Not surprisingly, it also has the fewest nurse scientists. This does not mean, however, that the field has few needs for research. Over 122 million of the U.S. population are in the labor force (Bulletin of Labour Statistics, 1995). In addition to addressing the hazards to health and safety that exist in the workplace, worksites offer the best access to adults to promote health. The challenge is to provide a research base for practice in this specialty.

Obviously, the research base for many clinical problems encountered in the worksite can be transferred from other specialties; for example, the care of the convalescent post-myocardial-infarction worker as he or she returns to the job, or the follow-up of diagnosed hyperten-

AUTHOR'S NOTE: The author wishes to acknowledge the assistance of Sandi Waite, research secretary, in the preparation of this chapter.

sives. However, there are additional needs related to the particular characteristics of workplaces and specific jobs that require specialized knowledge of occupational health and safety. It is beyond the purview of this chapter to identify the research transferable from other specialties or the worksite considerations specific to occupational health and safety. Instead, this chapter (a) provides a brief overview of research on health promotion and disease prevention interventions in the worksite, (b) describes the diversity of scholarly views, (c) focuses particularly on worksite health promotion and disease prevention intervention studies reported by nurses from 1990 through 1995, and (d) synthesizes the state of nursing science and makes recommendations for the advancement of nursing science relevant to worksite health promotion and disease prevention.

Conceptual and Theoretical Perspectives and Diversity of Views

Definition of Health Promotion

Identifying health promotion studies is not a clear-cut task, as no universally agreed-upon definition of health promotion programs exists. Pender (1987) made a distinction between health promotion, which is "directed toward *increasing* the level of well-being and self-actualization of a given individual or group . . . [and] focuses on movement toward a positively balanced state of enhanced health and well-being" (p. 57), and health protection, which is "directed toward decreasing the probability of experiencing illness by active protection of the body against pathological stressors or detection of illness in the asymptomatic stage" (p. 57). In contrast, *Healthy People 2000: National Health Promotion and Disease Prevention Objectives* (U.S. Department of Health and Human Services [USDHHS], 1991) categorizes programs as health promotion, health protection, or preventive services. The health promotion category is consistent with Pender's (1987) definition of health promotion programs by including fitness and nutrition, but *Healthy People 2000* (USDHHS, 1991) also includes as health promotion those programs focused on problem areas of tobacco, alcohol, drugs, family planning, mental disorders, and violence that would fit with Pender's definition of health protection. Health protection programs in *Healthy People 2000* include unintentional injuries, occupational health

and safety, environmental health, food and drug safety, and oral health. However, in the literature and in the survey of worksite health promotion programs (USDHHS, 1993), those programs to encourage seat belt use or to prevent back injuries (unintentional injuries) are identified as health promotion programs, not health protection programs. The preventive services category described by *Healthy People 2000* encompasses programs targeted to a specific population—that is, maternal and infant health—and to specific disease conditions—for example, cancer. Despite the lack of congruence of proposed definitions and categorizations of health promotion, operationally for this chapter, *health promotion programs* are defined as those designed to promote health or to reduce illness-producing behavior. Thus, workplace health promotion and disease prevention encompass a large and diverse body of programs offered to retirees, employees, and employees' families.

History of Health Promotion

Prior to the 1970s, there was little emphasis on health promotion. The preparation and publication of the USDHHS's (1979) *Surgeon General's Report on Health Promotion and Disease* and the first national objectives, *Promoting Health/Preventing Disease: Objectives for the Nation,* in 1980 (USDHHS, 1980), provided the impetus for attention to health promotion. Prior to that time, efforts had been directed toward improving environmental sanitation and development of vaccines to prevent infectious diseases to reduce the death rate. However, with the recognition that approximately one half of premature deaths could be prevented by lifestyle change, national attention shifted to changing individual behavior rather than focusing on communitywide clean-ups or immunization programs. Thus, with redirection to changing adult lifestyles, the workplace became the logical location for accessing adults to alter their behaviors.

Pros and Cons of Health Promotion in the Worksite

Almost everyone has the perception of health promotion in the worksite is a universal good, but there are detractors as well. Gordon (1987) has indicated that health promotion in the workplace is the right activity at the wrong place. Her concern is that emphasis on health promotion in the worksite will detract from the needed attention to solving occupational health and safety problems. Also, it often places the onus on the individual worker to change her or his behavior rather than on corporate responsibility for changing the environment to eliminate potential hazards. There is concern that such programs absolve the employer from any responsibility. Thus, Gordon suggests that only after all worksites have adequate programs to prevent illness and injury due to worksite exposures or hazards should health promotion activities be initiated.

This perspective is countered by many who support health promotion in the worksite and others who have noted the opportunity for synergistic effects between health promotion and occupational health and safety programs. Cohen (1987) has described ways in which these two types of programs can result in a stronger approach to preventing illness and injury. Examples he provided include:

a. improvement in lifestyle can lower risk of certain job hazards; for example, smoking and occupational respiratory disorders, drinking and workplace accidents, poor fitness and musculoskeletal stress in lifting;

b. emphasis on self-care in health promotion programs can translate to increased self-protection against workplace hazards; and

c. several of the 10 leading work-related disorders, specifically cancer, lung disease, traumatic injury, cardiovascular disease, and psychological disorders, would probably be affected by reducing behavioral risk factors through health promotion programs.

Regardless of the desirability of offering health promotion and risk reduction programs, worksites clearly offer the easiest access to adults. Because at least half of all waking hours are usually spent at the worksite and because it represents an area where groups congregate, it is the most accessible point for offering programs to adults. Where else are so many adults gathered for so much time to offer the opportunity to deliver interventions? In addition, families derive indirect benefit through programs offered to their working members.

Further, reviews of studies on the effects of worksite health promotion and risk reduction programs demonstrate positive effects. Pelletier (1991, 1993, 1996) has reviewed these studies for the *American Journal of Health Promotion,* noting positive effects in nearly all of the studies reported. These effects included changes in behavior, reduction in risk factors, improvement in morale and productivity, and reductions in both the utiliza-

tion and costs of health care. Business organizations regularly report dollars saved by specific health promotion programs (Tully, 1995; Bureau of Business Practice Center for Health Programs, 1993). Thus, reported scientific studies and press reports indicate benefits accruing to both employers and employees.

⬛ *Need for Programs*

As previously stated, the USDHHS Surgeon General's report (USDHHS, 1979) indicated that lifestyle habits are responsible for at least one half of premature deaths. More recently, a careful assessment of the effects of certain behaviors documented that about one half of all mortality can be attributed to nine factors, all affected by behavior (McGinnis & Foege, 1993). In descending order, these nine contributors to mortality are: tobacco use, diet and activity patterns, alcohol use, microbial agents, toxic agents, firearm use, sexual behavior, motor vehicle accidents, and illicit drug use.

Data in *Healthy People 2000* (USDHHS, 1991) clearly support the need for health promotion and risk reduction programs to alter such behaviors. Numerous objectives within that document identify the need and the opportunity for worksite programs. In the first 16 chapters of *Healthy People 2000* there are 45 objectives, specifically stated in terms of worksite programs. In addition, there are 105 objectives where the worksite represents an access point for adults or that deal with an activity that would take place as a part of work, for example, use of seat belts or institutional food service. Two specific goals of *Healthy People 2000* to increase health promotion activities in the worksite are:

• Goal 8.6: Provide employee health promotion activities in at least 85% of workplaces with 50 or more employees (a 31% increase) (p. 62).

• Goal 15.16: Increase to at least 50% the proportion of worksites with 50 or more employees that offer high blood pressure and/or cholesterol education and control activities to their employees (Baseline: 16.5% offered high blood pressure activities and 16.8% offered nutrition education activities in 1985) (p. 406).

In addition, worksite goals are identified for most of the diseases or conditions listed under the preventive services—for example, Heart Disease and Stroke. Surprisingly, *Healthy People 2000* does not include workplace goals for prevention or early diagnosis of cancer or for maternal and infant health activities. These areas should have worksite goals, and programs are already in place that offer health promotion programs in these areas—for example, mammography screening (Mayer et al., 1993) and prenatal education (Burton, Erickson, & Briones, 1991). Regardless of these omissions, the objectives for the nation clearly indicate a need for worksite programs, and data have been collected regarding the existence of such programs.

In 1985 and 1992, the USDHHS Office of Disease Prevention and Health Promotion (1993) surveyed worksites employing more than 50 persons regarding health promotion activities and progress toward the objectives in *Healthy People 2000*. Four types of approaches were assessed: policies, screening, information or activities, and facilities or services. From 1985 to 1992, programs (information or activities) on nutrition, weight control, physical fitness, high blood pressure, and stress management increased, while programs on back care and smoking cessation remained about the same. In the most recent survey, 81% of worksites surveyed offered at least one health promotion activity, up from 66% in 1985. Worksites with a greater number of employees were more likely to offer a program (99% with 750 or more employees offered a program; 75% of those with 50 to 99 employees did so). These proportions may appear impressive, but the limitations should be considered: (a) offering one single class session qualified the worksite as offering a program, (b) offering a single health promotion session is of limited benefit, (c) no data were collected regarding public sector employees or from small worksites, and (d) there was no attempt to measure the proportion of worksites offering comprehensive health promotion programs.

Questions regarding activities directed toward prevention of job hazards and injuries were first included in the 1992 survey. Surprisingly, only 64% of the worksites reported information or activities in that category. Given the Occupational Safety and Health Administration (OSHA) mandate to provide a safe and healthful workplace, nearly 100% would be a more appropriate number. There are numerous hazards associated with the occupational setting. Occupational medicine and occupational health textbooks delineate a myriad of potential hazards, and a separate discipline within engineering, safety engineering, further specifies safety hazards. It is beyond the scope of this chapter to deal with occupational health and safety hazards, but a brief summary of the categories of hazards is presented here to enhance understanding of the

risks and to help identify potential for integration of programs in health promotion, risk reduction, and occupational health and safety programs.

Workplace hazards can be classified as *physical,* for example, machinery, slippery floors, heat, noise, radiation, and lasers; *chemical,* including more than 30,000 routinely used substances with potentially adverse effects on humans; *biological,* for example, infectious agents; or *psychosocial,* for example, job stress (Levy & Wegman, 1988). With the increase in AIDS, biological hazards are receiving greater attention, but concern for costs has also focused on psychosocial factors. The greatest single source of stress is the workplace (Dear, 1995) and stress disorders are the most rapidly increasing occupational injury awarded workers compensation benefits (Larsen, 1995).

According to the Occupational Safety and Health Act (1970), every worker is to be provided a safe and healthful workplace. Clearly, that promise has not been kept. In 1992, the number of work-related injuries and illnesses surged to 6.8 million, the highest level on record and the highest rate since 1979. Three million of these injuries and illnesses resulted in a total of 60.4 million workdays lost ("Job Related Injuries," 1992). These figures underestimate the true count for two reasons: (a) underreporting of nonacute injuries and (b) exclusion of cumulative trauma disorders, which in and of themselves are estimated to cost $100 billion annually (National Safety Council, 1990). Although 2,900 work-related fatalities were reported for 1990, the Bureau of Labor Statistics (BLS) believed this to be a significant understatement. In 1992, for the first time, all 50 states participated in the BLS survey, and results showed that 6,083 workers had died as a result of occupational injuries (Castelli, 1994). The American Federation of Labor–Congress of Industrial Organizations (AFL-CIO) estimates that 10,000 workers die on the job each year (*Workplace Injuries,* 1991).

In addition, according to *Healthy People 2000,* "premature death, diseases, injuries, and other unhealthful conditions resulting from occupational exposures pose important national health problems" (USDHHS, 1991). Work-related illnesses and injuries appear to be increasing; during 1987, occupational illness and injury in manufacturing industries increased by 13.5% (USDHHS, 1991). Changes in the American workplace have increased the need for occupational health and safety services: (a) new technologies, including new chemicals, robots, and lasers, pose increased risks for workers; (b) hazardous substances are increasingly being used in the workplace, with the potential of negative effects on workers and the surrounding community; (c) certain types of work settings, such as agriculture and construction, typically have not received services but are now recognized as hazardous worksites; (d) growth in small businesses, office, and service industries has contributed to increasing cumulative trauma and stress disorders; and (e) until recently (National Institute for Occupational Safety and Health [NIOSH], 1988), little attention was directed to occupational risks for health care workers, yet nurses and personal care workers have the second highest rate of work-related injuries (construction workers are number one) (USDHHS, 1991).

Lifestyle factors are of great importance. In some cases, occupational exposures and unhealthy behaviors have a deleterious synergistic effect—for example, asbestos exposure and smoking. Changing lifestyles of the 122 million people in the workplace will have a significant impact on illness and its costs. Smoking-related illnesses cost more than $65 billion each year; avoiding one intervention, coronary bypass surgery, would save approximately $9 billion each year (USDHHS, 1991). Occupational health nurses (OHNs) are essential members of the team of occupational health specialists who implement control strategies, promote safe work practices and use of personal protective equipment, and provide monitoring for and surveillance of hazards. The OHN is the best-prepared professional at the worksite to provide health promotion activities and to integrate, through serial contacts with workers, occupational health and safety and health promotion interventions.

Individual Versus Environmental Focus

Regardless of the setting in which it occurs, the focus on how to change behavior and how to maintain positive changes is an important area of consideration. This is relevant for nursing research regardless of the setting in which the interventions are delivered. However, there are some special considerations for the worksite. The worksite offers both the need and the opportunity to simultaneously alter the environment while at the same time focusing on the behavior change of the individual. O'Donnell (1996) suggested that health promotion programs fail or fall short of their potential because they do not take a social ecological approach. This approach recognizes that changes in health behavior are part of a larger

social system; "Behavior changes do not take place in a vacuum" (O'Donnell, 1996, p. 244). Administrative and environmental factors can support an individual's efforts to change. A recent benchmark study elicited program strategies (awareness, behavior change, and supportive environment) used by those worksite health promotion programs identified as the best programs. Three fourths of these best programs used supportive environment strategies along with at least one of their awareness or behavior change programs. Most included these strategies in four out of five of their program topics (O'Donnell, 1996). As another example, in the largest study to date of effects of smoking bans, hospital workers had significantly higher quit rates than comparison groups (Longo et al., 1996). This result is attributed not only to the fact that the hospital industry was the first in the nation to prohibit smoking but also to the availability of smoking cessation assistance offered by 85% of the hospitals (Longo et al., 1996).

These supportive environmental factors have an important role in promoting the maintenance of behavior change as well. However, information provided in reports of the research often does not make explicit what, if any, social ecological strategies may have been operating.

Although from a programmatic basis multifaceted strategies are highly desirable and more likely to effect change in the desired behavior, these strategies can be troublesome from a research perspective. The researcher's goal is to be able to determine the effect of specific strategies. When multiple strategies are used, the research design, of necessity, must be more complex and typically requires a significantly larger sample. In regard to school-based health promotion programs, which in many ways are similar to worksite-based programs, Weissberg and Elias (1993) identified a gap between the comprehensive programs promoted by policy makers and the limited scope, duration, and intensity of programs studied by scientists. They also noted the absence of longitudinal field studies to assess the effects of comprehensive kindergarten to Grade 12 health promotion programs. Thus, there is a point of tension between clinical desirability and scientific rigor in regard to multifaceted program strategies. In fact, many of the criticisms of the studies by nurse and non-nurse scientists arise out of their failure to assess or control for factors outside their specific interventions that may have affected results.

An additional issue particularly relevant to the worksite is the time required to accomplish behavior changes and to insure their maintenance. High levels of participation in programs occur when workers are allowed to use work time for health promotion activities. However, use of work time represents a real cost to the employer. As is often the case, if changing the behavior requires long-term effort, time may become an important factor specific to the workplace.

Employer/Employee Responsibility and Incentives

The allocation for employer and employee responsibility has as many operationalizations as there are worksites. For example, Johnson and Johnson's Live for Life® (LFL) comprehensive health promotion program has six main components: (a) health screening on company time; (b) a 3-hour Lifestyle Seminar given on company time; (c) action programs on smoking cessation, weight control, stress management, nutrition, exercise, and high blood pressure control through groups, individual consultations, self-help kits, and telephone consultations or counseling; (d) shorter educational programs on breast self-exam, biofeedback, nutrition, and blood pressure; (e) promotion of participation by company leaders; and (f) a healthful environment, including shower and exercise facilities, linkage of food service and nutrition information, no-smoking policies, self-monitoring equipment for weight and blood pressure, flextime, and health fairs (Wilbur, 1983). The scope of a program is important because offering multifaceted programs expands the benefits of the individual programs. Shipley, Orleans, Wilbur, Piserchia, and McFadden (1988), in their analysis of LFL's smoking cessation program, found that participation in other programs on other topics contributed to smoking cessation, and those smokers who participated in the smoking clinic also participated in more health promotion programs.

In contrast, the majority of worksite health promotion programs are not so comprehensive and do not provide extensive services on work time or offer worksite facilities. Although one might expect the effects of smaller scale programs to be more difficult to demonstrate, these programs nevertheless do show positive effects (Lusk, 1995a). For example, relatively simple and inexpensive programs providing health promotion materials by mail to workers and retirees showed improvement in targeted health risk behaviors at a cost of $30 per participant and resulted in a decrease in medical claims costs (Fries, Fries, Parcel, & Harrington, 1992; Fries, Green, & Levine, 1989). Typically, the incentive for the employer to mount health promotion and risk reduction programs has been the desire to reduce costs for health care. For example, the Washington Business Group on Health's (WBGH) recent report (Jacobson, Kolarek, & Newton, 1996) indicates that childbirth-related costs are the single largest health care cost expenditure for many employers. Estimated costs for a normal health birth are $6,400; a problematic one can range from $20,000 to more than $1 million (Jacobson et al., 1996). This report highlights programs offered by seven corporations and one business group documenting their cost savings. These results have not yet been published in the peer-reviewed professional literature, suggesting the need for carefully controlled studies to validate the benefits of these interventions.

There is also a growing recognition that healthy employees are more productive (Fielding, 1990; Rosen, 1991), but effects on productivity have not received as much empirical study as the cost indicators. As previously indicated, for those studies that included cost outcomes, nearly all found positive effects of health promotion or risk reduction programs in the workplace. However, consideration of these effects should be tempered by realization of the fact that in all likelihood there are costs that have not been included in the calculations, such as increased longevity and, therefore, increased payouts for retirement and health care benefits (Lusk, 1992; Warner, Wickizer, Wolfe, Schildroth, & Samuelson, 1988). However, Keeler et al. (1989) have indicated that the increased duration of life (at most 10 to 12 months) results in negligible costs. Others (Fries, Green, et al., 1989) suggest that health promotion programs may not significantly increase longevity but will decrease morbidity, which would result in reduced costs. The point has been well made that the case for health promotion programs should not rest upon costs savings but on improved quality of life (Michigan Department of Public Health, 1987).

Integration of Worksite and Community Activities

Unfortunately, worksites, communities, and schools typically work in isolation from each other in developing and delivering health promotion programs. There is little doubt that collaboration and cooperation could enhance the efforts of each of these separate groups, resulting in synergistic effects. The large comprehensive worksite health promotion programs (Bertera, 1990; Breslow,

Fielding, Herrmann, & Wilbur, 1990) have not reported attempts to offer coordinated programs within local communities and schools. Although Weissberg and Elias (1993) discuss the importance of community-school linkages and of environmental support and reinforcement of school-based programs by members of the community, they do not address the potential for integration of school-based and worksite-based programs to achieve synergy in a given community. Although it is a community-based program, the Minnesota Healthy Heart Project (Gleason-Comstock, Lando, McGover, Pirie, & Rooney, 1994; Perry et al., 1990) has also offered programs in the schools and, to some extent, in worksites, but no research reports were found that reported tests of a collaborative model that included both schools and worksites in comprehensive health promotion programs.

Existing Research in the Field

A review of the studies of the health promotion and risk reduction interventions delivered in the worksite shows an increasing number of reported studies. Although the vast majority do not include nurse authors, a summary of these studies is presented as background for the existing nursing studies. Findings in the published reports have been overwhelmingly positive. Pelletier (1991, 1993) reported in his two reviews that 47 of the 48 reports obtained positive results in terms of health benefits or reducing costs. This must be tempered by the fact that positive results are more likely to result in manuscripts and are also more likely to be published.

Pelletier (1991, 1993) identified 24 reports from 1980 to 1991, and an additional 24 in the much shorter time period of 1991 to 1993, of health and cost outcomes of worksite comprehensive health promotion and disease prevention programs. Lusk (1997), through use of browsing and ancestry approaches, and through computerized database searches that included nursing journals, identified additional reports, resulting in the review of 73 reports published from 1990 through 1994. Because Pelletier (1991, 1993) did not describe procedures used in his literature searches, or the specific inclusion criteria for his review, his reviews should not be considered a comprehensive source.

From reviewing these reports, it is obvious that there are multiple and diverse foci for worksite intervention programs; in the schemata used by Lusk (1996), there

were at least 26 different categories of foci for programs. Outcomes measured included costs, health care utilization, and changes in the risk factors or behaviors of interest. Based on the reports, some worksites offered single-theme programs and others offered comprehensive health promotion programs with multiple foci of interventions, but the measurement of outcomes did not always directly track with the foci of the programs. For example, Shi (1993) measured changes in health risk appraisal scores and employee satisfaction after a back injury prevention program, as well as the expected prevalence of back injuries and pain and the costs in workers' compensation, medical care, and time lost. Additionally, stress management was often a component of comprehensive health promotion programs, but effects of that component were rarely measured directly. Further, although multiple foci programs may have been offered in a given worksite, the scope of outcomes reported in the publications was limited. This is not surprising given the limitations of presenting results in manuscript form.

In more than any other setting, worksite program outcomes have focused on cost-effectiveness or cost benefits, measuring program costs, injury and illness rates, medical care, medical care costs, disability, absenteeism, and turnover. In Pelletier's review (1993), all but 4 of the 24 studies reported on some aspect of costs. Although reporting on costs is common, as indicated in the previous section on incentives, the analyses in such reports are likely flawed because they do not take into consideration all the potential cost factors (Lusk, 1992). Warner et al. (1988) described cost factors that are not usually calculated, such as increased costs due to the greater number of years of expenditures and greater demands for health care by the elderly, because of greater longevity of participants. Regardless of the accuracy of the measures, worksite studies have been in the vanguard in attempting to measure the cost-effectiveness of programs.

In fact, Pelletier's (1996) latest review of 26 worksite studies reported from 1993 to 1995 included only those that reported both health and cost outcomes. Pelletier (1996) suggests that "the self-insured, self-administered health and medical plans of large corporations, with their emphasis on health promotion and disease prevention, were and are prototypes of managed care" (p. 380). The movement to managed care has increased the emphasis on costs and prevention activities. With considerable documentation that health promotion and disease prevention programs are cost-effective, they can be expected to continue to be supported in the managed care environment (Pelletier, 1996).

Critique of Existing Studies

Although Pelletier (1991) suggested that publication in peer-reviewed journals is an indicator of the quality of research, he recognized that there were methodological issues within the studies as well. As reported in the *Annual Review of Nursing Research* (Lusk, 1997), there were a number of inadequacies in the design, implementation, or reporting of health promotion and disease prevention studies. The most common problem with design was the lack of control or comparison groups, or if a comparison group was used, there were insufficient data and analyses to verify equivalency or to adjust for nonequivalency when it was found. It must be recognized that it is difficult to obtain control groups in worksite research. Implementation of the intervention must typically be done by worksite to avoid contamination, and worksites, even within the same division of a corporation, differ a great deal. As another example of the difficulty in using control groups, once Johnson and Johnson had implemented its comprehensive Live For Life® program in nearly all of the corporation's worksites, it discontinued the quasiexperimental studies of its effects because there were no longer comparison groups available (Breslow et al., 1990).

Other problems with the study designs were the duration and intensity of the intervention and the length of the postintervention evaluation period. One study, the Indiana Blue Cross/Blue Shield "Alive and Well" program (Conrad, Riedel, & Gibbs, 1990), offered multiple interventions for 8 years, evaluating effects at the end of that time period. Other than the large comprehensive programs offered by a few large corporations, many programs offer only a short, one-time, single-focus intervention; for example, a self-help smoking cessation guide (O'Hara, Gerace, & Elliott, 1993). Knowledge regarding the processes necessary for behavior change suggests the need for on-going or periodic interventions.

The literature is not clear regarding specific requirements for booster interventions (Goldenhar & Schulte, 1994; Lusk, 1995b), but there is recognition that one-time interventions can be expected to have only limited effects. A study not included in this chapter's analysis of research conducted by nurses because it preceded the specified time period (Sherman, Clark, & McEwen, 1989) evaluated effects of an intensive 3-day worksite wellness program on exercise, weight, smoking, and stress. Data were collected prior to the program, at the completion of the 30 days, and again at 3 months. The nonsignificant, but positive, changes made by participants decreased by 90 days, making differences between participants and nonparticipants negligible. The authors appropriately concluded that lifestyle changes are not made in 90 days and that short-term programs require periodic reinforcement. The importance of reinforcement was also supported in the previously described benchmark study of the best health promotion programs (O'Donnell, 1996), in which the social ecological approach of simultaneously including a supportive environment was a strategy of the best programs. Although the desirability of this strategy must be acknowledged, from the research perspective it must be noted that measuring the individual effects of components of multifaceted interventions requires large-scale studies with larger samples, and this may not be feasible for many investigators. Further, environmental changes suggested by the ecological approach may be more difficult for researchers external to the corporation to incorporate into intervention programs. However, existing large-scale programs may offer an opportunity for retrospective analyses of environmental factors such as the one reported by Conrad, Campbell, Edington, Faust, and Vilnius (1996). They deconstructed the total health-promoting program effects on posttest smoking to determine if the worksite environment served as a cue to smoking reduction. A total of 310 smokers was included in the analysis: 82 in the worksite that offered health promotion programs and 228 in another company site without such programs. Results suggested that exposure to a health-promoting worksite environment in and of itself reduced smoking behavior.

In terms of length of evaluation period, the Blue Cross/Blue Shield program evaluated effects after 8 years (Conrad, Riedel et al., 1990); another study evaluated an incentive program after only 2 weeks (Jasheway & Sirota, 1993). Obviously, a lengthy evaluation period presents its own problems, and an expectation for experimental studies to exceed 2 to 3 years is unrealistic. But, both physiological and behavioral factors need to be considered in determining the length of the evaluation period. For example, programs with a goal of reducing cholesterol levels must measure results after sufficient time has elapsed for changes in diet to yield changes in blood levels.

Implementation problems included lack of assessment of the needs of the population and selection bias of subjects in the studies. Dumka, Roosa, Michaels, and Suh (1995), in applying Coie et al.'s (1993) science of prevention treatise, emphasize the importance of defining the problem and identifying the risk and protective factors prior to designing an intervention. According to the published reports, most programs were offered without a determination of the particular needs and interests of the employee groups (Dupont's was a notable exception; see Bertera, 1990). Improved results would be expected when programs were specific to workers' needs and desires.

A concern regarding selection bias (self-selection of participants), that health promotion programs reach only the generally healthy group (Duffy & Pender, 1987), has already been expressed. The Indiana Blue Cross/Blue Shield study (Conrad, Riedel, et al., 1990) offers an illustration of this concern. The nonparticipant group in the analyses consisted of workers who had resisted participating in a single health promotion session over the 8 years of the program. No assessment of these "hard-core" nonparticipants was reported to determine if there were physical or medical factors that precluded their participation, which might also have affected their absenteeism from work (one of the major outcomes measured). Further, reports generally do not provide data regarding job categories of the subjects. There is evidence that health promotion programs enroll a smaller proportion of blue collar workers, and that future efforts need to be concentrated on that group (USDHHS, 1991).

Other inadequacies relate to interventions. Few of the written reports contained sufficient information regarding the intervention to permit evaluation of its theoretical base or appropriateness, and none, in and of themselves, provided enough information to permit replication. Seven of the 73 study reports made reference to constructs such as behavior change, behavior modification, social relationships, social support, self-efficacy, and efficacy of reinforcements. However, only two of the reports identified a theoretical model as the basis for the intervention (Demand Analysis Economic Theory, Pruitt, 1992; Social Learning Theory, Shi, 1992). Even in those two cases, the manner in which the theoretical base was translated into intervention content and outcome measures was not clear. The literature on study methods also lacks guidance for the translation of theoretical models into intervention content. Lusk, Ronis, and Kerr (1995) offer one approach, as they reported the method used to translate predictors of behavior identified through causal modeling to intervention content.

Rarely were the specific content, strategies (environmental and behavioral), and style of presentation of the intervention identified. Further, there was no mention of ensuring interintervenor reliability or intervention approaches that were culturally and educationally relevant (Lusk, 1997). All of these methodological issues have been identified by Muehrer and Koretz (1992) as "critical components of sound prevention research that allow interventions to be confidently linked to changes in outcomes" (p. 109).

Studies by Nurse Scientists

With only 13 worksite studies reported by nurse scientists in the 6 years from 1990 through 1995, it is difficult to generalize regarding nursing's contribution to worksite health promotion and disease prevention interventions, especially in light of the diverse foci represented in these studies. Outcomes measured in these studies include reducing cardiovascular risk factors, preventing musculoskeletal injuries, reducing absenteeism, reducing stress, improving attitudes toward breast cancer screening, and reducing medical costs. Because there are so few studies, those with nurse authors will be summarized here in Table 18.1 to depict the multiple foci and explain the lack of convergence of results. As is true for all specialties in nursing research to date, much of the focus has been on descriptive studies rather than intervention studies. This is even more of a problem for worksite research, as there are proportionately fewer investigators focusing on this area.

Reducing Cardiovascular Risk Factors

In the very broad field of reducing cardiovascular risk factors, there were only three studies of interventions in the worksite reported by nurse authors: "The Costs and Effects of a Nutritional Education Program Following Work-site Cholesterol Screening" (Byers et al., 1995), "Evaluating a Federal Health and Fitness Program" (Larsen & Simons, 1993), and "Cardiovascular Risk Factors in Textile Workers" (Harrell, Cornetto, & Stutts, 1992). As can be seen in Table 18.1, each of the studies reported some positive outcomes, but with the diverse approaches used, no firm conclusions regarding utilization of these research findings can be made. Two of these studies were limited by use of a single measure of cholesterol rather than an average of a series of measures as recommended by the Expert Panel (1988) on detection,

TABLE 18.1. Intervention Studies Reported by Nurses

Reducing Cardiovascular Risks

Authors and Title	Site, Subjects, and Sampling	Intervention	Outcome Measures	Results	Comments
Byers et al., 1995, "The Costs and Effects of a Nutritional Education Program Following Work-site Cholesterol Screening"	Workers with cholesterol levels of 200 mm Hg+; 40 small worksites in 4 states randomly assigned to "usual" or "special" intervention. Usual, $n = 464$; special, $n = 380$	Usual = American Heart Association Step 1 diet education and counseling; special = usual plus 2 hours of nutrition education over 1 month following cholesterol testing	Blood cholesterol levels (finger stick) at 6 and 12 months postintervention	No significant drop in cholesterol levels after 6 months. Significant decrease at 12 months. Additional 3.5% decrease attributable to special intervention	
Larsen and Simons, 1993, "Evaluating a Federal Health and Fitness Program"	Federal employees in 9 agencies in Chicago eligible for health fitness program. $n = 185$ who returned for rescreening. Subdivided into program participants, $n = 121$; nonparticipants, $n = 38$; and nonparticipants who reported exercising outside program, $n = 24$	Comprehensive health promotion program, including fitness facility, risk screening, health counseling, seminars, forums, and workshops.	Pre-post measure of cholesterol, HDL/cholesterol ratio, tryglyceride, systolic BP, diastolic BP, VO$_2$ max	Participants had significant reductions in all measures except triglyceride and significant improvements in health risk behaviors	Time period between measures not given; no adjustment for pretest scores
Harrell, Cornetto, and Stutts, 1992, "Cardiovascular Risk Factors in Textile Workers"	Textile workers, 70% from production, from 11 plants in one North Carolina corporation, $n = 1,390$, rescreened 6 months later, $n = 544$.	Provision of screening tests results and discussion of risks; additional counseling and classes for those with risk factors	At screening and 6 months later: BP, cholesterol, smoking, family history of heart disease	Significant decrease in blood pressure; significant increase in cholesterol levels	Differed by plants; compared to initial measures, those with high levels significantly decreased and those with low levels significantly increased

Musculoskeletal Injuries

Authors and Title	Site, Subjects, and Sampling	Intervention	Outcome Measures	Results	Comments
Sirles, Brown, and Hilyer, 1991, "Effects of Back School Education and Exercise in Back Injured Municipal Workers"	City workers, referred by physician, who had sustained a back injury, $N = 74$; with pre-post measures, $n = 50$	*Control group:* 6-week back school training program (exercise and education intervention); *Treatment group:* Back school plus counseling	Back strength, back flexibility, psychological well-being, anxiety, depression, pain	Significant improvements in all areas for all participants; no significant differences between treatment and control groups	
Brown, Sirles, Hilyer, and Thomas, 1992, "Cost-Effectiveness of a Back School Intervention for Municipal Employees"	Comparison of back school participants with 70 randomly selected back-injured city employees who had not participated in back school	Back school = exercise and education program	Lost work time, lost-time cost, medical cost, number of injuries	Back school participants had significant decrease in time and cost measures and significantly fewer injuries than comparison group	

348

Authors and Title	Site, Subjects, and Sampling	Intervention	Outcome Measures	Results	Comments
Galka, 1991, "Back Injury Prevention Program on a Spinal Cord Injury Unit"	Spinal cord injury nursing staff at a San Diego medical center	1 hour back school, 5 to 10 minutes stretching exercises at beginning of shift, use of lumbar-sacral back support	Low back injuries, number of lost work days	Favorable comparison with other units	Not given; not clear that *rates* were compared
Feldstein et al., 1993, "The Back Injury Prevention Project Pilot Study"	Nurses' aides and orderlies on 2 med/surg units at 2 medical centers in Portland, OR. Intervention, $n = 25$; control, $n = 30$; pre-post measures, $n = 37$	A didactic session on proper body mechanics, techniques of patient transfer, identification of environmental hazards, stretching exercises; 8 hours of personal assistance and feedback on unit	History of back pain, transfer evaluation, flexibility test, propriception pre- and 1 month postintervention	No significant decrease in back pain and fatigue in intervention group when compared with control group; significant improvement in quality of patient transfer for intervention group but not for control group.	
Scopa, 1993, "Comparison of Classroom Instruction and Independent Study in Body Mechanics"	Nursing personnel at 1 rural general med/surg hospital in southwest United States. 1. Classroom instruction, $n = 27$; 2. independent study, $n = 22$	1. A 2-hour classroom instruction in body mechanics and supervised practice; 2. Self-paced written learning module with practice encouraged	Pretest and 1-month posttest of body mechanics evaluation performing a patient transfer	No significant differences in posttest scores for the 2 groups	
Reducing Absenteeism					
Cohen and Mrtek, 1994, "Comparison of Maternal Absenteeism and Infant Illness Rates Among Breast-feeding and Formula-feeding Women in Two Corporations"	Convenience samples from 2 corporations, $N = 187$ women returning to work following maternity leave. Breast-feeding, $n = 59$; formula-feeding, $n = 42$	Facilities to collect and store milk; lactation counseling	Diary reports of infant illness and related absenteeism, verified by employee attendance records and health care provider reports.	Infants with no illnesses: 86% breast-fed, 14% formula-fed; maternal absences due to infant illnesses: 25% breast-fed, 75% formula-fed	
Conrad, Riedel, and Gibbs, 1990, "Effect of Worksite Health Promotion Programs on Employee"	Employees of Blue Cross/Blue Shield in Michigan, Indiana, and Ohio. Predominantly female white-collar workers, $n = 3,643$	Comprehensive health promotion program, differing by state, but all included health risk appraisal, screening, counseling, weight control, and smoking cessation.	Time lost, absenteeism frequency and duration	Participation in health promotion program associated with reduced time lost in 2 of the 3 states	
Pruitt, Bernheim, and Tomlinson, 1991, "Stress Management in a Military Health Promotion Program: Effectiveness and Cost Efficiency"; Pruitt, 1992, "Effectiveness and Cost Efficiency of Interventions in Health Promotion"	U.S. Army employees at Pentagon enrolled in "Fit To Win" program who had high-normal blood pressure	Stress management program	Stress-related symptoms, perceptions of stress, diastolic and systolic BP, program costs	Analyses with pretest scores as covariates found significant pre-post differences only in stress-related symptoms; cost per unit of change in measures reported	Some lack of clarity regarding cost-efficiency measures

(continued)

TABLE 18.1. *Continued*

Improving Attitudes Toward Breast Cancer Screening

Authors and Title	Site, Subjects, and Sampling	Intervention	Outcome Measures	Results	Comments
Kurtz, Kurtz, Given, and Given, 1994, "Promotion of Breast Cancer Screening in a Work Site Population"	Stratified sample of female employees from 7 diverse worksites, $n = 3,686$; response rate = 43%, $n = 1,585$	Mailed American Cancer Society brochures regarding breast cancer screening and guidelines for screening by age group	Questionnaire regarding screening intentions, practices, and attitudes, and barriers to mammography and clinical breast exam distributed 3 months prior to and 3 months after intervention	Significant improvement in perceptions regarding priority, importance, and discomfort of mammograms and regarding importance of breast exam; increased discussion at work	No control group, as precluded by funding agency

Reducing Medical Costs

Authors and Title	Site, Subjects, and Sampling	Intervention	Outcome Measures	Results	Comments
Harvey, Whitner, Hilyer, and Brown, 1993, "The Impact of a Comprehensive Medical Benefit Cost Management Program for the City of Birmingham: Results at Five Years"	Employees of city of Birmingham, AL	Annual medical screen for 5 years; health risk appraisal; health promotion programs in weight loss, stress management, smoking cessations, BP control, cholesterol reduction, fitness testing and training, and back care; incentives for participation.	Medical benefits expenses, program cost	Slower rate of increase in medical costs from 1985 to 1990: In 1985, costs were $397 higher than for State employees and, in 1990, $992 less than for State employees; program cost $100 per employee	

evaluation, and treatment of high blood cholesterol in adults. The report of the Larsen and Simons study (1993) was particularly difficult to evaluate, as it included no report of the time period in which the study took place nor the length of time between the Time 1 and Time 2 screenings, no comparison of participants' and nonparticipants' results, and use of a small volunteer sample. Further, this study compared pre/post mean scores without consideration of the covariation of initial scores. In the Harrell et al. (1992) study, cholesterol change scores differed significantly by plant, suggesting differences in implementation of the interventions or in physician practices in the local area; however, no mechanisms to ensure interintervenor reliability were reported. The large-scale study conducted by state health departments in 40 worksites (Byers et al., 1995) did not find significant changes in cholesterol levels until 12 months following the special intervention. This finding is important because 6 months has generally been considered a long enough time to observe changes in levels of cholesterol.

These three reports of studies to reduce cardiovascular risk factors, although generally achieving a positive outcome, also illustrated common deficiencies in worksite studies, specifically in the areas of interintervenor reliability, appropriate time periods for assessing change, adequate measures of the dependent variable, and appropriate analyses of effects of the interventions.

Reducing Musculoskeletal Injuries

As depicted in Table 18.1, five worksite studies assessed programs to reduce musculoskeletal injuries in municipal employees and in healthcare workers. The interventions varied from increasing strength and flexibility to specific training regarding prevention of back injuries. Various outcomes were measured, including flexibility, injuries, medical costs, health and psychological well-being, lost work time, back pain, fatigue, and observations of patient transfers. Authors of the first three studies in Table 18.1 reported methodological problems with subject selection and design and difficulty in controlling for possible Hawthorne effects. One study (Galka, 1991) did not provide essential information regarding the numbers of nurses on the study unit and other units, the rate of injuries on the units, the quantification of the exposures (lifts and transfers), and assessment of compliance with the intervention program, making it impossible to assess the effectiveness of the intervention. Feldstein, Valanis, Vollmer, Stevens, and Overton (1993) identified a common problem, the length of time for the

intervention, and suggested a need for a longer duration study (at least 2 years) to determine the maintenance of changes in patient transfer techniques. The Harvey, Whitmer, Hilyer, and Brown (1993) study compared medical costs per employee, demonstrating cost-effectiveness by lower costs for those employees in the intervention program. The authors did not report a cost-benefit analysis, but data reported were suggestive of a positive one. Although the outcomes of these studies were generally positive, the fact that the specific interventions, as well as the outcome measures, were so diverse makes it impossible, based on the results of these studies, to identify a research science base for this problem.

Reducing Absenteeism

As described in Table 18.1, the two studies focusing on reducing worksite absenteeism focused on two very different interventions and populations; specifically, maternal absenteeism based on the type of feeding of the infant and the effects of large-scale worksite health promotion programs on absenteeism. The first report suggested that if findings were replicated, a worksite lactation program would be economically beneficial for corporations (Cohen & Mrtek, 1994). Positive effects were found in the large-scale worksite health promotion programs in two of the three states involved (Conrad, Riedel, et al., 1990). These authors suggested that possible reasons for lack of positive effect in the third state were the unavailability of facilities for the physical conditioning program, insufficient assistance provided (e.g., stress management materials that helped to identify stressors but provided no assistance in handling them) insufficient management support, and a reorganization at the test site.

Reducing absenteeism is a high priority for corporations, due to the costs involved in sick pay, decreased productivity, and replacement workers. Based upon published reports, these nurse scientists are the only ones who have assessed the effects of a corporate lactation program. This is an important area, as corporations may reap significant benefits. The effects of comprehensive health promotion programs are more problematic to assess, with difficulties in ensuring consistent delivery of interventions, determining level of employee participation, and obtaining complete data regarding causes of absenteeism.

Other Studies

As can be seen in Table 18.1, other nursing research studies focused on worksite interventions to reduce stress, improve attitudes toward breast cancer screening, and reduce medical costs. Obviously, single studies provide limited generalizability and direction for practice. These studies illustrated further problems with worksite research. For example, the Pruitt (Pruitt, 1992; Pruitt, Bernheim, & Tomlinson, 1991) study of a stress management intervention used the terms *cost benefit, cost-effectiveness,* and *cost efficiency* interchangeably in their reports. Cost per unit of change is a cost-benefit analysis; cost-effectiveness is a comparison of costs of alternative programs (American Association of Occupational Health Nurses [AAOHN], 1996). In fact, what was actually presented was apparently cost-benefit analysis, but the manner in which it was presented made it very difficult to verify the appropriateness of the original regression analysis to obtain the beta weights used to determine the unit of change to calculate the cost per unit of change. Due to this concern regarding measurement of cost benefit and the conflicting results presented in the two reports of the single study, there is question about the contribution of this study to the nursing science base.

The lack of control groups in research on worksite interventions has already been identified as a problem common to all worksite studies. This problem pertains to studies conducted by nurse scientists as well. Kurtz, Kurtz, Given, and Given (1994), in their study to improve attitudes toward breast cancer screening, reported that the funding agency would not allow them to conduct the study using a control group. It is unfortunate that alternative arrangements could not have been made to allow a phased study of the effect of the intervention, ultimately still delivering the intervention to all subjects. This would have allowed for the attribution of the effect to the intervention.

Evaluation of Studies

These studies involving nurse scientists are representative of the larger body of research in the area and, not surprisingly, demonstrate similar inadequacies in design, implementation, and evaluation. Review of all of the studies by nurses suggests that in most cases they do not represent a program of research focused on *worksite* health promotion and disease prevention (Brown and Sirles are exceptions). Rather, in some cases, the worksite may be only one of a number of sites where the research of interest could be conducted. In others, the nurses may have been part of a team delivering services in a multisite study. All studies make a contribution to science, but it is the sustained and focused *programs* of worksite research

that are most likely to provide significant foundation for nursing practice in this area. Development of *programs* of research is usually only possible through sequential grant or contract funding.

Programs of Research

Three nurse scientists are known to be developing federally funded programs of research focusing on health promotion and disease prevention interventions in the worksite: Brown (1994), "Prevention of Back Injuries"; Lusk (1993), "Prevention of Noise Induced Hearing Loss"; and Conrad (1995), "Increasing Strength to Reduce Fatigue and Resulting Injuries." Sequential federal funding occurs only with critical peer review and offers evidence of the quality and significance of the research studies.

Prevention of Back Injuries

Back injuries are one of the most common health problems of workers, with expenditures for medical care, workers' compensation, and lost work time estimated to exceed $16 billion per year. Because it is the leading cause of early retirement of firefighters due to injury, Brown and colleagues (Brown, 1994) are comparing the effects of two worksite educational and exercise approaches (back school group, strength and flexibility group) with a control group on preventing back injuries (*n* = 180 firefighters from 21 fire stations in one municipal fire department). Outcomes to be measured at preintervention, 12 weeks, and 6 months postintervention include knowledge of functioning of the back and actual trunk performance. Comparisons of incidence of work-related back injuries, medical costs, lost time, and lost-time costs will be made among the three groups. When this study is completed, additional studies of firefighters and other worker groups will need to be conducted to determine the most effective interventions to prevent back injuries. No conceptual framework was specified in the abstract of the grant proposal, but the investigator indicated that the study is guided by an injury control perspective using Neuman's Systems Model (K. Brown, personal communication, January 23, 1997).

In addition to this currently funded study, Brown participated in two previously described studies of worksite interventions that provided a foundation for the current project: (a) to prevent back injuries in back-injured city workers (Sirles, Brown, & Hilyer, 1991) and to assess cost-effectiveness of the program (Brown, Sirles,

Hilyer, & Thomas, 1992) and (b) to prevent joint injuries in firefighters (Hilyer, Brown, Sirles, & Peoples, 1990). This latter study documented improvement in flexibility and lost time from work, but no differences in incidence of injuries between the experimental and control groups. The former study dealing with already-injured workers demonstrated significant improvement in 9 of 14 measures of health and psychological well-being in the intervention group, significant decreases in time and cost measures, and significantly fewer injuries in the intervention group than in the control group. Thus, the current study, contrasting tested interventions and building on experience gained in the previous studies, is expected to provide definitive information regarding preventing back injuries in this population. Further, many of their findings should be translatable to other worker groups.

Prevention of Noise-Induced Hearing Loss

Noise-induced hearing loss is an irreversible but preventable condition. It has been estimated that over 30 million workers are exposed to hazardous noise in the workplace (NIOSH, 1996). Consistent use of hearing protection devices (HPDs) reduces noise exposure, thus preventing hearing loss, but this requires specific actions by workers—in most cases, a new behavior to be performed by workers. Nearly all prior research on noise-induced hearing loss has focused on the efficacy of the HPDs rather than on the factors influencing workers' use of them (Lusk, 1989, 1993).

Lusk and colleagues (Lusk, 1989, 1993) began by testing the Health Promotion Model (HPM) as a causal model to explain auto workers' use of hearing protection devices (Lusk, Ronis, Kerr, & Atwood, 1994). The model had comparative fit indexes (CFI) of .98 (values of the CFI range from 0 to 1, with values over .95 indicating a good fit; Bentler, 1990) and accounted for from 47% to 64% of the variance in use of HPDs in the several convenience samples of auto factory workers ($n = 831$) (Lusk, Ronis, & Baer, 1997; Lusk, Ronis, Kerr, & Atwood, 1994).

In studies of several convenience samples of construction workers ($n = 359$) the model had good fit (CFI = .98) and accounted for 51% of the variance in use of HPDs (Lusk, Ronis, & Hogan, 1997). Although the strength of the relationship varied by worksite and job classification, across the groups, the most important factors were those specific to the behavior of interest: barriers to, self-efficacy of, benefits of, and interpersonal in-

fluences on use of hearing protection. Using the identified factors influencing workers' use, an intervention was designed to increase use of HPDs (Lusk et al., 1999; Lusk, Ronis, et al., 1995). The effectiveness of the theory-based intervention was tested using a Solomon Four Group design with construction workers (plumbers/pipefitters, carpenters, and operating engineers in the Midwest, and a national sample of plumber/pipefitter trainers) ($n = 1,143$). Using naturally occurring small groups assembled for training, these groups of workers were randomly assigned to one of the three experimental groups or the one control group. Ten- to 12-month postintervention data showed a significant increase in use of HPDs by the intervention groups as compared to the control group (Lusk et al., in press). A new project testing the effectiveness of an individually tailored, interactive multimedia intervention based on the dominant predictors of factory workers' use of HPDs was initiated in 1996 (Lusk, 1995b).

In summary, through use of a conceptual model, factors predicting workers' use of HPDs have been identified and used to design interventions. Similar results were obtained with multiple samples of workers in a number of settings and with different jobs: (a) although there were differences in relative importance, there was congruence in the factors from the HPM that were important predictors; and (b) the HPM had an excellent fit and accounted for a significant proportion of the variance in use of hearing protection. Results from these studies of various worker groups support the attention to factors influencing workers' use of HPDs, the use of the HPM as a causal model, and the importance of the identified factors in influencing use. Because the relative importance of some of the factors varied by worksite and job classification, further study is needed with other worker groups to determine important factors for different types of jobs and worksites and to test interventions with those groups.

Fitness Program to Decrease Physical and Mental Fatigue

Firefighters and paramedics are two groups who work extended shifts and shifts that are in opposition to circadian rhythms, resulting in fatigue. Fatigue has been associated with the occurrence of musculoskeletal injuries in these groups, whose rate is 4.3 times higher than the rate for private industry. Because most of the research investigating the linkage between fitness and fatigue has been conducted in the laboratory setting, Conrad and colleagues (Conrad, 1995) are determining the efficacy of an intervention, an intensive worksite fitness regimen, to increase resistance to fatigue and, ultimately, reduce musculoskeletal injuries. Twenty-four firefighters and paramedics from four fire departments will participate in the study, with 12 engaging in a program of aerobic conditioning, muscular isotonic strength training, and flexibility training for 12 weeks while 12 others will serve as the control group. The subjects are volunteers from four fire departments who have not participated in regular exercise in the past 6 months; who, through a series of physical screenings, are found to have acceptable coronary risk profiles; and who are willing and available to participate. Physical fitness measures will include aerobic fitness and heart rate measures, muscular strength and endurance, and body composition; fatigue measures will include measures of physical and mental fatigue. Individual day-to-day variations in workload will be treated as a critical covariate. Qualitative data will be obtained to evaluate the program from the perspective of the participants and from the departmental chiefs. Results will be used to develop a larger-scale nursing intervention study to assess the effects of fitness and fatigue on musculoskeletal injury.

State of Nursing Science

Although small in number, these three federally funded programs of research focusing on worksite interventions to prevent disease conditions illustrate important characteristics of worksite research. The hazards and needs of workers and the factors influencing their behaviors differ by type and site of work, and knowledge of the particular worksite settings is essential to the conduct of such studies. Therefore, researchers tend to focus on single worker groups, for example, firefighters or automotive plant workers. Auto plant workers can be considered a narrowly defined group, but differences were found in health behaviors and lifestyles and in the use of HPDs by different job categories within this worker group (Lusk, Kerr, & Ronis, 1995; Lusk, Ronis, Kerr, & Atwood, 1994). Thus, there is a greater need in this field to replicate studies with different worker groups, without assuming transferability of findings based on common demographic characteristics; for example, job categories or gender. This is to say that because an intervention was successful with middle-aged African-American blue-

collar females in one worksite, there is no assurance that it will be successful with this same population in a different worksite or with workers in different job categories. However, the studies assessing worksite health promotion interventions conducted by non-nurse and nurse scientists tended to treat all workers the same, regardless of worksite setting or job category. If greater attention were paid to characteristics of the worksite, and if analyses of effects were reported for different job categories, significant differences in effects may have been found.

In assessing the research base for practice, the Institute of Medicine report, *Nursing, Health, and Environment* (Pope, Snyder, & Mood, 1995), stated that "it is clear that scant research supports the clinical practice of nursing in environmental or occupational health" (p. 112). This report reiterates the National Institute for Nursing Research's (NINR's) focus on caregiving research, specifically the biological and behavioral elements of health rather than disease, and indicates that "non-nurse investigators in the area of environmental or occupational health do not appear to be conducting studies directly related to the knowledge base for nursing practice" (p. 111). Although the NINR focus is relevant to nurse scientists' worksite research, this latter statement does not seem to be true for worksite health promotion and disease prevention intervention research conducted by non-nurse investigators. The results of their studies do inform this aspect of occupational health nursing practice. Granted, there are many other areas of this specialty practice for which there is little research, but nursing science can and should use and build upon the worksite studies conducted by other disciplines.

Inherent in conducting research in the worksite are a number of issues in design and implementation of studies. First, comprehensive health promotion and occupational health and safety programs are very desirable due to their beneficial synergistic effects (Cohen, 1987; Lusk, 1997), but their complexity makes it very difficult to isolate and measure the effects of individual program components. To do so requires very large, multisite samples. However, once multiple worksites are included, differences peculiar to the individual worksites may influence effects of the intervention. More sophisticated research designs and multivariate analysis techniques are required to handle multisite studies, and difficult decisions must be made regarding the trade-offs for single-site versus multisite studies.

Worksite intervention studies reported in the literature across disciplines present almost uniformly positive effects (Lusk, 1997; Pelletier, 1991, 1993). This is also true for those with nurse scientist authors. It is not surprising that those involving nurse scientists also demonstrate inadequacies similar to those found in all worksite intervention studies. There are both commonalities and differences between worksite health promotion and disease prevention intervention studies conducted by nurse scientists and non-nurse scientists. Similar for both groups are the previously described issues in design, implementation, and reporting of results. Specifically, these include (a) lack of control or comparison groups; (b) assessment of needs of the group prior to designing intervention; (c) consideration of characteristics and needs of subgroups; (d) information regarding the intervention content, duration and intensity, and "dose" per subject; (e) indication of a theoretical base for the intervention; (f) specification of length of the evaluation period; and (g) nonbiased selection of subjects.

Although there are few differences in the issues or deficiencies in worksite research, whether conducted by nurse scientists or non-nurse scientists, there are some important differences in foci of interventions. In considering the contribution of studies by nurse scientists in light of the larger field of worksite interventions, there are several important points.

First, there are studies by nurse scientists addressing topics not studied by non-nurse scientists. The majority of the 73 worksite intervention studies conducted by nurse scientists and non-nurses reviewed by Lusk (1997) focused on some aspect of cardiovascular risk factors, an area of interest for researchers in many disciplines. Many of these studies also assessed some aspect of costs. A few reports addressed back injuries and effects of stress management programs, with a greater proportion of these studies being conducted by nurse scientists. In contrast, no other reports were found for worksite studies of attitudes toward breast cancer screening, predictors of workers' use of hearing protection, or effects of corporate lactation programs.

These unique foci for interventions are illustrative of nursing science's special contributions to the larger area of worksite interventions. The first two unique topics, the focus on attitudes toward breast cancer screening and predictors of use of hearing protection devices, are indicative of nursing's concern with individuals' perceptions as a basis for changing behavior. Consistent with the steps in the nursing process, clients' needs and desires are assessed prior to planning interventions.

In regard to the third foci, corporate lactation programs, there are three aspects of nursing's identification with the topic: (a) nursing has long had a very strong

presence in maternal-infant health; (b) nursing claims a holistic approach, thereby encompassing awareness of the effect of infant feeding on female employees' absenteeism; and (c) nursing brings to bear knowledge of medical, health, social, and environmental factors in identifying and solving problems.

Second, 2 of the 13 reports of studies by nurse scientists addressed worker attitudes or cognitive perceptual factors. This appears to represent a higher proportion of studies conducted by nurses, when contrasted with those in the larger field of worksite interventions. As an example, Lusk's (Lusk, 1989, 1993; Lusk, Ronis, & Hogan, 1997; Lusk, Ronis, Kerr, & Atwood, 1994) emphasis on workers' perceptions has altered the direction of federal research on HPDs (M. R. Stephenson, personal communication, August, 1995), as prior to this work, little attention had been directed to factors influencing workers' use of HPDs.

Third, some program foci, with their emphasis on serial behavioral interventions such as preventing back and other musculoskeletal injuries and noise-induced hearing loss, are particularly congruent to recognized strengths of professional nursing. Obviously, reducing cardiovascular risks also requires serial behavioral interventions and is congruent to nursing's role, but because this area is more crowded with researchers from other disciplines, there is less of a niche for nurse scientists (Lusk, 1997; Pelletier, 1991, 1993). Yet, most of the research in this area conducted by researchers from other disciplines would benefit from the involvement of nurse scientists. And the reciprocal holds true as well; studies conducted by nurse scientists are strengthened by contributions from scientists in other disciplines. Coie et al. (1993) has stated "that prevention research often will require collaborative efforts of interdisciplinary teams to achieve the diversity of expertise and breadth of intellectual focus that is necessary" (p. 1016). This is especially true for the worksite, with its diverse health problems.

Advances in worksite research will be made as more nurse scientists develop programs of research in fairly narrowly defined topic areas. A program of research also suggests direction and control of the study by nurse scientists. In at least two of the studies reviewed, nurses apparently did not direct the design and conduct of the studies. Conrad, Riedel, et al. (1990) retrospectively conducted a secondary analysis of effects of a health promotion program, having had no involvement in the design and conduct of the original study. In the large multistate program (Byers et al., 1995), the nurse authors were not prepared as nurse scientists but were employed by cooperating state health departments to coordinate a state program.

Clearly, worksite health promotion and disease prevention intervention research by nurse scientists can be seen as being in its infancy. An increasing number of studies are being reported in the literature, but such studies remain relatively few, particularly in relation to the size of the population of working adults. Nurse scientists have conducted studies and have been members of groups of researchers for only a relatively small number of studies with outcomes limited to reducing cardiovascular risk factors, preventing musculoskeletal injuries, reducing absenteeism, reducing stress, improving attitudes toward breast cancer screening, and reducing medical costs. Federally funded programs of worksite intervention research by nurse scientists were found in only three areas: preventing back injuries, preventing noise-induced hearing loss, and preventing fatigue leading to injuries.

Even though the identified programs of research were federally funded, the source of funding is not the critical factor. It is the nurse scientists' sustained and focused effort in worksite research and the control and direction of the studies that is essential to the progress of the science.

It is no surprise that, with so few studies and programs of worksite research, areas of substantiation of nursing science in this area cannot be clearly identified. In the preceding sections, strengths and weaknesses of nursing science in worksite intervention studies have been described, but it is not reasonable to identify specific gaps in research in this area; more studies need to be done in all areas. Worksite intervention research is an area of almost unlimited opportunity for nurse scientists.

Recommendations for Advancing Nursing Science

A number of deficiencies in worksite research conducted by nurse scientists and non-nurse scientists were identified. In addition to the need to correct those deficiencies and to develop programs of research, specific directions are suggested to capitalize on the opportunities for research by nurse scientists in this area. There are several approaches that could be used to facilitate advancing nursing science:

a. *Collaboration among nurse scientists in various clinical specialties with interests in adult health to focus on the particular concerns associated with worksite health promotion.* As examples, those scientists studying hypertension control could link with those studying effects of worksite health promotion programs, thereby furthering the goals of both groups of nurse scientists. Further, cancer screening is done in the worksite to monitor for exposures and as a part of health promotion programs, but these results are rarely integrated into a comprehensive cancer prevention program of which the effectiveness is carefully measured. This represents another example of opportunities for collaborative studies by nurse scientists in different specialties.

b. *Collaboration with practicing nurses in occupational health.* There is opportunity for nurse scientists to work with nurses in the clinical setting in occupational health to evaluate effects of existing worksite programs. Because these programs are already in place, scientists could use existing data and collect additional data as needed, thereby advancing nursing science at minimal cost. Further, retrospective analyses such as the study reported by Conrad, Riedel, et al. (1990) yield important data regarding effects of intervention programs.

c. *Continued attention to assessing cost-effectiveness and cost benefits, while recognizing the risks involved in focusing exclusively on cost benefits.* Previously, concerns were described that, with the emphasis on cost benefit, only those programs that can demonstrate a positive balance will be implemented, and those that contribute to positive effects on improved morale or quality of life but do not show dollar savings will be discarded. However, considering that proven cost benefits may promote the research and development of programs and result in an overall increase in support for programs, it is important to, whenever possible, attempt to demonstrate both cost-effectiveness and cost benefit. Further, medical costs, injury, and absenteeism records may already be available in corporate data bases, requiring only arrangements for access and interpretation.

d. *Continued focus on areas where nursing has strengths, but with involvement of other disciplines.* Nursing has long been recognized as having strengths in providing serial interventions to promote health and prevent disease. Because this emphasis is essential to worksite intervention research, nurse scientists can make important contributions to the science of the entire field. These strengths need to be built upon while simultaneously collaborating with interdisciplinary occupational safety and health team members in conducting research in the worksite. As previously stated, there is a need to integrate health promotion and occupational health and safety programs offered in the worksite. These integrated programs provide a myriad of opportunities for collaborative interdisciplinary research.

e. *Increased attention to social ecological factors.* O'Donnell (1996) and others have suggested the importance of including environmental supports for hearing protection interventions. Inclusion of interdisciplinary team members and collaboration with practicing nurses can facilitate the inclusion of environmental supports.

Summary

An increasing number of worksite health promotion and disease prevention intervention studies are being reported in the literature. A MacArthur Foundation paper (Kahn, 1993) emphasized the importance of collaboration in scientific discovery, due in part to increasing technological complexity, but also suggested that it is at the boundaries of the disciplines where progress is made. Further support for collaboration is the recogni-

tion that just as "it takes a village to raise a child," it takes a *group* to solve scientific problems (Harris, 1995). It is essential that the "group" working on scientific questions in worksite health promotion and disease prevention include nurse scientists. Even though health promotion and disease prevention have long been areas of expertise and focus for nursing, relatively few of the worksite studies are being conducted by nurse scientists or by teams that include nurse scientists. Based upon this review of the current literature, unique contributions of nurse scientists to this field may include greater attention to individuals' perceptions and attitudes as they relate to behavior change, a more holistic approach in defining and solving scientific problems, and a broader integration of knowledge and skills in health, disease, social, and environmental factors into health promotion interventions.

Because the worksite represents the best place to access the adult population, it behooves nurse scientists to take advantage of the opportunities that abound in this field. Achieving *Healthy People 2000* objectives for adult health requires changing adult behavior, and nurse scientists are especially well qualified to direct studies of health promotion and disease prevention interventions at worksites.

References

American Association of Occupational Health Nurses. (1996). Advisory: Cost benefit and cost occupational health. *American Association of Occupational Health Nurses Journal, 44.*

Bentler, P. M. (1990). Comparative fit indexes in structural models. *Psychological Bulletin, 107,* 238-246.

Bertera, R. L. (1990). Planning and implementing health promotion in the workplace: A case study of the DuPont Company experience. *Health Education Quarterly, 17*(3), 307-327.

Breslow, L., Fielding, J., Herrmann, A. A., & Wilbur, C. S. (1990). Worksite health promotion: Its evolution and the Johnson & Johnson experience. *Preventive Medicine, 19,* 13-21.

Brown, K. C. (1994). *Worksite education/exercise to prevent back injury* (Grant funded by National Institute for Nursing Research at National Institutes of Health, Grant No. RO1 NR03044-01A1).

Brown, K. C., Sirles, A. T., Hilyer, J. C., & Thomas, M. J. (1992). Cost-effectiveness of a back school intervention for municipal employees. *Spine, 17,* 1224-1228.

Bulletin of Labour Statistics. (1995). *1. General level of unemployment. 2. General level of unemployment.* Geneva: International Labour Office.

Bureau of Business Practice Center for Health Programs. (1993). *The health and economic impact of lifestyle behaviors.* Waterford, CT: Simon & Schuster.

Burton, W. N., Erickson, D., & Briones, J. (1991). Women's health programs at the workplace. *Journal of Occupational Medicine, 33,* 349-350.

Byers, T., Mullis, R., Anderson, J., Dusenbury, L., Gorsky, R., Kimber, C., Krueger, K., Kuester, S., Mokdad, A., Perry, G., & Smith, C. (1995). The costs and effects of a nutritional education program following work-site cholesterol screening. *American Journal of Public Health, 85,* 650-655.

Castelli, J. (1994, January). Safety and health watch: A digest of developments in occupational safety and health. *Safety and Health, 151*(7), 91-94.

Cohen, A. (1987). Perspectives on self-protective behaviors and work place hazards. In M. D. Weinstein (Ed.), *Taking care: Understanding and encouraging self-protective behavior* (pp. 298-322). Cambridge, England: Cambridge University Press.

Cohen, R., & Mrtek, M. B. (1994). The impact of two corporate lactation programs on the incidence and duration of breast-feeding by employed mothers. *American Journal of Health Promotion, 8,* 436-441.

Coie, J. D., Watt, N. F., West, S. G., Hawkings, J. D., Asarnow, J. R., Markman, H. J., Ramey, S. L., Shure, M. B., & Long, B. (1993). The science of prevention: A conceptual framework and some directions for a national research program. *American Psychologist, 48*(10), 1013-1022.

Conrad, K. M. (1995). *A nursing fitness intervention to reduce work fatigue* (Grant funded by Institute for Nursing Research at NIH, Grant No. 1 R15 NRO4035-01).

Conrad, K. M., Campbell, R. T., Edington, D. W., Faust, H. S., & Vilnius, D. (1996). The worksite environment as a cue to smoking reduction. *Research in Nursing and Health, 19*, 21-31.

Conrad, K. M., Riedel, J. E., & Gibbs, J. O. (1990). Effect of worksite health promotion programs on employee absenteeism. *American Association of Occupational Health Nurses Journal, 38*, 573-580.

Dear, J. A. (1995). Work stress and health '95: Creating healthier workplaces. *Vital Speeches of the Day, 62*, 39-42.

Duffy, M. E., & Pender, N. J. (Eds.). (1987). Conceptual issues in health promotion. In *Proceedings of a Wingspread Conference.* Indianapolis, IN: Sigma Theta Tau International.

Dumka, L. D., Roosa, M. W., Michaels, M. L., & Suh, K. W. (1995). Using research and theory to develop prevention programs for high risk families. *Family Relations, 44*, 78-86.

Expert Panel. (1988). Report of the national cholesterol education program expert panel on detection, evaluation, and treatment of high blood cholesterol in adults. *Archives of Internal Medicine, 148*, 36-39.

Feldstein, A., Valanis, B., Vollmer, W., Stevens, N., & Overton, C. (1993). The back injury prevention project pilot study. *Journal of Occupational Medicine, 35*(1), 114-119.

Fielding, J. E. (1990). Worksite health promotion programs in the United States: Progress, lessons, and challenges. *Health Promotion International, 5*(1), 75-84.

Fries, J. F., Fries, S. T., Parcel, C. L., & Harrington, H. (1992). Health risk changes with a low cost individualized health promotion program: Effects at up to 30 months. *American Journal of Health Promotion, 6*, 364-371.

Fries, J. F., Green, L. W., & Levine, S. (1989). Health promotion and the compression of morbidity. *Lancet, 1*(8636), 481-483.

Galka, M. L. (1991). Back injury prevention program on a spinal cord injury unit. *Spinal Cord Injury Nursing, 8*(2), 48-51.

Gleason-Comstock, J., Lando, H. A., McGover, P., Pirie, P., & Rooney, B. (1994). Promotion of worksite smoking policy in two Minnesota communities. *American Journal of Health Promotion, 9*, 24-27.

Goldenhar, L. M., & Schulte, P. A. (1994). Intervention research in occupational health and safety. *Journal of Occupational Medicine, 36*, 763-775.

Gordon, J. (1987). Point of view: Workplace health promotion: The right idea in the wrong place. *Health Education Research, 2*(1), 69-71.

Harrell, J. S., Cornetto, A. D., & Stutts, W. C. (1992). Cardiovascular risk factors in textile workers. *American Association of Occupational Health Nurses Journal, 40*, 581-589.

Harris, L. M. (1995). *Health and the new media: Technologies transforming personal and public health.* Hillsdale, NJ: Lawrence Erlbaum.

Harvey, M. R., Whitmer, R. W., Hilyer, J. C., & Brown, K. C. (1993). The impact of a comprehensive medical benefit cost management program for the city of Birmingham: Results at five years. *American Journal of Health Promotion, 74*, 296-304.

Hilyer, J. C., Brown, K. C., Sirles, A. T., & Peoples, L. (1990). A flexibility intervention to reduce the incidence and severity of joint injuries among municipal firefighters. *Journal of Occupational Medicine, 32*, 631-637.

Jacobson, M., Kolarek, M. H., & Newton, B. (1996). *Business, babies and the bottom line: Corporate innovations and best practices in maternal and child health.* Washington, DC: Business Group on Health.

Jasheway, L. A., & Sirota, H. (1993). Association for Worksite Health Promotion Practitioners' forum. *American Journal of Health Promotion, 7*, 165-166.

Job related injuries and illnesses rise. (1992, February). *Business and Health, 10*(2), 12.

Kahn, R. L. (1993). *An experiment in scientific organization* (MacArthur Foundation occasional paper). Chicago: John D. and Catherine T. MacArthur Foundation.

Keeler, E. B., Manning, W. G., Newhouse, J. P., Sloss, E. M., & Wasserman, J. (1989). The external costs of a sedentary life style. *American Journal of Public Health, 79*, 975-981.

Kurtz, M. E., Kurtz, J. C., Given, B., & Given, C. C. (1994). Promotion of breast cancer screening in a work site population. *Health Care for Women International, 15*, 31-42.

Larsen, P., & Simons, N. (1993). Evaluating a federal health and fitness program. *American Association of Occupational Health Nurses Journal, 41*, 143-148.

Larsen, R. C. (1995). Workplace psychiatry: Workers' compensation stress claims: Workplace causes and prevention. *Psychiatric Annals, 25*, 234-237.

Levy, B. S., & Wegman, D. H. (Eds.). (1988). *Occupational health: Recognizing and preventing work-related disease* (2nd ed.). Boston: Little, Brown.

Longo, D. R., Brownson, R. C., Johnson, J. C., Hewett, J. E., Kruse, R. L., Novotny, T. E., & Logan, R. A. (1996). Hospital smoking bans and employee smoking behavior. *Journal of the American Medical Association, 275*(16), 1252-1257.

Lusk, S. L. (1989). *Nursing model to prevent noise induced hearing loss* (Grant proposal). Funded by National Institute for Nursing Research, National Institute on Deafness and Other Communicable Disorders, Office of Research on Women and Health, National Institutes of Health, Grant No. R01 NRO 2050.

Lusk, S. L. (1992). Selling health promotion programs. *American Association of Occupational Health Nurses Journal, 40*, 414-418.

Lusk, S. L. (1993). *Preventing noise-induced hearing loss in construction workers* (Research grant proposal). Funded by National Institute for Occupational Safety and Health, Grant No. R01 OHO3136.

Lusk, S. L. (1995a). Linking practice and research: Health promotion by mail. *American Association of Occupational Health Nurses Journal, 43*, 346-348.

Lusk, S. L. (1995b). *Test of interventions to prevent workers' hearing loss* (Research grant proposal). Funded by National Institute for Nursing Research at National Institutes of Health, Grant No. 2R01 NR02050-04.

Lusk, S. L. (1996). Linking practice and research: Agency for Health Care Policy and Research clinical practice guidelines. *American Association of Occupational Health Nurses Journal, 44*, 151-153.

Lusk, S. L. (1997). Health promotion and disease prevention in the worksite. In J. J. Fitzpatrick & J. Norbeck (Eds.), *Annual review of nursing research, 15* (chap. 3). New York: Springer.

Lusk, S. L., Kerr, M. J., & Ronis, D. L. (1995). Health-promoting lifestyles of blue-collar, skilled trade, and white-collar workers. *Nursing Research, 44*, 20-23.

Lusk, S. L., Kerr, M. J., Ronis, D. L., & Eakin, B. L. (1999). Appying the Health Promotion Model to development of a worksite intervention. *American Journal of Health Promotion, 12*(4), 219-227.

Lusk, S. L., Ronis, D. L., & Baer, L. M. (1997). Gender differences in blue collar workers' use of hearing protection. *Women and Health, 25*(4), 69-89.

Lusk, S. L., Ronis, D. L., & Hogan, M. (1997). Test of the health promotion model as a causal model of construction workers' use of hearing protection. *Research in Nursing and Health, 20*, 183-194.

Lusk, S. L., Ronis, D. L., Hong, O. S., Early, M., & Eakin, B. L. (in press). Test of the effectiveness of an intervention to increase use of hearing protections among construction workers. *Human Factors.*

Lusk, S. L., Ronis, D. L., & Kerr, M. J. (1995). Predictors of hearing protection use among construction workers: Implication for training programs. *Human Factors, 37*(3), 635-640.

Lusk, S. L., Ronis, D. L., Kerr, M. J., & Atwood, J. R. (1994). Test of the health promotion model as a causal model of workers' use of hearing protection. *Nursing Research, 43,* 151-157.

Mayer, J. A., Jones, J. A., Eckhardt, L. E., Haliday, J., Bartholomew, S., Slymen, D. J., & Howell, M. F. (1993). Evaluation of a worksite mammography program. *American Journal of Preventive Medicine, 9,* 244-249.

McGinnis, J. M., & Foege, W. H. (1993). Actual causes of death in the United States. *Journal of the American Medical Association, 270,* 2207-2212.

Michigan Department of Public Health. (1987, October). *Health promotion can produce economic savings.* Lansing, MI: Department of Management and Budget, Office of Health and Medical Affairs, Center for Health Promotion.

Muehrer, P., & Koretz, D. S. (1992). Issues in preventive intervention research. *Current Directions in Psychological Science, 1*(3), 109-112.

National Institute for Occupational Safety and Health. (1988). *Guidelines for protecting the safety and health of health care workers.* Washington, DC: U.S. Government Printing Office.

National Institute for Occupational Safety and Health. (1996). *National occupational research agenda* (Pub. No. 95-115). Cincinnati, OH: Author.

National Safety Council. (1990). *Accident facts.* Chicago: Author.

Occupational Safety and Health Act of 1970. Pub. L. No. 91-596, § 1910.95, 29 CFR (1987).

O'Donnell, M. (1996). Editor's notes: Social ecological approach to health promotion. *American Journal of Health Promotion, 10,* 244.

O'Hara, P., Gerace, T. A., & Elliott, L. (1993). Effectiveness of self-help smoking cessation guides for firefighters. *Journal of Occupational Medicine, 35*(8), 795-799.

Pelletier, K. R. (1991). A review and analysis of the health and cost-effective outcome studies of comprehensive health promotion and disease prevention programs. *American Journal of Health Promotion, 5,* 311-313.

Pelletier, K. R. (1993). A review and analysis of the health and cost-effective outcome studies of comprehensive health promotion and disease prevention programs at the worksite: 1991-1993 update. *American Journal of Health Promotion, 8*(1), 50-62.

Pelletier, K. R. (1996). A review and analysis of the health and cost-effective outcome studies of comprehensive health promotion and disease prevention programs at the worksite: 1993-1995 update. *American Journal of Health Promotion, 10*(5), 380-388.

Pender, N. J. (1987). *Health promotion in nursing practice.* Norwalk, CT: Appleton & Lange.

Perry, C. L., Stone, E. J., Parcel, G. S., Ellison, R. C., Nader, P. R., Webber, L. S., & Luepker, R. V. (1990). School-based cardiovascular health promotion: The child and adolescent trial for cardiovascular health (CATCH). *Journal of School Health, 60*(8), 406-413.

Pope, A. M., Snyder, M. A., & Mood, L. H. (Eds.). (1995). *Nursing, health, and environment.* [Institute of Medicine]. Washington, DC: National Academy Press.

Pruitt, R. H. (1992). Effectiveness and cost efficiency of interventions in health promotion. *Journal of Advanced Nursing, 17,* 926-932.

Pruitt, R. H., Bernheim, C., & Tomlinson, J. P. (1991). Stress management in a military health promotion program: Effectiveness and cost efficiency. *Military Medicine, 156,* 51-53.

Rosen, R. (1991). *The healthy company: Eight strategies to develop people, productivity and profits.* Los Angeles: Tarcher.

Scopa, M. (1993). Comparison of classroom instruction and independnt study in body mechanics. *Journal of Continuing Education in Nursing, 24*(4), 170-173.

Sherman, J. B., Clark, L., & McEwen, M. M. (1989). Evaluation of a worksite wellness program: Impact on exercise, weight, smoking, and stress. *Public Health Nursing, 6,* 114-119.

Shi, L. (1992). The impact of increasing intensity of health promotion intervention on risk reduction. *Evaluation and the Health Professions, 15*(4), 3-25.

Shi, L. (1993). A cost-benefit analysis of a California county's back injury prevention program. *Public Health Reports, 108,* 204-211.

Shipley, R. H., Orleans, C. T., Wilbur, C. S., Piserchia, P. V., & McFadden, D. W. (1988). Effect of the Johnson & Johnson Live for Life® program on employee smoking. *Preventive Medicine, 17,* 25-34.

Sirles, A. T., Brown, K., & Hilyer, J. C. (1991). Effects of back school education and exercise in back injured municipal workers. *American Association of Occupational Health Nurses Journal, 39,* 7-12.

Tully, S. (1995, June 12). Managing: America's healthiest companies. *Fortune,* pp. 98-106.

U.S. Department of Health and Human Services, Public Health Service (1979). *Healthy people: The surgeon general's report on health promotion and disease prevention* (DHEW [PHS] Pub. No. 79-55071). Washington, DC: U.S. Government Printing Office.

U.S. Department of Health and Human Services, Public Health Service. (1980, Fall). *Promoting health/preventing disease: Objectives for the nation.* Washington, DC: U.S. Government Printing Office.

U.S. Department of Health and Human Services, Public Health Service. (1991). *Healthy people 2000: National health promotion and disease prevention objectives* (DHHS Pub. No. PHS 91-50212). Washington, DC: U.S. Government Printing Office.

U.S. Department of Health and Human Services, Public Health Service. (1993). 1992 national survey of worksite health promotion activities: Summary. *American Journal of Health Promotion, 7,* 452-464.

Warner, K. E., Wickizer, T. M., Wolfe, R. A., Schildroth, J. E., & Samuelson, M. H. (1988). Economic implications of workplace health promotion programs: Review of the literature. *Journal of Occupation Medicine, 30,* 106-112.

Weissberg, R. P., & Elias, M. J. (1993). Enhancing young people's social competence and health behavior: An important challenge for educators, scientists, policymakers, and funders. *Applied and Preventive Psychology, 2,* 179-190.

Wilbur, C. S. (1983). The Johnson & Johnson Program. *Preventive Medicine, 12,* 672-681.

Workplace injuries. (1991, November). *Atlanta Journal.*

Yearbook of Labour Statistics, (1995). Nos. 1 & 29, 54th ed. Geneva: International Labour Office.

PART
IIE

BIOBEHAVIORAL MANIFESTATIONS
OF HEALTH AND ILLNESS

Ada M. Lindsey
Joan L. F. Shaver

The six chapters in this section on biobehavioral manifestations of health and illness address the current state of nursing science and the clinical knowledge that has evolved for practice application. Each chapter also provides direction of future work required to advance the science.

In Chapter 19, "Management of Mobility and Altered Physical Activity," Barbara Smith and Mary MacVicar provide evidence of the importance of mobility and capacity for physical activity as outcome indicators for disease and illness recovery. With the more than 35 million Americans estimated to experience some functional limitations, and with the associated economic costs, nursing research has considerable potential to have an impact on this population. With an increasingly aging population and the concurrent increases in comorbidities, higher rates of functional decline are anticipated. Although interventions to improve physical activity are within the scope of nursing practice, some of these interventions do

not have sufficient empirical evidence to demonstrate their effectiveness. Smith and MacVicar suggest that intervention studies are needed to identify the physiological interactions of exercise and specific disease and treatment characteristics in particular patient populations.

Carrieri-Kohlman and Janson provide an overview of the science underpinning the management of dyspnea. Their review includes nursing research that has focused on theoretical models guiding the study of dyspnea, on the measurement of dyspnea, on factors or correlates of dyspnea, and on the management of dyspnea. Although the prevalence of dyspnea is not reported specifically, it is often a presenting symptom in pulmonary and heart disease, and is seen frequently in terminally ill patients. The authors acknowledge that nurse researchers have been leaders in studying descriptions of the sensation of dyspnea, the correlates of dyspnea, and in the development of measures of dyspnea. They suggest a number of areas for future study to strengthen the science.

Managing pain is described in the chapter by Ferrell as being integral to nursing practice; she acknowledges that pain is viewed as being a critical feature in chronic, acute, and terminal illness. As pain is a common clinical phenomenon, determining the effectiveness of interventions for the management of pain is considered a priority for nursing research. Ferrell describes the theoretical approaches used to guide pain research and reviews recent work by the Agency for Health Care Policy and Research and the National Institute of Nursing Research Priority Expert Panel on Symptom Management in synthesizing current work on pain management. Nursing research in the 1970s is credited with providing seminal efforts in contributing to the current advances in pain management. Ferrell suggests that future work is needed to address the management of pain in vulnerable populations and that more intervention studies are essential to advance the state of the science.

Dougherty and Jensen provide a review on the research base for managing urinary and fecal incontinence in adults. They acknowledge that the work in this field over the past two decades has provided support for improved nursing practice. Efforts of nurse researchers in the synthesis of current knowledge and development of clinical practice guidelines for urinary incontinence under the auspices of the Agency for Health Care Policy and Research are recognized. The authors include work on epidemiology and costs, present a revised paradigm of incontinence, and focus on clinical nursing research that has examined management strategies for incontinence. Less research has been completed on fecal incontinence, but the authors suggest that much research on urinary incontinence is at a state where it can be used to guide nursing practice. However, Dougherty and Jensen make a case that incontinence is underreported and undiagnosed, and there is inconsistent use of approaches that have been shown to be efficient in managing incontinence.

In "Managing Sleep and Waking Behaviors and the Symptom of Fatigue," Shaver recognizes that the quality and timing of sleep can have an impact on health and wellness and that fatigue may be an indicator of the quality of sleep/wake patterns. These manifestations are viewed from a biobehavioral science perspective in the review of research organized by design, populations studied, measures used, and conceptual basis. Shaver summarizes the state of the science as still being formulary, particularly in relation to sleep in disease and illness states. Understanding interventions for fatigue remains less clear, especially when fatigue is associated with particular disease and illness states. Shaver suggests that interdisciplinary research will be useful; however, she recognizes these phenomena as being of central interest to clinical nurse scientists.

Heitkemper reviews nursing research contributing to the understanding of nausea, vomiting, and anorexia. These symptoms, frequently experienced by individuals across the age span, are distressing side effects of some treatments and are assessed and managed in nursing practice. However, Heitkemper reports that little empirical work has been done to guide nursing therapies. The majority of nursing research in this field has been descriptive. However, a knowledge base about risk factors for symptom development and use of self-care strategies is emerging. Research has also included the development of instruments to quantify the symptom experience. Future efforts need to address the effectiveness of therapeutic interventions, including attention to person and environmental factors.

It is apparent from these six chapters that the state of the science dealt with in each requires more research to guide practice. Progress in some areas, such as management of pain and management of urinary incontinence, does provide a science base for some interventions. These reviews can serve to direct the next generation of studies necessary to advance the science base for practice.

19

MANAGEMENT OF MOBILITY AND ALTERED PHYSICAL ACTIVITY

Barbara Smith
Mary MacVicar

Introduction

Within the last decade, mobility and the capacity for physical activity have taken on increasing importance as indicators of outcomes related to disease and illness recovery. Functional loss occurs with many acute and chronic illnesses, although the more severe limitations are usually associated with cardiovascular, neuromuscular, and skeletal pathologies (Pope & Tarlov, 1991). Symptoms associated with some diseases and disease treatments, such as pain, nausea, and fatigue, are factors that may further alter mobility and physical activity. Advances in biomedical therapies and technology, although they have increased longevity, have also contributed to

an expanding population of physically impaired individuals. Examples are the recent advances in the treatment of HIV infection and associated opportunistic infections. New therapies have increased the life expectancy of infected individuals; however, symptoms related to these therapies cause them to live with challenges to their quality of life (Lenderking et al., 1994).

In the early 1990s, it was estimated that more than 35 million individuals in the United States experienced some degree of functional limitation (including problems associated with altered mobility and physical activity or activity intolerance), with economic costs calculated to be about 7% of the gross national product. The lowest incidence of activity limitations were in those under 18 years of age (10%) and the highest in women over 70 years (62%) (Pope & Tarlov, 1991; Task Force Report, 1990). African Americans experience activity limitations at a slightly higher rate than other racial groups, and there is an inverse relationship between activity limitations and family income (Pope & Tarlov, 1991; Task Force Report, 1990). There is every expectation that the occurrence of altered mobility and physical activity and the associated cost will increase in concert with an aging population. Comorbidities that increase with age and pharmacological treatments for many chronic diseases will contribute to higher rates of functional decline. Limitations in mobility and physical activity are associated with greater dependence upon family members, greater need for home services, and more admissions to hospitals and nursing homes (Boaz & Muller, 1994; Williams, Phillips, Torner, & Irvine, 1990).

In light of current economic and political pressures toward managed care with an emphasis on cost containment, it is expected that resources could become scarcer for those people with mobility and physical activity challenges (Lubeck & Yelin, 1988; Pope & Tarlov, 1991). Access to restorative and rehabilitation services will be more stringent and will require predictions of the functional levels that patients can expect to attain from a given intervention, at a given cost (Hoffman & Heller, 1995). There are pressures now for severely disabled individuals to receive rehabilitation treatments over a shorter period of time than previously (Johnston & Hall, 1994). Individuals without medically defined physical impairments or individuals with physical activity limitations and marginal mobility might not be considered for restorative training or rehabilitation services and therefore could be at risk for losing functional independence. Payers will be interested in interventions that exhibit decreased need for hospitalization, attendant care, and supportive services (Banja & Johnston, 1994).

Nurses are well prepared to respond to the challenge of providing appropriate restorative training and rehabilitation within a managed care environment. Although interventions aimed at improving mobility and increasing physical activity are within the scope of nursing practice, many nursing interventions lack the scientific underpinnings or empirical evidence necessary to document the desired outcomes. This chapter contains an overview of the concepts of mobility, impaired mobility, physical activity, activity intolerance, and related concepts; a review

and critique of the existing nursing research on mobility and physical activity; and an overview of the state of the science of mobility and physical activity research, with suggestions for future directions for nursing research.

Mobility, Physical Activity, Activity Intolerance, and Related Concepts

Although mobility and activity are related, there are important differences between the two phenomena that must be considered for research and practice. It is possible to be mobile but have little tolerance for sustained movement or physical activity. Conversely, physical activity is possible with significant mobility constraints, given appropriate prostheses and adaptive equipment. From a nursing perspective, *mobility* is defined as the ability to move freely within an environment (Cox et al., 1993). *Physical activity* refers to the capacity for sustained movement, typically involving the use of large muscle groups with increasing energy expenditure (Wilmore & Costill, 1994). This capability is needed to perform instrumental activities of daily living; that is, an expanded role in the home, in the community, and at work (Leon, 1989; Spector, Sidney, Murphy, & Fulton, 1987).

Carpenito (1997, p. 565) defines *impaired physical mobility* as a "state in which the individual experiences, or is at risk of experiencing, limitation of physical movement but is not immobile." Cox et al. (1997, p. 362) define it similarly as "a limitation of ability for independent movement." Carpenito defines *activity intolerance* as "a reduction in one's physiological capacity to endure activities to the degree desired or required" (p. 103). Cox et al. (1997) states that activity intolerance can result from reduced psychological, as well as physiological energy. Additionally, Cox et al. (1997) carefully differentiate between impaired mobility and activity intolerance. They point out that the nursing diagnosis of impaired mobility *without activity intolerance* (italics are the authors') implies that patients could move independently if "something were not limiting the motion." Conversely, the nursing diagnosis of activity intolerance *without impaired mobility* (italics are the authors') implies that individuals are freely mobile but unable to endure increased levels of movement or activity. Interventions aimed at improving mobility must focus on improving muscle strength, flexibility, balance, and coordination (Kottke, 1990b, 1990c). Physical activity, with its emphasis on sustained movement, may include the elements of mobility but also requires adequate cardiopulmonary endurance. Therefore, interventions aimed at improving physical activity tolerance must be focused on cardiopulmonary endurance through aerobic conditioning.

Strength is defined as the maximum force that can be generated by a muscle. It is closely related to muscular endurance, which is the ability of the muscle to perform repetitive movements. Improvements in strength are effected by overloading the muscle that is to be strengthened. Work with less weight and more repetitions trains slow-twitch oxidative fibers, produces an improvement in muscular endurance but does not produce much of an increase in strength. Higher intensity workouts with fewer repetitions train fast-twitch fibers, and produce the best chance for an increase in strength (Arheim & Prentice, 1993).

Flexibility refers to the range of joint motion and is influenced by the bones, muscles, tendons, and ligaments surrounding the joints. To improve flexibility, it is important to increase the extensibility of the muscles, tendons, and ligaments surrounding the joints. Flexibility can be enhanced using several stretching techniques. Static stretching is accomplished by stretching to the point of discomfort and then holding the stretch for several seconds (Brooks, Fahey, & White, 1996). More recently, a technique of alternating muscle contractions and stretching has been advocated. Ballistic stretching (repetitive bouncing or lunging while stretching) has fallen out of favor because the possibility of exceeding the functional extensibility of the muscle makes injuries more likely.

Balance and the coordination of ambulation represent complex phenomena. *Coordination* refers to the activation of one set of muscles, with concurrent inhibition of others (Kisner & Colby, 1990), to achieve relatively even and controlled movement. Assuming an intact nervous system, *balance*, body position, and motion all depend on adequate sensory and proprioceptive input from muscles, joints, tendons, and visual cues that serve as input to structures within the cerebellum that coordinate agonists and antagonists, adjust muscle tension, and correct position and movements (Schmitz, 1994; Van Wynsberghe, Noback, & Carola, 1995). The motor pattern that is essential for coordination is developed by repeating particular movements until a given activity can occur without conscious thought. Slow repetitive motion facilitates development of neuromuscular repatterning.

Once there is evidence that the activity can be performed with less mental concentration, that is, the task has become more automatic, the repetitions can be accelerated (Kottke, 1990b). Consider learning how to swing a golf club or how to ski. The movements of beginning golfers or skiers are uncoordinated compared to the almost effortless golf swing or ski run of professionals.

Aerobic exercise, strength training, and flexibility exercise are at the core of restorative training interventions. The production of energy for muscle activity requires high energy phosphate compounds. The energy release from the breakdown of these compounds can use oxygen (aerobic) or can occur without oxygen (anaerobic). Energy production without oxygen can provide energy for only 10 to 15 seconds when phosphocreatine is broken down, or 2 minutes when glucose is the substrate (Krisanda, Moreland, & Kushmerick, 1988). These pathways are used in sudden, highly intense exercise and are best improved through highly intense, short bursts of activity, such as sprint training. To persist in any sustained physical activity for longer than 2 to 3 minutes, an individual must generate large amounts of energy from the breakdown of carbohydrates and fats in the presence of oxygen (aerobic metabolism). The relative contribution of aerobic and anaerobic energy production depends upon the nature and intensity of the activity performed, and both are important to initiating and sustaining activity.

Exercise leading to improvements in aerobic power involves the rhythmic contraction of large muscle groups over a sustained period of time. This activity brings about central changes (increased stroke volume, decreased heart rate) and peripheral changes (increases in skeletal muscle mitochondria, increases in mitochondrial oxidative enzymes). Peripheral changes, which result in increased arterial/venous oxygen differences, are what account for training specificity. That is, if you train by walking, you bring about adaptations in the skeletal muscles associated with walking. If you train by cycling, you train only those muscles associated with cycling. Thus it is important to test the subjects in the same manner in which you trained them.

There has been an effort to make conceptual and clinical distinctions between disease-related and disuse or restricted-use functional limitations. Disease and disuse both represent deviations from normal physiological states and together have a cumulative effect, in some cases causing more severe functional limitations than would be caused by disease or disuse alone. In the late 1960s and 1970s, most individuals who experienced even an uncomplicated myocardial infarction were bed rested for several days to a week and hospitalized for several more days, up to 3 weeks. Clinicians believed their fatigue was due to the infarction, when in fact it was more likely due to the profound activity restriction. Traditionally viewed with skepticism by many health care professionals, impairments associated with prolonged disuse or a chronically sedentary lifestyle are gaining legitimacy. There is increasing recognition that physiological changes associated with disuse or sedentariness can tilt the scale toward more fragile, vulnerable physical and mental health states (Itoh & Lee, 1990; Leblanc et al., 1992; Vorhies & Riley, 1993). Functional decline can also accompany psychiatric disorders and the use of psychotropic medications. Older adults, especially, are at risk for increased functional loss, which threatens their independence.

The exact relationship between length of inactive time and level of activity intolerance (decreased cardiopulmonary endurance) is not clear from present studies. However, changes can be prevented or minimized to the extent permitted by the underlying disease, its treatment, and personal factors such as age, prior fitness level, genetic predisposition, and lifestyle habits. In general, disuse of large muscle groups will create more severe physiological changes in a shorter time, eventually affecting all organ systems and compounding the consequences of the primary disease (Vorhies & Riley, 1993). Halar and Bell (1990), citing earlier studies, estimated a decline in strength associated with bed rest to be between 13% and 15% per week, with a 50% loss by the 4th and 5th weeks of bed rest.

There is evidence that physical abilities decline in a predictable sequence (Itoh & Lee, 1990). Limited mobility can be observed earliest in the muscles of the lower extremities (those needed to overcome gravitational force), with postural instability indicated by poor balance and diminished coordination. This is followed by a decline in strength of the shoulder girdle muscles and biceps. With prolonged disuse, myogenic and connective tissue tightness can be detected, and without intervention, contractures develop. The capacity for sustained activity (endurance) is lost as a result of cardiopulmonary insufficiency secondary to decreased cardiac output, a corresponding drop in oxygen consumption, other ventilatory problems, and a decrease in skeletal muscle oxidative enzymes (Wenger, 1984). With continued disuse, decreased muscle contractibility; decreased bone density; autonomic lability; sensory motor deficits; and metabolic dysfunction such as insulin resistance, fluid and electrolyte imbalance, and changes in protein and carbohydrate metabolism are evident (Haller & Bell, 1990).

In a model for explaining the relationships between disease or pathology, impairment, functional limitations, and disability, Nagi (1969) postulated that disease or pathology involves mobilization of the body's defense systems and is characterized by objective signs and subjective symptoms that change over the course of the disease and its treatments. Impairments, whether temporary or permanent, are those disease-, treatment- or disuse-induced losses or abnormalities of the anatomy, physiology, or neurocognitive systems (e.g., organ removal, interrupted neural pathways, cardiopulmonary and metabolic defects, limited joint mechanics, decline in cognitive skills, negative affective states, and depression). Severity of impairments varies according to the underlying pathology, the systems affected, existence of comorbidities, and whether the underlying pathology is arrested, controlled, or progressive. Functional limitations become evident as the individual loses the ability to perform tasks or activities as they are normally performed by most people. There is a spectrum of functional limitations, from highly visible limitations, such as amputation of a limb or paralysis, to the more insidious limitations from diseases affecting the oxygen transport and energy-generating systems. When impairments are permanent, either as an inevitable consequence of the pathology or from lack of appropriate and timely intervention, functional limitations may result in disability. Disability is the difference between actual level of performance in a specific role and the social and cultural expectations of what constitutes appropriate performance of the role. Personal perceptions of disease and impairment, perceptions and reactions of significant others, the environment, and other psychosocial factors influence whether individuals are or become disabled (Granger, 1984; Guccione, 1994; Nagi, 1969, 1976; Pope & Tarlov, 1991).

Nursing Research Related to Mobility and Physical Activity

The initial strategy used to identify nursing research related to mobility and physical activity was a search of the past 10 years of both CINAHL and Medline using the keywords *mobility, physical activity, exercise, work performance, exertion, functional capacity, functional status, flexibility, strength, balance, endurance, self-care activities, impairment,* and *disability.* This search strategy resulted in over 21,000 articles by investigators across multiple disciplines, indicating a flourishing multidisciplinary interest in mobility, physical activity, and related areas. It was impossible to identify the studies that were conducted by nurses unless they were in traditional nursing journals or written by individuals known to the chapter authors. Therefore, the search was restricted to CINAHL, searching on the CD-Plus database using the keywords *mobility* and *physical activity.* The studies reviewed in this chapter covered the period from 1985 through 1996 and included all ages and disease categories. The selection of these dates permitted a comparison of nursing research prior to and after the Eighth Conference on the Classification of Nursing Diagnosis, in which characteristics of impaired physical mobility were defined (Creason, 1991). The search identified 142 citations, most of descriptive or correlational studies. The following review is based on the small number of intervention studies identified from the 142 citations.

Mobility Studies

Eight nursing studies related to improving alterations in one or more elements of mobility related to ambulation and one study involving finger and hand mobility were identified and reviewed. Seven of the eight ambulation-related studies tested protocols on community-dwelling elderly or elderly nursing home residents. In five of the studies, plus the finger and hand mobility study, stretching and flexibility exercises or resistance exercise were used. Three used walking protocols.

One study used an acute bout of exercise (i.e., a single exercise session) to assess the effects of range of motion and flexibility exercises on cognitive performance and independence in 20 cognitively impaired, institutionalized elderly using a pretest-posttest experimental design. Pre- and posttest results indicated that recall was improved for at least 30 minutes. No measure of improved independence was provided, and long-term effects were not examined (Dawe & Moore-Orr, 1995).

In another study, a 4-week program of lifting ankle weights to strengthen the quadriceps (thigh muscles) was tested for improvement of mobility, balance, gait velocity, and functional health status in 20 older adults, using a pretest-posttest design. An increase in the strength of the quadriceps as measured by an isokinetic dynamometer

and an increase in the number of pounds lifted at posttest were reported. In addition, the length of time necessary to complete a timed test was reduced, and subjects reported more confidence in walking, climbing stairs, and getting up from a chair (Noble, Salcido, Walker, Atchinson, & Marshall, 1994).

Using a two-group design, Hurwitz (1989) evaluated the effectiveness of a head-to-toe range of motion exercise protocol that was outlined in a manual for individuals with Parkinson's disease in improving self-care skills in 30 older adults with Parkinson's disease. Compared to controls, the experimental subjects showed improvements in recent memory, continence, and feeding habits following 1 year of participation in the protocol. Whether the subjects were randomly assigned or self-selected was not stated.

The effects of an 8-week stretching and lower extremity strength training protocol on balance, perception of balance, flexibility, and lower extremity strength in 47 elders who lived in senior housing complexes was tested using a pretest-posttest design. Physical activity journals were used to record subject self-report of compliance with the exercise protocol and other physical activities. Objective measures were made for ankle and knee flexion using a goniometer, and a hand-held manual muscle tester was used to evaluate muscle strength. Significant improvements in ankle flexibility and right knee flexibility were reported; however, no significant differences were found between the control and treatment groups on strength or balance (Mills, 1994).

The effects on balance and gait velocity of a 12-week strength training protocol was tested in a group of 63 community-dwelling elders with a pretest-posttest design. Surgical tubings of varying thickness were used to provide increments of resistance. One of the three weekly exercise sessions was supervised. Although results favored the experimental subjects, there were no statistically significant differences between groups on dependent measures (Topp, Mikesky, Wigglesworth, Holt, & Edwards, 1993).

The final study that used stretching and flexibility exercises or resistance exercise did so to improve hand and finger mobility, not ambulation. The effect of evening hand and finger exercises on elastic stiffness and metacarpophalangeal joint mobility was studied in 30 individuals diagnosed with rheumatoid arthritis using a nonexperimental, one-group design. Findings indicated significant improvement in finger mobility when the exercises were done the evening prior to testing. There was a correlation between subjective and objective arthrographic measures of stiffness (Byers, 1985).

In terms of walking protocols to improve mobility, a 6-week walking protocol, using age-adjusted heart rate to regulate exercise intensity, was tested for effects on balance and perceptions of balance in 52 elderly men and women using a comparative two-group design. There were significant differences between controls and experimental subjects on balance (time able to maintain different stances that challenge balance) but not on perception of balance (Roberts, 1989). A 12-week walking protocol to examine the effects on balance, mobility, and incontinence was tested using a pretest-posttest design with a single group of 15 cognitively impaired nursing home residents. No change in balance or walking speed was observed; however, the residents were able to walk an average of 23 additional feet following the 12-week program. The investigators also reported that daytime, but not overall, continence was improved (Jirovec, 1991).

Strengths and Weaknesses in Mobility Studies Reviewed

Conceptual definitions and theoretical links. A number of nurse-authored concept papers incorporated aspects of critical differences between mobility and activity (Catanzaro, 1993; Glick, 1992; Ouellet & Rush, 1992; Rush & Ouellet, 1993), but these distinctions were not made in some of the studies reviewed. However, what was most troublesome was that some studies did not carefully link the intervention and the outcome variables. For example, Dawe and Moore-Orr (1995) used one session of range of motion exercise to improve cognitive function. Although there have been some studies that have documented improvements in psychological variables such as depression and anxiety with aerobic training (10 to 12 weeks), these investigators did not provide the reader with evidence that links range of motion exercises with improved cognitive function. Roberts (1989) used walking to improve balance and perception of balance. Given the possible causes of balance disorders, walking would not be expected to improve balance.

Jirovec (1991) used walking to improve continence. Exercises that have demonstrated effectiveness in improving continence are exercises of pelvic floor musculature that is of an appropriate intensity and duration. No link was made for how walking might improve this variable.

Additionally, there are misunderstandings about which exercise interventions improve which functions. For example, Mills (1994) identifies her intervention as low-level aerobic exercise (which is generally used to increase cardiovascular endurance) but actually describes strength and flexibility exercises aimed at improving mobility. Certainly, the exercise she describes uses energy that is derived through aerobic metabolism; however, the primary purpose of the exercise she describes is to improve strength and balance, both elements of mobility, not aerobic power.

Methods (design). The studies reviewed varied considerably in study design. Three studies reviewed under "Mobility" used a single-group, nonexperimental design (Byers, 1985; Jirovec, 1991; Nobel et al., 1994). Threats to the internal validity of studies using a single-group design leave them open to criticism. Of the remaining mobility intervention studies, three equalized the groups by employing random assignment (Dawe & Moore-Orr, 1995; Hurwitz, 1989; Topp et al., 1993); others did not, allowing subjects to self-select the group or assigning the intervention by place of residence. Thus, only three of the eight studies reviewed may have had adequate controls over competing explanations for the data. Also, none of the eight studies related to mobility provided adequate information, from pilot work or the literature, for the reader to determine the adequacy of the sample size. Because many studies reported small samples, sample size may account for the investigators' inability to detect a difference between the groups in some studies.

Methods (intervention or independent variable). The exercise intervention studies varied dramatically by mode (type) of exercise used (finger and hand range of motion, whole-body range of motion, strength and flexibility, exercise using surgical bands of varying resistance, and walking). Still other exercise interventions were not described in a way that one could readily replicate the study. Further, they differed in the frequency of exercise sessions (one time per week to daily), duration of the individual exercise sessions (from a few minutes to 90 minutes), and overall duration or length of the intervention. Two studies examined subjects before and after a single bout of exercise (Byers, 1985; Dawe et al., 1995); other investigators trained subjects from 3 weeks to 12 months.

Some investigators relied on subjects' self-report that they had exercised at an appropriate intensity, frequency, and duration to bring about the desired physical adaptations to exercise (Topp et al., 1993). Other investigators did not adequately address the principle that for physiological adaptation to occur, the appropriate muscles must be overloaded or stressed, and this overloading must occur throughout the training period for continued adaptation to occur (Hurwitz, 1989; Topp et al., 1993).

Jirovec (1991) used a walking program to improve speed of walking, walking distance, balance, and ability to rise from a chair. She reported an improvement in distance walked (possibly indicating improved aerobic power, thus cardiovascular endurance) but no change in walking speed, balance, or ability to rise from a chair. It should have come as no surprise that balance and ability to rise from a chair were not changed, as walking would not be expected to improve either of these elements of mobility. Strength and flexibility exercises, targeting appropriate muscle groups and joints, would be necessary to improve these two variables. Exercise interventions, to be effective, must be targeted at the appropriate deficits.

In several studies, the training period was too brief (6 weeks or less) to attain the results sought (Byers, 1985; Nobel et al., 1994; Roberts, 1989). Resistive exercise (weight or strength training) produces initial improvement due to more efficient recruitment of motor units, but muscular hypertrophy (or an actual adaptation of the skeletal muscle to overload) occurs after a longer period of time (8 to 10 weeks) and represents a true increase in strength. Appropriate length of training times must be followed to bring about the desired physiological adaptation in strength.

Measurement (dependent variables). Some investigators reported precise measurement of the dependent variables through the use of state-of-the-art measurement techniques and stringent control of testing conditions. Only Nobel et al. (1994) used an isokinetic dynamometer to precisely measure improvements in muscle strength. Other investigators used field tests or intuitively appealing clinical tools that do not have a great deal of precision. For example, Topp and colleagues (1993) found no significant differences in gait velocity or balance following a 12-week dynamic resistive exercise training. Was the intervention not successful because the intervention was not appropriate, or were the investigators unable to detect a difference because they did not use a more precise laboratory measurement of balance and gait velocity?

Due to the myriad of measures used in the reviewed studies, psychological outcomes related to exercise were inconsistent and difficult to evaluate. Consistent use of well-known, thoroughly evaluated instruments measuring depression, anxiety, moods, quality of life, and other psychological outcomes must be employed.

Physical Activity Studies

In seven nursing intervention studies, a variety of aerobic exercise modes including cycle ergometry, treadmill, or aerobic dance were tested for improvement of cardiovascular endurance or other physical variables responsive to aerobic conditioning. Four studies employing inspiratory muscle training to improve cardiopulmonary endurance and pulmonary function are also reported.

Cycle ergometry was used to compare low and moderate aerobic exercise intensity levels on psychosocial variables (well-being, life satisfaction, health promotion, mental status) and physiological variables (maximal oxygen consumption [VO$_2$ max], resting, and submaximum and maximum heart rates and blood pressures) in 72 community-dwelling, healthy elders. Despite careful exercise prescription, both high and low intensity groups improved on most measures (Stevenson & Topp, 1990), with slight advantages gained by those with high attendance and effort scores in both groups (Topp & Stevenson, 1994).

A 12-week aerobic and strength training protocol was tested for effects on muscle mass, strength, and endurance in eight renal transplant subjects receiving corticosteroids. The protocol permitted subjects to select the mode of aerobic activity: treadmill walking or jogging, cycling, or walking. Outcomes indicated no significant differences between controls and experimental subjects (Leasure, Belknap, Burks, & Schlegel, 1995).

Cycle ergometry was used as the mode of exercise in a group of 24 Stage II breast cancer subjects, using maximal oxygen uptake as an indicator of functional capacity. Experimental subjects showed significant increases in maximal oxygen consumption over control subjects (MacVicar, Winningham, & Nickel, 1989). Additionally, experimental subjects did not gain as much weight as the control subjects and skinfold measurements revealed a small increase in lean mass versus fat mass (Winningham, MacVicar, Bondec, Anderson, & Minton, 1989).

Two types of aerobic dance exercise were used to assess effects on women's weight and indicators of physical fitness (VO$_2$, blood pressure, glucose, body composition, total cholesterol, HDL cholesterol, total cholesterol/HDL cholesterol ratio, endurance, and flexibility).

Pre- to posttest comparisons were based on treadmill testing, and both groups showed significant improvement in VO_2 max or oxygen uptake at maximal work. Differences in weight between groups were not significant (Gillett & Eisenman, 1987).

One study documented the benefits of a walking exercise program combined with support group meetings on performance status, a 12-minute-mile field test, psychosocial adjustment, and symptom intensity in 14 female breast cancer patients using a two-group quasiexperimental design (Mock et al., 1994). Distance walked in 12 minutes improved by 68 meters, which was statistically significant. Because of the use of both walking and a support group, the authors were unable to attribute the change solely to activity. Additionally, the number of chemotherapy cycles was considerably higher in the usual care group than in the treatment group and may explain the increased symptom burden.

A 6-week exercise program of calisthenics and low-impact movement (in-place stepping) reduced physical discomfort and depression and improved self-esteem in 58 ethnically diverse, exercising, pregnant, adolescent subjects when compared to nonexercising pregnant adolescents (Koniak-Griffin, 1994).

One investigator compared the effects of teaching, treadmill testing, and exercise training verses teaching and treadmill testing versus usual care on self-efficacy and the activity levels in 40 cardiac patients using a three-group design. Self-efficacy and activity performance improved for all groups, with the highest scores achieved by the group that received exercise training (Gulanick, 1991).

Improving ventilatory function and physical functioning (as measured by time on treadmill and 12-minute walks) through inspiratory muscle training in individuals with a chronic respiratory disease was the focus of four studies. Sawyer summarized the effects of 10 weeks of inspiratory muscle training on 20 children with cystic fibrosis. Pre- and posttest symptom-limited treadmill exercise tests showed significant gains in cardiopulmonary endurance (VO_2 max), vital capacity, and total lung capacity in those children who participated in the high-pressure load versus low-pressure load training (Sawyer & Clanton, 1993).

Investigators in another study compared the effects of 12 weeks of high- and low-resistance inspiratory muscle training in 20 subjects with COPD. Dependent variables included inspiratory muscle strength and endur-

ance, incremental inspiratory threshold loading, and the 12-minute distance walk. Subjects in both groups demonstrated significant improvement in inspiratory muscle strength, inspiratory muscle endurance, and distance walked in 12 minutes, but there were no significant differences in the effects of high- or low-resistance-level training (Preusser, Winningham, & Clanton, 1994).

Gift and Austin (1992) compared levels of depression and dyspnea in 10 subjects enrolled in the American Lung Association's program of systematic very-low-intensity movement with those of 10 subjects who were not enrolled in the program. Those who participated in the program reported lower levels of depression and less severe dyspnea than nonparticipants, and these differences were present at baseline and 8 weeks.

In another inspiratory muscle training study, 67 subjects with COPD were randomly assigned to either an inspiratory muscle or "sham" training group. Dependent variables included maximal inspiratory pressure, respiratory muscle endurance time, dyspnea, and health-related functional impairments. The 6 months of training involved using an inspiratory training device, with experimental subjects using a high-pressure load and control subjects receiving sham training (using light inspiratory pressure load). The subjects in both the experimental treatment and sham training groups improved on the dependent variables, but there were no significant differences between the groups (Kim et al., 1993).

Strengths and Weaknesses in Physical Activity Studies Reviewed

As in mobility, much of the nursing research related to physical activity and activity intolerence is descriptive. This descriptive work was an important step, but more intervention studies are needed to advance the science and explore this phenomenon from a nursing perspective.

Methods (design). Generally, the studies reviewed varied in the types of study design and the precision of the methods. All of the studies reviewed under physical activity used at least a two-group design. Most study investigators equalized the groups by employing random assignment; however, two studies did not, allowing subjects to self-select (Gift & Austin, 1992; Koniak-Griffin, 1994). These two studies may not have had adequate controls over competing explanations for the data. Also, of the reviewed studies, most did not provide adequate information from pilot work or the literature for the reader to determine the adequacy of the sample size. Because many studies reported small samples, sample size may account for some studies not being able to detect differences between the groups in key dependent variables.

Methods (intervention or independent variable). The exercise intervention studies varied dramatically by mode (type) of exercise used and included walking, treadmill walk or jog, cycling, or aerobic dance, and some of the studies allowed subjects to select the mode of exercise from a menu. Further, they differed in the frequency of exercise sessions, duration of the individual exercise sessions (from a few minutes to 90 minutes), and overall duration or length of the intervention (investigators trained subjects from 3 weeks to 12 months). In the studies comparing low-intensity (sham) and higher intensity inspiratory muscle exercise, the duration varied from 10 weeks (Sawyer & Clanton, 1993) to 6 months (Kim et al., 1993).

Some investigators relied on subjects' self-report that they exercised at an appropriate intensity, frequency, and duration to bring about the desired physical adaptations to exercise; however, some investigators rigorously controlled and monitored aerobic exercise (intervention) protocols (MacVicar et al., 1989; Gillett & Eisenman, 1987; Stevenson & Topp, 1990). The interventions in these well-controlled studies also used national standards, such as those published by the American College of Sports Medicine, American Heart Association, and so on. These same studies used individually prescribed exercise (mode, intensity, frequency, duration, and progression) and took into account the principle that for physiological adaptation to occur, the corresponding system must be overloaded or stressed. That is, if a person wants to improve aerobic power (thus cardiovascular endurance), the person must engage in aerobic exercise at a level that will overload the appropriate biochemical pathways.

Kim and colleagues (1993), Preusser et al. (1994), and Sawyer and Clanton (1993) reported devising protocols that were of the appropriate mode of exercise to bring about changes in inspiratory muscles. Gillett and Eisenman (1987), MacVicar et al. (1989), and Stevenson and Topp (1990) used appropriate modes of exercise to bring about improvements in aerobic power. However, some investigators seemed to confuse exercise protocols.

As mentioned earlier when addressing mobility related research, Mills (1994) identified her intervention as low-level aerobic exercise but actually described strength and flexibility exercises aimed at improving mobility. Jirovec (1991) used a walking program to improve speed of walking, walking distance, balance, and ability to rise from a chair. She reported an improvement in distance walked but no change in walking speed, balance, or ability to rise from a chair.

In several reports the training periods were too brief to attain significant physiological results. Although some studies reported an improvement in psychological variables, without a biological marker of training (and in the absence of an appropriate control group) it is not possible to attribute the change to exercise. Gift examined subjects already enrolled in a pulmonary exercise program at baseline and 8 weeks and compared them to a group who chose not to exercise. Besides the self-selection bias that existed, 8 weeks is insufficient time to bring about physiological adaptation in this population. Koniak-Griffin (1994) exercised pregnant adolescents twice each week for 6 weeks. Gulanick (1991) examined subjects at 4 and 9 weeks following a cardiac event. Research has shown that individuals with coronary artery disease require much longer exercise training to bring about sought after physiological change. Guidelines such as those advanced by the American College of Sports Medicine (1995) suggest that 10 to 12 weeks are necessary to bring about the appropriate physiological adaptations to chronic aerobic exercise training.

Measurement (dependent variables). Some investigators reported precise measurement of the dependent variables through the use of state-of-the-art measurement techniques and stringent control of testing conditions (Gillett & Eisenman, 1987; MacVicar et al., 1989; Stevenson & Topp, 1990); others did not. Measurement of dependent variables that is not precisely controlled threatens the internal validity of the study. Kim et al. (1993), Preusser et al. (1994), and Sawyer and Clanton (1993) reported rigorous control over the pulmonary end points in their inspiratory muscle-training study, but both Kim et al. and Preusser et al. used field tests to document improvements in aerobic power and found no differences between groups. It is not known if a more precise laboratory measure, such as a graded exercise test on a motor-driven treadmill or cycle ergometer (which is also more expensive than a field test), would have allowed these investigators to detect a difference. Sawyer and Clanton used a treadmill protocol to document improvements in aerobic power but allowed their subjects to hold on to the handrails (maybe enhancing safety during the test, but compromising the measurement of oxygen uptake or aerobic power).

Although non-nurses have recommended aerobic exercise as adjunct treatment for mild to moderate depression (Morgan & Goldston, 1987; Trine & Morgan, 1995), the findings in the nursing studies reviewed have been inconsistent and difficult to interpret in light of the great variations in conceptual designs, research protocols, methods, and inadequate sample size. Nevertheless, studies of psychological and immune response to therapeutic exercise are intriguing. Additionally, some studies did not document an exercise training effect and therefore were unable to attribute the change to exercise. Consistent use of well-known, thoroughly evaluated instruments measuring depression, anxiety, moods, quality of life, and other psychological outcomes must be employed.

Although much work is needed before sufficient empirical evidence is accumulated to serve as the foundation for clinical interventions, presently reported studies have produced interesting trends, and there is every expectation that future studies will continue to build on these efforts. Certainly, there is every indication that interventions to improve mobility and cardiovascular endurance can produce functional improvements, or at the very least, prevent or minimize impairments associated with a number of diseases.

Promising Approaches to Research

Intervention studies showing the effects of a variety of different exercise protocols on elements of mobility and physical activity are needed. Most promising are a number of recent studies by nurses that explore the mechanisms of impaired mobility (Kasper, St. Pierre, Fuchs, & Garfinkel, 1995; Kasper, White, & Maxwell, 1996), mechanisms of activity intolerance (Breslin & Garoutte, 1995), and the effects of aerobic conditioning on disease or pathology (Smith et al., 1992). Although limited in number, these intervention studies also illus-

trate a shift from a mostly psychosocial focus to a biobehavioral one, using both physiological and psychosocial outcome measures.

Addressing the activity limitations of COPD patients, Breslin and Garoutte (1995) examined respiratory responses (pattern of thoracoabdominal motion, dyspnea, and diaphragm recruitment) to unsupported arm lifts in normal subjects. Findings showed an increase on all measures over baseline resting measures. Despite the small sample, focusing on a functionally specific activity to isolate the physiological mechanisms of select movement lays the groundwork for intervention research.

Another study incorporated a rat model to induce skeletal muscle atrophy and to assess cellular level changes. In separate studies, Kasper and colleagues (Kasper, McNulty, Otto, & Thomas, 1993; Kasper, St. Pierre, et al., 1995) used a rodent hind-limb suspension model to simulate the conditions of bed rest. This model prohibits hind-limb weight bearing by the rodent while permitting torso movement and eating, drinking, and grooming activities. Findings were consistent with other studies on muscle atrophy, indicating a rapid onset and progression during the first 7 days under non-weight-bearing conditions. In an earlier study, Kasper, White, et al. (1990) characterized stages of muscle recovery from weightlessness-induced atrophy, which included initial injury primarily to myofibers with macrophage infiltration, followed by myogenesis and regeneration.

There is growing evidence that aerobic exercise may result in immunomodulation, although the underlying mechanisms remain unclear. Data from studies of healthy individuals, and especially those testing interventions to improve the health status of HIV+ and AIDS patients, show that moderate aerobic exercise appears to augment the immune system's surveillance capacity, evidenced by increased circulating peripheral monocular cells, as well as enhancement of resting immune function (Baigis-Smith, Coombs, & Larson, 1994; Nash, 1994). Natural killer cells (cells with CD5+ receptors) appear particularly sensitive to aerobic exercise interventions, resulting in an increase in both the number of NK cells and their cytotoxic activity (Pederson & Ullum, 1994; Watson, 1989). For women with breast cancer, a 7-month program of moderate exercise appeared to increase NK cell activity (Peters, Lotzerich, Hiemeier, Schule, & Uhlenbruck, 1994).

Motor performance deficits observed under controlled conditions in institutionalized elderly (Glick & Swanson, 1995) showed that three variables—turn balance, face wash, and finger dexterity—were most predictive of dependence. Improvement of these skills would require therapeutic exercises to increase lower extremity and trunk strength, finger dexterity, and coordination. Another investigation documenting the relationship between motor performance and falls used a 12-month intervention to test exercise effects on balance, strength, flexibility, and coordination of older women. Test measures conducted at baseline, 22 weeks, and 12 months included leg strength, reaction time, neuromuscular control, body sway, and reported falls. Results showed significant reduction of falls in those who attended 75% or more of the exercise sessions (Lord, Ward, Williams, & Strudwick, 1995). Although descriptive in nature, these studies illustrate the benefits of probing the mechanics of movement and give some insight into the kinds of intervention protocols that could be developed and the combinations of activities that would present adequate exercise challenges.

Strategies

For nurse scientists to advance knowledge in the area of impaired mobility and activity intolerance, a number of strategies must be developed. First, it will be necessary to construct more exacting conceptual models of these two related, yet distinct, phenomena. Precise operational definitions must be constructed. For example, physical activity has been defined as any bodily movements that involve skeletal muscles and result in energy expenditure (Casperson, 1989; Casperson, Powell, & Christenson, 1985). Although subsumed under physical activity, exercise is more structured and based on a prescribed frequency duration and intensity. Exercise can improve the capacity for physical activity, but the reverse is not necessarily true.

Interventions must be carefully tailored to the specific problem or impairments. For example, mobility has a great deal to do with flexibility and muscle strength, static and dynamic balance, postural stability, and coordination, all of which require the efficient integration of multiple physiological systems and the ability to interpret proprioceptive sensations (Kottke, 1990b; O'Sullivan, 1994). The centerpiece of an intervention to improve mobility would be to use resistance training to build strength, combined with exercises aimed at improving balance, postural stability, flexibility, and coordination. However, these exercises would not produce marked gains in the endurance necessary for sustained physical activity. This would require aerobic conditioning at a level of intensity to induce cardiopulmonary change.

Scientific advancement in the area of mobility and activity will require more sophisticated research models, state-of-the-art measurement equipment, protocols based on established exercise principles, and exploitation of our interdisciplinary colleagues. This interdisciplinary collaboration provides for effective and efficient shared use of facilities and other resources.

Multiple-site clinical trials would generate larger and more diversified samples of subjects and would be especially useful when attempting to intervene in rare conditions or gain reasonable size samples in a shorter period of time. With the speed of technological change and advancement, this is one way to ensure that nurses will keep pace.

Finally, important attention to exercise testing and measurement is key. Important information about testing that needs to be reported in published reports includes: environmental conditions, whether pre- and posttesting occurred at the same time of day, health history, demographics, exact testing procedures and protocols, reliability and validity checks on equipment prior to measurement, and whether or not the tester was blinded. An interesting study highlighting the importance of using exact protocols compared oxygen consumption (VO_2) and heart rates at submaximal and maximal levels when subjects held onto the treadmill siderails and when they did not hold on during testing. Those who did not hold on had higher heart rates and higher VO_2 at any given submaximal work load. Allowing the subject to hold on significantly alters the work load and the study results (Smith et al., 1986). Also, Christman et al. (1998) found that handrail support during the use of a stair-climber significantly reduced oxygen uptake and thus reduced caloric expenditure during the exercise.

Other variables that can affect exercise response and should be documented include physical activity outside the confines of the study, incentives, medications, and disease staging. For example, there is always the possibility that control subjects will become more active when exposed to the idea of exercise; thus the physical activity, especially of the control group, needs to be monitored. Also, it is important to document any differences in incentives provided to the control or exercise groups. For example, when children received modest financial incentives during a graded exercise test on a cycle ergometer, their mean VO_2 max and heart rate increased by 6% ($p < .05$) (Smith et al., 1995).

Prescribed and over-the-counter medication use is critical to document. There are a number of chemical substances such as diuretics; corticosteroids; nonsteroidal anti-inflammatory agents; and hormones such as insulin, antihistamines, and beta-blockers that can influence physiological responses to exercise, making it essential to consider medication-disease-exercise interactions (American College of Sports Medicine, 1995; Rosenberg, Fuentes, & Davis, 1992). In one study, the relationship between resting and exercise blood pressures in subjects with essential hypertension before and after propranolol treatment was evaluated. Propranolol reduced resting and maximal exercise blood pressure (Potempa, Folta, Braun, & Szidon, 1992).

Two studies used animal models to evaluate exercise-medication-disease interactions. In one, the effects of swimming on Bleomycin-treated mice compared to nonexercising controls showed significantly higher toxicity in exercising animals (Stone, Copelan, Weisbrode, & Rozmiarek, 1986). In the second study, comparing exercising and nonexercising rats, the deleterious consequences of aerobic exercise and cortisone injections on femoral articular cartilage were demonstrated (Gogia, Brown, & Al-Obaidi, 1993). Although there is reluctance to extrapolate data based on animal studies to humans, the findings send a cautionary signal about recommending exercise interventions for patient groups until more is understood about potential interactions. Additionally, when new medications are started, the timing of medication and other treatments relative to testing needs to be taken into account.

Disease staging is another important factor that must be documented not only to establish appropriate exercise parameters for each disease stage but also to compare data within and between clinical populations. Given the individualistic nature of human response to disease and treatment, disease stage is not necessarily a predictor of functional abilities, but empirical data would provide some insight into stage-specific limiting factors and associated precautions. The implications of timing interventions by stage were articulated in a study examining proximal lower extremity muscle strength training of patients with myotonic dystrophy and a second group of patients with hereditary motor and sensory neuropathy. Dependent measures included, in addition to strength, functional performance and serum myoglobin (Mb) to assess muscle fiber membrane permeability. On all measures, in both diagnostic categories, experimental groups showed slight, but statistically insignificant, gains over controls. The investigators speculated that in diseases where progression can be expected, late-stage strength training is not particularly effective and is costly. The investigators concluded that it would be more practical to initiate mobility and endurance interventions early in the disease (Lindeman et al., 1995).

In summary, in the past 5 years we have witnessed a significant increase in studies that represent explorations of the underlying mechanics and structures of mobility, disuse, and the efficacy of interventions, but progress has been very limited, and there are few intervention studies with patient populations. Interventions for those with progressive pathologies will present a particularly complex challenge, but with studies that identify the physiological interactions of exercise, disease, and treatment, significant gains in this area can be expected.

References

American College of Sports Medicine. (1995). *ACSM's guidelines for exercise testing and prescription* (5th ed.). Baltimore: Williams & Wilkins.

Baigis-Smith, J., Coombs, V. J., & Larson, E. (1994). HIV infection, exercise and immune function. *Image: The Journal of Nursing Scholarship, 26*(4), 277-281.

Banja, J., & Johnston, M. V. (1994). Part III: Ethical perspectives and social policy: Outcomes evaluation in TBI rehabilitation. *Archives of Physical Medicine and Rehabilitation, 75,* 19-28.

Boaz, F. R., & Muller, C. F. (1994). Predicting the risk of "permanent" nursing home residence: The role of community help as indicated by family helpers and prior living arrangements. *Health Services Research, 29*(4), 391-414.

Braun, L.T., Potempa, K., Holm, K., Fogg, L., & Szidon, J. P. (1994). The role of catecholamines, age, and fitness on blood pressure reactivity to dynamic exercise in patients with essential hypertension. *Heart and Lung: Journal of Critical Care. 23,*(5) 404-412.

Breslin, E. H., & Garoutte, B. C. (1995). Respiratory responses to unsupported arm lifts paced during expiration. *Western Journal of Nursing Research, 17*(1), 91-100.

Brooks, G. A., Fahey, T. D., & White, T. P. (1996). *Exercise physiology: Human bioenergetics and its applications* (2nd ed.). Mountain View, CA: Mayfield.

Byers, P. H. (1985). Effect of exercise on morning stiffness and mobility in patients with rheumatoid arthritis. *Research in Nursing and Health, 8*(3), 275-281.

Carpenito, L. J. (1997). *Nursing diagnosis: Applications to clinical practice* (7th ed.). Philadelphia: Lippencott.

Casperson, C. J. (1989). Physical activity epidemiology: Concepts, methods and applications to exercise science. In K. B. Pandolf (Ed.), *Exercise and sport sciences reviews 17* (pp. 423-473). Baltimore: Williams & Wilkins.

Casperson, C. J., Powell, K. E., & Christenson, G. M. (1985). Physical activity, exercise and physical fitness: Definitions and distinctions for health-related research. *Public Health Reports, 190*(2), 126-131.

Catanzaro, M. (1993). State of the science: Enhancing independence in physical activity. *Rehabilitation Nursing, 2*(1), 32-38.

Christman, S. K., Fish, A. F., Frid, D. J., Smith, B. A., & Bryant, C. X. (1998). Stepping as an exercise modality for improving fitness and function. *Applied Nursing Research, 11*(2), 49-54.

Cox, H. C. (1997). Clinical applications of nursing diagnosis: Adult, child, women's, psychiatric, gerontic, and home health considerations (3rd ed.). Philadelphi: F. A. Davis.

Cox, H. C., Hinz, M. D., Lubno, M. A., Newfield, S. A., Ridenour, N. A., Slater, M. M., & Sridaromont, K. (1993). *Clinical applications of nursing diagnosis* (2nd ed., pp. 313-460). Philadelphia: F. A. Davis.

Creason, N. S. (1991). Toward a model of clinical validation of nursing diagnosis: Developing conceptual and operational definitions of impaired physical mobility. In *Classification of nursing diagnosis: Proceeding of the ninth conference* (p. 241). Philadelphia: Lippincott.

Dawe, D., & Moore-Orr, R. (1995). Low intensity, range-of-motion exercise: Invaluable nursing care for elderly patients. *Journal of Advanced Nursing, 21*(4), 675-681.

Fox, E. L., & Matthew, D. K. (1980). *Interval training for lifetime fitness*. New York: Dial Press.

Gift, A. G., & Austin, D. J. (1992). The effects of a program of systematic movement on COPD patients. *Rehabilitation Nursing, 17*(1), 6-11.

Gillett, P. A., & Eisenman, P. A. (1987). The effect of intensity controlled aerobic dance exercise on aerobic capacity of middle-aged, overweight women. *Research in Nursing and Health, 10*(6), 383-390.

Glick, O. J. (1992). Interventions related to activity and movement. *Nursing Clinics of North America, 27*(2), 541-550.

Glick, O. J., & Swanson, E. A. (1995). Motor performance correlates of functional dependence in long-term care residents. *Nursing Research, 44*(1), 4-8.

Gogia, P., Brown, M., & Al-Obaidi, S. (1993). Hydrocortisone and exercise effects on articular cartilage in rats. *Archives of Physical Medicine and Rehabilitation, 74,* 463-467.

Granger, C. V. (1984). A conceptual model for functional assessment. In C. V. Granger & G. E. Gresham (Eds.), *Functional assessment in rehabilitation medicine* (pp. 14-25). Baltimore: Williams & Wilkins.

Guccione, A. A. (1994). Functional assessment. In S. B. O'Sullivan & T. J. Schmitz (Eds.), *Physical rehabilitation: Assessment and treatment* (3rd ed., pp. 193-208). Philadelphia: F. A. Davis.

Gulanick, M. (1991). Is phase 2 cardiac rehabilitation necessary for early recovery of patients with cardiac disease? A randomized, controlled study. *Heart and Lung: Journal of Critical Care, 20*(1), 9-15.

Haler, E. M., & Bell, K. R. (1990). Rehabilitation's relationship to inactivity. In F. J. Kottke & J. F. Lehman (Eds.), *Krusen's handbook of physical medicine and rehabilitation* (4th ed., pp. 1113-1133). Philadelphia: W. B. Saunders.

Hoffman, E. H., & Heller, J. (1995). The management challenge: Rehabilitation in a subacute environment. *Journal of Subacute Care, 1*(2), 11-15.

Hurwitz, A. (1989). The benefit of a home exercise regimen for ambulatory Parkinson's disease patients. *Journal of Neuroscience Nursing, 21*(3), 180-184.

Itoh, M., & Lee, H. M. (1990). The epidemiology of disability as related to rehabilitation medicine. In F. J. Kottke & J. F. Lehman (Eds.), *Krusen's handbook of physical medicine and rehabilitation* (4th ed., pp. 215-233). Philadelphia: W. B. Saunders.

Jirovec, M. M. (1991). The impact of daily exercise on mobility, balance and urine control of cognitively impaired nursing home residents. *International Journal of Nursing Studies, 28*(2), 145-151.

Johnston, M. V., & Hall, K. M. (1994). Part I: Outcomes evaluation in TBI rehabilitation: Overview and system principles. *Archives of Physical Medicine and Rehabilitation, 75,* 2-9.

Kasper, C. E., Maxwell, L. C., & White, T. P. (1996). Alterations in skeletal muscle related to short-term impaired physical mobility. *Research in Nursing and Health, 19*(2), 133-142.

Kasper, C. E., McNulty, A. L., Otto, A. J., & Thomas, D. P. (1993). Alterations in skeletal muscle related to impaired physical mobility: An empirical model. *Research in Nursing and Health, 16,* 265-273.

Kasper, C. E., St. Pierre, B., Fuchs, A., & Garfinkel, A. (1995). Spatial patterns of fiber types in atrophied skeletal muscle. *Western Journal of Nursing, 17*(1), 49-62.

Kasper, C. E., White, T. P., & Maxwell, K. C. (1990). Running during recovery from hindlimb suspension induces muscular injury. *Journal of Applied Physiology, 68,* 533-569.

Kim, M. J., Larson, J. L., Covery, M. K., Vitalo, C. A., Alex, C. G., & Patel, M. (1993). *Nursing Research, 42*(6), 356-361.

Kisner, C., & Colby, L. A. (1990). *Therapeutic exercise: Foundations and techniques* (2nd ed.). Philadelphia: F. A. Davis.

Koniak-Griffin, D. (1994). Aerobic exercise, psychological well-being and physical discomforts during adolescent pregnancy. *Research in Nursing and Health, 17,* 253-263.

Kottke, F. J. (1990b). Therapeutic exercise to develop neuromuscular coordination. In F. J. Kottke & F. Lehman (Eds.), *Krusen's handbook of physical medicine and rehabilitation* (4th ed., pp. 452-479). Philadelphia: F. A. Davis.

Kottke, F. J. (1990c). Therapeutic exercise to maintain mobility. In F. J. Kottke & J. F. Lehman (Eds.), *Krusen's handbook of physical medicine and rehabilitation* (4th ed., pp. 436-451). Philadelphia: W. B. Saunders.

Krisanda, J. M., Moreland, T. S., & Kushmerick, M. J. (1988). ATP supply and demand during exercise. In E. S. Horton & R. L. Terjung (Eds.), *Exercise, nutrition and energy metabolism.* New York: Macmillan.

Leasure, R., Belknap, E., Burks, C., & Schlegel, J. (1995). The effects of structured exercise on muscle mass, strength and endurance of immunosuppressed adult renal transplant patients: A pilot study. *Rehabilitation Nursing Research, 4*(2), 47-57.

Leblanc, A. D., Schneider, V. S., Evans, H. J., Pientok, C., Rowe, R., & Spector, E. (1992). Regional changes in muscle mass following 17 weeks of bed rest. *Journal of Applied Physiology, 73,* 2172-2178.

Lenderking, W. R., Gelber, R. D., Cotton, D. J., Cole, B. F., Golhirsch, A., Volberding, P. A., & Testa, M. A. (1994). Evaluation of the quality of life associated with zidovudine treatment in asymptomatic human immunodeficiency virus infection. *New England Journal of Medicine, 330,* 738-743.

Leon, A. S. (1989). Effects of physical activity and fitness on health. In T. F. Drury (Ed.), *Assessing physical fitness and physical activity in population-based surveys* (DHHS Pub. No. PHS 89-1253, pp. 509-525). Washington, DC: U.S. Government Printing Office.

Lindeman, E., Leffers, P., Spaans, F., Drukker, J., Reulen, J., Kerckhoffs, M., & Koke, A. (1995). Strength training in myotonic dystrophy and hereditary motor and sensory neuropathy: A randomized trial. *Archives of Physical Medicine and Rehabilitation, 76,* 612-620.

Lord, S. R., Ward, J. A., Williams, P., & Strudwick, M. (1995). The effect of a 12-month exercise trial on balance, strength, and falls in older women: A randomized controlled trial. *Journal of the American Geriatric Society, .43,* 1198-1206.

Lubeck, D. P., & Yelin, E. H. (1988). A question of value: Measuring the impact of chronic disease. *Milbank Quarterly, 66*(3), 444-463.

MacVicar, M., Winningham, M. L., & Nickel, J. (1989). Effects of aerobic interval training on cancer patients' functional capacity. *Nursing Research, 38*(6), 348-351.

Mills, E. M. (1994). The effect of low-intensity aerobic exercise on muscle strength, flexibility, and balance among sedentary elderly persons. *Nursing Research, 43*(4), 207-211.

Mock, V., Burke, M. B., Sheehan, P., Creaton, E. M., Winningham, M. L., McKenney-Tedder, S., Schwager, L. P., & Liebman, M. (1994). A nursing rehabilitation program for women with breast cancer receiving adjuvant chemotherapy. *Oncology Nursing Forum, 21*(5), 899-908.

Morgan, W. P., & Goldston, S. E. (1987). *Exercise and mental health.* Washington, DC: Hemisphere.

Nagi, S. Z. (1969). *Disability and rehabilitation.* Columbus: Ohio State University Press.

Nagi, S. Z. (1976). An epidemiology of disability among adults in the United States: Health and society. *Milbank Quarterly, 54,* 439-467.

Nash, M. S. (1994). Immune responses to nervous system decentralization and exercise in quadriplegia. *Medicine and Science in Sports and Exercise, 26*(2), 164-171.

Noble, L. J., Salcido, R., Walker, M. K., Atchinson, J., & Marshall, R. (1994). Improving functional mobility through exercise. *Rehabilitation Nursing Research, 3*(1), 23-29.

O'Sullivan, S. B. (1994). Motor control assessment. In S. B. O'Sullivan & T. J. Schmitz (Eds.), *Physical rehabilitation: Assessment and treatment* (3rd ed., pp. 111-131). Philadelphia: F. A. Davis.

Ouellet, L. L., & Rush, K. L. (1992). A synthesis of selected literature on mobility: A basis for studying impaired mobility. *Nursing Diagnosis, 3*(2), 72-80.

Pedersen, B. K., & Ullum, H. (1994). NK cell response to physical activity: Possible mechanisms of action. *Medicine and Science in Sports and Exercise, 26*(2), 140-146.

Peters, C., Lotzerich, H., Hiemeier, B., Schule, K., & Uhlenbruck, G. (1994). Influence of moderate exercise training on natural killer cytotoxicity and personality traits in cancer patients. *Anticancer Research, 14,* 1033-1036.

Pope, A. M., & Tarlov, A. R. (Eds.). (1991). *Disability in America: Toward a national agenda for prevention.* Washington, DC: National Academy Press.

Potempa, K. M., Folta, A., Braun, L. T., & Szidon, J. P. (1992). The relationship of resting and exercise blood pressure in subjects with essential hypertension before and after drug treatment with propranolol. *Heart and Lung: The Journal of Critical Care, 21*(6), 509-514.

Preusser, B. A., Winningham, M. L., & Clanton, T. L. (1994). High vs low intensity inspiratory muscle interval training in patients with COPD. *Chest: The Cardiopulmonary Journal, 106*(1), 110-117.

Roberts, B. L. (1989). Effects of walking on balance among elders. *Nursing Research, 38*(3), 180-182.

Rosenberg, J. M., Fuentes, R. J., & Davis, A. (Eds.). (1992). *Athletic drug reference.* Durham, NC: Allen & Hanaburys.

Rush, K. L., & Ouellet, L. L. (1993). Mobility: A concept analysis. *Journal of Advanced Nursing, 18,* 486-492.

Sawyer, E. H., & Clanton, T. L. (1993). Improved pulmonary function and exercise tolerance with inspiratory muscle conditioning in children with cystic fibrosis. *Chest, 104,* 1490-1497.

Schmitz, T. J. (1994). Coordination assessment. In S. B. O'Sullivan & Schmitz, T. J. (Eds.), *Physical rehabilitation: Assessment and treatment* (3rd ed., pp. 97-107). Philadelphia: F. A. Davis.

Smith, B. A., Hamlin, R. L., Bartels, R. L., Evans, R. G., Kirby, T. E., MacVicar, M. G., & Weisbrode, S. E. (1992). *Heart and Lung: The Journal of Critical Care, 21*(5), 440-447.

Smith, B. A., & Kirby, T. E. (1986). The effects of holding to the siderails during graded exercise testing. *Medicine and Science in Sports and Exercise, 18*(2), S36 (Abstract).

Smith, B., Schneider, B., & Franklin, W. (1995). Improving the performance of a child on a graded exercise test (GXT) using financial incentives. *Medicine and Science in Sports and Exercise, 27*(5), S116 (Abstract).

Spector, W. D., Katz, S., Murphy, J. B., & Fulton, J. P. (1987). The hierarchical relationship between activities of daily living and instrumental activities of daily living. *Journal of Chronic Disease, 40*(6), 481-489.

Stevenson, J. S., & Topp, R. (1990). Effect of moderate and low intensity long-term exercise by older adults. *Research in Nursing and Health, 13,* 209-218.

Stone, D. W., Copelan, E. A., Weisbrode, S. E., & Rozmiarek, H. (1986). Effects of exercise on Bleomycin-induced pulmonary toxicity in mice. *Cancer Treatment Reports, 70*(9), 1067-1071.

Task Force on Medical Rehabilitation Research. (1990). *Report to the National Institutes of Health.* Hunt Valley, MD: NIH.

Topp, R., Mikesky, A., Wigglesworth, J., Holt, W. Jr., & Edwards, J. E. (1993). The effect of a 12-week dynamic resistance strength training program on gait velocity and balance of older adults. *The Gerontologist, 33*(4), 501-506.

Topp, R., & Stevenson, J. S. (1994). The effects of attendance and effort on outcomes among older adults in a long-term exercise program. *Research in Nursing and Health, 17,* 15-24.

Trine, M. R., & Morgan, W. P. (1995). Influence of time of day on psychological responses to exercise. *Sports Medicine, 20*(5), 328-337.

Van Wynsberghe, D., Noback, C. R., & Carola, R. (1995). *Human anatomy and physiology* (3rd ed.). New York: McGraw-Hill.

Vorhies, D., & Riley, B. E. (1993). Deconditioning. *Geriatric Rehabilitation, 9*(4), 745-763.

Watson, R. R. (1989). Exercise, weightlessness and inactivity: Modifiers of immune functions. In J. F. Hickson, Jr., & I. Wolinsky (Eds.), *Nutrition in exercise and sport* (pp. 385-396). Boca Raton, FL: CRC.

Wenger, N. K. (1984). Early ambulation after myocardial infarction: Rationale, program components and results. In N. K. Wenger & H. K. Hellerstein (Eds.), *Rehabilitation of the coronary patient* (2nd ed., pp. 97-113). New York: Wiley.

Williams, B. C., Phillips, E. K., Torner, J. C., & Irvine, A. A. (1990). Predicting utilization of home health resources. *Medical Care, 28*(5), 379-391.

Wilmore, J. H., & Costill, D. L. (1994). *Physiology of sport and exercise.* Champaign, IL: Human Kinetics.

Winningham, M. L., MacVicar, M., Bondec, M., Anderson, J., & Minton, J. P. (1989). Effect of aerobic exercise on body weight and composition in patients with breast cancer on adjuvant chemotherapy. *Oncology Nursing Forum, 16*(5), 683-689.

20

MANAGING DYSPNEA

Virginia Carrieri-Kohlman
Susan Janson

Overview

Dyspnea is the subjective sensation of difficult, uncomfortable breathing and includes both the perception of labored breathing by the patient and the reaction to that sensation, rated solely by the patient (Comroe, 1965). Dyspnea is considered to be synonymous with the terms "shortness of breath" or "breathlessness" (Schwartzstein & Cristiano, 1996). Since 1965, when this early definition of dyspnea was proposed, there have been various new definitions suggested that include "increased respiratory effort needed to breathe," "uncomfortable and unpleasant feeling of inability to breathe," and "conscious awareness of increased commands to the inspiratory muscles." Most authors acknowledge that dyspnea includes an element of "distress" (Wright & Branscomb,

1954) or that it is "uncomfortable" (Comroe, 1965). These various definitions illustrate the variable aspects of the respiratory sensory experience and dyspnea as a multidimensional sensation.

There are no exact prevalence data about dyspnea, although it is the primary presenting symptom in patients with pulmonary and heart disease and is a major management problem in 25% to 78% of terminally ill patients (Roberts, Thorne, & Pearson, 1993; Reuben, 1986). Dyspnea also occurs in metabolic, infectious, and neuromuscular diseases and in normal pregnancy. Dyspnea is a frequent cause of emergency room visits and a common complaint in the general population; for example, dyspnea was reported by 6% to 27% of people of mixed ages and gender in the Framingham study (Stulbarg & Adams, 1994).

Mechanisms thought to be important in the origin of dyspnea are central (medullary) respiratory activity or drive and inputs from the chemoreceptors, respiratory muscle and chest wall receptors, lungs, and upper airways (Eldridge & Chen, 1996). Reviews of research related to physiological mechanisms are published elsewhere (Adams & Gun, 1991; Schwartzstein, Manning, Weiss, & Weinberger, 1990; Stulbarg & Adams, 1994; Tobin, 1990). Multidisciplinary clinical physiological research has focused on the following physiological mechanisms: ventilatory impedance, afferent-efferent disassociation, abnormal blood gas states, respiratory muscle dysfunction, and deconditioning of the cardiopulmonary system.

Only recently have nurse researchers conducted research related to the symptom of dyspnea. They have primarily concentrated on (a) theoretical *models* to guide the study of dyspnea, (b) *measurement* of dyspnea, (c) *factors or correlates* of dyspnea, and (d) *management* of dyspnea. The latter includes those strategies devised by patients themselves and strategies known to be clinically effective or likely to be effective based on theoretical soundness. These foci are used to summarize the research studies conducted solely by nurses or by nurses as members of multidisciplinary teams of researchers.

Theoretical Models

Theoretical models proposed by nurse investigators have emphasized sensory and affective dimensions of dyspnea and multifactorial aspects of the symptom. In an early framework, antecedent variables affecting the primary appraisal of dyspnea were categorized into personal, illness, and situational factors. These factors were conceptualized as affecting patient coping and self-care behaviors and therapeutic management strategies, which in turn modulate the intensity of dyspnea. Gift (1990a) articulated a framework with five components: (a) the sensation (physiological component), involving activation of receptors and transmission along nerve pathways; (b) the perception (cognitive component), involving interpretation of the sensation within the context of past experience and present expectation; (c) the distress (psychological component), including the psychological correlates of dyspnea; (d) the response, including the coping style and strategies used by the person; and (e) the reporting of dyspnea (social component), including the descriptors used as well as the decision to report or not to report the experience.

Steele and Shaver (1992) proposed a person-environment ecological framework profiling dyspnea as a nociceptive phenomenon and accounting for biopsychosocial factors that affect dyspnea. Dyspnea is seen as being similar to pain, with a cognitive-motivational-affective dimension in addition to a sensory dimension. Environmental factors and individual factors contribute to the biobehavioral dimensions of the dyspnea experience. Major concepts included in this model are *perceptual sensitivity* and *dyspnea tolerance*. Perceptual sensitivity is defined as the proportional increase in reported dyspnea magnitude accompanying an increased magnitude of a physical stimulus, and it represents a quantifiable estimate of sensitivity to dyspnogenic stimuli (Mahler, Rosiello, et al., 1987; Steele & Shaver, 1992). This model was used to direct a study in which two distinct sensations of perceived breathing effort and perceived breathing discomfort were measured in response to a threshold loading stimulus.

Following an investigation of the breathlessness experience in subjects with a history of emphysema and/or chronic bronchitis, West and Popkess-Vawter (1994) adapted a breathlessness model by Zelechowski (1977). The earlier model depicted individuals as having different nonaction (e.g., depression, apathy, and sleep) or action (e.g., anger, anxiety, and exercise). These reactions influenced dyspnea, which is affected by antecedent conditions such as degree of perceived threat and/or physiological change. Fatigue and congestion as antecedent conditions and positive and negative adaptive responses as outcomes were added to the model.

Lenz, Suppe, Gift, Pugh, and Milligan (1995) developed a middle-range theory, which they called the "Theory of Unpleasant Symptoms." This theory was developed from studies of fatigue during intrapartum and postpartum periods and dyspnea in populations of COPD and asthma patients. Using pain as an analogue, dyspnea was conceptualized as having physiological (sensory) and psychological (cognitive) components. The psychological aspects are similar to the distress components of pain. The important features of dyspnea were identified by comparing dyspnea in the same individual at times with and without dyspnea. In separate studies, the psychological or distress aspects of dyspnea were found to be similar to pain and to be related to anxiety, depression, and somatization (Gift, 1990b, 1991; Gift, Plaut, & Jacox, 1986). The basic structure outlined for the theory of unpleasant symptoms includes categories of factors (physiological, psychological, and situational) that affect one's disposition to or manifestation of the symptom, characteristics of the symptom, and the proposed performance variables affected by the symptom, including physical performance, functional status, and cognitive functioning.

Breslin, Roy, and Robinson (1992) proposed an integrated metaparadigm in which basic nursing science is seen as the understanding of the life processes and clinical science as the diagnosis and treatment of the patterning of life processes. In using this paradigm, Breslin has shifted from the usual examination of pulmonary function to pursuing the role of the respiratory pump and respiratory muscle function as a basic process contributing to dyspnea. Within this theoretical stance, the physiological mechanisms of dyspnea in COPD are related to intrinsic characteristics of the inspiratory muscles. Although COPD is characterized by reductions in expiratory airflow, dyspnea is perceived during inspiration and is usually associated with inspiratory muscle activity. Dyspnea is associated with the force generation required of the inspiratory muscles, their overall capacity to generate force, respiratory cycle temporal behaviors, and the specific pattern of respiratory muscle recruitment in ventilation. This schema is focused on the recruitment of the accessory respiratory muscles and the competitive roles of the respiratory muscles. Breslin's work has included concepts of basic nursing science: dyspnea and recruitment of rib cage and accessory muscles as a global model, dyspnea with unsupported arm exercise, dyspnea with mandibular and facial muscle activity, and the pattern of recruitment during pursed-lip breathing (Breslin, 1992; Breslin, Garoutte, & Celli, 1990). Clinical nursing science contributions include a tool to assess unsupported arm endurance and unsupported arm exercise training. Leg activity and unsupported arm activity with relationships to ventilatory demand and dyspnea have also been studied (Breslin, Roy, et al., 1992).

This metaparadigm presented by Breslin, Roy, et al. (1992) is similar to the general framework of selected biological and psychosocial life processes suggested by us and of pathophysiological concepts (Carrieri-Kohlman, Lindsey, & West, 1993). Dyspnea is presented as an alteration in the normal life process of sensation (Carrieri-Kohlman & Janson, 1993).

Based on findings related to the "desensitization" process for other symptoms and phobias, Carrieri-Kohlman and co-workers (1993) proposed a framework for the treatment of dyspnea distress. It was hypothesized that monitored exposure to higher than usual levels of dyspnea in a safe environment would produce more effective coping strategies and, therefore, increased confidence in controlling shortness of breath and a positive change in the appraisal of dyspnea. It was also hypothesized that change in appraisal from a threat to a benign challenge would decrease anxiety and distress and increase tolerance for dyspnea. This framework was tested in a randomized controlled trial with 51 patients with emphysema and chronic bronchitis who received either monitored or nurse-coached exercise training. Findings included a decrease in dyspnea and the anxiety and distress associated with it during laboratory exercise, an increase in self-efficacy for walking, and a decrease in dyspnea with activities of daily living (Carrieri-Kohlman, Gormley, Douglas, Paul, & Stulbarg, 1996).

A theoretical model was tested in patients with asthma in which it was hypothesized that three exogenous variable sets, representing personal, disease severity, and coping factors, exerted indirect effects on psychosocial and morbidity outcomes through dyspnea intensity (Janson-Bjerklie, Ferketich, Benner, & Becker, 1992). It was proposed that dyspnea had a direct effect on depression, life satisfaction, and number of emergency room visits. Early testing of dyspnea revealed complex relationships among dyspnea, dyspnea-related distress, and morbidity outcomes. Multiple regression analysis produced a respecified, more empirically based model in which 37% of the variance in depression was explained by the number of self-care strategies, amount of stressful life change within the past 6 months, nocturnal symptoms, and dyspnea-related distress during asthmatic episodes. High life stress, nocturnal asthma symptoms, and symptom distress were related to greater depression. Twenty-four percent of life satisfaction was explained by financial status and nocturnal symptoms, and 27% of emergency visits were explained by dyspnea-related distress during asthma episodes and perception of danger from asthma.

Carrieri-Kohlman and Gormley (1998) proposed classifying self-care strategies for dyspnea into overlapping categories of physiological, environmental-social, and cognitive-behavioral. They suggested that several coping strategies modulated dyspnea perception, primarily by affecting cognitive variables that influence dyspnea, rather than by affecting physiological mechanisms. Strategies can affect one or more cognitive variables or mediators of thought and action to alter the sensation of dyspnea, the interpretation of that sensation, and the behavioral response to manage that symptom. By modulating the cognitive variables, such as self-efficacy, mood, or perceived control of the symptom, the affective distress of the symptom is changed. The perceptual threshold for the symptom may increase and a concomitant decrease in the perceived intensity and distress of dyspnea may occur.

Measurement of Dyspnea

Qualitative Descriptions of Dyspnea

Individuals with dyspnea have been asked to describe the sensations of "shortness of breath." Verbal descriptors indicate many types of respiratory sensations across disease states, most probably a function of the pathophysiological mechanism involved (Schwartzstein & Cristiano, 1996). Phrases used by patients with various obstructive, restrictive, and vascular diseases included "I feel short of breath," "hard to breathe," "I feel chest tightness," "I can't get enough air," "I feel like I am suffocating," and "It feels like pain" (Janson-Bjerklie, Carrieri, & Hudes, 1986). These descriptors also have been given by patients with cancer of the lung (Brown, Carrieri, Janson-Bjerklie, & Dodd, 1986). Categorization of verbal descriptors for breathlessness has been extended primarily by medical researchers who have generated a list of 45 descriptors, which have been clustered into 12 groups that seem to describe different aspects of breathing discomfort according to pathophysiological categories. COPD patients chose distress more often, patients with asthma tended to indicate wheeziness, and people with restrictive disorders reported rapid breathing more often (Elliott et al., 1991; Simon et al., 1990). Qualitative descriptors of exertional breathlessness have been compared between normal subjects and patients with COPD. Only patients with COPD consistently chose descriptors denoting "increased inspiratory difficulty" (75%), "unsatisfied inspiratory effort" (75%), and "shallow breathing" (50%). These descriptors were attributed to thoracic hyperinflation and the resultant disparity between inspiratory effort and ventilatory output (O'Donnell, Bertley, Chau, & Webb, 1997).

Measurement of Dyspnea Intensity

Recent development of validated instruments has permitted evaluation of interventions for dyspnea. Nurse researchers have validated the Visual Analogue Scale

(VAS) in chronic COPD and asthma patients (Gift, 1989) and in critically ill ventilated patients (Bouley, Froman, & Shah, 1992; Knebel, Janson-Bjerklie, Malley, Wilson, & Marini, 1994; Lush, Janson-Bjerklie, Carrieri, & Lovejoy, 1988). Length of the scales varies from 100 to 300 mm (Carrieri-Kohlman et al., 1996; Reardon et al., 1994), and the anchor descriptors for the VAS vary (although the horizontal scale has been validated, other researchers have used vertical scales). Words used to guide rating of patients about dyspnea also differ across studies; examples include "shortness of breath," "breathing difficulty," "uncomfortable breathing," and "breathing effort." Evidence for concurrent and construct validity is indicated by data that the VAS correlates highly ($r = .90$) with the modified Borg (1982) scale for breathlessness in ventilated patients (Lush et al., 1988), the American Thoracic Society Grade of Breathlessness Scale (Janson-Bjerklie, Carrieri, et al., 1986), and with physiological measures of increasing airway resistance (Gift, Plaut, et al., 1986; Janson-Bjerklie, Ruma, Stulbarg, & Carrieri, 1987). In the laboratory setting, dyspnea has been measured at one point in time during a provocative stimulus (e.g., at maximum exercise) and has been estimated by the slope of the change related to a stimulus over time, such as with increasing minute ventilation (VE) during exercise (Carrieri-Kohlman et al., 1996), or with an increased ventilatory load administered in the laboratory (Steele et al., 1991). Nurses have refined instrumentation and used magnitude estimation as one methodology to measure dyspnea in the laboratory (Nield & Kim, 1991; Nield, Kim, & Patel, 1989). Magnitude estimation is used to scale the strength of an evoked perception given an applied stimulus.

Measurement of the Affective Components of Dyspnea

Steele and colleagues (1991) measured two dimensions of dyspnea with separate VAS scales. A sensory component (perceptual sensitivity to breathing effort) and an affective component (perceptual sensitivity to breathing discomfort) were measured in 27 subjects with COPD under added inspiratory muscle loads delivered through an inspiratory muscle trainer. "Effort" was rated higher than "discomfort" across all loads ($p = .05$); however, "perceptual sensitivity" was greater for discomfort than for effort (i.e., steeper slope for discomfort). Twelve out of 27 subjects were able to differentiate breathing discomfort from effort and 8 of those 12 had greater "perceptual sensitivity" for discomfort than for effort. The authors suggested that dyspnea does have separate affective and sensory dimensions and that both dimensions should be measured.

Whether patients could differentiate distress and anxiety associated with dyspnea from the intensity of dyspnea and the perceived effort of breathing was investigated in another study (Carrieri-Kohlman, Gormley, Douglas, et al., 1996). Fifty-two subjects with COPD rated their perception of four individual components of dyspnea: perceived work of breathing (JOB), intensity of shortness of breath (SOB), anxiety associated with dyspnea (DA), and distress associated with dyspnea (DD) on individual 200 mm visual analog scales at rest, after a 6-minute walk, and every 2 minutes during an incremental treadmill test. Intensity of shortness of breath was significantly related to perceived work of breathing ($p < .0001$), and distress was related to anxiety ($p < .0001$), suggesting overlap in the measurement of each pair. The ratings for JOB and SOB were significantly greater than and statistically different from the affective components of dyspnea (DD and DA) after the 6-minute walk and throughout a treadmill test. Subjects with COPD could rate and differentiate effort and intensity of dyspnea from the affective response (distress, anxiety). Although dyspnea distress and anxiety were closely related, the mean slope relating distress to ventilation was significantly larger than that for anxiety, suggesting that these two ratings (i.e., distress and anxiety) may reflect somewhat different aspects.

Instruments to Measure Dyspnea With Activities of Daily Living

In an early exploration of the phenomenon of dyspnea, Janson-Bjerklie, Ruma, and colleagues (1987) developed an open-ended interview questionnaire, the Dyspnea Interview, which included seven dimensions of the symptom, the symptom pattern, strategies used to manage dyspnea, and family support and education received related to shortness of breath. This was the first such questionnaire to be developed for exploring the impact of dyspnea on daily living.

Subsequently, nurse clinicians and researchers have developed instruments that measure the intensity of dyspnea with daily activities in the home. As part of a multidisciplinary team, Sassi-Dambron, Eakin, Ries, and Kaplan (1995) developed the University of California, San Diego (UCSD), Shortness of Breath Scale to measure the amount of dyspnea that patients have with selected daily activities. Patients indicate on a 6-point scale

how frequently they experience shortness of breath during 21 activities of daily living that are associated with varying levels of exertion. The questionnaire includes three additional questions about limitations caused by shortness of breath, fear of harm from overexertion, and fear of shortness of breath.

The Pulmonary Functional Status and Dyspnea Questionnaire (PFSDQ) (Lareau, Carrieri-Kohlman, Janson-Bjerklie, & Roos, 1994) is a 164-item self-administered questionnaire requiring 10 to 15 minutes to complete. The PFSDQ elicits ratings of 79 items in 6 categories: self-care (15 items), mobility (14), eating (8), home management (22), social (10), and recreational (10). The activities are evaluated for general performance as well as in association with dyspnea. Internal consistency of the instrument is reportedly $r = .91$. The PFSDQ has been shown to be responsive to symptoms, varying degrees of airway impairment, and clinical therapies. The numbers of activities in this instrument are being decreased with appropriate testing.

The Pulmonary Functional Status Scale (PFSS) developed by Weaver and Narsavage (1992) is a self-administered 56-item scale measuring the mental, physical, and social functions of the patient with COPD. Activities evaluated are in the categories of self-care, daily activities, household tasks, meal preparation, relationships, dyspnea, anxiety, and depression. This instrument has one scale measuring dyspnea; however, it primarily measures functional status and has been reported to have concurrent validity with the Sickness Impact Profile (SIP).

Correlates of Dyspnea

Nurse investigators have focused much of their research endeavors on factors that are hypothesized to influence the sensation of dyspnea. Naturally occurring and laboratory-induced dyspnea situations have been used to measure personal, physiological, psychological, and situational variables associated with it (Bouley et al., 1992; DeVito, 1990; Gift, 1991; Gift, Plaut, et al., 1986; Janson-Bjerklie, Ferketich, et al., 1992; Janson-Bjerklie, Ruma, et al., 1987; Knebel, 1989, 1994).

Dyspnea has been related to age (Carrieri, Kieckhefer, Janson-Bjerklie, & Sousa, 1991); physiological variables including minute ventilation (Bouley et al., 1992), work of breathing (Knebel, 1994), airway resistance

(Janson-Bjerklie, Ruma, et al., 1987); emotions such as anxiety (Gift, 1991; Knebel et al., 1998); self-efficacy (Carrieri-Kohlman, Gormley, & Stolberg, 1993; Gormley, Carrieri-Kohlman, Douglas, & Stolberg, 1994), and coping strategies (Kwiatkowski, Carrieri-Kohlman, Janson, Gormley, & Stolberg, 1995). These variables affect a symptom or the perception of a symptom and in turn affect the response to the symptom and the strategies patients use (Carrieri-Kohlman & Gormley, 1997; Jones & Wilson, 1996).

Fear, anxiety, and depression. Anxiety and depression are frequently associated with dyspnea. Patients in the hospital setting become more and more dyspneic as their anxiety increases, or anxiety may escalate as dyspnea increases. Clinically it has been observed that progressive breathlessness leads to a vicious "fear-dyspnea" cycle in which increasing dyspnea produces more fear and anxiety that in turn leads to more dyspnea (Carrieri-Kohlman & Janson-Bjerklie, 1993). Gift and colleagues (1991) measured emotional states during high, medium, and low dyspnea in hospitalized COPD patients. Anxiety was significantly higher during high or medium dyspnea when compared with low. Dyspnea severity was significantly related to the anxiety trait ($r = .34$) and depression trait ($r = .43$). In the emergency room, high dyspnea as rated by respiratory rate, the pulse, extent of wheezing, and accessory muscle use was higher; PEFR and oxygen saturation were lower. Anxiety has been reported as greater during high dyspnea than during low dyspnea in patients with asthma and COPD. When 30 adult lung cancer patients were asked to describe emotions experienced during dyspnea, they reported anxiety, depression, nervousness, and fear (Brown et al., 1986). Similarly, responses were gathered when 96 adults with COPD were asked during a nonacute phase of illness to recall their feelings associated with sensations of shortness of breath during hospitalizations for an acute episode (DeVito, 1990). Themes of fear, helplessness, loss of vitality, preoccupation, and legitimacy were identified. These reports corroborate the earlier findings of Janson-Bjerklie, Carrieri, and Hudes (1986), who found that patients' panic, anger, and worry were correlates of dyspnea and that at times of acute dyspnea, patients may want to be alone or isolate themselves in attempts to control their breathing. During acute dyspnea in critically ill patients, Knebel and colleagues (1998) found that anxiety was moderately related to dyspnea ($r = .55-.61$) in a group of 21 patients weaning from mechanical ventilation.

Fatigue. A most frequent physical correlate with dyspnea is fatigue. In a retrospective study of 68 patients with obstructive, restrictive and vascular pulmonary disease, fatigue, as measured by the Profile of Mood States (POMS), was correlated positively ($r = .41$) with usual dyspnea (Janson-Bjerklie, Carrieri, et al., 1986). In a correlational study relating dyspnea severity, functional status, and quality of life in 45 adults with chronic bronchitis, fatigue ($r = .47$) and depression increased ($r = .67$) and quality of life decreased ($r = -.75$) as dyspnea worsened (Moody, Fraser, & Yarandi, 1993). In nine ventilated acute respiratory failure patients, subjects with the highest dyspnea scores had the highest fatigue and tension scores (Knebel, 1989). Likewise, in the study by Gift (1991), fatigue, heart rate, somatization, and congestion were significantly higher during high dyspnea than during times of lower dyspnea in patients with asthma.

Social support. In an interview survey of patients with pulmonary disease, dyspnea was related to the number of persons in the social support network and the frequency of contact with others (Janson-Bjerklie, Carrieri, et al., 1986). The amount of material aid, affirmation, and affection was also positively related to the intensity of dyspnea. Although this research appears to be the only scientific investigation relating social support and dyspnea, many clinical observations have been published that indicate that for most patients, support and the presence of significant others are related to the level of functioning and ability to cope with symptoms.

Work of breathing. Many indicators of increased work of breathing have been shown in laboratory and clinical settings to be related to shortness of breath. Bouley and colleagues (1992) compared the degree of dyspnea to physiological variables in ventilator-dependent patients receiving synchronized intermittent mandatory ventilation (SIMV) with T-piece or pressure support ventilation (PSV) weaning. Although there were large interindividual differences, higher dyspnea was associated with increased heart rate, respiratory rate, and oxygen saturation. In a study of 21 patients mechanically ventilated for acute respiratory failure, lower dyspnea during synchronized intermittent mandatory ventilation (SIMV) predicted their ability to wean successfully (Knebel et al., 1998). Patients reported significant preweaning dyspnea and anxiety despite resting for 6 hours before any weaning attempts were made. Dyspnea and anxiety during weaning were not significantly different when SIMV was compared to PSV.

Accessory muscle use has been correlated with dyspnea in the laboratory and clinical settings. Healthy and COPD subjects who recruited accessory, neck, and rib cage muscles for ventilation were more likely to report higher sensations of dyspnea (Breslin et al., 1990). Clinically, the pattern of ventilation has been related to the sensation of dyspnea. An increase in minute ventilation (VE) is related to dyspnea in normal subjects and patients. An increase in respiratory rate alone has been associated with an increase in dyspnea in normal subjects and in hospitalized patients (Gift, 1991). The length of inspiratory time and asynchronous breathing, ranging from some lag between rib cage and abdominal movement to paradoxical breathing, has been associated with dyspnea (Breslin et al., 1990). Other physiological variables indicative of increased effort of breathing, such as hyperinflation, maximum inspiratory pressure (MIP), hypoxia, and hypercapnia, have been shown to be related to dyspnea in multidisciplinary studies and must be considered as important physiological factors in the initiation of acute and chronic dyspnea (Adams & Gun, 1991; Carrieri-Kohlman, 1991; O'Donnell, 1994).

Correlates of dyspnea have been identified during provoked dyspnea under experimental conditions. During induced airflow obstruction and induced cough, 31 adult subjects with mild to moderate asthma underwent methacholine challenge to induce bronchoconstriction, followed 24 hours later by cough induction with sodium gluconate inhalation (Janson-Bjerklie, Ruma, et al., 1987). Dyspnea was related to age ($r = -.41$) and cigarette smoking ($r = -.21$) but not to degree of airflow obstruction. Dyspnea at baseline, prior to methacholine inhalation, was correlated ($r = .44$) with dyspnea intensity during bronchoconstriction. The findings of this study explained some of the variability in perception of dyspnea in asthma.

Quality of Life

In several medical studies, dyspnea has been shown to be a greater predictor of quality of life than any of the gold-standard physiological variables, including measures of airflow such as forced expiratory volume in 1 second (FEV1) or disease severity (Curtis, Deyo, & Hudson, 1994; Mahler, Paryniarz, et al., 1992). This relationship has been varied in the predictive studies reported by nurse researchers. A group of nurse investigators used a path analysis model to examine interrelationships among significant variables related to dyspnea in 45 adults with chronic bronchitis and emphysema (Moody, McCormick, & Williams, 1990, 1991). Mastery (an individual's perceived ability to manage daily events), dyspnea, and depression mediated the effects of disease severity and environmental risk on quality of life in these subjects. Dyspnea severity had strong but separate effects on functional status ($r = -.40$) and quality of life ($r = -.23$). Mastery measured by the Quality of Life Questionnaire developed by the investigators was highly related to dyspnea severity ($r = -.71$). Because the relationship between dyspnea and mastery was greater than that between dyspnea and disease severity, these authors suggest that dyspnea can be considered more psychologically driven and that dyspnea might be responsive to direct psychological interventions to decrease depression and improve mastery. Improving dyspnea severity may improve quality of life and functional status.

Functional status. Weaver and colleagues (1997) tested an explanatory model of variables influencing functional status in 104 patients with COPD. Exercise capacity, dyspnea, and depressed mood significantly and directly influenced functional status. Dyspnea, depression, and pulmonary function indirectly influenced functional status through exercise capacity. These authors concluded that efforts to improve functional status of individuals with COPD should focus on interventions that influence exercise capacity, dyspnea, anxiety, and depressed mood, with strategies to minimize dyspnea and its antecedent anxiety being investigated in the future.

Graydon and colleagues (Graydon & Ross, 1995; Graydon, Ross, Webster, & Goldstein, 1995) examined the extent to which mood, symptoms, lung function and social support predicted the level of functioning of patients with COPD over a 30-month period. Dyspnea was measured, along with other symptoms, using the Bronchitis-Emphysema Symptom Checklist and with the Sickness Impact Profile as a measure of functioning. The best predictors of patients' functioning at 30 months were functioning at the initial visit, symptoms, forced expiratory volume in one second (FEV1), and age. The most prevalent symptoms were dyspnea and fatigue, both of which were highly correlated with functioning scores at 30 months.

Another researcher (Anderson, 1995) analyzed the relationships among several antecedent and mediator variables and the outcome variable of quality of life. Although dyspnea was hypothesized to have a direct effect on quality of life, the path analysis in a sample of 126 patients with COPD revealed that dyspnea had a direct effect on depression but only an indirect effect on quality of life. Variables having direct effects on quality of life were self-esteem, depression, social support, and age.

Management of Dyspnea

Without a precise understanding of the biobehavioral basis of breathlessness, management strategies at present are largely confined to interventions aimed at reducing ventilatory demand or improving ventilatory capacity. Management strategies for dyspnea are reviewed elsewhere (Altose, 1992; Carrieri-Kohlman & Gormley, 1997; O'Donnell, 1994; Tobin, 1990); therefore, only nurse researcher studies will be discussed in the following section.

Self-reported strategies for managing dyspnea. Strategies described by patients to self-manage dyspnea in chronic and terminal dyspnea and during an exacerbation of asthma are compared across nursing science studies, as summarized in Table 20.1 (Brown et al., 1986; Carrieri & Janson-Bjerklie, 1986; Janson-Bjerklie, Ferketich, et al., 1993; Kwiatkowski et al., 1995; Roberts et al., 1993). Other strategies have been added to these research-based treatments from a theoretical perspective (Carrieri-Kohlman & Janson-Bjerklie, 1990; Gift, 1990a). Environmental and social strategies included postponing, prioritizing and careful planning of activities, "breathing stations," avoiding precipitants, and making environmental alterations. Taking medications and using breathing strategies are some of the physiological strategies. Cognitive-behavioral strategies include focusing on the positive aspects of life, normalization or minimization, pacing activities, reminiscing, reflection, and problem solving. Subjects in all of these studies deny participating in any formal teaching programs and have learned these skills by themselves or from others with shortness of breath. Without formal education programs, people learn "skilled bodily responses to symptoms" such as relaxation or pursed lip breathing. They become experts in reading their own bodily states. They often develop accurate recognition of activities that will precipitate increased shortness of breath or bring on infections. Thus, patients become excellent "symptom managers" and

know their exercise tolerance relative to the amount of dyspnea, and they learn to regulate that activity. Patients learn to manage complex medication and activity regimens.

In a study of 30 adults, the effect of peak flow monitoring on selection of self-care strategies for asthma symptoms was studied (Janson-Bjerklie & Schnell, 1988). Feedback of physiological information to the subject was thought to alter self-management behavior. Subjects were randomly assigned to either a control or an experimental group. All subjects recorded episodes of asthma symptoms and self-care actions taken in an asthma episode diary, but only experimental group subjects recorded peak flow at the onset and resolution of each episode of asthma. Taking medication was reported by both groups as the most frequent strategy used to control symptoms and was rated significantly more efficacious than all other strategies tried. The experimental group with access to peak flow information used inhaled beta agonist medication significantly less often than the control group.

To explore dyspnea associated with HIV-related disease, patients' perceptions of pulmonary problems and nursing interventions were examined in a sample of 201 adults living with AIDS who were hospitalized for *Pneumocystis carinii* pneumonia. Out of a total of 601 identified problems, 61 instances of dyspnea and 83 other pulmonary problems were reported. Oxygen and medication administration were reported as nursing interventions. Contrary to expectations, dyspnea was reported by less than one third of the sample. Few independent nursing interventions were identified. Effective nursing management for dyspnea in HIV-related disease needs development (Janson-Bjerklie, Holzemer, & Henry, 1992).

Educational interventions. In one early study using nurse-administered teaching and counseling compared to nonspecific surveillance with psychotherapy, analytic psychotherapy, and supportive psychotherapy, the nurse-treated group was the only group to report a "sustained relief in breathlessness" (Rosser et al., 1983).

In a more recent investigation, 12 asthmatic adults participated in an open trial of an asthma educational intervention for effect on symptom intensity, pulmonary function, and sputum markers of airway inflammation. Symptom scores for dyspnea, chest tightness, wheezing, and cough decreased 25% over 8 weeks as a result of the intervention. Sputum and eosinophil cell counts and products decreased by 50% (Janson-Bjerklie, Fahy,

TABLE 20.1. Self-Care Strategies for Managing Dyspnea Reported by Patients in Selected Studies

	Brown et al., 1986: Adults, Lung Cancer (N = 30)	Carrieri and Janson-Bjerklie, 1986 (N = 68)	Carrieri Kieckhefer, et al., 1991: Children, Asthma (N = 39)	Janson-Bjerklie and Ferketich, 1992: Adults, Asthma (N = 95)	Kwiatkowski et al., 1995: Adults, COPD (N = 52)
Physiological					
Breathing strategies	x	x	x	x	
Pursed-lips breathing	x	x			x
Diaphragmatic breathing		x			x
Drink fluids		x	x	x	
Exercise	x	x			x
Medications	x	x		x	
Oxygen		x			
Positioning or posture	x	x		x	
Sit down		x	x		
Sit up			x		
Lie down		x			
Keep still		x	x	x	
Environmental and social					
Activity modification and energy conservation		x		x	
Advanced planning	x	x		x	
Decrease in activities	x	x		x	
Move slower	x				
Transfer ADLs to others	x	x			
Change in living arrangement	x				
Distancing from triggers	x	x		x	x
Fresh air		x	x	x	x
Seeking social support	x	x	x	x	x
Seeking medical care		x	x	x	
Cognitive and behavioral					
Self-monitoring					
Self-control of medication	x		x	x	
Stress reduction					
Distraction and diversion	x		x	x	x
Imagery				x	
Meditation, prayer	x	x			
Music				x	
Relaxation	x	x	x	x	x
Self-isolation	x	x			
Self-talk	x	x	x	x	

NOTE: ADL = activities of daily living.

Geaghan, & Golden, 1993; Janson-Bjerklie, Hardie, Fahy, & Boushey, 1994).

▬ *Pulmonary Rehabilitation Programs*

Dyspnea outcomes are often measured within the context of pulmonary rehabilitation or asthma self-management program evaluations. A recent meta-analysis of 14 randomized clinical trials for pulmonary rehabilitation indicated that both inpatient and outpatient pulmonary rehabilitation programs decreased the intensity of dyspnea measured in the laboratory and with activities of daily living, using a variety of instruments for measurement (Lacasse et al., 1996). Recently published evidence-based guidelines contain recommendations that pulmonary rehabilitation programs be the treatment of choice for improving the symptom of dyspnea in COPD patients (Ries, Carlin, et al., 1997). Similar to the findings of other randomized clinical trials (Fishman, 1994; O'Donnell, McGuire, Samis, & Webb, 1995; Ries, Kaplan,

Limberg, & Prewitt, 1995), Reardon and her colleagues (1994) showed that a 6-week outpatient comprehensive pulmonary rehabilitation program, compared to an untreated control group, resulted in significant improvement in dyspnea during incremental exercise testing and during daily functioning.

Structured pulmonary rehabilitation programs typically include a combination of physiological, social, and cognitive-behavioral strategies. Education about pulmonary disease is combined with breathing retraining and exercise. Coping strategies may include relaxation, imagery, use of social support resources, psychological support, contracting for goals, and energy conservation. Until future controlled trials examine the individual effects of specific components of multimodal programs, the individual contribution of each strategy remains unknown. In particular, exercise training does decrease the intensity and the distress of dyspnea. Selected small studies that have tested individual cognitive-behavioral strategies are discussed below.

Exercise training. In a recent study of 12 monitored exercise sessions, the intensity of dyspnea, as well as the anxiety and distress associated with it, was shown to decrease relative to ventilation in 51 subjects with COPD. Self-efficacy (for walking) also increased. These benefits occurred after patients with COPD exercised in a supervised safe environment with or without coaching by a nurse (Carrieri-Kohlman, Gormley, Douglas, et al., 1996). The decrease in dyspnea found in both of these studies was attributed in part to desensitization (Haas, Salazar-Schicchi, & Axen, 1993), increased muscle efficiency, and comfort on the treadmill, as there was little evidence for aerobic conditioning. A recent medical study to examine improvement in dyspnea as a result of exercise training revealed that dynamic hyperinflation and ventilatory impedance, desensitization to the symptom, mechanical efficiency, and aerobic conditioning were possible reasons for the reduced dyspnea (Ramirez-Venegas, Ward, Olmstead, Tosteson, & Mahler, 1997).

Cognitive behavioral strategies. Using small samples and uncontrolled designs, nurse researchers have studied the effect of cognitive behavioral distraction strategies; specifically, relaxation and guided imagery. These strategies decrease dyspnea while the intervention is administered; however, the long-term effect is unknown. Cognitive behavioral strategies alone, without exercise, have not been found to decrease dyspnea in the long term. In a recent randomized clinical trial, a program of education

and practice of coping strategies for dyspnea was compared to a control group who heard lectures about health (Sassi-Dambron et al., 1995). The education program consisted of breathing, anatomy and physiology and description of COPD, a dyspnea-function model (panic and discomfort that lead to a decrease in activities, deconditioning, dyspnea on exertion), breathing strategies (diaphragmatic and PLB), progressive muscle relaxation, pacing and energy-saving techniques, self-talk and panic control, and stress management with suggested coping strategies. There were no significant differences between treatment and control groups in outcomes including measurement of dyspnea with six different instruments, a 6-minute walk, quality of well-being, and psychological functioning, with the exception that one measure of dyspnea decreased more significantly for the group receiving the strategies and practice.

Relaxation. Most investigators who have systematically studied relaxation have included patients with asthma; they have measured respiratory rate, flow rates, and lung volumes but not dyspnea as an outcome variable. One investigator studied the effect of relaxation on dyspnea in 10 COPD patients, compared with a control group that was instructed to relax but was not given specific instructions. Although dyspnea was significantly reduced for the experimental group only during treatment sessions, group differences were lacking after 4 weeks (Renfroe, 1988). Other researchers found that the use of relaxation techniques by patients with COPD decreased state anxiety as well as the perception of dyspnea intensity at rest (Gift, Moore, & Soeken, 1992).

These preliminary studies exhibited immediate and significant decreases in dyspnea that did not persist beyond the experimental sessions. The effect of relaxation techniques on dyspnea is not well established. If relaxation decreases respiratory rate, increases concentration, and reduces tension or stress, a logical assumption is that dyspnea will be reduced, at least temporarily. Relaxation might also increase feelings of control of breathing, slow respiratory rate, and increase tidal volume. These physiological variables have been related to dyspnea in the laboratory and in critically ill patients (Bouley et al., 1992; Carrieri-Kohlman, 1991).

Guided imagery. In an uncontrolled study of the effect of guided imagery on dyspnea, depression, quality of life, anxiety, and functional status, 19 patients with COPD met weekly for 1 hour of practice for 4 weeks. While a standard guided imagery script was read, subjects were asked to visualize the scene described. Audiotapes of the script were provided for twice-daily patient practice. Reported dyspnea did not change significantly (Moody, Fraser, et al., 1993).

Distraction. Music has been tested by investigators from other disciplines and been found to increase exercise performance in patients with COPD. Decreased breathlessness was suggested as a reason for this improvement. (Thornby, Haas, & Axen, 1995).

Recommendations for Knowledge Development

A published framework developed at the University of California at San Francisco (UCSF) for the study of symptom management incorporates the dimensions of *symptom perceptions, symptom responses, symptom management,* and *outcomes.* It is used along with considerations of measurement as follows to summarize the state of the science for dyspnea in terms of recommendations for furthering the science (Larson et al., 1994).

Symptom Perceptions

Knowledge related to understanding dyspnea is in the early stages of development. The physiological mechanisms are barely known. Neurophysiological pathways are now being identified, and mechanical muscle contributions are being investigated in more depth. New theories are demonstrating the significant role that dynamic hyperinflation, which places ventilatory muscles at a mechanical disadvantage, plays in dyspnea. The convergence of neuroventilatory coupling with the classic theory of length-tension theory is also exciting (Belman, Botnick, & Shin, 1996; O'Donnell & Webb, 1993). For example, while using positron emission tomography (PET) during CO_2-stimulated breathing at a level sufficient to induce dyspnea, it was shown that regional cerebral blood flow (as an index of regional change in neuronal synaptic activity) is increased in the upper brainstem and midbrain and in structures that are closely associated with the limbic system. This finding is suggestive of physiological pathways underlying emotional responses to dyspnea (Corfield et al., 1995). Future studies should continue according to a variety of proposed mechanisms including mechanical, chemical, and neurological pathways.

As depicted in the UCSF Symptom Management Model, the experience of dyspnea is thought to involve three components: perception of the sensation, evaluation of its meaning, and response. Perception, evaluation, and response may not have temporal or linear dimensions but, rather, overlap in a consensual or dynamic fashion. This conceptualization requires further study and development. Factors that affect perception of dyspnea and require further exploration are ethnic differences, age-related changes, hormonal flux, and variations in dyspnea during special physiological states, such as pregnancy, menopause, and puberty. Some imposed conditions, such as smoking, may actually decrease dyspnea while worsening the overall disease state. This phenomenon presents a paradox that requires a completely different conceptual approach.

Symptom Responses

Acute or chronic dyspnea is the source of multidimensional responses strongly influenced by the meaning attached to having the symptom. For example, if having dyspnea imposes the threat of death, the response may be extreme anxiety and panic, but dyspnea that signals exertion and work carries a completely different meaning and may be interpreted differently. These different interpretations carry different meanings and undoubtedly influence behavior, yet little is known about why patients with chronic symptoms behave the way they do. Behaviors associated with symptoms are observable to others and have been described, but the mechanisms linking symptom, meaning, response, and behavior require much more study.

Symptom Management

At the present time, treatments for dyspnea are directed toward decreasing ventilatory impedance, improving respiratory muscle function, decreasing respiratory drive, and/or decreasing the central perception of dyspnea by targeting psychological and behavioral variables that modulate the perception of dyspnea. There are many strategies that patients use and nurses observe clinically that seem to improve the perception of dyspnea. Some of these therapies have a physiological or psychological basis and have been tested in the laboratory with normal subjects (i.e., cold air on the face) or in small uncontrolled studies with patients (relaxation). As yet, nurses have not been involved in the study of pharmacological therapies for dyspnea, such as oxygen and opiates with terminal illness. Future study of the strategies known to decrease dyspnea for the patient requires emphasis. Nothing is known about the individual variations of differing treatments on different individuals. What strategies work with different types of illnesses? Most of the research has been with COPD patients, but little is known about the types and use frequency of dyspnea management strategies in other diseases such as cardiac, interstitial disease, neuromuscular disease, or normal pregnancy. Because it is known that dyspnea and distress accompanying dyspnea are modulated by other psychosocial factors (e.g., self-efficacy and mood), alteration of these factors may influence dyspnea. For example, if self-efficacy for walking can be increased, walking more often or for longer periods of time in turn may affect the intensity of dyspnea with a certain level of work. Exercise training has been found to be a powerful treatment for dyspnea and the distress associated with it. However, little is known about the dose (i.e., intensity, frequency, mode) of the exercise needed to bring about changes in the intensity of dyspnea with a given amount of work.

Outcomes of Dyspnea

Dyspnea has been shown to be a greater predictor of quality of life than any physiological variable, including measures of airflow (FEV1) or arterial blood gases (Curtis et al., 1994). There is a shift in the study of dyspnea across disciplines to emphasize a multifactorial approach. Examples include studies of the descriptions of breathlessness provoked by varied physiological stimuli; determining which neuroreceptors in the airways, nasopharynx, and face are activated; and the pursuit of therapies that are targeted to both physiological and psychological mechanisms, such as exercise, opiates, oxygen, and relaxation (Carrieri-Kohlman, 1992). The effect of differing levels of dyspnea on outcome variables such as quality of life, functional status, health care utilization, and emotional response deserves more study. Improvements in the perception of dyspnea and the distress associated with it that may result by targeting moderator variables including self-efficacy, feelings of control, and mood should be investigated. Discrete components of pulmonary rehabilitation programs need to be studied for their individual effects on the symptom of dyspnea.

Measurement of Dyspnea

Dyspnea is most often measured for research; its measurement in clinical settings is infrequent. The symp-

tom may be monitored but is rarely documented. Measurement of symptoms such as dyspnea is influenced by individuals' beliefs so that ratings can reflect sensory and cognitive/emotional elements. Measurement tools require individuals to evaluate the symptom or sensation to rate it, so repeated measurement may influence subsequent ratings of dyspnea in unknown ways. The repeated measurement of dyspnea within short time intervals may enhance perceptions and lead to inflated ratings. The influence on rating scores of time and duration between measurements is poorly understood. Dyspnea, or shortness of breath, is only one of a variety of respiratory sensations that are felt by people with respiratory illness. The variety of respiratory sensations has been clustered according to physiological mechanisms. Different mechanisms may provoke different sensations that heretofore have been labeled "shortness of breath." In addition, different cultures may use different words for the same sensation of shortness of breath, and these differences need to be explored. There is beginning evidence that gender and culture may affect the perception, rating, and language that people use to describe dyspnea.

There are many measurement tools published for dyspnea, but there is little direction in the literature about how to use them appropriately to measure the dimension of greatest interest in any one study. As examples, when is it best to use a visual analogue scale? Does a numerical scale provide more significant advantages over the VAS, and, if so, how many numbers should be used? When is the use of a Borg scale more appropriate? What is the best dyspnea instrument to use in randomized clinical trials where outcomes of the intervention need to be measured precisely? Although there is beginning work on the measurement of dyspnea with daily activities, study in this area needs to be enhanced. There are few if any studies by nurses in the documentation and study of dyspnea in patients with terminal illness.

Conclusions

An enormous amount of progress has been made in the past few years in the study of theoretical mechanisms, measurement techniques, and therapeutic management of dyspnea in patients with pulmonary disease, especially those with chronic obstructive pulmonary disease. Focus finally has been directed toward the symptom rather than toward the physiological mechanisms of pulmonary disease that result in shortness of breath. Nurse researchers have been at the forefront in the description of the sensation, the study of related correlates, and in the development of measures of the sensation in both the laboratory and clinical setting. Future research directions should include all areas of study described here. Nursing research efforts should go beyond the study of dyspnea with respiratory illness. The measurement and treatment of dyspnea in patients with other illnesses such as interstitial, cardiac, terminal cancer or pulmonary disease, and/or musculoskeletal diseases should be emphasized. There is a need to expand the study of mechanisms, especially those that are physi-

ological and neurobiological. Measurements and treatments for acute dyspnea in people who are ventilated and those who are spontaneously breathing need to be studied and tested. The study of cultural and gender differences in the perception, language, and rating of dyspnea is needed to better inform practice. Treatments targeted to the affective response or distress and anxiety associated with the symptom should be tested. To date, the evidence for the usefulness of education and/or cognitive-behavioral strategies in coping with dyspnea is conflicting. Nursing investigators need to target these strategies and use randomized clinical trials to determine the true effectiveness of these interventions for modulating the symptom of dyspnea.

References

Adams, L., & Gun, A. (1991). Dyspnea on exertion. In B. J. Whip & K. Wasserman (Eds.), *Exercise: Pulmonary physiology and pathology* (pp. 449-494). New York: Marcel Dekker.

Altos, M. (1992). Management of breathlessness. In N. L. Jones & K. J. Killian (Eds.), *Breathlessness: The Campbell symposium* (pp. 162-169). Hamilton, Ontario: Boehringer Ingelheim.

Anderson, K. L. (1995). The effect of chronic obstructive pulmonary disease on quality of life. *Research in Nursing and Health, 18,* 547-556.

Belman, M. J., Botnick, W. C., & Shin, J. W. (1996). Inhaled bronchodilators reduce dynamic hyperinflation during exercise in patients with chronic obstructive pulmonary disease. *American Journal of Respiratory and Critical Care Medicine, 153,* 967-975.

Borg, G.A.V. (1982). Psychophysical basis of perceived exertion. *Medicine and Science in Sports and Exercise, 14,* 377-381.

Borson, S., McDonald, G., Gayle, T., Deffebach, M., Lakshminarayan, S., & VanTuinen, C. (1992). Improvement in mood, physical symptoms, and function with nortryiptyline for depression in patients with chronic obstructive pulmonary disease. *Psychosomatics, 33* (2), 190-201.

Bouley, G. H., Froman, R., & Shah, H. (1992). The experience of dyspnea during weaning. *Heart and Lung, 21,* 471-476.

Breslin, E. H. (1992). The pattern of respiratory muscle recruitment during pursed-lip breathing. *Chest, 101*(7), 5-78.

Breslin, E. H., Garoutte, B. C., Carrieri, V. K., & Celli, B. R. (1990). Correlations between dyspnea, diaphragm, and sternomastoid recruitment during respiratory resistive breathing in normal subjects. *Chest, 98,* 298-302.

Breslin, E. H., Garoutte, B. C., & Celli, B. R. (1990). Respiratory muscle and dyspnea responses to unsupported upper extremity exercise in normal subjects. In S. G. Funk, E. M. Tornquist, M. T. Champagne, L. A. Copp, & R. Wiese (Eds.), *Key aspects of recovery: Improving nutrition, rest and mobility* (pp. 239-247). New York: Springer.

Breslin, E. H., Roy, C., & Robinson, C. R. (1992). Physiological nursing research in dyspnea: A paradigm shift and a metaparadigm exemplar. *Scholarly Inquiry for Nursing Practice: An International Journal, 6,* 81-104.

Brown, M., Carrieri, V. A., Janson-Bjerklie, S., & Dodd, M. (1986). Lung cancer and dyspnea: The patient's perception. *Oncology Nursing Forum, 13,* 19-24.

Carrieri, V. K., & Janson-Bjerklie, S. (1986). Strategies patients use to manage the sensation of dyspnea. *Western Journal of Nursing Research, 8,* 284-305.

Carrieri, V. K., Janson-Bjerklie, S., & Jacobs, S. (1984). The sensation of dyspnea: A review. *Heart and Lung, 13,* 436-447.

Carrieri, V. K., Kieckhefer, G., Janson-Bjerklie, S., & Souza, J. (1991). The sensation of pulmonary dyspnea in school-age children. *Nursing Research, 40,* 81-85.

Carrieri-Kohlman, V. (1991). Dyspnea in the weaning patient: Assessment and intervention. *AACN Clinical Issues in Critical Care Nursing, 2,* 462-473.

Carrieri-Kohlman, V. (1992). Response to "Physiological Nursing Research in Dyspnea: A Paradigm Shift and a Metaparadigm Exemplar." *Scholarly Inquiry for Nursing Practice: An International Journal, 6,* 105-109.

Carrieri-Kohlman, V., Douglas, M. K., Gormley, J., & Stolberg, M. S. (1993). Desensitization and guided mastery: Treatment approaches for the management of dyspnea. *Heart and Lung, 22,* 226-2234.

Carrieri-Kohlman, V., & Gormley, J. M. (1998). Coping strategies for dyspnea. In D. Mahler (Ed.), *Dyspnea.* New York: Marcel Dekker.

Carrieri-Kohlman, V., Gormley, J. M., Douglas, M. K., Paul, S. M., & Stolberg, M. S. (1996a). Differentiation between dyspnea and its affective components. *Western Journal of Nursing Research, 18,* 626-642.

Carrieri-Kohlman, V., Gormley, J. M., Douglas, M. K., Paul, S. M., & Stolberg, M. S. (1996b). Exercise training decreases dyspnea and the distress and anxiety associated with it. *Chest, 110,* 1526-1535.

Carrieri-Kohlman, V., Gormley, J. M., & Stolberg, M. S. (1993, November). The perception of dyspnea is related to self-efficacy for walking during 12 treadmill treatment sessions in subjects with chronic obstructive pulmonary disease (COPD). *ANA Council of Nurse Researchers: 1993 Scientific Sessions* (p. 373). Washington, DC.

Carrieri-Kohlman, V., & Janson-Bjerklie, S. (1993). In V. Carrieri-Kohlman, A. M. Lindsey, & C. M. West (Eds.), *Pathophysiologi-*

cal phenomena in nursing: Human responses to illness (2nd ed., pp. 247-278). Philadelphia: W. B. Saunders.

Carrieri-Kohlman, V., Lindsey, A. M., & West, C. M. (1993). The conceptual approach. In V. Carrieri-Kohlman, A. M. Lindsey, & C. M. West (Eds.), *Pathophysiological phenomena in nursing: Human responses to illness* (2nd ed., pp. 1-10). Philadelphia: W. B. Saunders.

Comroe, J. H. (1965). Some theories of the mechanisms of dyspnea. In J. B. Howell & E.J.M. Campbell (Eds.), *Breathlessness* (pp. 1-7). Boston: Blackwell Scientific.

Corfield, D. R., Fink, G. R., Ramsay, S. C., Murphy, K., Harty, H. R., Watson, J.D.G., Adams, L., Frackowiak, R.S.J., & Gun, A. (1995). Evidence for limbic system activation during CO_2-stimulated breathing in man. *Journal of Physiology, 488,* 162-170.

Curtis, J. R., Deyo, R. A., & Hudson, L. D. (1994). Health-related quality of life among patients with chronic obstructive pulmonary disease. *Thorax, 49,* 162-170.

DeVito, A. J. (1990). Dyspnea during hospitalizations for acute phase of illness as recalled by patients with chronic obstructive pulmonary disease. *Heart and Lung, 19,* 186-191.

Eldridge, F. L., & Chen, Z. (1996). Respiratory sensation: A neurophysiological perspective. In L. Adams & A. Gun (Eds.), *Respiratory sensation* (pp. 19-67). New York: Marcel Dekker.

Elliott, M., Adams, L., Cockroft, A., MacRae, K. D., Murphy, K., & Gun, A. (1991). The language of breathlessness. *American Review of Respiratory Disease, 144,* 826-832.

Fishman, A. P. (1994). Pulmonary rehabilitation research: NIH workshop summary. *American Journal of Respiratory and Critical Care Medicine, 149,* 825-833.

Gift, A. (1989). Validation of a vertical visual analogue scale as a measure of clinical dyspnea. *Rehabilitation Nursing, 14,* 323-325.

Gift, A. (1991). Psychologic and physiologic aspects of acute dyspnea in asthmatics. *Nursing Research, 40,* 196-199.

Gift, A. G. (1990a). Dyspnea. *Nursing Clinics of North America, 25,* 955-965.

Gift, A. G. (1990b). Psychophysiologic aspects of dyspnea in chronic obstructive pulmonary disease: A pilot study. *Heart and Lung, 19,* 252-257.

Gift, A. G., Moore, T., & Soeken, K. (1992). Relaxation to reduce dyspnea and anxiety in COPD patients. *Nursing Research, 41,* 242-246.

Gift, A. G., Plaut, M., & Jacox, A. (1986). Psychologic and physiologic factors related to dyspnea in subjects with chronic obstructive pulmonary disease. *Heart and Lung, 15,* 595-601.

Gift, A. G., & Pugh, L. C. (1993). Dyspnea and fatigue. *Nursing Clinics of North America, 28,* 373-383.

Gormley, J. M., Carrieri-Kohlman, V., Douglas, M. K., & Stolberg, M. (1994). Treadmill self-efficacy and walking performance in COPD patients. *Journal of Cardiopulmonary Rehabilitation, 13,* 424-431.

Graydon, J. E., & Ross, E. (1995). Influence of symptoms, lung function, mood, and social support on level of functioning of patients with COPD. *Heart and Lung, 24,* 369-375.

Graydon, J. E., Ross, E., Webster, P. M., Goldstein, R., & Avendano, M. (1995). Predictors of functioning of patients with chronic obstructive pulmonary disease. *Heart and Lung, 24,* 369-375.

Haas, F., Salazar-Schicchi, J., & Axen, K. (1993). Desensitization to dyspnea in chronic obstructive pulmonary disease. In R. Casaburi & T. Petty (Eds.), *Principles and practice of pulmonary rehabilitation* (pp. 241-251). Philadelphia: W. B. Saunders.

Harver, A., & Mahler, D.A. (1990). The symptom of dyspnea. In D.A. Mahler (Ed.), *Dyspnea* (pp. 1-53). Mt Kisco, NY: Futura.

Janson-Bjerklie, S., Carrieri, V. K., & Hudes, M. (1986). The sensation of pulmonary dyspnea. *Nursing Research, 35,* 154-159.

Janson-Bjerklie, S., Fahy, J., Geaghan, S., & Golden, J. (1993). Disappearance of eosinophils from bronchoalveolar lavage fluid after patient education and high-dose inhaled corticosteroids: A case report. *Heart and Lung, 22,* 235-238.

Janson-Bjerklie, S., Ferketich, S., Benner, P., & Becker, G. (1992). Clinical markers of asthma severity and risk: Importance of subjective as well as objective factors. *Heart and Lung, 21,* 265-272.

Janson-Bjerklie, S., Ferketich, S., Benner, P., & Becker, G. (1993). Predicting the outcomes of living with asthma. *Research in Nursing and Health, 16,* 241-250.

Janson-Bjerklie, S., Hardie, G., Fahy, J., & Boushey, H. A. (1994). Effects of an asthma education intervention on markers of airway inflammation, peak flow, and symptoms [Abstract]. *American Journal of Respiratory and Critical Care Medicine, 149,* A1078.

Janson-Bjerklie, S., Holzemer, W., & Henry, S. B. (1992). Patients' perceptions of pulmonary problems and nursing interventions during hospitalization for *Pneumocystis carinii* pneumonia. *American Journal of Critical Care, 1,* 114-121.

Janson-Bjerklie, S., Ruma, S. S., Stolberg, M., & Carrieri, V. K. (1987). Predictors of dyspnea intensity in asthma. *Nursing Research, 36,* 179-183.

Janson-Bjerklie, S., & Schnell, S. (1988). Effect of peak flow information on patterns of self-care in adult asthma. *Heart and Lung, 17,* 543-549.

Jones, P. W., & Wilson, R. C. (1996). Cognitive aspects of breathlessness. In L. Adams & A. Gun (Eds.), *Respiratory sensation* (pp. 311-339). New York: Marcel Dekker.

Knebel, A. R. (1989). Patient perceptions of the weaning experience following prolonged mechanical ventilation [Abstract]. *American Review of Respiratory Disease, 13,* A97.

Knebel, A. R. (1998). Dyspnea in the ventilator-assisted patient: evaluation and treatment. In D. A. Mahler (Ed.), *Dyspnea* (pp. 363-390). New York: Marcel Dekker.

Knebel, A. R., Janson-Bjerklie, S. L., Malley, J. D., Wilson, A. G., & Marini, J. J. (1994). Comparison of breathing comfort during weaning with two ventilatory modes. *American Journal of Respiratory and Critical Care Medicine, 149,* 14-18.

Kohlman-Carrieri, V., & Janson-Bjerklie, S. (1990). Coping and self-care strategies. In D. A. Mahler (Ed.), *Dyspnea* (pp. 201-230). Mt. Kisco, New York: Futura.

Kwiatkowski, M., Carrieri-Kohlman, V., Jansen, S., Gormley, J. M., & Stolberg, M. S. (1995, March 12-15). *Patients with chronic obstructive pulmonary disease (COPD) increase coping strategies for dyspnea after an exercise program.* Paper presented at the International Conference on Pulmonary Rehabilitation and Home Ventilation, Denver, CO.

Lacasse, Y., Wong, E., Guyatt, G. H., King, D., Cook, D. J., & Goldstein, R. S. (1996). Meta-analysis of respiratory rehabilitation in chronic obstructive pulmonary disease. *Lancet, 348,* 1115-1119.

Lareau, S. C., Breslin, E. H., Anholm, J. D., & Roos, P. J. (1992). Reduction in arm activities in patients with severe obstructive pulmonary disease. *American Review of Respiratory Disease, 145,* A476.

Lareau, S. C., Carrieri-Kohlman, V., Janson-Bjerklie, S., & Roos, P. J. (1994). Development and testing of the Pulmonary Functional Status and Dyspnea Questionnaire (PFSDQ). *Heart and Lung, 23,* 242-250.

Larson, P., Carrieri-Kohlman, V., Dodd, M., Douglas, M., Faucett, J., Froehlicher, E., et al. (1994). A model for symptom management. *Image: The Journal of Nursing Scholarship, 26,* 272-276.

Lenz, E. R., Suppe, F., Gift, A. G., Pugh, L. C., & Milligan, R. A. (1995). Collaborative development of middle-range nursing theories: Toward a theory of unpleasant symptoms. *Advances in Nursing Science, 17,* 1-13.

Lush, M., Janson-Bjerklie, S., Carrieri, V., & Lovejoy, N. (1988). Dyspnea in the ventilator-assisted patient. *Heart and Lung, 17,* 528-535.

Mahler, D. A., Paryniarz, K., Tomlinson, D., Colice, G., Robins, A. G., Olmstead, E. M., & O'Connor, G. T. (1992). Impact of dyspnea on physiologic function on general health status in patients with chronic obstructive pulmonary disease. *Chest, 102,* 395-401.

Mahler, D., Rosiello, R., Harver, A., Lentine, T., McGovern, J., & Daubenspeck, J. (1987). Comparison of clinical dyspnea ratings and psychophysical measurements of respiratory sensation on obstructive airway disease. *American Review of Respiratory Disease, 135,* 1229-1233.

Moody, L. E., Fraser, M., & Yarandi, H. (1993). Effects of guided imagery in patients with chronic bronchitis and emphysema. *Clinical Nursing Research, 2,* 476-478.

Moody, L., McCormick, K., & Williams, A. (1990). Disease and symptom severity, functional status, and the quality of life in chronic bronchitis and emphysema (CBE). *Journal of Behavioral Medicine, 13,* 297-306.

Moody, L., McCormick, K., & Williams, A. R. (1991). Psychophysiologic correlates of quality of life in chronic bronchitis and emphysema. *Western Journal of Nursing Research, 13,* 336-352.

Nield, M., & Kim, M. J. (1991). The reliability of magnitude estimation for dyspnea measurement. *Nursing Research, 40,* 17-19.

Nield, M., Kim, M. J., & Patel, M. (1989). Use of magnitude estimation for estimating the parameters of dyspnea. *Nursing Research, 38,* 77-80.

O'Donnell, D. E. (1994). Breathlessness in patients with chronic airflow limitation: Mechanisms and management. *Chest, 106,* 904-912.

O'Donnell, D. E., Bertley, J. C., Chau, L.K.L., & Webb, K. A. (1997). Qualitative aspects of exertional breathlessness in chronic airflow limitation. *American Journal of Respiratory and Critical Care Medicine, 155,* 109-115.

O'Donnell, D. E., McGuire, M., Samis, L., & Webb, K. (1995). The impact of exercise reconditioning on breathlessness in severe chronic airflow limitation. *American Journal of Respiratory and Critical Care Medicine, 152,* 2005-2013.

O'Donnell, D. E., & Webb, K. A. (1993). Exertional breathlessness in patients with chronic airflow limitation: The role of lung hyperinflation. *American Review of Respiratory Disease, 148,* 1351-1357.

Ramirez-Venegas, A., Ward, J. L., Olmstead, E. M., Tosteson, A. N., & Mahler, D. A. (1997). Effect of exercise training on dyspnea measures in patients with chronic obstructive pulmonary disease. *Journal of Cardiopulmonary Disease, 17,* 103-109.

Reardon, J., Awad, E., Normandin, E., Vale, F., Clark, B., & ZuWallack, R. L. (1994). The effect of comprehensive outpatient pulmonary rehabilitation on dyspnea. *Chest, 105,* 1046-1052.

Renfroe, K. L. (1988). Effect of progressive relaxation on dyspnea and state anxiety in patients with chronic obstructive pulmonary disease. *Heart and Lung, 17,* 408-413.

Reuben, D. B. (1986). Dyspnea in terminally ill cancer patients. *Chest, 89,* 234-236.

Ries, A. L., Carlin, B. W., Carrieri-Kohlman, V., Casaburi, R., Celli, B. R., Emery, C. F., Hodgkin, J., Mahler, D. A., Make, B., & Skolnick, J. (1997). Pulmonary rehabilitation: Joint ACCP/AACVPR evidence based guidelines. *Chest, 112,* 1363-1396.

Ries, A. L., Kaplan, R. M., Limberg, T. M., & Prewitt, L. M. (1995). Effects of pulmonary rehabilitation on physiologic and psychosocial outcomes in patients with chronic obstructive pulmonary disease. *Annals of Internal Medicine, 122,* 823-832.

Roberts, D. K., Thorne, E., & Pearson, C. (1993). The experience of dyspnea in late-stage cancer. *Cancer Nursing, 16,* 310-320.

Rosser, R., Denford, J., Heslop, A., Kinston, W., Macklin, D., Minty, K., Moynihan, C., Muir, B., Rein, L., & Gun, A. (1983). Breathlessness and psychiatric morbidity in chronic bronchitis and emphysema: A study of psychotherapeutic management. *Psychology Medicine, 13,* 93-110.

Sassi-Dambron, D. E., Eakin, E. G., Ries, A. L., & Kaplan, R. M. (1995). Treatment of dyspnea in COPD: A controlled clinical trial of dyspnea management strategies. *Chest, 107,* 724-729.

Schwarzstein, R. M., & Cristiano, L. M. (1996). Qualities of respiratory sensation. In L. Adams & A. Gun (Eds.), *Respiratory sensation* (pp. 125-154). New York: Marcel Dekker.

Schwarzstein, R. M., Manning, H. L., Weiss, J. W., & Weinberger, S. T. (1990). Dyspnea: A sensory experience. *Lung, 168,* 185-199.

Simon, P. M., Schwartzstein, R. M., Weiss, J. W., Fencl, V., Teghtsoonian, M., & Weinberger, S. E. (1990). Distinguishable types of dyspnea in patients with shortness of breath. *American Review of Respiratory Disease, 142,* 1009-1014.

Steele, B., & Shaver, J. (1992). The dyspnea experience: Nociceptive properties and a model for research and practice. *Advances in Nursing Science, 15,* 64-76.

Steele, B., Shaver, J., Hildebrandt, J., Schoene, R., Tyler, M., & Betrus, P. (1991). Dimensions of dyspnea during inspiratory threshold loading (ITL) in chronic obstructive pulmonary disease (COPD) [Abstract]. *American Review of Respiratory Disease, 143,* A595.

Stulberg, M., & Adams, L. (1994). Dyspnea. In J. Murray & J. Nadel (Eds.), *Textbook of respiratory medicine* (2nd ed., pp. 511-528). Philadelphia: W. B. Saunders.

Thornby, M. A., Haas, F., & Axen, K. (1995). Effect of distractive auditory stimuli on exercise tolerance in patients with COPD. *Chest, 107,* 1213-1217.

Tobin, M. J. (1990). Dyspnea: Pathophysiologic basis, clinical presentation and management. *Archives of Internal Medicine, 150,* 1604-1613.

Weaver, T. E., & Narsavage, G. L. (1992). Physiological and psychological variables related to functional status in chronic obstructive pulmonary disease. *Nursing Research, 41,* 286-291.

Weaver, T. E., Richmond, T. S., & Narsavage, G. L. (1997). An explanatory model of functional status in chronic obstructive pulmonary disease. *Nursing Research, 46,* 26-31.

West, N., & Popkess-Vawter, S. (1994). The subjective and psychosocial nature of breathlessness. *Advanced Nursing, 20,* 622-626.

Wilson, R. C., & Jones, P. W. (1989). A comparison of the visual analogue scale and modified Borg scale for the measurement of dyspnea during exercise. *Clinical Science, 76,* 277-282.

Wright, G. W., & Branscomb, B. V. (1954). The origin of the sensations of dyspnea. *Transactions of the American Clinical and Climatological Association, 1966,* 116-125.

Zelechowski, G. P. (1977). Physiological and psychological implications of dyspnea. *Respiratory Therapy, 7,* 18-21, 105-107.

21

MANAGING PAIN

Betty R. Ferrell

Introduction

Management of pain is integral to nursing practice, and there has, fortunately, been a wealth of nursing research in this area. Pain is one of the most distressing aspects of illness; it transcends all clinical settings, patient populations, and ages. Pain is a critical problem in acute, chronic, and terminal illness care.

The significance of pain to the core of nursing is evident in professional code4s and philosophies. Medical care is primarily focused on diagnosis and treatment of disease, but nursing care is focused on the patient experience of illness and relief of symptoms. Nursing care is also family centered, providing recognition of the profound impact of illness on the family unit. Pain represents a symptom that creates great distress for family caregivers in addition to the patient experiencing it. For example, alleviating procedure-related pain in premature infants provides comfort both to the infant and to the parents.

In 1968, Margo McCaffery introduced the modern definition of pain as a subjective phenomenon by identifying pain as "what the experiencing person says it is and existing whenever s/he says it does" (p. 95). Almost 30 years later, professional organizations and societies have adopted similar definitions. For example, the American Pain Society (APS) (1992) defines pain as "an unpleasant sensory and emotional experience associated with actual or potential tissue damage, or described in terms of such damage" (p. 2).

Members of the American Nurses Association (ANA) Council on Nursing Research (1985) stressed the importance of building nursing science to encompass the spectrum of human responses to actual and potential health problems. Pain, as a common experience of acute and chronic illness, is an important area of nursing research and a priority area for nursing intervention in clinical practice.

TABLE 21.1.   Summary of Recommendations by the National Institute of Nursing Research Priority Expert Panel on Symptom Management: Acute Pain

1. Investigate the six dimensions of pain (physiological, sensory, affective, cognitive, behavioral, and sociocultural), exploring their individual components as well as the contribution of each dimension to pain as a dynamic process; focus in particular on the affective, cognitive, behavioral, and sociocultural-cultural dimensions, with special attention to vulnerable populations.
2. Determine the critical assessment components for each dimension and test across patient populations.
3. Design and test strategies for management of pain that address the dimensions of pain, are multimodal and interdisciplinary in nature, influence the dimensions of pain in predicted directions, and result in positive patient outcomes.
4. Determine appropriateness and adequacy of existing approaches for assessing the six dimensions of pain, with particular attention to the needs of culturally diverse populations; develop tools to meet their needs if necessary.
5. Test the dynamic interplay of the multidimensional nature of pain, assessment, management, and outcomes.
6. Expand the basic understanding of the neural pathways for pain in preverbal children.
7. Explore the consequence of invasive procedures on the development of neural pathways.
8. Differentiate pain response from irritability and agitation.
9. Develop developmentally appropriate tools to measure different types of pain.
10. Focus studies on older infants and toddlers in addition to preterm and term neonates and infants under 6 months.
11. Specify pain issues for children with special needs, such as those with multiple handicaps, disorders of sensory mechanisms, cognitive impairments, a history of abuse, and those requiring multiple invasive procedures such as high-risk premature infants, or children of substance abusers.
12. Examine the socioeconomic and cultural issues that affect pain expression and management, especially for children of different ethnicities.
13. Test the effectiveness of pharmacological and nonpharmacological strategies simultaneously and singly for relieving pain.
14. Examine the roles and effectiveness of parents and other family members in caring for children with pain.
15. Examine the integration of pain assessment and management procedures into clinical practice.
16. Document the prevalence of pain related to trauma, treatment, diagnostic tests, and procedures.
17. Develop and test instruments to assess the behavioral dimensions of pain.
18. Evaluate the use of a standardized tool and/or protocol to assess pain.
19. Validate clinical impressions that influence pain assessment and management strategies.
20. Examine the link between physiological indicators of pain and behavioral and self-report responses.
21. Document the incidence of analgesic side effects and evaluate the extent to which opiates can be used safely.
22. Examine the synergistic effect of nonpharmacological strategies when used in conjunction with each other or with pharmacological strategies for managing pain.
23. Evaluate high-technology methods for delivering analgesics, including variables influencing effectiveness of use.
24. Examine attitudes and the decision-making process related to safe and effective analgesic management.
25. Evaluate the effectiveness of preparing children and adolescents for anticipated pain experiences.
26. Test patient-centered variables, including satisfaction with pain relief, preference for assessment and management approaches, self-efficacy beliefs, fears and concerns regarding taking drugs, gender, and ethnicity as they relate to assessment and management strategies.
27. Evaluate strategies for assisting parents to prepare and support children for painful experiences and for assessing and managing pain.
28. Address pain management issues for under-represented populations, including the developmentally disabled, multiple handicapped, substance abusers, those with other socially stigmatizing conditions, and culturally diverse populations.
29. Identify the factors, including beliefs and attitudes, that impede effective pain management; test strategies for changing or modifying beliefs and attitudes that hinder effective pain management; test strategies for changing or modifying beliefs and attitudes that hinder effective pain management in children and adolescents.
30. Design and test approaches to pain assessment that are culturally sensitive and can be useful for both clinical research and clinical practice.
31. Develop and test interventions for the suffering component of pain.
32. Test approaches for the application of currently available guidelines for the clinical management of pain. This may take the form of demonstration projects or dissemination projects but would necessitate inclusion of patient pain outcomes as a component of evaluation.
33. Test appropriateness and adequacy of nonpharmacological approaches to pain, including the impact of these approaches on the dimensions of pain and the relationship of nonpharmacological to pharmacological approaches. Emphasis on cognitive and physical approaches provides a beginning scientific foundation on which to build the clinical testing of specific nonpharmacological approaches.
34. Investigate the physiological dimension of pain, exploring physiological mechanisms involved, neurotransmitters, opioid receptors, and the impact of pain and pain relief on the immune system.
35. Test assessment tools to determine if they are cognitively appropriate, practical, reliable, and valid.

In this chapter, I describe the various conceptualizations of pain and theoretical approaches used to guide pain research, and I synthesize current knowledge based upon recent work by the Agency for Health Care Policy and Research (AHCPR) (1994) and the National Institute of Nursing Research (NINR) (1994) Priority Expert Panel on Symptom Management: Acute Pain. Further, I identify future areas of research and describe opportunities for translating the abundant knowledge into direct care of people in pain.

TABLE 21.1. (Continued)

36. Identify behavioral indexes of pain in cognitively impaired elderly.	44. Evaluate the interaction among patients, physicians, and nurses within the organizational context on patient outcomes such as pain, anxiety, satisfaction with care, length of stay, and costs.
37. Develop and test measures of the effectiveness of nonpharmacological pain management strategies in the elderly and the effects of combined nonpharmacological and pharmacological interventions.	45. Identify organizational variables that affect the effectiveness of pain management programs on patient outcomes such as pain, anxiety, satisfaction with care, length of stay, and costs.
38. Develop and test methods to examine age-related differences in the meaning of pain.	46. Evaluate the effectiveness of programs designed to change pain management practices.
39. Identify factors in caregivers' (spouse, family members, friends, significant others) attitudes and knowledge about pain that influence their management of the individual's pain and the pain behavior of the individual.	47. Examine ways to address the education-practice gap related to pain management.
40. Develop assessment tools that are applicable to various ethnic groups.	48. Determine the effects of informal unit standards that guide pain management practices in clinical units.
41. Develop a research base on the effects of acculturation on various ethnic groups and whether the length of time immigrants spend in this country influences their pain experience and manifestations.	49. Evaluate the effectiveness of formalized standards, policies, and guidelines for managing pain on patient outcomes such as pain, anxiety, satisfaction with care, length of stay, and costs.
42. Develop nursing care strategies in pain assessment issues: effectiveness of pharmacological interventions and nonpharmacological interventions alone and in combination and pain education for patients, caregivers, and patients' families.	50. Evaluate programs for educating the public about pain.\n51. Examine the costs, benefits, and harms of pain management programs in various settings such as the hospital, day surgery, clinics, and home care.
43. Determine the effects of innovative pain management educational programs on patient and health-care provider behaviors, attitudes, and knowledge.	52. Evaluate the effectiveness of acute-pain management services on patient outcomes such as pain, anxiety, satisfaction with care, length of stay, and costs.\n53. Evaluate the effectiveness of societal programs such as state-level cancer pain initiatives and the World Health Organization pain management initiatives on the undertreatment of pain.

SOURCE: National Institute of Nursing Research (1994).

State of the Science

A surge of nursing research activity in the 1970s can be credited for many of the current advances in pain management. Nurse researchers such as Benoliel and Crowley (1977), Copp (1974), and Jacox (1977) conducted seminal studies emphasizing the importance of pain and symptom control to well-being. Professional nursing organizations, also, have advanced the science of pain relief by identifying comfort as a basic goal of nursing care. Work by scientists such as Benoliel and McCorkle (1978) is recognized not only for initiating nursing research in pain management but also for the development of instruments such as the Symptom Distress Scale, still used by investigators across many disciplines.

Most writers who have synthesized pain knowledge have concluded that the previous descriptive work should now be extended to experimental studies to evaluate pain management interventions; however, such intervention testing is still scarce. When Smith, Holcombe, and Stullenbarger (1994) conducted a meta-analysis of intervention effectiveness for symptom management in oncology nursing, only 28 experimental studies were isolated from 428 published and unpublished nursing research reports, and only five were related to pain. The results indicated effectiveness of the interventions in relieving symptoms, but the authors acknowledged the many deficiencies in the literature with regard to intervention research. These included small samples, lack of a theoretical perspective, and wide variation in instruments used.

Similar deficits have been identified in knowledge about pain in pediatrics. Guardiola and Banos (1993) identified 2,193 published articles on pediatric pain, although the number of these citations by nurses was not known. These authors report a 91% increase in articles on pediatric pain over the past 20 years, including a fourfold increase in neonatal literature, a threefold increase regarding infants, and double the information on school and preschool children. However, these authors identified little literature on adolescent pain. In a meta-analysis of interventions for pediatric pain, Broome, Lillis, and Smith (1989) revealed only 28 studies over 22 years and across disciplines. Broome (1995) later reported that 58 intervention studies on pediatric pain were published between 1990 and 1994.

Despite the abundance of literature, many areas of additional research have been identified as necessary to advance the relief of pain. Table 21.1 presents a synthesis by the National Institute for Nursing Research (1994) Priority Expert Panel on Symptom Management: Acute Pain. Based on an extensive review of literature and analysis of knowledge, this panel summarized 53 recommendations for future research.

Analysis of these recommendations reveals several major areas for future research. The NINR panel identified the need for additional research in *pain assessment* (recommendations 2, 4, 9, 17, 18, 27, 30, 35, 36, 40, and 42), increased knowledge of the *physiological mechanisms* of pain (recommendations 6, 7, and 34), and conceptual or theoretical knowledge (recommendation 1). Three areas (recommendations 8, 20, and 31) addressed the need for *biobehavioral research.* The panel synthesis of future research needs includes several suggestions for *intervention studies* (recommendations 3, 5, 13, 15, 19, 21-23, 25, 27, 33, 37, and 42), encompassing both pharmacological and nonpharmacological interventions. Another area emphasized in the recommendations was the need for increased research in *special populations* such as children, the elderly, culturally diverse, and vulnerable groups (recommendations 1, 2, 4, 6, 10-12, 14, 28, 30, 36-38, 40, and 41). Research needs were identified in the area of *family or public education* (recommendations 39, 42, 50) and in the area of addressing both patients' and professionals' *knowledge and beliefs* related to pain management (recommendations 24, 26, 29, 43, and 47). The final area identified in these recommendations was the need for *translational research* to improve the quality of pain management (recommendations 32, 44-46, 48, 49, 51-53).

Many important advances have occurred in pain assessment and management based on the work of nurse researchers. Nurses have developed pain assessment instruments for pediatrics using graphic pain rating scales such as the Wong-Baker Faces Scales (Whaley & Wong, 1987) or the Oucher Scale (Beyer, Denyes, & Villarruel, 1992). Other techniques in pediatric pain assessment evolving from nursing research include the Poker Chip technique developed by Hester and colleagues, which had several behavioral assessment scales (Hester, Jacox, Miaskowski, & Ferrell, 1992) and word scales adapted for children (Tesler et al., 1991). These pain assessment scales measure only pain intensity but are important attempts to establish children's perspectives of pain.

Nurse researchers have used pain intensity instruments for adults such as the Visual Analogue Scale (Cline, Herman, Shaw, & Morton, 1992; Gift, 1989) and verbal descriptor scales (De Conno et al., 1994). In recent years, nurses have also used behavioral assessment tools to observe behaviors in acute or chronic pain (Ahles,

Coombs, Jensen, & Martin, 1990; Fordyce et al., 1984). This technique often includes videotapes of patients in pain and evaluation of the taped activity with the behavioral assessment scales.

Nursing intervention in pain management often involves patient and family education. Two instruments, the Patient Pain Questionnaire (PPQ) and the Family Pain Questionnaire (FPQ), assess knowledge and beliefs about pain and experiences in managing pain and are useful to assess outcomes of pain education (Ferrell, Grant, Chan, Ahn, & Ferrell, 1995; Ferrell, Rhiner, & Rivera, 1993). Nurse investigators have also relied on multidimensional pain instruments such as the McGill Pain Questionnaire (Melzack, 1987) or Brief Pain Inventory (Daut, Cleeland, & Flanery, 1983). Dr. Jo Ann Dalton developed a multidimensional pain questionnaire, the Biobehavioral Pain Profile, which has been extensively used (Dalton, Feuerstein, Carlson, & Roghman, 1994).

A more thorough review of pain instruments can be found in McGuire (1997). Review of nursing research literature also reveals that investigators commonly use instruments measuring related constructs, such as quality of life tools or coping instruments, in pain research. Items assessing pain are also included in other instruments, such as the Symptom Distress Scale (Benoliel & McCorkle, 1978).

Description and Comparison of Conceptual and Theoretical Perspectives

For a more comprehensive synthesis of the conceptual and theoretical approaches to pain, readers are referred to the *Report of the NINR Priority Expert Panel on Symptom Management: Acute Pain* (1994). However, a brief review of conceptual approaches follows.

Physiological theories have been derived from other disciplines and applied by nurse researchers. In the specificity theory, nociception was addressed in the main. Muller (1942) postulated that specific cutaneous pain receptors are activated to relay pain sensations to the brain. Pain was identified as a specific entity with unique peripheral and central components. The pattern theory embodied the notion of free nerve endings versus specific nerve fibers responding to painful stimuli (Wilkie, 1995). This theory has contributed to our understanding of various pain patterns and characteristics, such as the pattern of neuropathic pain amenable to the use of adjuvant pharmacological approaches in opioid addiction. Perhaps the most widely known theory is the Gate Control Theory (Melzack & Wall, 1965), which incorporated gating mechanisms at the level of the spinal cord for modulating sensory transmission of pain messages and the influence of higher brain (psychological or cognitive) factors on the pain experience. The Gate Control Theory has provided a framework for understanding the importance of cognitive factors on the physiological mechanisms of pain transmission. Much research continues regarding these theories and other approaches to understanding the physiological mechanisms of pain.

More recently, multidimensional frameworks have been articulated that incorporate variables affecting pain experience. Multidimensional frameworks of pain, such as one developed by Loeser (1982), include domains of nociception, pain, suffering, and pain behaviors. Ahles, Blanchard, and Ruckdeschel's (1983) framework of cancer pain includes physiological, sensory, affective dimension, cognitive, and behavioral influences.

McGuire (1997), a nurse researcher, described physiological, sensory, behavioral, cognitive, affective, and sociocultural components of pain. Nurse researchers have addressed these dimensions and contributed significantly to the state of knowledge in pain management. The physiological component includes such aspects as the location, onset, duration, etiology, and associated symptoms. The sensory component includes the intensity, quality, and pattern of the pain. The behavioral component includes communication about pain, interpersonal aspects, physical activity, pain behaviors, medications, interventions, and sleep. The cognitive component includes the meaning of pain, the view of pain, coping strategies, previous therapy, attitudes and beliefs, influencing factors, and prior experience of pain. The affective component refers to the mood state and includes anxiety, depression, anger, and feelings of powerlessness. Finally, the sociocultural component of pain includes the ethnic component, family and social life, work and home roles, recreation and leisure factors, and social behaviors and activities.

At the City of Hope National Medical Center, our program of research has resulted in a conceptual model of the impact of pain on quality of life (QOL) (Figure 21.1). The model was developed and refined over the past decade as a result of many studies involving patients, family caregivers, and nurses, and it had a range of subjects, from children in pain to the frail elderly. The model depicts four dimensions of QOL: (a) physical well-being, (b) psychological well-being, (c) social well-being, and (d) spiritual well-being (Ferrell, 1995).

The dimension of physical well-being captures the impact of pain on physical function and related symptoms. Pain is also closely associated with overall physical function, with evidence that many physical symptoms, such as fatigue, anorexia, sleeplessness, constipation, and nausea, are increased when pain is not controlled. Of important note, however, is that nursing care to improve pain relief also improves each of these aspects of physical well-being. Particularly striking is the extent to which pain results in extreme fatigue, another significant symptom affecting QOL (Ferrell, 1995; Ferrell, Dow, & Grant, 1995; Ferrell, Ferrell, Ahn, & Tran, 1994).

The dimension of psychological well-being depicts the impact of pain on symptoms such as depression and anxiety as well as related psychological constructs such as fear or coping. Social well-being is affected by pain through the impact on roles and relationships, employment, intimacy, and other aspects of life. Aspects such as the spiritual dimension of QOL is influenced by pain through the individual's sense of hope, religiosity, and uncertainty.

Review of existing frameworks demonstrates that there is consensus that pain is multidimensional and there is some consensus on the type of dimensions. Future research should involve exploration of less-developed dimensions, and investigators will use these frameworks to guide intervention studies in pain relief.

There is an important opportunity to use these frameworks to demonstrate the importance of nursing intervention for patients in pain. Use of multidimensional frameworks allows clinicians to capture the outcomes of effective pain management, not only on reduced pain intensity, but also on other aspects of the patient's life. Novel routes of analgesic administration, new analgesics, and use of nondrug interventions require adequate evaluation based on these conceptual frameworks.

Areas for Future Inquiry

Based on the review of literature and synthesis of the recommendations by the guideline panels cited above, the following eight areas of inquiry are recommended to build the science of pain management.

Physical Well-Being	**Psychological Well-Being**
Fatigue/Strength	Anxiety
Appetite	Depression
Sleep	Coping
Constipation	Control
Nausea	Concentration
Function	Sense of Usefulness
	Fear
	Enjoyment/Happiness

Pain

Social Well-Being	**Spiritual Well-Being**
Family Distress	Religiosity
Family Support	Uncertainty
Sexuality/Affection	Positive Changes
Employment	Sense of Purpose
Isolation	Hopefulness
Financial Burden	Suffering
Appearance	Meaning of Pain
Roles and Relationships	Transcendence

Figure 21.1. The Impact of Pain on Quality of Life
SOURCE: Ferrell, Grant, et al. (1995).

Conceptualization of Pain

Nurse researchers such as Dalton (1987) and McGuire (1997) have explored biobehavioral factors and affective states associated with pain in an attempt to explore further the relationship between variables influencing pain. Although a number of models exist, further work is needed to refine these models, to explore the relationships between variables within the frameworks and influencing variables, and to test these models in intervention research.

Barriers to Pain Management

Issues that serve as barriers to effective pain relief have been extensively identified and categorized by the AHCPR cancer pain panel according to patient barriers, professional barriers, and system barriers (Table 21.2). Studies of professional knowledge and attitudes provide strong evidence of the need for improved pain assessment and understanding of analgesic pharmacology on the part

of health care professionals (Ferrell, McCaffery, & Rhiner, 1992; Ferrell, McGuire, & Donovan, 1993; Jacox et al., 1994; McCaffery & Ferrell, 1991, 1992, 1995). This research has been descriptive in nature and has contributed to current efforts to overcome professional barriers. Patient barriers include patient reluctance to report pain or to use opioids due to unfounded fears such as addiction (Dalton, 1987; Ferrell, Ferrell, Ahn, et al., 1994; Jacox et al., 1994; Madison & Wilkie, 1995; Rimer, Kedziera, & Levy, 1992). The study of system barriers has not been a priority in research but is clearly an area of need. Nurses are centrally involved in each of these areas, and much research is needed now to test interventions that can overcome those barriers.

Pain Assessment

Nurse researchers have identified major obstacles to accurate and comprehensive pain assessment (Grossman, Sheidler, Swedeen, Mucenski, & Piantadosi, 1991) and the importance of obtaining patient reports of pain while

TABLE 21.2. Barriers to Cancer Pain Management

Problems related to health care professionals
Inadequate knowledge of pain management
    Poor assessment of pain
    Concern about regulation of controlled substances
    Fear of patient addiction
    Concern about side effects of analgesics
    Concern about patients becoming tolerant to analgesics

Problems related to patients
Reluctance to report pain
    Concern about distracting physicians from treatment of
      underlying disease
    Fear that pain means disease is worse
    Concern about not being a "good" patient
Reluctance to take pain medications
    Fear of addiction or of being thought of as an addict
    Worries about unmanageable side effects
    Concern about becoming tolerant to pain medications

Problems related to the health care system
Low priority given to cancer pain treatment
Inadequate reimbursement
    The most appropriate treatment may not be reimbursed or
      may be too costly for patients and families
Restrictive regulation of controlled substances
Problems of availability of treatment or access to it

SOURCE: Jacox et al. (1994).

studying pain assessment in special contexts, including postoperative (Zalon, 1993). Critical contributions have also been made in describing the needs of special populations such as neonates (Stevens, Johnston, & Horton, 1993) and the elderly (Ferrell, Ferrell, & Rivera, 1995).

Further pain assessment research is needed to adapt pain assessment tools to special populations (e.g., various ethnic groups) and settings of care (e.g., intensive care, ambulatory care settings). Nurses have been at the forefront of establishing the reliability and validity of pain assessment instruments and making these accessible for research and for clinical practice (Beyer et al., 1992; Savedra, Tesler, Holzemer, Wilkie, & Ward, 1989). An additional area for furthering the knowledge base in pain assessment is in behavioral observation, for those patients who are unable to provide verbal reports of pain, such as neonates (Stevens et al., 1993) and the cognitively impaired elderly (Ferrell, Ferrell, & Rivera, 1995).

Pharmacological Intervention

Nursing research is needed to advance the science of pharmacological interventions for pain. Consistent with the mission of nursing in assessing human responses to illness and treatment, nurse investigators should evaluate patient response to the myriad of analgesic treatments available for pain. Nurse investigators have explored top-

ics such as patterns of opioid use, routes of administration, and side effects of analgesics (Coyle, Adelhardt, Foley, & Portenoy, 1990; Coyle, Mauskop, Maggard, & Foley, 1986). New methods such as intraspinal delivery of analgesics (Paice, 1984; Penn & Paice, 1987) also require nursing research to determine the impact of the intervention. There is vast opportunity for nursing collaboration in interdisciplinary research in the area of pharmacology (Puntillo, 1994).

Nursing Knowledge Regarding Pain

The current emphasis on pain as a priority topic is due in part to research that revealed inadequacies in professional knowledge and attitudes about pain (Grossman et al., 1991; McCaffery & Ferrell, 1991). Inadequacies in professional education and texts (Ferrell, McCaffery, et al., 1992) and major obstacles in areas such as understanding addiction or principles of equianalgesia (McCaffery & Ferrell, 1992) are evident. Descriptive research is needed to explore other areas that should be targeted for intervention. It is also important to implement novel educational approaches to overcome these barriers and to evaluate these educational approaches.

Nondrug Interventions

Previous consensus conferences and panels have consistently identified a relative paucity of studies in the area of interventions outside of drug interventions for pain (Barbour, McGuire, & Kirchoff, 1986; Ellis & Spanos, 1994). Nurse investigators have explored patient education (Dalton, 1987; Ferrell, Ferrell, Ahn, et al., 1994), cognitive behavioral approaches with children, and use of nondrug interventions during painful procedures (Ellis & Spanos, 1994). Nondrug interventions have been recognized as inexpensive, simple, and valuable adjuncts to pharmacological approaches; having few side effects; and ideal interventions for independent nursing practice (Hyman, Feldman, Harris, Levin, & Malloy, 1989). In a review of nursing science related to pain, Gaston-Johansson and Fall-Dickson (1995) emphasized the need for future research to include randomized clinical trials of both drug and nondrug interventions.

Health Policy Issues

A critical yet virtually unexplored territory is the health policy implications of pain management. The AHCPR Cancer Pain Panel initiated preliminary work in identifying cost issues related to pain (Ferrell & Griffith, 1994). Nurse investigators have challenged the use of "high-tech" pain treatments and associated costs and ethical issues associated with their use (Whedon & Ferrell, 1991).

In initial research, Holcombe and Griffin (1993) reported significant differences in the pain medications prescribed for patients, depending on payor status. It will be important to document the effect of future health care financing and providers (e.g., managed care) on patient access to pain relief. Nurse investigators also have great opportunity to participate in the evaluation of pain clinics and pain specialty services. Yet another area for inquiry will be the evaluation of the role of the advanced practice nurse in pain management.

Nurses should also evaluate the financial impact of nursing interventions for pain. Grant, Ferrell, Rivera, and Lee (1995) have studied the costs of hospital readmission related to uncontrolled pain and the resultant costs savings following implementation of an aggressive pain management quality improvement program. Nurses have great opportunity to demonstrate the cost savings of improved pain relief through nursing care.

▬ *Pain and Quality Improvement*

Literature and clinical experience have demonstrated that pain management is best achieved when it becomes part of the institutional philosophy of an organization. Nurse researchers have pioneered efforts to integrate pain management within quality improvement programs (Ferrell, Whedon, & Rollins, 1995; Miaskowski, Jacox, Hester, & Ferrell, 1992; Miaskowski, Nichols, Brody, & Synold, 1994). Future research opportunities exist to evaluate quality assurance efforts based on patient and institutional outcomes and to further refine strategies.

Translation of Knowledge Into Practice

Because of the wealth of knowledge regarding pain, it is timely to focus efforts on transferring knowledge into practice. Table 21.3 is an example of specific strategies that have been suggested for clinical practice based on synthesis of scientific data regarding pain from the nurse members of the AHCPR Guideline Panel (Ferrell, Jacox, Miaskowski, Paice, & Hester, 1994).

Nursing research in pain management should continue the tradition of the nursing profession by maintaining a focus on the entire family rather than only on single individuals in pain (Clipp & George, 1992; Dar, Beach, Barden, & Cleeland, 1992; Ferrell, Rhiner, Cohen, & Grant, 1991). The tradition of nursing as a caring discipline sustains the interest of nursing scientists in pain as a priority area for research.

Madison and Wilkie (1995) addressed the need for increased research related to family perceptions of pain, as the family contributes to the social context of the pain experience. McIlveen and Morse (1995) conducted a historical analysis of the role of "comfort" in nursing care from 1900 to 1980. A total of 621 journal articles and 17 textbooks written by nurses were coded for key words such as *comfort, discomfort,* and *pain.* Content analysis revealed 12 categories explicating comfort roles in nursing. The authors observe that the prominance of providing patient "comfort" in nursing practice over time has changed from a central focus and moral imperative to a less important emphasis. They suggest that comfort has consistently been a significant goal for patients for whom there was no medical treatment.

From a methodological perspective, we have found in our research that it is very helpful to assess not only the *intensity* of symptoms but also the *distress* associated with symptoms. For example, in measuring pain, we ask, "How much pain do you have?" to assess pain intensity on a scale of 0 to 10, with 0 as no pain and 10 as severe pain. We then ask the patient to tell us, "How distressing is the pain to you?" This technique enables the patient to express how bothersome or distressing that particular symptom is. This technique assists us in appreciating the importance of individual problems to patients. For example, we often find that although patients may rate their pain as "fairly mild," they often describe it as "extremely distressing" because it limits them from participating in important activities. This is an example of ensuring that nursing research not only focuses on the presence of a symptom such as pain, but also on the impact on quality of life.

Previous research has benefited from the use of both qualitative and quantitative methods to capture the human dimension of pain and suffering (Ferrell, 1995; Polit & Hungler, 1995). As Benoliel (1995) noted in her review of nursing research in pain management, the meaning of pain and lived experience of the person in pain are often best understood through personal narrative. Qualitative research methods can provide a mechanism for understanding the patient's experience of symptoms and physical status in a way not achievable through quantitative scales or methods. Most of the nursing studies conducted

TABLE 21.3. Examples of Strategies to Implement Pain Knowledge in Clinical Practice

1. Obtain copies of the AHCPR guidelines and distribute them widely to your staff.
2. Perform a pain audit, including review of charts and patient interviews. The first step toward change is demonstrating that a problem exists.
3. Create an awareness of the status of pain management in your institution. Inform physicians, nursing staff, and administrators of the status of pain control and areas in need of improvement.
4. Designate an "expert nurse" on each shift as the consultant to colleagues on pain. Support that nurse in getting additional pain education and in becoming the unit "watchdog" for untreated pain.
5. Educate the physicians. Circulate articles, monographs, or audiotapes of interest. Work to sponsor a continuing medical education offering on pain management.
6. Adopt a uniform pain assessment tool for use during admission to the unit of any patient whose pain is a significant problem.
7. Adopt a uniform system for pain assessment (e.g., a 0-10 pain rating scale).
8. Establish standards of care. (Nurses do not accept uncontrolled infection rates, extravasations, and falls, so why accept uncontrolled pain?)
9. Involve others in pain management. Develop an army of supporters, such as volunteers and personnel from physical therapy, occupational therapy, social services, and the pharmacy.
10. Educate the patients. Patients must know that pain is preventable and treatable. Pain management should become a consumer issue, and patients should not settle for unrelieved pain.
11. Involve families in every aspect of pain management. Family members can be the greatest asset to pain relief or the greatest barrier.
12. Develop a "bag of tricks" of nondrug interventions for pain management, such as heat and cold therapy, instructions for breathing exercises, music and videotapes used for relaxation, and audiotapes used for imagery or relaxation.
13. Educate the nursing staff about basic principles of pain management.
14. Post equianalgesic charts on the unit. They are required nursing knowledge.
15. Develop a working relationship with someone in the pharmacy who can advocate for pain management.
16. Include pain management philosophy and strategies in new employee orientation.
17. Develop a pocket card for every nurse that includes the pain assessment scale and equianalgesia guides.
18. Make pain management accessible. Ensure that the pharmacy stocks appropriate medications and doses of drugs.
19. Develop an expectation in the unit that pain can be relieved. Nurses and patients often believe that cancer pain is inevitable and uncontrollable.
20. Plan for continuity in pain management. Coordinate pain efforts between inpatient units, the outpatient area, physician offices, and home or hospice services.
21. Document pain assessment. The patient's pain experience must be effectively communicated among all disciplines involved.
22. Evaluate your efforts.
23. Ask the patient. The patient is the best authority on his or her pain and our treatment of it.
24. Educate yourself, your professional organizations, and your institution regarding regulatory barriers to pain relief and work to overcome these barriers.
25. Sponsor a public education forum on pain.
26. Incorporate pain content into patient support groups.
27. Provide the kind of pain management that you would seek for your own family members.

SOURCE: Ferrell, Jacox, et al. (1994, p. 30). Used by permission of Oncology Nursing Press, Inc.

at the City of Hope National Medical Center have combined quantitative and qualitative methods to obtain the most complete descriptions of pain from cancer patients.

Conclusions

Nurse scientists and clinicians have made a major contribution to the science of pain management. Research initiated by nurses in the 1970s has culminated in the development of clinical practice guidelines to direct the care of patients in pain. There is consensus in the literature that future pain research should address gaps in knowledge such as the experience and management of pain in vulnerable populations and the transition to intervention studies. The nursing profession's proud tradition of bringing pain management to the forefront of literature and public policy should serve as an inspiration to continue our leadership in this critical health care need.

References

Agency for Health Care Policy and Research. (1994). *Management of cancer pain.* Washington, DC: U.S. Department of Health and Human Services.

Ahles, E T. A., Blanchard, E. B., & Ruckdeschel, J. C. (1983). The multidimensional nature of cancer-related pain. *Pain, 17,* 277-288.

Ahles, T. A., Coombs, D. W., Jensen, L., & Martin, J. B. (1990). Development of a behavioral observation technique for the assessment of pain behavior in cancer patients. *Behavioral Therapy, 21,* 449-460.

American Nurses Association Council on Nursing Research. (1985). *Directions for nursing research: Toward the twenty-first century.* Kansas City, MO: American Nurses Association.

American Pain Society. (1992). *Principles of analgesic use in the treatment of acute pain and chronic cancer pain.* Skokie, IL: Author.

Barbour, L. A., McGuire, D. B., & Kirchoff, K. T. (1986). Nonanalgesic methods of pain control used by cancer outpatients. *Oncology Nursing Forum, 13,* 56-60.

Benoliel, J. Q. (1995). Multiple meanings of pain and complexities of pain management. *Nursing Clinics of North America, 30*(4), 583-596.

Benoliel, J. Q., & Crowley, D. M. (1977). The patient in pain: New concepts. *Nursing Digest, 5,* 41-48.

Benoliel, J. Q., & McCorkle, R. (1978). A holistic approach to terminal illness. *Cancer Nursing, 1,* 143-149.

Beyer, J., Denyes, M., & Villarruel, A. (1992). The creation, validation and continuing development of the Oucher: A measure of pain intensity in children. *Journal of Pediatric Nursing, 7,* 335-346.

Broome, M., Lillis, P., & Smith, M. (1989). Pain interventions in children: A meta-analysis of the research. *Nursing Research, 38,* 154-158.

Broome, M. E. (1995). Pain intervention research with children. *American Pain Society Bulletin, 5*(6), 1-4.

Cline, N. E., Herman, J., Shaw, E. R., & Morton, R. D. (1992). Standardization of the Visual Analogue Scale. *Nursing Research, 41,* 378-380.

Clipp, E. C., & George, L. K. (1992). Patients with cancer and their spouse caregivers: Perceptions of the illness experience. *Cancer, 69,* 1074-1079.

Copp, L. (1974). The spectrum of suffering. *American Journal of Nursing, 74,* 63-67.

Coyle, N., Adelhardt, J., Foley, K., & Portenoy, R. (1990). Character of terminal illness in the advanced cancer patient: Pain and other symptoms during the last four weeks of life. *Journal of Pain and Symptom Management, 5,* 83-93.

Coyle, N., Mauskop, A., Maggard, J., & Foley, K. (1986). Continuous subcutaneous infusions of opiates in cancer patients with pain. *Oncology Nursing Forum, 13,* 53-57.

Dalton, J. (1987). Education for pain management: A pilot study. *Patient Education Counsel, 9,* 155-165.

Dalton, J. A., Feuerstein, M., Carlson, J., & Roghman, K. (1994). Biobehavioral Pain Profile: Development and psychometric properties. *Pain, 57,* 95-107.

Dar, R., Beach, C. M., Barden, P. L., & Cleeland, C. S. (1992). Cancer pain in the marital system: A study of patients and their spouses. *Journal of Pain and Symptom Management, 7,* 87-93.

Daut, R. L., Cleeland, C., & Flanery, R. C. (1983). Development of the Wisconsin Brief Pain Questionnaire to assess pain in the cancer and other diseases. *Pain, 17,* 197-210.

De Conno, F., Caraceni, A., Gamba, A., Abbatista, A., Brunelli, C., La Mura, A., & Ventafridda, V. (1994). Pain measurement in cancer patients: A comparison of six methods. *Pain, 57,* 161-166.

Ellis, J. A., & Spanos, N. P. (1994). Cognitive-behavioral interventions for children's distress during bone marrow aspirations and lumbar punctures: A critical review. *Journal of Pain and Symptom Management, 9,* 96-108.

Ferrell, B., Rhiner, M., & Rivera, L. (1993). Development and evaluation of the Family Pain Questionnaire. *Journal of Psychosocial Oncology, 10*(4), 21-35.

Ferrell, B., Whedon, M., & Rollins, B. (1995). Pain and quality assessment/improvement. *Journal of Nursing Care Quality, 9*(3), 69-85.

Ferrell, B. A., Ferrell, B. R., & Rivera, L. (1995). Pain in cognitively impaired nursing home patients. *Journal of Pain and Symptom Management, 10*(8), 591-598.

Ferrell, B. F., McGuire, D. B., & Donovan, M. I. (1993). Knowledge and beliefs regarding pain in a sample of nursing faculty. *Journal of Professional Nursing, 9*(2), 79-88.

Ferrell, B. R. (1995). The impact of pain on quality of life: A decade of research. *Nursing Clinics of North America, 30*(4), 609-624.

Ferrell, B. R., Dow, K. H., & Grant, M. (1995). Measurement of the quality of life in cancer survivors. *Quality of Life Research, 4,* 523-531.

Ferrell, B. R., Ferrell, B. A., Ahn, C., & Tran, K. (1994). Pain management for elderly cancer patients at home. *Cancer, 74,* 2139-2146.

Ferrell, B. R., Grant, M., Chan, J., Ahn, C., & Ferrell, B. A. (1995). The impact of cancer pain education on family caregivers of elderly patients. *Oncology Nursing Forum, 22*(8), 1211-1218.

Ferrell, B. R., & Griffith, H. (1994). Cost issues related to pain management: Report from the cancer pain panel of the Agency for Health Care Policy and Research. *Journal of Pain and Symptom Management, 9*(4), 221-234.

Ferrell, B. R., Jacox, A., Miaskowski, C., Paice, J. A., & Hester, N. O. (1994). Cancer guidelines: Now that we have them, what do we do? *Oncology Nursing Forum, 21*(7), 1229-1238.

Ferrell, B. R., McCaffery, M., & Rhiner, M. (1992). Pain and addiction: An urgent need for changing nursing education. *Journal of Pain and Symptom Management, 7*(2), 117-124.

Ferrell, B. R., Rhiner, M., Cohen, M., & Grant, M. (1991). Pain as a metaphor for illness. Part I: Impact of cancer pain on family caregivers. *Oncology Nursing Forum, 18*(8), 1303-1309.

Fordyce, W. E., Lansky, T., Calsyn, D. A., Shelton, J. L., Stolov, W. C., & Rock, D. L. (1984). Pain measurement and pain behavior. *Pain, 18*(1), 53-69.

Gaston-Johansson, F., & Fall-Dickson, J. M. (1995). The importance of nursing research design and methods in cancer pain management. *Nursing Clinics of North America, 30*(40), 597-606.

Gift, A. G. (1989). Visual analogues scales: Measurement of subjective phenomena. *Nursing Research, 38,* 286-288.

Grant, M., Ferrell, B., Rivera, L., & Lee, J. (1995). Unscheduled readmissions for uncontrolled symptoms. *Nursing Clinics of North America, 30*(4), 673-682.

Grossman, S., Sheidler, V. R., Swedeen, K., Mucenski, J., & Piantadosi, S. (1991). Correlation of patient and caregiver ratings of cancer pain. *Journal of Pain and Symptom Management, 6,* 53-57.

Guardiola, E., & Banos, J. (1993). Is there an increasing interest in pediatric pain? Analysis of biomedical articles published in the 1980s. *Journal of Pain and Symptom Management, 8,* 449-450.

Hester, N. O., Jacox, A., Miaskowski, C., & Ferrell, B. R. (1992). The management of pain in infants, children and adolescents. *Maternal Child Nursing, 17*(3), 146-152.

Holcombe, R. F., & Griffin, J. (1993). Effect of insurance status on pain medication prescriptions in a hematology/oncology practice. *Southern Medical Journal, 86,* 151-156.

Hyman, R. B., Feldman, H. R., Harris, R. B., Levin, R. F., & Malloy, G. B. (1989). The effects of relaxation training on clinical symptoms: A meta-analysis. *Nursing Research, 38,* 216-229.

Jacox, A., Carr, D. B., Payne, R., et al. (1994). *Management of cancer pain: Clinical practice guideline* (AHCPR Pub. No. 94-0592). Rockville, MD: Agency for Health Care Policy and Research, Public Health Service, U.S. Department of Health and Human Services.

Jacox, A. K. (1977). *Pain: A source book for nurses and other health professionals.* Boston: Little, Brown.

Loeser, J. D. (1982). Concepts of pain. In M. Stanton-Hicks & R. Boas (Eds.), *Chronic low back pain* (pp. 145-148). New York: Raven.

Madison, J. L., & Wilkie, D. J. (1995). Family members' perceptions of cancer pain. *Nursing Clinics of North America, 30*(4), 625-644.

McCaffery, M. (1968). *Cognition bodily pain in man-environment interactions* [syllabus]. Los Angeles: University of California.

McCaffery, M., & Ferrell, B. (1991, June). How would you respond to these patients in pain? *Nursing 1991,* pp. 34-37.

McCaffery, M., & Ferrell, B. R. (1992, March/April). Opioid analgesics: Nurses' knowledge of doses and psychological dependence. *Journal of Nursing Staff Development,* pp. 77-84.

McCaffery, M., & Ferrell, B. R. (1995). Nurses' knowledge about cancer pain: A survey of five countries. *Journal of Pain and Symptom Management, 10*(5), 356-369.

McGuire, D. (1997). Measuring pain. In M. Stromborg & S. Olsen (Eds.), *Instruments for clinical health care research* (pp. 528-564). Sudbury, MA: Jones & Bartlett.

McIlveen, K. H., & Morse, J. M. (1995). The role of comfort in nursing care: 1900-1980. *Clinical Nursing Research, 4*(2), 127-148.

Melzack, R. (1987). The short-form McGill Pain Questionnaire. *Pain, 30,* 191-197.

Melzack, R., & Wall, P. D. (1965). Pain mechanisms: A new theory. *Science, 150,* 971-979.

Miaskowski, C., Jacox, A., Hester, N. O., & Ferrell, B. R. (1992). Interdisciplinary guidelines for the management of acute pain: Implications for quality improvement. *Journal of Nursing Care Quality, 7*(1), 1-6.

Miaskowski, C., Nichols, R., Brody, R., & Synold, T. (1994). Assessment of patient satisfaction utilizing the American Pain Society's quality assurance standards on acute and cancer-related pain. *Journal of Pain and Symptom Management, 9,* 5-11.

Muller, J. (1942). *Elements of physiology.* London: Taylor.

National Institute of Nursing Research. (1994). *Report of the NINR priority expert panel on symptom management: Acute pain.* Washington, DC: U.S. Department of Health and Human Services.

Paice, J. A. (1984). Intrathecal morphine sulfate for intractable cancer pain. *American Association of Neuroscience Nursing, 16,* 237-240.

Penn, R. D., & Paice, J. A. (1987). Chronic intrathecal morphine for intractable pain. *Journal of Neurosurgery, 67,* 182-186.

Polit, D. F., & Hungler, B. P. (1995). *Nursing research principles and methods.* Philadelphia: J. B. Lippincott.

Puntillo, K. A. (1994). Dimensions of procedural pain and its analgesic management in critically ill surgical patients. *American Journal of Critical Care, 3,* 116-122.

Rimer, B. K., Kedziera, P., & Levy, M. H. (1992). The role of patient education in cancer pain control. *Hospice Journal, 8(2),* 171-191.

Savedra, M., Tesler, M., Holzemer, W., Wilkie, D., & Ward, J. (1989). Pain location: Validity and reliability of body outline markings by hospitalized children and adolescents. *Research in Nursing and Health, 12,* 207-214.

Smith, M. C., Holcombe, J. K., & Stullenbarger, E. (1994). A meta-analysis of intervention effectiveness for symptom management in oncology nursing research. *Oncology Nursing Forum, 21*(7), 1201-1210.

Stevens, B. J., Johnston, C. C., & Horton, L. (1993). Multidimensional pain assessment in premature neonates: A pilot study. *Journal of Obstetric, Gynecologic and Neonatal Nursing, 22,* 531-541.

Tesler, M., Sevedra, M., Holzemer, W., Wilkie, D., Ward, J., & Paul, S. (1991). The word-graphic rating scale as a measure of children's and adolescents' pain intensity. *Research Nursing Health 14,* 361-371.

Whaley, L., & Wong, D. (1987). *Nursing care of infants and children* (3rd ed.). St. Louis, MO: Mosby.

Whedon, M., & Ferrell, B. R. (1991). Professional and ethical considerations in the use of high-tech pain management. *Oncology Nursing Forum, 18,* 1135-1143.

Wilkie, D. J. (1995). Neural mechanisms of pain: A foundation for cancer pain assessment. In D. B. McGuire, C. H. Yarbro, & B. R. Ferrell (Eds.), *Cancer pain management* (2nd ed., pp. 61-87). Boston: Jones & Bartlett.

Zalon, M. L. (1993). Nurses' assessment of postoperative patients' pain. *Pain, 54,* 329-334.

22

MANAGING URINARY
AND FECAL INCONTINENCE

Molly C. Dougherty
Linda L. Jensen

Introduction

Knowledge development about adulthood urinary and fecal incontinence has grown steadily in the past two decades and provides a basis for improved nursing practice. Urinary incontinence is defined as the involuntary loss of urine in sufficient amounts that it is a problem (Fantl, Newman, Colling, et al., 1996). Fecal incontinence is defined as the involuntary loss of gas, liquid, or solid stool (Tuckson & Fazio, 1989). The Clinical Practice Guidelines for urinary incontinence sponsored by the Agency for Health Care Policy and Research (AHCPR) (Fantl, Newman, et al., 1996; Urinary Incontinence Guideline Panel [UIGP], 1992) provide a comprehensive review and evaluation of the research literature and are valuable

to nurses with interests in urinary incontinence. Nurses were members of the panels for both guideline panels and, in addition, served as co-chairpersons. No such guidelines exist for fecal incontinence, however. This chapter serves as a summary and critical examination of clinical nursing research in these two areas. Research literature from nursing, medicine, and other health professions was examined. However, emphasis is placed on the nursing research literature and research from related fields in which nurses were authors or co-authors.

The review is organized around major themes in the research literature, beginning with an epidemiology overview and costs of incontinence. A brief physiological

AUTHORS' NOTE: The extensive editing and manuscript preparation by Valerie Parham are gratefully recognized.

407

review of relevant organ systems provides background for a discussion of the revised paradigm of incontinence published in the 1990s. Clinical nursing studies supporting nursing management strategies are emphasized, with careful attention to interventions and outcomes relevant to incontinence.

Background

Epidemiology and Costs

Incontinence accounts for considerable morbidity, especially in late adulthood. Although incontinence of either type is not usually life-threatening, it is prevalent, associated with social stigma, and contributes to high health care costs. Urinary incontinence affects approximately 13 million people in the United States, the majority of whom are elderly in community and nursing home settings (National Kidney and Urologic Diseases Advisory Board, 1994). Among those 15 to 64 years of age, the prevalence of urinary incontinence in men is from 1.5% to 5% and among women, 10% to 30% (Fantl, Newman, et al., 1996). As well, between the ages of 25 and 64 years, approximately 29% of women experience urinary incontinence (Herzog & Fultz, 1990). For persons over 60 years of age living outside of institutions, the prevalence is 15% to 35%, with the prevalence in women twice that in men (Diokno, Brock, Brown, & Herzog, 1986). Incontinence is a leading cause of placement of individuals in long-term care. Urinary incontinence affects approximately 50% of institutionalized elderly, and risk factors include physical and mental impairment (National Center for Health Statistics, 1979; Palmer, German, & Ouslander, 1991). Among care recipients living at home, 53% were incontinent (Noelker, 1987).

There are few published reports on the prevalence of fecal incontinence. This may be because (a) physicians and nurses do not recognize it to be a problem or (b) the population is reluctant to discuss the problem. Nelson, Norton, Cautley, and Furner (1995), using a telephone survey with questions regarding fecal incontinence embedded in general health questions, reported that the incidence of fecal incontinence in the community setting was 2.2%. Using questionnaires in family practice or gastroenterologist offices, 18.4% of the patients admitted to having some form of fecal incontinence and 7% said they had it on a daily basis (Johanson & Lafferty, 1996). Fecal incontinence in a long-term care facility was reported in approximately 46% of residents (Borrie & Davidson, 1992). Fecal incontinence in men and women at home was said to be 3% to 5% in individuals 65 to 84 years and 30% in nursing homes (Norton, 1996). This variability in reported prevalence of fecal incontinence implies that it is a subject not easily discussed by those experiencing it.

Costs associated with incontinence are high and are expected to increase as the population in the United States gets steadily older. Costs for urinary incontinence increased more than 60% from 1990 to 1994 (Hu, 1990, 1994). In 1994, estimated direct annual costs for all people with incontinence was $11.2 billion in the community and $5.2 billion in nursing homes. Because incontinence is often a dual problem, the cost of fecal incontinence alone is difficult to assess. One study revealed that 52.5 minutes per day per institutionalized patient was spent dealing with fecal incontinence, for an estimated total annual cost per patient of $10,000 (Borrie & Davidson, 1992).

Incontinence affects millions of Americans across adulthood. In spite of concentrated efforts to educate professionals and the public, incontinence remains underreported and underdiagnosed (Fantl, Newman, et al., 1996). It is often stated, and merits repeating, that incontinence is not an inevitable consequence of aging. Although incontinence cannot always be cured, it can be managed. Clinical research results provide the foundation for prevention and management of this costly problem that takes a toll on psychological and physical health. The prevalence and costs associated with incontinence, particularly in the dependent elderly, establish incontinence as a major health problem that merits the attention of nurses.

Related Physiology

Continence, although controlled by the central nervous system, requires the coordination of somatic (skeletal muscle of the pelvic muscles) and autonomic (smooth muscle of the bowel, bladder, and urethra) components of the peripheral nervous system. Intact efferent and afferent pathways are necessary for normal bowel and bladder function. Useful overviews of the neurological control of micturition and bowel function are available in a number of medical texts (Sagar & Pemberton, 1996; Wall, Norton, & DeLancey, 1993; Walters & Karram, 1993).

Anatomical or physiological factors or factors external to the individual may contribute to problems with incontinence. Commonly, multiple factors contribute to function, particularly in frail elders. The etiology of urinary and fecal incontinence, genital prolapse, and bowel retention are interrelated and complex. In the literature of the 1990s, a revised paradigm of incontinence has emerged and is contributing to improved interdisciplinary collaboration in research (Wall et al., 1993). Factors that are considered in the revised paradigm are genetic endowment, connective tissue, muscle fiber types, and alterations in the function of these structures. The number and fiber types of skeletal muscle cells are determined before birth. Individuals are born with a certain physiological potential, which they activate and can maximize. Genetic endowment determines the quantity and type of collagen (the primary component of fascia and ligaments) and the number and type of striated muscle cells. These factors, and habitual practices such as physical exercise and work-related physical activity, contribute to wide individual variations in bowel and bladder function among normal individuals.

A number of factors contribute to the anatomical support of the structures that control continence (bladder, urethra, and rectum). The striated pelvic muscles (levator ani, puborectalis, ischiocavernous, compressor urethrae, pubovesical ligament [muscle], and urethrovaginal sphincter) are different from other skeletal muscles in important ways. Most striated muscles have clear points of origin and insertion, and often fine motor control is provided by nerve plexus. Some of the pelvic muscles have bony attachments, but others are supported by fascia or ligaments and motor control is less precise. These distinctions affect the development of incontinence and influence training and rehabilitation.

It is important, also, to consider the fiber type and composition of the pelvic muscles. There is increasing awareness of the importance of the distribution of Type I and Type II fibers, which make up the pelvic muscles. The composition of fiber types in striated muscle is established early in life and is stable, generally. Muscle fiber types are usually described as Types I, IIa, and IIb fibers, but Type IIb fibers rarely occur in humans. Type I fibers (slow twitch fibers) have high endurance capacity, have low contraction speed, and are fatigue resistant. Type II fibers (fast twitch fibers) have low endurance, have high contractions, and fatigue quickly.

Type I fibers increase with age, and there is selective atrophy of Type II fibers, not necessarily accompanied by changes in Type I fibers. In studies specific to the pelvic muscles, denervation appears to progress during a period of many years and functional disorders usually first appear in middle or late life. Partial denervation of the pelvic muscle cells, with subsequent reinnervation, may be a normal process. The recuperative response of motoneurons to injury of their axons (Bishop, 1982) is an important but poorly understood process in continence mechanisms.

In normal individuals, the pelvic muscles are composed of 66% to 90% of Type I fibers (Critchley, Dixon, & Gosling, 1980), suggesting the supportive role of Type I fibers in maintenance of continence. Type II fibers appear to be important in quickly increasing urethral and anal sphincter pressure and maintaining urinary continence during points of increased intra-abdominal pressure.

Fecal continence is achieved by a combination of several pelvic floor mechanisms, including a competent, closed anal sphincter; normal anorectal sensation and sampling reflex; adequate rectal capacity; and compliance and conscious control. Maintenance of fecal continence when the anal sphincter is under maximum strain is associated with marked electrical activity in the sphincter complex and puborectalis muscle. According to the flap valve theory of fecal continence, when intra-abdominal pressure increases, the anterior rectal mass is pressed down onto the upper anal canal, preventing rectal contents from moving into the anal canal. The compliance of the rectum also aids in fecal continence.

Histological samples from two groups of women, those with and without stress urinary incontinence or genital prolapse, showed that with dysfunction there was a decrease in the proportion of Type II fibers and an increase in the proportion of Type I fibers. These changes, concentrated in the posterior portion of the pelvic muscles, suggest denervation and reinnervation from a shared motor axon (Gilpin, Gosling, Smith, & Warrell, 1989).

Histochemical studies of biopsies from the pelvic floor and external and sphincter muscles have demonstrated that individuals with rectal prolapse and fecal incontinence exhibit evidence of partial denervation of the striated muscle. Electromyography (EMG) and histochemical studies in women with genitourinary prolapse, stress urinary incontinence (SUI), or both, exhibit partial denervation of the pelvic muscles and striated urethral sphincter muscles (Smith, 1994). A growing body of research focuses on vaginal childbirth and chronic straining during defecation as activities that injure the pudendal nerve and the motor unit axons supplying striated pelvic muscles.

Other factors also contribute to the development of problems with incontinence. Although the role of fascia and ligaments in supporting the pelvic organs is not fully understood, it is recognized as important. Tension placed on endopelvic fascia is relieved by the pelvic muscles.

Damage to the pelvic muscles is interrelated with failure of the ligaments. Normally, the ligaments do not need to be strong, but if the muscles are damaged, the ligaments are required to carry an increased load. In such a case, strong ligaments will maintain normal support, but in the presence of weak ligaments, prolapse is likely. Usually, it is not possible to determine whether prolapse is caused by damage to the muscles or ligaments because these components of pelvic support are closely interrelated (DeLancey, 1994).

Within this revised paradigm, habitual behaviors and events in adulthood are viewed as important in the development of incontinence. This perspective provides support for research on interventions to prevent and manage incontinence during adulthood and with elders. In this review, the revised paradigm is the conceptual foundation and organizing framework for the examination of nursing research on incontinence.

▬ *Definition and Classification of Incontinence and Bowel Retention*

A number of classifications of urinary incontinence based on diagnosis appear in the literature, but the classification of urinary incontinence by types based on symptoms is useful to guide nursing practice and thus is used in the organization of this chapter. The most commonly described types of urinary incontinence are *urge, stress, mixed,* and *overflow* incontinence.

Urge incontinence is the involuntary loss of urine associated with a strong desire to void, referred to as urgency. *Stress urinary incontinence* is associated with urine loss during coughing, sneezing, laughing, or other physical activities that increase intra-abdominal pressure. *Mixed incontinence* is the combined presence of symptoms of stress incontinence and urge incontinence. *Overflow incontinence* is involuntary urine loss associated with an overdistended bladder. Other types and causes of urinary incontinence are classified as *functional* and *unconscious* or *reflex* incontinence. Factors contributing to *functional incontinence* are beyond the lower urinary tract and may result from chronic impairment— cognitive or physical—and relate to environmental context. *Unconscious* or *reflex incontinence* occurs without any warning or sensory awareness. It occurs most commonly in paraplegics and occasionally in others for poorly understood reasons. *Sleep enuresis* is defined as persistent bedwetting after 3 or 4 years of age in the absence of organic pathology accounting for the wetting.

Urine alarm treatments for sleep enuresis based on research literature in psychology have been refined (Schwartz, 1995) and are beyond the scope of this chapter.

Fecal incontinence is considered *severe* when there is intermittent, involuntary elimination of large volumes of stool; *mild* when the leakage is confined to passage of small amounts of stool visible on the underclothing, sometimes called staining, or when a person is unable to voluntarily control the discharge of gas from the rectum. *Bowel retention* occurs when the stool is of an appropriate consistency and passes to the rectum and sphincter mechanism in a regulated fashion. Loss of sensory awareness of rectal filling to warn of impending defecation, to determine the nature of the rectal contents (gas, liquid, or solid), or to initiate increased contraction of the striated sphincters that brings about evacuation can lead to retention.

Excellent research-based information on evaluation and diagnosis of urinary incontinence in adults is available in the AHCPR guidelines (Fantl, Newman, et al., 1996; UIGP, 1992) and in other sources (Jirovec, 1991; McCormick & Palmer, 1992; McCormick, Scheve, & Leahy, 1988; Wyman, 1988). Wyman (1991) provided a detailed outline on the causes and nursing assessment of fecal incontinence. MacLeod's (1991) chapter on the assessment of patients with fecal incontinence provides an excellent overview of the laboratory assessments used to evaluate fecal incontinence.

Nursing Management: Interventions and Application

▬ *Long-Term Care Settings*

Much of the research on nursing management of incontinence has concentrated on dependent individuals, particularly those in nursing homes or long-term care settings. This is synchronous with the epidemiology and costs of incontinence and is examined first. Other interventions more appropriate for mobile and cognitively intact adults who are able to follow through on behavioral changes are reviewed subsequently.

The value of timely and appropriate incontinence evaluation cannot be overstated. An overview of urinary incontinence is provided in the AHCPR guidelines (Fantl, Newman, et al., 1996; UIGP, 1992), taking into account health and severity factors. The recommended basic evaluation includes a history, physical examination, estimation of postvoid residual volume, and urinalysis. In individuals who require further testing before interventions, specialized tests (urodynamic, endoscopic, and/or imaging) may be indicated.

Fecal incontinence and/or bowel retention may be present in patients with a rectal neoplasm or rectal prolapse or intussusception as well as an altered bowel transit or deficient sphincter mechanism. Careful assessment is also important. In addition to the history and physical examination and standard flexible sigmoidoscopy or colonoscopy, physiological tests including anal manometry, anal EMG, defecography, and endorectal or endoanal ultrasound should also be carried out (Jensen, 1997).

Environmental assessment in settings for disabled individuals is important to nursing management of incontinence. Access to toileting is necessary for frail, older individuals to remain continent. A short distance to the toilet, minimal elevation changes en route to the toilet, adequate height of the toilet (at least 17 inches), and grab bars to aid mobility are important factors. Obstacles such as poor lighting, throw rugs, furniture, and stairs contribute to the inability of frail elders to reach the toilet in time (Wells & Brink, 1980). In very disabled, cognitively intact older adults, cognitive assessment, environmental assessment including the accessibility of the toilet, assistive devices, and the availability of a caregiver, as well as interventions tailored to the capabilities of the individual, require emphasis (McDowell, Engberg, Weber, Brodak, & Engberg, 1994).

Physical restraints and sedation contribute to incontinence, especially among cognitively impaired individuals (Ouslander, 1990). In a longitudinal secondary analysis of nursing home data, neurological risk factors for urinary incontinence showed that age was not associated with prevalence or incidence of urinary incontinence. However, male gender, urinary incontinence, poor behavioral adjustment, cognitive impairment, and impaired mobility were risk factors. Residents who were not cognitively impaired, had adjusted to the nursing home environment, and were independently mobile had lower risks of incontinence (Palmer et al., 1991).

Research on nursing home residents who are cognitively impaired and immobile showed that urinary incontinence is improved by interventions to enhance mobility. The best predictor of urinary incontinence was the inability to walk unassisted. Among cognitively impaired nursing home residents, mobility and urinary continence were improved by daily walking. Research results indicate that emphasizing residents' mobility and de-emphasizing restraints are important to improving urinary control in cognitively impaired residents (Jirovec, 1991; Jirovec & Wells, 1990). Research indicates that risk and environmental assessment is an important early step in continence management.

Prompted voiding and timed toileting are effective strategies for management of urinary incontinence in long-term care and home settings. These require staff implementation and adherence to a specific protocol. The goal of timed voiding is to avoid incontinence by providing voiding opportunities at regular intervals. Prompted voiding differs from timed voiding by teaching individuals to be sensitized to their continence status and to request toileting assistance. There are three major elements in prompted voiding. Wet status is monitored and individuals are asked to report wet or dry status on a scheduled basis. Individuals are reminded (prompted) to use the toilet and are praised for continence and using the toilet (UIGP, 1992).

Nursing home residents of advanced age (average age 85 years) with urge or mixed urinary incontinence have been studied with respect to individuals' voiding patterns (Colling, Ouslander, Hadley, Eisch, & Campbell, 1992). A nursing intervention was tested involving (a) a 4-hour in-service to nursing staff on how to apply the intervention, (b) constructing an individual toileting schedule for each subject based on the electronic monitoring data, and (c) positive reinforcement for patients and staff for adhering to the toileting program and for successful toileting outcomes (Harke & Richgels, 1992). Overall, the intervention significantly decreased incontinence for the treatment group, with one third of the group improving more than 20%. Residents with greater bladder capacity and less mental impairment responded best. Yet, there was resistance to changing nursing staff routines because of staff shortages. Nursing staff complied with the treatment regimen approximately 70% of the time. Tailoring tested strategies to individual needs and environmental context are important considerations for success.

Toileting individuals according to their individual voiding habits (Colling et al., 1992) is supported by research. Approximately 35% of nursing home residents are poor candidates for prompted voiding, especially those with frequent incontinence or those who do not respond to prompts and are unable to cooperate with toileting (Schnelle, Newman, Fogarty, Wallston, & Ory,

1991). Yet, up to 40% respond well. Responders can be identified by assessing their responsiveness to a 3-day trial of prompted voiding (Ouslander et al., 1995). Any interventions are difficult if staff are untrained, undersupervised, or inadequate in number. Caregivers of home-bound individuals might find some treatments to be viable options for management of urinary incontinence that are more difficult to apply within institutions.

The research indicates that toileting interventions are effective, but they may be compromised by lack of adherence by nursing staff (Campbell, Knight, Benson, & Colling, 1991; Schnelle, 1990). Nursing staff often expect total continence and are disappointed when this does not occur (Colling et al., 1992; Schnelle, Newman, & Fogarty, 1990).

A number of clinical trials in nursing homes using prompted voiding have documented significant reductions in incontinence episodes. For example, an average reduction of 1.0 to 2.2 incontinence episodes per patient per day has been reported (Engel et al., 1990; Hu et al., 1989; Schnelle, 1990). Selection of individuals is important to the success of prompted voiding. Residents with lower voiding frequencies (fewer than four in a 12-hour period) and those who toilet appropriately over 75% of the time were most likely to show long-term benefits from prompted voiding. Although nursing staff compliance is cited as a barrier to success of these techniques (Schnelle, Newman, & Fogarty, 1990; Schnelle, Newman, Fogarty, Wallston, et al., 1991), nursing staff were able to maintain improved resident continence levels for 6 months among residents who were highly responsive to prompted voiding (Colling et al., 1992).

In disabled but cognitively intact home-bound samples, behavioral techniques resulted in reductions in urine loss episodes. In the two groups studied, the nursing intervention involved counseling on habit training, relaxation training, diet modifications, bowel regimens, and instruction in performance of pelvic muscle exercise (PME). In Group 1, referred by a visiting nurses association ($n = 18$), biofeedback on performance of PME was provided. In Group 2, obtained from the health department ($n = 21$), verbal feedback on PME performance was provided. In both groups there was a significant decrease in the number of accidents per week between the initial visit and the end of the focused treatment. The average number of urinary accidents per week in Group 1 and Group 2 was 16 and 19.3, respectively; improvement was 78% and 79%, respectively. Although it was not possible to determine which components of the nursing intervention accounted for the improvement, the focus of the in-

tervention was on PME with biofeedback. The use of behavioral techniques to reduce urinary incontinence in frail, older adults in their homes was supported (Rose, Baigis-Smith, Smith, & Newman, 1990).

▬ Prevention and Early Intervention: Diet and Elimination

One barrier to prevention and early intervention is the relative inattention by health professionals to incontinence. A secondary impediment is the reluctance of individuals to address mild incontinence with health care providers, often based on the belief that little can be done. However, bladder and bowel control problems generally begin gradually and intermittently and can be managed with elementary strategies. There is growing interest in preventive strategies to manage frequency and urgency before urine loss begins.

Some nursing investigators have integrated elementary strategies in an early phase of a urine loss intervention protocol. For example, Rose et al. (1990) counseled on various ways to improve incontinence (habit training, relaxation training, diet modification, and bowel regimens) before introducing PME. The effect of the strategies introduced early in the protocol was not measured separately but was accounted for by measurement after PME performance. Similarly, McDowell et al. (1994) introduced urine control measures and PME with biofeedback. Their protocol emphasized environmental assessment and tailoring the treatment to the individual needs of participants. The effect of specific elements of the treatment were not measured, but the combined effect of the elements was tapped in the measurement of urine loss at the end of the protocol. Thus, in many studies, counseling and changes in daily patterns of intake may account for important increases in urine control but often are not measured because they are not the primary intervention under study.

Maintaining adequate, timely, and appropriate fluid intake is widely recognized as important to continence (Pearson & Droessler, 1988). Many individuals attempt to control urine loss by decreasing fluid intake, which tends to concentrate urine. Concentrated urine is believed to make the urine more irritating to the bladder, leading to urgency and frequency. A minimum fluid intake of at least 1,500 cc should be maintained (Subcommittee on the Tenth Edition, 1989). Depending on climate and activity level, it can be more but should not exceed 4,000 cc (Tomlinson et al., 1997).

Caffeine aggravates urine control problems in many individuals. Creighton and Stanton (1990) found that women with urge incontinence had significant increases in detrusor pressure (associated with the symptom of urge incontinence) after ingestion of 200 mg of caffeine, a finding not observed in controls with normal detrusor pressure. A 6-oz cup of brewed coffee contains 85 to 100 mg of caffeine (Etherton & Kochar, 1993). Reduction of caffeinated beverages to two or fewer servings per day is recommended. Alcoholic beverages, which retard motor and sensory activity and impair continence mechanisms, should be minimized. These recommendations increase in importance with increasing age. The diminished thirst and the slowing of physiological responses with age make adequate fluid intake and the reduction of alcoholic beverages especially important for elders.

For individuals with nocturia twice or more nightly, concentrating intake of fluids in the early part of the day is supported by research. Generally, the recommendation is to limit fluids after 6 p.m. In individuals who retain fluid in the lower extremities during the day, elevation of the feet and lower legs for 1 to 2 hours midday helps to diminish nocturia.

An excessive voiding interval is most commonly found in those in physically active employment. In individuals with a voiding interval over 4 hours, reducing the voiding interval to 2 to 3 hours is an elementary prevention strategy for control of urine loss.

In a behavioral management for continence (BMC) program, the components of (a) self-monitoring, (b) bladder training, and (c) PME with biofeedback have been tested. Urine loss measures were obtained at the end of each phase (Bear, Dwyer, Benveneste, Jett, & Dougherty, 1997). Forty-one participants completed the self-monitoring phase. The majority (83%, $n = 34$) decreased their dietary caffeine, half (51%, $n = 21$) increased their fluid intake, and fewer than half (44%, $n = 18$) decreased their voiding interval to less than 4 hours during the day. Additionally, two individuals decreased their daily fluid intake to under 4,000 cc. In this group, a 42% reduction in volume of urine loss was achieved by these steps tailored to their daily activities (Tomlinson et al., 1997).

Fecal incontinence to which behavioral patterns contribute can be prevented. This includes lifelong dietary habits that may later lead to diverticular disease or carcinoma and, subsequently, incontinence. Altered fiber and fluid intake and limited physical activity may lead to impaction, and avoidance of straining at stool may preserve the integrity of the pelvic floor musculature. Excessive straining may lead to rectal intussusception or prolapse, which is often associated with incontinence. A common cause of fecal incontinence is obstetrical injury. Although injury to the pelvic floor is not always preventable during childbirth, qualified obstetrical care during pregnancy reduces risk of birth injury.

At the onset of fecal incontinence, medical help should be sought to evaluate the cause of the incontinence. Patients require reassurance about the prevalence and medical treatment options. Interventions include environmental manipulations, medications, proper bowel regimen, and PME. Surgical interventions include correction of an existing prolapse, repair of the sphincter muscle, or augmentation of the sphincter muscle with new investigational surgeries (Basch & Jensen, 1991).

The limited research base for elementary strategies to maintain continence stems from the difficulty in measuring outcomes. Measurement of involuntary urinary and fecal loss and bladder and bowel symptoms is difficult, and in those without quantifiable involuntary loss, objective demonstration of improvement is problematic. Yet, the literature supports the effectiveness of elementary strategies.

Bladder and Bowel Training

Definitive research has demonstrated the effectiveness of bladder training for urge incontinence. There are a number of variations on the basic elements of bladder training—education, scheduled voiding, and positive reinforcement. Bladder training is noninvasive and reduces urine loss in women with stress incontinence (Burton, Pearce, Burgio, Engel, & Whitehead, 1988; Fantl, Wyman, Harkins, & Hadley, 1990; Rose et al., 1990).

The educational component of bladder training customarily combines written, visual, and verbal instructions that address the physiology and pathophysiology of the lower urinary tract. The voiding schedule incorporates a progressively increased interval between prescribed voiding with the use of distraction or relaxation to delay voiding off schedule. If the individual is unable to delay voiding or experiences incontinence, the scheduled voiding interval is shortened to eliminate urine loss and unscheduled voids. The voiding schedule is progressively lengthened as urgency and urine loss is controlled, and the interval can usually be lengthened to 2 to 3 hours.

Bladder training requires the individual to resist or inhibit the sensation of urgency, to postpone urination, and to void according to a schedule rather than according to the urge to void (McCormick & Burgio, 1984). Bladder training incorporates techniques to help distend the bladder. Fluid intake is maintained, voiding is delayed by controlling the scheduled interval, and strategies to control urge are used. Initially, the voiding interval is set at 1 hour during waking hours and progressively lengthened weekly until an interval of 2 to 4 hours is achieved. Generally, bladder training is completed in 6 to 8 weeks. A carefully described approach to bladder training based on research is available (Wyman & Fantl, 1991). In a randomized, controlled study, 123 women with stress and/or urge incontinence completed bladder training. Of those in the treatment group, 12% became dry and 75% had at least a 50% reduction in number of incontinent episodes. The reductions were of a greater magnitude for those with urge incontinence, and effect of the treatment was sustained at a 6-month follow-up in the treatment group (Fantl, Wyman, McClish, et al., 1991).

Several authors have discussed the necessity and components of bowel retraining (Basch & Jensen, 1991; Doughty, 1996; Takano-Stone, 1991). Successful bowel retraining requires that there be some rectal sensory and sphincter function. Assessments should be made as to the functional ability, cognitive status, motivation, and current bowel function. Key components include a bowel cleansing regimen, a return to normal stool consistency, and good patient education regarding normal bowel function and the importance of defecation at the urge to defecate. Although all authors provide excellent guidelines for bowel retraining, what is lacking is sound research on the effectiveness of a well-conceptualized bowel training program.

Pelvic muscle exercise. PME is often recommended to childbearing and perimenopausal women, for childbirth rehabilitation, control of SUI, and sexual responsiveness promotion. Brought into public awareness by Kegel (1948) in the early 1950s, PME is integrated into nursing and childbirth education. For many years PME was not convincingly recommended by health care professionals because definitive research to support it was not published.

In recent years, a substantial body of research on PME has been published. A number of weaknesses are found in early PME studies, but a number of recent well-designed studies demonstrate that PME is effective for mild to moderate SUI. Additionally, PME is recommended in conjunction with bladder training for urge incontinence (Fantl, Newman, et al., 1996). A few nursing studies that have made contributions to the knowledge base and are the foundation for clinical nursing are summarized below.

To evaluate the effect of PME with or without an intravaginal device to provide training resistance, 20 women with stress incontinence were randomly assigned to the PME with resistance device or PME alone. After 6 weeks of exercise, the PME with resistance group and the PME alone group achieved reduction in urine loss volume of 71% and 66%, respectively. The use of the resistance device did not improve performance of the pelvic muscles or decrease urine loss significantly more than the PME alone group (Ferguson et al., 1990). The results indicated that significant reductions in urine loss occur in as little as 6 weeks of PME in women with mild to moderate stress incontinence.

To compare PME to pharmacological treatment of stress incontinence, a sample of 157 older women were randomly assigned to either PME or phenylpropanolamine hydrochloride, a drug commonly used to manage stress incontinence. After 6 months, self-reported wetting did not differ significantly between the groups, and PME was comparable in benefit to phenylpropanolamine in reducing urine loss (Wells, Brink, Diokno, Wolfe, & Gillis, 1991).

In a randomized controlled trial, 135 older women with stress incontinence who got biofeedback (with PME), used PME only, or were part of a control group were studied. Number of urine loss episodes was monitored over 8 weeks and at 3 and 6 months after the intervention. For all incontinence severity subgroups, a significant decrease in incontinent episodes occurred in the biofeedback and PME subjects, but not in the control group. There was a significant correlation between pelvic muscle activity measured by EMG and incontinent episodes, but only the biofeedback group demonstrated significant improved EMG measures. There was a 61% urine loss reduction in the biofeedback and a 54% reduction in the PME groups, respectively (Burns et al., 1993).

The effect of PME on stress incontinence was studied with a wait-list control design in 65 women engaging in 16 weeks of exercise three times per week. The primary outcome measure was grams of urine loss on a 24-hour pad test. No significant changes were found after the control period, but significant reductions in grams of urine loss (55%) were found after 16 weeks of PME. Significant reductions in urine loss were found with PME three times per week at an intensity less than usually recommended in clinical literature (Dougherty, Bishop, Mooney, Gimotty, & Williams, 1993).

With these nursing and other well-designed studies, the question For whom is PME effective? has been answered reasonably well. PME is effective for women with mild to moderate SUI, with a more than 50% reduction in urine loss episodes reported in controlled studies.

Many studies report that approximately 25% of women achieve 100% improvement.

A corollary question, For whom is PME not effective? is more complex. It is recognized that central nervous system defects and spinal cord injuries are among the reasons that PME is not effective. An interesting but unresolved issue is the role of injuries to the pudendal nerve, muscle cell loss, and damage to connective tissue on PME performance.

Another issue related to PME is the process by which PME affects SUI. Principles of exercise training have been the foundation for several investigations of PME (Bo, Hagen, Kvarstein, Jorgensen, & Laarsen, 1990; Boyington, 1997; Boyington, Dougherty, & Kasper, 1995; Dougherty, Bishop, Abrams, Batich, & Gimotty, 1989; Dougherty, Bishop, Mooney, & Gimotty, 1989; Dougherty, Bishop, Mooney, Gimotty, & Williams, 1992; Miller, Kasper, & Sampselle, 1994). Because muscle hypertrophy is the primary mechanism for most gains in skeletal muscle training, it is inferred that muscle hypertrophy occurs with PME. Other factors appear to be important also.

It is logical to surmise that improvements in SUI occur because of pelvic muscle contractions used naturally in daily life at moments of increased abdominal pressure. Appropriate timing combined with the intensity of pelvic muscle contractions is essential. Because no significant relationship between improvement in urine loss and pelvic muscle characteristics has been documented (Dougherty, Bishop, Mooney, Gimotty, & Williams, 1993: Rose et al., 1990), decreases in urine loss are likely to be related to improved neuromuscular coordination rather than improvements in pelvic muscle strength. With careful instruction, improvements in SUI are observed after 1 week in women with mild SUI (Miller, Aston-Miller, & DeLancey, 1996).

Specific features of PME protocols are important, including (a) frequency, (b) number of repetitions, (c) duration of pelvic muscle contraction, (d) duration of rest phase between repetitions, and (e) length (number of weeks) of PME. A related issue is a maintenance regimen after the period of intensive training is completed. Research to specifically compare alternative protocols are few; an exception is the Bo et al. (1990) study, which is discussed later.

For successful PME outcomes, it is essential that the pelvic muscles and not adjacent muscle groups (abdomen, buttocks, thighs) are contracted. Afferent activity from substituting abdominal and gluteal muscle contractions can easily mask the weaker signals from the pelvic floor muscles. The amplitude of the pelvic muscle contraction is related to proprioceptive feedback; that is, weak pelvic muscle contractions provide diminished proprioceptive feedback. In individuals with weak contractions, it becomes more important to provide opportunities for contraction and relaxation of the pelvic muscles during PME. The physical exam, pelvic exam, and practice in the clinical setting are necessary for optimal PME prescription.

The stop test (Sampselle, 1993) provides some assurance that the woman is activating the pelvic muscles. Five seconds after initiating voiding, a pelvic muscle contraction is used to halt the urine stream. Many women with pelvic muscle dysfunction cannot stop the urine stream after it has started. Some investigators recommend the stop test weekly, others daily. Consistently, it is recommended that the stop test not be performed more than once a day because it contributes to dysfunctional voiding.

Self-assessment of pelvic muscle performance is important to self-monitoring PME performance, and it can be done a number of ways. Most urinary incontinence episodes occur in the upright posture; thus self-exam in this position provides a more accurate assessment of pelvic muscle activity than in a recumbent posture. A digital exam is carried out in the standing position, with one foot elevated and supported. Palpated intravaginally, the characteristics of the muscle during repeated efforts can be discerned. Additionally, a mirror may be used to observe the characteristics of the clitoris, introitus, and anus during pelvic muscle contractions. Correct performance of a pelvic muscle contraction results in the movement of the clitoris downward, the movement inward of the introitus and the tightening of the anus. These changes during pelvic muscle contraction help to confirm that the pelvic muscles are activated. Importantly, these changes do not occur during increases in abdominal pressure or Valsalva. It is reinforcing to the woman to carry out steps that assure activation of the pelvic muscles during PME training. Steps to assure contraction of the pelvic muscle and the resting state of related muscles of the abdomen, buttocks, and thighs are essential in PME protocols.

The literature varies somewhat on the frequency of PME. Most protocols call for daily exercise; some break the total number of pelvic muscle contractions into two or three exercise sessions within the day. Others recommend carrying out the pelvic muscle contractions in different postures, reclining, standing, and sitting. Daily PME enhanced with group exercise with a physiotherapist resulted in significant improvement in urine loss over

PME alone (Bo et al., 1990). PME prescribed three times per week, graded to begin with 15 repetitions and ending with 45 in a 16-week protocol, resulted in significant reductions in urine loss and improvements in pelvic muscle pressure characteristics in women with SUI (Dougherty, Bishop, Mooney, Gimotty, & Williams, 1993). This protocol may be at the low end of PME intensity needed to obtain significant improvements. However, daily PME is not essential to achieve significant reductions in urine loss in women with mild to moderate stress incontinence. Relatively little information is available about adherence to PME protocols, an area of high importance to understanding why PME is not effective in some women.

The intensity of PME is recommended to be between 30 and 60 repetitions per day, although more are prescribed by some clinicians (Tries & Eisman, 1995). A PME protocol that includes 30 to 60 repetitions is supported by the research literature (Dougherty, Bishop, Mooney, Gimotty, & Williams, 1993; Ferguson et al., 1990; McDowell, Engberg, et al., 1994; Rose et al., 1990) and results in significant reductions in urine loss. Further, it seems to be a PME routine that many women can incorporate into their lives.

Most of the research literature is based on pelvic muscle contractions of 10-second duration. Although not clearly demonstrated, a 10-second contraction is assumed to recruit Type II fibers and activate Type I fibers, also. In skeletal muscles generally, the proportion of Type II fibers activated during heavy activity is greater than the proportion of Type I fibers. A 10-second contraction probably activates Type II fibers first. Type II fibers fatigue quickly. Type I fibers sustain the contraction and represent muscle effort during most of the contraction. This would suggest that contractions of shorter duration (1 to 2 seconds) would be more effective in training Type II fibers, and this is recommended by Tries and Eisman (1995). Some PME protocols feature pelvic muscle contractions of shorter duration and include longer duration contractions to develop endurance. However, differential results from shorter (1- to 2-second) contractions have not been clearly demonstrated. Neuromuscular control and coordination may be enhanced by having the individual gradually increase intensity up to a stable maximum or ramping. This technique is reported to establish the ability to sustain an extended pelvic muscle contraction without effort (Tries & Eisman, 1995).

The period of relaxation between contractions is an essential feature in PME protocols. A 10-second relaxation phase is most commonly reported and individuals with dysfunctional voiding may need longer. The rationale for the relaxation phase is found in the characteristics of the muscle fibers. The Type II fibers tire quickly during contraction, which suggests the need for relaxation between efforts. Additionally, during early learning, many tighten related muscle groups (abdomen, thighs, buttocks), and a relaxation phase permits time to recognize this proscribed behavior and correct it. Further, the desired activity is concentration on the pelvic muscle. Often, if relaxation is not sufficient, a proprioceptive sense of the pelvic muscle on which to form the next pelvic muscle contraction is not achieved. This enhances the ability to discriminate the relaxed state in contrast to the contracted state.

The coordination of the striated pelvic muscles with the smooth muscle of the bladder and bowel are necessary to normal bowel and bladder function. Research on the coordinated relaxation of the pelvic muscles and the contraction of the smooth muscle of the bladder and bowel is not well addressed in PME research but has received attention in bowel and bladder biofeedback training and is discussed later.

There is considerable variability within the research literature on recommended durations (number of weeks) for PME protocols, which vary from 4 to 20 weeks; most are between 6 and 12 weeks. The major gain in pelvic muscle pressures is observed during the first 6 to 8 weeks, but continued increases in pelvic muscle pressures are found through 16 weeks (Dougherty et al., 1993). Clear directions to guide nursing practice do not emerge from the research at this time. However, if a woman does not make improvements within 6 to 8 weeks with appropriate monitoring by the nurse and consistent adherence to the protocol, other approaches should be considered. There is no consensus of opinion on the maintenance protocol for PME. However, it is generally understood that sustained effectiveness from PME requires continued exercise.

Within the PME protocol it is important to have memory cues. Written records of PME are frequently used. Audiotapes to guide PME at home and videotapes are available and help to promote adherence.

A final, commonly considered feature of PME protocols is motivation. Successful PME requires adherence to a regimen. Relatively little research has been conducted in this area specifically, but most investigators include steps to encourage motivation and adherence to PME protocols. Frequent contact with the clinician appears to be important in maintaining motivation (Bo et al., 1990; Burns et al., 1993; Dougherty, Bishop, Mooney, Gimotty, & Williams, 1993; McDowell, Engberg, et al., 1994). Wells et al. (1991) commented specifically on issues related to adherence to PME protocols. Achieving the desired effect from PME (decreased urine loss) is also a powerful motivator. Clearly, integrating pelvic muscle contractions into daily life to achieve the desired effect is helpful.

There is consensus in much of the research that PME results in significant changes in urine loss and that the effects are long lasting. Five published studies in which women were evaluated 2 to 8 years after completion of a PME protocol showed that improvement in incontinence was sustained over those years in most women (Bo & Talseth, 1996; Cammu & Van Nylen, 1995; Dougherty, Bishop, Mooney, Gimotty, & Williams, 1993; Hahn, Milsom, Fall, & Ekelund, 1993; Klarskov, Nielsen, Kromann-Andersen, & Maegaard, 1991). The research literature supports PME in the management of mild to moderate SUI in women.

The literature lacks any good work on PME for fecal incontinence. Most institutions model their programs to mirror the treatment elements demonstrated for urinary incontinence.

PME with biofeedback. Biofeedback is a powerful modality to enhance the coordination of the contraction and relaxation of the bowel, bladder, and pelvic muscles. Additionally, biofeedback in conjunction with PME enhances the consistency and amplitude of pelvic muscle contractions and may be used to assist individuals in gaining improved relaxation of the pelvic muscle in the management of chronic constipation (Tries, 1990a, 1990b; Tries & Eisman, 1995). Biofeedback is defined as techniques using equiPMEent (usually electronic) to reveal to individuals their internal physiological events, normal and abnormal, in the form of visual and auditory signals to teach them to manipulate these events by manipulating the signals displayed (Basmajian & De Luca, 1985). Biofeedback requires equiPMEent that (a) monitors signals representing relevant physiological processes (pelvic muscle, bladder, bowel, abdominal, or gluteal activity) and (b) provides the individual with auditory or visual information that varies with the signal produced.

When used in nursing interventions for urinary incontinence, biofeedback may be used to monitor (a) pelvic muscle activity; (b) abdominal muscle activity; (c) gluteal muscle activity; and, (d) in some cases, bladder pressure. Monitoring bladder pressure is more invasive than monitoring abdominal and pelvic muscles because it involves insertion of a catheter into the bladder, and this is not well accepted by some individuals.

Three different approaches to biofeedback for urinary incontinence have been investigated over the past two decades: (a) simultaneously measuring and reinforc-ing stable intra-abdominal and bladder pressures during pelvic muscle contractions, (b) reinforcing pelvic muscle contraction to improve force and muscle tone, and (c) reinforcing bladder inhibition (Tries & Eisman, 1995).

Biofeedback in urinary incontinence therapy relays information to individuals about their physiological activity and provides information to modify activity and change bladder and pelvic muscle performance. Although biofeedback typically employs a single measurement (pelvic muscle or bladder), multimeasurement feedback is necessary for reliable results. Changes in abdominal pressure are referred to the bladder and rectum; if abdominal activity is not monitored, measurement of pelvic muscle and bladder pressure is confounded by abdominal activity. In biofeedback for fecal incontinence, the gluteal muscles should also be monitored in addition to the pelvic floor muscles. Isolation of the pelvic floor muscles during contraction of the external anal sphincter is a key component in the success of biofeedback. The anatomy, physiology, and coordinated function of elimination are complex. With biofeedback, functional behaviors are substituted for dysfunctional behavior. In most cases, single method measurement techniques do not provide the individual with sufficient information to restore continence.

In a major controlled trial, Burns et al. (1993) studied older women with primarily stress incontinence who were randomly assigned to PME with biofeedback, PME, or a control group. The two treatment groups demonstrated significant improvement in incontinent episodes over the control group, but significant differences between the two treatments were not found. Additionally, a study designed to compare bladder-sphincter biofeedback with behavioral training that does not use biofeedback resulted in significant reductions in urinary accidents (79% for biofeedback and 82% for behavioral training without biofeedback) 1 month following treatment (Burton et al., 1988). Despite variable results with biofeedback in research, clinicians who employ biofeedback recognize its value. In individuals with urine loss problems and poor coordination of striated and smooth muscle controlling elimination, biofeedback is often the therapy needed to restore the coordination necessary to achieve continence.

In groups where urge incontinence is the dominant symptom, multimeasurement biofeedback, including monitoring bladder pressure, has shown greater reductions in urine loss than PME or than PME with pelvic muscle and abdominal biofeedback alone. However, it may be noted that these studies involved small numbers of subjects and possibly more controlled subject recruitment procedures. Multimeasurement biofeedback studies reveal 75.9% to 82% reductions in urine loss (Burgio, Robinson, & Engel, 1986; McDowell, Burgio, Dombrowski, Locher, & Rodriguez, 1992). Multimeasurement biofeedback in combination with other behavioral techniques, such as bladder training, has shown significant reduction in incontinence in samples with neurological disease and frail elders (McDowell, Engberg, et al., 1994; Middaugh, Whitehead, Burgio, & Engel, 1989; O'Donnell & Doyle, 1991).

Multimeasurement biofeedback provides specific reinforcement for pelvic muscle contraction and control of abdominal and gluteal activity. It appears to improve awareness of pelvic muscle contraction and relaxation. PME addresses improving coordination and increasing the amplitude of pelvic muscle contractions, and biofeedback enhances relaxation of the bladder and the contraction and relaxation of the bowel and pelvic muscles. This is achieved with multimethod biofeedback by reinforcing a short latency to contract in response to urgency. Neurological injury to the pudendal nerve and terminus axons interferes with the normal coordination between the smooth muscle of the bladder and the striated muscles during voiding. Hence, the striated urethral sphincter does not fully relax and/or the bladder does not effectively contract, leading to incomplete bladder emptying. To manage this suboptimal voiding pattern, emphasis is placed on pelvic muscle relaxation at rest and during voiding (Middaugh et al., 1989; Tries, 1990a, 1990b).

Biofeedback is an effective technique in the management of incontinence. Appropriate training and equiPMEent are important considerations. Because biofeedback is ideally suited to be individually modified to each specific situation, and the dysfunctions that lead to incontinence are molded in subtle ways with biofeedback, definitive research in well-controlled studies is gradually increasing.

Measurement and Outcomes in Urinary and Fecal Incontinence Research

Measurement of urinary and fecal incontinence has presented special challenges to investigators. Bowel and bladder function involve the coordinated action of somatic and autonomic components of the peripheral nervous system and the respective striated and smooth muscles. These systems are complex, and in some cases injury to these systems is not well understood. Nonetheless, substantial progress has been made in measurement of outcomes in bowel and bladder research. Research on bowel and bladder function with urodynamics, multimeasurement EMG, and pressure systems has appeared primarily in the medical literature and, with few exceptions, is beyond the scope of this chapter.

Quality of Life and Symptom Distress

Nursing interventions are complemented by methodological research that assesses the experiences and perceptions of incontinence. Research on the impact of urinary incontinence on life has developed simultaneously with quality of life research in cancer and other areas. A series of studies over the past 10 years on the Incontinence Impact Questionnaire (IIQ) (Wyman, Harkins, Choi, Taylor, & Fantl, 1987) established the reliability and validity of the IIQ. Further work resulted in a short form (IIQ-7), which has desirable psychometric properties and is useful in clinical applications. Parallel research has been completed with the Urogenital Distress Inventory to evaluate symptom distress, which is useful in research and clinical settings (Uebersax et al., 1995). Other instruments to assess knowledge, adjustment, coping, or personal acceptance of urinary incontinence have been developed and tested and may be appropriate in specific clinical situations (Lee, Reid, Saltmarche, & Linton, 1995; Wagner, Patrick, Bavendam, Martin, & Buesching, 1996).

Several instruments to score fecal incontinence have been published. Although these instruments attempt to measure incontinence and its impact on quality of life, no universal instrument has been accepted, making comparison of results difficult. The American Society of Colon and Rectal Surgeons is currently completing the validation of such an instrument, which will enable uniformity in the scoring of fecal incontinence and its impact on patients.

Clinical Evaluation of Incontinence

Measurement of incontinence events has been an outcome for which reliable and valid measures have been sought. Approaches in many clinical studies include (a) bladder records, (b) pad tests, and (c) the urine stream interruption test. Bladder records are used to document the frequency, timing, and amount of voiding. Episodes of urine loss are often the focus of the bladder record. Additionally, fluid intake, including caffeinated and alcoholic beverages, may be included on the bladder record. Documentation of intake and urine loss is used as outcome measures in urinary incontinence research (Burns et al., 1993; Fantl, Wyman, Harkins, et al., 1990; McDowell, Engberg, et al., 1994; Rose et al., 1990; Wells et al., 1991). Although a number of bladder records are found in the literature, particularly careful work has been done on the urinary diary (Wyman, Choi, Harkins, Wilson, & Fantl, 1988). Generally, bladder records available in the literature are adapted to the needs of specific settings.

Measuring the loss of bowel function should focus on the type (gas, liquid, mucous, and/or solid stool) and the frequency of the incontinence. Bowel diaries should include whether or not the patient was able to sense the oncoming incontinence, a record of any bowel-altering medication, and any other factors that may contribute to incontinence. Having patients record their food and fluid intake as well as physical activity helps the clinician understand what may be contributing to the incontinence (Wyman & Fantl, 1991).

Bladder records are considered as objective measures (Elser, Fantl, & McClish, 1995), but they are dependent on the diligence and memory of the individual keeping the record. The importance of carefully instructing individuals in the use of bladder records is recognized (Robinson, McClish, Wyman, Bump, & Fantl, 1996). Urine loss quantity is not captured well by self-report but is needed for determining management strategies (Fantl, Newman, et al., 1996).

Pad tests that provide information on the quantity of urine loss have been used in clinic and home settings. Absorbent pads are pre-weighed and weighed after the intervention to indicate the quantity of urine loss. Pad tests of urine loss conducted in a clinic setting involve the individual undertaking a series of activities designed to provoke urine loss with a full bladder. Bladder filling is accomplished by having the individual drink a known quantity of fluid and wait a specified period of time before the provocative maneuvers, or the bladder is filled to capacity during urodynamics (Fantl, Harkins, Wyman, Choi, & Taylor, 1987; Pierson, 1984).

Pad tests conducted at home may provide more complete information on the quantity of urine loss that is occurring during daily life activities. Home pad tests have been used as outcome measures in addition to bladder diaries in some studies (Dougherty, Bishop, Mooney, Gimotty, & Williams, 1993; Ferguson et al., 1990). Both clinic and home pad tests provide an objective measure of urine loss. Voiding and urine loss are highly variable within and between individuals; these characteristics limit the reliability of measurement and remain a challenge to clinicians and researchers.

Characteristics of the Pelvic Muscles

Measures of urine loss have been the primary outcome measure in urinary incontinence research. However, considerable attention has been directed to independent variables that monitor components of the intervention. Significant relationships between pelvic muscle characteristics and episodes of urine loss have not been reported. It is not clear whether this is because of weaknesses in the measurement of urine loss or measurement of pelvic muscle characteristics or the high interindividual variability in these measures. Three approaches to measurement of pelvic muscle characteristics are useful in the nursing management of urinary incontinence. Assessment of the pelvic muscles during physical examination is widely used in PME prescription and to track the progress of PME (Brink, Sampselle, Wells, Diokno, & Gillis, 1989; Sampselle, Brink, & Wells, 1989; Worth, Dougherty, & McKey, 1986). Based on a series of studies, the Pelvic Muscle Strength Rating Scale is used to rate on a scale of 1 to 4 the three dimensions—pressure, duration, and displacement of vertical plane—during vaginal examination. Strong relationships between muscle strength and the ability to control urine flow and significant positive correlations were found between EMG measures of pelvic muscle strength and PME Rating Scale scores (Brink et al., 1989; Sampselle et al., 1989). Some experience with vaginal examinations and instruction is needed to use the PME Rating Scale. However, it is relatively simple, easily used in clinical settings, and provides important information needed to guide PME.

The urine stream interruption test is based on the relationship between urinary control and the strength of the pelvic muscles. For this test, the woman is seated on a commode and is informed that she will be given a verbal signal to stop the urinary flow and that she should attempt to interrupt the flow of urine by contracting the pelvic muscles. The signal to stop is given 5 seconds into the void because maximum flow is usually attained at this point. A stop watch is used to time the number of seconds required to interrupt the urine stream. The length of time required to interrupt correlates well with clinical rating scale scores and with intravaginal EMG measures of pel-

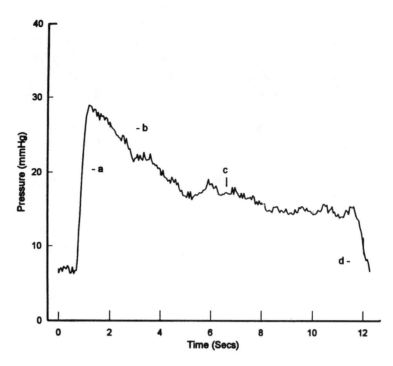

Figure 22.1. Pelvic Muscle Contraction, Showing (a) Recruitment, (b) Decay, (c) Tonus, and (d) Relaxation

vic muscle strength (Sampselle, 1993; Sampselle et al., 1989). The urine stream interruption test is a simple assessment technique and is useful in establishing the relationship between the pelvic muscle contractions and urine flow for the individual, reinforcing correct PME technique, and monitoring the progress of PME.

EMG and pressure multimeasurement systems, with devices placed intravaginally, have been developed to evaluate the characteristics of the pelvic muscles during rest and contraction. Measurement of the pelvic muscle characteristics provides objective evidence of pelvic muscle contractions that are used to teach PME and is an independent variable in PME research on incontinence. A series of studies have provided an understanding of pressures developed during pelvic muscle contractions with pressure-sensitive intravaginal devices and surface EMG (Abrams et al., 1986; Boyington et al., 1995; Dougherty, Bishop, Abrams, et al., 1989; Dougherty, Bishop, Mooney, & Gimotty, 1989; Dougherty, Bishop, Mooney, Gimotty, & Williams, 1993; Ferguson et al., 1990; McKey & Dougherty, 1986). During pelvic muscle contractions in women with normal pelvic muscle function, a resting muscle tone is present in the resting state. When the woman contracts voluntarily, the pressure increases dramatically and quickly. Although she may be instructed to sustain the contraction, there is a point of decay 1 to 2

seconds after the voluntary effort reaches its maximum. Following this moment of pressure decay, considerable pressure is maintained, but at a lower level than the burst of activity at the beginning of the contraction. After relaxation, the pressure decrement is rapid but not as great as the initial moment of activation (see Figure 22.1).

The pressure curves are related to pelvic muscle function, PME, and continence. The pelvic muscles are fully relaxed only during voiding and defecation. During rest, electrical activity is always present in the pelvic muscles; tonus is present and is represented by resting pressure or low-level EMG activity. Based on research on skeletal muscle function, it may be inferred that, initially, early activation of Type II fibers results in dramatic pressure increase. The pelvic muscle contraction involves coordinated response of Type I and Type II fibers. In women with dysfunction and a preponderance of Type I fibers, this process may be modified. In normal women, the pelvic muscle pressure curves are generally similar to that shown in Figure 22.1. In dysfunction, more variable patterns are observed. Further research is needed to better understand the variable patterns and their relationship to denervation injury.

Monitoring pelvic muscle characteristics is valuable in assessment, teaching PME, and providing feedback to women on pelvic muscle characteristics. Digital assessment and urine stream interruption tests are important develoPMEents in managing incontinence that are easily adapted to a variety of clinical settings.

The measurement of independent and dependent variables in the management of incontinence is essential for research, and many of the approaches that have been developed can be easily adapted to clinical settings for continence management.

State of the Science

The revised paradigm of urinary and fecal incontinence provides the basis for expansion of research relevant to nursing management and nursing practice. Urinary and fecal incontinence in healthy adults appear to begin in adulthood, with vaginal childbirth being a signal event for many women. Research on health practices to prevent or delay dysfunctional voiding and urinary and fecal incontinence is an increasingly important focus. Studies that examine the role of dietary interventions for the prevention and early intervention for urinary and fecal incontinence are of special interest, particularly the effects of fiber, caffeine, and alcohol. The roles of physical activity and rehabilitation of the pelvic muscles after childbirth in the prevention of incontinence are not well understood.

The compelling body of literature on PME in the management of mild and moderate SUI suggests that other interventions will be supported by a scientific base as this research develops. The research support for biofeedback with bladder inhibition for urge incontinence is strong, but its applicability is diminished by the urethral catheterization required. Bladder training is clearly an approach that has proven effective for urge and stress urinary incontinence. The use of bladder training techniques for dysfunctional voiding, particularly urgency and frequency, not necessarily accompanied by urinary incontinence, has not been well investigated but may be important in prevention of urinary incontinence.

PME with biofeedback does not have sufficient support at this time to merit widespread investment in multimeasurement biofeedback systems. However, clinical evidence of its value in teaching PME to women with pelvic muscle dysfunction suggests that well-controlled research in this area is needed. The importance of adapting biofeedback to the individual suggests that research will need to include ways to tailor interventions to specific needs, situations, and populations. Individualizing approaches within carefully described interventions is an important step in demonstrating the effectiveness of interventions that require the active participation of the individual (Coffman et al., 1996).

The advances in successfully treating urinary and fecal incontinence have come because a body of research validating sound scientific principles is available. Research that does not have appropriate control groups is, perhaps, useful for concept develoPMEent and pilot study, but of note is that improvement in incontinence has often been observed in untreated, comparative groups (Fantl, Wyman, Harkins, et al., 1990; Nygaard, Kreder, Lepic, Fountain, & Rhomberg, 1996).

Research to guide nursing practice with elders and in long-term care is an especially important develoPMEent. The long-term care environment is a setting in which nursing has long had a prominent role. The importance of environmental assessment to promote continence, and the use of timed voiding and prompted voiding, suggest that future research will build on these successes. Multiple components of interventions in this area, such as staff develoPMEent and monitoring and individualizing the voiding schedule based on objective information about individuals, suggest directions needed in future research.

Incontinence occurs in individuals across adulthood and in highly varied health conditions; the severity of incontinence differs greatly within and between individuals. Research is needed to better clarify the effect that chronic conditions have on incontinence and to better focus interventions based on health status and other factors. Relatively little research is available on ethnic minorities, but tailoring nursing interventions to specific populations is recognized as important. At this time, there is little research to support modification in nursing interventions for special populations.

Knowledge develoPMEent on incontinence has expanded dramatically in the past two decades, although the majority of this information deals with urinary incontinence. Much of the research has reached a point in develoPMEent where it can be used to guide nursing practice. Yet, incontinence remains under-reported and underdiagnosed, and the application of current knowledge is hampered by the lack of success in encouraging the consistent use of proven approaches within health care settings. Among the greatest challenges that lie ahead are the dissemination and application of this research by nurses, including staff in long-term care settings, and the dissemination of information on prevention and management to the public.

References

Abrams, R. M., Batich, C. D., Dougherty, M. C., McKey, P. L., Lin, Y. C., & Parker, J. (1986). Custom-made vaginal balloons for strengthening circumvaginal musculature. *Biomaterials, Medical Devices and Artificial Organs, 14,* 239-248.

Basch, A., & Jensen, L. (1991). Management of fecal incontinence. In D. B. Doughty (Ed.), *Urinary and fecal incontinence: Nursing management* (pp. 235-268). St. Louis, MO: Mosby.

Basmajian, J. V., & De Luca, C. J. (1985). *Muscles alive: Their functions revealed by electromyography* (5th ed.). Baltimore: Williams & Wilkins.

Bear, M., Dwyer, J. W., Benveneste, D., Jett, K., & Dougherty, M. (1997). Home-based management of urinary incontinence: A pilot study with both frail and independent elders. *Journal of Wound, Ostomy, and Continence Nursing, 24*(3), 163-171.

Bishop, B. (1982). Neural plasticity: Part 3. Responses to lesions in the peripheral nervous system. *Physical Therapy, 62*(9), 1275-1282.

Bo, K., Hagen, R. H., Kvarstein, B., Jorgensen, J., & Laarsen, S. (1990). Pelvic floor muscle exercise for the treatment of female stress urinary incontinence: III. Effects of two different degrees of pelvic floor muscle exercises. *Neurourology and Urodynamics, 9,* 489-502.

Bo, K., & Talseth, T. (1996). Long-term effect of pelvic floor muscle exercise five years after cessation of organized training. *Obstetrics and Gynecology, 87*(2), 261-265.

Borrie, M. J., & Davidson, H. A. (1992). Incontinence in institutions: Cost and contributing factors. *Canadian Medical Association Journal, 147,* 322-328.

Boyington, A., Dougherty, M. C., & Kasper, C. E. (1995). Pelvic muscle profile types in response to pelvic muscle exercise. *International Journal of Urogynecology, 6,* 68-72.

Boyington, A. R. (1997). The effect of pelvic muscle exercise on pelvic muscles in women with and without pelvic muscle dysfunction. (Doctoral dissertation, University of Florida). *Dissertation Abstracts International.*

Brink, C. A., Sampselle, C. M., Wells, T. J., Diokno, A. C., & Gillis, G. L. (1989). A digital test for pelvic muscle strength in older women with urinary incontinence. *Nursing Research, 38*(4), 196-199.

Burgio, K. L., Robinson, J. R., & Engel, B. T. (1986). The role of biofeedback in Kegel exercise training for stress urinary incontinence. *American Journal of Obstetrics and Gynecology, 154,* 58-64.

Burns, P. A., Pranikoff, K., Nochajski, T. H., Hadley, E. C., Levy, K. J., & Ory, M. G. (1993). A comparison of effectiveness of biofeedback and pelvic muscle exercise treatment of stress incontinence in older community-dwelling women. *Journal of Gerontology, 48*(4), M167-M174.

Burton, J., Pearce, L., Burgio, K., Engel, B., & Whitehead, W. (1988). Behavioral training for urinary incontinence in elderly ambulatory patients. *Journal of the American Geriatrics Society, 36,* 693-698.

Cammu, H., & Van Nylen, M. (1995). Pelvic floor muscle exercises: 5 years later. *Urology, 45*(1), 113-117.

Campbell, E. B., Knight, M., Benson, M., & Colling, J. (1991). Effect of an incontinence training program on nursing home staff's knowledge, attitudes, and behavior. *Gerontologist, 31,* 788-794.

Coffman, M. A., Francis-Felsen, L., Tomlinson, B. U., Yoon, S. J., Boyington, A. R., Dougherty, M. C., & Dwyer, J. W. (1996). Program fidelity in a community-based clinical trial. *Gerontologist, 36*(Special Issue 1), 295.

Colling, J., Ouslander, J., Hadley, B. J., Eisch, J., & Campbell, E. (1992). The effects of patterned urge response toileting (PURT) on urinary incontinence among nursing home residents. *Journal of the American Geriatrics Society, 40,* 135-141.

Creighton, S. M., & Stanton, S. L. (1990). Caffeine: Does it affect your bladder? *British Journal of Urology, 66*(6), 613-614.

Critchley, H.O.D., Dixon, J. S., & Gosling, J. A. (1980). Comparative study of the periurethral and perianal parts of the human levator ani muscle. *Urologia Internationalis, 35,* 226-232.

DeLancey, J.O.L. (1994). The anatomy of the pelvic floor. *Current Opinion in Obstetrics and Gynecology, 6,* 313-316.

Diokno, A. C., Brock, B. M., Brown, M. B., & Herzog, A. R. (1986). Prevalence of urinary incontinence and other urological symptoms in the noninstitutionalized elderly. *Journal of Urology, 136*(5), 1022-1025.

Dougherty, M., Bishop, K., Mooney, R., Gimotty, P., & Williams, B. (1993). Graded pelvic muscle exercise: Effect on stress urinary incontinence. *Journal of Reproductive Medicine, 38*(9), 684-691.

Dougherty, M. C., Bishop, K. R., Abrams, R. A., Batich, C. D., & Gimotty, P. A. (1989). The effect of exercise on the circumvaginal muscles in postpartum women. *Journal of Nurse-Midwifery, 34*(1), 8-14.

Dougherty, M. C., Bishop, K., Mooney, R., & Gimotty, P. (1989). The effect of circumvaginal muscle (CVM) exercise. *Nursing Research, 38*(6), 331-335.

Dougherty, M. C., Bishop, K. R., Mooney, R., Gimotty, P. A., & Williams, B. (1992). Graded exercise: Effect on pressures developed by the pelvic muscles. In S. G. Funk, E. M. Tornquist, M. T. Champagne, & R. E. Wiese (Eds.), *Key aspects of elder care: Managing falls, incontinence, and cognitive impairment* (pp. 214-232). New York: Springer.

Doughty, D. (1996). A physiologic approach to bowel training. *Journal of Wound, Ostomy, and Continence Nursing, 23,* 46-56.

Elser, D. M., Fantl, J. A., & McClish, D. K. (1995). Comparison of "subjective" and "objective" measures of severity of urinary incontinence in women. Program for Women Research Group. *Neurology and Urodynamics, 14*(4), 311-316.

Engel, B. T., Burgio, L. D., McCormick, K. A., Hawkins, A. M., Scheve, A. A., & Leahy, E. (1990). Behavioral treatment of incontinence in the long-term care setting. *Journal of the American Geriatrics Society, 38*(3), 361-363.

Etherton, G. M., & Kochar, M. S. (1993). Coffee: Facts and controversies. *Archives of Family Medicine, 2*(3), 317-322.

Fantl, J. A., Harkins, S. W., Wyman, J. F., Choi, S. C., & Taylor, J. R. (1987). Fluid loss quantitation test in women with urinary incontinence: A test-retest analysis. *Obstetrics and Gynecology, 70*(5), 739-743.

Fantl, J. A., Newman, D. K., Colling, J., et al. (1996, March). *Urinary incontinence in adults: Acute and chronic management* (Clinical Practice Guidelines No. 2, 1996 update). Rockville, MD: U.S. Department of Health and Human Services, Public Health Service, Agency for Health Care Policy and Research.

Fantl, J. A., Wyman, J. F., Harkins, S. W., & Hadley, E. C. (1990). Bladder training in the management of lower urinary tract dysfunction in women: A review. *Journal of the American Geriatrics Society, 38*(3), 329-332.

Fantl, J. A., Wyman, J. F., McClish, D. K., Harkins, S. W., Elswick, R. K., Taylor, J. R., & Hadley, E. C. (1991). Efficacy of bladder training in older women with urinary incontinence. *Journal of the American Medical Association, 265*(5), 609-613.

Ferguson, K. L., McKey, P. L., Bishop, K. R., Kloen, P., Verheul, J. B., & Dougherty, M. C. (1990). Stress urinary incontinence: Effect of pelvic muscle exercise. *Obstetrics and Gynecology, 75,* 671-675.

Gilpin, S. A., Gosling, J. A., Smith, A.R.B., & Warrell, D. W. (1989). The pathogenesis of genitourinary prolapse and stress incontinence of urine: A histological and histochemical study. *British Journal of Obstetrics and Gynaecology, 96*(1), 15-23.

Hahn, I., Milsom, I., Fall, M., & Ekelund, P. (1993). Long-term results of pelvic floor training in female stress urinary incontinence. *British Journal of Urology, 72*(4), 421-427.

Harke, J. M., & Richgels, K. (1992). Barriers to implementing a continence program in nursing homes. *Clinical Nursing Research, 1,* 158-168.

Herzog, A. R., & Fultz, N. H. (1990). Prevalence and incidence of urinary incontinence in community-dwelling populations. *Journal of the American Geriatrics Society, 38,* 273-281.

Hu, T. (1994). *The cost impact of urinary incontinence on health care services.* Paper presented at the National Multi-Specialty Conference on Urinary Incontinence, Phoenix, AZ.

Hu, T. W. (1990). Impact of urinary incontinence on health-care costs. *Journal of the American Geriatrics Society, 38*(3), 292-295.

Hu, T. W., Igou, J. F., Kaltreider, D. L., Yu, L. C., Rohner, T. J., Dennis, P. J., Craighead, W. E., Hadley, E. C., & Ory, M. G. (1989). A clinical trial of a behavioral therapy to reduce urinary incontinence in nursing homes: Outcome and implications. *Journal of the American Medical Association, 261*(18), 2656-2662.

Jensen, L. L. (1997). Fecal incontinence: Evaluation and treatment. *Journal of Wound, Ostomy, and Continence Nursing, 24*(5), 277-282.

Jirovec, M. M. (1991). The impact of daily exercise on the mobility, balance and urine control of cognitively impaired nursing home residents. *International Journal of Nursing Studies, 28*(2), 145-151.

Jirovec, M. M., & Wells, T. J. (1990). Urinary incontinence in nursing home residents with dementia: The mobility-cognition paradigm. *Applied Nursing Research, 3*(3), 112-117.

Johanson, J. F., & Lafferty J. (1996). Epidemiology of fecal incontinence: The silent affliction. *American Journal of Gastroenterology, 91*(1), 33-36.

Kegel, A. (1948). Progressive resistance exercise in the functional restoration of the perineal muscles. *American Journal of Obstetrics and Gynecology, 56,* 238-248.

Klarskov, P., Nielsen, K. K., Kromann-Andersen, B., & Maegaard, E. (1991). Long-term results of pelvic floor training and surgery for female genuine stress incontinence. *International Urogynecology Journal, 2,* 132-135.

Lee, P. S., Reid, D. W., Saltmarche, A., & Linton, L. (1995). Measuring the psychosocial impact of urinary incontinence: The York Incontinence Perceptions Scale (YIPS). *Journal of the American Geriatrics Society, 43,* 1275-1278.

MacLeod, J. H. (1991). Assessment of patients with fecal incontinence. In D. B. Doughty (Ed.), *Urinary and fecal incontinence: Nursing management* (pp. 203-233). St. Louis, MO: Mosby.

McCormick, K. A., & Burgio, K. L. (1984). Incontinence: An update on nursing care measures. *Journal of Gerontological Nursing, 10*(10), 16-19, 22-23.

McCormick, K. A., & Palmer, M. H. (1992). Urinary incontinence in older adults. In J. J. Fitzpatrick, R. L. Taunton, & A. K. Jacox (Eds.), *Annual review of nursing research* (Vol. 10, pp. 25-53). New York: Springer.

McCormick, K. A., Scheve, A., & Leahy, E. (1988). Nursing management of urinary incontinence in geriatric inpatients. *Nursing Clinics of North America, 23,* 231-264.

McDowell, B. J., Burgio, K. L., Dombrowski, M., Locher, J. L., & Rodriguez, E. (1992). An interdisciplinary approach to the assessment and behavioral treatment of urinary incontinence in geriatric outpatients. *Journal of the American Geriatric Society, 40,* 370-374.

McDowell, B. J., Engberg, S., Weber, E., Brodak, I., & Engberg, R. (1994). Successful treatment using behavioral interventions of urinary incontinence in homebound older adults. *Geriatric Nursing, 15*(6), 303-307.

McKey, P. L., & Dougherty, M. C. (1986). The circumvaginal musculature: Correlation between pressure and physical assessment. *Nursing Research, 35*(5), 307-309.

Middaugh, S. J., Whitehead, W. E., Burgio, K. L., & Engel, B. T. (1989). Biofeedback in treatment of urinary incontinence in stroke patients. *Biofeedback and Self Regulation, 14*(1), 3-19.

Miller, J., Aston-Miller, J. A., & DeLancey, J.O.L. (1996). The knack: A precisely-timed pelvic muscle contraction can be used within a week to reduce leakage in stress urinary incontinence. *Gerontologist, 36*(Special Issue 1), 328-329.

Miller, J. M., Kasper, C., & Sampselle, C. M. (1994). Review of muscle physiology with application to pelvic muscle exercise. *Urologic Nursing, 14,* 92-97.

National Center for Health Statistics. (1979). *The national nursing home survey: 1977 summary for the United States by Van Nostrand, et al.* (DHEW Pub. No. 79-1794; Vital and Health Statistics, Series 13, No. 43). Washington, DC: Health Resources Services Administration, Government Printing Office.

National Kidney and Urologic Diseases Advisory Board. (1994, March 7-9). *Barriers to rehabilitation of persons with end-stage renal disease or chronic urinary incontinence* (Workshop summary report). Bethesda, MD: Author.

Nelson, R., Norton, N., Cautley, E., & Furner, S. (1995). Community-based prevalence of anal incontinence. *Journal of the American Medical Association, 274,* 559-561.

Noelker, L. S. (1987). Incontinence in elderly cared for by family. *Gerontologist, 27*(2), 194-200.

Norton, C. (1996). Providing appropriate service for continence: An overview. *Nursing Standard, 10*(40), 41-45.

Nygaard, I. E., Kreder, K. J., Lepic, M. M., Fountain, K. A., & Rhomberg, A. T. (1996). Efficacy of pelvic floor muscle exercises in women with stress, urge, and mixed urinary incontinence. *American Journal of Obstetrics and Gynecology, 174*(1), 120-125.

O'Donnell, P. D., & Doyle, R. (1991). Biofeedback therapy technique for treatment of urinary incontinence. *Urology, 37,* 432-436.

Ouslander, J. (1990). Urinary incontinence in nursing homes. *Journal of the American Geriatrics Society, 34,* 83-90.

Ouslander, J. G., Schnelle, J. F., Uman, G., Fingold, S., Nigam, J. G., Tuico, E., & Bates-Jensen, B. (1995). Predictors of successful prompted voiding among incontinent nursing home residents. *Journal of the American Medical Association, 273,* 1366-1370.

Palmer, M. H., German, P. S., & Ouslander, J. G. (1991). Risk factors for urinary incontinence one year after nursing home admission. *Research in Nursing and Health, 14,* 405-412.

Pearson, B., & Droessler, D. (1988). Continence through nursing care. *Geriatric Nursing, 9*(6), 347-349.

Pierson, C. A. (1984). Assessment and quantification of urine loss in incontinent women. *Nurse Practitioner, 9*(2), 18-30.

Robinson, D., McClish, D. K., Wyman, J. F., Bump, R. C., & Fantl, J. A. (1996). Comparison between urinary diaries completed with and without intensive patient instructions. *Neurourology and Urodynamics, 15*(2), 143-148.

Rose, M. A., Baigis-Smith, J., Smith, D., & Newman, D. K. (1990). Behavioral management of urinary incontinence in homebound older adults. *Home Healthcare Nurse, 8*(5), 10-15.

Sagar, P. M., & Pemberton, J. H. (1996). Anorectal and pelvic floor function: Relevance to continence, incontinence and constipation. *Gastroenterology Clinics of North America, 25*(1), 163-182.

Sampselle, C. M. (1993). Using a stopwatch to assess pelvic muscle strength in the urine stream interruption test. *Nurse Practitioner: American Journal of Primary Health Care, 18,* 14-16, 18-20.

Sampselle, C. M., Brink, C. A., & Wells, T. J. (1989). Digital measurement of pelvic muscle strength in childbearing women. *Nursing Research, 38*(3), 134-138.

Schnelle, J. F. (1990). Treatment of urinary incontinence in nursing home patients by prompted voiding. *Journal of the American Geriatrics Society, 38*(3), 356-360.

Schnelle, J. F., Newman, D. R., & Fogarty, T. (1990). Management of patient continence in long-term care nursing facilities. *Gerontologist, 30*(3), 373-376.

Schnelle, J. F., Newman, D. R., Fogarty, T. E., Wallston, K., & Ory, M. (1991). Assessment and quality control of incontinence care in long-term nursing facilities. *Journal of the American Geriatrics Society, 39*(2), 165-171.

Schwartz, M. S. (Ed.). (1995). *Biofeedback: A practitioner's guide.* New York: Guilford.

Smith, A.R.B. (1994). Role of connective tissue and muscle in pelvic floor dysfunction. *Current Opinion in Obstetrics and Gynecology, 6,* 317-319.

Subcommittee on the Tenth Edition of the RDAs, Food and Nutrition Board, National Research Council. (1989). *Recommended dietary allowances* (10th ed.). Washington, DC: National Academy Press.

Takano-Stone, J. (1991). Managing bowel function. In W. C. Chenitz, J. Takano-Stone, & S. A. Salisbury (Eds.), *Clinical gerontological nursing: A guide to advanced practice* (pp. 217-232). Philadelphia: Saunders.

Tomlinson, B. U., Dougherty, M. C., Pendergast, J. F., Boyington, A. R., Coffman, M. A., & Pickens, S. M. (1997). Dietary caffeine, fluid intake, and urinary incontinence in older, rural women. *International Urogynecology Journal and Pelvic Floor Dysfunction.* Manuscript submitted for publication.

Tries, J. (1990a). Kegel exercises enhanced by biofeedback. *Journal of Enterostomal Therapy, 17*(2), 67-76.

Tries, J. (1990b). The use of biofeedback in the treatment of incontinence due to head injury. *Journal of Head Trauma Rehabilitation, 5,* 91-100.

Tries, J., & Eisman, E. (1995). Urinary incontinence: Evaluation and biofeedback treatment. In M. S. Schwartz (Ed.), *Biofeedback: A practitioner's guide.* New York: Guilford.

Tuckson, W. D., & Fazio, V. W. (1989). Anal incontinence. In V. W. Fazio (Ed.), *Therapy in colon and rectal surgery* (pp. 83-87). Philadelphia: B. C. Decker.

Uebersax, J. S., Wyman, J. F., Shumaker, S. A., McClish, D. K., Fantl, J. A., & the Continence Program for Women Research Group.

(1995). Short forms to assess life quality and symptom distress for urinary incontinence in women: The Incontinence Impact Questionnaire and the Urogenital Distress Inventory. *Neurourology and Urodynamics, 14*(2), 131-139.

Urinary Incontinence Guideline Panel. (1992). *Urinary incontinence in adults: Guideline report* (AHCPR Pub. No. 92-0039). Rockville, MD: Agency for Health Care Policy and Research.

Wagner, T. H., Patrick, D. L., Bavendam, T. G., Martin, M. L., & Buesching, D. P. (1996). Quality of life of persons with urinary incontinence: Development of a new measure. *Urology, 47*(1), 67-72.

Wall, L. L., Norton, P. A., & DeLancey, J.O.L. (1993). *Practical urogynecology.* Baltimore, MD: Williams & Wilkins.

Walters, M. D., & Karram, M. (1993). *Practical urogynecology.* St. Louis, MO: Mosby.

Wells, T., & Brink, C. (1980). Urinary continence/incontinence. Helpful equiPMEent: What's available to make life pleasanter for patients and staff. *Geriatric Nursing, 1*(4), 264-269, 276.

Wells, T. J., Brink, C. A., Diokno, A. C., Wolfe, R., & Gillis, G. L. (1991). Pelvic muscle exercise for stress urinary incontinence in elderly women. *Journal of the American Society, 39*(8), 785-791.

Worth, A. M., Dougherty, M. C., & McKey, P. L. (1986). DeveloPMEent and testing of the circumvaginal muscles rating scale. *Nursing Research, 35*(3), 166-168.

Wyman, J. F. (1988). Nursing assessment of the incontinent geriatric outpatient population. *Nursing Clinics of North America, 23,* 169-187.

Wyman, J. F. (1991). Incontinence and related problems. In W. C. Chenitz, J. Takano-Stone, & S. A. Salisbury (Eds.), *Clinical gerontological nursing: A guide to advanced practice* (pp. 181-201). Philadelphia: Saunders.

Wyman, J. F., & Fantl, J. A. (1991). Bladder training in ambulatory care management of urinary incontinence. *Urologic Nursing, 11*(3), 11-17.

Wyman, J. F., Choi, S. C., Harkins, S. W., Wilson, M. S., & Fantl, A. J. (1988). The urinary diary in evaluation of incontinent women: A test-retest analysis. *Obstetrics and Gynecology, 71*(6), 812-817.

Wyman, J. F., Harkins, S. W., Choi, S. C., Taylor, J. R., & Fantl, J. A. (1987). Psychosocial impact of urinary incontinence in women. *Obstetrics and Gynecology, 70*(3), 378-381.

23

MANAGING NAUSEA AND VOMITING

Margaret Heitkemper

Overview

Nausea, vomiting, and loss of appetite (anorexia) are among the most prevalent symptoms experienced by patients across all age groups. In addition, they are frequently rated as the most distressing and feared side effects of treatment such as chemotherapy (Rhodes, Watson, McDaniel, Hanson, & Johnson, 1995; Griffin et al., 1996). Decreased caloric and fluid intake can be related to a number of pathophysiological processes and symptoms, including lack of appetite (anorexia), nausea, and vomiting. There are situations in which decreased oral intake may be advantageous to the individual, such as during times of gastrointestinal tract inflammation, but prolonged decreases in oral nutrient intake will have adverse consequences. Nursing practice involves the assessment of nutritional status, as well as symptoms accountable for decreased nutrient intake, and the implementation of strategies to alleviate symptoms and subsequently increase caloric intake.

Nausea and Vomiting

Despite the significance and frequency of nausea and vomiting (N/V), there is surprisingly little empirical study to guide nursing therapies. Knowledge regarding the mechanisms of N/V has been generated by multiple disciplines (e.g., nursing, pharmacy, medicine, neuroscience, psychology), sometimes collaboratively. The majority of studies published in the nursing literature have been descriptive in nature—for example, determining the prevalence and severity of these symptoms in select patient groups. There is an emerging knowledge base related to risk factors for symptom development, cultural and age variations in susceptibility and consequences, use of self-care strategies, and therapeutic management. Nursing scientists have also played an important role in the development of measurement instruments to quantify symptom experiences and their impact on functional outcomes and self-care activities.

425

Definition

Vomiting is the rapid evacuation of gastric or intestinal contents through the mouth. Retching is similar to vomiting but without evacuation of gastric contents. Both are often accompanied by the sensation of nausea, which is an unpleasant feeling of impending vomiting. With both N/V there is a decrease in gastric motility and tone and retrograde movement of duodenal contents into the stomach. N/V and retching are considered autonomic symptoms and are often accompanied by other autonomic signs or symptoms such as increased salivation, sweating, tachycardia, pallor, diarrhea, and dizziness.

Vomiting is a centrally mediated action, in that abdominal and respiratory muscle coordination are controlled by the "vomiting center" in the brain. This center or group of neurons is located in the lateral reticular formation. The vomiting center receives neural input from the vestibular apparatus, higher brainstem, and cortical structures, as well as the periphery, including the visceral organs. In addition, biochemical factors circulating in the cerebrospinal fluid and the blood can also stimulate the chemoreceptor trigger zone (CTZ), which is in the area postrema. The area postrema is a specialized area at the bottom of the fourth ventricle, which lacks a blood/brain barrier; thus, the cells are exposed to biochemical constituents of the circulating blood as well as cerebrospinal fluid. Once stimulated, the CTZ sends input to the vomiting center to initiate the act of vomiting. There is no clearly delineated "nausea center."

There are a variety of physical and biochemical factors known to elicit N/V. Psychological factors acting through the cortical areas of the brain can also stimulate the vomiting center. Clinically, this is exemplified by the anticipatory N/V, which can accompany chemotherapy. Trauma or inflammation of peripheral tissues can stimulate afferent fibers, primarily the vagus nerve, and transmit stimuli to the vomiting center to elicit vomiting. Distention of the organs of the GI tract (e.g., gastroparesis) can also result in nausea. Nausea is often cited as an extragastrointestinal symptom of patients with functional gastrointestinal problems such as irritable bowel syndrome. Thus, N/V may serve as indicators of organic pathological conditions as well as psychological disturbances and functional problems.

From a biochemical perspective, there are a variety of neurotransmitters (e.g., serotonin, histamine, acetylcholine, dopamine) and neuropeptides (e.g., somatostatin, substance P) involved in the sensation of nausea and the act of vomiting. An understanding of the roles of the neurotransmitters has resulted in current pharmacological therapies to manage symptom experiences. For example, serotonin (5-HT) receptor antagonists (5-HT3 receptor antagonists) may act directly on the vomiting center or at the level of the gastrointestinal tract to decrease afferent nerve stimulation to decrease N/V. Serotonin is present in the central nervous system as a neurotransmitter and also in the periphery. The largest peripheral stores of 5-HT are the enterochromaffin (EC) cells of the gastrointestinal tract. Release of 5-HT from EC cells results in stimulation of peripheral afferent vagal fibers and subsequent stimulation of brain areas involved in N/V (Gale, 1995). Both radiation treatment and certain types of chemotherapy result in EC cell release of 5-HT stores.

Adverse outcomes associated with prolonged vomiting include potential fluid and electrolyte imbalances, malnutrition, esophageal tears, esophagitis, and aspiration pneumonia. The risk of fluid imbalance is much greater in pediatric patients, because their body fluid content is proportionately higher, and in elderly patients who have less cardiovascular reserve and decreased ability to respond to volume deficits. Prolonged nausea can result in psychological distress, anorexia, disruption of normal lifestyle activities, and decreased quality of life. When symptoms of N/V are the result of therapy (e.g., antineoplastic therapy), they can result in decreased compliance with the therapeutic regimen. Thus, the study of N/V and strategies for their alleviation is an important area for nursing investigation.

Scientific Evidence

Nursing studies of N/V have focused primarily on three clinical patient groups: pediatric and adult oncology patients, women during the first trimester of pregnancy, and postsurgical patients, because it is well known that these patient groups have high rates of N/V. With respect to these groups, there has been emphasis on the development of tools to measure these symptoms (Rhodes, Watson, & Johnson, 1984), patterns of N/V relative to treatment (Rhodes, Watson, Johnson, Madsen, & Beck, 1987), interventions to reduce the symptoms (Cotanch, Hockenberry, & Herman, 1985), and the identification of characteristics of patients likely to experience N/V or respond to therapies (Dodd, Onishi, Dibble, & Larson, 1996). There are studies in the nursing literature related to nurses' perceptions of patient experiences (Burish & Jenkins, 1992). Studies on the basic physiology of N/V have been performed only to a limited degree by nurse scientists.

Measurement

In general, it is difficult to compare clinical studies of N/V because of the variety of measures used to quantify N/V episodes and severity. In addition, timing of measurements often varies considerably among studies. Other related variables, such as pain and distress, if measured at all, are also measured using a variety of tools. For the purpose of research, it is important that tools distinguish between nausea, vomiting, and retching episodes. Vomiting episodes are counted to determine frequency and, when possible, volume.

On the other hand, nausea is a subjective experience and thus has multiple dimensions. In a survey by Rhodes (Rhodes, Watson, & Johnson, 1984), it was noted that approximately two thirds of oncological, surgical, gynecological, and medical patients did not understand the term "nausea." The term "sick at stomach" was the most commonly selected descriptor for nausea. The ideal tool measures the intensity of the symptom, its frequency and distress quality, its duration, its impact on activities of daily living, and its impact on self-care strategies (Rhodes, 1995). Scales commonly used include self-report instruments such as visual analog scales (VAS), which measure severity or intensity (Syrjala, Donaldson, Davis, Kippes, & Carr, 1995). The VAS may be anchored with "no nausea at all" and "worst nausea possible." Rhodes, Johnson, and McDaniel (1995) state that "when used properly, the VAS is a reliable, valid, and sensitive self-report tool, yet many respondents find the VAS confusing and difficult to complete." As noted by Jenns (1994), the duration of the symptom experience, which may be equally important in terms of patient distress, is not often measured. Other tools include the Symptom Experience Scale (SES), which was developed to measure women's experiences with symptoms associated with treatment for breast cancer (Samarel et al., 1996). The SES is a modification of the McCorkle Symptom Distress Scale (SDS), another tool that is frequently used in studies of oncology patients and includes items related to nausea and vomiting. Another commonly used tool is the Rhodes Index of Nausea and Vomiting (INV), which is a 9-item, 5-point, Likert-type self-report tool (Headley, 1987; Rhodes, Watson, & Johnson, 1984). Form 2 of this tool was later developed and has been used by investigators (Rhodes, Watson, Johnson, Madsen, & Beck, 1987; Troesch, Rodehaver, Delaney, & Yanes, 1993). Quality of life tools used in clinical trials for oncology patients often contain measures related to N/V. More indirect measures of nausea include caloric intake records, antiemetic medication

use, and self-report of appetite or anorexia. Some studies also incorporate nurses' observations of patients' nausea and vomiting episodes (Burish & Jenkins, 1992).

Although most studies do not include physiological indicators of N/V, some include measures of autonomic nervous system function such as blood pressure and heart rate. Nausea and vomiting are difficult to study in animal models (e.g., rats do not vomit). In animal models, anorexia measured as a decrease in food intake is often used as an indirect measure of nausea. For example, nursing scientists have used this model (food intake) to explore the potential role of cytokines on food intake (see "Anorexia" section for further discussion).

Intervention Testing

There have been a number of nursing and non-nursing studies performed to explore the effectiveness of nonpharmacological therapies. However, these studies vary on the timing and frequency of outcome measures (e.g., pre-post treatment, daily log, weekly summaries), the instruments used, criteria for "optimal or good control" (Furst et al., 1992), and the examination of important covariates, such as person and environmental factors. Another important variable is antiemetic medication use, which is frequently not measured when studying the effectiveness of nonpharmacological interventions for nausea and vomiting.

Nausea and vomiting can be viewed as human responses that are modulated by person (vulnerability) and environment (risk) factors. The literatures related to these factors are described below.

Person (vulnerability) factors. Disease, physical condition and treatment (surgery, radiation, antineoplastic drugs) are all important risk factors for nausea and vomiting. Of these, cancer and its treatment as vulnerability factors for the development of N/V have been addressed in the nursing and related literatures.

Cancer therapy. Nausea and vomiting are commonly reported symptoms in patients with cancer, particularly in those undergoing therapy. In addition to symptoms related to the disease and its treatment, constipation and N/V are also common symptoms accompanying opioid treatment. Chemotherapy-induced N/V are well-recognized clinical problems that can impinge on compliance with therapy as well as affect the patient's functional ability and quality of life (Osoba et al., 1997). In studies of side effects associated with cancer therapy, N/V are frequently cited by patients as those most distressing (Rhodes, Watson, & McDaniel, 1995). There is considerable variability in cytotoxic drugs with respect to their ability to elicit N/V.

In cancer therapy, there are two types of N/V. The first is the acute episode associated directly with the cancer chemotherapy. It generally occurs within 2 hours of the start of therapy and may last for up to 24 hours. Patients who have not been well managed during the acute treatment episodes may go on to develop the second type of N/V, which is anticipatory N/V (ANV). Thus, treatment and posttreatment N/V are related to the development of ANV. ANV is defined as the presence of symptoms prior to treatment or at a time when symptoms would not be expected. It is estimated that by the fourth treatment cycle, approximately 25% of patients receiving chemotherapy develop ANV (Morrow & Rosenthal, 1996). The development of ANV is viewed as classical Pavlovian conditioning (Morrow & Rosenthal, 1996), in which an unconditioned response (N/V) that typically results from an unconditioned stimulus (chemotherapy) can be elicited by a conditioned stimulus (thinking about therapy, sights or smells of treatment room). There appear to be several factors predictive of the development of ANV, including psychological distress (i.e., anxiety and depression) (Razavi et al., 1993). In addition, there is a positive association between number of treatments and ANV (Morrow & Rosenthal, 1996; Tomoyasu, 1996).

In the past decade, pharmacological antiemetic therapy has markedly reduced the frequency and severity of acute nausea and vomiting associated with cancer chemotherapy (Fernández-Marcos et al., 1996; Morrow & Rosenthal, 1996). The newer 5-HT3 receptor antagonists have fewer central nervous system side effects (e.g., drowsiness) as compared to the older centrally acting antiemetic drugs (e.g., phenothiazines) (Gale, 1995). Antiemetic therapy for chemotherapy-induced nausea and vomiting frequently involves multiple drugs (e.g., dexamethasone, phenothiazines, 5-HT3 antagonists) in combination. However, despite these pharmacological advances, an estimated 25% of patients continue to experience nausea and 10% vomiting (Morrow & Rosenthal, 1996). In a prospective study of 12 symptoms using the SDS in bone marrow transplant patients ($N = 28$), Lawrence, Gilbert, and Peters (1996) noted that mild intermittent nausea persisted in the outpatient setting for up to 9 days after bone marrow transplant despite continuous combination antiemetic therapy. Once in place, ANV can be refractory to antiemetic therapy (Tavorath & Hesketh, 1996). It has been suggested that behavioral management strategies might be more effective than pharmacological

agents in reducing ANV symptoms (Morrow & Rosenthal, 1996). One approach is to use systematic desensitization. This involves counterconditioning, a response (e.g., muscle relaxation) that is incompatible with the stimuli that elicit the ANV (Morrow & Rosenthal, 1996). Thus, additional adjunct therapies need to be studied.

Pregnancy. N/V during the first trimester of pregnancy are estimated to occur in 50% to 80% of pregnant women (DiIorio, 1985; Gadsby, Barnie-Adshead, & Jagger, 1993). The severity ranges from mild nausea upon awakening to hyperemesis gravida in which nutritional interventions are warranted. Approximately 11% of pregnant women experience severe vomiting episodes (Zhang & Cai, 1991). Despite the prevalence of the problem, the pathophysiological mechanisms accountable for N/V remain poorly understood. A number of potential mechanisms include psychological distress, hormone changes (e.g., thyroid dysfunction), afferent nerve stimulation, and dysmotility of the gastrointestinal tract. There is descriptive information regarding the presence of gastric dysrhythmias in pregnant women (Walsh, Hasler, Nugent, & Owyang, 1996).

There is also limited information on the impact of N/V episodes on quality of life or self-care activities. Using a semistructured interview of 27 women who experienced varying degrees of N/V, O'Brien and Naber (1992) noted that these symptoms imposed substantial lifestyle limitations on the individual and family. In addition, therapeutic interventions (e.g., dietary) remain to be empirically tested.

Nonpharmacological interventions for women with pregnancy-related N/V are particularly important because of the desire to avoid antiemetic agents. In a review of nursing textbooks, DiIorio, van Lier, and Manteuffel (1994) listed commonly recommended therapies such as eating crackers, eating small meals, providing reassurance that N/V were normal, avoiding odors, taking vitamin B, avoiding greasy foods, using acupuncture, and taking antiemetic medications. DiIorio and colleagues conducted a descriptive exploratory study of clinicians to answer the following questions: (a) What relief measures for N/V are recommended most by clinicians? (b) Are different relief measures recommended based on symptom severity? (c) How effective are the therapies as perceived by clinicians? and (d) What factors guide the clinician in determining the therapeutic intervention? Results showed that clinicians ranked taking prescription medications, eating small meals, eating when one feels nauseated, avoiding certain foods or drinks, and acupressure as higher on the list of relief measures recommended.

Although descriptive studies contribute to our understanding of current practice related to N/V during pregnancy, they do not provide clear guidelines for the care and management of patients with this condition. Clearly, additional work is needed, particularly with respect to therapeutic interventions for women experiencing N/V.

Postsurgery. With the increased number of outpatient surgeries and shorter hospital stays for inpatient surgery patients, control of postoperative N/V has become increasingly important. Postoperative N/V is thought to decrease patient comfort, put undue stress on surgical incisions, alter fluid and electrolyte status, and place the patient at risk for aspiration. In general, postoperative N/V episodes are of a shorter duration than those associated with chemotherapy. Non-nursing studies of postoperative N/V episodes suggest that patient characteristics and surgical factors (e.g., anesthetic agent, length of surgery, type of surgery) are predictive of postoperative N/V (Haynes & Bailey, 1996; Chung, Lee, & Su, 1996).

Additional person factors. In the scientific literature, there has been increased attention to person factors that may predispose to N/V, as well as increased refractoriness to therapeutic interventions. Women appear to be more likely to self-report N/V (Furst et al., 1992; Grebenik & Allman, 1996). There is evidence to suggest that age may dampen the likelihood of developing N/V or retching with cancer chemotherapy. Dodd and colleagues compared younger (< 65 years; $n = 102$) and older (> 65 years; $n = 25$) patients receiving chemotherapy. Younger patients were found to have more problems with N/V after the first 24 hours of treatment, despite few group differences in self-care strategies. The investigators hypothesized that such differences were related to higher trait anxiety and the expectation for being ill in the younger patient group as compared to the older patient group (Dodd et al., 1996). Similar age-related differences in N/V frequency were found in a study of postcardiac surgery patients (Grebenik & Allman, 1996).

Other characteristics that may contribute to increased vulnerability to N/V include a history of motion sickness and/or food aversions, few coping strategies, and high trait anxiety (Fallowfield, 1992). In a study of relaxation training and distraction, Vasterling, Jenkins, Tope, and Burish (1992) found that high levels of base-

line anxiety were associated with increased nausea levels through the chemotherapy experience.

Coping style may also contribute to the individual's response to therapeutic interventions. Lerman and colleagues (1990), in a study of 58 cancer patients, examined coping style with respect to the efficacy of a relaxation program to reduce nausea in patients undergoing chemotherapy. These investigators noted that in the group whose coping style was described as "monitoring," there were higher levels of self-reported anxiety and nausea before chemotherapy and nausea during treatment as compared to the group whose coping style was described as "blunting." Limitations to this study included inability both to determine compliance with the relaxation intervention and to determine differences in antiemetic medication use. However, the results do support the notion that understanding patient characteristics, including coping style, may enhance the ability to match appropriate interventions to reduce N/V.

Whether nausea is affected by the menstrual cycle is unclear. In a retrospective study of 85 female patients who underwent middle ear surgery, reports of N/V during the periovulatory phase (days 11 to 24) were compared to perimenstrual (days 25 to 10) phase (Honkavaara, Lehtinen, Hovorka, & Korttila, 1996). The investigators noted that the incidence of N/V after middle ear surgery was less during the perimenstrual period. No efforts were made in this study to determine the ovarian hormone levels or the subjects' ovulation status. Other studies have shown inconsistent results relative to the influence of menstrual cycle phase on postoperative N/V (Gratz, Allen, Afshar, Joslyn, Buxbaum & Prilliman, 1996).

Environmental (risk) factors. Environmental factors, including unpleasant sights and smells, may contribute to N/V. Common nursing recommendations to patients include small frequent meals, eating slowly to avoid gastric distention, reducing emotional stress at mealtime, and reducing strong odors and unpleasant sights in the dining environment. Although intuitively logical, such interventions packaged as a comprehensive environmental intervention remain to be tested. The role of environment in terms of placing patients at risk for greater symptom intensity or compliance with therapies to manage the therapies also needs to be studied in patient groups.

Therapeutic Management

The majority of nursing studies have focused on nonpharmacological management of N/V. Nonpharmacological management strategies for N/V include modification of dietary intake, alterations in the physical environment (e.g., smells, sights), relaxation therapy, systematic desensitization, and distraction (e.g., playing video games during therapy), including guided imagery. Such therapies are often viewed as adjunct therapies to pharmacological management. In addition to the measurement issues described above, other problems plague the comparison of intervention trials. For example, there are differences in the timing of the intervention, intensity of the intervention, and the qualifications of the person delivering the intervention. In addition, the generalizability of most studies is limited because of the small samples used and the relatively short-term follow-up.

A variety of nonpharmacological approaches has been studied, including relaxation, guided imagery, biofeedback, music, and hypnosis. In a small sample of oncology patients ($N = 28$) receiving antineoplastic treatment, Troesch and colleagues (1993) found no group differences in the reporting of N/V or retching in those who received guided imagery as compared to a control group who did not. However, patients receiving guided imagery did report a greater sense of control and relaxation than patients in the control group as measured with the Chemotherapy Experience Survey. In a study of eight Japanese patients (four in each group) undergoing chemotherapy, Arakawa (1995) was unable to detect the effectiveness of progressive muscle relaxation, in part because both the treatment and control groups reported a decrease in N/V over time.

Syrjala and colleagues (1995) noted that psychological interventions (relaxation with imagery, cognitive-behavioral skills) for cancer pain relief in bone marrow transplant patients were effective in reducing pain but had little effect on nausea. This study consisted of four groups ($N = 94$): (a) treatment as usual, (b) therapist support, (c) relaxation and imagery training, and (d) relaxation training as a package of cognitive-behavioral skills. The failure to find group differences in self-report of nausea level was supported by the patient's report on the lack of helpfulness of the therapies for N/V. In 1985, Frank (1985) reported on a study of music therapy with guided imagery to reduce anxiety and N/V in a small sample ($N = 15$) of patients receiving chemotherapy. The results supported a beneficial effect of music on reducing the patients' self-report of their vomiting severity but did not support a beneficial effect on self-report of nausea. In this study, N/V were measured with an 8-item tool developed by the investigator, but no reliability or validity data regarding the tool were provided.

Several studies have demonstrated a beneficial effect of relaxation and imagery and distraction on N/V during chemotherapy. In a non-nursing study of 81 adult ambulatory patients receiving intravenous chemotherapy, Burish and Jenkins (1992) compared the effectiveness of two forms of electromyography (EMG) biofeedback with and without relaxation training on both patient-rated and nurse-rated N/V episodes. The relaxation group showed a significant reduction in nausea (both patient and nurse rated) after the second chemotherapy session as compared to EMG biofeedback and no-treatment groups. Neither of the biofeedback groups showed any difference in nausea levels as compared to controls. Although nurses were unaware of the patients' ratings, they were not blinded to the patient treatment group, suggesting potential bias in their observations. Another methodological concern is that antiemetic medication use was examined prior to group assignment but not during therapy. As this study only monitored the acute effects of chemotherapy, it is not possible to determine any potential long-term effectiveness of the treatments. Of note in this study is that patients were able to apply the relaxation procedure on their own during the fifth session.

Vasterling et al. (1993) found that distraction (i.e., video games) was equal to relaxation training as compared to a control group in reducing the report of nausea before and during chemotherapy in a group of adult patients ($n = 60$). Both treatments were more effective during the initial part of the therapy as compared to later in therapy. Similarly, Morrow (1989) found that video games reduced both ANV and posttreatment N/V in children receiving chemotherapy.

Using a multimodal and multidisciplinary approach to chemotherapy-induced N/V management, Furst et al. (1995) compared two groups of women with ovarian cancer receiving cisplatin, a highly emetic chemotherapeutic agent. Patients were treated on two separate wards, one receiving usual antiemetic pharmacological treatment ($n = 34$) and the other an experimental unit ($n = 44$), in which patients received training in progressive muscle relaxation, nutritional advice, and "continuity in nursing care in an attempt to optimize the antiemetic measures." Marked group differences were noted, with those in the experimental group showing consistently lower levels of N/V as compared to the control group.

Exercise as an intervention for N/V has not been extensively studied by nurse investigators. In a review of eight studies examining the effects of exercise on physical and psychological symptoms in women with breast cancer, N/V were found to be two symptoms that could be reduced through exercise (Friedenreich & Courneya, 1996). However, as pointed out in this review, there were considerable methodological issues across the eight studies. A randomized clinical trial design to determine the efficacy of this therapy as an adjuvant therapy remains to be performed.

Hypnosis is another form of behavioral management that has been used to reduce symptoms in chemotherapy and surgical patients (Cotanch et al., 1985). Studies of hypnosis related to N/V have been conducted primarily by non-nurse investigators. In a pediatric oncology patient population, Zeltzer, Dolgin, LeBaron, and LeBaron (1991) found that children in the hypnosis group (imagination focused) had reduced the duration but not severity of symptoms associated with therapy when compared to a control group receiving a similar amount of time with the therapist before and during chemotherapy but with no hypnosis. A third group of children received generalized support and distraction. However, not all children in the hypnosis group benefited from the treatment. This study emphasizes the need to consider patient characteristics (e.g., age, disease, treatment, anxiety, history) that might predict improvement with hypnosis. In a study of hypnosis as an adjunct therapy in conscious sedation surgical procedures, Faymonville et al. (1995) found that postoperative N/V were reported by 1.2% of the hypnosis group (*n* = 172) as compared to 26.7% of those in the intravenous sedation group (n = 137). There were no group differences in the amounts of anxiolytic and analgesic medications administered during the procedure. A major limitation of this study was the lack of detail regarding the actual measures (i.e., tool used and timing of measurement) for N/V.

Overall, these studies support some positive effects of nonpharmacological therapies to reduce N/V associated with cancer therapy. Differences in the study findings support the need to consider differences in the intervention (e.g., components, timing, who delivers it), disease conditions, and treatment protocols as well as person characteristics of the sample.

Recommendations for Advancing the Science

Nursing science has contributed to our understanding of the prevalence and impact of N/V on patient distress and quality of life, primarily in oncology patients undergoing therapy. In addition, self-care strategies related to these symptoms have been explored, although much remains to be done. As reflected in the literature, there is evidence that patients at risk can be identified for symptom development and refractoriness to therapeutic interventions. There is a need to clarify the demographic, medical, psychological, and physiological predictors of N/V and the probable effectiveness of specific therapeutic interventions.

There is a clear need for the conduct of intervention trials. Such trials need to be performed with emphasis on person and environmental factors that may be predictors of compliance with therapies and response. Randomized clinical trials of behavioral interventions, including distraction, relaxation training with and without guided imagery, and hypnosis, with emphasis on their cost-effectiveness as adjunct therapy to pharmacological antiemetic therapy, are warranted.

With the continuing development of pharmacological therapies and increased use of nonpharmacological therapies as adjuncts, it is necessary for nurse scientists to gather descriptive information on the frequency and severity of N/V in clinical practice settings. Evidence from patients receiving chemotherapy demonstrates that interventions for N/V need to be instituted early and their effectiveness monitored. Greater emphasis also needs to be placed on physiological measures, including the use of noninvasive measures of gastrointestinal motility and measurement of peripheral stimulants such as cytokines.

Anorexia

Definition

Anorexia is defined as a lack of appetite. Appetite regulation is primarily a function of the central nervous system. However, there are neurohormonal signals from the periphery that act to modulate feeding behavior. In the central nervous system, there are numerous brain areas, especially the hypothalamus nuclei (e.g., lateral hypothalamus, ventro-medial hypothalamus), which are involved in the complex function of eating. Food intake is modified by psychological, sociocultural, and physiological conditions. Pharmacological agents can also significantly increase or decrease appetite. Most agents work by influencing central neurotransmitter systems, including serotonin, dopamine, or norepinephrine. Feeding behavior is also modulated by peripheral (e.g., cholecystokinin) and central neuropeptides and hormones. Most recently, attention has focused on chemical mediators called cytokines, which are produced and released by immune system cells during both inflammation and tumor growth and which can decrease appetite either directly or through stimulation of other chemical mediators.

Scientific Evidence

Studies related to anorexia have provided descriptive information on the prevalence of the problem in select patient groups such as those with cancer and the elderly (Morley & Kraenzle, 1994; Sarna, Lindsey, Dean, Brecht, & McCorkle, 1993) as well as data regarding the pathophysiological mechanisms that might account for this problem. (A discussion of the psychiatric condition anorexia nervosa is beyond the scope of this chapter.) Another symptom closely related to feeding behavior is hunger. Hunger has been studied in a variety of patient groups, including neonatal intensive care unit patients (Kinneer & Beachy, 1994), where the emphasis has been on understanding feeding cues, and patients with cancer (Sarna et al., 1993).

Measurement

Issues previously described under N/V apply to the measurement of anorexia or hunger in patient groups. Clinical research studies often use visual analogue scales to evaluate the sensation of hunger or appetite. To quantify the degree to which dietary intake is affected by the sensations of hunger or appetite, 24-hour food recall, 3-day food records, or food frequency questionnaires are used.

Person (Vulnerability) Factors

Like N/V, the human response anorexia is modulated by person and environment factors. Important person factors include disease, treatment, psychological distress, and age. As stated above, anorexia in response to tumors and inflammation has been studied by nurse investigators.

In cancer patients, anorexia is a component of cachexia, which is characterized by both body mass wasting and loss of appetite. It has been well established that tumor growth is associated with a decrease in food intake and body weight (Nelson, Walsh, & Sheehan, 1994). The etiology of this syndrome has been explored by nurse investigators. In a series of animal (Fischer 344 rats) experiments, Smith, Conn, and Kluger (1993) demonstrated that tumor growth induced significant anorexia as measured by decreased food intake, weight loss, and decreased motor activity. These changes were associated with an increase in blood interleukin-6 (IL-6) levels but

not tumor necrosis factor-cachectin (TNF-C) levels. A strength of the study design was the use of a pair-fed control group to demonstrate that the observed effects in activity and IL-6 levels were independent of decreased food intake or weight loss. Despite the lack of change in TNF-C levels, the investigators hypothesized that this cytokine may still play a role in cancer anorexia and cachexia via stimulation of IL-6 production. In another experiment to clarify the role of TNF-C, Smith and Kluger (1993) administered anti-TNF antibodies to cachetic tumor-bearing rats. The antibodies to TNF only partially reversed the decrease in food intake in the tumor-bearing rats, and this result was transient. These results suggest that in this model of cancer-induced anorexia, TNF-C does not play a major role.

Another proposed mechanism for cancer-induced anorexia is an alteration in gastrointestinal motility. Delayed gastric emptying rate and gastric stasis may contribute to early satiety and subsequent lack of appetite. In an initial attempt to explore the relationship between food intake, gastric emptying, and tumor growth, McCarthy and Daun (1992a) used Sprague-Dawley rats implanted with Walker 256 carcinosarcoma. They noted that growth of the tumor was associated with a decrease in food intake but not with a change in gastric emptying. However, gastric emptying was measured immediately after and 3 hours after gavage administration of a 7-ml liquid diet, which may not be a sensitive indicator of differences with respect to the initial rate of emptying or the emptying of solids. Additional measures might include gastric motor activity (motility) and geometric center determinations for gastric and intestinal transit to further clarify the potential impact of delayed GI motor function on appetite.

In a follow-up study, McCarthy and Daun (1992b) examined the role of prostaglandins in mediating appetite and gastric emptying alterations associated with tumor growth in rats. Ibuprofen, a prostaglandin synthesis inhibitor, attenuated tumor growth but not tumor-induced anorexia. In 1992, McCarthy and Daun reported that rats treated with interleukin-1 (IL-1) had both decreased food intake and decreased rate of gastric emptying. Pretreatment with ibuprofen prior to IL-1 increased the rate of gastric emptying and appetite but did not achieve values similar to that observed in placebo-treated rats. These results suggested that IL-1 effects on gastric emptying were mediated at least in part by prostaglandins.

In an early experiment with nonhuman fasted primates, Metzger and Hansen (1983) administered the octapeptide cholecystokinin (CCK) intravenously at the time of food presentation. In this model, CCK temporarily suppressed caloric intake. A decade later, Daun and McCarthy (1993) also conducted experiments to examine the role of the CCK in the rats treated with IL-1C. In their model, Sprague-Dawley rats were fasted overnight and then injected with IL-1C in the morning. Rats receiving IL-1C had significantly increased plasma CCK-LI levels, along with reduced food intake and decreased gastric emptying. Pretreatment of the rats with a CCK receptor antagonist significantly but not completely improved food intake and the emptying of gastric contents in the IL-1C-treated rats. Thus, CCK, in addition to prostaglandins, works peripherally to affect feeding behavior. There are likely to be other factors that work either peripherally or centrally to modulate feeding behavior. Thus, more work, including the use of healthy volunteers and select patient groups, needs to be done to determine the roles of these factors and whether modulation of their levels pharmacologically will affect nutritional intake.

Inflammation produces a number of physiological responses that may account for the subsequent anorexia associated with it. Inflammation produces substantial increases in IL-6 levels. Using a model of acute inflammation (turpentine subcutaneous injection) in an animal model (Sprague-Dawley rats), Lennie, McCarthy, and

Keesey (1995) found that the metabolic responses (i.e., anorexia, weight loss, fever, increased metabolic rate, synthesis of acute-phase proteins) were dependent on the animal's initial weight. That is, rats who were overfed prior to inflammation exhibited a longer period of anorexia and greater weight loss; those who were underfed ingested food in amounts adequate to promote weight gain. These results suggest that body weight, and thus perhaps genetic predisposition, may be important factors in determining the impact of inflammation on appetite and weight changes.

State of the Science

Understanding the physiological responses to injury and tumor growth as exemplified by these nursing studies is likely to provide valuable information upon which to build intervention studies. It is clear that both peripheral and central neurohormonal factors must be considered in the etiology of altered feeding behavior. Additional work is clearly needed to build on these findings and to expand our understanding of how disease influences nutritional intake and metabolism. The importance of anorexia and nutritional intake in terms of quality of life or functional outcomes needs to be carefully explored.

References

Arakawa, S. (1995). Use of relaxation to reduce side effects of chemotherapy in Japanese patients. *Cancer Nursing, 18,* 60-66.

Burish, T. G., & Jenkins, R. A. (1992). Effectiveness of biofeedback and relaxation training in reducing the side effects of cancer chemotherapy. *Health Psychology, 11,* 17-23.

Chung, F., Lee, V., & Su, J. (1996) Postoperative symptoms 24 hours after ambulatory anesthesia. *Canadian Journal of Anaesthesia, 43,* 1121-1127.

Cotanch, P., Hockenberry, M., & Herman, S. (1985). Self-hypnosis as antiemetic therapy in children receiving chemotherapy. *Oncology Nursing Forum, 12,* 41-45.

Covino, N.A., & Frankel, F.H. (1993). Hypnosis and relaxation in the medically ill. *Psychotherapy Psychosom, 60,* 75-90.

Daun, J. M., & McCarthy, D. O. (1993). The role of cholecystokinin in interleukin-1-induced anorexia. *Physiology and Behavior, 54,* 237-241.

DiIorio, C. (1985). First trimester nausea in pregnant teenagers: Incidence, characteristics, intervention. *Nursing Research, 34,* 372-374.

DiIorio, C., van Lier, D., & Manteuffel, B. (1994). Recommendations by clinicians for nausea and vomiting of pregnancy. *Clinical Nursing Research, 3,* 209-227.

Dodd, M. J., Onishi, K., Dibble, S. L., & Larson, P. J. (1996). Differences in nausea, vomiting, and retching between younger and older outpatients receiving cancer chemotherapy. *Cancer Nursing, 19,* 155-161.

Fallowfield, L. J. (1992). Behavioural interventions and psychological aspects of care during chemotherapy. *European Journal of Cancer, 28A,* S39-S41.

Faymonville, M. E., Fissette, J., Mambourg, P. H., Roediger, L., Joris, J., & Lamy, M. (1995). Hypnosis as adjunct therapy in conscious sedation for plastic surgery. *Regional Anesthesia, 20,* 145-151.

Fernández-Marcos, A., Martín, M., Sanchez, J., Rodriguez-Lescure, A., Casado, A., López-Martin, J., & Diaz-Rubio, E. (1996). Acute and anticipatory emesis in breast cancer patients. *Supportive Care in Cancer, 4,* 370-377.

Fitch, M.I. (1992). Managing treatment-induced emesis: A nursing perspective. *Oncology, 49, 312-316.*

Frank, J. M. (1985). The effects of music therapy and guided visual imagery on chemotherapy induced nausea and vomiting. *Oncology Nursing Forum, 12,* 47-52.

Friendenreich, C. M., & Courneya, K. S. (1996). Exercise as rehabilitation for cancer patients. *Clinical Journal of Sports Medicine, 6,* 237-244.

Furst, C. J., Johansson, S., Fredrikson, M., Hursti, T., Steineck, G., & Peterson, C. (1992). Control of cisplatin induced emesis Cd: A multidisciplinary intervention strategy. *Medical Oncology and Tumor Pharmacotherapy, 9,* 81-86.

Gadsby, R., Barnie-Adshead, A. M., & Jagger, C. (1993). A prospective study of nausea and vomiting during pregnancy. *British Journal of General Practice, 43,* 245-248.

Gale, J. D. (1995). Serotonergic mediation of vomiting. *Journal of Pediatric Gastroenterology and Nutrition, 21,* S22-S28.

Gratz, I., Allen, E., Afshar, M., Joslyn, A. F., Busbaum, J., & Prilliman, B. (1996). The effects of menstrual cycle on the incidence of emesis and efficacy of ondansetron. *Anesthesia and Analgesia, 83,* 565-569.

Grebenik, C. R., & Allman, C. (1996). Nausea and vomiting after cardiac surgery. *British Journal of Anaesthesia, 77,* 356-359.

Griffin, A. M., Butow, P. N., Coates, A. S., Childs, A. M., Ellis, P. M., Dunn, S. M., & Tattersall, M. H. (1996). On the receiving end: V. Patient perceptions of the side effects of cancer chemotherapy in 1993. *Annals of Oncology, 7,* 189-195.

Haynes, G. R., & Bailey, M. K. (1996). Postoperative nausea and vomiting: Review and clinical approaches. *Southern Medical Journal, 89,* 940-949.

Headley, J. A. (1987). The influence of administration time on chemotherapy-induced nausea and vomiting. *Oncology Nursing Forum, 14,* 43-47.

Heitkemper, M.M. & Shaver, J.F. (1989). Research opportunities in enteral nutrition. *Nursing Clinics of North America, 24,* 415-426.

Honkavaara, P., Lehtinen, A. M., Hovorka, J., & Korttila, K. (1996). Effect of transdermal hyoscine on nausea and vomiting during and after middle ear surgery under local anaesthesia. *Canadian Journal of Anaesthesia, 38,* 876-879.

Jenns, K. (1994). Importance of nausea. *Cancer Nursing, 17,* 488-493.

Keller, V.E. (1995). Management of nausea and vomiting in children. *Journal of Pediatric Nursing, 10*(5), 280-286.

Kinneer, M. D., & Beachy, P. (1994). Nipple feeding premature infants in the neonatal intensive-care unit: Factors and decisions. *Journal of Obstetric, Gynecologic, and Neonatal Nursing, 23,* 105-112.

Lawrence, C. C., Gilbert, C. J., & Peters, W. P. (1996). Evaluation of symptom distress in a bone marrow transplant outpatient environment. *Annals of Pharmacotherapy, 30,* 941-945.

Lennie, T. A., McCarthy, D. O., & Keesey, R. E. (1995). Body energy status and the metabolic response to acute inflammation. *American Journal of Physiology, 269,* R1024-R2031.

Lerman, C., Rimer, B., Blumberg, B., Cristinzio, S., Engstrom, P. F., MacElwee, N., O'Connor, K., & Seay, J. (1990). Effects of coping style and relaxation on cancer chemotherapy side effects and emotional responses. *Cancer Nursing, 13*(5), 308-315.

Marin, J., Ibanez, M.C., & Arribas, S. (1990). Therapeutic management of nausea and vomiting. *General Pharmacology, 21,* 1-10.

McCarthy, D. O., & Daun, J. M. (1992a). The effect of diet consistency on food intake of anorectic tumor-bearing rats. *Research in Nursing and Health, 15,* 433-437.

McCarthy, D. O., & Daun, J. M. (1992b). The role of prostaglandins in interleukin-1 induced gastroparesis. *Physiology and Behavior, 52,* 351-353.

Metzger, B. L., & Hansen, B. C. (1983). Cholecystokinin effects on feeding, glucose, and pancreatic hormones in rhesus monkeys. *Physiology and Behavior, 30,* 509-518.

Morley, J. E., & Kraenzle, D. (1994). Causes of weight loss in a community nursing home. *Journal of the American Geriatrics Society, 42,* 583-585.

Morrow, G. R. (1989). Chemotherapy side effects and cancer patient nutrition. *Nutrition, 5,* 119-121.

Morrow, G. R., & Rosenthal, S. N. (1996). Models, mechanisms and management of anticipatory nausea and emesis. *Oncology, 53,* 4-7.

Nelson, K. A., Walsh, D., & Sheehan, F. A. (1994). The cancer anorexia-cachexia syndrome. *Journal of Clinical Oncology, 12,* 213-225.

O'Brien, B., & Naber, S. (1992). Nausea and vomiting during pregnancy: Effects on the quality of women's lives. *Birth, 19,* 138-143.

Osoba, D., Zee, B., Pater, J., Warr, D., Latreille, J., & Kaizer, L. (1997). Determinants of postchemotherapy nausea and vomiting in patients with cancer. *Journal of Clinical Oncology, 15,* 116-123.

Razavi, D., Delvaux, N., Farvacques, C., De Brier, F., Van Heer, C., Kaufman, L., Derde, M.-P., Beauduin, M., & Piccart, M. (1993). Prevention of adjustment disorders and anticipatory nausea secondary to adjuvant chemotherapy: A double-blind, placebo-controlled study assessing the usefulness of alprazolam. *Journal of Clinical Oncology, 11*(7), 1384-1390.

Rhodes, V. A., Watson, P. M., & Johnson, M. A. (1984). Development of a reliable and valid measure of nausea and vomiting. *Cancer Nursing, 7,* 31-41.

Rhodes, V. A., Watson, P. M., Johnson, M. A., Madsen, R. W., & Beck, N. C. (1987). Patterns of nausea, vomiting, and distress in patients receiving antineoplastic drug protocols. *Oncology Nursing Forum, 14,* 35-44.

Rhodes, V. A., Watson, P. M., & McDaniel, R. W. (1995). Nausea, vomiting, and retching: The management of the symptom experience. *Seminars in Oncology Nursing, 11,* 256-265.

Rhodes, V. A., Watson, P. M., McDaniel, R. W., Hanson, B. M., & Johnson, M. H. (1995). Expectation and occurrence of postchemotherapy side effects: Nausea and vomiting. *Cancer Practice, 3,* 247-253.

Samarel, N., Leddy, S. K., Greco, K., Cooley, M. E., Torres, S., Tulman, L., & Fawcett, J. (1996). Development and testing of the Symptom Experience Scale. *Journal of Pain and Symptom Management, 12,* 221-228.

Sarna, L., Lindsey, A. M., Dean, H., Brecht, M. L., & McCorkle, R. (1993). Nutritional intake, weight change, symptom distress, and functional status over time in adults with lung cancer. *Oncology Nursing Forum, 20,* 481-489.

Smith, B. K., Conn, C. A., & Kluger, M. J. (1993). Experimental cachexia: Effects of MCA sarcoma in the Fischer rat. *American Journal of Physiology, 265,* R376-R384.

Smith, B.K. & Kluger, M.J. (1992). Human IL-1 receptor antagonist partially suppresses LPS fever but not plasma levels of IL-6 in Fischer rats. *American Journal of Physiology, 263,* R653-R655.

Smith, B. K., & Kluger, M. J. (1993). Anti-TNF-alpha antibodies normalized body temperature and enhanced food intake in tumor-bearing rats. *American Journal of Physiology, 265,* R615-R619.

Syrjala, K. L., Donaldson, G. W., Davis, M. W., Kippes, M. E., & Carr, J. E. (1995). Relaxation and imagery and cognitive-behavioral training reduce pain during cancer treatment: A controlled clinical trial. *Pain, 63,* 189-198.

Tavorath, R., & Hesketh, P. J. (1996). Drug treatment of chemotherapy-induced delayed emesis. *Drugs, 52,* 639-648.

Tomoyasu, N., Bovberg, D. H., & Jacobsen, P. B. (1996). Conditioned reactions to cancer chemotherapy: Percent reinforcement predicts anticipatory nausea. *Physiology and Behavior, 59,* 273-276.

Troesch, L. M., Rodehaver, C. B., Delaney, E. A., & Yanes, B. (1993). The influence of guided imagery on chemotherapy-related nausea and vomiting. *Oncology Nursing Forum, 20,* 1179-1185.

Vasterling, J., Jenkins, R. A., Tope, D. M., & Burish, T. G. (1992). Cognitive distraction and relaxation training for the control of side effects due to cancer chemotherapy. *Journal of Behavioral Medicine, 16*(1), 65-80.

Walsh, J. W., Hasler, W. L., Nugent, C. E., & Owyang, C. (1996). Progesterone and estrogen are potential mediators of gastric slow-wave dysrhythmias in nausea of pregnancy. *American Journal of Physiology, 270,* G506-G514.

Zeltzer, L. K., Dolgin, M. J., LeBaron, S., & LeBaron, C. (1991). A randomized, controlled study of behavioral intervention for chemotherapy distress in children with cancer. *Pediatrics, 88,* 34-42.

Zhang, J., & Cai, W. W. (1991). Severe vomiting during pregnancy: Antenatal correlates and fetal outcomes. *Epidemiology, 2,* 454-457.

24

MANAGING SLEEP AND WAKING BEHAVIORS AND THE SYMPTOM OF FATIGUE

Joan L. F. Shaver

Overview

Sleep is a periodic behavior that oscillates with periods of waking on a daily basis. Its quality and timing can affect health and wellness in ways that are only beginning to be revealed through research. Fatigue is a symptom that can be indicative of poor sleep/wake patterns, manifested in concert with recognized disease or illness, or it can occur for unexplained reasons. Each phenomenon represents an area ripe for the development of biobehavioral science with central relevance to the practice of nursing. Biobehavioral science incorporates the attempt to understand (on the whole human level) how mental (psychological, cognitive, emotional, affective) elements

435

interact with bodily (physicochemical) elements to drive behaviors and how behaviors of human interaction with the environment influence mental and physical function. Within this chapter, nursing research related to each of these phenomena is reviewed first according to design, populations studied, measures used, and theoretical or conceptual perspectives. Secondly, summative comments regarding the state of the science emanating from individual studies of sleep and fatigue are made. Finally, some recommendations are posited for advancing nursing science regarding sleep/wake behaviors and the symptom of fatigue.

A literature search of the CINAHL index was done, and articles from 1980 to the present were reviewed. A search was also done of the major authors in the field who are known to the author, as well as members of a nurse sleep-interest group, to locate publications of nurse investigators reporting their work in interdisciplinary journals. Because work is published across many types of journals, the review is not necessarily completely exhaustive. The majority of articles included are databased; a few review articles are cited. There were 61 articles in which *sleep* was the major focus of the study and 44 articles in which the focus was *fatigue*.

Sleep and Waking Behaviors

Only within the past three to four decades has sleep emerged as a phenomenon of study for its relationship to health. The study of sleep is a highly trans- and interdisciplinary science. Biological scientists seek to understand the molecular biological, genetic, and physicochemical regulation of sleep/wake behavior. Behavioral scientists seek to understand the function of sleep and its effects on waking behaviors and function and the normative patterns of sleep across age groups or across animal species. The close association of sleep disturbance with affective disorder has spawned the scientific interest of those in mental health, particularly psychiatry. The association of functional disturbances during sleep, such as sleep apnea (cessation of breathing during sleep), provokes study by scientists affiliated with respiratory health. Abnormal behaviors in concert with sleep, such as gross muscle movements or abnormal patterns of sleep like narcolepsy, spark the interest of those who seek to diagnose and treat neurological dysfunction. Inadequate or disrupted sleep is commonly a concomitant

of major stressful life conditions, including disease and illness, and thereby draws the interest of nursing scientists. Nursing scientists seek to understand those dimensions most relevant to their practice, especially how sleep (more precisely sleeplessness) or daytime sleepiness affect health and what contributes to sleeplessness, good sleep, and daytime alertness. This particularly includes how sleep is affected by environments (e.g., critical care units or longer-term care centers) and by life contexts (e.g., with enduring pain, injury, diseases, or major transitions).

Sleep and waking behaviors oscillate relative to one another, generally on a regular basis within 24 hours, with sleep taking up one quarter to one third of each day or night (i.e., 6 to 8 hours) for most people. During sleep, a consistent pattern of physiological state changes occurs, in the face of relative unconsciousness. Physically, sleep is seen as a series of predictable cycles through non-rapid eye movement (NREM) and rapid eye movement (REM) sleep stages. Normally, sleep is entered through a transitional stage (stage 1), moves into a light stage (stage 2), with progressive descent into slow wave sleep (SWS) or deep sleep (stages 3 and 4). Deep sleep is followed by a period of REM sleep to complete one sleep cycle, taking about 60 to 90 minutes. Consequently, a night of sleep consists of 3 to 6 cycles of sleep, depending on sleep duration. The NREM/REM cycle is an ultradian characteristic described early in somnographic sleep work. Of note is that early sleep cycles contain proportionally more SWS than later cycles. Alternately, REM sleep shows a progressive increase from the first to the last third of the night, with the majority in the latter third of the night. Slow wave sleep is believed to be crucial to the body and brain restitution; REM sleep has been associated most often with emotional and mental functions.

Sleep as a behavior can be measured physiologically using technology and behaviorally by observation or by self-report. Physiological measurement includes somnography, wherein patterns of brainwaves are assessed using electroencephalogram (EEG), muscle tension is tracked by electromyogram (EMG), and eye movements are detected using electrooculogram (EOG). Specific conventions for scoring the somnogram are used by the clinical and scientific community to describe sleep according to stages, the series of predictable cycles through NREM and REM sleep stages. Somnography is considered the "gold standard" for assessing physical sleep patterns because it reveals the structure of sleep, but it is time consuming, expensive, and runs the risk of interfering with natural sleep because of added instrumentation. Activity monitors can be used to estimate overall sleep, but they do not reveal the structure of sleep, have inaccuracy to the extent that they detect quiet resting rather than sleeping, and are not suitable for certain types of subjects (e.g., those with tremors or who are paralyzed).

Behavioral observations of sleep do not reveal the structure of sleep and are tedious to perform, time consuming, and potentially inaccurate. Self-report methods can involve retrospective recall of specific or global impressions in the form of histories or concurrent reporting in the form of diaries or logs. Self-report methods are prone to subjects giving "desired" answers. Further, some people have a propensity to report negative impressions on almost any element of their lives about which they are asked that can skew self-reported responses. Experience has shown that recall modalities frequently generate a higher prevalence of problems than concurrent measures. It is a well-known observation that what people report about the quality of their sleep and what is documented through somnography do not always match. This is not to imply that either self-report or somnography is more "correct" or accurate. Rather, data must be interpreted with the limitations of each method in mind, and measures of both types might best reveal the science to underlie our assessments and treatments.

Sleep and Waking Behaviors: Science in Nursing

Sixty-one articles were reviewed for this topic and are summarized in Table 24.1. Three methods, one meta-analysis, and six review-type papers were included in the table. Articles appeared in *Journal of Community Health, Research in Nursing and Health, Journal of Advanced Nursing, Journal of Clinical Nursing, Progress in Cardiovascular Nursing, Oncology Nursing Forum, Journal of Pediatric Nursing, Journal of Perinatal and Neonatal Nursing, Sleep, Clinical Nursing Research, Heart-Lung, Science, Applied Nursing Research, Journal of Neuroscience Nursing, Family Practice Research Journal, Nursing Research,* and *Advances in Nursing Science,* among others. The implication is that no preferred journal exists for reporting nursing research issues in this domain, making it a challenge to track and summarize the development of nursing-related science in this area.

With respect to design types, 38 of the 51 databased articles (60.7%) displayed descriptive, often correla-

tional designs. Thirty-one studies (50.8%) involved single group design; in 7 studies, comparisons to control groups were done; in 4 of those, subjects were compared at two or more time points. Thirteen reports (21.3%) represented tests of interventions. Of these, 9 reports represented an intersubject design whereby subjects were assigned to a test or control group; 4 involved an intrasubject design whereby subjects were tested prior to and after an intervention with no control groups.

With respect to populations and methods for the 51 databased articles, 38 (74.5%) were reports using adults as subjects, and 4 of these were of older adults or seniors. Seven reports were of subjects in childhood or adolescence, and 4 were reports that used infants as the target population. Twenty-three (45%) of the databased articles were focused on subjects with disorders or illness, including 7 studies of postcardiac surgery, mostly coronary artery bypass grafting (CABG), one exclusively with women. Others were single studies of renal dialysis patients, postabdominal surgery, hospitalized patients with tumors, older women with Parkinson's disease, and people with HIV. Four reports were of women examined under mock intensive care conditions, 2 of women with inflammatory conditions or chronic fatigue conditions, and 5 of individuals with narcolepsy. Overall, 22 of the 51 reports (43.1%) addressed exclusively women subjects. In 8 of the studies, pregnant or postpartum women were the subjects; 4 were about midlife women; 1 was about menstruating women; 1 was of nurses; and the remaining 8 were about women with disorders or illness.

The measures varied significantly across studies. Of the 13 infant and children/adolescent studies, most used observation to detect behaviors of and associated with sleep ($n = 8$), 2 used self-report by adolescents, 2 used self-report by parents, and 1 used somnography. Of the 4 studies with older adults, 2 involved solely self-report, 1 incorporated self-report with wrist actigraphy, and only 1 involved somnography. Within the studies of adults not specifically older in age, 29 incorporated solely self-reported measures, and 7 incorporated somnography, albeit by four investigators; 2 reported on sleep using wrist actigraphy. Consequently, it is evident that in nearly three quarters of the studies, self-report was used to assess quality of sleep (i.e., from the subjects' perspective).

There is evidence from the studies reviewed that a few investigators have developed a focused research program in this area. Multiple reports were evident for Becker et al. (Becker, Chang, Kameshima, & Bloch, 1991; Becker, Grunwald, Motorman, & Stuhr, 1993; Becker & Thoman, 1981), who studied low birth weight infants and

(text continued on page 442)

TABLE 24.1.   Summary of Sleep Studies in Nursing Science

Authors	Journal	Subjects	Sleep Measures	Results	Study Type
1. Campbell	Midwifery, 1986	Adults, 9 primiparas postpartum, in homes	Nursing child assessment sleep activity record, 2 to 4 postpartum weeks	Sleep duration same as prior, interrupted often, reported feeling less rested and more tired	Correlative/ descriptive
2. Clark et al.	Journal of Advanced Nursing, 1995	Adults, 23 midlife women, 40-55 years old, home	7-day sleep diary	13/23 reported sleep disturbance	Correlative/ descriptive
3. Closs	Journal of Clinical Nursing, 1992	Adults, 100 patients postabdominal surgery, hospital	Interview questionnaire	Pain disturbed sleep, 1/2 had worse pain during sleep, believed sleep helped	Correlative/ descriptive
4. Cohen et al.	Holistic Nursing Practice, 1996	Adults, 50 HIV/AIDS subjects	Questionnaire	Variety of sleep problems unrelated to HIV status	Correlative/ descriptive
5. Cohen, Nehring, and Cloninger	Holistic Nursing Practice, 1996	Adults, narcolepsy	Questionnaire	High use of nonpharmacological symptom management	
6. Dowling	Journal of Neuroscience Nursing, 1995	Adults, 21 older women with PD and 21 controls, home	Stanford Sleepiness Scale, nighttime sleep questions	PD women = more day sleepiness, less at night, poorer mood, more affected	
7. Evans and Rogers	Applied Nursing Research, 1994	Adults, 14 seniors, home	Wrist actigraphy × 48 hrs.	Spent 7.5 hrs. in bed, slept 6.0, napped × 1 hr.	Correlative/ descriptive
8. Evans et al.	Clinical Nursing Research, 1995	Adults, 99 pregnant women, home and hospital	Visual Analogue Scale of sleep in a.m.	High sleep disturbance, no relationship between sleep perceptions and labor and delivery	Correlative/ descriptive
9. Knapp- Spooner and Yarcheski	Heart and Lung, 1992	Adults, 24 post-CABG, preadmission and 3rd and 6th post-op a.m., hosp.	VSH sleep scale	Difference in sleep variables over time	Correlative/ descriptive
10. Lee	Sleep, 1992	Adults, 760 RNS, 22 to 64 years old, at work	Health survey		Correlative/ descriptive
11. Lee and DeJoseph	Birth, 1992	Adults, 25 pregnant women, 29 postpartum, home	Questionnaire	Pregnant: Difficulty initiating and maintaining sleep; postpartum B: Difficulty maintaining sleep	Correlative/ descriptive, comparative pre- to postpartum
12. Lee et al.	Sleep, 1990	Adults, 18-year-old menstruating women, laboratory	Somnography	Luteal: Shorter REM latency, if negative affect processes; less deep sleep in both phases	Correlative/ descriptive, comparative menstrual
13. Lentz and Killien	Journal of Perinatal and Neonatal Nursing, 1991	Adults, 34 postpartum women, hospital	Sleep observation, Q 15 min. X 8 hrs.	Few sleep opportunities; awake 1/2 of observations	Correlative/ descriptive
14. Mead- Bennett	Journal of Obstetric, Gynecologic and Neonatal Nursing, 1990	Adults, 28 primigravidae, home	Questionnaire	Increased 3rd trimester sleep, intrapartal sleep loss, no sleep loss, and mood relationship	Correlative/ descriptive, comparative — trimesters

TABLE 24.1. *Continued*

Authors	Journal	Subjects	Sleep Measures	Results	Study Type
15. Parker	*American Nephrology Nurses Association Journal,* 1996	Adults, 8 on hemodialysis, 8 peritoneal, 8 control outpatients	Sleep quality inventory, interviews re: dreams, post-REM wakening	Both dialysis groups = poor sleep quality, no difference in dream content	Correlative/ descriptive, controls
16. Redeker, Mason, Wykpisz, and Glica	*Applied Nursing Research,* 1996	Adults, 22 women post-CABG, hospital and home	Actigraphy, sleep-rest subscale of Sickness Impact Profile	Initial sleep disturbances normalize over time	Correlative/ descriptive
17. Rodgers and Aldrich	*Nursing Research,* 1993	Adults, 16 narcoleptics, home and laboratory	Logs: Frequency and timing of sleep attacks, naps, and night sleep	3 timed naps, SOL improved	Correlative/ descriptive
18. Rogers and Rosenberg	*Sleep,* 1990	Adults, 30 narcoleptic, 30 controls, laboratory	Memory tests	No deficits in memory but difficulty with attention	Correlative/ descriptive, controls
19. Rogers, Aldrich, and Caruso	*Sleep,* 1994	Adults, 25 narcoleptic, 25 controls, laboratory	Somnography	Shorter SOL, more disturbed sleep, more naps	Correlative/ descriptive, controls
20. Schaefer	*Journal of Obstetric, Gynecologic and Neonatal Nursing,* 1995	Adults, 63 women, 13 CFS, 50 FM, community	Fatigue and sleepiness	Strong relationship between fatigue and sleepiness	Correlative/ descriptive
21. Schaefer, Swavely, Rothenberger, Hess, and Williston	*Progressive Cardiovascular Nursing,* 1996	Adults, 49 post-CABG, home	Telephone interview, 1 week, 1 month, 3 months, 6 months	< ½ had sleep disturbance in 1st month due to incisional pain, positioning, and nocturia	Correlative/ descriptive
22. Schumacher, Merritt, and Cohen	*Journal of Neuroscience Nursing,* 1997	Adults, narcolepsy	Perceived symptoms	No association between CNS stimulant intake and ADL abilities	Correlative/ descriptive
23. Shaver and Paulsen	*Family Practice Research Journal,* 1993	Adults, 135 midlife women, laboratory and home	Somnography	⅓ reported poor sleep, menopausal status not related, poor sleep associated with more fatigue and musculoskeletal symptoms	Correlative/ descriptive, premeno- pausal women used as controls
24. Shaver, Giblin, Lentz, and Lee	*Sleep,* 1988	Adults, 76 pre-, peri-, and postmenopausal women, laboratory	Somnography	Decreased sleep efficiency associated with hot flashes	Correlative/ descriptive, premeno- pausal women used as controls
25. Shaver, Giblin, and Paulsen	*Sleep,* 1991	Adults, 82 midlife women classed as poor or good sleepers, laboratory and home	Somnography of poor sleepers by self-report	12 (15%) showed no physiological sleep disturbance, 7 (8.5%) did	Correlative/ descriptive, good sleepers as controls
26. Sheely	*Oncology Nursing Forum,* 1996	Adults, 50 hospitalized patients, 58% women, hospital	VSH sleep scale, observation (nocturnal disturbances)	Positive correlation between environmental disturbances and sleep quality	Correlative/ descriptive

(continued)

TABLE 24.1. *Continued*

Authors	Journal	Subjects	Sleep Measures	Results	Study Type
27. Simpson and Lee	*American Journal of Critical Care,* 1996	Adults, 102 postcardiac surgery, hospital	Questionnaire	Slept fewer hours in hospital than at home, no difference in perceived sleep before or after	Correlative/descriptive
28. Simpson, Lee, and Cameron	*Research in Nursing and Health,* 1996	Adults, 97 hospitalized patients (cardiac surgery), 75 men, 22 women, hospital	VSH sleep scale, Factors Influencing Sleep Questionnaire	Perceived brief sleep, disturbed	Correlative/descriptive
29. Walker and Best	*Women and Health,* 1991	Adults, 148 mothers of infants, home	Questionnaire	Most frequently mentioned: Return-to-work conflicts, sleep and fatigue, lack of time	Correlative/descriptive
30. Waters and Lee	*Journal of Nurse-Midwifery,* 1996	Adults, 31 pre- and postpartum women, home	Sleep efficiency, fatigue	Primiparae had more disturbed sleep and fatigue than multiparae	Correlative/descriptive
31. Corser	*Issues in Comprehensive Pediatric Nursing,* 1996	12 infants and toddlers, PICU and home	Observation Questionnaire	Loss of sleep, REM sleep loss, sleep changes persisted postdischarge, recovered total sleep time faster than usual awakes	Correlative/descriptive
32. Lane and Fontaine	*Heart and Lung,* 1992	9 children, mean age 4.7 years, PICU	Observation (Echols tool) Q 5 minutes over night, sound and light meters	Slept 4.7 hours, 9.8 hours awake, sleep episode = 28 min., noise average = 55 decibels	Correlative/descriptive
33. White et al.	*Maternal-Child Nursing Journal,* 1988	40 children, 3 to 8 years old, hospital	Observation (SOL), distress, self-soothing behavior	Behaviors little related to family or environmental variables	Correlative/descriptive
34. Williams, White, Powell, Alexander, and Conlon	*Computers in Nursing,* 1988	40 children, 3 to 8 years old, hospital	Actigraphy and observation	Validated use of actigraph to determine sleep onset	Correlative/descriptive
35. Mahon	*Public Health Nursing,* 1995	106 age 12-to-14 years olds, 111 age 15- to-17 years olds, 113 age 18-to-21 years old, home	VSH sleep scale	Middle adolescents: sleep disturbance, sleep effectiveness, amount of sleep correlated with general health rating index	Correlative/descriptive
36. Yarcheski	*Journal of Pediatric Nursing,* 1994	116 each early, middle, and late adolescents, home	VSH sleep scale	Middle adolescents had most sleep disturbance, females had less sleep effectiveness, males slept more	Correlative/descriptive, compared ages and gender
37. Becker and Thoman	*Science,* 1981	15 newborns, weeks 2 to 5 and 3, 6, and 12 months, NICU	Somnography (REM activity)	REM storms inversely related to developmental status (Bayley)	Correlative/descriptive
38. Becker et al.	*Research in Nursing and Health,* 1991	23 adolescent and 23 adult mothers of newborns, 15 to 37 years old	Sleep patterns	Percentage sleep at night related to parenting stress	Correlative/descriptive

TABLE 24.1. *Continued*

Authors	Journal	Subjects	Sleep Measures	Results	Study Type
39. Johnson	*Journal of Community Health Nursing,* 1991a	176 seniors < 65 years old, home	Sleep pattern questionnaire (Baekland and Hay)	Relaxation improved state of mind, SOL, soundness of and satisfaction with sleep	Intervention, intra-individual muscle relaxation
40. Johnson	*Applied Nursing Research,* 1991b	55 women, 65 years old, laboratory	Somnography	Shorter SOL, fewer arousals, more SWS in first 3 hours	Intervention, intra-individual muscle relaxation
41. Topf and Davis	*Heart and Lung,* 1993	70 women, laboratory	Somnography (REM)	Noise conditioned poorer REM sleep	Intervention, inter-individual, posttest, control
42. Topf	*Behavioral Medicine,* 1992b	105 females, laboratory, conditioned noise with control, instructions, noise without instructions, and quiet	Physiological stress	No effect on stress	Intervention, inter-individual
43. Topf	*Research in Nursing and Health,* 1992a	Same as above, laboratory	Same	No sleep improvement	Intervention, inter-individual
44. Topf, Bookman, and Arand	*Journal of Advanced Nursing,* 1996	60 women randomly assigned to simulated CCU noise or not, laboratory	Self-rated subjective	Sleep noise: longer to fall asleep, less sleep time, awake more, poor quality compared to home	Intervention, inter-individual
45. Williamson	*American Journal of Critical Care,* 1992	Adults, 60 CABG patients, hospital	Richards-Campbell sleep questionnaire	Differences in sleep depth, awakes, quality, total sleep	Intervention, inter-individual, control group, ocean sounds
46. Zimmerman, Nieveen, Barnason, and Schmaderer	*Scholarly Inquiry for Nursing Practice,* 1996	Adults, 98 post-CABG, hospital	Richards-Campbell sleep questionnaire	Video group had better sleep scores 3rd a.m. than control	Intervention, inter-individual, music, audio and video
47. Kerr, Jowett, and Smith	*Journal of Advanced Nursing,* 1996	86 children test, 83 children control, 3 to 12 months old, home	Parent reporting	Smaller percentage of test group had sleep difficulties	Intervention, sleep education, inter-individual
48. White, Wear, and Stephenson-Gordon	*Research in Nursing and Health,* 1983	18 children, 3 to 8 years old, hospital	Observation and behavioral coding	Bedtime story more sleepy	Intervention, parent tape-recorded story, intra-individual

(continued)

TABLE 24.1. *Continued*

Authors	Journal	Subjects	Sleep Measures	Results	Study Type
49. White et al.	*Nursing Research,* 1990	94 children, 3 to 8 years old, hospital	Observation	Increased SOL and distress with parent-read story	Intervention, intra-individual, none, parent, or stranger story
50. Becker et al.	*Nursing Research,* 1993 (also reported 1991)	Infants < 1500 gms, 21 pre- and 24 post-NICU	Observation during 18 min–Q 30 seconds, 2 times per week	Postintervention more alert wake, higher O_2, fewer movements	Intervention, inter-individual, staff training to reduce stressors
51. Holditch-Davis et al.	*Journal of Obstetric, Gynecologic and Neonatal Nursing,* 1995	46 preterm infants, NICU	Observation of states: quiet awake, active, and sleep	At 3 weeks, infants had less quiet waking and longer sleep bouts	intervention, inter-individual, applied 4 standard rest periods
52. Rediehs, Reis, and Creason	*Sleep,* 1990	Adults, older	Meta-analysis, sleep in old age, 29 studies	Gender differences small to moderate	Meta-analysis
53. Floyd	*ANS,* 1993	84 healthy seniors		Methods comparison	Methods
54. Merritt, Keegan, and Mercer	*Nursing Research,* 1994	Adults, narcolepsy	Pupillometry	Managing artifacts	Methods
55. Rogers et al.	*Nursing Research,* 1993	Adults, narcolepsy, laboratory	Somnography	.87 kappa agreement, high sensitivity, and specificity	Methods
56. Jensen	*Nursing Clinics of North America,* 1993	General			Review
57. Kedas, Lux, and Amodeo	*Western Journal of Nursing Research,* 1989	Adults, older			Review
58. Spenceley	*Image,* 1993	Adults, critically ill			Review
59. Wood	*Critical Care Nursing,* 1993	Adults, critically ill			Review
60. Glod	*Archives of Psychiatric Nursing,* 1992	Children			Review
61. Kerr and Jowett	*Journal of Advanced Nursing,* 1996	Children			Review

NOTE: ADL = activities of daily living; NICU = neonatal intensive care unit; PD = Parkinson's disease; PICU = pediatric intensive care unit; SOL = sleep onset latency; SWS = slowwave sleep; VSH = Verran-Snyder-Halpern.

manipulated the environment to reduce stressors; White et al. (White, Powell-Gail, Alexander, Williams-Phoebe, et al., 1988; White, Wear, & Stephenson-Gordon, 1983; White, Williams, Alexander, Powell-Cope, & Conlon, 1990), who looked at hospitalized young children and manipulated the environment; Topf (1992a, 1992b, 1993), who has simulated ICU noise to relate to stress

and tested sound modulation interventions for improving sleep; Lee et al. (Lee, 1992; Lee & DeJoseph, 1992; Lee, Hicks, & Nino-Murcia, 1991; Lee, Shaver, Giblin, & Woods, 1990), who looked at sleep in women during the menstrual cycle, in pregnancy and postpartum, and in nurses working shifts; Rogers et al. (Rogers & Aldrich, 1993; Rogers, Aldrich, & Caruso, 1994; Rogers, Caruso,

& Aldrich, 1993; Rogers & Rosenberg, 1990), with a program of research investigating subjects with narcolepsy; and Shaver et al. (Shaver, Giblin, Lentz, & Lee, 1988; Shaver, Giblin, & Paulsen, 1991; Shaver & Paulsen, 1993), who have focused on midlife women and, particularly, insomnia.

Besides these program studies, 13 studies involved assessment of sleep in conjunction with health threats: for example, postabdominal surgery (Closs, 1992); after cardiac surgery, especially CABG (Knapp-Spooner & Yarcheski, 1992; Redeker, Mason, Wykpisz, & Glica, 1996; Schaefer, Swavely, Rothenberger, Hess, & Williston, 1996; Simpson & Lee, 1996; Simpson, Lee, & Cameron, 1996; Williamson, 1992; Zimmerman, Nieveen, Barnason, & Schmaderer, 1996); in renal dialysis groups (Parker, 1996); in women with chronic fatigue and fibromyalgia (Schaefer, 1995); with Parkinson's disease (Dowling, 1995); with cancer (Sheely, 1996); with narcolepsy (Cohen, Nehring, & Cloninger, 1996); with HIV (Cohen, Ferrans, Vizgirda, Kunkle, & Cloninger, 1996); and in hospitalized adults and children (Lane & Fontaine, 1992; Holditch-Davis, Barham, O'Hale, & Tucker, 1995). As well, Evans and Rogers (1994) and Floyd (1993) have published studies related to sleep in seniors, and Johnson (1991a, 1991b) has published regarding interventions to promote sleep in seniors. Sleep associated with pregnancy, mostly the postpartum phase, has been studied by several investigator groups (Campbell, 1986; Evans, Dick, & Clark, 1995; Lee & DeJoseph, 1992; Lentz & Killien, 1991; Mead-Bennett, 1990; Waters & Lee, 1996). Clark, Flowers, Boots, and Shettar (1995) reported on sleep in midlife women. Mahon (1995) and Yarcheski (1994) have reported on preteen and teenaged individuals and sleep.

Sleep and Waking: State of the Nursing Science

Within nursing science, few theoretical viewpoints about sleep, sleeplessness, or sleepiness have been tested. Clear conceptual perspectives are only beginning to emerge from the science attributable to nursing scientists. Overall, much work seems built on the premises that transitions for women such as menstrual cycle, pregnancy, menopause, or chronic illness affect sleep and that personal or individual stress affects sleep/wake behavior. The general notion that illness and disease interfere with

normal sleep/wake behavior is prominent, and the hospital environment constitutes, in and of itself, a stressful environment associated with disrupted sleep. Interventions fall in the realms of changing individuals within their environments or changing the environments. In the remainder of this section, reviews of some results associated with these features are summarized and other studies are noted in Table 24.1.

With regard to sleep in women during transitions and associated stress, Lee, Shaver, et al. (1990) reported that over the luteal phase, using two menstrual cycles, REM latency was shorter compared to the follicular phase. Women with negative affect premenstrually had less deep sleep during both menstrual cycles compared to asymptomatic women. The meaning of these results is not entirely clear. Shorter REM latency has been associated with dysphoria, depression in particular, and could represent brain biochemical changes that affect both REM sleep and mood. Such observations provoke the question of whether interventions to improve sleep would ameliorate menstrual-related symptoms or whether treatments for menstrual symptoms improve sleep.

Like sleep during the menstrual cycle, sleep during pregnancy has received only sparse study. Using self-report, women in the third trimester have been found to have problems initiating and maintaining sleep; women in the first month postpartum have problems maintaining sleep but not falling asleep (Lee & DeJoseph, 1992). Primipara women were found to experience more disturbed sleep and fatigue postpartum than multipara women (Waters & Lee, 1996). The authors suggest that these descriptive data could inform anticipatory guidance interventions for women who are dealing with pregnancy. In other studies of sleep and pregnancy, perceptions of sleep interruptions, tiredness, or impact of tiredness were not related to length of time in hospital for delivery (Carty, Bradley, & Winslow, 1996), an outcome probably due to inadequate variability in hospital stay duration to see a relationship. Furthermore, a relationship of perceptions of sleep quality related to length of labor was found lacking (Evans et al., 1995).

In midlife women, Shaver's group found that sleep, measured by somnography, was not tightly related to menopausal status, as corroborated using self-report data by Clark et al. (1995). However, lower sleep efficiency was associated with more hot flash activity (Shaver, Giblin, Lentz, et al., 1988). In looking at midlife women with insomnia (perceived poor or inadequate sleep quality) in relation to somnographic sleep, two patterns have been identified. Some women report insomnia without evidence of disturbed somnographic sleep. These women tend to score high on psychological distress and somatic symptoms but not on menopausal symptoms such as hot flashes or sweats. Other women report insomnia with evidence of poor somnographic sleep quality. This group of women tends to have high menopausal symptom activity but does not have high psychological distress or somatic symptom scores. Treatment options can be implied in light of these data. For example, women with perceived and somnographic disturbed sleep, hot flashes, and low psychological distress might incur benefits from treatment for hot flashes in combination with sleep hygiene or sleep-enhancement strategies. Women with perceived but not somnographic poor sleep accompanied by high psychological distress and few hormonally modulated symptoms such as hot flashes might benefit from education about sleep as a behavior and learning strategies to cope with excess distress or possible changing of life events (Shaver & Paulsen, 1993).

Sleep disturbances are a relatively ubiquitous feature of many chronic conditions, although in-depth studies of sleep in particular conditions remain to be done, and only highlights of findings are presented here. For example, in single studies in the home environment, women with fibromyalgia and chronic fatigue syndrome mentioned "trouble staying asleep" as the most frequently rated sleep problem, and "fatigue" as the most commonly reported symptom (Schaefer, 1995). More than half of patients post-CABG reported sleep disturbances at 1 week, 1 month, 3 months, and 6 months following and attributed sleep problems to incisional pain, inability to assume comfortable positions, and nocturia (Schaefer, Swavely, et al., 1996). Patients on hemodialysis or continuous ambulatory peritoneal dialysis report poor sleep compared to those with no illness (Parker, 1996).

One would expect that people with various neurological disregulations might have difficulties with sleep, yet study from a nursing perspective is meager. In general, nurse researchers typically document the nature of the sleep pattern perceptions and incorporate investigation of the impact of the disease or illness on sleep patterns by identifying associated mental or somatic functionality changes. As examples, Dowling (1995) has reported that women with Parkinson's disease were sleepier than controls during the day and less sleepy at night, had more dysphoria consistent with borderline depression, and were more impaired in carrying out activities of daily living. In comparing people with narcolepsy to controls using home somnography, Rogers, Aldrich, and Caruso (1994) found that those with narcolepsy had

more disturbed nocturnal sleep and averaged significantly more daytime sleep than controls. Earlier, Rogers's group had reported that people with narcolepsy had more difficulty in maintaining attention but no striking memory deficits as compared to those without narcolepsy matched for age and gender (Rogers & Rosenberg, 1990).

To date, most studies of chronic illness and disease are descriptive mainly to the point of documenting sleep as a problem. Most investigators have used self-report measures of sleep, but few have used somnographic measures. It is difficult to determine whether physical sleep changes might be (a) a consequence of the disease or illness' biochemical or physiological fundamental mechanisms, (b) an outcome of associated physical sensations and discomfort, or (c) concomitant with psychosocial adjustments to illness or disease or part of "suffering"—that is, cognitive-emotional coping dimension of illness and disease or combinations thereof.

Having or potentially having an illness or disease and also being hospitalized for diagnosis or treatment are likely to compound stress activation in individuals and certainly affect usual sleep patterns. Overall in this context, it is difficult to separate out factors contributing to sleep disruptions that are due to the illness from those due to the environment. In a study of patients immediately following CABG, analyses indicated that hospital and illness-related stress, duration of cardiopulmonary bypass, anesthesia time, and sleep medication were related to patients' sleep disturbance, effectiveness, or supplementation in different ways and at different times during the study periods (Knapp-Spooner & Yarcheski, 1992). Other studies of CABG patients have revealed that sleep problems occur beyond intensive care (Simpson et al., 1996) but improve with time through 24 weeks (Redeker et al., 1996). Music as an intervention for this population needs further testing (Zimmerman et al., 1996).

Several studies of the intensive care environment have been done and have invariably indicated that time available for sleep is inadequate to complete sleep cycles and that noise and care-related interruptions mainly contribute to disturbed sleep patterns. In a pediatric intensive care environment, children were found to sleep a mean of 4.69 hours ($SD = 0.49$) in 24 hours, with 9.8 awakenings ($SD = 2.48$) and an average sleep episode lasting only 27.6 minutes ($SD = 25.85$). This indicates highly fragmented sleep, as a full sleep cycle takes 60 to 90 minutes. The mean noise level was 55 decibels. Time series multiple regression indicated that noise ($p = .001$), light ($p = .05$), and caregiver contact ($p = .001$) were significantly related to sleep state (Lane & Fontaine, 1992).

Manipulation of the environment to improve sleep and stress in adults has been reported by Topf (1992a, 1992b), using a simulated hospital critical care environment and healthy subjects. Subjects were randomly assigned to instructions for personal control over the noise (a sound conditioner to block unwanted sounds), no such instruction, or a quiet condition. Measures of stress perceptions and stress hormones, as well as sleep perceptions and somnography, were done. Results indicated a positive relationship of noise to perceived stress but not stress hormones, and the intervention failed to affect either perceived stress or stress hormones or somnographic or perceived sleep quality.

Manipulation of the environment is a logical sleep improvement intervention, tested some in infants and children. For example, White's group tested an intervention of bedtime story-telling, comparing a live parent, parent-recorded, stranger-recorded, and no story situation in hospitalized children 3 to 8 years old for effects on sleep onset latency, self-soothing behaviors, and incidence of distress. They found that the longest sleep onset latency and highest prevalence of distress behaviors occurred in the children hearing a parent-recorded story. The story read by the parent present was associated with longer sleep onset latencies than the no story or stranger story group. Self-soothing behaviors were not affected by the story situation.

Recommendations for Advancing Nursing Science Regarding Sleep and Waking

Sleep quality is inextricably linked to mood and mental and physical function and is thereby a biobehavioral phenomenon that can be assessed using physical, perceptual, or behavioral measures. Perceptually, individuals can describe their sleep according to length and quality, but somnographic features do not necessarily match with perceptions. In the main, nursing scientists have used descriptive methodology and self-report measures to document sleep disturbances within groups of people undergoing significant transitions, with specific diseases and illness, and within the context of hospitalization. Movement of scientific discovery beyond description is warranted to the testing of interventions

and effects on outcomes. This necessitates the use of experimental and quasiexperimental designs. Emerging knowledge from descriptive studies done across many disciplines can form the basis for intervention testing.

Sleep in relation to waking is distinctly a rhythmic phenomenon. In the American or Canadian culture, most people maintain a sustained period of wakefulness (approximately 16 hours), mostly during the light hours of the day, and sleep for a single period during the dark hours. This is likely a pattern driven by social pressures because when humans have been assessed for sleepiness over the day/night, a bimodal distribution of sleepiness is evident. A pinnacle of sleepiness is reached at night but also in the early afternoon, implying a natural pattern for sleep to occur twice in 24 hours. The bimodal rhythm for sleep tendency is seen across age groups, and daytime sleep is likely to emerge in older adults not subject to the dynamics of work life.

Studies of extended sleep and naps at various times of the day indicate a pressure for SWS to emerge in the afternoon. Afternoon naps, compared with morning or evening naps, contain higher amounts of SWS, and the probability of REM sleep is high in morning naps. Furthermore, there is a period in the early evening of an inability to fall asleep that has been referred to as the *wake maintenance* zone. From these observations, the natural tendency to have bimodal sleep is obvious. The relative dominance of SWS and REM sleep depending on time of day for naps is suggestive that timed naps should be tested for therapeutic outcomes in certain contexts, such as those when nighttime sleep is marginal or inadequate (e.g., older adults with Parkinson's disease, Alzheimer's disease, or painful arthritis conditions).

It is now evident from studies in time-cue free environments that there is an endogenous circadian rhythm of biological functions as measured by the body temperature (BT) with a period of 24.5 to 25 hours. Subjective alertness or sleep tendency and performance on tests (minus memory testing) tend to cycle in concert with the BT rhythm, and BT is believed to be the major determinant of the timing of sleep onset or duration. The BT falls about 1.0 to 1.5 hours before bedtime and begins its ascent 0.5 to 2.0 hours prior to waking. A morning increase in BT is earlier in time for people who are designated "larks" and perform best in the morning, and the increase is later in people designated "owls" and who function best late in the day. Disturbed sleep is concomitant with disturbed endogenous BT rhythms. Consequently, interventions to alter the timing of the temperature rhythm, for example, using light or warming (passively with the application of heat or cold or actively using exercise), warrant testing in appropriate contexts. Where one tries to sleep on the BT curve is important (on the falling phase improves probability of sleep), so matching opportunities for sleep with the BT rhythm is an important therapeutic considerations. Another factor regulating sleep tendency is the duration of prior wakefulness. It is believed that some hypnogogic factor(s) accumulate(s) during wakefulness to a threshold inducing sleep and dissipates over the course of sleep. Amount of prior wakefulness can be manipulated to improve sleep.

A common concept that transcends the contexts of life transitions, illness, and hospitalization is that of *stress.* It is clear from many studies that exposure to catastrophic and major challenging events (i.e., experiencing high life strain) is associated with perceived sleeplessness or poor sleep. A strong link between emotional distress and sleep has been implicated in studies of both non- and psychiatric cases, particularly depressed and anxious individuals. Of note is that continuing insomnia has been linked to high rates of new cases of major depression and anxiety. If valid, at issue is whether sleep disturbance is a precursor to depression and treatment for poor sleep will prevent progression or development of depression or whether sleep is a manifestation of depression and treatment for depression is necessary to improve sleep.

Poor sleep, termed *insomnia,* has been conceptualized as a *tension-anxiety disorder.* It can be temporary, but some individuals exhibit enduring manifestations. Classically, insomnia is believed to represent overactive arousal as seen in both mental and emotional excitement and muscle tension. Developing personal control over the stress activation state using stress management techniques is a potential intervention mode for improving sleep or reducing sleeplessness. A number of behavioral treatments are based on learning to dampen cognitive and physiological activation (e.g., learning deep relaxation and thought-stopping techniques).

Besides personal factors, environmental features or contexts influence sleep. A belief about factors contributing to insomnia includes the tendency on the part of some individuals to be conditioned not to sleep in their bed due to engaging in opposing behaviors. Therefore, learning to control stimuli associated with going to sleep is the root of some behavioral therapies to improve sleep (e.g., *stimulus control*). As previously mentioned, it is clear from the majority of studies in hospitals that the environment is not conducive to sleep and that environmental manipulation is warranted in the direction of reducing excess noise, excess light, and unnecessary inter-

actions. Caregiving procedures can be grouped to allow time for naps (sleep cycle completion) and the timing of naps studied for effects on mood, mental processing, and physical recovery.

It is most likely that a constellation of factors contributes to sleep disturbance. Therefore, interventions are likely to be more powerful if they combine features of manipulating both person and environment elements. Few studies of environmental manipulation that also incorporate sleep-promoting elements have been done for adults. In addition, much literature exists revealing that the anxiety and uncertainty of having a major illness and poor symptom management, especially pain control, are factors altering usual sleep/wake patterns. Strategies to better manage symptoms and the emotional activation that constitutes stress should be tested in combination with manipulations that reduce the impact of environmental features.

In summary, the repertoire of studies in sleep science done by nursing scientists is addressed to understanding sleep related to health and illness, thus supporting a central focus for nursing practice. It is imperative to the development of nursing sleep science that more sustained study be done on vulnerable populations, specifically, those who are acutely ill, chronically ill, suffering from sleep disorders for which behavioral treatments are prominent (e.g., insomnia, narcolepsy), and in high-risk environments (e.g., hospitals, high stress factors). Within these populations and environments, sustained intervention studies are needed that combine personal behavioral modifications based on relevant and likely contributing factors and environmental stimulus control features. Such studies should incorporate methods to reveal dose response elements, titration, timing, individualized responses, and the factors affecting behavioral choice and adherence. Furthermore, the application of biobehavioral methods that involve combined physiological and perceptual measures to determine the effects of such interventions will do much to develop our future knowledge of sleep and its role in alleviating symptoms, preventing illness and disease, and promoting health.

Fatigue as a Symptom

Fatigue is an ill-defined and used term. In the main, it has been used in terms of whole human beings to refer to the sensations experienced and behaviors noted after enduring physical and mental challenges or after sleep deprivation and as a symptom accompanying many illness or disease states and with certain therapies. Apart from a whole human being attribute, fatigue has been used to describe physical systems and subsystems. One example is in reference to the inability of muscles to generate force through contractile mechanisms after intense use. The fatigue of biological systems or subsystems is of lesser importance to this discussion because the majority of nursing investigators have focused on applied clinical science rather than basic biological science.

Considering fatigue as a biobehavioral phenomenon or symptom makes its definition complex. It might be considered to be a symptom like *pain,* with a sensory component; that is, one experiences a sensation of fatigue. However, the sensation of fatigue has less of a discriminatory component than the sensation of pain. Fatigue is more likely to be a generalized sensation rather than being regionally or specifically located. Like pain, fatigue might also be considered to have a cognitive/emotional/motivational component. Fatigue often covaries with depressed mood and suppressed vitality. Like insomnia, fatigue can be viewed as acute (short term or temporary) or chronic (long term or sustained). Connotatively, fatigue is linked with feelings of lessened energy and inability to perform both mental and physical activities. It is difficult to distinguish from *tiredness.* Tiredness might be used to describe a state of depleted energy that is subject to recovery following rest, but fatigue may or may not be associated with clear excess energy expenditure and recovery. Fatigue can be classed according to context or main contributory factors and, as such, have descriptor labels such as *pathological, situational, psychologically based, physiological, exertional,* or *pain related.*

Presently, there is little consensus on how fatigue should be viewed within health and nursing science, but various definitions of the fatigue associated with illness, and particularly chronic illness, have been advanced. Piper (1986) defined fatigue as the perception of a complex interplay of both somatic and psychological factors. Belza (1990) specified fatigue as a subjective sensation of generalized tiredness or exhaustion. The North American Nursing Diagnosis Association (NANDA) definition of fatigue is "an overwhelming sustained sense of exhaustion and decreased capacity for physical and mental work" (NANDA, 1996). It is clear that the fatigue is manifested in noticeable physical and mental negative impact and consequential suffering. It accompanies many illness conditions and deserves much more study than it has heretofore received.

Fatigue as a Symptom: Science in Nursing

Fifty articles were reviewed for this topic and are summarized in Table 24.2. Seventeen review-type or concept papers were included in the table, and two reports by the same pair of authors seemed so alike that they were considered one report, leaving 32 data-based articles (three of these were methods papers). Articles appeared in *Applied Nursing Research, Research in Nursing and Health, Journal of Advances in Nursing, Oncology Nursing Forum, Cancer Nursing, Heart and Lung, Nursing Research, Advances in Nursing Science,* and *Arthritis Care Research,* among others. As with the nursing science of sleep, it is a challenge to track and summarize the development of nursing science regarding fatigue. It should be noted that fatigue as a concept is often a major dimension in studies beyond the ones reviewed here. Particular examples include studies of quality of life, general symptoms, and what predicts functionality and self-care in various types of chronic illness.

With respect to design types, of the 32 data-based articles (minus the 3 methods papers), all exhibited a descriptive design except one study, which was an intervention study. Twenty-five studies incorporated quantitative methods, three used a qualitative methodology, and one had both qualitative and quantitative measures. All involved a single group design except for four studies in which healthy controls were used.

With respect to populations and methods, all of the studies had samples of adults, with about 38% ($n = 12$) having exclusively women subjects. These included pregnant or postpartum women ($n = 5$ studies), healthy women ($n = 2$ studies) or women with illness, mostly cancer ($n = 5$ studies). Twenty-four studies were focused on subjects with disorders or illness, including 12 papers about people with cancer, 4 dealing with rheumatoid arthritis, 2 studies of heart disability, 1 dealing with chronic renal disease (2 reports), and 1 each dealing with HIV, multiple sclerosis, and sleep disturbance.

Like measuring sleep quality, the measures for fatigue varied significantly across studies. As with most symptom phenomena, the measurement of fatigue is based on self-report and consists of assessing descriptors of sensations, coexisting symptoms, extent of bothersomeness (suffering), and impact on quality of life, including effects on activities of daily living and ability to fulfill role functions. Two instruments originally developed for workplace fatigue studies are Yoshitake's Fa-

(text continues on page 451)

TABLE 24.2.   Summary of Fatigue Studies in Nursing Science

Authors	Journal	Subjects	Sleep Measures	Results	Study Type
1. Belza et al.	*Nursing Research,* 1993	Adults, RA	Fatigue Scale	Fatigue model: Variance explained by pain rating, functional status, sleep quality; in females, cormorbidities and disease duration	Correlative/ descriptive
2. Tack	*Arthritis Care Research,* 1990a	Adults, 20 patients, RA	Fatigue interview schedule	Descriptors, conditions, and self-management	Correlative/ descriptive, qualitative
3. Tack	*Arthritis Care Research,* 1990b	Adults, 20 patients, RA	POMS, fatigue and pain VAS, assessment	Fatigue associated with depression, pain, and poor mood, 3 measures congruent	Correlative/ descriptive
4. Blesch et al.	*Oncology Nursing Forum,* 1991	Adults, 77 with lung or breast cancer	Rhoten Fatigue Scale, checklist	Correlates of fatigue: pain and POMS scores	Correlative/ descriptive
5. Brunier and Graydon	*American Nephrology Nurses Association Journal,* 1992	Adults, 43 patients with end stage renal disease	POMS, VAS, hematocrit, nonspecific Sx and physical activity	Low physical activity and frequent Sx related to more fatigue	Correlative/ descriptive
6. Brunier and Graydon	*American Nephrology Nurses Association Journal,* 1993	Adults, 43 patients with end stage renal disease	POMS, VAS, hematocrit, nonspecific Sx and physical activity	Low physical activity and frequency of symptoms related to fatigue	Correlative/ descriptive
7. Carty, Bradley, and Winslow	*Clinical Nursing Research,* 1996	Adults, postpartum women whose hospital stay = 3 or < 3 days	Rest and activity questionnaire	Few differences in fatigue and sleep, depending on stay	Correlative/ descriptive
8. Cimprich	*Research in Nursing and Health,* 1992	Adults, 32 women who had surgery for breast cancer, Stage I or II	Attentional scores	Manifested attention deficits	Correlative/ descriptive
9. Crosby	*Journal of Advanced Nursing,* 1991	Adults, 100 people with RA, 15 RA (5 in flare), 12 controls	Factors contributing to fatigue	Factors: disease activity, poor sleep, physical effort, fatigue negatively correlated to pain (McGill), somnography, walking time, grip strength	Correlative/ descriptive
10. Dean et al.	*Cancer Practice,* 1995	Adults, 30 with melanoma	Piper Fatigue Scale, Symptom Distress Scale	Most extreme scores in affective domain	Correlative/ descriptive
11. Friedman and King	*Heart and Lung,* 1995	Adults, 80 women postheart failure, hospital	Interview	Fatigue most common symptom	Correlative/ descriptive
12. Gardner	*Applied Nursing Research,* 1991	Adults, 35 postpartum women	Survey	Mildly fatigued: situational/psychological	Correlative/ descriptive
13. Glaus, Crow, and Hammond	*European Journal of Cancer Care,* 1996	Adults, 20 cancer, 20 healthy	Grounded theory		Correlative/ descriptive, qualitative
14. Graydon et al.	*Cancer Nursing,* 1995	Adults, women, 54 radiation, 45 chemotherapy	Pearson-Byars Fatigue Feeling Checklist, Fatigue Relief Scale	Sleep and exercise most often used to cope	Correlative/ descriptive
15. Irvine et al.	*Cancer Nursing,* 1994	Adults, 54 radiotherapy, 47 chemotherapy, women, healthy controls	Pearson-Byars Fatigue Feeling Checklist and Relief Scale done at start and end	More fatigue on second time; sleep and exercise used to combat	Correlative/ descriptive, controls

TABLE 24.2. *Continued*

Authors	Journal	Subjects	Sleep Measures	Results	Study Type
16. Jensen and Given	*Support Care Cancer,* 1993	Adults, 248 caregivers for cancer	Survey	No relationship of fatigue to caregiver age, employment status, hours of care, or duration of role, did affect daily schedule	Correlative/ descriptive
17. Lee	*Image,* 1994	Adults, community women	Secondary analysis	Fatigue associated with mood and less with external demands	Correlative/ descriptive
18. Libbus et al.	*Women and Health,* 1995	Adults, 155 women	Piper Fatigue Scale	Fatigue related to depression (Beck Depression Inventory), sleep, rest, and perceived stress	Correlative/ descriptive
19. Pearce and Richardson	*Journal of Clinical Nursing,* 1994	Adults, cancer	Phenomenological		Correlative/ descriptive, qualitative
20. Pickard-Holley	*Cancer Nursing,* 1991	Adults, 12 women with ovarian cancer getting chemotherapy	Rhoten Fatigue Scale	No relation to age, stage, course of treatment, or depression	Correlative/ descriptive
21. Pugh	*Journal of Nursing Measures,* 1993	Adults, women in labor, 2 studies	Modified Fatigue Feeling Checklists, VAS	Measures validity and reliability, multidimensions	Correlative/ descriptive
22. Pugh and Milligan	*Applied Nursing Research,* 1995	Adults, childbearing women			Correlative/ descriptive
23. Ream and Richardson	*International Journal of Nursing Studies,* 1997	Adults, cancer and chronic obstructive airway disease	Phenomenological		Correlative/ descriptive, qualitative
24. Reeves, Potempa, and Gallo	*Journal of Nurse-Midwifery,* 1991	Adults, 30 women, 20 to 35 years old, less than 20 weeks gestational		Relationship between physiological variables and fatigue and psychological, not environmental	Correlative/ descriptive
25. Richardson and Ream	*International Journal of Nursing Studies,* 1997	Adults, 109 chemotherapy patients	Structured diaries, self-care behaviors	Rest activity modification, psychosocial changes	Correlative/ descriptive
26. Richardson and Ream	*International Journal of Palliative Nursing,* 1996	Adults, cancer patients	Fatigue	Fatigue increases as cancer progresses	Correlative/ descriptive
27. Robinson and Posner	*Seminars in Oncology Nursing,* 1992	Adults, 16 patients receiving biological response modifiers, family and nurses	Interview	No correlation between fatigue and therapy dose, identified self-care	Correlative/ descriptive
28. Sears and Hubsky	*Kansas Nurse,* 1993	Adults, MS			Correlative/ descriptive
29. Schaefer and Potylycki	*Journal of Advanced Nursing,* 1993	Adults, congestive heart failure	Qualitative and quantitative	Resulted from stress, physical activity, and disease; used Levine's conservation model	Correlative/ descriptive, qualitative

(continued)

TABLE 24.2.   *Continued*

Authors	Journal	Subjects	Sleep Measures	Results	Study Type
30. Reillo	*Journal of the Association of Nurses in AIDS Care,* 1993	Adults, 25 HIV-infected treated with 100% O_2 at 2 atmospheres 3 times per week for 2 months, 2x/m0 ongoing	Fatigue	Relief from debilitating fatigue	Intervention, no controls
31. Brunier and Graydon	*International Journal of Nursing Studies,* 1996	Adults, 43 patients on chronic hemodialysis	POMS fatigue subscale, VAS-F single item	$R = .80$, shared variance = 64%	Methods
32. Lee, Hicks, and Nino-Murcia	*Psychiatry Research,* 1991	Adults, 75 healthy, 57 patients with sleep disorders	VAS-F, 18 items	Compares favorable with POMS and Stanford Sleepiness Scale	Methods
33. Troy and Dalgas-Pelish	*Applied Nursing Research,* 1995	Adults, women	self-care guide developed	Postpartum	Methods
34. Hart, Freel, and Wilde	*Nursing Clinics of North America,* 1990	General			Review
35. Ream and Richardson	*International Journal of Nursing Studies,* 1996	General	concept analysis		Review
36. Pugh and Milligan	*ANS,* 1993	Childbearing			Review
37. Milligan and Pugh	*Annual Review of Nursing Research,* 1994	Childbearing			Review
38. Gift and Pugh	*Nursing Clinics of North America,* 1993	Dyspnea			Review
39. Ingersoll	*Applied Nursing Research,* 1989	Inspiratory muscle fatigue			Review
40. Potempa	*Annual Review of Nursing Research,* 1993	Chronic fatigue			Review
41. Hubsky and Sears	*Rehabilitation Nursing,* 1992	MS			Review
42. Belza	*Arthritis Care and Research,* 1994	RA			Review
43. Irvine et al.	*Cancer Nursing,* 1991	Cancer			Review
44. Nail and King	*Seminars in Oncology Nursing,* 1987	Cancer			Review
45. Nail and Winningham	*Seminars in Oncology Nursing,* 1995	Cancer			Review
46. Piper, Rieger, et al.	*Oncology Nursing Forum,* 1989	Biotherapies for cancer			Review
47. Piper, Lindsey, and Dodd	*Oncology Nursing Forum,* 1987	Cancer			Review
48. Richardson	*European Journal of Cancer Care,* 1995	Cancer			Review
49. St. Pierre, Kasper, and Lindsey	*Oncology Nursing Forum,* 1992	Cancer			Review
50. Winningham et al.	*Oncology Nursing Forum,* 1994	Cancer			Review

NOTE: MS = multiple sclerosis; POMS = Profile of Mood States; RA = rheumatoid arthritis.

tigue Scale (Yoshitake, 1971) and the Pearson and Byars Fatigue Feeling Tone Checklist (Pearson & Byars, 1956). The latter one was used in a few of the reviewed studies. Several of the studies used more recent clinical measures, including the McCorkle and Young Symptom Distress Scale (McCorkle & Young, 1978), the Rhoten Fatigue Scale and Fatigue Observation Checklist (Rhoten, 1982), the Piper Fatigue Self-Report Scale (Piper, Rieger, et al., 1989), the Lee visual analogue scale for fatigue, (Lee, Hicks, et al., 1991), and the Multidimensional Assessment of Fatigue Questionnaire (Belza, Henke, Yelin, Epstein, & Gilliss, 1993). Measures such as the Fatigue Severity Scale (Krupp, LaRocca, Muir-Nash, & Steinberg, 1989), a newer scale (Schwartz, Jandorf, & Krupp, 1993), or the Fatigue Symptom and Distress Scale (Sears & Hubsky, 1993) did not appear in the studies reviewed for this chapter.

Programs of research related to fatigue were evident in the multiple publications of Graydon's group in Canada, which reported on fatigue across medical disease categories, including women with cancer and people with chronic obstructive pulmonary disease or end stage renal disease (Brunier & Graydon, 1992, 1993, 1996; Graydon, Bubela, Irvine, & Vincent, 1995; Irvine, Vincent, Bubela, Thompson, & Graydon, 1991; Irvine, Vincent, Graydon, Bubela, & Thompson, 1994). Fatigue in cancer is the subject of multiple data-based reports by Richardson, along with Ream, in Britain (Richardson, 1995; Richardson & Ream, 1996, 1997). Belza (Belza, 1994; Tack, 1990a, 1990b; Tack & Gilliss, 1990) has developed a multidimensional assessment instrument and has reported across studies of fatigue in subjects with rheumatoid arthritis. Pugh, along with Milligan, has reported on the fatigue of childbearing (Pugh, 1993; Pugh & Milligan, 1993, 1994, 1995).

Fatigue: State of the Nursing Science

The majority of studies in the nursing science literature are addressed to fatigue associated with cancer and its treatments. In looking across the 12 studies of fatigue with cancer patients, 2 papers were from the Graydon group in Canada and 4 were from the Richardson group in Great Britain, leaving 6 singular studies, 1 published in Europe and the others in the United States. Patient samples included individuals with a broad variety of types of cancer.

In 5 studies, investigators described the trajectory of fatigue during medical treatments with equivocal results. In one study of women receiving chemotherapy or radiation therapy for cancer, the fatigue became progressively worse over time (Irvine, Vincent, Graydon, et al., 1994). Richardson and Ream (1996) corroborated progressive worsening of fatigue in a study of patients undergoing chemotherapy. Yet in melanoma patients receiving interferon therapy, the pattern of fatigue was reported as consistent over the five points of time during treatment (Dean et al., 1995). In women undergoing chemotherapy for ovarian cancer (Pickard-Holley, 1991) and in patients receiving biological response modifier therapy (Robinson & Posner, 1992), there were no relationships between fatigue and course of treatment.

Control group comparisons were sparse, but Irvine, Vincent, Graydon, and collaborators (1994) reported that women with cancer did not differ in fatigue levels with the control women prior to treatment. In one other qualitative study done in Europe, both cancer patients and control subjects described fatigue using physical and affective or cognitive terms. For both groups, physical descriptors were used more than affective or cognitive ones, but themes varied between the groups. For the cancer patients, fatigue was extreme, and unusual "need to rest" was expressed (Glaus, Crow, & Hammond, 1996). One qualitative study from the Richardson group in Britain was a comparison of fatigue descriptions in patients with cancer and chronic obstructive airway disease (Ream & Richardson, 1997). The authors revealed that the two groups shared thematic structures that related to the experience of fatigue that included physical and mental sensations embodied in fatigue, the impact of fatigue on functionality and perceived control, and the emotional effects on disease management. Shared themes also related to the capacity to manage the fatigue, including the importance of fatigue recognition and understanding, significance of setting and reaching goals, and self-care effectiveness to alleviate fatigue.

Several investigators have pursued the correlates of fatigue with some convergence of evidence. In the Irvine, Vincent, Graydon, et al. (1994) study of women, fatigue reportedly covaried with weight, symptom distress, mood disturbance, and physical alterations. However, symptom distress and mood disturbances were the strongest covariates (Irvine, Vincent, Graydon, et al., 1994). This is in synchrony with a study of people with breast or lung cancer in which fatigue correlated with pain level and mood scores using the Profile of Mood States instrument (Blesch et al., 1991). In women being treated for ovarian cancer, however, no relationship between fatigue and depression was found (Pickard-Holley, 1991). It should be noted that self-reported data are likely subject to influence by negative affectivity. When individuals are experiencing negative affect, the tendency might be to report negatively about any domain of self. In the Dean et al. (1995) study, the most extreme scores regarding symptom reporting were in the affective domain, followed by the sensory, temporal, total fatigue, and fatigue severity scores. These data collectively imply that the cognitive and emotional components of fatigue are substantial with patients managing cancer and its medical therapies, and this should be a platform on which to consider innovative nursing therapies.

Some studies have looked at the strategies with which patients cope with fatigue. In one study, a large number of strategies was used, particularly reducing or ceasing activity, increasing physical or social activity, and distraction, among others. Sleep and rest manipulations were seen to be among the most effective (Graydon et al., 1995). Sleep and rest manipulations and psychological techniques were mentioned most often in another study of people undergoing chemotherapy along with social interventions, preservation of normality, nutritional interventions, and symptom relief and comfort strategies. However, strategies were viewed to be largely ineffective (Ream & Richardson, 1997). It is very striking that nursing scientists have studied self-care strategies for fatigue but have published little in regard to developing and testing interventions for fatigue.

In singular studies of cancer patients, a variety of concepts were studied that are difficult to compare or that represent unreplicated outcomes. Cimprich (1992) found that women discharged postmastectomy manifested attentional deficits labeled as attentional fatigue of varying intensity. In a study of fatigue in the family caregivers of cancer patients, it was reported that severity of fatigue was not related to caregiver age, employment status, daily hours, or overall duration of caregiving but was related to the reported impact of the care demand on the daily schedule (Jensen & Given, 1993).

Of the four papers published with rheumatoid arthritis (RA) subjects, three were done by Belza and colleagues (Belza et al., 1993; Tack, 1990a, 1990b) and one by Crosby (1991). Belza has outlined multiple dimensions of fatigue that include descriptors, context for, consequences of, and strategies to manage or prevent fatigue (Tack, 1990a). She and her colleagues also developed an instrument based on what subjects have revealed about the fatigue associated with RA (Belza et al., 1993).

Belza's group has noted that fatigue was significantly associated with depression, pain, and overall poor mood (Tack, 1990b) and that fatigue is persistent and reported daily and affects walking and abilities to do household chores (Belza et al., 1993). Crosby (1991) reported that subjects with RA most often attributed their fatigue to disease activity, disturbed sleep, and increased physical effort. Subjects with a flare-up of their condition had significantly more joint pain, more fragmented sleep, and reduced functional capacity, as measured through walking time and grip strength, when compared to nonflare and control subjects.

The remaining studies of disease- and illness-related fatigue for which some detail could be obtained were addressed to heart failure, end-stage renal failure, and HIV/AIDS. Of note is that in these conditions, pain might not be as prominent a feature as in cancer or chronic rheumatoid conditions. In the descriptive studies of heart failure and renal patients, physical rather than psychological factors seemed to emerge as more closely tied to fatigue. In two separate studies of fatigue in heart failure, fatigue was reported to result from stress, physical activity, and disease, with significant correlations of fatigue with age and O_2 saturation in one (Schaefer & Potylycki, 1993). In the other study, sleep difficulties, chest pain, and weakness contributed most to the variance in fatigue within 1 year of hospitalization, and dyspnea was the only variable contributing by 18 months later (Friedman & King, 1995). In the same study, reported twice by Brunier and Gratin (1992, 1993) regarding patients in end-stage renal disease, it was reported that low levels of physical activity and frequent nonspecific uremic symptoms were related to high levels of fatigue, but the degree of anemia was not. Inactivity contributed to fatigue scores more than symptoms. Level of physical activity and frequency of symptoms together accounted for 52% of the variance in the fatigue scores.

In the only intervention study, hyperbaric oxygen therapy was used to relieve the debilitating fatigue associated with HIV/AIDS. Patients were treated with 100% oxygen at two atmospheres of absolute pressure three times per week for 2 months, then two times per week on an ongoing basis. According to the author, all patients experienced relief of debilitating fatigue within 1 month of hyperbaric oxygen therapy (Reillo, 1993).

Five studies were addressed to the intra- and postpartum phases of pregnancy, with two studies reported by Pugh (1993) and Pugh and Milligan (1993). Reeves, Potempa, and Gallo (1991) found in 30 women less than 20 weeks postpartum and 20 to 35 years old that 90%

reported feeling fatigued, and there was significant impact on the abilities to maintain personal and social activities. Fatigue was significantly related to nausea, poor sleep, and mood states (depression, anger, anxiety, and confusion). It was not related to number of children at home or hours worked. Gardner (1991) reported that women postpartum were mildly fatigued with situational and psychological fatigue. Using a rest and activity questionnaire, Carty et al. (1996) could find no evidence that postpartum women discharged from hospital within 3 days differed in reported sleep and tiredness. These studies are difficult to compare in terms of results, but obvious conclusions are that fatigue is a major symptom of pregnancy throughout its stages and that fatigue is related most prominently to negative mood or psychological challenges.

In sum, the science of fatigue is less developed in the nursing literature than the science of sleep. Like sleep science, to date, most studies of fatigue associated with chronic illness and disease are descriptive, documenting fatigue as highly prevalent in many chronic illness conditions. The data derived to date on the experience of fatigue in cancer patients are insubstantial for understanding the trajectory of fatigue in relation to disease severity or treatment factors such as type, route, and dose response.

Recommendations for Advancing Nursing Science Regarding Fatigue

Like sleep, fatigue is inextricably linked to mood and mental and physical function and is thereby a biobehavioral phenomenon for which assessments using physical, perceptual, or behavioral measures should be considered. Almost exclusively, investigators have used self-report measures of fatigue, with little or no use of behavioral observations, mental or physical performance evaluations, or physiological markers in individuals perceiving fatigue.

Part of nursing science should incorporate clear approaches to the understanding of fatigue according to potential mechanisms (contributing factors) for the sake of basing interventions on such understandings. Like the science of sleep disturbances, it is difficult to determine whether disease- or illness-related fatigue should be viewed as emanating from the pathology or biochemical and physiological fundamental mechanisms, or as concomitant with other disease or illness physical sensations

and discomfort. However, careful sorting out of major contributing factors as linked to context is needed. Physical factors may predominate in some circumstances and psychosocial ones might predominate in others. Careful accounting for possible competing explanations for variations in fatigue needs to be done. Because fatigue is so closely linked to pain, depression, dyspnea, oxygenation capacity, and physical fitness, to name a few factors, studies that incorporate multimodal measures are likely to be more instructive in understanding fatigue.

It can be seen from the review summarized in Table 24.2 that the nursing science related to fatigue is even less well developed than that for sleep. In the field of fatigue, studies of weaker design methodology dominate in nursing science. Investigators have failed to use a control group or control for confounding variables such as clinical depression, have used measures without multimodal scope, and have not derived the studies from clearly articulated conceptual or theoretical perspectives. These observations warrant recommending an increase in studies using more robust methodologies. Moving scientific discovery beyond description to the testing of interventions and effects on outcomes necessitates the use of experimental and quasiexperimental designs.

A recurrent theme reiterated by most authors is that the research on fatigue is fragmented. Fatigue associated with disease and illness states or unusual physiological states like pregnancy is studied by most as a context-specific entity. More study of the concept of fatigue across conditions and contexts is needed, along with studies that focus on specific conditions.

Summary of Comments on Nursing Science Related to Sleep and Fatigue

The research related to sleep/wake done by nursing scientists, although still formulary, is contributing substantially to our understanding of sleep in various contexts. This is particularly in relation to sleep related to states of disease and illness and institutionalization; it is congruent with the historical majority practice of nursing within hospitals. Within contemporary health care delivery, the study of sleep in relation to remaining healthy, during major life transitions, and as a public health (population-based) behavioral issue deserves more emphasis. A nursing approach of intervening at an environmental level as well as behaviorally at an individual person level is bound to be generative in relation to sleep, as the mainstay medical therapies such as pharmacology and surgery are not relevant as treatment in most sleep/wake actual or potential disturbances. The behavioral nature of promoting sleep and preventing and treating sleep-related disturbances suggests that working with other behavioral scientists will advance the science.

Fatigue is still an ill-defined concept that probably needs multimodal classification. To date, the science base

instructive to understanding how to intervene is unclear. As with sleep, nursing scientists are focusing on fatigue in relation to recognized disease and illness situations. Nursing scientists skilled in eliciting and analyzing the experiential aspects are likely to advance our understanding of this phenomenon. However, the physiological basis deserves attention. Much of what is likely to modify this symptom promises to be behavioral, making it a phenomenon of central interest to nursing clinical scientists and across clinical disciplines.

References

Becker, P. T., Chang, A., Kameshima, S., & Bloch, M. (1991). Correlates of diurnal sleep patterns in infants of adolescent and adult single mothers. *Research in Nursing and Health, 14*(2), 97-108.

Becker, P. T., Grunwald, P. C., Motorman, J., & Stuhr, S. (1993). Effects of developmental care on behavioral organization in very-low-birth-weight infants. *Nursing Research, 42*(4), 214-220.

Becker, P. T., & Thoman, E. B. (1981). Rapid eye movement storms in infants: Rate of occurrence at 6 months predicts mental development at 1 year. *Science, 212*(4501), 1415-1416.

Belza, B. (1994). The impact of fatigue on exercise performance. *Arthritis Care and Research, 7*(4), 176-180.

Belza, B. L., Henke, C. J., Yelin, E. H., Epstein, W. V., & Gilliss, C. L. (1993). Correlates of fatigue in older adults with rheumatoid arthritis. *Nursing Research, 42*(2), 93-109.

Blesch, K. S., Paice, J. A., Wickham, R., Harte, N., Schnoor, D. K., Purl, S., Rehwalt, M., Kopp, P. L., Manson, S., Coveny, S. B., McHale, M., & Cahill, M. (1991). Correlates of fatigue in people with breast or lung cancer. *Oncology Nursing Forum, 18*(1), 81-87.

Brunier, G., & Graydon, J. (1992). The relationship of anemia, non-specific uremic symptoms, and physical activity to fatigue in patients with end stage renal disease on hemodialysis. *American Nephrology Nurses Association Journal, 19*(2), 157.

Brunier, G., & Graydon, J. A. (1996). A comparison of two methods of measuring fatigue in patients on chronic dialysis: Visual Analogue vs. Likert Scale. *International Journal of Nursing Studies, 33*(3), 338-348.

Brunier, G. M., & Graydon, J. (1993). The influence of physical activity on fatigue in patients with ESRD on hemodialysis. *American Nephrology Nurses Association Journal, 20*(4), 457-462, 521.

Campbell, I. (1986). Postpartum sleep patterns of mother-baby pairs. *Midwifery, 2*(4), 193-201.

Carty, E. M., Bradley, C., & Winslow, W. (1996). Women's perceptions of fatigue during pregnancy and postpartum: The impact of length of hospital stay. *Clinical Nursing Research, 5*(1), 67-80.

Cimprich, B. (1992). Attentional fatigue following breast cancer surgery. *Research in Nursing and Health, 15*(3), 199-207.

Clark, J., Flowers, J., Boots, L., & Shettar, S. (1995). Sleep disturbance in mid-life women. *Journal of Advanced Nursing, 22*(3), 562-568.

Closs, S. J. (1992). Post-operative patients' views of sleep, pain and recovery. *Journal of Clinical Nursing, 1*(2), 83-88.

Cohen, F. L., Ferrans, C. E., Vizgirda, V., Kunkle, V., & Cloninger, L. (1996). Sleep in men and women infected with human immunodeficiency virus. *Holistic Nursing Practice, 10*(4), 33-43.

Cohen, F. L., Nehring, W. M., & Cloninger, L. (1996). Symptom description and management in narcolepsy. *Holistic Nursing Practice, 10*(4), 44-53.

Corser, N. C. (1996). Sleep of 1- and 2-year-old children in intensive care. *Issues in Comprehensive Pediatric Nursing, 19*(1), 17-31.

Crosby, L. J. (1991). Factors which contribute to fatigue associated with rheumatoid arthritis. *Journal of Advanced Nursing, 16*(8), 974-981.

Dean, G. E., Spears, L., Ferrell, B. R., Quan, W.D.Y., Groshon, S., & Mitchell, M. S. (1995). Fatigue in patients with cancer receiving interferon alpha. *Cancer Practice: A Multidisciplinary Journal of Cancer Care, 3*(3), 164-172.

Doling, G. A. (1995). Sleep in older women with Parkinson's disease. *Journal of Neuroscience Nursing, 27*(6), 355-357.

Evans, B. D., & Rogers, A. E. (1994). 24-hour sleep/wake patterns in healthy elderly persons. *Applied Nursing Research, 7*(2), 75-83.

Evans, M. L., Dick, M. J., & Clark, A. S. (1995). Sleep during the week before labor: Relationships to labor outcomes. *Clinical Nursing Research, 4*(3), 238-252.

Floyd, J. A. (1993). The use of across-method triangulation in the study of sleep concerns in healthy older adults. *ANS, 16*(2), 70-80.

Friedman, M. M., & King, K. B. (1995). Correlates of fatigue in older women with heart failure. *Heart and Lung, 24*(6), 512-528.

Gardner, D. L. (1991). Fatigue in postpartum women. *Applied Nursing Research, 4*(2), 57-62.

Gift, A. G., & Pugh, L. C. (1993). Dyspnea and fatigue. *Nursing Clinics of North America, 28*(2), 373-384.

Glaus, A., Crow, R., & Hammond, S. (1996). A qualitative study to explore the concept of fatigue/tiredness in cancer patients and in healthy individuals. *European Journal of Cancer Care (English), 5*(2 Suppl.), 8-23.

Glod, C. A. (1992). Circadian dysregulation in abused individuals: A proposed theoretical model for practice and research. *Archives of Psychiatric Nursing, 6*(6), 347-355.

Graydon, J. E., Bubela, N., Irvine, D., & Vincent, L. (1995). Fatigue-reducing strategies used by patients receiving treatment for cancer. *Cancer Nursing, 18*(1), 23-28.

Hart, L. K., Freel, M. I., & Milde, F. K. (1990). Fatigue. *Nursing Clinics of North America, 25*(4), 967-976.

Holditch-Davis, D., Barham, L. N., O'Hale, A., & Tucker, B. (1995). Effect of standard rest periods on convalescent preterm infants. *Journal of Obstetric, Gynecologic and Neonatal Nursing, 24*(5), 424-432.

Hubsky, E. P., & Sears, J. H. (1992). Fatigue in multiple sclerosis: Guidelines for nursing care. *Rehabilitation Nursing, 17*(4), 176-180.

Ingersoll, G. L. (1989). Respiratory muscle fatigue research: Implications for. *Applied Nursing Research, 2*(1), 6-15.

Irvine, D. M., Vincent, L., Bubela, N., Thompson, L., & Graydon, J. (1991). A critical appraisal of the research literature investigating fatigue in the individual with cancer. *Cancer Nursing, 14*(4), 188-199.

Irvine, D., Vincent, L., Graydon, J. E., Bubela, N., & Thompson, L. (1994). The prevalence and correlates of fatigue in patients receiving treatment with chemotherapy and radiotherapy: Comparison with the fatigue experienced by healthy individuals. *Cancer Nursing, 17*(5), 367-378.

Jensen, S., & Given, B. (1993). Fatigue affecting family care givers of cancer patients. *Support Care Cancer, 1*(6), 321-325.

Johnson, J. E. (1991a). A comparative study of the bedtime routines and sleep of older adults. *Journal of Community Health Nursing, 8*(3), 129-136.

Johnson, J. E. (1991b). Progressive relaxation and the sleep of older noninstitutional women. *Applied Nursing Research, 4*(4), 165-170.

Johnson, J. E. (1993). Progressive relaxation and the sleep of older men and women. *Journal of Community Health Nursing, 10*(1), 31-8.

Kedas, A., Lux, W., & Amodeo, S. (1989). A critical review of aging and sleep research. *Western Journal of Nursing Research, 11*(2), 196-206.

Kerr, S. J. S. (1994). Sleep problems in pre-school children: A review of the literature. *Child: Care, Health and Development, 6,* 379-391.

Knapp-Spooner, C., & Yarcheski, A. (1992). Sleep patterns and stress in patients having coronary bypass. *Heart and Lung, 21*(4), 342-349.

Krupp, L. B., LaRocca, N. G., Muir-Nash, J., & Steinberg, A. D. (1989). The Fatigue Severity Scale: Application to patients with multiple sclerosis and systemic lupus erythematosus. *Archives of Neurology, 46*(10), 1121-1123.

Lane, R. C., & Fontaine, D. (1992). Sleep in the pediatric intensive care unit. *Heart and Lung, 21*(3), 287.

Lee, K. A. (1992). Self-reported sleep disturbances in employed women. *Sleep, 15*(6), 493-498.

Lee, K. A., & DeJoseph, J. F. (1992). Sleep disturbances, vitality, and fatigue among a select group of employed childbearing women. *Birth, 19*(4), 208-213.

Lee, K. A., Hicks, G., & Nino-Murcia, G. (1991). Validity and reliability of a scale to assess fatigue. *Psychiatry Research, 36*(3), 291-298.

Lee, K. A., Shaver, J. F., Giblin, E. C., & Woods, N. F. (1990). Sleep patterns related to menstrual cycle phase and premenstrual affective symptoms. *Sleep, 13*(5), 403-409.

Lentz, M. J., & Killien, M. G. (1991). Are you sleeping? Sleep patterns during postpartum hospitalization. *Journal of Perinatal and Neonatal Nursing, 4*(4), 30-38.

Mahon, N. E. (1995). The contributions of sleep to perceived health status during adolescence. *Public Health Nursing, 12*(2), 127-133.

McCorkle, R., & Young, K. (1978). Development of a symptom distress scale. *Cancer Nursing, 1*(5), 373-377.

Mead-Bennett, E. (1990). The relationship of primigravid sleep experience and select mood on the first postpartum day. *Journal of Obstetric, Gynecologic and Neonatal Nursing, 19*(2), 146-152.

Milligan, R. A., & Pugh, L. C. (1994). Fatigue during the childbearing period. *Annual Review of Nursing Research, 12,* 33-49.

Nail, L. M., & King, K. B. (1987). Fatigue: A side effect of cancer treatments. *Seminars in Oncology Nursing, 3*(4), 257-262.

Nail, L. M., & Winningham, M. L. (1995). Fatigue and weakness in cancer patients: The symptom experience. *Seminars in Oncology Nursing, 11*(4), 272-278.

North American Nursing Diagnosis Association. (1996). *North American Nursing Diagnosis Association taxonomy II* (Rev.). St. Louis: Author.

Parker, K. P. (1996). Dream content and subjective sleep quality in stable patients on chronic dialysis. *American Nephrology Nurses Association Journal, 23*(2), 201-213.

Pearson, P. G., & Byars, G. E. (1956). (Report No. 56-115). Randolf Air Force Base, TX: School of Aviation, United States Air Force.

Pickard-Holley, S. (1991). Fatigue in cancer patients: A descriptive study. *Cancer Nursing, 14*(1), 13-19.

Piper, B. (1986). Fatigue. In *Pathophysiological phenomena in nursing: Human response to illness* (pp. 219-234). Philadelphia: W. B. Saunders.

Piper, B. F., Lindsey, A. M., & Dodd, M. J. (1987). Fatigue mechanisms in cancer patients: Developing nursing theory. *Oncology Nursing Forum, 14*(6), 17-23.

Piper, B. F., Rieger, P. T., Brophy, L., Haeuber, D., Hood, L. E., Lyver, A., & Sharp, E. (1989). Recent advances in the management of biotherapy-related side effects: Fatigue. *Oncology Nursing Forum, 16*(Supp. 6), 27-34.

Potempa, K. M. (1993). Chronic fatigue. *Annual Review of Nursing Research, 11,* 57-76.

Pugh, L. C. (1993). Childbirth and the measurement of fatigue. *Journal of Nursing Measures, 1*(1), 57-66.

Pugh, L. C., & Milligan, R. M. (1993). A framework for the study of childbearing fatigue. *ANS, 15*(4), 60-70.

Pugh, L. C., & Milligan, R. A. (1995). Patterns of fatigue during childbearing. *Applied Nursing Research, 8*(3), 140-143.

Ream, E., & Richardson, A. (1996). Fatigue: A concept analysis. *International Journal of Nursing Studies, 33*(5), 519-529.

Ream, E., & Richardson, A. (1997). Fatigue in patients with cancer and chronic obstructive airways disease: A phenomenological study. *International Journal of Nursing Studies, 34*(1), 44-53.

Redeker, N. S., Mason, D. J., Wykpisz, E., & Glica, B. (1996). Sleep patterns in women after coronary artery bypass surgery. *Applied Nursing Research, 9*(3), 115-122.

Rediehs, M. H., Reis, J. S., & Creason, N. S. (1990). Sleep in old age: Focus on gender differences. *Sleep, 13*(5), 410-424.

Reeves, N., Potempa, K., & Gallo, A. (1991). Fatigue in early pregnancy: An exploratory study. *Journal of Nurse-Midwifery, 36*(5), 303-339.

Reillo, M. R. (1993). Hyperbaric oxygen therapy for the treatment of debilitating fatigue associated with HIV/AIDS. *Journal of the Association of Nurses in AIDS Care, 4*(3), 33-38.

Rhoten, D. (1982). Fatigue and the postsurgical patient. In C. M. Norris (Ed.), *Concept clarification in nursing* (pp. 277-300). Rockville, MD: Aspen.

Richardson, A. (1995). Fatigue in cancer patients: A review of the literature. *European Journal of Cancer Care, 4*(1), 20-32.

Richardson, A., & Ream, E. (1996). Research and development: Fatigue in patients receiving chemotherapy for advanced cancer. *International Journal of Palliative Nursing, 2*(4), 199-204.

Richardson, A., & Ream, E. K. (1997). Self-care behaviours initiated by chemotherapy patients in response to fatigue. *International Journal of Nursing Studies, 43*(1), 35-43.

Robinson, K. D., & Posner, J. D. (1992). Patterns of self-care needs and interventions related to biologic modifier therapy: Fatigue as a model. *Seminars in Oncology Nursing, 8*(4), 17-22.

Rogers, A. E., & Aldrich, M. S. (1993). The effect of regularly scheduled naps on sleep attacks and excessive daytime sleepiness associated with narcolepsy. *Nursing Research, 42*(2), 111-117.

Rogers, A. E., Aldrich, M. S., & Caruso, C. C. (1994). Patterns of sleep and wakefulness in treated narcoleptic subjects. *Sleep, 17*(7), 590-597.

Rogers, A. E., Caruso, C. C., & Aldrich, M. S. (1993). Reliability of sleep diaries for assessment of sleep/wake patterns. *Nursing Research, 42*(6), 368-372.

Rogers, A. E., & Rosenberg, R. S. (1990). Tests of memory in narcoleptics. *Sleep, 13*(1), 42-52.

Schaefer, K. M. (1995). Sleep disturbances and fatigue in women with fibromyalgia and chronic fatigue syndrome. *Journal of Obstetric, Gynecologic and Neonatal Nursing, 24*(3), 229-233.

Schaefer, K. M., & Potylycki, M.J.S. (1993). Fatigue associated with congestive heart failure: Use of Levine's Conservation Model. *Journal of Advanced Nursing, 18*(2), 260-268.

Schaefer, K. M., Swavely, D., Rothenberger, C., Hess, S., & Williston, D. (1996). Sleep disturbances post coronary artery bypass surgery. *Progressive Cardiovascular Nursing, 11*(1), 5-14.

Schwartz, J. E., Jandorf, L., & Krupp, L. B. (1993). The measurement of fatigue: A new instrument. *Journal of Psychosomatic Research, 37*(7), 753-762.

Sears, J., & Hubsky, E. (1993). Effectiveness of strategies to cope with fatigue in multiple sclerosis. *Kansas Nurse, 68*(5), 5.

Shaver, J., Giblin, E., Lentz, M., & Lee, K. (1988). Sleep patterns and sleep stability in midlife women. *Sleep, 11*(6), 556-561.

Shaver, J., Giblin, E., & Paulsen, V. (1991). Sleep quality subtypes in midlife women. *Sleep, 14*(1), 18-23.

Shaver, J., & Paulsen, V. (1993). Sleep, psychological distress and somatic Symptoms in perimenopausal women. *Family Practice Research Journal, 13*(4), 373-384.

Shaver, J.L.F., Lentz, M., Landis, C. A., Heitkemper, M. M., Buchwald, D. S., & Woods, N. F. (1997). Sleep, psychological distress, and stress arousal in women with fibromyalgia. *Research in Nursing and Health, 20*(3), 247-257.

Sheely, L. C. (1996). Sleep disturbances in hospitalized patients with cancer. *Oncology Nursing Forum, 23*(1), 109-111.

Simpson, T., & Lee, E. R. (1996). Individual factors that influence sleep after cardiac surgery. *American Journal of Critical Care, 5*(3), 182-189.

Simpson, T., Lee, E. R., & Cameron, C. (1996). Relationships among sleep dimensions and factors that impair sleep after cardiac surgery. *Research in Nursing and Health, 19*(3), 213-223.

Spenceley, S. M. (1993). Sleep inquiry: A look with fresh eyes. *Image: Journal of Nursing Scholarship, 25*(3), 249-256.

St. Pierre, B. A., Kasper, C. E., & Lindsey, A. M. (1992). Fatigue mechanisms in patients with cancer: Effects of tumor necrosis factor and exercise on skeletal muscle. *Oncology Nursing Forum, 19*(3), 419-425.

Tack, B. B. (1990a). Fatigue in rheumatoid arthritis: Conditions, strategies, and consequences. *Arthritis Care and Research, 3*(2), 65-70.

Tack, B. B. (1990b). Self-reported fatigue in rheumatoid arthritis. *Arthritis Care and Research, 3*(3), 154-157.

Tack, B. B., & Gilliss, C. L. (1990). Nurse-monitored cardiac recovery: A description of the first 8 weeks. *Heart and Lung, 19*(5, Pt. 1), 491-499.

Topf, M. (1992a). Effects of personal control over hospital noise on sleep. *Research in Nursing and Health, 15*(1), 19-28.

Topf, M. (1992b). Stress effects of personal control over hospital noise. *Behavioral Medicine, 18*(2), 84-94.

Topf, M. (1994). Theoretical considerations for research on environmental stress and health. *Image: Journal of Nursing Scholarship, 26*(4), 289-93.

Topf, M., Bookman, M., & Arand, D. (1996). Effects of critical care unit noise on the subjective quality of sleep. *Journal of Advanced Nursing, 24*(3), 545-551.

Topf, M., & Davis, J. E. (1993). Critical care unit noise and rapid eye movement (REM) sleep. *Heart and Lung, 22*(3), 252-258.

Troy, N. W., & Dalgas-Pelish, P. (1995). Development of a self-care guide for postpartum fatigue. *Applied Nursing Research, 8*(2), 92-96.

Walker, L. O., & Best, M. A. (1991). Well-being of mothers with infant children: A preliminary comparison of employed women and homemakers. *Women and Health, 17*(1), 71-89.

Waters, M. A., & Lee, K. A. (1996). Differences between primigravidae and multigravidae mothers in sleep disturbances, fatigue, and functional status. *Journal of Nurse-Midwifery, 41*(5), 364-367.

White, M. A., Powell-Gail, M., Alexander, D., Williams-Phoebe, D., et al. (1988). Distress and self-soothing bedtime behaviors in hospitalized children with non-rooming-in parents. *Maternal-Child Nursing Journal, 17*(2), 67-77.

White, M. A., Wear, E., & Stephenson-Gordon, R. (1983). A computer-compatible method for observing falling asleep behavior of hospitalized children. *Research in Nursing and Health, 6*(4), 191-198.

White, M. A., Williams, P. D., Alexander, D. J., Powell-Cope, G. M., & Conlon, M. (1990). Sleep onset latency and distress in hospitalized children. *Nursing Research, 39*(3), 134-139.

Williamson, J. W. (1992). The effects of ocean sounds on sleep after coronary artery bypass graft surgery. *American Journal of Critical Care, 1*(1), 91-97.

Winningham, M. L., Nail, L. M., Burke, M. B., Brophy, L., Cimprich, B., Jones, L. S., Pickard-Holley, S., Rhodes, V., St. Pierre, B., Beck, S., Glass, E. C., Mock, V. L., Mooney, K. H., & Piper, B. (1994). Fatigue and the cancer experience: The state of the knowledge. *Oncology Nursing Forum, 21*(1), 23-36.

Wood, A. M. (1993). A review of literature relating to sleep in hospital with emphasis on the sleep of the ICU patient. *Critical Care Nursing, 9*(2), 129-136.

Yarcheski, A.M.N.E. (1994). A study of sleep during adolescence. *Journal of Pediatric Nursing, 9*(6), 357-367.

Yoshitake, H. (1971). Relations between the symptoms and the feeling of fatigue. *Ergonomics, 14*(1), 175-186.

Zimmerman, L., Nieveen, J., Barnason, S., & Schmaderer, M. (1996). The effects of music interventions on postoperative pain and sleep in coronary artery bypass graft (CABG) patients. *Scholarly Inquiry for Nursing Practice, 10*(2), 153-174.

PART

IIF

WOMEN'S HEALTH

Nancy Fugate Woods

This section addresses selected topics in women's health of particular relevance to nursing practice: sexuality, menstrual cycle, infertility, women's roles, and violence against women. Nurse researchers have made significant contributions to understanding women's sexuality across the lifespan and in relation to a variety of health problems. Moreover, nurse researchers have contributed to explaining and predicting contraceptive efforts and sexually risky and protective behavior. Additional work is needed about normative experiences and attention to diversity of ethnic and social class among study populations. Measurement of sexual attitudes and knowledge of sexual health, as well as risky behaviors, has been advanced, but measurement of normative experiences lags behind problem-oriented measures.

Nurses have also made significant contributions to understanding menarche, menstruation and menstrual symptoms, and menopause. In this arena, measurement research has led other disciplines' efforts, especially in regard to symptoms. Nurses have studied normative experiences and symptoms, but more research is needed about symptom management, especially use of nonpharmacological measures.

Infertility has been addressed in a variety of studies, but most have focused on charting women's experiences. Measurement issues have not been addressed, and trials of interventions to promote fertility and health for those seeking infertility care are needed.

Research about women's roles and their health has focused on women's experiences with parenting, partnering, working outside the home, and caregiving. This body of literature has emphasized the complement of women's roles and their health effects. Spillover of work effects to family and family effects to work could provide the impetus for interventions to promote role sufficiency and reduce role strain, but this area has not been well developed. Efforts to measure relevant concepts such as role strain are needed.

Violence against women, particularly male battery of women, has been the focal point for nursing research, supported by a network of nurse investigators working in a consortium mode. This body of work informs practice

457

about risk situations for women and promotes screening for violence and identification of women who have been battered. Preventive interventions to empower women to protect themselves and their children are being tested.

Nursing research has made a substantial contribution to knowledge for clinical practice in these five areas. Taken together, this body of work has informed the science of practice and is beginning to guide therapeutic efforts.

25

WOMEN'S WORK, WOMEN'S HEALTH

Marcia Gruis Killien

Overview

Women have always worked. However, the widespread entry of women across all socioeconomic groups into the paid labor force has occurred only since World War II. Accompanying this demographic trend has been increasing scientific interest in the effects of employment on women's health and how women's health influences their working lives. Major areas of research have included gender differences in work performance and health outcomes, environmental workplace hazards (especially reproductive hazards), and working and stress. Nurse investigators, along with other health scientists, psychologists, and sociologists, have explored many of these areas. Their contributions have especially focused on research that describes women's predominant work-related symptoms and illnesses, women's work experiences during biological transitions such as pregnancy and menopause, workplace stress, and experiences of balancing work and family responsibilities. This review is based on citations identified through a search of Medline and CINAHL from 1980 onward on the topics of women, work, and health; primary emphasis was placed on published reports of research in nursing journals or from authors identified as nurses.

To examine the state of the science with regard to women and work, it is first important to understand the changing demographic patterns and future projections with respect to women in the workforce. This understanding assists us in targeting groups of women vulnerable to health problems currently and in the future and increases our awareness of new challenges faced by women at work.

Perspectives on Women and Work

Historical and Demographic Perspectives

Labor Force Participation

World War II brought women into the U.S. labor force as never before, providing them with unprecedented exposure to new job skills, work experience, and the rewards of both economic and intrinsic satisfaction. Married women, with and without young children, from all socioeconomic groups joined the labor force. For the substantial majority of these new workers, the end of the war also signaled the end of their employment lives; women returned to traditional family roles focusing on unpaid household and family work. Women considered (and were encouraged to consider) it their patriotic duty to free up jobs for returning male veterans and also set about the work of childbearing to replenish the population and stabilize family lives. In the 1960s, there began a dramatic movement of women into the paid labor force in the United States, which continues to the present. The needs of a growing industrial nation for more workers again created employment opportunities for women, and the baby boom generation reached working age. During the subsequent two decades, new female workers were primarily married women without children and mothers whose children had entered elementary school. In 1950, 23% of women participated in the labor force, comprising less than one third of all workers; by 1978, 50% of women were in the labor force, comprising 42% of all workers. In the 1980s and 1990s, societal changes again influenced the complexion of the labor force. Increases in marital separation and divorce, smaller family size, and economic necessity brought women with infants and preschool-age children into the workplace, accounting for the greatest increase in labor force participation among women. In 1994, women's labor force participation rate rose to 58.8%, with women representing 46% of the total labor force (Herz & Wootten, 1996; U.S. Department of Labor, 1990, 1995; Women's Bureau, 1994). It has been projected that by 2005 women's labor force participation will reach 63%; in contrast, men's labor force participation rate has been slowly but steadily declining during the past 20 years, from 78% in 1975 to a projected 75.4% in 2005 (Costello, Stone, & Dooley, 1994; Women's Bureau, 1994).

Employment Patterns

Women's employment patterns have increasingly come to resemble those of men. In the 1960s, women's employment tended to be intermittent; they entered the labor force upon completing their education, remaining employed during the early years of marriage but dropping out to bear and rear children and re-entering when the youngest child entered school or had left the family nest. In the 1980s, women's employment was more likely continuous, with only brief interruptions for childbearing. Thus, in 1960 and 1970, the highest rates of labor force participation were in women 20 to 24 and 45 to 54 years old; since 1990, women 25 to 44 years old have had the highest rate (Costello et al., 1994). The proportion of older women (55 to 64 years) in the labor force increased from one quarter in 1948 to over one half in 1994. Between 1972 and 1994, the labor force participation of women with children under age 18 increased from 39.5% to 68.4%. The greatest increase in the proportion of working mothers during these two decades was among women with young children (under 6 years), from 29% to 60.3%.

Economic conditions, women's commitment to labor force participation after long years of educational investment, and access to upward job mobility were among the factors contributing to this pattern (Costello et al., 1994; Herz & Wootten, 1996; Wolf & Rosenfeld, 1978; Women's Bureau, 1994). Women's employment is now likely to span 30 or more years of their adult lives.

Although marriage and child-rearing responsibilities no longer preclude labor force participation, they do influence women's employment patterns. Based on data from 1994 (Herz & Wootten, 1996), marital status was shown to affect labor force participation, with divorced (74%) and never married (65%) women having the highest rates of participation; 61% of married women with spouses present were employed. Among married couples with children, in 20.3% of families, only the father was employed; in 2.2%, only the mother was employed; and in 48%, both parents were employed. Parenthood also influences labor force participation. In general (again based on data from 1994), women with children under age 18 are more likely to be employed (68.4%) than women who are not parents (53.1%). Women are more likely to be employed as their children get older. Labor force participation rates for women with children under 1 year (54.6%) is only slightly higher than that for women with no children; employment rates increase steadily with the age of the youngest child: under 3 years (57.1%), under 6 years (60.3%), 6 to 17 years (76%). Seventy-one percent of working mothers reported that they worked to support the family (Herz & Wootten, 1996; Women's Bureau, 1994).

Women in general are more likely than men to work part-time, comprising two thirds of all part-time workers. However, the number of women employed full-time, year-round doubled between 1971 and 1991. Nearly three quarters of all women employed in 1992 were working full-time, compared to 89% of men. When women worked part-time, they were more likely than men to do so voluntarily; however, in 1994, 12% of women working less than 35 hours per week indicated that they would work full-time if the opportunity were available. African American and Hispanic women were more likely to work part-time involuntarily, with a quarter of both groups preferring to work full-time, compared to 11% of White women (Herz & Wootten, 1996). Women with children under age 6 are most likely to be employed part-time. Women are increasingly adopting a male-dominant work pattern in the number who hold multiple paid jobs simultaneously. In 1970, for every woman who worked multiple jobs, there were more than five men who did. By 1991, there were three multiple-job women for every four multiple-job men (Costello et al., 1994; Women's Bureau, 1994).

Occupations of Women

Women are employed in a diverse array of occupations, with the largest numbers of women employed as secretaries, managers and administrators, cashiers, bookkeepers, registered nurses, nursing aides, and elementary teachers. Women are disproportionately represented in the lower paying service sector occupations; gender segregation in occupations continues. Of the 20 leading occupations of women (7 of which are listed above) 11 are known as traditionally female jobs. Occupations that are female dominant include secretarial/clerical (98.5% female), dental hygiene (99.8%), receptionist (97.1%), child care work (97%), and nursing (95%). The largest increase in female employment in the past decade has been in professional and managerial positions; in 1994, men and women were nearly equally represented in this occupational group. Women are more likely than men to be in the entry and middle levels of management, and the future may see women entering higher level management positions in greater numbers. Within professional health

care occupations, women account for three fourths of those employed in health assessment and treatment (e.g., nurses, dietitians, therapists) and two thirds of health and medical management positions. Women dominate preschool though secondary education, accounting for three fourths of all teachers during these years; however, men outnumber women among college and university teachers. The most extreme differences in gender representation occur in precision production, craft, and repair occupations, with women comprising only 1% of carpenters and 2% of electricians in 1994 (Herz & Wootten, 1996; Women's Bureau, 1994).

Racial and ethnic differences exist in occupational employment of women. Although 30% of White women held professional and managerial positions in 1994, 21% of African-American and 17% of Hispanic women were represented in these groups. These latter two groups are over-represented among service and labor occupations; all three groups are equally represented (approximately 25% of women) among administrative support personnel. Occupational opportunities reflect differences in educational attainment among racial and ethnic groups; 25% of White women in the labor force had completed 4-year college degrees, compared to 17% of African-American women and 13% of Hispanic women (Herz & Wootten, 1996).

Although the income gap between men and women has been narrowing in the past decade, employed women continue to earn less than men. In 1994, median earnings for women working full-time was 76% of the median for men. Occupations with the highest gender parity (90% or more) in earnings were bookkeepers, registered nurses, and precision mechanics and repairers. Older women experience a larger earnings gap with men than do younger women; this difference reflects to some extent differences in educational attainment and employment experience but may also be a reflection of age or gender discrimination. Among all racial and ethnic groups, women with more education are more likely to have higher earnings; differences in earnings between women of different races within each educational level are small (Herz et al., 1996).

Conceptual Perspectives

The research to date examining women, work, and health has focused almost exclusively on how work, added to women's other roles and responsibilities, influences their health. This research has derived from two main theoretical perspectives: the role stress perspective and the health benefits perspective (Barnett, 1996; Frankenhaeuser, Lundberg, & Chesney, 1991; Killien, 1990; Sorensen & Verbrugge, 1987). However, new frameworks are currently being proposed that offer promise for moving the state of the science forward by focusing on the synchrony of the work and family spheres of women's lives, person-environment fit, and biobehavioral perspectives of health (Barnett, 1996).

Role Stress and Illness Perspectives

The role stress perspective posits that specific roles (e.g., parent, partner, worker) are sources of unique stressors that are harmful to individuals' physical and mental well-being. Further, simultaneously maintaining multiple roles compounds health problems through cumulative stress (role overload) and competing demands (role conflict) (Haw, 1982; McBride, 1990; Sorensen & Verbrugge, 1987; Woods, 1985). Research from this perspective has focused on the direct effects of workplace stress on health, as well as the stress associated when employment roles are combined with family roles. Investigators have suggested that stressful aspects of workplace environments account for decreased emotional well-being, increased acute morbidity and absenteeism, elevated rates of cardiovascular disease, and chronic health problems associated with exposure to environmental hazards (Frankenhaeuser, Lundberg, & Chesney, 1991; Institute of Medicine, 1995; Moos, 1980; Moos, Fenn, & Billings, 1988). Research that documented these effects on men's health has more recently been extended to women, with the belief that women's exposure to the job stressors previously felt largely by men is likely to increase their health risks in a similar manner (Frankenhaeuser, Lundberg, & Chesney, 1991; Sorensen & Verbrugge, 1987; Waldron, 1991). Specific characteristics of the workplace that have documented effects on health include task characteristics (e.g., workload, pacing, deadlines, repetition), organizational aspects (e.g., job ambiguity, decision control), interpersonal relations with coworkers and supervisors, and physical and environmental hazards (Frankenhaeuser, Lundberg, & Chesney, 1991; Stellman, 1978). Research on employed women further documents that stress associated with interference of dual responsibilities at home and job compound women's health risks (Hock, 1992; McBride, 1990). Such research employs a scarcity hypothesis that presumes that individual re-

sources of time and energy have an upper limit that can be exhausted by multiple role responsibilities (Sorensen & Verbrugge, 1987). Even when women assume responsibilities outside the home, their responsibility for household maintenance, child care, and spousal support continues at high levels (Hochschild, 1989; Pleck, 1985). The role of parent has been found to be particularly stressful when combined with other roles (Capell, 1995; Gruis, 1977; Mercer, 1986; Woods, 1985).

Health Benefits Perspectives

The health benefits perspective counterposes that social roles provide resources to individuals that directly or indirectly maintain or enhance health. Employment provides access to income, health care benefits, and social support; it also provides an expansion of opportunities for building knowledge, skills, and self-esteem, as well as alternative sources of reward and satisfaction, thereby promoting health (Billings & Moos, 1982; Froberg, Gjerdingen, & Preston, 1986; Gjerdingen, Froberg, & Fontaine, 1991; Hibbard & Pope, 1992; Sorensen & Verbrugge, 1987). Verbrugge (1986) ranked women with various role configurations by health status as indicated by incidence of acute illness, illness-restricted days, chronic illness limitations, and self-rated health status. Employed, married women, with or without children, were found to have the best health outcomes. In contrast, women with the absence of these roles fared increasingly less well. In the more recent Commonwealth Fund Survey (Hartmann, Kuriansky, & Owens, 1996), employed women of all ages and all racial and ethnic groups were also found to have better health than nonworking women on three measures of health status: incidence of hypertension, heart disease, arthritis, anxiety/depression; incidence of disability; and self-assessment of health. Hibbard and Pope (1992, 1993) used longitudinal medical record and interview data from a large, randomly selected sample of HMO members to establish that differences in morbidity and mortality between employed and nonemployed women were significantly related to social support at work. Employment appears to offer the strongest health benefits to those women with limited alternative sources of social support, self-esteem, and satisfaction (Nathanson, 1980). In a longitudinal, prospective survey of a random sample of 403 employed women who varied in occupation, race, and family role characteristics, Barnett, Marshall, and Singer (1992) found that declines in the quality of the employment role were associated with increases in psychological distress among single women and women without children; women who were partnered or who were parents were psychologically unaffected by these changes in their employment quality. Meisenhelder (1986) found that self-esteem of homemakers was significantly more predicted by their husbands' appraisals of them than was that of employed women. Hall, Williams, and Greenberg (1985) found that being unmarried, unemployed, and having a low income were positively related to depressive symptoms in mothers of young children. In the Commonwealth Fund Survey, the least healthy women were those who did not work, but would have liked to (Hartmann et al., 1996).

Emerging Frameworks and Perspectives

Difficulties in evaluating these two perspectives regarding the effects of employment on health are related to insufficient understanding or control of several factors. First, healthier people may acquire and maintain employment more easily than those who are less healthy (i.e., the healthy worker effect). Second, multiple roles may be incompatible with sick-role behavior and thus decrease sensitivity to symptoms or willingness to respond to symptoms. Third, the interactive effects of work and family roles and individual characteristics have only recently been recognized and studied. Individuals vary in their resilience, and thus some may be more able than others to manage the stress associated with multiple roles (Lambert & Lambert, 1987; Rose & Killien, 1983; Rutter, 1987). Further, work and family roles are interactive and cannot be studied as separate spheres. Stress experienced at work may have a contagious effect on family life, stimulating marital or parenting stress, or the positive effects of supportive family relationships may spill over into the workplace, moderating the negative relationship between workplace stress and health (Barnett, 1996). Thus, the transmission of both stress and resilience among women's multiple environments is an important emerging perspective to guide future research.

The research to date has not sufficiently clarified these issues because of reliance on cross-sectional designs, use of global measures of health and functioning such as absenteeism, and focus on the demands rather than the benefits of multiple roles. Emerging conceptual frameworks to guide research in this area will focus increased attention on the individual characteristics that might mediate the effects of employment on health outcomes and provide a more unified conceptualization of women's lives and health that integrates not only physical and psychological dimensions of health but also decompartmentalizes work and family experiences.

State of the Science on Women, Work, and Health

Nursing research contributions to knowledge on women, work, and health have emerged from two dominant branches of the discipline: women's health and occupational health. Research from the occupational health perspective has a strong base within environmental health and has made contributions to the literature on environmental hazards in the workplace, especially reproductive hazards, and the effects of workplace stress on employee health. Women's health researchers bring sociocultural and feminist perspectives to contributions focusing on the interrelationship of employment and other dimensions of women's lives, including work and family balance and gender influences on health. The literature suggests that women workers are more vulnerable than their male counterparts to several health problems: stress-related disorders, violent death, and repetitive strain injuries. Additionally, women's reproductive role and traditional caregiving responsibilities present unique challenges in the workplace.

Health Concerns of Women Workers

Working and Stress

Chronic stress has become one of the most serious occupational health hazards of our times. Stress, in relation to women and their work, is both a public health and a political issue. It is the number one problem for working women, identified by almost 60% of women (Dear, 1995; Lusk, 1997). A 1984 survey on women and stress, sponsored by the National Association of Working Women, provided important descriptive information on the relationship between general categories of workplace stress and the outcomes of major and minor illnesses and absenteeism (National Association of Working Women, 1984). This survey documented women workers' experiences of stress in three major areas. One area was job design, including the rapid pace of work, lack of control over time pressures and workload, physical immobility (such as sitting or standing for long periods), boredom or monotony, lack of adequate rest breaks, long hours, underuse of skills, lack of decision-making authority, and working under productivity and time standards. A second area of stress was problematic work relations; conflicting demands from supervisors; ineffective grievance procedures; age, race, or sexual discrimination; sexual harassment; and discord between coworkers. The third type was socioeconomic stressors such as low pay, job immobility, job insecurity, lack of child care support, and reduction in workforce or wages. Survey results indicated that jobs were rated as very stressful by one third of women respondents and as somewhat stressful by an additional 62%. Stress was associated with the occurrence of conditions such as heart disease, hypertension, and gastrointestinal disorders. Specific job conditions found to be significantly associated with these illnesses were lack of clout, never finding work interesting or challenging, having too much work, facing constant deadlines, and having to work very fast. Minor illness episodes were associated with experiencing high job pressure and responsibility without concurrent decision-making authority. Absenteeism was associated with boredom and insufficient challenge and lack of power and decision authority. Negative work relations were also associated with major and minor health problems and absenteeism. These factors were also identified by the National Institute for Occupational Safety and Health (NIOSH) as a major contributor to workplace stress (NIOSH, 1996).

Martocchio and O'Leary (1997) reported the results of a meta-analysis of 15 studies of the effects of workplace stress on males and females. They concluded that there were no gender differences in either physiological or psychological stress; however, none of the studies reviewed included measures of family or home stress, an important factor in women's lives. Several occupational groups have been identified as showing the highest rates of job stress. Managers report the highest rates of very stressful jobs, followed by clerical and sales workers. The health care industry also ranked as very stressful, with nurses, other health care workers, and social workers rating their jobs as very stressful more often than the norm, independent of the number of hours worked (National Association of Working Women, 1984).

Clerical workers experience both mental and physical stress in their jobs; common symptoms include depression, muscular fatigue, visual discomfort, and stress from deadlines, demands, and poor environmental conditions. These experiences have been described using qualitative methodologies in a series of reports of studies of female clerical workers in various organizational settings (Hall, Stevens, & Meleis 1992a, 1992b; Meleis, Messias, & Arruda, 1996; Meleis, Norbeck, Laffrey, Solomon, & Miller, 1989b; Stevens, Hall, & Meleis, 1992). Although data gathered in the 1960s for the Framingham Heart Study (Haynes & Feinleib, 1980) revealed a high rate of coronary heart disease and emotional distress among clerical women, data from a subsequent National Health Interview Survey (Verbrugge, 1984) suggested that clerical workers were not disadvantaged for poor health outcomes; the authors suggested that changes in the work environment and societal values over time might change the pressures on clerical workers. However, in a random sample of 3,484 women employed full-time, women employed in clerical positions were significantly more depressed and more likely to miss work than women in other occupations (Garrison & Eaton, 1992). Henning, Sauter, Salvendy, and Krieg (1989) tested the effects of frequent, short work breaks on occupational fatigue in an experimental study in a NIOSH laboratory of 20 female data entry personnel. The microbreaks were initiated by a computerized cue, but participants stopped the microbreak at their own discretion. The mean length of the microbreak was 27.4 seconds; the investigators concluded that these breaks were not sufficiently long to achieve performance recovery. The work environment for nurses and other health care workers includes not only exposure to infectious and toxic agents, but also a stressful work environment. For example, Topf and Dillon (1988) found that noise-induced stress was a statistically significant predictor of emotional exhaustion and burnout in a sample of 100 critical care nurses. Shiftwork is another stressor for many health care workers that has been examined. Lee (1992) surveyed 760 registered nurses about their sleep patterns and sleep quality; women working night and rotating shifts had a higher incidence of sleep disturbances and excessive sleepiness. Gordon, Cleary, Parker, and Czeisler (1986) found that women working rotating shifts used more alcohol and sleeping and tranquilizing drugs, had weaker social networks, and perceived more severe job and emotional problems than women working consistent (straight) shifts. Gold and associates' (1992) study of 635 nurses found that nurses working either the night shift or rotating shifts had twice the number of accidents or errors compared to nurses working day or evening shifts. In a prospective study of female nurses between 1988 and 1992, Kawachi and associates (1995) found an increased relative risk of coronary heart disease among participants who worked rotating shifts as compared to those who never rotated shifts; this risk increased among women who had experienced shiftwork for over 6 years.

Few studies were found that examined the effectiveness of interventions to reduce stress among health care workers. However, Thomas, Riegel, Gross, and Andrea (1992) tested differences in job-related stress among emergency department nurses after implementing staff-generated strategies. Sources of stress were identified by staff, and interventions included a problem-focused task force, classes in conflict resolution, assertive communication, and situational leadership. There were no significant posttest differences on staff burnout, but other predictors of burnout (e.g., low social support) were identified for future research. Staats and Staats (1983) compared stress levels, responses, and stressors of male and female managers. They found that women reported a higher level of stress and their stressors were primarily family, not job related. Women responded with more illness, medical consultations, work loss, and mental health consultations. Men consumed more alcohol and had a greater incidence of hypertension.

Age has been related to ratings of job stress, with women in their 30s reporting more stress than either their younger or older counterparts (National Association of Working Women, 1984). Griffith (1983) surveyed 579 women between 25 and 65 years old and found that women's stressors differed significantly by age groups. Women between 25 and 34 indicated that finding personal time and personal success were major stressors.

Women over 35 also identified finding personal time as a major stress, but physical health was their primary stressor. Other researchers have referred to women in these middle years as the sandwich generation, responsible not only for the care of young children but also that of aging parents (National Association of Working Women, 1984).

Efforts have been made to identify strategies and approaches beneficial in reducing or managing stress. In general, negative coping mechanisms have been found to have a more powerful impact on health outcomes than have positive coping mechanisms. Negative coping strategies related to poor health include always apologizing, blaming, and using alcohol. Two positive coping strategies found to be significantly related to the absence of health problems are regular exercise and blowing off steam (National Association of Working Women, 1984). This latter finding supports earlier reports from the Framingham Study that difficulty or inability to express anger or frustration was one of the three strongest predictors of the development of coronary heart disease among clerical workers (Haynes & Feinleib, 1980). Griffith found that

women's coping strategies varied by age group, with younger women (between 25 and 34 years old) using talking, food consumption, and rest and relaxation more often than older women. Women between 35 and 54 years were more likely to use exercise as a coping strategy than other groups of women. Working was a common coping strategy used by nearly one third of women under age 45 and by over half of women over age 45 (Griffith, 1983).

Sexual harassment. Women workers have identified sexual harassment as one source of stress they experience in the workplace (National Association of Working Women, 1984). The legal community seeks to establish a standard of what the reasonable person or reasonable woman would identify as harassment in the workplace, but men and women have been found to differ in their perceptions of what constitutes a hostile and harassing work environment. Women perceive behaviors by male perpetrators as more threatening than those by female perpetrators (Baird, Bensko, Bell, Viney, & Woody, 1995). Large surveys of working women suggest that half of all working women will be harassed at some point during their working lives (Fitzgerald, 1993). Harassment has been reported by workers in all types of environments, ranging from community workers for the elderly in rural communities (Rogers & Maurizio, 1993) to medical residents in universities (Komaromy, Bindman, Haber, & Sande, 1993). In a study of internal medicine residents, 73% of female respondents (compared to 22% of male respondents) indicated having encountered sexual harassment during medical school or residency; women were more likely than men to have been physically harassed, and the harassers were of higher professional status. The majority of victims believed their experience created a hostile work environment or interfered with their work performance, but few reported their experiences to an authority. Women cited a lack of belief they would be helped as the primary barrier to reporting. In a study of job stressors among male and female firefighters, Murphy, Beaton, Cain, and Pike (1994) found that, although there were few gender differences in either job stressors or symptoms of stress, female firefighters were more likely to report job discrimination. A study comparing job stress of male and female law enforcement officers (Norvell, Hills, & Murrin, 1993) revealed that women experienced lesser degrees of perceived stress and more promotional opportunities than their male colleagues; however, sexual harassment was not specifically addressed in this study.

Sexual harassment is experienced as degrading and frightening and may be physically violent; it may extend over a long period of time and can have major health- and job-related consequences for the victim (National Association of Working Women, 1984). Support from others, including coworkers and employers, as well as organizational support, has been found to improve the health outcomes of women who experience sexual harassment at work (Fitzgerald, 1993; Gutek & Koss, 1993; Komaromy et al., 1993).

Violence in the Workplace

Homicide is the leading cause of worksite mortality for women (followed by motor vehicle injuries); homicide ranks third as the cause of worksite mortality for men (Bell, 1991; Dannenberg, Baker, & Li, 1994; Felton, 1993; Freda, 1994; Jenkins, Layne, & Kisner, 1992; Levin, Hewitt, & Misner, 1992; Lusk, 1992). Findings from the National Traumatic Occupational Fatality database (Bell, 1991) showed that although only 6% of U.S. victims of work-related injury deaths were female, 41% of these women were murdered; the leading cause of death was handgun wounds. Homicide rates were highest among women over 65 years of age, women of non-White races, and women employed in retail trade. Worksite violence includes business disputes, customer disputes, disputes involving relatives, and robbery or crime, with the latter category accounting for 80% of homicides (Lusk, 1997; Windau et al., 1994). Women working in retail trade represent the largest group of homicide victims (43%); women in law enforcement occupations and health care workers are also highly vulnerable, due to the prevalence of handguns on site and inadequate care for mentally ill and disturbed persons (Lusk, 1997). The nursing literature includes descriptions of the problem of workplace violence and urges the implementation of programs to reduce violence; however, no research evaluating violence prevention programs was found (Felton, 1993; Levin et al., 1992; Lusk, 1997).

Repetitive Strain Disorders

Hand, arm, and neck symptoms associated with repetitive movements at work have been termed repetitive strain or cumulative trauma disorders. Higher rates of these disorders have been reported in females. Risk factors may include differences in stature, physiology, and the nature of jobs performed by women. For example, tools and work equipment are frequently designed for men and may be inappropriate for women's anatomical characteristics. Occupations in which women may be especially exposed to these disorders include secretarial and clerical positions, assembly line workers, hairdressers, and cleaners or domestics (Carson, 1993; English et al., 1995; Fransson-Hall, Bystrom, & Kilbom, 1995; Lusk, 1997; Reid, Ewan, & Lowy, 1991). One interview study (Reid et al., 1991) indicated that women diagnosed with repetitive strain injuries had difficulty establishing the validity of their condition, suggesting the need for additional research to describe these symptoms as well as to develop and test effective preventive and treatment strategies.

Special Concerns for Working Women

Women's biology, developmental transitions, and social roles present them with special challenges and concerns in relation to work. Among those issues that have been addressed by nursing research are menstruation and menopause, reproductive hazards in the workplace, working during pregnancy, and the balancing of work and family caregiving responsibilities.

Menstruation and Menopause

During the past decade, there has been a dramatic increase in research and popular interest in the phenomenon of premenstrual symptomatology among women. Concern about the ability of women to function in responsible employment positions while menstruating has in the past been a basis for gender discrimination in employment. In a 1982 survey of a healthy population of U.S. women, Woods, Dery, and Most (1992) found that although 30% of women reported perimenstrual symptoms, for the most part their symptoms were mild. Brown and Woods (1986) found that employment was unrelated to premenstrual symptoms, but those in traditional female occupations experienced more severe negative affect symptoms premenstrually, such as depression, irritability, and mood disturbance. Lee and Rittenhouse (1991b) examined the prevalence of perimenstrual symptoms in a cross section of professionally employed women; these women did not differ from other cross sections of the population in their reports of symptoms. Perimenstrual symptoms produce variable responses among women, ranging from modest effects on well-being to major disruption of daily activities. Woods, Most, and Longenecker (1985) found that women with the most severe symptoms were most likely to rest in bed or decrease their activities. The greatest disability was associated with negative affect symptoms. O'Rourke (1983) found that among employed women, nonmenstrual symptom experiences affected general psychological well-being, but perimenstrual symptoms, although sometimes causing short-term disruption of usual activities, were unrelated to general psychological well-being. In contrast, Lee and Rittenhouse (1992a) found that employed women with premenstrual symptoms were less satisfied with their social lives, had less social support, lower psychological well-being, and more physical health problems than nonsymptomatic women. These data suggest that although a small proportion of women experience severe distress and related disruption of activities, for the most part, menses-related absenteeism or work disruption is low (Roberts & Garling, 1981).

It appears that employment can be a source of stress but may also be protective against symptoms and symptom-related responses in midlife. In a randomly selected sample of 8,114 Massachusetts women aged 45 to 54, employment was associated with positive self-assessed health status, fewer psychological symptoms, and decreased use of medications. When compared with women who were unemployed or homemakers, employed women had fewer health problems and reported the fewest illness behaviors (Jennings, Mmazaik, & McKinlay, 1984). Uphold and Susman (1985) found that within a sample of 185 healthy, midlife women, the more roles women enacted, the less likely they were to experience climacteric symptoms. The number of hours worked was unrelated to number or severity of menopausal symptoms. Wilber and Dan (1989) found that work patterns during the careers of nurses were unrelated to their psychological well-being at midlife. In a study by Woods and Mitchell (1996) of depressed mood in a population-based sample of 508 midlife women, employment status failed to discriminate women experiencing patterns of depressed mood from those not experiencing depression.

Reproductive Health and Work

Historically, the focus of concern for women's occupational health and safety has been on hazards to women's reproductive health. Research on women's reproductive outcomes continues to dominate the occupational health literature (Misner, Levin, & Hewitt, 1993). In the past, social norms and workplace policies forced U.S. women to leave their jobs when they announced their pregnancies or when physical signs of pregnancy became noticeable. American legislation was protectionist, restricting prenatal and postpartum employment yet offering little protection of income, benefits, or job security. In 1964, the passage of Title VII of the Federal Civil Rights Act disallowed employment discrimination on the basis of gender, but various interpretations prevented full protection of the rights of pregnant workers. Additional protection was provided in 1978 by an amendment to Title VII, the Pregnancy Discrimination Act. This amendment formed the legal basis for ensuring that benefits from health insurance plans for sickness or temporary physical disability must be extended to female employees disabled by pregnancy, miscarriage, abortion, childbirth, or recovery from these conditions. It also prohibits refusing to hire pregnant women, requiring mandatory leaves due to pregnancy, or denying benefits, promotions, or reinstatement of employees after pregnancy leaves. These laws enabled women to continue working throughout pregnancy (Killien, 1990). Today, two thirds of women in the labor force are of childbearing age, and more than 1 million infants are born each year to women who are employed during pregnancy. It has been estimated that 85% of the female labor force will be pregnant at some point during their working years (Killien, 1990; Paul, 1994).

Considerable research has been conducted by scientists from many disciplines on the effects of employment during pregnancy on fetal health; less attention has been paid to the effects of work on maternal health and well-being. Possible exposure to potentially harmful substances at work can be a great source of concern for the woman who is attempting to become or is pregnant. The growth of the petrochemical industry has resulted in a vast increase in the number of synthetic chemicals in the workplace. Consequences of human exposure to agents such as thalidomide changed the prevailing view of the placenta as a protective barrier for the fetus. In the mid-1980s, the National Institute for Occupational Safety and Health (NIOSH) ranked reproductive disorders among the 10 leading work-related illnesses and injuries in the nation (Paul, 1994). However, because there are so many potential toxic substances within the work environment, research on many has not been conducted.

In general, pregnant workers can be reassured by the findings of research on the relationship between maternal employment during pregnancy and reproductive outcomes. These investigations have focused on common reproductive outcomes such as fertility, spontaneous abortion, low birth weight, prematurity, birth defects, and infant mortality. Studies conducted prior to the 1970s frequently reported detrimental effects of working on infant birth weight and mortality; these findings have no doubt contributed to prohibitions and concerns about pregnant women continuing to work until term. However, these early studies failed to take into account other important variables such as socioeconomic status; maternal age and parity; and work conditions, such as the number of hours worked, type of employment, and specific work activity. Studies also tended to be retrospective and rely on recall (Killien, 1990; Launer, Villar, Kestler, & De Onis, 1990; U.S. Department of Labor, 1990). The 1988 National Maternal and Infant Health Survey, a stratified random sample of 9,953 live births selected from the vital statistics records of 48 states and the District of Columbia, demonstrated that women employed during pregnancy were advantaged with respect to the socio-demographic and behavioral characteristics associated with good perinatal outcomes (the healthy worker effect) (Moss & Carver, 1993; Wen, Tsai, & Gibson, 1983). Compared to nonemployed women, women who worked during pregnancy were of lower parity, higher income, higher educational level, had health insurance, obtained early prenatal care, were less likely to smoke, and had a desired pregnancy. However, among pregnant workers, those employed in professional and managerial occupations were more likely than those in skilled and unskilled occupations to obtain early prenatal care and have lower rates of preterm birth (Gabbe & Turner, in press; Moss & Carver, 1993).

Research conducted since the 1970s has accounted for some of these variables in the study designs and, taken together, shows no direct association between employment per se during pregnancy and outcomes such as spontaneous abortion, preterm birth, infant birth weight, and infant mortality (Ferketich & Mercer, 1989; Marbury et al., 1984; Meyer & Daling, 1985). However, several work conditions have been identified as contributing to reproductive disorders.

Strenuous work has been associated with decreased fertility as well as preterm labor and low birth weight (Berkowitz, 1981; Berkowitz, Kelsey, Holford, & Berkowitz, 1983; Florack, Zielhuis, & Rolland, 1994; Klebanoff, Shiono, & Carey, 1990). Occupations involving strenuous exercise, such as that experienced by professional athletes and dancers, may suppress the hypo-thalamicpituitary axis, leading to amenorrhea and difficulty with conception (Cummings & Rebar, 1993). During pregnancy, moderate exercise has been shown to be beneficial for perinatal outcome, but intense exercise has been associated with preterm labor, although women in strenuous occupations typically decrease their level of exertion as pregnancy advances. During pregnancy, work

involving prolonged standing and lifting heavy loads are the two conditions most consistently associated with preterm delivery and infants of low birth weight (Henriksen, Savitz, Morten, & Niels, 1994; Klebanoff et al., 1990; Luke et al., 1995; Naeye & Peters, 1982; Mamelle, Bertucat, & Munoz, 1989; Mamelle, Laumon, & Lazar, 1984; Ramirez, Grimes, Annegers, Davis, & Slater, 1990; Saurel-Cubizolles & Kaminski, 1987; Teitleman, Welch, Hellenbrand, & Bracken, 1990). For example, data from a recent questionnaire survey of members of the Association of Women's Health, Obstetric, and Neonatal Nurses (AWHONN) showed that the risk of pre-term birth increased for female nurses working more than 36 hours per week, more than 10 hours per shift, and standing for 4 to 6 hours per shift (Luke et al., 1995). A recent prospective study of the relationship between occupational stress and fatigue on preterm labor in Black and White low-income multiparous women found that being able to take rest breaks when tired was associated with a significantly lower preterm delivery rate (Hickey et al., 1995).

High levels of mental and emotional stress have also been associated with preterm delivery (Lederman, 1986; Nuckolls, Cassel, & Kaplan, 1972; Wadhwa, Sandman, Porto, Dunkel-Schetter, & Garite, 1993; Willeamson, Le-Fevre, & Hector, 1989), although few studies have focused specifically on work-related stress. In their classic study of 170 women, Nuckolls and colleagues (1972) documented that women with high levels of life stress prior to and during pregnancy who also had fewer psychosocial assets experienced increased rates of pregnancy complications. In a more recent study of 513 women, Willeamson and associates (1989) also documented a significant relationship between increases in life stress in midpregnancy and neonatal complications; this relationship remained after controlling for socioeconomic status, medical risk factors, or social support. These studies failed to independently examine work-related stress. However, Mamelle and colleagues constructed a measure of occupational fatigue that included posture, work on industrial machines, physical exertion, mental stress, and work environment; preterm birth was associated with higher occupational fatigue scores, with mental stress independently associated with delivery before 37 weeks (Gabbe & Turner, in press; Mamelle, Laumon, et al., 1984; Mamelle & Munoz, 1987). Homer, James, and Siegel (1990) studied 786 young working women and found no relationship between preterm labor and occupational stress as measured by job title, but for women who did not wish to remain in the workforce, work-related stress increased the risk of poor perinatal outcomes.

Exposure to toxic substances, including chemicals and biohazards, in the workplace has also been associated with reproductive difficulties. The effect on pregnancy of various exposures varies with the time during gestation when exposure occurs as well as with the intensity and duration of exposure. In addition, current research suggests that women may be exposed to workplace hazards through transmission from their male partners (Paul, 1994). Women exposed to certain chemicals may have difficulty becoming pregnant. For example, dental workers exposed to high levels of nitrous oxide were found to have a 60% lower probability of conception in each menstrual cycle than nonexposed workers (Rowland, Baird, & Weinberg, 1992). Standards have been issued by the Occupational Safety and Health Administration (OSHA) for four substances that have potential hazardous impact on reproduction: lead, dibromochloropropane (DBCP), ethylene oxide, and ionizing radiation (Kaczmarczyk & Paul, 1996; U.S. Congress, 1998).

Health care workers, in particular, face increased exposure to harmful substances (Adler, 1989; DiBenedetto, 1995; Hellman & Gram, 1993). The practice of universal precautions and preventive care such as immunizations and handwashing can reduce the risk of exposure to biological or infectious agents (Centers for Disease Control and Prevention, 1988). Risks from exposure to anesthetic gases and antineoplastic drugs can be reduced though appropriate ventilation and following handling precautions (Cohen et al., 1974; Gabbe & Turner, in press; Kaczmarczyk & Paul, 1996; Selevan, Lindbohm, Hornung, & Hemminki, 1985; Vessey & Nunn, 1980). However, these preventive health measures are often not optimally practiced by health care personnel (Larson & Killien, 1982; Lund et al., 1994; Zimakoff, Stormark, & Larsen, 1993).

Nurse scientists' efforts in the study of reproductive outcomes associated with work is not easily identifiable; research in this area tends not to be published in the nursing literature except in review format. Within the occupational health nursing literature can be found examples of studies of the impact of pregnant workers on workplace policies, procedures, and outcomes. Mahone and Wilkinson (1985) studied work adjustments made for pregnant employees and the consequences of those adjustments for the employees and the work environment. Such research needs to be extended and repeated under current legal and social contexts for pregnant workers. Brown (1987) compared employed and nonemployed

women's health at midpregnancy; pregnant workers were distinguished from their homemaker counterparts by higher fatigue, feelings of stress, and euphoria. Women employed in occupations with greater prestige had fewer somatic symptoms, less depression, and greater well-being; women who planned to return to employment within the first postpartum year reported fewer somatic and psychological symptoms than those intending to remain at home. Fatigue during pregnancy is a symptom with potential impact on work productivity and safety. Lee and DeJoseph (1992) found that pregnant women have problems initiating and maintaining sleep, primarily due to the common pregnancy symptom of urinary frequency.

Employment Issues for Mothers of Young Children

Although the rapid increase in the employment rates of mothers is a recent phenomenon, considerable research has been conducted on employed mothers. Past research, primarily conducted within the psychology field, has largely been child centered. Such research has focused mainly on the relationship between the mother's employment status and the child's development and behavior, based on the implicit, if not explicit, assumption that maternal absence is harmful to children. More recent research has addressed the processes by which maternal employment might affect children, focusing on such mediating variables as role satisfaction, infant gender, quality of nonmaternal care, and the characteristics of maternal interaction (Gottfried, 1988; Hock, 1992; Owen & Cox, 1987; Riesch, 1984). Although few consistent differences in children have been directly attributable to maternal employment per se, many experts are reluctant to conclude that maternal employment has little relevance to children's development and continue to advocate that mothers remain at home for varying periods after birth (Belsky, 1986; Belsky & Rovine, 1988; Brazelton, 1985; Bronfenbrenner & Crouter, 1982). Rubin's (1984) suggestion that the process of maternal identity formation as distinct from that of the child does not begin until 3 months postpartum and is not stabilized until 8 to 9 months after birth is congruent with these recommendations. Such recommendations contrast with the actual decisions to return to work that mothers are making. Over half (54.6%) of women with infants under 1 year of age are employed (Herz & Wootten, 1996). Surveys document that, on the average, mothers have returned to work by 12 to 16 weeks postpartum, with up to 85% of mothers returning to work by 3 months postpartum (Brown, 1987; Killien, 1993; Mercer, 1986; Tulman & Fawcett, 1990). The majority of research on employment of women with young children has focused on individual (especially child or maternal) outcomes. Little research has occurred from a family perspective. Sund and Ostwald (1985) surveyed dual-earner parents of preschool children and found that family stress was moderate compared to national stress level norms calculated for families at a similar developmental stage. Hall (1991, 1992) compared the experiences of men and women in dual-earner families following the birth of their first child; she found that although each partner's experience was a process of redefining roles, women more than their male partners experienced role strain and placed lower priority on meeting their own needs.

Studies that have described values influencing maternal employment decisions cite financial need, the desire and commitment to work, attitudes about the maternal role, and the degree of egalitarianism in the marriage as major factors associated with maternal employment (Hall, 1987; Killien, 1993; Mercer, 1986; Owen & Cox, 1987; Tulman & Fawcett, 1990). The decision to return to work has been identified as one of the predominant concerns and sources of stress for mothers of infants (Gruis, 1977; Mercer, 1986; Walker & Best, 1991). Yet, research literature offers little knowledge on decision aids or decision outcomes for nurses who counsel women during the perinatal period regarding employment decisions.

Studies conducted from a qualitative perspective have described the process of returning to work following childbirth. Using grounded theory methodology, Hall (1987) generated a substantive theory for this process that she called the process of role definition, comprising the stages of taking on multiple roles, experiencing role strain, and reducing role strain. Recent research, using both cross-sectional and longitudinal designs, has focused on the health outcomes of women who return to work while their children are infants. Despite the common belief that physical restoration is completed by 6 weeks postpartum, women continue to experience illness episodes and symptoms during the first postpartum year; these symptoms interfere with functioning in work and family roles.

Fatigue during the childbearing period has been a particular focus of descriptive research in the past decade (Gardner, 1991; Killien & Jarrett, 1994; Milligan & Pugh, 1994; Pitzer & Hock, 1989; Poole, 1986; Tulman & Fawcett, 1988). Several longitudinal surveys have docu-

mented changes in health during the first postpartum year. Mercer (1986) conducted a longitudinal survey of 294 women from three age cohorts (teens, 20s, 30s), gathering data through structured and open-ended interviews at 1, 4, 8, and 12 months postpartum. At 4 months postpartum, 20% to 50% of women in each cohort were employed. Between two thirds and three fourths of postpartum mothers reported one or more recent illness episodes when surveyed at each measurement occasion; maternal well-being decreased at 8 months postpartum. Gardner (1991) explored fatigue at 2 days, 2 weeks, and 6 weeks postpartum among 35 healthy women. Reports of fatigue declined during the study period; employment status of participants was not reported. Tulman and Fawcett (1990) gathered questionnaire data from 92 women at 3 and 6 weeks and 3 and 6 months postpartum; 58% were employed by 6 months postpartum. By this time, many still had not returned to their usual level of energy; however, employed women were more likely to report that they had fully regained their usual level of physical energy than were nonemployed mothers. Still, 60% reported they had not yet fully resumed usual occupational activities (Tulman, Fawcett, Groblewski, & Silverman, 1990). This finding is consistent with that of Mike, McGovern, Kochevar, and Roberts (1994), who surveyed a stratified, random sample of postpartum women who had been employed during pregnancy. Among their small sample of 26 women who were at least 6 months postpartum, 82% reported one or more work or activity limitations due to feeling tired or unwell. Killien (1992) surveyed 141 employed women at 1, 4, 8, and 12 months postpartum, using questionnaires and open-ended interviews. In this sample, the highest reports of fatigue were at 1 month postpartum, with a steady decline through 12 months postpartum. A similar pattern was documented by Gjerdingen, Froberg, and Fontaine (1990), who gathered data using a mailed questionnaire from 436 recently or currently employed women at 1, 3, 6, 9, and 12 months postpartum; physical symptoms generally declined throughout the study. In each of these studies, the most common health problems during the first postpartum year are fatigue, respiratory illnesses, breast problems, and depression (Gardner, 1991; Gjerdingen, Froberg, & McGovern, 1993; Killien, 1992; Lee & DeJoseph, 1992; Mercer, 1986; Milligan & Pugh, 1994; Tulman et al., 1990).

Proposed explanations for these health problems have focused on the context of employed mother's lives: stress related to multiple role demands, infectious diseases contracted from children placed in group care settings, and increased vulnerability to illness as a result of poor health maintenance practices. For example, Gjerdingen, Froberg, and McGovern (1993) found that respiratory symptoms were experienced by more than 40% of mothers from 3 months postpartum onward; these symptoms were more frequent for women who returned to the workforce than for those who remained at home. These authors suggested that exposures in both work and child-care settings, as well as work stress, contributed to this vulnerability to infectious diseases. These illnesses were unrelated to absenteeism, however, with mothers' reported illness days greatest at 1 month postpartum and remaining stable from 3 to 12 months postpartum.

These longitudinal studies of employed women's postpartum health (Gjerdingen, Froberg, & McGovern, 1993; Killien, 1992; Tulman et al., 1990) have contributed to a better understanding of the impact of childbearing and returning to work on both maternal health and on absenteeism. Several studies were limited to surveys of women only following childbirth, but Killien's (1992) study began with prospective data collection during mid-pregnancy and continued through 12 months postpartum. From this additional data point came the findings that not only were women's symptom reports highest during pregnancy but that a subset of women could be identified who consistently reported poorer health throughout the perinatal period. Similarly, Lenz, Parks, Jenkins, and Jarrett (1986) found that illness prior to childbirth was a stronger predictor of mothers' illnesses at 6 months postpartum than was life change during the 6-month postpartum period. Such information can assist in the development of early prevention and health promotion programs.

Breast-feeding can be a major challenge for women returning to work following childbirth. Kearney and Cronenwett (1991) found that mothers who planned to work after giving birth both anticipated and experienced shorter duration of breast-feeding than those who remained at home. Ryan and Martinez (1989) examined responses from a sample of 83,985 women with 6-month-old infants from the Ross Laboratories Mothers Survey. Comparable proportions of employed and nonemployed women reported breast-feeding immediately postpartum, but employed mothers were less likely to be breast-feeding at 6 months (24.3% vs. 10%). Similarly, Piper and Parks (1996) analyzed data from a sample of 2,372 breast-feeding women who participated in the National Maternal-Infant Health Survey between 1989 and 1991; duration of breast-feeding beyond 6 months was significantly correlated with delay of return to work postpartum. In a prospective survey of employment and

duration of breast-feeding among 558 Black and 511 White women, women of both racial groups who returned to professional employment following childbirth had a longer duration of breast-feeding than women who returned to sales or technical positions (Kurinij, Shiono, Ezrine, & Rhoads, 1989). These studies suggest that continuing to breast-feed while employed is challenging, especially in positions with limited flexibility. Morse, Bottorff, and Boman (1989) documented the challenges and coping strategies working women used to manage breast-feeding and working in a sample of 61 Canadian postpartum women who were interviewed monthly by telephone. Women who were able to successfully work and breast-feed were either able to breast-feed on demand at work because of the proximity of the infant or were able to change their pattern of breast-feeding to some combination of breast and bottle feeding; few expressed breast milk at work. One of the more difficult problems identified in this study was that of leaking breasts; at 6 months postpartum, 66% of the 61 women interviewed still experienced leaking (Morse & Bottorff, 1989). Williams and Morse (1990) subsequently surveyed by telephone 100 primiparas on the process of weaning. These two studies contribute practical knowledge to assist working mothers.

Nurse scientists have studied several interventions to assist working mothers who wish to breast-feed while working. The first approach focuses on interventions that combine breast and bottle feeding. Morse, Harrison, and Prowse (1986) followed 30 mothers (including 11 who were returning to work) who implemented a program of minimal breast-feeding; the descriptive findings indicated that this is one method that may assist women to continue breast-feeding when their workplace cannot more fully accommodate their needs. Cronenwett and colleagues (1992) conducted a prospective experimental study of the effects of planned bottle use during early postpartum on breast-feeding outcomes. Women ($n = 121$) who were committed to breast-feed for at least 6 weeks were randomly assigned either to a group that avoided bottle feeding for the first 6 weeks postpartum or to a group that offered one bottle daily between 2 and 6 weeks postpartum in addition to breast-feeding. Group assignment had no effect on breast-feeding problems, achievement of breast-feeding duration goals, or breast-feeding duration of at least 6 months postpartum. Although the planned bottle group weaned somewhat earlier than the total breast-feeding group, the differences were not statistically significant. Women who returned to work by 2 months postpartum weaned faster than those who did not. A second approach has focused on anticipatory guidance and individual problem-solving. Duckett (1992) described the outcomes of an experimental study in which 50 primiparas who planned to return to work were randomly assigned to either a control group or an experimental group that received videotaped and 1:1 anticipatory guidance on breast-feeding and working as well as an opportunity to use a breast pump. Although women in the experimental group breast-fed longer, on average, than controls, the differences were not statistically significant. Additional strategies for further testing and workplace accommodations to support breast-feeding have been described by Duckett (1992) and Katcher and Lanese (1985).

The majority of recent studies of maternal employment have focused on mothers of infants, but the challenges of juggling multiple roles continues with preschool-age children. Rankin (1993) interviewed 118 mothers of preschoolers who were employed at least 30 hours per week about the stresses and rewards of their experiences. Sixty-two percent reported a high level of stress; major stresses included lack of time, child problems, and guilt. Employment among mothers of vulnerable children was the subject of a longitudinal investigation by Youngblut, Loveland-Cherry, and Horan (1993, 1994). They followed two-parent families with preterm infants from birth through 18 months postpartum and found no differences in family cohesion or adaptability related to employment status or number of hours worked by mothers. Youngblut, Singer, Madigan, and Swegart (1997) examined data from single-mother families in this same database when the infants were preschoolers. They found that birth weight was unrelated to employment status at the time of birth, to the time of returning to work postpartum, and to current employment status. However, preschoolers with employed mothers were hospitalized more often than preschoolers with nonemployed mothers, though the number of children with health problems was unrelated to mothers' employment status. The authors speculated that maternal employment might have increased the children's exposure to infectious diseases or that maternal employment might provide health care insurance coverage that influenced hospital admissions.

Despite the numerous studies describing the challenges of employed mothers of infants, very few projects have examined strategies to assist these women. One of the few is a program developed by Collins and Tiedje (1988). In a quasiexperimental study (Collins, Tiedje, & Stommel, 1992), the effects of this six-session small group intervention on the well-being of mothers who were returning to work within 6 months of their infants' births were tested. The group intervention was based on Lazarus and Folkman's (1984) stress and coping framework. At 1 year after delivery, participants in the intervention reported increased levels of marital satisfaction, parenting satisfaction, and work satisfaction; however, only the difference in marital satisfaction reached statistical significance.

Caregiving for Ill and Elderly Family Members

In 1988, slightly less than 2% (approximately 1.5 million) of the U.S. population were employed full-time and providing care to a disabled elder. Employed women were four times more likely to be caregivers than men (Stone & Stone, 1990). Brody and Schoonover (1986) compared employed and nonemployed daughters of elderly disabled widows. They found no difference in the hours of help provided by caregiving daughters based on employment status. Findings from a nationally representative sample of over 1,000 elder caregivers (Stone & Stone, 1990) indicated that 23% of caregivers had to make job accommodations (e.g., reduced hours, unpaid leave, change work schedule), and 7% quit their jobs to meet caregiving demands. About 20% of working mothers also provide elder care. Stueve and O'Donnell (1984) studied 81 working women aged 30 to 60 years old and found that variation in their own family patterns shaped how they responded to the needs of aging parents. Although employment per se made little difference in caregiving responsibilities, job characteristics such as flexibility and hours worked did affect caregiving. They also found that women were involved in caregiving for multiple elders, not just their own parents. A recent prospective study of 2,000 seriously ill adults (Covinsky et al., 1994) revealed that one third of patients required considerable caregiving from family members upon hospital discharge. In 20% of these families, a family member had to quit work or make another major life change to provide the needed home care. Subsequently, 12% of families experienced negative health effects for the caregiver, including stress-related illnesses. Krach and Brooks (1995) similarly reported that caregivers of the elderly report a variety of personal health care problems related to caregiver burden and miss an average of 8 days of work annually related to caregiving responsibilities. The stress associated with family caregiving may be especially problematic when added to caregiving that is a woman's occupational responsibility. Ross, Rideout, and Carson (1994) conducted a qualitative study of 40 nurses employed full-time who also cared for others in their private lives. Analysis of diary and interview data indicated that most participants experienced high levels of stress while also experiencing rewards from dual caregiving. McKinlay, Triant, McKinlay, Brambilla, and Ferdock (1990) found that 25% of their random sample of 2,000 midlife women cared for a parent or in-law; of these, half reported that this caregiving caused stress. Caregiving stress was significantly associated with physical symptoms, psychological symptoms, and depression. Similar findings have been reported by nurse investigators examining caregiving (England & Roberts, 1996; Phillips et al., 1995).

Although family caregiving responsibilities may increase the stress of working women, employment has been shown to protect women from negative health effects following bereavement. In a study of 157 widows 55 to 75 years old, Aber (1992) found that work history and work attitude were statistically significant predictors of women's health 2 years after the death of a spouse. The quality of the relationship between daughters and their elderly mothers was also found by Patsdaughter (Patsdaughter & Killien, 1990) to be predictive of the daughters' health status, suggesting that the stressors of caregiving are modified by relationship factors.

Home care for the elderly and chronically ill in need of long-term care is often cited to be less costly. To challenge that assumption, Ward and Brown (1994) studied 53 primary caregivers for a person with AIDS (PWA). Caregivers reported an average of 8.5 hours daily performing personal care tasks and 5 hours weekly performing household tasks. Using a market valuation method, they calculated the cost of unpaid care for one PWA as in excess of $25,000 annually. Ward's (1990) discussion of five valuation methods applied to determining the costs of kin care shows much promise for documenting the cost of women's caregiving, often devalued in policy analyses on the economics of home care. The devaluing of the unpaid caregiving of women was discussed by Angus (1994) as an ideology of separate spheres that designates paid activity in the public sphere as work and therefore valued, while unpaid activities pursued in the private sphere of the home are overlooked. Not only is this unpaid work at home a source of stress that interacts with or compounds workplace stress to affect women's health, but this work is often done to promote the health of others.

Current research in nursing is testing interventions to support families caring for ill and elderly members. Archbold (1995) pilot-tested an intervention system to increase preparedness, enrichment, and predictability in families providing care to older members. Results indicated positive responses from families and lower hospital costs, warranting future research on intervention.

Balancing Multiple Roles: Challenges and Strategies

Challenges of Balancing Work and Family

The majority of American women juggle employment responsibilities with family responsibilities; over two thirds of women in the workforce have dependent children, and others care for dependent adult family members. Women are less likely to share these responsibilities with a spouse than are men—for example, 23% of working women are single parents; only 4% of employed fathers are. Working mothers are more likely than working fathers to be employed part-time, to earn less, and to have less access to employment benefits. Both men and women agree that women carry a larger share of the responsibility for at-home work in addition to paid employment (Galinsky & Bond, 1996).

Employment has important effects on the health of women who attempt to juggle work and family responsibilities. In one widely quoted study, Haynes and Feinleib (1980) found that of women who participated in the Framingham Study, women who worked at home had the lowest incidence of heart disease, whereas women who were currently employed and those who had been employed previously had higher rates of disease. The incidence of heart disease was highest among women who were clerical workers, who were married to blue-collar husbands, and who had children, suggesting that the combination of work and family demands may lead to stress that is harmful to women's physical and emotional well-being. In a survey of 103 business and professional women with and without children, McEntee and Rankin (1983) found that more than half of the respondents reported gastrointestinal problems, fatigue, mood swings, and tension headaches; one third of the women reported sleep difficulties and musculoskeletal discomforts. In 1987, the National Institute of Mental Health (NIMH) identified the mental health effects of women's multiple roles as a priority research area (Eichler & Parron, 1987).

Meleis and colleagues (Meleis, Norbeck, & Laffrey, 1989; Meleis, Norbeck, Laffrey, Solomon, et al., 1989) proposed that the construct of role integration or balance could account for variance in health and psychological symptoms. That is, the number and constellation of roles assumed by a women are less predictive of her well-being than is the integration among the roles she enacts. A related hypothesis suggests that the conflict between women's traditional social role as wife and mother and the more contemporary role of worker contributes to stress. A traditional sex role orientation has been found to be associated with depression (Napholz, 1994; Woods, 1985). Thomas (1995) examined correlates of health outcomes among 238 midlife women employed in occupations varying in occupational prestige. Physical health was associated with perceptions of stress and locus of control. However, dimensions of marital and parental roles were stronger predictors of health than were employment variables. The least healthy women were employed in low-prestige occupations and were responsible for the care of young children; these women had the most concerns regarding their work, marital, and child-rearing roles. Role-related concerns were more salient to women's health than were role rewards. These findings correspond with those of Woods (1985), who studied young women a decade earlier. Gender differences in the experiences of stress at work and at home were documented in a Swedish study of male and female managers and clerical workers (Frankenhaeuser, Lundberg, Fredrikson, et al., 1989). Groups were similar in physiological measures of stress at work, but at home in the evening after work, females, especially female managers, had elevated catecholamine and blood pressure levels compared with their male colleagues. These responses were attributed to higher levels of stress from unpaid work, especially the responsibilities for children at home (Lundberg, 1996). The ability of women to unwind after a stressful work day may be related to the support available at home. These studies provide evidence that supports the importance of the construct of role integration and balance.

The relationship between symptomatology and impaired functioning in work and family roles remains unclear. Physical and emotional illness are believed to be associated with absenteeism, and McEntee and Rankin (1983) found that working mothers, especially those who were single, were less likely than women without children to be absent from work due to illness or to spend time in bed due to illness. The low rate of absenteeism may not be indicative of good health; as suggested by Woods (1985), women's multiple role demands and expectations may be incompatible with sick-role behavior. Such lack of self-care when ill was found to have long-term negative consequences by Berkman and Syme (1979), who observed that adults who had no illness-related absences from work during a 1-year period had a higher mortality rate in the subsequent 5 years than those adults who were absent 3 to 5 days. It may also be that the types of symptoms and illnesses experienced most often by working mothers affect the level of functioning in work and family roles but do not result in work absenteeism.

Strategies for Promoting Health

Individual self-care strategies. The focus of much research on strategies to promote working women's health is to supplement individual resistance to the effects of stress through leading a health-promoting lifestyle and enhancing individual coping. Such strategies include practices related to self-actualization, taking responsibility for one's health, exercise, nutrition, seeking and using interpersonal support, and stress management (Walker, Sechrist, & Pender, 1987). Women juggling multiple roles, especially during the first postpartum year, consistently report a lack of time for self (Gruis, 1977; Mercer, 1986). In an effort to meet family and work responsibilities, they may neglect the self-care behaviors that promote and maintain their own health (Brown & Killien, 1987; Killien & Brown, 1987). In a comparison of 148 employed women and homemakers with young infants, Walker and Best (1991) found that employed women reported less healthy lifestyles than homemakers. They suggested that employed women's lifestyles were characterized by overload and that self-neglect was a result. However, Pender, Walker, Sechrist, and Frank-Stromborg (1990) found that women employees had healthier lifestyles than did males. The physical exercise involved in daily work routines varies among occupations, with clerical workers identified as having lower levels of energy expenditure at work than other groups, such as nurses and teachers (Wilbur & Dan, 1989). These findings suggest that health promotion programs need to take into account differences in occupational activities.

Much attention has also been paid to describing and enhancing the coping behaviors used by women to modify role-related stressors. Lazarus and Folkman identified three major approaches to the conceptualization and measurement of coping, including coping as ego processes or defenses, coping as personality trait or style, and coping as situation-specific responses. The latter perspective on coping accounts for the individual's intentional efforts and contextual determinants of the coping process and has been used most often in research on coping strategies on employed women (Lazarus & Folkman, 1984). Multiple coping strategies used by employed women have been identified (Collins & Post, 1986; Hall, Williams, et al., 1985; Harrison & Minor, 1982; Skinner, 1987), but attempts to link coping strategies and women's well-being have been few. Several studies found that coping strategies such as structural role redefinition, personal role redefinition, and role expansion were not associated with life satisfaction (Hall, 1972; Harrison & Minor, 1978). However, Grey (1983) reported that coping strategies such as having time to pursue personal interests, organization and planning, increasing family sharing of household chores, and awareness of limitations were positively associated with life satisfaction; in contrast, lack of conscious strategies for meeting multiple role demands and striving to meet everyone's expectations were negatively associated with life satisfaction.

Family strategies. A consistent finding is that women assume a greater share of the burdens of balancing work and family than do men. Many voices (e.g., Hochschild, 1989) urge more egalitarian division of work and family responsibilities within the family unit, but Jordan's (1990) work suggests that there may be more partner and societal support for mothers to assume the employment role than there is for men to assume an active family role. Data from the Wisconsin Maternity Leave and Health Project, a longitudinal study of 570 women and 550 male partners, document that men holding the most egalitarian gender role attitudes took the longest leaves after their children's birth. Women who took postpartum leaves of less than six weeks duration and who had high marital concerns had the highest depression scores (Hyde, 1995; Hyde, Klein, Essex, & Clark, 1995). Gjerdingen and Chaloner's (1994) longitudinal data from 436 married, employed, postpartum mothers indicated that the women assumed primary responsibility for the majority of household and family tasks and that they perceived declines over time in their husbands' participation in these tasks. Lennon, Wasserman, and Allen (1991) found the most consistent predictor of husbands' involvement in

child care and housework was the wives' relative income; also, lower levels of husbands' participation were associated with increases in wives' depressive symptoms. Similarly, Ozer (1995) reported that a woman's belief in her capability to enlist the help of her spouse for child care was the most consistent predictor of both well-being and distress among full-time professional women.

Social support during transitions in and out of employment was the subject of a qualitative, prospective study by Harrison, Neufeld, and Kushner (1995). Women returning to work following an extended absence or retiring from full-time employment were interviewed about access and barriers to social support. These transitions often took as long as 2 years to complete, and accessing desired support was found to be difficult for some women.

Programs, policies, and environmental strategies. Workplace policies and programs can be instrumental in promoting the health of women employees. Access to health insurance is a major benefit of employment that is positively associated with indicators of women's health (Hartmann et al., 1996). Employed mothers are significantly less likely than fathers to have access to job-related health insurance; 16% of mothers, compared to 10% of fathers, had no access through their jobs. However, working mothers are no more likely than fathers to be uninsured, because more women have health coverage through their spouse's employer (Galinsky & Bond, 1996).

The workplace is increasingly being seen as a site of health promotion. Salazar and Carter (1994) interviewed 19 employed women to identify a taxonomy of issues and concerns about breast self-examination (BSE), and Salazar (1994) surveyed 52 employed women about their beliefs and behaviors related to BSE; 29% of participants were found to perform BSE. These findings were used to develop and test the effects of a workplace program to increase BSE among employees. Following participation in a cancer risk appraisal program, women's beliefs about the usefulness of early detection and intentions to engage in preventive health behaviors (e.g., mammography, BSE) significantly increased (Salazar et al., 1994).

Employers have increasingly become sensitive to the family needs of employees, and many find it beneficial for their productivity outcomes to implement family-friendly policies. Based on data from a survey of 69 companies in New York, companies with more female employees were found to have more policies and programs to accommodate caregiver needs (Warshaw, Barr, & Schachter, 1987). The size of an employer may affect the benefits available to women employees. The most notable example is the federal Family and Medical Leave Act (FMLA) of 1993, which exempts employers with fewer than 50 employees.

A 1992 survey of a random sample of men and women in the U.S. labor force, conducted by the Families and Work Institute, highlighted several important findings related to employer benefits to assist women to manage work and family stressors (Galinsky & Bond, 1996). Although women were as likely as men to be employed by FMLA-covered employers (about 50% of all employed mothers and fathers), they were less likely to meet the eligibility requirements for these benefits because they work part-time; 41% of working mothers (compared to 49% of working fathers) were covered by FMLA benefits. This survey also documented the effects of home-to-work spillover of stress. Employed women were significantly more likely than men to report that they were distracted and less productive at work due to worries about children or family. Employed mothers were twice as likely as employed fathers to be absent from work to care for a sick child (0.64 days in the past 3 months compared to 0.29 days). However, few employers provided on-site child care, sick-child care, or other child care benefits to address these concerns. The average employed parent paid 8.5% of his or her annual household income for child care; federal or employer assistance was available for fewer than 5% of working parents. This same survey indicated that lower job burnout for women was associated with better policies for leave and dependent care benefits, more control over work schedules, a more supportive work environment, and more opportunities for advancement (Galinsky et al., 1996). The promotion of women's health will involve activism in the selection of benefits packages that address the unique needs of women workers (Conway-Welch et al., 1997).

Corporate practices have been found to directly influence individual health and safety. A recent study by the Minnesota Nurses Association (MNA) found a positive relationship between reductions in nursing staff in hospitals in the state and the incidence of workplace injury and illness among registered nurses (Canavan, 1996). OSHA logs from health care facilities showed a 65.2% increase in injuries for nurses between 1990 and 1994; this corresponded to a 10.2% decrease in the number of RN positions and a 19.3% increase in RN FTEs to

patient days. These data were used to add health promotion measures into MNA-negotiated contracts.

Recommendations for Advancing Nursing Science

Research in the past decade has contributed greatly to our understanding of women's health as it intersects with employment and other critical dimensions of their lives. The primary focus of this past research has been to describe the nature of women's work, to compare health status of women workers to nonemployed women and to working men, and to identify areas in which women are vulnerable to health problems because of their employment.

What emerges from this research, taken as a whole, is that work per se presents no particular risk to women's health and is more likely a resource that promotes women's health. However, certain occupations, work environments, work tasks, or combinations of contextual factors present risks for some or all women exposed to them. We have an emerging understanding of these conditions, but research to date has typically failed to sufficiently incorporate the complexity of work and family variables in study measures and designs to generate promising interventions for promoting, maintaining, or restoring health to working women. There is a paucity of research to guide interventions to improve the health of employed women at the individual, group, worksite, or policy level. The majority of research, in nursing and other disciplines, has been descriptive or factor-relating in nature, using either small, selective samples or large, population-based samples. This research has identified variables associated with both health-promoting and health-damaging consequences for employed women. However, studies that incorporate these variables into intervention and outcomes studies are rare. It is in this area that nurse scientists, in partnership with scientists from other disciplines, can make major contributions in the coming years. The unique perspective of nurse scientists, with their focus on developing clinical therapeutics to promote human health, is likely to place nursing research at the forefront of this endeavor in the decades to come. Nurse scientists are at the forefront of efforts to link the

perspectives and findings of occupational health research, women's health research, and family health research. Additionally, the efficacy of individual, family,
workplace, and policy strategies in relation to health outcomes is of particular importance to nursing science, as
it is likely that these will be the basis for interventions
with individuals to promote positive health outcomes.

This chapter began with a description of recent
changes in the female workforce; projected future
changes will also influence important areas for consideration by nurse scientists. Women will continue to enter
the labor force and gender segregation of occupations
will likely disappear, especially in those occupations traditionally dominated by men. We could expect disparity
in pay, non-opportunities for advancement, and sexual
harassment to dissipate also. It is anticipated that the
workforce will exhibit more age and ethnic diversity
(Walcott-McQuigg, 1994). As mandatory retirement
policies evaporate, economic needs increase, and the
population ages, the average age of workers will increase.
These changes will have implications for common health
concerns of women in the workplace. For example, management of chronic conditions and the benefits of programs such as flexible work schedules will be of increasing importance.

In 1982, Haw reviewed the literature on women,
work, and stress and suggested an agenda for future research. Among her recommendations were that future
research should include (a) longitudinal studies of
women's experiences before, during, and after cessation
of employment, (b) specificity in measurement of job
environment and family responsibilities, (c) measurement of the length and continuity of exposure to potentially stressful and hazardous conditions, and (d) examination of individual perceptions of and coping responses
to stress. Evident from this review of research on women,
work, and health is that although some progress has been
made in implementing these recommendations, much remains to be done. Future research must emerge from new
conceptual frameworks, use more strategic methodologies, and be targeted toward those conditions, populations, and questions most in need of new knowledge to
promote women's health.

Existing research clearly illustrates that neither a
health-risk nor a health-benefits perspective has been
adequate in answering questions related to women and
work. Future research needs to be guided by more complex and holistic frameworks that account for the full

complexity of women's lives. Such research would not
be limited to examining only women's lives as workers
without acknowledging the complex interconnections
between work and nonwork (e.g., family) influences on
health, as well as the contextual factors in the environment (Barnett, 1996). The next phase of research on work
and women needs to focus on these questions: Under
what specific environments and conditions are women
placed at risk for health problems? Which environments
are most beneficial for health? Which groups or communities of women are particularly vulnerable to work-
associated health problems or benefits? What interventions
are the most efficacious in promoting the health of women
workers? Despite a massive literature that describes the
experiences of women workers, specific risk and protective factors for various health conditions have not been
sufficiently identified to guide the development of interventions to promote health. Research is needed that focuses on groups of women that have been underrepresented or unidentified in the past, especially minority
women, older women, and women with fewer socioeconomic resources. In addition to studying special health
issues for occupational groups in which the largest numbers of women are represented, it will be important to
identify areas of concern in occupations in which women
were previously underrepresented. In these occupations,
existing equipment, environments, and policies may
place women at particular risk for injury or negative
health consequences. One example of such research is
that of studies of women in the military (Committee on
Military Nursing Research, 1996; Poth, 1997; Wahl &
Randall, 1996).

Various units of analysis will need to be employed
in the future. Most research to date on women, work, and
health considers the individual as the principal unit of
analysis. Yet family and organizational outcomes are
equally important to consider in the future. Our knowledge would be extended if variables were more exqui-
sitely conceptualized and measured. For example, work
needs to be considered as a more complex variable, considering the research question that is the focus of the
particular study. Such consideration would mean, for example, that a respondent is categorized not just as employed (yes/no), but that data are gathered on the number
and pattern of work hours, including the shift worked.
This will become even more important as flexible work
options become more prevalent. The nature of work demands may need to be described and measured more

fully than can be represented merely by job title. Similarly, family must be conceptualized and measured as more than the variables of married and/or parent. For example, work and family balance issues might vary with the developmental stage of a child or the women or as a combination of a woman's stage of career development and the family's stage of development. Women in varying family constellations (e.g., lesbian families) need to be represented in research rather than excluded or inappropriately categorized as single or not married.

The need for research that evaluates preventive and health promotion strategies is critical. In this research, a variety of outcomes should be measured. Individual health outcomes such as physical and emotional symptoms continue to be important outcomes for study. However, the focus on women's reproductive health must be extended to other areas of concern for women's health, including cardiovascular health, cancer, and emotional well-being. In addition, indicators of the impact of health on the ability to function in work and family roles should be considered. Family outcomes to be considered include indicators of family relationship quality, such as marital and parenting quality. Organizational outcomes might include measures of productivity and cost/benefit analysis of workplace policies and programs.

Consideration needs to be given to the interpretation and dissemination of results. In the past, research findings from studies using samples of working women have frequently been based on the experiences of White, middle-class working women but generalized to all women workers. These findings may not be useful or applicable for the workforce of the future. A critical challenge will be the framing and interpretation of research results in a way to effectively inform policy makers.

Summary

Women will continue to work, both in home and employment settings. As these environments change, both in biophysical and sociocultural dimensions, women's health will be affected. The challenge for nursing science is not only to continue to identify characteristics of women workers and critical dimensions of their environments and their relationship to women's health but also to bring our disciplinary perspective on concern about human health to the development of effective clinical interventions to promote health.

References

Aber, C. S. (1992). Spousal death, a threat to women's health: Paid work as a "resistance resource." *Image: The Journal of Nursing Scholarship, 24*(2), 95-99.

Adler, S. P. (1989). Cytomegalovirus and child day care: Evidence for an increased infection rate among day care workers. *New England Journal of Medicine, 321,* 1290-1296.

Angus, J. (1994). Women's paid/unpaid work and health: Exploring the social context of everyday life. *Canadian Journal of Nursing Research, 26*(4), 23-42.

Archbold, P. (1995). The PREP system of nursing interventions: A pilot test with families caring for older members. *Research in Nursing and Health, 18,* 3-16.

Baird, C. L., Bensko, N. L., Bell, P. A., Viney, W., & Woody, W. D. (1995). Gender influence on perceptions of hostile environment sexual harassment. *Psychological Reports, 77*(1), 79-82.

Barnett, R. C. (1996). *Toward a review of the work/family literature: Work in progress.* Wellesley, MA: Wellesley Center for Research on Women.

Barnett, R. C., Marshall, N. L., & Singer, J. D. (1992). Job experiences over time, multiple roles, and women's mental health: A longitudinal study. *Journal of Personality and Social Psychology, 62*(4), 634-644.

Bell, C. A. (1991). Female homicides in United States workplaces, 1980-1985. *American Journal of Public Health, 81*(6), 729-732.

Belsky, J. (1986). Infant day care: A cause for concern? *Zero to three: Bulletin of the National Center for Clinical Infant Programs, 6*(5), 1-7.

Belsky, J., & Rovine, M. J. (1988). Nonmaternal care in the first year of life and the security of infant-parent attachment. *Child Development, 59*(1), 157-167.

Berkman, L. F., & Syme, L. (1979). Social networks, host resistance, and mortality: A nine-year followup study of Alameda County residents. *American Journal of Epidemiology, 109,* 186-204.

Berkowitz, G. S. (1981). An epidemiologic study of preterm delivery. *American Journal of Epidemiology, 113,* 81-92.

Berkowitz, G. S., Kelsey, J. L., Holford, T. R., & Berkowitz, R. L. (1983). Physical activity and the risk of spontaneous preterm delivery. *Journal of Reproductive Medicine, 28,* 581-588.

Billings, A. G., & Moos, R. H. (1982). Social support and functioning among community and clinical groups: A panel model. *Journal of Behavioral Medicine, 5*(3), 295-311.

Brazelton, T. B. (1985). *Working and caring.* Reading, MA: Addison Wesley.

Brody, E. M., & Schoonover, C. (1986). Patterns of parent-care when adult daughters work and when they do not. *Gerontologist, 26,* 372-381.

Bronfenbrenner, U., & Crouter, A. C. (1982). Work and family through time and space. In S. G. Kamerman & C. D. Hayes (Eds.),

Families that work: Children in a changing world (pp. 39-84). Washington, DC: National Academy Press.

Brown, M. A. (1987). Employment during pregnancy: Influences on health and social support. *Health Care for Women International, 8*(2), 151-168.

Brown, M. A., & Killien, M. G. (1987). Coping with daily hassles: Influence of women's roles [Abstract]. *Communicating Nursing Research, 20,* 117.

Brown, M. A., & Woods, N. F. (1986). Sex role orientation, sex typing, occupational traditionalism, and perimenstrual symptoms. In V. L. Olsen & N. F. Woods (Eds.), *Culture, society, and menstruation* (pp. 25-38). Washington, DC: Hemisphere.

Canavan, K. (1996). Minnesota study supports link between hospital downsizing and workplace injury/illness. *American Nurse,* 15.

Capell, P. (1995). The stress of relocating. *American Demographics, 17,* 15-16.

Carson, R. (1993). Proper health management can reduce cumulative trauma disorder incidence. *Occupational Health and Safety, 62*(12), 41-44.

Centers for Disease Control and Prevention. (1988). Update: Universal precautions for prevention of transmission of human immunodeficiency virus, hepatitis B virus, and other blood-borne pathogens in health care settings. *Morbidity and Mortality Weekly Report, 337,* 377-388.

Cohen, E., Brown, B., Bruce, D., Cascorbi, H., Corbett, T., Jones, T., & Whitcher, C. (1974). Occupational disease among operating room personnel: A national study. *Anesthesiology, 41,* 321-340.

Collins, C., & Post, L. (1986). An instrument to measure coping responses in employed mothers: Preliminary results. *Research in Nursing and Health, 9,* 309-316.

Collins, C., & Tiedje, L. B. (1988). A program for women returning to work after childbirth. *Journal of Obstetric, Gynecologic, and Neonatal Nursing, 17*(4), 246-253.

Collins, C., Tiedje, L. B., & Stommel, M. (1992). Promoting positive well-being in employed mothers: A pilot study. *Health Care for Women International, 13*(1), 77-85.

Committee on Military Nursing Research. (1996). *The program for research in military nursing: Progress and future direction.* Washington, DC: National Academy Press.

Conway-Welch, C., Fogel, C., Holm, K., Killien, M., Marion, L., McBride, A. B., Shaver, J., Simms, L., Swanson, K., Taylor, D., & Woods, N. (1997). Women's health and women's health care: Recommendations of the 1996 AAN Expert Panel on Women's Health. *Nursing Outlook, 45*(1), 7-15.

Costello, C., Stone, A. J., & Dooley, B. (1994). *The American woman, 1994-95, where we stand: Women and health.* New York: W. W. Norton.

Covinsky, K., Goldman, L., Cook, E., Oye, R., Desbiens, N., Reding, D., Fulkerson, W., Connors, A., Lynn, J., & Phillips, R. (1994). The impact of serious illness on patients' families. *Journal of the American Medical Association, 272,* 1839-1844.

Cronenwett, L., Stukel, T., Kearney, M. H., Barrett, J., Covington, C., DelMonte, K., Reinhardt, R., & Rippe, L. (1992). Single daily bottle use in the early weeks postpartum and breastfeeding outcomes. *Pediatrics, 90*(5), 760-766.

Cummings, D., & Rebar, R. (1993). Exercise and reproductive function in women. *American Journal of Industrial Medicine, 4,* 113-125.

Dannenberg, A. L., Baker, S. P., & Li, G. (1994). Intentional and unintentional injuries in women: An overview. *Annals of Epidemiology, 4*(2), 133-139.

Dear, J. A. (1995, November 1). Work stress and health '95. *Vital Speeches of the Day, 62,* 39-42.

DiBenedetto, D. V. (1995). Occupational hazards of the health care industry: Protecting health care workers. *American Association of Occupational Health Nurses Journal, 43*(3), 131-137.

Duckett, L. (1992). Maternal employment and breastfeeding. *NAACOG's Clinical Issues in Perinatal and Women's Health, 3*(4).

Eichler, A., & Parron, D. L. (1987). *Women's mental health: Agenda for research.* Rockville, MD: National Institute of Mental Health.

England, M., & Roberts, B. (1996). Theoretical and psychometric analysis of caregiver strain. *Research in Nursing and Health, 19,* 499-510.

English, C., Maclaren, W., Court-Brown, C., Hughes, S., Porter, R., Wallace, W., Graves, R., Pethick, A., & Soutar, C. (1995). Relation between upper limb soft tissue disorders and repetitive movements at work. *American Journal of Industrial Medicine, 27*(1), 75-90.

Felton, J. S. (1993). Occupational violence: An intensified work concomitant. *OEM Report, 7*(12), 101-103.

Ferketich, S. L., & Mercer, R. T. (1989). Men's health status during pregnancy and early fatherhood. *Research in Nursing and Health, 12*(3), 137-148.

Fitzgerald, L. F. (1993). Sexual harassment: Violence against women in the workplace. *American Psychologist, 48*(10), 1070-1076.

Florack, E., Zielhuis, G., & Rolland, R. (1994). The influence of occupational physical activity on the menstrual cycle and fecundability. *Epidemiology, 5*(1), 14-18.

Frankenhaeuser, M., Lundberg, U., & Chesney, M. (1991). *Women, work, and health: Stress and opportunities.* New York: Plenum.

Frankenhaeuser, M., Lundberg, U., Fredrikson, M., Melin, B., Tuomisto, M., Myrsten, A., Hedman, M., Bergman-Losman, B., & Wallin, L. (1989). Stress on and off the job as related to sex and occupational status in White-collar workers. *Journal of Organizational Behavior, 10,* 321-346.

Fransson-Hall, C., Bystrom, S., & Kilbom, A. (1995). Self-reported physical exposure and musculoskeletal symptoms of the forearm-hand among automobile assembly-line workers. *Journal of Occupational Medicine, 37*(9), 1136-1144.

Freda, M. C. (1994). Childbearing, reproductive control, aging women, and health care: The projected ethical debates. *Journal of Obstetric, Gynecologic and Neonatal Nursing, 23*(2), 144-152.

Froberg, D., Gjerdingen, D. K., & Preston, M. (1986). Multiple roles and women's mental and physician health: What have we learned? *Women and Health Review, 11*(2), 79-96.

Gabbe, S. G., & Turner, L. P. (in press). Reproductive hazards of the American lifestyle: Work during pregnancy. *American Journal of Obstetrics and Gynecology.*

Galinsky, E., & Bond, J. (1996). Work and family: The experiences of mothers and fathers in the U.S. labor force. In C. Costello, B. Krimgold, & B. Dooley (Eds.), *The American woman, 1996-97, where we stand: Women and work* (pp. 79-103). New York: W. W. Norton.

Gardner, D. L. (1991). Fatigue in postpartum women. *Applied Nursing Research, 4*(2), 57-62.

Garrison, R., & Eaton, W. W. (1992). Secretaries, depression and absenteeism. *Women & Health, 18*(4), 53-76.

Gjerdingen, D. K., & Chaloner, K. (1994). Mothers' experience with household roles and social support during the first postpartum year. *Women & Health, 21*(4), 57-74.

Gjerdingen, D. K., Froberg, D. G., & Fontaine, P. (1990). A causal model describing the relationship of women's postpartum health to social support, length of leave, and complications of childbirth. *Women & Health, 16*(2), 71-87.

Gjerdingen, D. K., Froberg, D. G., & Fontaine, P. (1991). The effects of social support on women's health during pregnancy, labor and delivery, and the postpartum period. *Family Medicine, 23*(5), 370-375.

Gjerdingen, D. K., Froberg, D. G., & McGovern, P. M. (1993). Changes in women's physical health during the first postpartum year. *Archives of Family Medicine, 2*(3), 277-283.

Gold, D., Rogacz, S., Bock, N., Tosteson, T., Baum, T., Speizer, F., & Czeisler, C. (1992). Rotating shift work, sleep, and accidents related to sleepiness in hospital nurses. *American Journal of Public Health, 82,* 1011-1014.

Gordon, N. P., Cleary, P. D., Parker, C. E., & Czeisler, C. A. (1986). The prevalence and health impact of shiftwork. *American Journal of Public Health, 76*(10), 1225-1228.

Gottfried, A. (1988). *Maternal employment and children's development: Longitudinal research.* New York: Plenum.

Grey, J. D. (1983). The married professional woman: An examination of her role conflicts and coping strategies. *Psychology of Women Quarterly, 7*(3), 235-243.

Griffith, J. W. (1983). Women's stressors according to age groups: Part 1. *Issues in the Health Care of Women, 6,* 311-326.

Gruis, M. (1977). Beyond maternity: Postpartum concerns of mothers. *MCN: The American Journal of Maternal/Child Nursing, 2*(3), 182-188.

Gutek, B. A., & Koss, M. P. (1993). Effects of sexual harassment on women and organizations. *Occupational Medicine, 8*(4), 807-819.

Hall, D. (1972). A model of coping with role conflict: The role behavior of college-educated women. *Administrative Science Quarterly, 7,* 471-486.

Hall, J. M., Stevens, P. E., & Meleis, A. I. (1992a). Experiences of women clerical workers in patient care areas. *Journal of Nursing Administration, 22*(5), 11-17.

Hall, J. M., Stevens, P. E., & Meleis, A. I. (1992b). Developing the construct of role integration: A narrative analysis of women clerical workers' daily lives. *Research in Nursing and Health, 15*(6), 447-457.

Hall, L. A., Williams, C. A., & Greenberg, R. S. (1985). Supports, stressors, and depressive symptoms in low-income mothers of young children. *American Journal of Public Health, 75*(5), 518-522.

Hall, W. (1987). The experience of women returning to work following the birth of their first child. *Midwifery, 8,* 187-195.

Hall, W. (1991). The experience of fathers in dual-earner families following the births of their first infants. *Journal of Advanced Nursing, 16*(4), 423-430.

Hall, W. (1992). Comparison of the experience of women and men in dual-earner families following the birth of their first infant. *Image: The Journal of Nursing Scholarship, 24*(1), 33-37.

Harrison, A. O., & Minor, J. H. (1978). Interrole conflict, coping strategies, and satisfaction among Black working wives. *Journal of Marriage and the Family, 40*(4), 799-805.

Harrison, A. O., & Minor, J. H. (1982). Interrole conflict, coping strategies, and role satisfaction among single and married employed mothers. *Psychology of Women Quarterly, 6*(3), 354-360.

Harrison, M. J., Neufeld, A., & Kushner, K. (1995). Women in transition: Access and barriers to social support. *Journal of Advanced Nursing, 21*(5), 858-864.

Hartmann, H., Kuriansky, J., & Owens, C. (1996). Employment and women's health. In M. Falik & K. Collins (Eds.), *Women's health: The Commonwealth Fund Survey* (pp. 296-323). Baltimore: Johns Hopkins University Press.

Haw, M. A. (1982). Women, work and stress: A review and agenda for the future. *Journal of Health and Social Behavior, 23*(2), 132-144.

Haynes, S. G., & Feinleib, M. (1980). Women, work and coronary heart disease: Prospective findings from the Framingham heart study. *American Journal of Public Health, 70*(2), 133-141.

Hellman, S. L., & Gram, M. C. (1993). The resurgence of tuberculosis: Risk in health care settings. *American Association of Occupational Health Nurses Journal, 40*(2), 66-72.

Henning, R., Sauter, S., Salvendy, G., & Krieg, C. (1989). Microbreak length, performance, and stress in a data entry task. *Ergonomics, 32,* 855-864.

Henriksen, T. B., Savitz, D., Morten, H., & Niels, J. S. (1994). Employment during pregnancy in relation to risk factors and pregnancy outcome. *British Journal of Obstetrics and Gynaecology, 101,* 858-865.

Herz, D., & Wootton, B. (1996). Women in the workforce: An overview. In C. Costello, B. Krimgold, & B. Dooley (Eds.), *The American woman, 1996-97, where we stand: Women and work* (pp. 44-78). New York: W. W. Norton.

Hibbard, J. H., & Pope, C. R. (1992). Women's employment, social support, and mortality. *Women and Health, 18*(1), 119-133.

Hibbard, J. H., & Pope, C. R. (1993). The quality of social roles as predictors of morbidity and mortality. *Social Science and Medicine, 36*(3), 217-225.

Hickey, C. A., Cliver, S. P., Mulvihill, F. X., McNeal, S. F., Hoffman, H. J., & Goldenberg, R. L. (1995). Employment-related stress and preterm delivery: A contextual examination. *Public Health Reports, 110*(4), 410-418.

Hochschild, A. R. (1989). *The second shift: Working parents and the revolution at home.* New York: Viking.

Hock, E. (1992). Maternal separation anxiety: Its developmental course and relation to maternal mental health. *Journal of Marriage and the Family, 63*(1), 93-102.

Homer, C., James, S., & Siegel, E. (1990). Work-related psychosocial stress and risk of preterm, low birthweight delivery. *American Journal of Public Health, 80,* 173-177.

Hyde, J. S. (1995). Women and maternity leave: Empirical data and public policy. *Psychology of Women Quarterly, 19*(3), 299-314.

Hyde, J. S., Klein, M. H., Essex, M. J., & Clark, R. (1995). Maternity leave and women's mental health. *Psychology of Women Quarterly, 19*(2), 257-286.

Institute of Medicine. (1995). *Nursing, health and the environment: Strengthening the relationship to improve the public's health.* Washington, DC: National Academy Press.

Jenkins, E. L., Layne, L. A., & Kisner, S. M. (1992). Homicide in the workplace: The U.S. experience, 1980-1988. *American Association of Occupational Health Nurses Journal, 40*(5), 215-218.

Jennings, S., Mmazaik, C., & McKinlay, S. (1984). Women and work: An investigation of the association between health and employment status in middle-aged women. *Social Science and Medicine, 19,* 423-431.

Jordan, P. L. (1990). Laboring for relevance: Expectant and new fatherhood. *Nursing Research, 39*(1), 11-16.

Kaczmarczyk, J. M., & Paul, M. E. (1996). Reproductive health hazards in the workplace: Guidelines for policy development and implementation. *International Journal of Occupational and Environmental Health, 2*(1), 48-57.

Katcher, A., & Lanese, M. (1985). Breast-feeding by employed mothers: A reasonable accommodation in the workplace. *Pediatrics, 75*(4), 644-647.

Kawachi, I., Colditz, G., Stampfer, M., Willett, W., Manson, J., Speizer, F., & Hennekens, C. (1995). Prospective study of shift work and risk of coronary heart disease in women. *Circulation, 92*(11), 3178-3182.

Kearney, M. H., & Cronenwett, L. (1991). Breastfeeding and employment. *Journal of Obstetric, Gynecologic, and Neonatal Nursing, 20*(6), 471-480.

Killien, M. (1992). Transitions in the well-being of working mothers. [Abstract]. *Communicating Nursing Research, 25.*

Killien, M., & Brown, M. A. (1987). Work and family roles of women: Sources of stress and coping strategies. *Health Care for Women International, 8*(2/3), 169-184.

Killien, M., & Jarrett, M. (1994). Predictors of postpartum fatigue. [Abstract]. *Communicating Nursing Research, 27*, 287.

Killien, M. G. (1990). Working during pregnancy: Psychological stressor or asset? *NAACOG's Clinical Issues in Perinatal and Women's Health, 1*(3), 325-332.

Killien, M. G. (1993). Returning to work after childbirth: Considerations for health policy. *Nursing Outlook, 41*(2), 73-78.

Klebanoff, M., Shiono, P., & Carey, J. (1990). The effect of physical activity during pregnancy on preterm delivery and birth weight. *American Journal of Obstetrics and Gynecology, 163*, 1450-1456.

Komaromy, M., Bindman, A. B., Haber, R. J., & Sande, M. A. (1993). Sexual harassment in medical training. *New England Journal of Medicine, 328*(5), 322-326.

Krach, P., & Brooks, J. A. (1995). Identifying the responsibilities and needs of working adults who are primary caregivers. *Journal of Gerontological Nursing, 21*(10), 41-50.

Kurinij, N., Shiono, P. H., Ezrine, S. F., & Rhoads, G. G. (1989). Does maternal employment affect breast-feeding? *American Journal of Public Health, 79*(9), 1247-1250.

Lambert, C. E., & Lambert, V. A. (1987). Hardiness: Its development and relevance to nursing. *Image: The Journal of Nursing Scholarship, 19*(2), 92-95.

Larson, E., & Killien, M. (1982). Factors influencing handwashing behavior of patient care personnel. *American Journal of Infection Control, 10*, 93-99.

Launer, L., Villar, J., Kestler, E., & De Onis, M. (1990). The effect of maternal work on fetal growth and duration of pregnancy: A prospective study. *British Journal of Obstetrics and Gynaecology, 97*, 62-70.

Lazarus, R., & Folkman, S. (1984). *Stress, appraisal and coping.* New York: Springer.

Lederman, R. (1986). Maternal anxiety in pregnancy: Relationship to fetal and newborn health status. *Annual Review of Nursing Research, 4*, 3-20.

Lee, K. A. (1992). Self-reported sleep disturbances in employed women. *Sleep, 15*(6), 493-498.

Lee, K. A., & DeJoseph, J. F. (1992). Sleep disturbances, vitality, and fatigue among a select group of employed childbearing women. *Birth, 19*(4), 208-213.

Lee, K. A., & Rittenhouse, C. A. (1992a). Health and perimenstrual symptoms: Health outcomes for employed women who experience perimenstrual symptoms. *Women & Health, 19*(1), 65-78.

Lee, K. A., & Rittenhouse, C. A. (1991b). Prevalence of perimenstrual symptoms in employed women. *Women & Health, 17*(3), 17-32.

Lennon, M. C., Wasserman, G. A., & Allen, R. (1991). Infant care and wives' depressive symptoms. *Women & Health, 17*(2), 1-23.

Lenz, E. R., Parks, P. L., Jenkins, L. S., & Jarrett, G. E. (1986). Life change and instrumental support as predictors of illness in mothers of 6-month-olds. *Research in Nursing and Health, 9*, 17-24.

Levin, P. F., Hewitt, J. B., & Misner, S. T. (1992). Female workplace homicides: An integrative research review. *American Association of Occupational Health Nurses Journal, 40*(5), 229-236.

Luke, B., Memelle, N., Keith, L., Monuz, F., Minogue, J., Papiernik, E., & Johnson, T. (1995). The association between occupational factors and preterm birth: A United States nurses' study. *American Journal of Obstetrics and Gynecology, 173*, 849-862.

Lund, S., Jackson, J., Leggett, J., Hales, L., Dworkin, R., & Gilbert, D. (1994). Reality of glove use and handwashing in a community hospital. *American Journal of Infection Control, 22*(6), 352-257.

Lundberg, U. (1996). Influence of paid and unpaid work on psychophysiological stress responses of men and women. *Journal of Occupational Health Psychology, 1*(2), 117-130.

Lusk, S. L. (1992). Violence in the workplace. *American Association of Occupational Health Nurses Journal, 40*(5), 212-213.

Lusk, S. L. (1997). Workers and worker populations. In M. K. Salazar (Ed.), *Core curriculum for occupational health nursing.* Philadelphia: W. B. Saunders.

Mahone, M. E., & Wilkinson, W. E. (1985). Women, work and pregnancy: Implications for occupational health nursing. *Occupational Health Nursing, 33*(7), 343-348.

Mamelle, N., Bertucat, I., & Munoz, F. (1989). Rest periods to prevent preterm birth? *Paedia Perinatal Epidemiology, 3*, 19-28.

Mamelle, N., Laumon, B., & Lazar, P. (1984). Prematurity and occupational activity during pregnancy. *American Journal of Epidemiology, 119*, 309-322.

Mamelle, N., & Munoz, F. (1987). Occupational working conditions and preterm birth: A reliable scoring system. *American Journal of Epidemiology, 126*, 150-152.

Marbury, J., Linn, S., Monson, R., Wegman, D., Schoenbaum, S., Stubblefield, P., & Ryan, K. (1984). Work and pregnancy. *Journal of Occupational Medicine, 26*, 415-421.

Martocchio, J., & O'Leary, A. (1997). Sex differences in occupational stress: A meta-analytic review. *Applied Psychology, 74*, 495-501.

McBride, A. B. (1990). Mental health effects of women's multiple roles. *American Psychologist, 45*(3), 381-384.

McEntee, M. A., & Rankin, D. S. (1983). Multiple role demands, mind-body distress disorders, and illness-related absenteeism among business and professional women. *Issues in Mental Health Nursing, 4*, 177-190.

McKinlay, S. M., Triant, R. S., McKinlay, J. B., Brambilla, D. J., & Ferdock, M. (1990). Multiple roles for middle-aged women and their impact on health. In M. G. Ory & H. R. Warner (Eds.), *Gender, health and longevity: Multidisciplinary perspectives* (pp. 119-136). New York: Springer.

Meisenhelder, J. B. (1986). Self-esteem in women: The influence of employment and perception of husband's appraisals. *Image: The Journal of Nursing Scholarship, 18*(1), 8-14.

Meleis, A. I., Messias, D. K., & Arruda, E. N. (1996). Women's work environment and health: Clerical workers in Brazil. *Research in Nursing and Health, 19*(1), 53-62.

Meleis, A., Norbeck, J. S., & Laffrey, S. C. (1989). Role integration and health among female clerical workers. *Research in Nursing and Health, 12*(6), 335-364.

Meleis, A. I., Norbeck, J. S., Laffrey, S., Solomon, M., & Miller, L. (1989). Stress, satisfaction, and coping: A study of women clerical workers. *Health Care for Women International, 10*(4), 319-334.

Mercer, R. T. (1986). *First-time motherhood: Experiences from teens to forties.* New York: Springer.

Meyer, B., & Daling, B. (1985). Activity level of mother's usual occupation and low infant birth weight. *Journal of Occupational Medicine, 27*, 841-847.

Mike, D., McGovern, P., Kochevar, L., & Roberts, C. (1994). Role function and mental health in postpartum working women: a pilot study. *American Association of Occupational Health Nurses Journal, 42*(5), 214-229.

Milligan, R. A., & Pugh, L. C. (1994). Fatigue during the childbearing period. *Annual Review of Nursing Research, 12*, 33-49.

Misner, S. T., Levin, P. F., & Hewitt, J. B. (1993). Occupational issues in women's health. In B. McElmurry & R. Parker (Eds.), *Annual review of women's health* (pp. 31-65). New York: National League for Nursing Press.

Moos, R. H. (1980). *Work Environment Scale manual.* Palo Alto, CA: Consulting Psychologists Press.

Moos, R. H., Fenn, C. B., & Billings, A. G. (1988). Life stressors and social resources: An integrated assessment approach. *Social Science and Medicine, 27*(9), 999-1002.

Morse, J. M., & Bottorff, J. L. (1989). Leaking: A problem of lactation. *Journal of Nurse Midwifery, 34,* 15-20.

Morse, J. M., Bottorff, J. L., & Boman, J. (1989). Patterns of breast-feeding and work: The Canadian experience. *Canadian Journal of Public Health, 80*(3), 182-188.

Morse, J. M., Harrison, M. J., & Prowse, M. (1986). Minimal breast-feeding. *Journal of Obstetric, Gynecologic, and Neonatal Nursing, 15*(4), 333-338.

Moss, N., & Carver, K. (1993). Pregnant women at work: Sociodemographic perspectives. *American Journal of Industrial Medicine, 23,* 541-557.

Murphy, S. A., Beaton, R. D., Cain, K. C., & Pike, K. C. (1994). Gender differences in fire fighter job stressors and symptoms of stress. *Women & Health, 22*(2), 55-69.

Naeye, R., & Peters, E. (1982). Work during pregnancy: Effects on the fetus. *Pediatrics, 69,* 724-727.

Napholz, L. (1994). Indices of psychological well-being and sex role orientation among working women. *Health Care for Women International, 15*(4), 307-316.

Nathanson, C. (1980). Social roles and health status among women: The significance of employment. *Social Science and Medicine, 14A,* 463-471.

National Association of Working Women. (1984). *The 9 to 5 national survey on women and stress.* Cleveland, OH: Author.

National Institute for Occupational Safety and Health. (1996). *National occupational research agenda.* Atlanta: U.S. Department of Health and Human Services.

Norvell, N., Hills, H., & Murrin, M. (1993). Understanding stress in female and male law enforcement officers. *Psychology of Women Quarterly, 17,* 289-301.

Nuckolls, K., Cassel, J., & Kaplan, B. (1972). Psychosocial assets, life crises and the prognosis of pregnancy. *American Journal of Epidemiology, 95,* 431-441.

O'Rourke, M. W. (1983). Subjective appraisal of psychological well-being and self-reports of menstrual and nonmenstrual symptomatology in employed women. *Nursing Research, 32*(5), 288-292.

Owen, M. T., & Cox, M. J. (1987). Maternal employment and the transition to parenthood. In A. E. Gottfried & A. W. Gottfied (Eds.), *Maternal employment and children's development: Longitudinal research.* New York: Plenum.

Ozer, E. M. (1995). The impact of childcare responsibility and self-efficacy on the psychological health of professional working mothers. *Psychology of Women Quarterly, 19*(3), 315-336.

Patsdaughter, C. A., & Killien, M. (1990). Developmental transitions in adulthood: Mother-daughter relationships. *Holistic Nursing Practice, 4*(3), 37-46.

Paul, M. E. (1994). Disorders of reproduction. *Occupational Health, 21*(2), 367-385.

Pender, N. J., Walker, S. N., Sechrist, K. R., & Frank-Stromborg, M. (1990). Predicting health-promoting lifestyles in the workplace. *Nursing Research, 39*(6), 326-332.

Phillips, L., Morrison, E., Steffl, B., Chae, Y., Cromwell, S., & Russell, C. (1995). Effects of the situational context and interactional process on the quality of family caregiving. *Research in Nursing and Health, 18,* 205-216.

Piper, S., & Parks, P. L. (1996). Predicting the duration of lactation: Evidence from a national survey. *Birth, 23*(1), 7-12.

Pitzer, M. S., & Hock, E. (1989). Employed mothers' concerns about separation from the first- and second-born child. *Research in Nursing and Health, 12*(2), 123-128.

Pleck, J. (1985). *Working wives, working husbands.* Beverly Hills, CA: Sage.

Poole, C. J. (1986). Fatigue during the first trimester of pregnancy. *Journal of Obstetric, Gynecologic, and Neonatal Nursing, 15,* 375-379.

Poth, M. (1997). Forum on the health of women in the military: Executive summary. *Women's Health Issues, 6*(6), 311-314.

Ramirez, G., Grimes, R., Annegers, J., Davis, B., & Slater, C. (1990). Occupational physical activity and other risk factors for preterm birth among US Army primigravidas. *American Journal of Public Health, 80,* 728-730.

Rankin, E. D. (1993). Stresses and rewards experienced by employed mothers. *Health Care for Women International, 14,* 527-537.

Reid, J., Ewan, C., & Lowy, E. (1991). Pilgrimage of pain: The illness experiences of women with repetition strain injury and the search for credibility. *Social Science and Medicine, 32*(5), 601-612.

Riesch, S. K. (1984). Occupational commitment and the quality of maternal infant interaction. *Nursing and Health, 7,* 295-303.

Roberts, S. J., & Garling, J. (1981). The menstrual myth revisited. *Nursing Forum, 20*(3), 267-273.

Rogers, J. L., & Maurizio, S. L. (1993). Prevalence of sexual harassment among rural community care workers. *Home Healthcare Nurse, 11*(4), 37-40.

Rose, M. H., & Killien, M. (1983). Risk and vulnerability: A case for differentiation. *Advances in Nursing Science, 5*(3), 60-73.

Ross, M. M., Rideout, E., & Carson, M. (1994). Nurses' work: Balancing personal and professional caregiving careers. *Canadian Journal of Nursing Research, 26,* 43-59.

Rowland, A. D., Baird, D. D., & Weinberg, C. R. (1992). Reduced fertility among women employed as dental assistants exposed to high levels of nitrous oxoide. *New England Journal of Medicine, 327,* 993-997.

Rubin, R. (1984). *Maternal identity and the maternal experience.* New York: Springer.

Rutter, M. (1987). Psychosocial resilience and protective mechanisms. *Journal of Orthopsychiatry, 57*(3), 316-331.

Ryan, A., & Martinez, G. (1989). Breast-feeding and the working mother. *Pediatrics, 83,* 524-531.

Salazar, M. K. (1994). Breast self-examination beliefs: A descriptive study. *Public Health Nursing, 11*(1), 49-56.

Salazar, M. K., & Carter, W. B. (1994). A qualitative description of breast self-examination beliefs. *Education Research, 9*(3), 343-354.

Salazar, M. K., Wilkinson, W. E., DeRoos, R. L., Lee, C. Y., Lyons, R., Rubadue, C., & Fetrick, A. (1994). Breast cancer behaviors following participation in a cancer risk appraisal. *Health Values: Achieving High Level Wellness, 18*(3), 41-49.

Saurel-Cubizolles, M., & Kaminski, M. (1987). Pregnant women's working conditions and their changes during pregnancy: A national survey. *British Journal of Industrial Medicine, 44,* 236-243.

Selevan, S., Lindbohm, M. L., Hornung, R., & Hemminki, K. (1985). A study of occupational exposure to antineoplastic drugs and fetal loss in nurses. *New England Journal of Medicine, 313,* 1173-1178.

Skinner, D. (1987). The stressors and coping patterns of dual-career families. In H. McCubbin & A. Thompson (Eds.), *Family assessment inventories for research and practice.* Madison: University of Wisconsin.

Sorensen, G., & Verbrugge, L. M. (1987). Women, work, and health. *Annual Review of Public Health, 8,* 235-251.

Staats, M. B., & Staats, T. E. (1983). Differences in stress levels, stressors, and stress responses between managerial and professional males and females in the stress vector analysis-research edition. *Issues in the Health Care of Women, 4,* 165-176.

Stellman, J. (1978). Occupational health hazards of women: An overview. *Preventive Medicine, 7,* 281-293.

Stevens, P. E., Hall, J. M., & Meleis, A. I. (1992). Examining vulnerability of women clerical workers from five ethnic/racial groups. *Western Journal of Nursing Research, 14*(6), 754-774.

Stone, R., & Stone, P. (1990). The competing demands of employment and informal caregiving to disabled elders. *Medical Care, 28,* 513-529.

Stueve, A., & O'Donnell, L. (1984). The daughter of aging parents. In G. Baruch & N. Brooks-Gunn (Eds.), *Women in midlife* (pp. 203-226). New York: Plenum.

Sund, K., & Ostwald, S. (1985). Dual-earner families' stress levels and personal and life style related variables. *Nursing Research, 34*(6), 357-361.

Teitleman, A., Welch, L., Hellenbrand, K., & Bracken, M. (1990). Effect of maternal work activity on preterm birth and low birth weight. *American Journal of Epidemiology, 131,* 104-113.

Thomas, L., Riegel, B., Gross, D., & Andrea, J. (1992). Job stress among emergency department nurses [Abstract]. *Heart and Lung, 21*(3), 294.

Thomas, S. P. (1995). Psychosocial correlates of women's health in middle adulthood. *Issues in Mental Health Nursing, 16,* 285-314.

Topf, M., & Dillon, E. (1988). Noise-induced stress as a predictor of burnout in critical care nurses. *Heart and Lung, 17,* 567-573.

Tulman, L., & Fawcett, J. (1988). Return of functional ability after childbirth. *Nursing Research, 37,* 77-81.

Tulman, L., & Fawcett, J. (1990). Maternal employment following childbirth. *Research in Nursing and Health, 13,* 181-188.

Tulman, L., Fawcett, J., Groblewski, L., & Silverman, L. (1990). Changes in functional status after childbirth. *Nursing Research, 39*(2), 70-75.

Uphold, C. R., & Susman, E. J. (1985). Child-rearing, marital, recreational and work role integration and climacteric symptoms in midlife women. *Research in Nursing and Health, 8,* 73-81.

U.S. Congress. (1998). *Reproductive health hazards in the workplace* (OTA-BA-266). Washington, DC: U.S. Government Printing Office.

U.S. Department of Labor, Women's Bureau. (1990). *Facts on working women* (Bull. 95-485). Washington, DC: U.S. Government Printing Office.

U.S. Department of Labor. (1995). *BLS releases new 1994-2005 employment projections* (Bull. 95-485). Washington, DC: U.S. Government Printing Office.

Verbrugge, L. M. (1984). Physical health of clerical workers in the U.S., Framingham, and Detroit. *Women and Health, 9*(1), 17-41.

Verbrugge, L. M. (1986). Role burdens and physical health of women and men. *Women & Health, 11,* 47-77.

Vessey, M. P., & Nunn, J. F. (1980). Occupational hazards of anesthesia. *British Medical Journal, 281,* 696-698.

Wadhwa, P., Sandman, C., Porto, M., Dunkel-Schetter, C., & Garite, T. (1993). The association between prenatal stress and infant birth weight and gestational age at birth: A prospective investigation. *American Journal of Obstetrics and Gynecology, 169,* 858-865.

Wahl, C., & Randall, V. (1996). Military women as wives and mothers. *Women's Health Issues, 6*(6), 315-319.

Walcott-McQuigg, J. A. (1994). Worksite stress: Gender and cultural diversity issues. *American Association of Occupational Health Nurses Journal, 42*(11), 528-533.

Waldron, I. (1991). Effects of labor force participation on sex differences in mortality and morbidity. In M. Frankenhaeuser, U. Lundberg, & M. Chesney (Eds.), *Women, work, and health: Stress and opportunities* (pp. 17-35). New York: Plenum.

Walker, L. O., & Best, M. A. (1991). Well-being of mothers with infant children: A preliminary comparison of employed women and homemakers. *Women & Health, 17*(1), 71-89.

Walker, S. N., Sechrist, K. R., & Pender, N. J. (1987). The health promoting lifestyle profile: Development and psychometric characteristics. *Nursing Research, 36*(2), 76-81.

Ward, D. (1990). Gender, time, and money in caregiving. *Scholarly Inquiry for Nursing Practice, 4*(3), 223-236.

Ward, D., & Brown, M. A. (1994). Labor and cost in AIDS family caregiving. *Western Journal of Nursing Research, 16*(1), 10-22.

Warshaw, L. J., Barr, J. K., & Schachter, M. (1987). Care givers in the workplace: Employer support for employees with elderly and chronically disabled dependents. *Journal of Occupational Medicine, 29*(6), 520-525.

Wen, C., Tsai, S., & Gibson, R. (1983). Anatomy of the healthy worker effect: A critical review. *Journal of Occupational Medicine, 25,* 283-289.

Wilbur, J. E., & Dan, A. J. (1989). The impact of work patterns on psychological well-being of midlife nurses. *Western Journal of Nursing Research, 11*(6), 703-716.

Wilbur, J., Miller, A., Dan, A. J., & Holm, K. (1989). Measuring physical activity in midlife women. *Public Health Nursing, 6*(3), 120-128.

Willeamson, H., LeFevre, M., & Hector, M. (1989). Association between life stress and serious perinatal complications. *Journal of Family Practice, 29,* 489-496.

Williams, K. M., & Morse, J. M. (1990). Weaning patterns of first-time mothers. *MCN: The American Journal of Maternal/Child Nursing, 14,* 188-192.

Windau, J., & Toscano, G. (1994). *Workplace homicides in 1992.* Washington, DC: U.S. Department of Labor, U.S. Government Printing Office.

Wolf, W., & Rosenfeld, R. (1978). Sex structure of occupations and job mobility. *Social Forces, 56,* 823-844.

Women's Bureau, U. S. Department of Labor. (1994). *1993 handbook on women workers: Trends and issues.* Washington, DC: U.S. Department of Labor.

Woods, N. (1985). Employment, family roles, and mental ill health in young adult married women. *Nursing Research, 34*(1), 4-9.

Woods, N. F., Dery, G. K., & Most, A. (1992). Recollections of menarche, current menstrual attitudes, and perimenstrual symptoms. *Psychosomatic Medicine, 44,* 285-293.

Woods, N. F., & Mitchell, E. S. (1996). Patterns of depressed mood in midlife women: Observations from the Seattle midlife women's health study. *Research in Nursing and Health, 19,* 111-123.

Woods, N. F., Most, A., & Longenecker, G. (1985). Major life events, stressors, and perimenstrual symptoms. *Nursing Research, 34,* 263-267.

Youngblut, J. M., Loveland-Cherry, C. J., & Horan, M. (1993). Maternal employment, family functioning, and preterm infant development at 9 and 12 months. *Research in Nursing and Health, 16,* 33-43.

Youngblut, J. M., Loveland-Cherry, C. J., & Horan, M. (1994). Maternal employment effects on families and preterm infants at 18 months. *Nursing Research, 43*(6), 331-337.

Youngblut, J., Singer, L. T., Madigan, E., & Swegart, L. A. (1997). Mother, child, and family factors related to employment of single mothers with LBW preschoolers. *Psychology of Women Quarterly, 21,* 247-263.

Zimakoff, J., Stormark, M., & Larsen, S. O. (1993). Use of gloves and handwashing behaviour among health care workers in intensive care units. *Journal of Hospital Infection, 24*(1), 63-67.

26

FROM MENARCHE TO MENOPAUSE

Contributions From Nursing Research and Recommendations for Practice

Nancy Fugate Woods
Ellen Sullivan Mitchell
Diana Taylor

Introduction

Nurses have made a significant contribution to understanding the menstrual cycle, having studied menarche, menstruation, and menopause. Since the late 1970s, nursing research has contributed in a unique way to understanding menarche, menstruation, and menopause as normative experiences and symptoms related to the menstrual cycle and menopause as illness experience. In contrast, during the same period, biomedical research has contributed to understanding the problems related to menstruation and menopause as disease or risk factors for disease. Nurse investigators have explored phenomena such as beliefs and attitudes among menarcheal girls, menstrual cycle characteristics and premenstrual changes among adult women, and experiences typical of meno-

pausal transition among midlife women. They have also contributed to work complementing biomedical research in developing diagnostic categories and criteria for phenomena such as premenstrual syndrome and premenstrual dysphoric disorder and therapies for problems related to menstruation and menopause.

Because of the breadth of concern of the nursing discipline and the multiple disciplines in which nurses have pursued their research training, there is a wide range of research interests reflected in this review. As a result, tracking published work across a range of disciplines was necessary. Medline and CINAHL searches provided primary sources of literature reviewed from 1980 onward. The Society for Menstrual Cycle Research has shaped much of the research by nurses about the menstrual cycle. Since 1977, the society has held a series of 10 conferences. Over the past 20 years, the published proceedings of these conferences have provided an invaluable chronology of research on the menstrual cycle and advanced thinking across several disciplines: nursing, psychology, sociology, epidemiology, anthropology, biostatistics, physiology, medicine, and literature. The proceedings of these conferences were also reviewed and are cited for reference in Table 26.1.

The body of published nursing research about menstruation and menopause stands to benefit over half of the population who receive nursing services over the course of their reproductive and postreproductive years. Therefore, continuing development of this knowledge has significant implications for health promotion, prevention of health problems, and symptom management.

This chapter focuses on nursing research about menarche, menstruation, and menopause. The purposes of this chapter are to

1. review the development of nursing science regarding the menstrual cycle, dating from the late 1970s to the present;

2. identify models for understanding the menstrual cycle advanced by nurse scientists;

3. evaluate the contributions of nurse scientists and gaps remaining in knowledge to guide practice; and

4. recommend directions for advancing nursing science regarding the menstrual cycle to guide nursing practice.

Menarche

The Normative Experience

Studies of menarche have been more limited than those of other aspects of menstruation and menopause. Indeed, Doan and Morse (1985) reviewed the challenges to studying menarche, emphasizing the current protective attitudes toward discussing menstruation with adolescents that impede research by limiting access of scientists to menarcheal girls. Nonetheless, published works by nurses have addressed images of menstruation presented to menarcheal girls, menstrual attitudes, symptoms, and the relationship of recalled menarcheal experiences and attitudes to adult women's subsequent experiences of symptoms.

TABLE 26.1.   Published Proceedings of the Society for Menstrual Cycle Research

Conference Year and Site	Title of Proceedings
1977: Chicago, IL	Dan, A., Graham, E., & Beecher, C. (Eds.). (1980). *The menstrual cycle: Volume 1. A synthesis of interdisciplinary research.* New York: Springer.
1978: St. Louis, MO	Komnenich, P., McSweeney, M., Noack, J., & Elder, N. (Eds.). (1981). *The menstrual cycle: Volume 2. Research and implications for women's health.* New York: Springer.
1979: Tucson, AZ	Voda, A., Dinnerstein, M., & O'Donnell, S. (Eds.). (1982). *Changing perspectives on menopause.* Austin: University of Texas Press.
1981: New Rochelle, NY	Golub, S. (Ed.). (1982). *Menarche: The transition from girl to woman.* Lexington, MA: Lexington Books.
1983: San Francisco, CA	Olesen, V., & Woods, N. (Eds.). (1986). *Culture, society, and menstruation.* Washington, DC: Hemisphere.
1985: Galveston, TX	Dan, A., & Lewis, L. (Eds.). (1992). *Menstrual health in women's lives.* Chicago: University of Illinois Press.
1987: Ann Arbor, MI	Taylor, D., & Woods, N. (Eds.). (1992). *Menstruation, health, and illness.* Washington, DC: Hemisphere.
1989: Salt Lake City, UT	Voda, A., & Conover, R. (Eds.). (1991). *Proceedings of the Eighth Conference of the Society for Menstrual Cycle Research.* Society for Menstrual Cycle Research, University of Utah.
1991: Seattle, WA	Society for Menstrual Cycle Research. (1994). *Mind-body rhythmicity: A menstrual cycle perspective. Proceedings from the Society for Menstrual Cycle Research Ninth Conference.* Seattle, WA: Hamilton & Cross.
1993: Boston, MA	Society for Menstrual Cycle Research. (1993). *Building a science of menstruation based on women's experiences.*
1995: Montreal, Quebec	Chrisler, J. *Broadening our vision: Class and cultural issues in women's health.*
1997: Chicago 20th anniversary	Berg, D. *Looking forward, looking back: The place of women's everyday lives in health research.*
1999: Tucson, AZ	"Cycling towards the millennium: Interdisciplinary research on women's health."

Images of menstruation. Havens and Swenson (1988) reviewed advertisements for sanitary products and products to relieve menstrual discomfort from issues of a magazine targeting adolescent girls. They found themes of menstruation as a hygienic crisis to be managed by an effective security system necessary to prevent revelation of her menses. At the same time, menstruating women were portrayed as dynamic, energetic, and functioning at their optimum level. Patterson and Hale (1985) interviewed 25 adult women about their self-care practices related to menstruation. They found that women observed patterns of self-care similar to that of other eliminative problems, such as those for dealing with ostomies or incontinence. Menstruation was viewed by adult women as a hygienic challenge, consistent with the images presented to adolescents.

Menstrual attitudes. Menke (1983) studied the menstrual beliefs and experiences of Caucasian mother-daughter dyads. Daughters ranged in age from 12 to 16 years and their mothers from 31 to 50 years of age. She found that these mothers and daughters had similar beliefs about menstruation. They saw menstruation as slightly debilitating, bothersome, predictable, positive, and affecting one's behavior. They also had similar beliefs about what was bad about menstruation and activities one should or should not participate in during menstruation, such as physical activities. Stoltzman (1986) also studied menstrual attitudes, beliefs, self-care practices, communication patterns, and symptom experiences among four groups of women: 30 adolescent volunteers, 19 of their close girlfriends, 46 mothers of the adolescents, and mothers of their daughters' friends. There were significant differences between the scores of mothers and their daughters, but no differences among the scores of the adolescents. Adolescents were more likely to view menstruation as debilitating, bothersome, and unsanitary, and less likely than their mothers to view it as a positive event. Williams (1983) studied 74 fourth-, fifth-, and sixth-grade midwestern girls' knowledge of reproductive anatomy and menstrual physiology, finding that they were not knowledgeable. They had a wide variety of beliefs about menstruation, including three taboos: communication about menstruation with boys and in public, failure to conceal menstruation, and activities such as swimming during menstruation. Girls attributed changes in emotion to menstruation, such as being more nervous and upset during menses. Dashiff and Buchanan (1995) found no significant differences in menstrual attitudes among Black and White premenarcheal girls aged 10 to 12 years (N = 55).

Symptoms among menarcheal girls. Menke (1983) found that mothers and daughters resembled one another with respect to symptom experiences and attitudes. Mothers had significantly more severe water retention symptoms than their daughters, but there were no other differences. Menke pointed out the important influence of socialization in shaping young women's menstrual experiences. Stoltzman (1986) found that adolescents reported significantly more acute pain, water retention, and arousal symptoms than their mothers. Girls' symptoms resembled those of their peers.

Consequences of menarcheal experiences. Woods, Dery, and Most (1982) interviewed 193 adult women from a southern community about their current perimenstrual symptoms and menstrual attitudes and their recollections of menstruation. Recollections of menarcheal experiences had little relationship to women's experiences of symptoms or their adult attitudes toward menstruation. Sveinsdottir (1993) also found little relationship between Icelandic women nursing students' recollection of menarche and characteristics of their current menstruation.

Preparation for Menarche

Preparation for menarche has been studied most by investigators from other disciplines, such as psychologists. Despite nurses' involvement in practices with school-age girls, such as in school-based clinics, there has been little nursing research to guide health education about menarche. Bloch (1978) interviewed over 100 mothers of seventh-grade girls. She found that 20% of the mothers had never told their daughters about menstruation. Only 16% had provided an explanation of hygiene to their daughters. Twenty-six percent of the mothers had explained the physiology of menstruation and the relationship between menstruation and pregnancy. This study needs to be replicated in the 1990s to determine if mothers and daughters have become more comfortable discussing menstruation.

Family relationships. Danza (1983) studied premenarcheal and postmenarcheal girls' relationships with their mothers and fathers in a convenience sample of middle-class families. She found that menarche affected limits, responsibilities, closeness, distance, conflict, and roles the daughter experienced and served as a point for changing the mother's and father's relationship with their developing daughter. Because of changing social relationships between menarcheal girls and their parents, frank discussions about menarche and sexuality may be difficult for both.

Health Promotion

Menarche presents nurses with a unique opportunity to address health promotion issues, particularly those related to reproductive and sexual health of school-age girls. To date, there have been no published studies of health promotion activities specifically linked to the developmental opportunity presented by menarche. Studies are needed of how to facilitate mother-daughter communication about menarche, sexuality, and other health promotion issues and to test whether communication by a nurse would be more successful than that by a parent. Because monitoring biological rhythms and symptoms, such as sleep patterns and symptoms across the menstrual cycle, has been found to be an important component of health promotion for adult women, young women may benefit from monitoring their health and functional changes related to the menstrual cycle.

Measurement

Development of instrumentation for studying menarche has been pursued by Morse and associates. Morse and Doan (1987) identified five dimensions of adolescents' responses to menarche, including negative responses, natural and accepting responses, excited responses, responses to symptoms, and managing menstruation. Janes and Morse (1990) studied 141 girls (Grades 6 to 8) regarding their feelings about menarche, preparation for menarche, symptoms related to menses, information about menarche, and school facilities to help them cope with menstruation. Morse, Kieren, and Bottorff (1993) then developed an age-appropriate, 58-item instrument (the Adolescent Menstrual Attitude Questionnaire) and presented the factor structure for the instrument and established known groups' validity and reliability. Six factors included positive feelings, negative feelings, living with menstruation, openness, menstrual symptoms, and acceptance of menarche. Morse and Kieren (1993) published norms for 860 pre- and 1,013 postmenarcheal girls, presented by age and grade. They refined the scale by creating a separate version for premenarcheal and postmenarcheal girls. The complete scale and reliability estimates are published in Morse and Kieren (1993).

Menstruation

Normative Experiences

Early efforts to understand the normative experience of menstruation and menstrual symptoms as illness experiences have included studies of healthy community-based populations of women. From these studies, we have been able to estimate the normative experiences of women and identify some that are idiosyncratic.

The Tremin Trust Database, currently administered by Ann Voda at the University of Utah, represents a national resource of information about women's menstrual cycles that now includes data from over 5,000 women and spanning three generations (Voda et al., 1991). Currently 1,316 women are actively recording their cycles. From the Tremin Trust Database it is possible to follow women from menarche through menopause and in some instances to do so for three generations. This database has provided important information about menstrual cyclicity across the reproductive years, length of cycles and bleeding episodes, regularity, and estimates of menopause. Currently this database includes a menstrual calendar card and health report form completed annually. In 1987, women completed a five-page health update. Many special surveys have been conducted on a variety of topics.

Menstrual Changes and Menstrual Symptoms

Studies of nonclinical populations of women have revealed an array of experiences ranging from premenstrual changes (sometimes called molimina) to premenstrual syndromes. Most women who monitor their experiences on a daily basis over more than one menstrual cycle notice changes in their bodies and moods that seem to vary with the course of the menstrual cycle. These premenstrual changes, or molimina, have been attributed to changing ovarian steroid levels and their widespread effects on physiological function. Most women who experience changes such as swelling of their breasts, increased attentiveness and sensitivity, or bursts of energy do not consider themselves sick or ill. Instead, they view such changes as a "natural" part of being a woman (Woods, Lentz, Mitchell, Lee, et al., 1992). Although most attention has been directed at understanding the changes that women perceive as negative or troubling, it is important to notice that some women describe positive experiences associated with menstrual cyclicity, including an increasing energy level that enables them to accomplish more work or to be more creative (Woods, Lentz, Mitchell, Taylor, et al., 1987).

Premenstrual symptoms. Studies of women's premenstrual symptoms have included samples of women representing a cross section of a population as well as women seeking health care. As a result, a variety of labels now appear in the menstrual cycle literature. Premenstrual symptoms refer to cyclic changes that a woman perceives as troublesome or problematic and that escalate before menstruation and then subside after menses begins. Premenstrual symptoms, particularly those of low or moderate intensity, usually do not interfere with a woman's ability to function or perform her typical roles (Woods, Lentz, Mitchell, Lee, et al., 1992).

Premenstrual syndrome (PMS) is a diagnostic term used to indicate cyclical recurrence of distressing physical, affective, and behavioral experiences that often affect interpersonal relationships and personal health. A PMS symptom pattern can be discerned by the absence of symptoms or low severity symptoms after menses (postmenses, defined as approximately days 6 through 10 of the cycle), followed by an escalation in symptoms premenses (days -1 to -7 of the cycle, counting backward from the next menses, that is, the 7 days preceding the next menses). Premenstrual magnification (PMM) is a variant of the premenstrual syndrome pattern in which women experience moderately severe symptoms postmenses, and more severe symptoms premenses (Mitchell, Woods, & Lentz, 1991). This variant (PMM) may represent an exacerbation of an existing mental health problem. Both premenstrual syndrome and premenstrual magnification are symptom patterns that may interfere with women's usual functioning.

Premenstrual dysphoric disorder (PDD) is a diagnostic label, now included in the *Diagnostic and Statistical Manual IV* (*DSM-IV*) of the American Psychiatric Association (APA) (1994), which replaces the earlier label of late-luteal-phase dysphoric disorder. This disorder represents a more severe form of PMS, with an emphasis on the emotional symptoms. To make a diagnosis of PDD, clinicians need to establish that a woman experiences multiple symptoms premenses, with at least one of the symptoms being depression, anxiety, affective/lability, or persistent and marked anger or irritability (APA, 1994). Criteria for PDD also specify that symptoms have occurred in most menstrual cycles during the past year, that more than five symptoms were present for most of the time during the last week of the luteal phase, that symptoms begin to remit within a few days after the onset

of the follicular phase, and were absent in the week after menses.

Most women who seek treatment for self-defined premenstrual symptoms will not meet the *DSM-IV* criteria for premenstrual dysphoric disorder. Their symptoms may not meet the severity criteria or criteria for cycle phase difference (amount of change in severity of symptoms between postmenses and premenses), and comorbidity may make it impossible to differentiate their symptoms from another underlying disorder without a psychological assessment. Nursing research has contributed to understanding the experiences of the majority of women seeking care—those who have bothersome symptoms, including a range of bodily symptoms such as swelling or sensation of weight gain, seen among women with a PMS or PMM symptom pattern, but who do not have a psychiatric disorder.

Measurement

One of the most important challenges to researchers, clinicians, and the women with whom they work is classification of women's experiences in a way that is accurate and foundational to studies of etiology and efficacious treatment. Because nearly 200 different symptoms have been associated with menstrual cyclicity, classification is not an insignificant problem. Over the past two decades, nurses have studied the classification and measurement of premenstrual symptoms and syndromes. In early efforts, nurses used retrospective administration of questionnaires such as the Menstrual Distress Questionnaire, initially developed with a graduate student population (Logue & Moos, 1986), in studies of women seeking health care for their symptoms (York, Freeman, & Strauss, 1989) and in studies of a cross section of the general population (Woods, Most, & Dery, 1982c). Based on these early studies, investigators modified these measures to include a greater range of symptoms, reflecting women's idiosyncratic presentation.

The Washington Women's Health Diary (WWHD) is an instrument designed to measure prospectively perimenstrual symptoms; it has been used in a series of studies by Woods, Mitchell, and Lentz, and their associates (see Mitchell, Woods, & Lentz, 1994; Woods, Mitchell, Lentz, & Kogan, 1995; Woods, Mitchell, & Lentz, 1996), and collaborative groups led by Reame (Reame, Marshall, & Kelch, 1993), and Cahill (1998). The diary includes nearly 60 different symptoms and feelings. Embedded in this list are 33 symptoms that the investigators term the Menstrual Symptom Severity List (MSSL). Also included in the diary are items related to illness behavior, stressful experiences, dietary and alcohol intake, smoking, exercise, and menses.

Clusters of Symptoms

As the number of symptoms included in measures expanded to reflect individual variations in experience, investigators have focused on identifying symptom clusters, such as negative affect or fluid retention, using techniques such as factor analysis (Woods, Most, & Dery, 1982a, 1982b; York et al., 1989) to aid in data reduction to simplify analyses and as a basis for profile analysis for directing symptom management. Ratings of the 57 symptoms commonly reported in studies about PMS by 345 women from a community-based sample have been factor analyzed. Four factors accounted for most of the variance: emotional turmoil, fluid retention, somatic symptoms, and arousal symptoms (Woods, Mitchell, & Lentz, 1998). This factor structure was similar to that obtained by Woods, Most, and Dery (1982b) using the Moos Menstrual Distress Questionnaire (negative affect, water retention, pain, and behavioral changes) and to that obtained by Monagle, Dan, and Chatterton (1986) in a study using the Menstrual Symptoms Questionnaire (premenstrual negative affect, menstrual pain, premenstrual pain, gastrointestinal/prostaglandin, water retention, and asymptomatic).

In the study by York et al. (1989) of women diagnosed with PMS who were seeking clinical services, the factor structure differed across menstrual cycle phases. One hundred women recorded scores daily on 18 symptoms for one menstrual cycle in a calendar. Two factors predominated throughout the cycle, the first including emotional and behavioral symptoms and the second, physical and cognitive symptoms. Emotional symptoms clustered together throughout the menstrual cycle but loaded on both factors during the postmenstrual phase. Behavioral symptoms loaded on the first factor throughout the cycle but were prevalent during the latter half of the intermenstrual and premenstrual phases. Cognitive symptoms loaded on the second factor during premenses.

Retrospective measurement of symptoms, the most commonly used approach during the 1970s and early 1980s, has given way to prospective measurement of symptoms. Symptom tracking using a daily health diary (Woods, Lentz, Mitchell, Taylor, et al., 1987; Woods, Most, & Dery, 1982a, 1982b, 1982c) has been applied to document the time course of symptoms and to support analyses of cycle phase differences in symptom experiences

(Mitchell, Woods, & Lentz, 1991). Mitchell has developed a scannable diary form that enables use of a computer scanner for data entry, saving significant effort for the research team. Although it is not always feasible to collect data from more than one menstrual cycle using daily recording, prospective recording has been used for multiple cycles to determine eligibility for participation in studies of PMS or PMM (Mitchell, Woods, & Lentz, 1994; Reame, 1993; Woods, Mitchell, & Lentz, 1995) and for diagnosis in a clinical setting. Prospective recordings appear to be more accurate than retrospective reporting of symptoms in a community-based sample (Woods, Dery, & Most, 1982). For women selected with severe premenstrual symptomatology, however, retrospective recording for the past cycle does approximate the results obtained with daily recording (Gallant, Popiel, Hoffman, Chakraborty, & Hamilton, 1992).

Another approach to measuring premenstrual symptoms has involved timing observations to women's individual symptom pattern so that measures are made during the time women are actually symptomatic rather than on a specific cycle day. This approach has merit, particularly when studying factors associated with symptom onset (Lewis, 1989).

Prevalence

Nurse researchers have investigated the prevalence of perimenstrual symptoms in community-based populations as well as the prevalence of specific symptom severity patterns such as PMS and PMM. When the frequency of symptoms is analyzed, results suggest that premenstrual symptoms of low and moderate severity are common, with prevalence estimates ranging from 30% to 50%, dependent on the specific symptom (Woods, Most, & Dery, 1982c). The most prevalent premenstrual symptoms rated retrospectively on the MDQ by a population-based sample of women from a southeastern U.S. city ($N = 193$) were cramps, mood swings, fatigue, swelling, irritability, tension, skin disorders, headache, depression, backache, painful or tender breasts, weight gain, anxiety, and crying. When only symptoms that women rated as severe or disabling were considered, the prevalence of symptoms was a much lower 10% to 20% (Woods, Most, & Dery, 1982c). This study was replicated in Jerusalem, with different prevalence estimates, suggesting the importance of ethnicity and sociocultural context (Most, Woods, Dery, & Most, 1981).

In a more recent study of a population-based multiethnic sample from Seattle, prevalence estimates for premenstrual symptoms were obtained from ratings of symptoms in a daily health diary (WWHD) kept for at least one menstrual cycle. The symptoms that women ($N = 345$) most frequently rated as moderate or extreme during premenses days -1 to -3 were fatigue (26%), sensation of weight gain (14%), awakening during the night (13%), depression (11%), painful or tender breasts (11%), and bloating (10%). Symptoms were most severe during menses (Woods, Lentz, Mitchell, Taylor, et al., 1987). Prevalence estimates were comparable to some of the symptoms reported by Monagle from her study with Italian women (Monagle et al., 1986).

Sveinsdottir and Marteinsdottir (1991) studied premenstrual symptoms among Icelandic women. They found that Icelandic women experienced premenstrual changes similar to those of women of other countries. The most common symptoms were bloating, mood swings, irritability, abdominal discomfort, intolerance, and impatience. Women who had premenstrual symptoms also had symptoms at other times. Consistency of symptoms across more than one cycle was estimated by Shaver and Woods (1985). They found that selected symptoms were consistently reported.

In a study of the prevalence of specific premenstrual symptom severity pattern, Mitchell, Woods, and Lentz (1991) used the Menstrual Symptom Severity List (MSSL). To develop criteria for classifying women into one of three symptom severity patterns, the severity of 33 symptoms in the MSSL was tallied for cycle days 4 to 10 to estimate postmenses severity of symptoms and days -1 to -7 to estimate premenses severity. The investigators identified population-based criteria for critical levels of symptom severity and cycle phase differences that formed the classification rule for identifying PMS and PMM symptom patterns, as well as the low symptom severity (LS) group. Criteria for LS, PMS, and PMM are given in Table 26.2. These criteria were then used to determine the prevalence of the PMS, PMM, and LS patterns. The criteria have since been used in subsequent studies by Reame (1993) and Cahill (1998) to identify women with PMS, PMM, and LS patterns.

When the daily MSSL was used for two to three complete cycles to estimate prevalence of premenstrual symptom patterns (PMS and PMM) from symptoms recorded daily in a health diary over two complete cycles, the prevalence estimates were much lower than was the case for premenstrual symptoms. Approximately 9% of the women not using oral contraceptives or hormone preparations had a symptom pattern consistent with PMS (no symptoms or low-severity symptoms postmenses,

TABLE 26.2. Criteria for LS, PMS, and PMM: 5-Day Mean Symptom Severity Scores for the 33-Symptom MSSL

	Cycle Phase Difference	Postmenses Severity	Premenses Severity
PMS	> 6.2	< 6.5	> 7.8
PMM	> 6.2	> 6.6	> 12.1
LS	< 3.6	< 6.5	< 7.8

SOURCE: Adapted from Mitchell, Woods, and Lentz (1991).
NOTE: LS = low-severity symptoms; PMS = premenstrual syndrome; PMM = premenstrual magnification; MSSL = Menstrual Symptom Severity List.

moderate- to high-intensity symptoms premenses). Approximately 8% of the women had a symptom pattern consistent with criteria for PMM (moderate-severity symptoms postmenses, with a cycle phase difference resulting in significantly increased intensity premenses) (Mitchell, Woods, & Lentz, 1991; Mitchell et al., 1992).

In another study to illustrate the time course of premenstrual symptoms, Sveinsdottir and Reame (1991) identified seven different variants of the PMS symptom pattern. In four of these, women recorded increased severity at ovulation as well as premenses. The PMS and LS patterns accounted for the symptoms of 65% (399) of the women studied.

Consistency of premenstrual symptom patterns across multiple cycles has been estimated. Shaver and Woods (1985) explored consistency of symptoms across two menstrual cycles. Concordance was significant for backache, headache, and cramps during menses and for backache, cold sweats, fatigue, depression, and tension premenses. Mitchell, Woods, and Lentz (1994) found that 78% of women classified over several cycles with a low-severity symptom pattern had the same pattern during a subsequent cycle, whereas only 53% of women with a PMM pattern and 40% of those with a PMS pattern were likely to have the same pattern during a subsequent cycle. This points out the importance of assessing symptom severity for more than one cycle to make a diagnosis of PMS and also supports the use of stringent sampling criteria for studies of PMS.

Lewis (1995) followed one woman with PMS for one year (13 menstrual cycles). She found a significant predictive cycle-to-cycle symptom pattern. She also found that symptoms altered the woman's interpretations of her environment and herself.

To date, there have been no published longitudinal studies to determine whether women who experience premenstrual symptoms continue to experience distress during their 40s and whether their symptoms persist throughout the transition to menopause. Results of one group of women studied in their 30s who were restudied in their 40s revealed they had similar symptom patterns and physiological responses (Woods, Lentz, Mitchell, Heitkemper, & Shaver, 1997). Mitchell and Woods (1996) found that among midlife women, symptoms persisted from one year to the next. Data from women followed at four different points in time over a 3-year period revealed that dysphoric mood symptoms and neuromuscular symptoms were relatively stable across 3 years. Vasomotor and somatic symptoms were the least stable during this period.

Studies of Menstrual Cycle in Context

Another feature of nursing research about the menstrual cycle is the attempts of investigators to study menstrual phenomena in the context of everyday life. A common criticism of women's health research by feminist theorists and scientists is that work not grounded in an understanding of the fabric of women's lives is unlikely to be informative or serve emancipatory ends for women (Harding, 1991). Locating the problem of symptoms within the woman herself, rather than acknowledging the simultaneous influences of women's social experiences, perpetuates the belief that biological events that are experienced only by women can be associated with premenstrual symptoms. A model that incorporates the social context in which menstruation occurs may more accurately reflect the realities of women's lives and suggest possibilities for caring for women who find their symptoms distressing.

A woman's social context may contribute to and be affected by her experiences of affective and bodily changes, perceptions of and responses to her environments, and perceived personal and behavioral changes associated with her menstrual cycle. Dimensions of a woman's social context include socialization about being a woman and, more specifically, her expectations about how she will experience menstruation. Another important dimension is everyday stresses and strains and women's resources with which to respond to them.

Socialization About Menstruation

Social constructions about menstruation and premenstrual symptomatology influence women through social transmission of beliefs, attitudes, and expectations by health professionals, media, and their families and peers. Young girls learn about symptoms from observing their mothers, sisters, and peers, including expectations regarding menstrual experiences and effects of menstruation on feelings and behavior (Menke, 1983; Stoltzman, 1986). In addition, young girls learn from the communications media that menstruation is a hygienic crisis to be concealed, and this model persists into adulthood (Patterson & Hale, 1985). Woods (1986) found that the attitudes of adult women ($N = 179$) who viewed menstruation as debilitating were related to the subjects' socialization as women and also influenced their own symptom experiences and need to reduce their activities during the perimenstruum.

Mothers' experiences with premenstrual symptoms appear linked to daughters' subsequent symptom experiences and illness behavior (Menke, 1983; Stoltzman, 1986; Taylor, Woods, Lentz, Mitchell, & Lee, 1991). Indeed, exposure to a mother with premenstrual symptoms and teachings about negative effects of menstruation were associated with negative affect symptomatology during the premenses and menses for adult women (Taylor et al., 1991). Moreover, women with PMS and PMM symptom patterns were more likely to have had a mother with more premenstrual symptomatology than women with an LS pattern (Mitchell, Woods, & Lentz, 1994). Whether these findings reflect only social learning or also genetic or physiological similarity between mothers and daughters remains unclear.

Expectations about having symptoms are transmitted through socialization about menstruation. Menke (1983) proposed that women's attitudes are a function of their own experiences as well as their socialization, including reciprocal mother-daughter influence. Although stereotypic biases in information processing about menstrual symptom cyclicity may influence symptom reporting, it is likely that lived experiences with symptoms come to influence expectancy. Women who have perimenstrual symptoms may come to anticipate having them and perceive events around the time of menstruation as more stressful.

Socialization about women's roles in society provides a general cognitive orientation that may support more specific socialization about menstruation and its debilitating effects. A negative attributional style, in turn, could adversely affect women's self-esteem. Hamilton, Alagna, and Sharpe (1985) pointed out that many women experience learned helplessness as an extension of life experiences related to their economic inequality, subordinate group status, vulnerability to victimization, situational stressors related to their roles, and the internalization of stereotypes that devalue women. Thus women who have been exposed to difficult life circumstances that underscore how women are devalued may be more vulnerable to learning negative aspects about menstruation and may have their negative experiences reinforced by the social context. Woods (1986) found that women ($N = 179$) socialized to traditional sex role norms had more negative affect symptoms premenses and also had more negative attitudes about menstruation being debilitating.

Stressors. Since the 1970s, researchers have examined relationships between naturally occurring stressors and perimenstrual symptoms. Early efforts demonstrated that major life stressors and daily hassles were related to perimenstrual symptoms, especially negative affect (Taylor et al., 1991; Woods, Dery, & Most, 1982; Woods, Most, & Longenecker, 1985).

In more recent studies in which stringent criteria were used to select women with specific perimenstrual symptom patterns, findings are mixed. Brown and Lewis (1993) did not find a cycle phase difference in perceived stress among women with high levels of premenstrual symptomatology. Woods and colleagues found that in a stress-testing laboratory manipulation, women with LS or PMS patterns did not rate cognitive stressors (the Stroop test and solving anagrams) as more stressful premenses than postmenses (Woods et al., 1992), but these same stressors produced different physiological responses among women with PMS, PMM, and LS patterns (Woods et al., 1995).

Although most investigators have assumed that stressors caused or exacerbated perimenstrual symptomatology, women asserted that their symptoms precipitated stressful experiences such as interpersonal conflict or increased sensitivity to their impact (Woods, Taylor, Lentz, & Mitchell, 1992). Cycle phase differences in women's perceptions of stressors could be explained by stressors occurring as a result of PMS and intensifying women's symptom experiences.

Of note is the absence of work exploring whether women see their social situations more clearly premenses than at other times of the cycle. The ability to perceive situations more sharply when aroused has been demonstrated as an adaptive component of stress response. Perhaps premenstrual arousal enhances women's perceptions of situations such that their clearer perception premenses may be more accurate than their perceptions

at other times. Thus, if there are dimensions of a woman's life about which she is unhappy, she may become more aware of the situation premenstrually and experience more distress.

To date, little work has focused on how dimensions of women's life context such as employment, social relationships, education, and income influence symptoms and stress during the premenstruum. Employment does not seem related to premenstrual symptoms (Brown & Woods, 1986), but women in traditional occupations had more severe negative affect premenstrually. Lee, Lentz, Taylor, Mitchell, and Woods (1994) have studied a cross section of professionally employed women ($N = 594$, unselected with respect to their premenstrual symptom status) to determine the prevalence of perimenstrual symptoms. Symptoms that were most frequent were weight gain, swelling, anxiety, tension, irritability, fatigue, cramps, breast pain, mood swings, and food cravings, not different from the symptoms seen in cross sections of the population. Fewer Asian than Caucasian women reported symptoms. Single women and those younger than 30 years reported food cravings and depression more frequently than others. Weight gain and swelling were reported by more than 60% of the sample. Parity, cycle regularity, menses duration, and endometriosis diagnosis were associated with more severe cramps (Lee & Rittenhouse, 1991). Rittenhouse and Lee (1993) found that premenstrual weight gain was related to caffeine consumption, weight, exercise, depression and anxiety, menses flow days, clots, number of children, social support, and satisfaction with the work environment. Lee and Rittenhouse (1992) found that employed women with premenstrual symptoms were less satisfied with their social lives, had less social support, lower psychological well-being, and more physical health problems. The investigators recommended consideration of lifestyle change for therapy rather than drugs.

Other studies suggest the importance of a woman's social relationships are associated with symptoms. In one study, women who used social support as a coping strategy experienced less severe premenstrual symptoms (Warren & Baker, 1992). In another study, women with PMS reported lower satisfaction with marital and sexual relationships than women with LS patterns (Winter, Ashton, & Moore, 1991). Icelandic women with premenstrual symptoms reported negative effects on their children and partners (Sveinsdottir & Martiensdottir, 1991).

Ornitz and Brown (1993) examined how families coped with a woman who had PMS. Couples ($N = 104$) were asked to described how they coped. Those with

PMS used more spiritual coping than LS families. Husbands of women with PMS believed the problem would go away if they waited long enough. These data suggest that family dynamics should be considered as part of the context for women's PMS experiences.

The relationship between education and PMS is puzzling, with those with a PMS pattern having more formal education (Mitchell, Woods, & Lentz, 1994; Taylor et al., 1991). No relationship between income and PMS has been reported.

Multivariate studies of social factors differentiating women with PMS, PMM, and LS demonstrate the importance of social stress, socialization for menstrual symptoms, and expectations about having perimenstrual symptoms. Women with PMS and PMM were more likely to have been exposed to mothers with more premenstrual symptoms than the LS group. Women with PMM had more stress than those with LS. Women with PMS had more education and more nontraditional attitudes toward women (Mitchell, Woods, & Lentz, 1994). In another study comparing women with PMS, PMM, and LS, women with PMS had greater expectation of having perimenstrual symptoms, more stress, more pregnancies, and less education than the LS group. Those with PMM demonstrated greater expectation of perimenstrual symptoms, and higher stress levels than the LS group. Both the PMS and PMM groups had higher depression scores than the LS group and saw themselves as less healthy (Woods, Mitchell, & Lentz, 1995).

▭ Biological Correlates of Menstrual Symptoms

In the search for the etiology of perimenstrual symptoms, investigators have studied the relationship between a variety of neuroendocrine factors and symptoms. One of the earliest lines of inquiry focused on the role of the hypothalamic-pituitary-ovarian (HPO) axis hormones. Another line of inquiry has emphasized the potential role of the hypothalamic-pituitary-adrenal (HPA) axis and the autonomic nervous system in mediating perimenstrual symptomatology. To date, studies of ovarian and stress hormone patterns across the menstrual cycle in women with and without symptoms have been limited by problems of classifying women with various premenstrual symptom patterns. Moreover, investigators have not focused on the relationship among hormones of the HPO and HPA axis across the menstrual cycle phases.

HPO-axis hormones. Lentz and colleagues (1998) found no differences in levels of ovarian steroids measured in daily late afternoon urine samples across one cycle for women with PMS, PMM, and LS pattern. Intraindividual analysis demonstrated that changing progesterone levels led symptom severity. Thus, progesterone may orchestrate the events associated with PMS. Taylor compared 10 women with PMS and 10 women with an LS pattern with respect to their salivary progesterone levels over one menstrual cycle. Women with PMS had slightly lower progesterone levels during the luteal phase (Taylor, 1994).

Reame et al. (1993) found that LH pulsatility patterns among women with PMS and LS were similar. The only difference between groups was higher FSH levels in the PMS group. She concluded that HPO axis function among women with PMS was normal. Lewis, Greenblatt, Rittenhouse, Veldhuis, and Jaffe (1995) studied coupling of LH and progesterone pulses among women with PMS during the luteal phase. In the PMS group, significant coincident pulsing occurred; it was especially noted at symptom onset. The length of time between LH and P pulses increased across the luteal phase. This suggests some disregulation of the LS and P pulse patterns at the onset of symptoms. Lewis is currently studying stress challenge effects on LH and progesterone pulsatility patterns.

Lee, Shaver, Giblin, and Woods (1990) studied sleep patterns in relation to the menstrual cycle and to symptoms. They found that REM latency was significantly shorter during the luteal phase compared to the follicular phase, but there was no significant difference in latency to sleep onset or the percentage of REM sleep. Women with negative affect symptoms during premenses demonstrated significantly less delta sleep during both menstrual cycle phases when compared with the asymptomatic women. These findings suggest that women with premenstrual symptoms experience less deep sleep than those who are asymptomatic. These findings are in agreement with other studies of physiological arousal among women with PMS.

Physiological arousal and stress reactivity. In a study of women with an LS pattern ($n = 28$) and a PMS symptom pattern ($n = 15$), women with the PMS pattern exhibited accentuated arousal and physiological responses to stressors, especially premenses. Women with a PMS pattern experienced premenses elevation of skin conductance at rest and in response to cognitive stressors (Woods, Lentz, Mitchell, & Kogan, 1994). In addition, women with a PMS symptom pattern exhibited premenstrual elevation of muscle tension (EMG) at rest and in response to cognitive and symptom imagery stressors (Woods, Lentz, Mitchell, & Kogan, 1994). These findings suggest that women with PMS experience heightened arousal as well as stress reactivity, especially premenses. Woods, Lentz, Mitchell, Shaver, and Heitkemper (1998) examined the relationship between perceived stress, ovarian steroids (estradiol and pregnanediol), stress arousal indicators (cortisol, catecholamines), and premenstrual syndrome (turmoil, fluid retention). Women ($N = 74$) with LS, PMS, or PMM symptom patterns provided daily urine samples over one cycle and recorded their symptoms and perceived stress levels in a health diary. Multiple regression analysis was used to test models of premenstrual symptoms in separate analyses for women with the LS and PMS symptom patterns and the LS and PMM symptom patterns. Analyses indicated that greater stress ratings accounted for turmoil symptoms and higher luteal phase cortisol levels for fluid retention symptoms in analyses including women with PMS. In contrast, lower luteal phase norepinephrine levels, higher global stress ratings, and a more gradual drop in estradiol premenses accounted for turmoil symptoms and premenses norepinephrine and epinephrine levels, and premenses stress ratings accounted for fluid retention in the analysis that included women with PMM pattern. These findings support an important relationship among perceived stress, stress arousal indicators, and premenstrual symptoms that differ for women with a PMS and PMM symptom pattern.

Intraindividual analyses of cortisol, catecholamines, stress levels, and symptoms revealed that (a) women with PMS and PMM patterns reported higher stress levels than LS women, and their stress levels increase premenses, and (b) there were no cycle phase, group, or group × phase differences in cortisol or catecholamines, but epinephrine levels dropped significantly from postmenses to premenses for the PMS group. Intraindividual analyses with cross correlations revealed a positive time-lagged relationship between perceived stress and norepinephrine and cortisol for women in all groups. Only women with a PMS pattern demonstrated that perceived stress led epinephrine levels. Cortisol, epinephrine, and norepinephrine led symptoms in all three groups, with one exception: There was no cross correlation between epinephrine and turmoil symptoms for the PMS group. Perceived stress led symptoms in all groups and symptoms also led stress (Woods, Lentz, Mitchell, Heitkemper, Shaver, & Henker, 1998).

Among women 40 years old and older, in a comparison of those with PMS and LS symptom patterns, Woods, Lentz, Mitchell, Heitkemper, et al. (1997) found increased phsiological arousal and stress responses (skin conductance and muscle tension levels) and relatively higher norepinephrine levels among women with PMS than among women with an LS pattern, but this group also showed dampened cardiovascular responses to stressors.

Taylor (1994) compared 10 women with PMS and 10 women with an LS pattern with respect to salivary assays for cortisol and progesterone across three complete menstrual cycles. She found that salivary cortisol did not change with cycle phase but was significantly higher in the PMS group during the premenstrual phase only.

Cahill studied basal levels of cortisol to differentiate women with low severity symptoms of turmoil from women with PMS patterns and those with PMM patterns. Symptoms and cortisol patterns were monitored for three consecutive menstrual cycles. Significant differences in symptom severity were seen as predicted. There were no statistically significant differences in cortisol among groups for the follicular phase, but for the luteal phase cortisol levels were lower for the PMS group, suggesting altered regulation of the stress axis in PMS.

Taylor and Bledsoe (1986a, 1986b) studied the use of a support group intervention with 22 women volunteers with moderate to severe perimenstrual symptoms. A nonprofessional volunteer convened the support group as part of a treatment program developed by a menstrual disorders clinic. The women were studied before and after 8 weeks of group sessions. Twenty-two women were matched to controls from the same clinic by age, marital status, pregnancy history, and occupation. Results of this intervention showed that peer support indirectly affected symptoms by informing women about lifestyle changes and facilitated their making those changes.

In another symptom management study, Taylor (1994) emphasized an individualized approach and used an intraindividual approach to study treatment effectiveness. She used an interrupted time series design with replications ($N = 5$) to test a system of nonpharmacological strategies involving self-monitoring, personal choice, self-regulation, and self-modification of environment, administered within a group format of peer support and professional guidance. Her purpose in using a multimodal approach was to provide a therapeutic environment in which women could incorporate nonpharmacological treatments, learn to adhere to difficult treatment plans, and be part of milieu in which behavioral, cognitive, and environmental change strategies could be modeled.

A group facilitated by a nurse met for 2 hours for 7 weeks. Knowledge was exchanged about nonpharmacological remedies for PMS, including specific dietary changes (lower caffeine and sugar, higher complex carbohydrate intake, small frequent meals, vitamin supplementation), aerobic and relaxation or stretching exercise, behavioral stress reduction techniques (stress identification, thought stopping, affirmations, self-esteem enhancements, and lifestyle alterations), and environmental control (time and role management, communication, and social competency training). Women rated their symptoms daily for 3 menstrual cycles prior to treatment, during treatment, and for 3 menstrual cycles after treatment. Each woman had been screened for and met criteria for PMS based on cycle phase differences and symptom severity criteria.

Taylor used time series analysis to identify patterns within each woman's daily symptom data. Baseline time series (for 90 days) were compared to post-treatment series (120 days), and data were analyzed as an interrupted time series. Taylor identified 3 treatment response patterns from correlograms that included a "normalizing" treatment effect in which the cyclic determinants of symptoms became predictable and regular (like molimina) but the severity of symptoms was markedly reduced. This effect was evident in three women. A second pattern was an "unstable" treatment effect characterized by high variability of negative affect across all menstrual cycle phases during baseline that did not respond to the therapy. This woman was referred for psychotherapy for a major life event that caused her to become severely depressed during the course of the study. Finally, one woman had a nonmenstrual cycle symptom pattern combined with a social week (effect on day of the week) symptom pattern that was reduced in severity after treatment. The advantages of the small N experimental design included an opportunity to analyze which treatment strategies women actually used and found helpful, modify strategies throughout the course of treatment, and assess effects of the changes women actually made as a result of the therapy.

Taylor (1998) conducted a clinical trial of professional-peer group treatment for perimenstrual symptoms to assess the short-term and long-term effectiveness of treatment on stress and symptom experiences. She treated 91 women with severe PMS who were randomized to an early treatment or a delayed treatment control group (treated 5 to 6 months later). The PMS symptom mangement program reduced symptom severity by 75%, premenstrual depression and general distress by 30-54%, and increased well-being and self-esteem. The results compared favorably with studies of antidepressant drug therapy. Effects of treatment persisted at 12 and 18 months. Women with limited incomes (25%) had underlying depression but used the program as a complement to psychotherapy.

In a recent trial of a positive reframing social support intervention on perceptions of permenstrual changes, Morse (1997) found that perimenstrual impairment decreased for women who completed the intervention (N = 18). This program used a comprehensive health promotion plan and a variety of educational and behavioral methods in each 42-hour unit, which included an overview of PMS, nutritional theories of PMS, exercise benefits, and stress reduction. Positive reframing was embedded in each.

Brown and Zimmer (1986a, 1986b) found widespread dissatisfaction with treatment among women with PMS symptoms. Women reported being treated disrespectfully and not being taken seriously. Eighty-three women attending a seminar on PMS rated their treatment. Sixty-seven percent rated their care by nurse practitioners as positive and 33% rated their care by physicians as positive.

Exercise has been proposed as a health-promoting behavior, yet there is evidence that certain exercise regimens affect menstrual cyclicity. Estok, Rudy, Kerr, and Menzel (1993) studied 146 women who participated in different levels of running. They found that runners reported a shorter luteal phase than nonrunners. There were no significant differences in ovulatory disturbances among groups, but runners versus nonrunners had more ovulatory disturbances. Uses of exercise for symptom management remain to be explored.

Despite the frequency with which nurses care for women with disability, only one study has addressed the relationship between disability and menstruation. Reame (1992) studied 67 menstrual cycles in 20 women (13 were quadriplegic, 7 paraplegic). Level of injury did not affect cycle length, menses duration, or concentration of gonadotropins and ovarian hormones. Ovulatory cycles were experienced by 93% of women, according to their progesterone levels. Cyclic dysmenorrhea was reported by 13 women with C5 to T-12 injuries. The need for contraception among this group was stressed. Better understanding of menstrual management for women with disabilities is needed.

Dysmenorrhea

Despite the prevalence of dysmenorrhea, nursing research has been limited. Aside from a few research papers published by nurses during the 1980s, only one research team has published multiple reports addressing the problem. Jordan and Meckler (1982) studied the relationship of life stress and social support among women with dysmenorrhea. They found a positive relationship between life change and dysmenorrhea among women not using oral contraceptives. Life change and social support together accounted for 16% of the variance in menstrual distress.

Brown and Woods (1984) assessed the correlates of dysmenorrhea among 193 women. They found that the strongest correlates were attitudes toward menstruation, although associations between dysmenorrhea and items reflecting traditional or feminist dimensions were absent. Shaver, Woods, Wolf-Wilets, and Heitkemper (1985) compared 55 women with dysmenorrhea to 98 women without dysmenorrhea. Women with dysmenorrhea had greater menstrual flow, more menstrual symptoms, and saw menstruation as more debilitating than those without dysmenorrhea but believed menstruation was a natural event. They perceived themselves as healthy.

Heitkemper, Shaver, and Mitchell (1988) have conducted a program of studies focusing on dysmenorrhea. Their earliest work involved a comparison of women with dysmenorrhea and without dysmenorrhea, including women using oral contraceptives and not using oral contraceptives. They found that menstrual cycle phase influenced gastrointestinal (GI) symptoms and stool consistencies in the sample as a whole. GI symptoms were more prevalent among the women with dysmenorrhea, especially nausea and decreased food intake; the loosest stools coincided with menses. In a subsequent study, Heitkemper, Jarrett, Bond, and Turner (1991) assessed stool characteristics, GI symptoms, and anxiety level daily. They also obtained early-morning urinary catecholamines and blood levels of ovarian steroids and cortisol at menses, follicular, and luteal phases. They replicated earlier findings of greater prevalence of gastrointestinal symptoms during menses. Cycle phase differences in serum cortisol, urine catecholamines, and anxiety were noted, especially in dysmenorrheic women. GI symptoms were not correlated with ovarian hormones or indicators of psychophysiological arousal. In a related study, Jarrett, Heitkemper, and Shaver (1995) investigated symptoms and self-care among women with and without dysmenorrhea. Despite significant differences in gastrointestinal, perimenstrual symptoms, there were no significant differences in smoking, alcohol use, exercise, and stressors. Few self-care strategies were reported aside from medications for cramps.

Heitkemper and Bond (1995) investigated gastric motility in rats in basal and thyrotropin-releasing hormone (TRH)-stimulated states. Ovariectomized rats were implanted with progesterone pellets, estrogen pellets, or both for 26 days. Gastric tension was measured via an implanted transducer. Estrogen- and estrogen-plus-progesterone-implanted rats had greater contractility than did the progesterone-implanted rats.

Menopause

The Experience of Menopause

The typical experience of menopause has been described in nursing research from two perspectives: the personal and social perspective and the bodily changes perspective. The work focusing on the former has addressed meanings of menopause, attitudes toward menopause, and the experiences of women from different ethnic and social class groups.

Meanings of Menopause

Several nurse researchers have studied the meanings women associated with menopause. McKeever (1991) studied 30 women who experienced irregularity or change in the menstrual cycle, hot flashes, or night sweats or who believed they were in menopause. She found women used four explanatory models to account for menopause. Some viewed menopause from a developmental perspective that depicted menopause positively as a process within women's adult development. Others saw menopause as symbolic of aging. Some had a rational view of menopause, believing that one experienced menopause as a function of how one thought about it. Others had the perspective of failed expectations or being let down. These models influenced the course of action women took in dealing with symptoms and how they viewed themselves as women.

Quinn (1991) conducted a grounded theory study of 12 middle-class women 40 to 60 years of age. "Integrating a changing me" was the conceptual model that included four categories of their menopausal experience. "Tuning in to me, my body and my moods" reflected women's awareness that they were in menopause. Facing a paradox of positive and negative feelings about menopause, aging, reproduction, vulnerability, and uncertainty comprised the second category. Some expressed contrasting impressions, concerned with processing and tempering information about menopause. Others described making adjustments, reflecting changes they made in their bodies and their emotions.

Cooksey, Imle, and Smith (1991) studied 10 postmenopausal women and developed a conceptual framework for viewing women's experiences of menopause that consisted of the following components: sorting it out, searching for meaning, coping, and integrating the transition with the self. Sorting it out was affected by the woman's expectations about menopause in combination with her own experiences. Searching for meaning concerned the significance of menopause. Coping was influenced by support from others.

Common to these studies is a central process women experience involving clarifying what the changes they perceived in their bodies and feelings meant and attributing them to menopause or to other midlife events. Women's experiences were quite heterogeneous, and their responses to menopause were a function of the significance they assigned to menopause within the broader context of their lives.

Attitudes Toward Menopause

Nurse researchers have also studied women's attitudes toward menopause. Bowles (1992) developed a semantic differential scale to assess menopausal attitudes. This scale has established validity and reliability and has been used in several nursing studies. Its brevity (20 items) makes it attractive for use in studies with multiple measures. Theisen, Mansfield, Seery, and Voda (1995) studied 287 women aged 35 to 55 years using Bowles' Menstrual Attitudes Scale. They found that both individual and contextual factors were related to women's attitudes. Menopausal stage, age, health status, menopause-related changes women experienced, and number of people to whom women could talk and the ease with which they could talk about menopause were examined as correlates of attitudes. Menopausal status, emotional health, ease with discussing menopause, number of family members the women could talk to about menopause, and menopause-related changes were all related to menopausal attitudes. In a study of low-income clinic patients ($N = 66$), Standing and Glazer (1992) found that women had a somewhat positive attitude toward menopause, with younger women being less positive than older women.

Woods, Saver, and Taylor (1998) explored the relationship among women's attitudes toward menopause and hormone therapy and paradigms of menopause as a natural life event versus a biomedical phenomenon.

Women ($N = 2,092$) selected from physicians' practices in Washington completed mailed questionaires. Women's atitudes toward menopause were unrelated to their adoption of a biomedical versus developmental paradigm of menopause. In contrast, women's adoption of the view that menopause was an endocrine deficiency and that symptoms could be treated with hormones were correlated. Women who endorsed the endocrine deficiency model had attitudes toward use of hormone therapy as more effacious, less risky and requiring daily use of a drug. Women's experiences of hysterectomy and use of hormone therapy were also associated with their attitudes toward hormone threrapy. Women embraced menopause as part of life and simultaneously accepted changes in their endocrine production.

Woods and Mitchell (1999) asked participants in the Seattle Midlife Women's Health Study about their definitions of menopause, and their expectations and concerns about their own menopausal experiences during in-person interviews conducted at the beginning of the study between late 1990 and early 1993. Women ranged in age from 35 to 55 years and were premenopausal or had begun the transition to menopause. Women defined menopause as cessation of their periods, end of their reproductive ability, a time of hormonal changes, a change of life, a changing body, changing emotions, an aging process. Few women defined menopause as a time of symptoms or disease risk or a time for medical care. Women were most likely to be uncertain of their expectations of their own menopause and many had no expectations.

Ethnicity and Class: Menopausal Experiences

Jackson studied African-American women ($N = 522$), who often experience menopause due to hysterectomy at an earlier age than do White women. She found that when a woman experiences menopause is a critical factor. Those who experienced menopause between 25 and 34 years of age had the most severe physical and mental health symptoms, compared to those experiencing menopause between 35 and 44 years of age (Jackson, 1992; Jackson, Taylor, & Pyngolil, 1991). Although timing of menopause was important, women's relationships were significant predictors of their life satisfaction (Jackson, 1990).

Berg and Taylor examined the symptom experiences of Filipino American midlife women. In a cross-sectional study of a community-based sample of 165 Filipina Americans between the ages of 35 and 56, women provided data about their symptoms believed to be related to changing estrogen levels and their management. Women's use of non-pharmacologic remedies exceeded their use of either over the counter medications or hormones. Filipina American women considered the perimenopausal transition in a positive light and reported little distress associated with the presumably estrogen-related symptoms. Their choice of remedies for symptoms is consistent with their posititve attitudes toward the perimenopausal transition and sends a strong message to health care providers about culturally appropriate care.

Transition to Menopause

Voda and colleagues' (1994) studies of bleeding patterns during perimenopause have begun to clarify what women can expect as they make the transition to menopause. Women 45 years and younger had fewer bleeding and clotting days than women who were older. For a subset of women over 45, bleeding increased beyond 6 days. Women between 44.4 and 47.6 years were more likely than those who were older or younger to say they were in the menopausal transition. For these women, heaviest flow and heavy clotting were most likely to occur on Day 2, with both decreasing until bleeding stopped. Women who had irregular cycles were more likely to be 25 to 49 years old and to have slightly heavier bleeding and more clots. Voda's use of the menstrual calendar to track bleeding patterns has been adopted by several investigators, including Woods and Mitchell and Reame and associates.

Symptoms

Although there have been many studies of menopausal symptoms, the earliest nursing studies were those of Voda, whose careful description of the menopausal hot flash from both a physiological and personal perspective is a classic. Recordings revealed the time of day, length, origins, spread, and intensity of the hot flash and strategies women used to deal with them. There was no common trigger for the hot flash, and timing of occurrence was unpredictable. The origin and spread were predictable. Severity was related to length of time the flash lasted and the discomfort women linked to its experience. The most common strategy for dealing with hot flashes was applying an external coolant or doing nothing (Voda, 1981, 1982).

A subsequent epidemiological study of the prevalence of menopausal hot flashes revealed that the prevalence was highest in women between 46 and 50 years of age and that 86% of women who experience natural menopause experienced hot flashes, but the frequency was highly variable (Feldman, Voda, & Gronseth, 1985). Current work on the hot flash is being conducted by Kronenberg and Barnard (1992), who have found that hot flashes increase in warm environments but decrease with fever (Barnard, Kronenberg, & Downey, 1992; Kronenberg & Barnard, 1992).

Sleep problems become more common as women age, but the relationship between menopausal stage and sleep patterns remains unclear. Although there are few differences in sleep among premenopausal, perimenopausal (defined as women experiencing changes in bleeding patterns prior to menopause), and postmenopausal women, perimenopausal and postmenopausal women who experience hot flashes have lower sleep efficiencies and longer REM latency than those without hot flashes (Shaver, Giblin, Lentz, & Lee, 1988). Shaver and Paulsen (1992) found that a larger proportion of postmenopausal women than premenopausal or perimenopausal women rated themselves as poor sleepers. There was a trend for the perimenopausal and postmenopausal women to take longer to fall asleep and to have less deep sleep (Shaver & Paulsen, 1994). Polysomnographic recordings of sleep did not agree with women's self-ratings. A subset of the midlife women ($n = 135$) reported distressing symptoms and poor sleep despite having fairly stable and efficient sleep in the laboratory. These women were also likely to be psychologically distressed. Those who perceived poor sleep and whose sleep was unstable in the laboratory did not differ in psychological distress from women with good sleep. Their unstable sleep may have coincided with physiological instability, such as hot flashes and sweats. Most of the women in this sample demonstrated and perceived good sleep. The lack of congruence between perception of sleep quality and lab measures suggested the importance of environmental effects on sleep (Shaver, Giblin, & Paulsen, 1991). Paulsen and Shaver (1991) determined that psychological distress, as influenced by negative life events and nonsupportive contacts with one's social network, influenced perceived sleep ratings but not somnographic recordings of sleep in the lab setting.

Depression is prevalent among women, and investigators have been interested in how depression is linked to menopause. Nurse researchers have investigated the prevalence of depressed mood among midlife women and have found, like researchers from other fields, little evidence that menopause causes depression. Woods and Mitchell (1997) studied 347 women enrolled in the Seattle Midlife Women's Health Study, a population-based longitudinal study. Using LISREL-VII to test a multidimensional causal model comparing effects of a stressful life context pathway, health status pathway, and menopausal changes pathway, Woods and Mitchell (1997) found that the stressful life context pathway was most influential in accounting for depressed mood. Health status (measured as chronic illnesses and perceived health) had a direct effect on depressed mood and an indirect effect through stress. The menopausal changes pathway had little explanatory power. These results support the need for clinicians to look beyond menopausal status to the broader context of midlife women's lives. Depression was assessed over each subsequent year of the study. Patterns of depressed mood over the first 2 years of the study were classified to reveal four different patterns: absence of depression in both years, consistent depression in both years, emerging depression (not depressed in year 1, but depressed in year 2), and recovering depression (depressed year 1, not depressed year 2). They found that women's patterns of depressed mood were related to stressful life context, past and present health status, and social learning about midlife. Having a PMS history, poorer health status, being socialized negatively for midlife, having fewer family resources, and having less social support differentiated women with emerging depression from those with absence of depression over the 1-year period. More stress, fewer family resources, and poorer health status differentiated women recovering from depression from those with absence of depression. Having more stress, a PMS history, and a postpartum blues history differentiated women with consistent depressed mood from those with absence of depression. Menopausal status did not differentiate women with patterns of emerging depression, recovering depression, and consistent depression from women who were not depressed on either occasion. Vasomotor symptoms, history of premenstrual syndrome, postpartum blues history, and midlife socialization helped differentiate women with consistently depressed mood from those recovering from depressed mood.

Mitchell and Woods (1996) also asked women to keep daily health diaries over an 80-day period each year. From women who returned at least one cycle of daily data ($n = 301$), the investigators have been able to establish the prevalence of symptoms as well as the factor structure describing how symptoms cluster. Five premenstrual factors emerged: dysphoric mood and vasomotor, somatic, neuromuscular, and insomnia symptoms explaining 51.7% of the variance. Test-retest internal reliability estimates over 3 years indicated that the most reliable clusters were dysphoric mood and somatic symptoms. When stability across the 3 years was examined, the most stable were dysphoric mood, neuromuscular, and insomnia symptoms. Somatic symptoms were the least stable. This work will complement completed, large, population-based studies of menopausal symptoms that have relied on single-point measures of symptoms rather than on daily recordings.

Health Consequences of Menopause

Consequences of menopause for subsequent perceived health have been explored. Engel (1987) found that among women 40 to 55 years old ($N = 249$), completing menopause was associated with slightly poorer perceived health. Women with more stressful lives had poorer perceived health status. Bareford (1991) found that midlife women had more symptoms when they had more difficult life events and negative attitudes toward menopause. Positive attitudes buffered effects of life stress on symptoms.

Symptom Management

Hormone replacement therapy (HRT) has received most attention in the medical literature about menopausal symptoms. In contrast to studying whether HRT produces beneficial health outcomes, nurse researchers have focused on how women decide to adopt hormone therapy. In response to hypothetical case studies focusing on estrogen use, women were influenced largely by symptom distress associated with hot flashes and, to a lesser extent, by risk of osteoporosis and side effects of estrogen therapy. Although health professionals tend to emphasize risk reduction, women themselves were concerned about the immediate effects of estrogen on symptoms they perceived as distressing (Rothert et al., 1990).

In a later study (Schmitt et al., 1991) of midlife women's decisions to use estrogen or combined hormone therapy to alleviate menopausal symptoms, again based on hypothetical cases, women's decision patterns sorted into four distinct groups. One group of women based their decision to take hormones on whether their hot flashes were severe. A second would use hormones if hot flashes were severe but would also consider the risk of osteoporosis and cancer in making their decision. A third were most influenced by the unpleasant effects of adding progestin to the hormone therapy because they did not want to resume menses or spotting. The fourth considered health risks, particularly the risk of cancer. These groups were distinguished by several factors: educational level, perceived stress, and attitudes toward menopause and use of medications. Women in the second group (who considered severity of hot flashes and risks of osteoporosis and cancer) had the most formal education, had higher stress levels, and were more likely to use vitamins to control menopausal symptoms. Women in group three (dissuaded by resumption of menses) had the most positive attitudes toward menopause. In all cases, prediction of willingness to take estrogen was related to the perception that hormone treatment might be helpful in controlling menopausal symptoms and knowledge about menopause and its effects on women. Expectations that menopause would be difficult were related to lower likelihood of taking hormone therapy. Current comfort level, as indicated by hot flashes, was an overriding concern in women's decisions.

In a study of women 40 to 60 years of age, Logothetis (1991) compared over 200 users and nonusers of estrogen therapy, controlling for perceived menopausal distress, with respect to elements of the health belief model (perceived susceptibility, seriousness, benefits, barriers) and philosophical orientation to menopause. Women who did not feel highly susceptible to menopausal problems did not perceive menopausal problems as serious, had stronger perceptions of barriers to using estrogen than benefits, and were undecided about whether or not menopause was a medical event. Combined health beliefs accounted for about 30% of the variance in estrogen use. Perceptions of estrogen's benefits and barriers to use accounted for most of the difference between users and nonusers, followed by philosophy of menopause and seriousness of menopausal problems.

Woods, Falk, Saver, Stevens, Taylor, Moreno, and MacLaren (1997) studied the decision process in which women engaged as they committed to use and continue to use postmenopausal hormone therapy. Data collected from midlife women in a series of six focus groups encompassing multiple ethnic and social groups. Participants identified five phases of a decision process: precontemplation, contemplation, commitment, critical evaluation, and continuance of therapy. Health care providers had significant opportunities to interact with women during the transitional points between these phases. Woods and associates validated this model in subsequent individual in-depth interviews with midlife women at varying stages in their decision processes (Woods et al., 1998).

O'Connor and colleagues (1998) developed a self-administered hormone replacement therapy (HRT) decision aid and evaluated it with 94 women from six family practices who participated in a before-after study. An audiotape guided women through an illustrated booklet that contained detailed information about HRT benefits and risks that were tailored to a women's clinical risk and a values clarification exercise to promote informed decision-making that was consistent with the women's own values. Women who completed the decision aid had better general knowledge and more realistic personal expectations of HRT benefits. They also felt more certain, informed, clear about their values, and supported in decision making. Women with strong preferences at the beginning did not change their minds, but felt better informed. Changes in preferences occurred among women who were uncertain.

Shaver (1994) proposed that nonpharmacological therapies for menopausal symptoms warranted investigation. Among these are dietary modification, exercise, and stress management. Although such therapies are frequently recommended, intervention studies using these strategies are scarce in the nursing literature. One published intervention study focused on women's uncertainty before and after a class on menopause. Using a pretest-posttest ipsitive control design, Lemaire and Lenz (1995) found that uncertainty decreased significantly after the program. Age and perceived level of knowledge were related to preprogram uncertainty. Postprogram uncertainty was a function of preprogram uncertainty, perception of knowledge gained, and level of postprogram knowledge. The consequences of programs such as this for women's experiences of symptoms will be important to assess in future studies.

Wilbur, Holm, and Dan (1992) studied exercise patterns of 279 midlife women 37 to 64 years of age. They found that leisure activity exercise was correlated negatively with menopausal symptoms. Fewer than 30% of women had vasomotor symptoms, but more than 50% complained of symptoms such as fatigue, headaches, and irritability. Perimenopausal women reported more symptoms than pre- and postmenopausal groups or women who had hysterectomies.

McElmurry and Huddleston (1991) studied self-care response patterns of 146 perimenopausal women. Two clusters were evident. The first cluster of women did not use self-care, although they recognized that changes were occurring in their bodies. The second cluster included women who used a broad repertoire of self-care responses and used them frequently in an attempt to manage the changes they were experiencing. Education encouraged greater use of self-care.

Discourse Analysis

A final area of investigation has been analysis of the discourse about menopause. MacPherson (1981, 1985, 1990, 1992) has traced the conceptions of menopause as a deficiency disease to the current notion of menopause as the cause of other diseases, such as heart disease and osteoporosis. Her work continues to challenge the medicalization of menopause. Dickson's (1991) interpretive analyses of the scientific literature about menopause and midlife women's own knowledge of menopause revealed women's differing images of menopause. The manipulation of women's bodies arose as a theme in discussion of hormone therapy and hysterectomy. Displacement of knowledge was a theme reflecting the professionals' use of medical knowledge to displace women's experiences of their own bodies. The cloak of silence surrounding menopause reflected women's experiences of limited communication about their experiences.

Critique

Nurses have made a significant contribution to understanding the menstrual cycle and symptoms related to menstruation and menopause and have begun to contribute to understandings of therapeutics. In particular, nurses have contributed careful descriptions of women's everyday experiences rather than restricting their focus to the pathological or abnormal. As a result, there is a great deal of knowledge available to clinicians regarding the typical experiences of menarche, menstruation (including PMS and dysmenorrhea), and menopause.

Much of the nursing research has been stimulated and nurtured by the Society for Menstrual Cycle Research.[1] This multidisciplinary society has provided nurse investigators with opportunities for exchange of perspectives about the menstrual cycle and collegial support and collaboration. Nurses have enriched the society by their sustained and significant contributions to the science about the menstrual cycle.

Most research conducted in other fields has emphasized the abnormal or pathological aspects of the menstrual cycle and menopause. Support for menstrual cycle research in general has been directed toward biomedical explorations, with lesser amounts of funding having been directed toward studies of the menstrual cycle and menopause as normative events in women's lives. Nonetheless, nursing research over the past two decades has provided a rich complement to that from other fields.

Models Guiding the Research

Central to models guiding the research have been images of women as whole human beings, with body-mind-emotions-social relationships. Attention to a holistic perspective has bound findings about women's biology together with those about the social context in which women live their lives. Related to this perspective is an attempt to recontextualize women's experiences by addressing symptoms in the broader context of women's lives. Although nurse investigators give credence to the importance of a woman's biology seen in context, the majority of studies have not included measures of biological indicators. Artificial distinctions in types of symptoms being studied, such as isolating emotional and cognitive symptoms, as is done in the diagnosis of premenstrual dysphoric disorder, are not commonly encountered in nursing research. Creative tensions between those investigators who recognize and those who contest the existence of premenstrual syndrome and menopausal syndromes seem to have been de-emphasized in the nursing literature in favor of more encompassing theories about how a woman's social context and her biology together account for her symptoms.

Women's health primary care practice has received increasing emphasis in nursing education, but research to support it has lagged behind the curricular efforts. Nonpharmacological trials for symptom management are sparse in the literature on premenstrual syndrome, dysmenorrhea, and menopause symptoms. Moreover, there is little discussion of health education and health promotion interventions for premenarcheal girls and adult women related to their menstrual experiences.

Measurement Advances

In the areas of menarche, menstruation, and menopause, nurse investigators have contributed to the development and validation of measurement instruments that have utility in both research and practice. Questions such as what symptoms to measure; how much variability within and across cycles to expect; when to measure; and use of continuous versus interrupted sampling, time- or event-based sampling, and retrospective versus prospective recording have been addressed. In addition, criteria have been developed for explicating the severity of symptoms and cycle phase differences to define PMS and PMM and have been contributed to literature that is currently cited by investigators within and beyond the field. Important advances have come from daily sampling of symptoms, pulsatile sampling of gonadotropins, and use of urinary assays to allow frequent measurement without harming participants. Use of symptom-related sampling instead of cycle-phase-determined sampling has been a unique contribution. Future development of indirect indicators (for example, an indirect indicator of CNS function, such as platelet uptake of serotonin) will enhance studies relating biological changes across the menstrual cycle to symptoms.

Samples

Nursing research results reflect studies with women seeking care in clinical settings as well as community-based populations of women. Comorbidity in these samples remains a challenge, as does accounting for the influences of oral contraceptives, other drugs, psychiatric history, age, ovulatory status, and characteristics of the menstrual cycle. Criteria for the menopausal transition will contribute to more precise sampling for studies of menopause. Development of these criteria await further progress in analyzing data related to women's bleeding patterns during perimenopause.

Treatment Trials

This area of the literature is the most underdeveloped. Controlled trials and crossover trials assessing the efficacy of treatments prescribed by nurses are needed to guide primary care delivery. These therapies should be compared to currently used drug therapy, not only to placebo controls. Use of small *N* experiments as pilot studies would enhance progress in this area.

Menarche

Most work about menarche has focused on the event as a normative experience, and nurses have attempted to contextualize menarche in their work by focusing on the social context surrounding the experience. There has been little work focusing on biological changes surrounding menarche and in relation to symptoms. Studies of menarcheal preparation are needed to provide young girls with optimum preparation for healthy experiences of menstruation and their sexuality. The difference between mother-daughter communication and communication with a health professional needs to be clarified. Which types of messages, including information about anticipated experiences, feelings, and values, are best communicated by a nurse or by a girl's mother remain uncertain. The type of information girls need, beyond how to cope with the hygienic challenge of menstruating, is yet to be defined. Psychoeducational interventions for school-age girls provided by school nurses is an area for fruitful study.

Menstruation

Nurses have studied menstruation as a normative experience. Their work includes careful description of the experience of women with molimina, as well as symptoms. Patterns of premenstrual symptoms, including PMS and PMM, and dysmenorrhea symptoms have been described carefully as the basis for treatment. The existence of a symptom pattern consistent with definitions of PMS has been described, and the possibility for its idiosyncratic experience has been discussed. Definitions and criteria for clinical assessment based on daily recordings as well as retrospective assessment have been established.

Attention to the context in which menstruation occurs has been an important part of nursing research into the menstrual cycle. Studies have documented the importance of stressful life circumstances in association with symptoms, as well as the importance of socialization for menstruation. Nurse researchers have made clear the consequences for women of a social context in which menstrual symptoms such as PMS are invalidated or used to invalidate women's complaints and abilities.

Although there has been less emphasis on the biological basis for menstrual cycle symptoms, studies of ovarian steroids, gonadotropins, and stress hormones (cortisol and catecholamines), as well as other stress response indicators (skin conductance, EMG), have been published. Taken together, these indicate the importance of considering both the HPO and HPA axes in understanding women's experiences of symptoms.

One important aspect of nursing research about symptom patterns such as PMS has been emphasis on bodily symptoms as well as symptoms with only emotional or cognitive referents. This is a significant difference in emphasis from that assumed by the American Psychiatric Association's definition of premenstrual dysphoric disorder, in which mental health is emphasized almost to the exclusion of concern for bodily symptoms that women associate with PMS. Thus the nature of diagnoses nurses use in practice will be important in defining women as having a mental illness or as having a symptom pattern that includes both bodily and cognitive-emotional dimensions.

For purposes of diagnostic specificity, some investigators have ignored symptoms with bodily referents, for example, swelling and cramps, thus treating dysmenorrhea symptoms and fluid retention as if they were not part of a woman's perimenstrual experience. Although this approach may simplify studies such as those of PDD, it compromises the validity of the women's lived experience and may blind investigators and clinicians to the underlying mechanisms responsible for a woman's distress. Bancroft (1993) thus pointed out that investigators studying PMS have chosen to ignore the role of prostaglandins in symptom experience, choosing instead to proceed as if the uterus and brain were disconnected.

As more nurses assume roles as primary care providers for women, the need to develop and test therapeutic models for primary care for women is becoming more acute. Tests of treatment models, coupled with health education interventions to promote understanding of menstruation, symptoms, and self-care options, should be aggressively pursued.

Dysmenorrhea

Despite its prevalence, nursing research about dysmenorrhea has been limited. Perhaps the advent of non-steroidal anti-inflammatory drugs (NSAIDs) has reduced clinicians' urgency to find new treatments. Because NSAIDs will not be an appropriate solution for all women, it is important for nurses to continue to test alternative treatments to NSAIDs. Use of self-care strategies, including self-management protocols for dysmenorrhea, should be explored. In addition, nurse investigators need to consider the joint prevalence of PMS and dysmenorrhea in designing intervention trials that could effectively address these menstrual cycle problems that frequently co-occur.

Menopause

Nursing research on menopause, like that on the menstrual cycle, has emphasized studies of normative experiences. The literature contains rich descriptions of symptoms associated with menopause, including studies of hot flashes, sleep problems, and depression—problems of great significance to the women who experience them. In addition, nurses have focused on the meanings of menopause, women's attitudes toward the experience, and the social context in which it occurs and how the social context modifies the experience. What is needed are studies of health education interventions, such as those designed to reduce women's uncertainty about the experience. In addition, primary care models of therapeutics for menopause are needed. Of high priority should be studies of the decision processes women use in arriving at a commitment to use (or not use) hormone therapy and development and testing of decision support models and aids. In addition, there is acute need to find nonpharmacological options for symptom management for symptoms such as hot flashes and sleep disturbances.

Note

1. To order copies of proceedings of past meetings, e-mail pkm@psu.edu or contact Phyllis Mansfield, 13 Sparks Bldg., Penn State University. University Park, PA 16802.

References

American Psychiatric Association. (1994). *Diagnostic and statistical manual IV.* Washington, DC: Author.

Bancroft, J. (1993). The premenstrual syndrome: A reappraisal of the concept of the evidence. *Psychological Medicine,* (Suppl. 24), 1-47.

Bareford, C. (1991). An investigation of the nature of the menopausal experience: Attitude toward menopause, recent life change, coping method, and number and frequency of symptoms in menopausal women. In D. Taylor & N. Woods (Eds.), *Menstruation, health and illness* (pp. 223-236). New York: Hemisphere.

Barnard, R., Kronenberg, F., & Downey, J. (1992). Effect of fever on menopausal hot flashes. *Maturitas, 14,* 181-188.

Berg J., & Taylor, D. (in press-a). The Symptom Experiences of Filipino American Midlife Women. *Menopause.*

Berg. J., & Taylor, D. (in press-b). Symptom Responses of Midlife Filipina Americans. *Menopause.*

Bloch, D. (1978). Sex education practices of mothers. *Journal of Sex Therapy, 4,* 7-12.

Bowles, C. (1992). The development of a measure of attitude. In A. J. Dan & L. L. Lewis (Eds.), *Menstrual health in women's lives* (pp. 206-212). Urbana and Chicago: University of Illinois Press.

Brown, M., & Woods, N. (1984). Correlates of dysmenorrhea: A challenge to past stereotypes. *Journal of Obstetric, Gynecologic and Neonatal Nursing, 13,* 259-265.

Brown, M. A., & Lewis, L. L. (1993). Cycle-phase changes in perceived stress in women with varying levels of premenstrual symptomatology. *Research in Nursing and Health, 16,* 423-429.

Brown, M. A., & Woods, N. F. (1986). Sex role orientation, sex typing, occupational traditionalism, and perimenstrual symptoms. In V. L. Olesen & N. F. Woods (Eds.), *Culture, society, and menstruation* (pp. 25-38). Washington, DC: Hemisphere.

Brown, M. A., & Zimmer, P. A. (1986a). Help-seeking for premenstrual symptomatology: A description of women's experiences. *Health Care for Women International, 7,* 173-184.

Brown, M. A., & Zimmer, P. A. (1986b). Help-seeking for premenstrual symptomatology: A description of women's experiences. In V. L. Olesen & N. F. Woods (Eds.), *Culture, society, and menstruation* (pp. 173-184). Washington, DC: Hemisphere.

Brown, M. A., & Zimmer, P. A. (1986c). Personal and family impact of premenstrual symptoms. *Journal of Obstetric, Gynecologic, and Neonatal Nursing, 15,* 31-38.

Cahill, C. A. (1998, Sept.-Oct.). Differences in cortisol, a stress hormone, in women with turmoil-type premenstrual symptoms. *Nursing Research, 47*(5), 278-284.

Cooksey, S., Imle, M., & Smith, C. (1991). An inductive study of the transition of menopause. In A. Voda & R. Conover (Eds.), *Proceedings of the Society for Menstrual Cycle Research, Eighth Conference* (pp. 75-111). Scottsdale, AZ: Society for Menstrual Cycle Research.

Danza, R. (1983). Menarche: Its effects on mother-daughter and father-daughter interactions. In S. Golub (Ed.), *Menarche* (pp. 99-105). New York: Lexington.

Dashiff, C. J., & Buchanan, L. A. (1995). Menstrual attitudes among Black and White premenarcheal girls. *Journal of Child and Adolescent Psychiatric Nursing, 8,* 5-14.

Dickson, G. (1991). Menopause: Language, meaning, and subjectivity: A feminist poststructuralist analysis. In A. Voda & R. Conover (Eds.), *Proceedings of the Society for Menstrual Cycle Research, Eighth Conference* (pp. 112-125). Scottsdale, AZ: Society for Menstrual Cycle Research.

Doan, H. M., & Morse, J. M. (1985). The last taboo: Roadblocks to researching menarche. *Health Care for Women International, 6,* 277-283.

Engel, N. S. (1987). Menopausal stage, current life change, attitude toward women's roles, and perceived health status. *Nursing Research, 36,* 353-357.

Estok, P., Rudy, E., Kerr, M., & Menzel, L. (1993). Menstrual response to running: Nursing implications. *Nursing Research, 42,* 158-165.

Feldman, B. M., Voda, A., & Gronseth, E. (1985). The prevalence of the hot flash and associated variables among perimenopausal women. *Research in Nursing and Health, 8,* 261-268.

Gallant, S. J., Popiel, D. A., Hoffman, P. K., Chakraborty, P. K., & Hamilton, J. A. (1992). Using daily rating to confirm premenstrual syndrome/late luteal phase dysphoric disorder. Part 1: Effects of demand characteristics and expectations. *Psychosomatic Medicine, 54,* 149-166.

Hamilton, J., Alagna, S., & Sharp, K. (1985). Cognitive approaches to understanding and treating premenstrual depression. In H.

Ofofsky (Ed.), *Premenstrual syndrome* (pp. 382-392). Washington, DC: American Psychiatric Association.

Harding, S. (1991). *Whose science? Whose knowledge? Thinking from women's lives.* Ithaca, NY: Cornell University Press.

Havens, B., & Swenson, I. (1988). Imagery associated with menstruation in advertising targeted to adolescent females. *Adolescence, 23,* 89-97.

Heitkemper, M., & Bond, E. (1995). Gastric motility in rats with varying ovarian hormone status. *Western Journal of Nursing Research, 17,* 9-19.

Heitkemper, M., Jarrett, M., Bond, E., & Turner, P. (1991). GI symptoms, function, and psychophysiological arousal in dymenorrheic women. *Nursing Research, 40,* 20-26.

Heitkemper, M., Shaver, J., & Mitchell, E. (1988). Gastrointestinal symptoms and bowel patterns across the menstrual cycle in dysmenorrhea. *Nursing Research, 37,* 108-113.

Jackson, B. (1990). Social support and life satisfaction of Black climacteric women. *Western Journal of Nursing Research, 12,* 9-27.

Jackson, B. (1992). Black women's responses to menarche and menopause. In A. Dan & L. Lewis (Eds.), *Menstrual health in women's lives* (pp. 178-190). Chicago: University of Illinois Press.

Jackson, B., Taylor, J., & Pyngolil, M. (1991). How age conditions the relationship between climacteric status and health symptoms in African American women. *Research in Nursing and Health, 14,* 1-9.

Janes, B. A., & Morse, J. M. (1990). Adolescent girls' perceptions of and preparation for menarche. *Canadian Journal of Nursing Research, 22,* 47-58.

Jarrett, M., Heitkemper, M., & Shaver, J. (1995). Symptoms and self-care strategies in women with and without dysmenorrhea. *Health Care for Women International, 16,* 167-178.

Jordan, J., & Meckler, J. (1982). The relationship between life change events, social supports, and dysmenorrhea. *Research in Nursing and Health, 5,* 73-79.

Kronenberg, F., & Barnard, R. (1992). Modulation of menopausal hot flashes by ambient temperature. *Journal of Termal Biology, 1,* 43-49. Ann Arbor, MI: University of Michigan.

Lee, K., & Rittenhouse, C. (1991). Prevalence of perimenstrual symptoms in employed women. *Women and Health, 17,* 17-32.

Lee, K. A., Lentz, M. J., Taylor, D., Mitchell, E. S., & Woods, N. F. (1994). Fatigue as a response to environmental demands in women's lives. *Image: The Journal of Nursing Scholarship, 26,* 149-154.

Lee, K. A., & Rittenhouse, C. A. (1992). Health and perimenstrual symptoms: Health outcomes for employed women who experience perimenstrual symptoms. *Women and Health, 19,* 65-78.

Lee, K. A., Shaver, J. F., Giblin, E. C., & Woods, N. F. (1990). Sleep patterns related to menstrual cycle phase and premenstrual affective symptoms. *Sleep, 13,* 403-409.

Lemaire, G. S., & Lenz, E. R. (1995). Perceived uncertainty about menopause in women attending an educational program. *International Journal of Nursing Studies, 32,* 39-48.

Lentz, M., Henker, R., Heitkemper, M., Mitchell, E., Woods, N., & Shaver, J. (1998). The relationship between ovarian steroids and perimenstrual symptoms: A comparison of group differences and intra-individual patterns. Submitted.

Lewis, L. (1989). Premenstrual syndrome. In C. J. Leppa & C. Miller (Eds.), *Women's health perspectives: An annual review* (Vol. 2, pp. 81-108). Phoenix, AZ: Oryx.

Lewis, L. (1992). PMS and progesterone: The ongoing controversy. In A.J. Dan & L.L. Lewis (Eds.), *Menstrual health in women's lives* (pp. 61-74). Urbana and Chicago: University of Illinois Press.

Lewis, L. L. (1995). One year in the life of a woman with premenstrual syndrome: A case study. *Nursing Research, 44,* 111-116.

Lewis, L. L., Greenblatt, E. M., Rittenhouse, C. A., Veldhuis, J. D., & Jaffe, R. B. (1995). Pulsatile release patterns of luteinizing hormone and progesterone in relation to symptom onset in women with premenstrual syndrome. *Fertility and Sterility, 64,* 288-292.

Logothetis, M. (1991). Women's decisions about estrogen replacement therapy. *Western Journal of Nursing Research, 13,* 458-474.

Logue, C. M., & Moos, R. H. (1986). Perimenstrual symptoms: Prevalence and risk factors. *Psychosomatic Medicine, 48,* 388-414.

MacPherson, K. (1981). Menopause as disease: The social construction of a metaphor. *Advances in Nursing Science, 3,* 95-114.

MacPherson, K. (1985). Osteoporosis and menopause: A feminist analysis of the social construction of a syndrome. *Advances in Nursing Science, 7,* 11-22.

MacPherson, K. (1990). Nurse researchers respond to the medicalization of menopause. In M. Flint, F. Kronenberg, & W. Utian (Eds.), *Multidisciplinary perspectives on menopause* (pp. 180-184). New York: New York Academy of Sciences Press.

MacPherson, K. (1992). Cardiovascular disease in women and non-contraceptive use of hormones: A feminist analysis. *Advances in Nursing Science, 14,* 34-49.

Martin, E. (1987). *The woman in the body: A cultural analysis of reproduction.* Boston: Beacon.

McElmurry, B. J., & Huddleston, D. S. (1991). Self-care and menopause: Critical review of research. *Health Care for Women International, 12,* 15-26.

McKeever, L. (1991). Informal models of women's perimenopausal experiences: Implications for health care. In A. Voda & R. Conover (Eds.), *Proceedings of the Society for Menstrual Cycle Research, Eighth Conference* (pp. 232-255). Scottsdale, AZ: Society for Menstrual Cycle Research.

Menke, E. (1983). Menstrual beliefs and experiences of mother-daughter dyads. In S. Glub (Ed.), *Menarch* (pp. 133-137). New York: Lexington.

Mitchell, E., & Woods, N. (1996). Symptom experiences of midlife women: Observations from the Seattle Midlife Women's Health Study. *Maturitas, 25,* 1-10.

Mitchell, E., Woods, N., & Lentz, M. (1994). Differentiating women with premenstrual syndrome and premenstrual magnification of symptoms: The development of a predictive model. *Nursing Research, 43,* 25-30.

Mitchell, E.S., Lentz, M.J., Woods, N.F., Lee, K., & Taylor, D. (1992). Methodological issues in the definition of premenstrual syndrome. In A.J. Dan & L.L. Lewis (Eds.), *Menstrual health in women's lives* (pp. 7-14). Urbana and Chicago: University of Illinois Press.

Mitchell, E. S., Woods, N. F., & Lentz, M. J. (1991). Recognizing PMS when you see it: Criteria for PMS sample selection. In D. Taylor & N. Woods (Eds.), *Menstruation, health and illness* (pp 89-102). Washington, DC: Hemisphere.

Monagle, L. A., Dan, A. J., & Chatterton, R. (1986). Toward delineating menstrual symptom groupings: Examination of factor analytic results of menstrual symptom instruments. In V. L. Olesen & N. F. Woods (Eds.), *Culture, society, and menstruation* (pp. 131-144). Washington, DC: Hemisphere.

Morse, G. G. (1997). Effect of positive reframing and social support on perception of perimenstrual changes among women with premenstrual syndrome. *Health Care for Women International, 18,* 175-193.

Morse, J. M., & Doan, H. M. (1987). Adolescents' response to menarche. *Journal of School Health, 57,* 385-389.

Morse, J. M., & Kieren, D. (1993). The Adolescent Menstrual Attitude Questionnaire: Normative scores, part 2. *Health Care for Women International, 14,* 63-76.

Morse, J. M., Kieren, D., & Bottorff, J. (1993). The Adolescent Menstrual Attitude Questionnaire: Scale construction, part 1. *Health Care for Women International, 14,* 39-62.

Most, A., Woods, N. F., Dery, G., & Most, B. (1981). Distress associated with menstruation among Israeli women. *International Journal of Nursing Studies, 18,* 61-71.

Napholz, L. (1994). The relationship of age and attitudes toward menopause among three age groups of college educated American women. *International Journal of Psychiatric Nursing Research, 1,* 50-62.

O'Connor, A., Tugwell, P., Wells, G., Elmslie, T., Jolly, E., Hollingworth, G., McPherson, R., Bunn, H., Graham, I., & Drake, E. (1998). A decision aid for women considering hormone therapy after menopause: Decision support framework and evaluation. *Patient Education and Counseling, 33,* 267-279.

Ornitz, A. W., & Brown, M. A. (1993). Family coping and premenstrual symptomatology. *Journal of Obstetric, Gynecologic, and Neonatal Nursing, 22,* 49-55.

Patterson, E. T., & Hale, E. S. (1985). Making sure: Integrating menstrual care practices into activities of daily living. *Advances in Nursing Science, 7,* 18-31.

Paulsen, V., & Shaver, J. (1991). Stress, support, psychological states and sleep. *Social Science and Medicine, 32,* 1237-1243.

Quinn, A. A. (1991). A theoretical model of the perimenopausal process. *Journal of Nurse-Midwifery, 36,* 25-29.

Reame, N. (1992). A prospective study of the menstrual cycle and spinal cord injury. *American Journal of Physical Medicine and Rehabilitation, 71,* 15-21.

Reame, N. E., Marshall, J. C., & Kelch, R. P. (1993). Pulsatile LH secretion in women with premenstrual syndrome (PMS): Evidence for normal neuroregulation of the menstrual cycle. *Psychoneuroendocrinology, 17,* 205-213.

Rittenhouse, C., & Lee, K. (1993). Biopsychosocial correlates of perceived perimenstrual weight gain. *Journal of Women's Health, 2,* 145-148.

Rothert, M., Rover, D., Holmen, M., Schmitt, N., Talarczyk, G., Knoll, J., & Gogato, J. (1990). Women's use of information regarding hormone replacement therapy. *Research in Nursing and Health, 13,* 355-366.

Schmitt, N., Gogate, J., Rothert, M., Rovner, D., Holmes, M., Talarcyzk, G., Given, B., & Kroll, J. (1991). Capturing and clustering women's judgment policies: The case of hormonal therapy for menopause. *Journal of Gerontology: Psychological Sciences, 46,* 92-101.

Shaver, J. (1994). Beyond hormonal therapies in menopause. *Experimental Gerontology, 29,* 469-476.

Shaver, J., Giblin, E., Lentz, M., & Lee, K. (1988). Sleep patterns and stability in perimenopausal women. *Sleep, 11,* 556-561.

Shaver, J., Giblin, E., & Paulsen, V. (1991). Sleep quality subtypes in midlife women. *Sleep, 14,* 18-23.

Shaver, J., & Paulsen, V. (1993) Sleep quality, psychological distress and somatic symptoms in menopausal women. *Journal of Family Practice Research, 13,* 373-384.

Shaver, J., & Paulsen, V. (1994). Sleep, psychological distress and somatic symptoms in perimenopausal women. *Menopause Digest, 1994,* 21-24.

Shaver, J., & Woods, N. F. (1985). Concordance of perimenstrual symptoms across 2 cycles. *Research in Nursing and Health, 8,* 313-319.

Shaver, J., Woods, N. F., Wolf-Wilets, V. W., & Heitkemper, N. (1987). Menstrual experiences: Comparison of dysmenorrheic and non-dysmenorrheic women. *Western Journal of Nursing Research, 9,* 423-439.

Standing, T. S., & Glazer, G. (1992). Attitudes of low-income clinic patients toward menopause. *Health Care for Women International, 13,* 271-280.

Stoltzman, S. M. (1986). Menstrual attitudes, beliefs, and symptom experiences of adolescent females, their peers, and their mothers.

In V. L. Olesen & N. F. Woods (Eds.), *Culture, society, and menstruation* (pp. 97-114). Washington, DC: Hemisphere.

Sveinsdottir, H. (1993). The attitudes towards menstruation among Icelandic nursing students: Their relationship with menstrual preparation and menstrual characteristics. *Scandinavian Journal of Caring Sciences, 7,* 37-41.

Sveinsdottir, H., & Marteinsdottir, G. (1991). Retrospective assessment of premenstrual changes in Icelandic women. *Health Care for Women International, 12,* 303-315.

Sveinsdottir, H., & Reame, N. (1991). Symptom patterns in women with premenstrual syndrome complaints: A prospective assessment using a marker for ovulation and screening criteria for adequate ovarian function. *Journal of Advanced Nursing, 16,* 689-700.

Taylor, D. (1994). *Stress & PMS: Biobehavioral responses.* Proceedings of the Society for Psychosomatice OB-GYN, Houston, TX.

Taylor, D. (1995). *Stress & PMS: Biobehavioral factors.* Society for Menstrual Cycle Research Abstracts. Toronto, Quebec, Canada: McGill University.

Taylor, D. (in press). Effectiveness of professional-peer group treatment: Clinical trial results of the perimenstrual symptom management program. *Research in Nursing and Health.*

Taylor, D., & Bledsoe, L. (1986b). Peer support, PMS, and stress: A pilot study. *Health Care for Women International, 7,* 159-171.

Taylor, D., Woods, N. F., Lentz, M., Mitchell, E. S., & Lee, K. (1991). Perimenstrual negative affect: Development testing of an explanatory model. In D. Taylor & N. Woods (Eds.), *Menstruation, health and illness* (pp. 103-118). Washington, DC: Hemisphere.

Taylor, D. L. (1994). Evaluating therapeutic change in symptom severity at the level of the individual woman experiencing severe PMS. *Image: The Journal of Nursing Scholarship, 26,* 25-33.

Theisen, S., Mansfield, P., Seery, B., & Voda, A. (1995). Predictors of midlife women's attitude toward menopause. *Health Values: Achieving High Level Wellness, 19,* 22-31.

Voda, A. (1981). Alterations of the menstrual cycle: Hormonal and mechanical. In P. Komnenich, M. McSweeney, J. Noack, & N. Elder (Eds.), *The menstrual cycle* (pp. 145-163). New York: Springer.

Voda, A. (1982). Menopausal hot flash. In A. Voda, M. Dinnerstein, & S. O'Donnell (Eds.), *Changing perspectives on menopause* (pp. 136-159). Austin: University of Texas Press.

Voda, A. (1991). The Tremin Trust: An intergenerational research program on events associated with women's menstrual and reproductive lives. In D. Taylor & N. Woods (Eds.), *Menstruation, health, and illness* (pp. 5-18). Washington, DC: Hemisphere.

Voda, A. M., & Mansfield, P. K. (1994). Menstrual bleeding patterns in premenopausal women. In N. Woods (Ed.), *Mind-body rhythmicity: A menstrual cycle perspective.* Seattle: Hamilton & Cross.

Warren, C. J., & Baker, S. (1992). Coping resources of women with premenstrual syndrome. *Archives of Psychiatric Nursing, 6,* 48-53.

Williams, L. (1983). Beliefs and attitudes of young girls regarding menstruation. In S. Golub (Ed.), *Menarche* (pp. 139-148). New York: Lexington.

Winter, E.J.S., Ashton, D. J., & Moore, D. L. (1991). Dispelling myths: A study of PMS and relationship satisfaction. *Nurse Practitioner: American Journal of Primary Health Care, 16,* 34, 37-40, 45.

Woods, N. (1986). Socialization and social context: Influence on perimenstrual symptom, disability and menstrual attitudes. *Health Care for Women International, 7,* 1-2.

Woods, N., Dery, G., & Most, A. (1982). Recollections of menarche, current menstrual attitudes, and perimenstrual symptoms. *Psychosomatic Medicine, 44,* 285-293.

Woods, N., Falk, S., Saver, B., Stevens, N., Taylor, T., Moreno, R., & MacLaren, A. (1997). Deciding against using hormone therapy for prevention of diseases of advancing age. *Menopause, 4*(2), 105-114.

Woods, N., Falk, S., Saver, B., Taylor, T., Stevens, N., & MacLaren, A. (1998). Deciding about hormone therapy: Validation of a model. *Menopause, 5*(1), 52-100.

Woods, N., Lentz, M., Mitchell, E., Heitkemper, M., & Shaver, J. (1997). PMS after 40: Persistence of a stress-related symptom pattern. *Research in Nursing and Health, 20,* 329-340.

Woods, N., Lentz, M., Mitchell, E., Heitkemper, M., Shaver, J., & Henkor, R. (1998). Perceived stress, physiologic stress arousal, and premenstrual symptoms: Group differences and intra-individual patterns. *Research in Nursing & Health, 21,* 511-523.

Woods, N., Lentz, M., Mitchell, E., & Kogan, H. (1994). Arousal and stress response across the menstrual cycle in women with three perimenstrual symptom patterns. *Research in Nursing and Health, 17,* 99-110.

Woods, N., Lentz, M., Mitchell, E., Lee, K., Taylor, D., & Allen-Barash, N. (1992). Perimenstrual symptoms and the health-seeking process: Models and methods. In A. J. Dan & L. L. Lewis (Eds.), *Menstrual health in women's lives* (pp. 155-168). Urbana and Chicago: University of Illinois Press.

Woods, N., Lentz, M., Mitchell, E., Shaver, J., & Heitkemper, M. (1998). Luteal phase ovarian steroids, stress arousal, premenses perceived stress and premenstrual symptoms. *Research in Nursing and Health, 21,* 129-142.

Woods, N., Lentz, M., Mitchell, E., Taylor, D., Lee, K., & Allen-Barash, N. (1987, July-August). Premenstrual symptoms: Another look. *Public Health Reports* (Suppl.), pp. 106-112.

Woods, N. & Mitchell, E. (1996). Midlife depression: Patterns of depressed mood in midlife women: Observations from the Seattle Midlife Women's Health Study. *Research in Nursing and Health, 19,* 111-123.

Woods, N., & Mitchell, E. (1997). Pathways to depressed mood in midlife women: Observations from the Seattle Midlife Women's Health Study. *Research in Nursing and Health, 20,* 119-129.

Woods, N., & Mitchell, E. (1999). Anticipating menopause: Observations from Seattle Midlife Women's Health Study. *Menopause, 6*(1).

Woods, N., Mitchell, E. S., & Lentz, M. J. (1995). Social pathways to premenstrual symptoms. *Research in Nursing and Health, 18,* 1-13.

Woods, N., Mitchell, E. S., & Lentz, M. J. (1998, submitted). *Premenstrual symptoms delineating symptom clusters.*

Woods, N., Most, A., & Dery, G. K. (1982a). Estimating perimenstrual distress: A comparison of two methods. *Research in Nursing and Health, 5,* 81-91.

Woods, N., Most, A., & Dery, G. K. (1982b). Prevalence of perimenstrual symptoms. *American Journal of Public Health, 72,* 1257-1263.

Woods, N., Most, A., & Dery, G. K. (1982c). Toward a construct of perimenstrual distress. *Research in Nursing and Health, 5,* 123-136.

Woods, N., Most, A., & Longenecker. (1985). Major life events, daily stressors, and perimenstrual symptoms. *Nursing Research, 34,* 263-267.

Woods, N., Saver, B., & Taylor, T. (1998). Attitudes toward menopause and hormone therapy among women with access to health care. *Menopause 5*(3), 178-188.

Woods, N., Taylor, D., Lentz, M., & Mitchell, E. (1992). Perimenstrual symptoms and health seeking behavior. *Western Journal of Nursing Research, 14,* 418-443.

York, R., Freeman, Lowery, B., & Strauss, J. F. (1989). Characteristics of premenstrual syndrome. *Obstetrics and Gynecology, 73,* 601-605.

27

INFERTILITY

Ellen Olshansky

The phenomenon of infertility has been a topic of great interest to clinicians, researchers, and the lay public for more than two decades, since the birth of the first baby born as a result of *in vitro* fertilization (IVF) in 1978. With advances in the diagnostic and treatment approaches to infertility and, in particular, with the burgeoning of assisted reproductive technology (ART), the scientific community and the consumers of infertility care have significantly increased their attention toward infertility. This surge of interest is reflected in both the scientific and the lay literature. This chapter focuses on the scientific literature, with specific emphasis on the nursing scientific literature that addresses infertility. An overview of the various perspectives and viewpoints is presented; an evaluation, synthesis, and critique of the literature are presented; and recommendations for advancing our scientific knowledge in the area of infertility are included.

Overview of Description and Comparison Across Various Perspectives

The majority of nursing research on infertility has focused on psychosocial responses to infertility, with various perspectives included in the findings of such research. Some nurse researchers have described infertility as chronic sorrow (Unruh & McGrath, 1985); others have described it as similar to the color grey, where much uncertainty and ambiguity exists (Sandelowski & Pollock, 1986); and infertility has also been described as affecting one's identity or sense of self (Olshansky, 1987a).

Some of the nursing research has examined clinical aspects of infertility, including counseling approaches and assisting with the actual intervention procedures, such as IVF and other kinds of assisted reproductive technology. There are also articles written by nurses, although these are not necessarily research based, that explain the basic infertility work-up.

Evaluation, Synthesis, and Critique of the Literature

Psychosocial Literature

Psychosocial Responses to Infertility

The literature on psychological aspects centers on women's, to a lesser extent couples', and to an even lesser extent men's emotional responses to the experience of infertility. The psychological experience of infertility has been described as similar to a grief response (Menning, 1988), as being composed of a series of stages (Blenner, 1990), as a chronic experience of sorrow (Hainsworth, Eakes, & Burke, 1994; Unruh & McGrath, 1985), as encompassing one's identity of self (Olshansky, 1987a), and as a cultural experience (Sandelowski, 1988).

Barbara Eck Menning (1980, 1988), the founder of RESOLVE, an infertility support and information organization, is considered a pioneer in her work on the psychosocial aspects of infertility. Through her analysis of interviews with infertile women and men, she detailed a grief response associated with infertility. This grief response was explained as a response to a potential loss: Infertility was not an actual loss of a child but instead represented what could have been. A similar theory of "passage through infertility treatment" was described by Blenner (1990) as including three concepts of engagement, immersion, and disengagement, which comprise the process persons undergo in their experiences of infertility from prediagnosis to posttreatment. These three concepts included a total of eight stages, identified as experiencing a dawning of awareness, facing a new reality, having hope and determination, intensifying treatment, spiralling down, letting go, quitting and moving out, and shifting focus.

A different perspective of the psychological response to infertility has been described as chronic sorrow (Hainsworth et al., 1994; Unruh & McGrath, 1985). Chronic sorrow refers to women's ongoing sense of loss or despair, often triggered by specific events such as menses, visits with friends who have children, baby showers, and encountering babies and their mothers in grocery stores. Thus, the response is not linear but is ongoing and accentuated by cycles of hope and despair (Woods, Olshansky, & Draye, 1991).

Olshansky (1987a) described a theoretical model of taking on and managing an identity of self as infertile. According to this model, those persons who are distressed by infertility often take on infertility as a central identity of themselves, pushing to the periphery other important identities. Not only do individuals take on an identity of self as infertile, but often married couples take on an identity of their marriages as infertile (Olshansky, 1988a). In the same vein, women's career identities are affected by their infertile identities, with many women pushing aside their career identities by "putting their careers on hold" while they focus on infertility (Olshansky, 1987b).

Sandelowski and Pollock (1986) described three major concepts that are salient to women's experiences of infertility, which they referred to as "ambiguity," "temporality," and "otherness." Ambiguity encompassed feelings of uncertainty, ambivalence, floundering, doubtfulness, and suspicion. Temporality consisted of setting and extending time limits, including planning and wasting time. Otherness referred to a sense of feeling separated or different from the majority of others; in this case, the fertile others. These concepts are even better understood when viewed as constructed realities that represent one's "culture" (Sandelowski, 1988). In other words, from the vantage point of the constructed realities of infertile women, these women viewed themselves within a social or cultural context that was different from or other than those women who resided within the context of fertility.

Psychosocial Aspects of Assisted Reproductive Technology (ART)

ART has a profound influence on individuals' and couples' psychosocial and emotional responses to infertility. Olshansky's (1988b) qualitative analysis of human responses to ART revealed several concepts. One important concept was the "drivenness" experienced by individuals as they pursued their infertility treatments, particularly as they became involved in the highly technological procedures, such as IVF, which entail precisely timed and often invasive treatments. Drivenness is exemplified by a "tunnel vision," whereby the goal of pregnancy was pursued to the exclusion of most other things in their lives. Along with the drivenness was, paradoxically, a desire to "get on with life." Individuals and couples described their frustration with their inability to pursue other aspects of their lives, even those aspects that previously gave them much pleasure. Because of the extreme drivenness, they were unable to get on with other aspects of their lives. Human responses to ART also involved a disruption of a couple's sexual relationship, as they experienced interference in the most intimate parts of their lives. The infertility treatments often included prescriptions for when and when not to have sex, making it very difficult to maintain a spontaneous and loving sexual relationship.

One important consequence of ART is the effect on a person's sense of self. Olshansky (1992) described how infertile persons often internalized failure of the infertility treatment to mean personal failure. Because infertility clinics emphasize their "success rates" and the focus of treatments such as IVF is on achieving a pregnancy, which is considered a successful outcome, those persons who do not achieve a pregnancy through IVF tend to consider themselves "failures." Olshansky (1992) suggested that nursing interventions to assist persons coping with infertility should be directed at helping them redefine their concepts of success and failure. In other words, by helping persons reframe their sense of themselves, they may be able to separate out treatment failure from personal failure.

Psychosocial Aspects of the Infertile Couple

Some of the literature on psychosocial aspects of infertility focuses specifically on the couple relationship, and some of the research emphasizes gender differences between women's and men's responses to and experiences of infertility. Draye, Woods, and Mitchell (1988) found that women and men are affected differently by infertility and its treatment. For the most part, women experience a greater sense of vulnerability, a greater assault on their self-esteem, and a greater sense of loss than do men. These responses among women seem to occur regardless of whether the physiological cause of the infertility is in the male or the female. Most of the men do not experience these responses to the same extent as the women. When the infertility is caused by a male physiological problem, however, there is a greater sense of loss and a lowered self-esteem in those men as compared to men who do not have a physiological cause for the infertility. Even men who do have a physiological infertility problem do not usually experience the same extent of disruption in their lives as do their female counterparts (Draye, 1995).

Hirsch and Hirsch (1989) examined married couples' experiences of infertility and found that infertility is a stress on the self-concept of the spouses within the marital relationship. Olshansky (1988a) reported that spouses sometimes experienced a "mismatch" in their views and perceptions of their infertility, creating increased stress in their relationship. For some couples, infertility took on a central identity in their views of their marriage, whereas for other couples, infertility was a significant portion of their definition of their marriage but did not take over this definition to such a large degree.

Psychosocial Aspects of Pregnancy and Parenting After Infertility

Another category research related to psychosocial aspects of infertility addresses the experiences of pregnancy and parenting after infertility. The past 10 years have witnessed the development of research on women's (and to a lesser extent, men's) perspectives of pregnancy after experiencing infertility. Garner (1985) and Shapiro (1986) reported clinical findings that reveal the significant influence of prior infertility on a woman's experience of pregnancy. Concepts such as disbelief, apprehension, euphoria, anxiety, and ambivalence are mentioned in these clinical reports. Salzer (1991) addressed the complex feelings experienced by previously infertile pregnant women in her description of how these women often anticipate pregnancy as not being accompanied by "fireworks" but instead, although it is joyful, as being accompanied by fear and mistrust.

Glazer (1990) aptly delineated five major concerns that are evident in couples who are pregnant after infertility. These concerns are (a) fear of loss of the pregnancy, (b) fear of having a baby with birth defects, (c) difficulty in becoming an obstetrical patient (as opposed to an infertility patient), (d) feeling neither fertile nor infertile (in "no-person's land," as noted by Glazer, p. 13), and (e) fear of having a high-risk pregnancy.

Sandelowski (1993) insightfully described pregnancy after infertility as being, in many ways, a "reversal in the normal transition to parenthood" (p. 138), as she suggested that couples have already gone through labor before conception. Sandelowski found that couples go back and forth between identities of self as infertile and identities of self as expectant parents. The important influence of ART is evident in that the majority of the couples Sandelowski studied had become pregnant through ART and, thus, remained physically infertile despite being pregnant. Olshansky (1987a) described this process as "circumventing" rather than "overcoming" infertility. Besides the persistent physical infertility, Sandelowski also emphasized that the persistent psychological effects of the infertility struggle remained during and after the pregnancy (and even with the delivery of a healthy baby).

Olshansky (1990) described a process referred to as attempts to "normalize one's pregnancy," in which women struggle to view themselves as normal pregnant women rather than as "infertile pregnant woman." The women, in effect, experience a complex and difficult "identity shift" to that of a fertile woman. Many women find this shift difficult due to their own history of infertility and its contribution to their construction of their own identities. Not all women, in fact, actually make this shift completely. The ability to make this shift, however, enables them to eventually begin to "normalize" their views of themselves as pregnant rather than as infertile women.

Research on psychological aspects of parenting is extensive (Johnson, 1986; Mercer, 1986; Rubin, 1984), but research is extremely scarce on parenting after infertility. The research that has been done in this area has mostly been directed toward couples who have become parents through adoption (Hallenbeck, 1984; Johnston, 1984).

Few authors have written about the phenomenon of parenting after infertility (Glazer, 1990; Salzer, 1991). Glazer (1990) noted that the experience of infertility may influence how new parents consider the ramifications of the following five questions: (a) how and when they may have a second child; (b) what about career, particularly for new mothers; (c) how will the couple focus on their current relationship with each other, accounting for changes in their relationship due to parenting; (d) how new and renewed friendships will be affected; and (e) the feeling of being obligated to be "superparents" (p. 38). These questions probably reflect concerns of many new parents, regardless of prior infertility, but the fact of the

experience of prior infertility may add another dimension of concern to the issues raised by these questions.

Salzer (1991) identified several potential problems that previously infertile parents may encounter. One of these potential problems is being overprotective of the child, resulting in interference with the child's own development of independence. Another potential problem is difficulty disciplining the child because of the inability or reluctance to become angry with the child due to the guilt surrounding the anger. A third potential problem is that parents may put excessive and unrealistic pressure on themselves to be "perfect parents," an unattainable expectation.

Historical Perspective on the Literature

In synthesizing the literature on psychosocial aspects of infertility, it is evident that the recent focus has been directed toward psychosocial consequences of infertility, with much less emphasis on the possible psychosocial causes or contributing factors to infertility. One major reason for this focus is that the earlier literature (during the 1940s, 1950s, and 1960s) reflected a tone of "blaming" women for infertility because the explanations put forth for women's infertility centered on women's unresolved psychological problems. Male infertility was rarely, if ever, discussed, and infertility that did not have a known physiological cause was termed "psychogenic infertility," with explanations for the cause directed at women rather than men. Thus, the more recent scientific work on infertility has consciously moved away from assuming a psychological cause as a diagnosis of exclusion and from explaining infertility as due to women's unresolved psychological problems. With the technological and diagnostic advances, it is possible to determine more physiological causes of infertility so that "psychogenic infertility" is rarely diagnosed. There remain, however, about 10% of infertility diagnoses attributed to unexplained causes, and questions persist regarding whether or not and, if so, to what degree psychological factors contribute to infertility. Therefore, scientific literature is again beginning to focus on potential psychological causes or contributors to infertility. Much more work is needed in this area.

Recommendations for Advancing Our Scientific Knowledge

Despite the recent surge of research on infertility, much remains to be studied. This section addresses recommendations for future research in the area of psychosocial aspects of infertility.

Research has been and is continuing to be conducted on the phenomenon of pregnancy after infertility, but many gaps remain in our knowledge. A particularly valuable research endeavor would be to delineate the differences in experiences of infertility and correlate those different experiences with subsequent experiences of pregnancy. For example, differences may be explained by whether pregnancy was achieved through ART or through more conventional infertility treatment, or differences may be explained by whether spontaneous abortions had been experienced. Differences may also be explained by the women and men themselves. In other words, it would be helpful to follow specific men and women longitudinally even before pregnancy is achieved. This suggestion, however, is difficult to follow as it is not possible to predict which persons will achieve pregnancy a priori.

Another suggestion for future research is to include a more diverse sample in the study. Because infertility treatment is expensive and often requires missing days at work, many people are precluded from such treatment. Most infertility research studies reflect that limitation, with the noted exception of the work of Sandelowski and Jones (1986), although the problem of infertility is certainly not limited to those persons who can afford such treatment. And, despite access to some of the infertility treatments, pregnancy may still not be achieved. Thus, it would be helpful to make a better effort to achieve greater diversity in sampling.

Specifically examining gender differences in responses to pregnancy after infertility would also add valuable information to our understanding of this phenomenon. Although it is only women who physiologically experience pregnancy, men clearly experience it psychologically (Jordan, 1990) and may, in fact, even have physiological responses. Including specific attention to men's experiences of pregnancy after infertility would contribute to our understanding and to our clinical approaches.

Attention to the phenomenon of parenting after infertility has only begun. A dearth of information exists in this important area. Many questions are raised from both clinical experience and the beginning research in this area. For example, if it can be verified that children of previously infertile persons are viewed as more vulnerable than other children, to what extent does this occur? If these children are viewed as more vulnerable, how does such a perspective influence the parenting styles and what are the consequences to the children? If it can be verified that previously infertile parents feel a lack of entitlement to complain about factors normally associated with parenting, such as fatigue and frustration, to what extent does this feeling occur, and what are the consequences to their parenting styles and to the children? What are the effects of parenting via ART on the relationship between the parents, particularly in the situation of a donor (whether it be donor sperm or donor egg)? What are the consequences of telling or not telling children about how they were conceived? What is the incidence of postpartum depression in previously infertile mothers?

An ideal study would be a longitudinal examination of parents who were previously infertile as compared with a comparable group of parents who had no prior experience with infertility. It would be very interesting to examine these two groups of parents over time to gain more in-depth insight and understanding of their experiences of parenthood and how those experiences may or may not be correlated with their previous fertility issues.

An important area of research that would contribute to health care that fosters high-level wellness is the long-term consequences of infertility even after the infertility itself is "resolved." Only a very few studies have addressed long-term consequences. If we had a better understanding of these potential consequences, we might be better able to assist previously infertile parents in the parenting process and beyond, or we might be better able to assist infertile persons who never become pregnant or become parents to live highly fulfilling lives.

Depression in new mothers with a history of infertility is an important area of study. The series of studies conducted by Olshansky (1996) explored the emotional consequences of infertility, including the effects on a marital relationship, on women's careers, on pregnancy, and on parenting. A major concept generated from these studies is that of identity as infertile. Infertility often becomes the central focus of persons' lives as they struggle with the "work of fertility." As a result, important parts of themselves and their identities are suppressed or pushed aside in favor of focusing most of their energies on this work. The scholars at the Stone Center (Jordan, Kaplan, Miller, Stiver, & Surrey, 1991; Miller, 1986) developed a theoretical perspective termed "relational theory" that emphasizes the importance of connected, reciprocal, empathic relationships. Jack (1991) described how women who silence themselves in an effort to maintain relationships that are not connected, reciprocal, and empathic eventually develop depression. It is plausible that previously infertile mothers have suffered prolonged and profound interpersonal losses and have, as a result of infertility, suppressed parts of themselves. Their sense of self and their relationships with others may have been strongly affected by the infertility. The long-term consequences of this phenomenon could be depression.

Indeed, Bernstein, Mattox, and Kellner (1988) found that women who were infertile had slightly elevated mean scores on depression, measured by the 90-item Symptom Checklist (SCL-90), and after the infertility was resolved these scores did not improve. Research also reveals that anxiety or depressive symptoms often occur during or after infertility treatment (Baram, Tourtelot, Muechler, & Huang, 1988; Freeman, Boxer, Rickels, Tureck, & Mastroianni, 1985; Greenfeld, Diamond, & DeCherney, 1988; Mahlstedt, MacDuff, & Bernstein, 1987). It has been demonstrated that concurrent preexisting psychological symptoms may be present in patients undergoing infertility treatment (Klock & Maier, 1991). Mahlstedt and her colleagues (1987) noted that 80% of those infertile persons in their sample described infertility as stressful or extremely stressful, with 63% stating that infertility was more stressful than divorce for those who had experienced divorce as well as infertility. Another study by Freeman and others (1985) revealed that 49% of the women described infertility as the most upsetting experience in their lives. Berg and Wilson (1990) administered the SCL-90 to 104 infertile couples, finding that 44% of the males and 52% of the females demonstrated psychiatric symptoms, including tension, depressive symptoms, worry, and interpersonal alienation. In the same sample of infertile couples, these same researchers (Berg & Wilson, 1991) looked cross-sectionally at different stages of medical investigation and treatment for infertility, focusing on each of 3 years of treatment. Findings revealed that psychological distress was moderate during the first year, decreased to more normal levels during the second year, and markedly increased during the third year. Thus the experience of infertility may cause significantly greater stress as it continues over time, and for infertility to continue for several years is quite common.

Synthesizing the literature on emotional aspects of infertility in women and the literature on depression in women, it is plausible that there is an association between a history of infertility and the development of depression in new mothers. The literature has demonstrated that women who are infertile do become depressed during the infertility experience, and it suggests that these women may experience depression during pregnancy, although further study is needed in this area. Extrapolating the ideas of relational theory and depression to previously infertile mothers, it is plausible that these women may have experienced repeated and sustained losses of actual and potential relationships over the course of their infertility and, despite the recent new role as mother to their very own infant, the deep-rooted influences of the previous losses may continue to exert a profound effect on their current mood state. Such losses may have been experienced in the form of marital discord and stress; stress in relationships with family and friends, particularly friends who have become mothers and who represented the losses experienced by the infertile woman or friends who have remained infertile as the woman becomes pregnant and feels uncomfortable with her still infertile friends.

Summarizing the current literature on long-term psychological effects of infertility, there are several things that are known. First, it is clear that infertility is more than a one-time event; it is an experience that occurs over time and in a chronic manner, leading to what Unruh and McGrath (1985) describe as "chronic sorrow." Second, infertility is a confrontation with one's own mortality, as persons are forced to make decisions based on the proverbial "biological clock." Third, infertility may create a feeling of dependence upon technology and a resulting disbelief in one's own bodily competence. Fourth, infertility is a direct threat to one's interpersonal relationships and sense of self, as infertile persons often construct their worlds in such a way as to exclude much of the fertile world, thus constricting their social context of interpersonal relationships.

Another major area that is deserving of research is the interrelationship between physiological and psychological variables in potential long-term consequences of infertility. Herz (1992) reported that clinical observation indicates that more previously infertile women may develop postpartum psychiatric illness than may women without a history of infertility. She stated that one hypothesis is that this phenomenon is perhaps due to endocrinological problems associated with idiopathic infertility. Another important question is how physiological effects of treatment for infertility may influence physiological variables. It would be interesting to study any potential correlations among previous infertility, perimenstrual stress, and menopause. No such studies have been conducted.

With the advent of more complex technology to diagnose and treat infertility, it is not surprising that persons often undergo the stresses of infertility treatment over a longer time period and have greater difficulty discontinuing treatment. Thus, more people are likely to experience infertility as a long-term event. Once this long-term event is resolved, in whatever way, the psychological sequelae do not simply vanish. It may be that the losses associated with infertility are accompanied by unresolved grieving. Sometimes, in fact, couples may give birth to a "replacement child" after losing a child to miscarriage and may have distorted views of the child and his or her abilities (Burns, 1990). Sustained infertility treatments may have had an untoward effect on the couple's sexual relationship, making it difficult for them to resume normal sexual activity despite the fact that they may have resolved their infertility. In addition, marital conflict may become exacerbated by the stress of infertility. Friendships may have been deeply affected, as infertile women found it difficult to maintain friendships with their fertile friends.

If we, as nurses, understand the potential for these psychological sequelae to occur, perhaps we can take measures to prevent them or to mitigate them. Psychological interventions during the infertility work-up, during a subsequent pregnancy and early parenting, as well as possibly during later life events, may be very helpful.

Questions for future scientific inquiry include the following:

1. What are the psychological consequences for the children conceived after infertility? How do the various forms of conception affect the child?

2. What are the long-term consequences to the marital relationship, particularly as these consequences are related to specific forms of conception, such as donor sperm or donor egg?

3. What are the long-term consequences for the family as a unit, including extended family members?

4. What is the occurrence of postpartum depression and depression beyond postpartum in previously infertile mothers?

5. What potential relationship exists between physiological and biological effects of infertility and infertility treatment and its psychological sequelae?

6. What is the experience of menopause like for previously infertile women?

7. What factors influence decisions regarding tubal ligation or vasectomy among couples who have conceived after infertility?

8. What is the experience of parents who have a history of infertility, when their own grown children conceive?

9. How do the long-term psychological losses associated with infertility compare to the long-term psychological losses associated with miscarriage?

Conducting studies of long-term consequences of infertility raises several methodological issues. First, many intervening or extraneous variables may occur over time, making it difficult to draw conclusions about cause and effect relationships between infertility and particular dependent variables. Second, it is not always feasible to conduct longitudinal studies, and often the alternative is to conduct retrospective studies. Retrospective studies, although they may yield important information, are plagued with problems of lack of memory and perceptions being altered by intervening variables. Third, it may be very difficult to obtain accurate results on psychological tests, many of which are pencil-and-paper tests that rely on the respondent's accuracy. Because so many previously infertile persons may feel that they are not "entitled" to complain after finally becoming parents, they may in fact "censor" their true psychological feelings, thus influencing their responses to the pencil-and-paper tests. Efforts need to be made to develop accurate ways of measuring chronic sorrow and stress as it relates specifically to infertility.

Summary

This chapter has presented an overview of the nursing research on infertility. Directions for future research have been suggested. Nurses are in key positions to conduct research and to intervene with patients who are experiencing infertility.

References

Baram, D., Tourtelot, E., Muechler, E., & Huang, K. (1988). Psychological adjustment following unsuccessful in vitro fertilization. *Journal of Psychosomatic Obstetrics and Gynecology, 9,* 181-190.

Berg, B. J., & Wilson, J. F. (1990). Psychiatric morbidity in the infertile population: A reconceptualiztion. *Fertility and Sterility, 53*(4), 654-661.

Berg, B. J., & Wilson, J. F. (1991). Psychological functioning across stages of treatment for infertilitiy. *Journal of Behavioral Medicine, 14*(1), 11-25.

Bernstein, J., Mattox, J. H., & Kellner, R. (1988). Psychological status of previously infertile couples after a successful pregnancy. *Journal of Obstetric, Gynecologic and Neonatal Nursing, 17*(6), 404-408.

Blenner, J. L. (1990). Passage through infertility treatment: A stage theory. *Image: The Journal of Nursing Scholarship, 22*(3), 153-158.

Burns, L. (1990). An exploratory study of perceptions of parenting after infertility. *Family Systems Medicine, 8*(2), 177-189.

Draye, M. A. (1995). Emotional aspects of infertility. In D. Lemcke & J. Pattison (Eds.), *Primary care of women* (pp. 506-510). Norwalk, CT: Appleton and Lange.

Draye, M. A., Woods, N. F., & Mitchell, E. (1988). Coping with infertility in couples: Gender differences. *Health Care of Women International, 9,* 163-175.

Freeman, E., Boxer, A., Rickels, K., Tureck, R., & Mastroianni, L., Jr. (1985). Psychological evaluation and support in a program of in vitro fertilization and embryo transfer. *Fertility and Sterility, 43,* 48-53.

Garner, C. H. (1985). Pregnancy after infertility. *Journal of Obstetric, Gynecologic and Neonatal Nursing, 14s,* 58s-62s.

Glazer, E. F. (1990). *The long-awaited stork: A guide to parenting after infertility.* Toronto: Lexington Books.

Greenfeld, D., Diamond, M., & DeCherney, A. (1988). Grief reactions following in vitro fertilization treatment. *Journal of Psychosomatic Obstetrics and Gynecology, 8,* 169-174.

Hainsworth, M. A., Eakes, G. G., & Burke, M. L. (1994). Coping with chronic sorrow. *Issues in Mental Health Nursing, 15*(1), 59-66.

Hallenbeck, C. A. (1984). *Our child: Preparation for parenting in adoption—instructor's guide.* Wayne, PA: Our Child Press.

Herz, E. K. (1992). Prediction, recognition, and prevention. In J. A. Hamilton & P. N. Harberger (Eds.), *Postpartum psychiatric illness.* Philadelphia: University of Pennsylvania Press.

Hirsch, A. M., & Hirsch, S. M. (1989). The effect of infertility on marriage and self-concept. *Journal of Obstetric, Gynecologic and Neonatal Nursing, 18*(1), 13-20.

Jack, D. C. (1991). *Silencing the self: Women and depression.* Cambridge, MA: Harvard University Press.

Johnson, S. H. (1986). *Nursing assessment and strategies for the family at risk: High risk parenting.* Philadelphia: J. B. Lippincott.

Johnston, P. I. (1984). *An adopter's advocate.* Indianapolis, IN: Perspectives.

Jordan, J. V., Kaplan, A. G., Miller, J. B., Stiver, I. P., & Surrey, J. L. (Eds.). (1991). *Women's growth in connection.* New York: Guilford.

Jordan, P. L. (1990). Laboring for relevance: Expectant and new fatherhood. *Nursing Research, 39*(1), 11-16.

Klock, S. C., & Maier, D. (1991). Guidelines for the provision of psychological evaluations for infertile patients at the University of Connecticut Health Center. *Fertility and Sterility, 56*(40), 680-685.

Mahlstedt, P., MacDuff, S., & Bernstein, J. (1987). Emotional factors and the in vitro fertilization and embryo transfer process. *Journal of in Vitro Fertilization and Embryo Transfer, 4,* 232-236.

Menning, B. E. (1980). The emotional needs of infertile couples. *Fertility and Sterility, 34*(4), 313-319.

Menning, B. E. (1988). *Infertility: A guide for the childless couple* (2nd ed.). New York: Prentice Hall.

Mercer, R. T. (1986). *First-time motherhood: Experiences from teens to forties.* New York: Springer.

Miller, J. B. (1986). *Toward a new psychology of women.* Boston: Beacon.

Olshansky, E. F. (1987a). Identity of self as infertile: An example of theory-generating research. *Advances in Nursing Science, 9*(2), 54-63.

Olshansky, E. F. (1987b). Infertility and its influence on women's career identities. *Health Care for Women International, 8*(2,3), 185-196.

Olshansky, E. F. (1988a). Married couples' experiences of infertility [abstract]. *Communicating Nursing Research, 21,* 47.

Olshansky, E. F. (1988b). Responses to high technology infertility treatment. *Image: The Journal of Nursing Scholarship, 20*(3), 128-131.

Olshansky, E. F. (1990). Psychosocial implications of pregnancy after infertility. *NAACOG's Clinical Issues in Women's Health and Perinatal Nursing, 1*(3), 342-347.

Olshansky, E. F. (1992). Redefining the concepts of success and failure in infertilitiy treatment. *NAACOG's Clinical Issues in Women's Health and Perinatal Nursing, 3*(2), 343-346.

Olshansky, E. F. (1996). Theoretical issues in building a grounded theory: Application of a program of research on infertility. *Qualitative Health Research, 6*(3), 394-405.

Rubin, R. (1984). *Maternal identity and the maternal experience.* New York: Springer.

Salzer, L. P. (1991). *Surviving infertility.* New York: Harper Perennial.

Sandelowski, M. (1988). Without child: The world of infertile women. *Health Care for Women International, 9,* 147-161.

Sandelowski, M. (1993). *With child in mind: Studies of the personal encounter with infertility.* Philadelphia: University of Pennsylvania Press.

Sandelowski, M., & Jones, L. (1986). Social exchanges of infertile women. *Issues in Mental Health Nursing, 8*(3), 173-189.

Sandelowski, M., & Pollock, C. (1986). Women's experiences of infertility. *Image: The Journal of Nursing Scholarship, 18*(4), 140-144.

Shapiro, C. H. (1986). Is pregnancy after infertility a dubious joy? *Social Casework, 67*(5), 306-313.

Unruh, A. M., & McGrath, P. J. (1985). The psychology of female infertility: Toward a new perspective. *Health Care for Women International, 6*(5,6), 369-381.

Woods, N. F., Olshansky, E., & Draye, M. A. (1991). Infertility: Women's experiences. *Health Care for Women International, 12,* 179-190.

WOMEN AND SEXUALITY

Contributions From Nursing Research and Practice Recommendations

Catherine Ingram Fogel

The nursing profession has long recognized the legitimacy of nursing's role in sexual health promotion. Issues relating to human sexuality are a part of every nursing specialty, and clinicians consistently address individuals' health care needs. No review of nursing research in women's sexuality has ever been published, and nursing research in human sexuality has not been summarized since the early 1980s (Hott & Ryan-Merrit, 1982). Nursing research in the area of women and sexuality reflects the wide range of clinical interests and concerns of nurses caring for women. Although individual nurse researchers have conducted studies whose findings may inform specific practice needs for over two decades, it is only within the past 10 years that nurses have made significant contributions in the understanding of two areas of women's sexuality: sexual risk practices and sexual orientation.

Because of the breadth of issues related to the sexuality of women and the multiple disciplines within which nurses conduct their research, the range of research interests reflected in this review is extensive. As a result, a number of strategies were used to identify published studies. CINAHL and Medline provided primary sources of literature reviewed. In addition, the ancestry approach outlined by Cooper (1984), in which reference citations are also reviewed for research reports, was used. Finally, research reported in dissertations was reviewed when available. Some studies that included both men and women as respondents were identified; only those studies in which responses of women were clearly differentiated

517

were included in this review. The global and complex nature of the sexuality of women necessitated that decisions regarding the scope and breadth of this review be made. Broad categories established for this review by the author included normative experiences, clinical interruptions, and health promotion and disease prevention. The earliest nursing research regarding sexuality examined nurses' knowledge and attitudes about their own and their patients' sexuality. A brief review of the most recent studies in this area is also included. As previously indicated, there is a considerable body of nursing research in the area of sexual orientation and lesbian health care. Because this body of research addresses many issues relevant to lesbian health care and does not focus on sexual activity, functioning, or practices, it will not be reviewed here.

This chapter will focus on nursing research about women and sexuality, specifically normative experiences, clinical interruptions, and health promotion and prevention of disease. The purposes of the chapter are (a) to review the development of nursing science about women's sexuality from the late 1970s through the mid-1990s, (b) to evaluate the contributions of nurse scientists and gaps remaining in knowledge to guide practice, and (c) to make recommendations for advancing nursing science about women and sexuality to guide nursing practice.

Normative Experiences

Normative experiences of sexuality include the impact of life transitions and events on sexual experiences and function. Nurses have studied the effect of life transitions such as adolescence and aging and life events such as childbearing on sexuality and sexual function.

Adolescence

Nurses have explored adolescent sexual activity and teenage pregnancy in a number of descriptive, correlational studies. Recognizing the vulnerability of young women to sexually transmitted diseases (STDs) and unintended pregnancy, many of the studies have identified factors associated with teenage sexual activity and/or pregnancy.

Sexual Activity

Epidemiological analyses conducted by nurses have identified factors associated with early age at first inter-

course (Coker et al., 1994) and adolescent female sexual activity (Coray, 1991). Analysis of the 1991 Center for Disease Control (CDC) Youth Risk Behavior Survey revealed that 5% of White females and 12% of Black females were sexually active before age 13. Carrying a weapon to school, fighting, and early (< age 13) experimentation with cigarettes and alcohol were associated with early initiation of sexual activity (Coker et al., 1994). Further, young women who initiated sexual activity early had greater numbers of sexual partners, were less likely to use condoms regularly, and were more likely to have had an STD and to have been pregnant. Analyzing data from an adolescent health risk survey of 879 female, multiethnic high school students in Northern California, Coray (1991) found that sexually active females were more likely to use alcohol, cigarettes, and illegal drugs; to have thought about and attempted to harm themselves; to have felt less hopeful; to receive lower grades; to have lower educational aspirations; and to have parents who were separated or divorced. Age and ethnic differences were also noted by Coray: Younger sexually active females had experienced earlier menarche; reported feeling less good about themselves; and reported feeling more nervous, scared, or bored than abstinent students. Asian students (19.9% of sample) were more likely to remain abstinent than other ethnic groups.

Tucker (1989, 1990) examined familial patterns in the amounts and sources of information received about sex, contraception, and the menstrual cycle among 179 Black adolescent daughters, mothers, and grandmothers and the impact of this information on the sexual behavior of adolescent women. Using data collected through surveys and in-depth interviews, she found that family members played an important role in the sexual socialization of teenage females, with mothers being the major source of sex-related information. Familial triads and dyads were more likely to have discussed the menstrual cycle than either sex or contraception. Information about sex was generally focused on avoidance of sexual liaisons, and discussions regarding contraception centered on the purpose of birth control and accessibility. No significant relationships between amounts of information received and age at first intercourse, pregnancy before age 18, or giving birth as a teenager were noted.

Influential Factors

Recognizing that sociodemographic characteristics, although useful for risk identification, are often immutable, nurse researchers have sought to identify other factors that might respond to intervention. Social factors related to sexual practices and pregnancy in adolescent women found to be protective against teenage pregnancy included employed parents, parental control of behavior, two-parent families, and strong parent-child communication; protective psychological factors included internal locus of control, group membership, and future aspirations (Rhodes, 1990). Recognizing the influence of parental attitudes about teenage sexuality on behavior, De-Santis and Thomas (1987) identified differences in child-rearing practices, including views on sex roles and sexuality, among Cuban and Haitian mothers. Cuban females learned about menstruation and intercourse from their mothers or sex education classes in school; information provided was of a scientific nature. In contrast, only 26% of Haitian mothers knew where their daughters learned about menstruation and 50% did not know when or how their daughters learned about intercourse. What information was provided to Haitian adolescents was cautionary.

Childbearing

No nursing studies of sexual activity or sexuality during pregnancy were located. However, two early studies (Ellis & Hewat, 1985; Fischman, Rankin, Soeken, & Lenz, 1986) documented changes and adjustments during the postpartum period. Women reported declines in the frequency of and desire for sexual activity when compared to sexual activity before birth (Fischman et al., 1986) and decreased sexual interest over the 6 months following the birth of the infant (Ellis & Hewat, 1985). Reasons mothers gave for the decline in activity and interest were physical discomfort with intercourse, decline in physical strength, dissatisfaction with bodily appearance, and fatigue that interfered with sex. Breast-feeding was not significantly related to the negative changes in either study.

Aging

Nurses have documented older women's knowledge and attitudes about sexuality and sexual activity in aging (Portonova, Young, & Newman, 1984; Steinke, 1988, 1994). In general, elderly women held positive attitudes toward sexuality (Steinke, 1994) and sexual activity in their peers; however, attitudes were found to be more positive toward married sexually active older adults regardless of gender (Portonova et al., 1984). Further, elderly women appear to have a moderate amount of sexual

knowledge, with married and widowed women being more knowledgeable than separated or divorced women (Steinke, 1994).

Steinke (1988, 1994) has provided information on the sexual activity of older (60 to 84 years) women. Although 28% of women in one sample and 40% in a second reported their sexual activity to be zero to four times per month, up to 3% reported they were sexually active between 11 and 30 times a month.

Clinical Interruptions

Reflecting nursing's heritage as a practice discipline, nurses have studied the effects of various health problems or clinical conditions on the sexuality of women. Several nurse researchers have studied women's sexuality in relation to illness and health problems, but these efforts have been largely fragmented. In only a few cases—diabetes, reproductive system, and, more recently, drugs—has more than one study been conducted on the effect of the same health problem or condition on sexual functioning or sexuality. Approximately half of the studies of clinical interruptions of sexuality employ an orienting framework. The majority of the studies are descriptive or comparative, with convenience samples; none are interventions.

Diabetes

Recognizing that diabetes is a serious health problem for women and that the sexuality of diabetic women has been poorly understood, nurse researchers have provided much information about sexual functioning in diabetic women (LeMone, 1991, 1993; Shah, 1989; Watts, 1994; Young, Koch, & Bailey, 1989). Conceptualizing sexuality as the "totality of expression," Shah (1989) examined the psychosocial adjustment, self-concept, and sexual satisfaction of women with diabetes. For the 106 diabetic women who volunteered, high levels of sexual satisfaction were positively related to duration of diabetes, positive psychosocial adjustment, and high self-concept. Women reported that the fatigue associated with a chronic illness such as diabetes and the scheduling demands necessitated by diabetes negatively affected their lives. However, they did not report that diabetes affected their sexuality or intimate relationships.

When the dyadic relationships of White diabetic women and matched control nondiabetic women were compared, Young and associates (1989) found no statistically significant differences in overall marital adjustment. However, diabetic women were significantly more concerned about specific sexual functioning areas: frequency of feeling repulsed, difficulties with vaginal lubrication, difficulty reaching orgasm, and impact of genital discomfort. Diabetic women experienced more performance anxiety and were bothered more by performance anxiety than nondiabetic women. Levels of sexual concerns and overall dyadic adjustment were not related in either group. Watts (1994) explored differences in sexual function of African-American diabetic and nondiabetic women. Like LeMone (1993), she found that diabetic women disclosed low levels of sexual desire; further, levels of desire were significantly lower than those of women without diabetes. In contrast to other studies, both groups reported similar levels of sexual arousal, orgasm, and satisfaction. Additionally, clinical indexes of diabetes were not significantly related to sexual function in these diabetic women. Significant negative relationships between age and sexual arousal were found for both groups; additionally, age was negatively associated with sexual desire and orgasm for the diabetic.

Using grounded theory methodology, LeMone (1991, 1993) explored patterns of sexual function and meeting intimacy needs in adults (6 men, 5 women) with insulin-dependent diabetes. Women reported that sexual function was affected by alterations in glucose levels and that monilial vaginal infections affected interest in and comfort during sexual intercourse. Supporting earlier finding by Young and associates, women experienced decreases in vaginal lubrication, necessitating use of lubricants during intercourse. In contrast to earlier research (Young et al., 1989), none of the women reported changes in orgasm. A consistent theme for all women regardless of their sexual experiences was the importance of maintaining their relationship in meeting their intimacy needs.

The cumulative findings of these studies suggest that sexual performance problems are associated with diabetes for both Caucasian and African-American women, specifically in areas of sexual arousal, interest, and comfort. Whether or not diabetes affects orgasm is less clear. Further, diabetes appears to have less effect on women's than on men's intimate relationships.

Reproductive System

Nurses have investigated the effect of hysterectomy on women's sexuality, women's sexual adaptation following treatment for endometrial cancer, and the rela-

tionship between premenstrual tension (PMS) and sexual relationships.

Hysterectomy

Krueger and associates (1979) noted that sexual patterns after hysterectomy were significantly and positively related to sexual patterns prior to surgery in a convenience sample of 80 premenopausal women. Thus women who reported more frequent sexual intercourse prior to surgery expressed more positive sexual satisfaction following surgery. These researchers also found that nurse counseling of hysterectomy patients and sexual adjustment following surgery were not significantly related 8 weeks postsurgery.

Bernhard's (1992) study of adult, premenopausal, low-income women who underwent hysterectomies provides longitudinal information about the sexuality and sexual experiences of women experiencing hysterectomies. Consequences of hysterectomy for the women's sexuality involved personal appearance, sexual intercourse, and the relationship with the sexual partner. Women commented about the surgical scar and gaining (12) or losing (7) weight. At 4 weeks after surgery, very few of the women had resumed sexual intercourse, and many were anxious about resumption. Within 3 months after hysterectomy, most women had resumed sexual intercourse. Although the first experience was a time of anxiety for the women, most women reported that intercourse returned to normal after they had engaged in it a few times. Overall sexual functioning scores (Derogatis Sexual Functioning Inventory) increased significantly in the 3 months after surgery. However, 2 years following surgery, women reported considerable variation in sexual functioning and interest. For example, a minority of women reported decreased sex drive and taking longer to climax.

Other Reproductive Problems

Lamb and Sheldon (1994) exploring the process of sexual adaptation in 19 women treated for endometrial cancer found that recovery of an intimate relationship after endometrial cancer is a trajectory that begins with onset of symptoms and extends well past completion of treatment. Most women reported satisfaction with their current sexual functioning but stated that this had been achieved slowly in the period of time since they completed their cancer treatment. Women emphasized the overwhelming aspects of onset of symptoms (commonly vaginal bleeding) and their negative effect on sexual expression. During the treatment phase, lethargy was common and adversely affected sexual function. Although partners' reactions to the illness did influence sexual adaptation, women reported that their own internal reactions to the disease and its treatment had the most effect.

Recognizing the lack of research on the relationship of women's roles and development with the psychoemotional symptoms of PMS, Winter, Ashton, and Moore (1991) compared marital-, sexual-, and family-relationship satisfaction in women with PMS (26) and women who did not have PMS (26). Women with a diagnosis of PMS reported statistically significantly more dissatisfaction with marital and sexual relationships than did control women. No significant differences between the groups were noted for family relationship satisfaction; further, no effects linked to age were found. Given the great differences regarding how PMS is defined and diagnosed by researchers and clinicians (Fogel, 1995), the lack of description of how the diagnosis of PMS was made in this sample limits the applicability of the findings.

Chemical Dependency

As nursing and society recognized that chemical dependency was a major health problem for women, nurses have begun to study issues of special concern for chemically dependent women. In recent years, nurse researchers have provided important information about the sexuality of women who use drugs. Using group observations and content notes generated from meetings held in a halfway house, Teets (1990) identified sexual issues of recovering chemically dependent women. Concerns documented included experiences of incest, childhood sexual abuse, and rape as well as violent relationships as adults. Many of the women had never had sex while sober and were uncertain and anxious as to how they would feel. Women expressed a desire for a good sexual relationship.

Kearney, Murphy, and Rosenbaum (1994) explored women crack users' experiences and views on sexuality, fertility, contraception, and pregnancy-related decisions. Some women believed they were controlled by sex; others perceived sex to be controllable. Women crack users who were young, who were caught in violent relationships, and those who had been sexually abused were likely to report viewing sex as controlling; others viewed sex as a given part of their relationships with men. Most of the women in Kearney et al.'s study reported a history of serial monogamy rather than the promiscuous, sexually careless stereotype often suggested. Although

women in this study knew of women who had traded sex for drugs and some had done this, few reported continuing the practice.

The sexual feelings and sexual functioning of women who used large amounts of crack has been described (Henderson, Boyd, & Whitmore, 1995). Using a structured interview with 100 African-American women, the researchers found that commonly held notions of crack as an aphrodisiac or stimulant to sexual desire were not supported. The women in this study described the effects of crack on their sexual feelings negatively. Sexual dysfunction was also common, with almost half reporting having an orgasm less than half the time or never.

Other Health Problems

A number of single-effort studies have been conducted to examine the effects of various illnesses and health problems on women's sexuality. These studies can provide a base for further research to build upon. Although nurse researchers have studied the effect of cardiac disease on sexuality, the published studies include small numbers of women compared to men (Froelicher, Kee, Newton, Lindskog, & Livingston, 1994); do not report the number of women in the sample, only that women were included (Watts, 1982); or do not report study findings by gender (Froelicher et al., 1994). Watts (1982), comparing sexual functioning in hypertensive and nonhypertensive men and women, found that females in the two groups did not report significant differences in sexual desire, arousal, satisfaction, or orgasm. Hypertensive men reported significantly more drug-related sexual problems than did women with hypertension.

White, Rintala, Hart, and Fuhrer (1994) compared the sexuality of a sample of randomly selected women (40) and men (79) with spinal cord injury (SCI) and found no significant gender differences in the percentage of subjects reporting having had a physical sexual relationship in the past 12 months or those reporting having had intercourse during that period. Women rated having a sex life as less important than men, but there were no gender differences in the ratings of satisfaction with sex life. Areas of highest sexual concern differed for men and women. Three contributing factors related to sexual behaviors of women with SCI were identified: age, age at onset of injury, and time since injury. Younger women were more likely to have had intercourse; women injured at an earlier age were more likely to have resumed sexual activity; and the more time since the injury, the more likely the woman was to have resumed sexual activity.

Sexual adjustment following ostomy surgery and the influence of surgery on individual body image was explored by Gloeckner (1984). Although the sample included men and women, only one finding was differentiated by gender. Findings suggested that men and women perceived themselves differently after surgery than before surgery, with women perceiving themselves as more sexually attractive than men after more than 1 year following surgery.

Self-perceptions of sexual functioning in women with mood disorders have been described (Pollack, 1993). A convenience sample of 34 in-patient and outpatient women were interviewed using a structured questionnaire developed by the researcher. More than half (19, 55.9%) of the women perceived that they were currently experiencing sexual disruptions, and more than three quarters (27, 79.4%) reported that their mood disorder adversely affected their sexual relationships.

Health Promotion and Disease Prevention

Promoting sexual health and assisting women to prevent unanticipated and/or unwanted consequences of sexual activity are legitimate roles for health professionals and important nursing functions. Research regarding women's sexual behaviors, expressions of sexuality, and sexual functioning is an essential foundation upon which to base sexual health promotion activities. Two areas of research into the prevention of the unwanted consequences of sexual behavior that nurses have focused on are contraception and sexual protective or risky behaviors.

Sexual Experiences

A few nurse researchers have documented how women experience sexuality in the normalcy of their lives or the diversity of these experiences. Two early studies documented isolated sexual experiences of healthy community-based women (Bullough et al., 1984; Whitley, 1978). Whitley (1978) studied the prevalence of expectation of bleeding and pain with the first coital experience of 100 randomly selected family planning clients. Almost half reported expecting bleeding and pain. The majority (54%) of women reported some slight bleeding with initial coitus; more than half of the women (55%) experienced little or no pain. Several of the women who experienced no bleeding at initial coitus expressed concern

that they were "abnormal" in some way. Whitley also reported that 11 women in her study were noted to have vaginismus (criteria for diagnosis not reported) during their physical examination; 8 of the 11 women reported experiencing moderate to severe pain at first vaginal intercourse.

Bullough and associates (1984) documented women's subjective awareness of ejaculation, finding that 54% of their sample of 233 gay and heterosexual women reported that they had experienced ejaculation, which was defined as orgasmic expulsion of fluid. Most women reported that ejaculation did not occur with every orgasm; the major stimulation associated with all orgasms as well as ejaculation was a combined vaginal and clitoral stimulation. More women who had had sexual experience with a woman partner reported experiencing ejaculation than did those who had no sexual experience with a woman. More recently, researchers, including nursing researchers (Darling, Davidson, & Conway-Welch, 1990), surveyed 1,230 heterosexual professional women in health-related fields regarding their perception of the existence of female ejaculation. Further, the researchers examined factors associated with this fluid release, including the Grafenberg spot or sensitive area, orgasmic response, and sexual satisfaction. Forty percent ($n = 463$) of respondents reported having a fluid release at the moment of orgasm; further, almost two thirds of the women perceived an especially sensitive area that upon stimulation during sexual arousal produced an orgasm.

Contraception

Efforts of nurse researchers to understand the contraceptive decisions of women have contributed to a growing knowledge of the factors that influence or shape contraceptive decision making and use, particularly in adolescents. Less information is available on contraceptive practices of young adult or midlife women. Further, not all investigators obtained information on the sexual behavior or activities of women using contraception.

Perception of risk and seriousness of unwanted pregnancy have been suggested as influential factors in contraceptive initiation and use. White and Kellinger (1989) found that adolescents seeking contraception for the first time viewed an unplanned pregnancy as serious and believed that they were susceptible yet had been sexually active for an average of 15 months. Further, only 30% of their sample of 50 adolescents had used anything to prevent pregnancy at their first or last sexual encounters. Being concerned about pregnancy did not mean that the young women felt good about using oral contraceptive pills (OCPs); barriers such as using OCPs meant that they were planning to have intercourse, and concern about the potential side effects of OCPs were described. Further, the perception that she could get pregnant and that this would have serious consequences did not necessarily mean that an adolescent would continue to use contraception; 6 weeks after initiation of oral contraception, 13% were no longer using or had not begun to use OCPs. In support of these findings, Sullivan (1989) found that feelings of invulnerability were a significant predictor of contraceptive risk taking.

Three studies have examined how cognitive development affected contraceptive decision making among female adolescents (Hughes & Torre, 1987; Sachs, 1985; Sullivan, 1989). In Sachs' study, the adolescents' stage of cognitive ability was the single best predictor of contraceptive decision making for her sample of Black, urban teens. Sullivan found that although level of cognitive development contributed to the prediction of contraceptive risk taking in suburban, predominantly White adolescent females it was not the most important predictor. In contrast, cognitive development was not significantly related to use of effective contraception in 60 freshman and senior women seen at the university health center (Hughes & Torre, 1987).

Contraceptive knowledge frequently has been thought to be significantly related to contraceptive practices; however, study findings are mixed. Contraceptive knowledge was found to be the most significant predictor of risk taking (Sullivan, 1989) and to contribute significantly to the prediction of contraceptive decision-making abilities (Sachs, 1985). In contrast, effective and ineffective users of contraception did not differ in level of knowledge in a sample of 112 teenage subscribers, 13-18 years, to a prepaid health plan located in the Northwest (Marcy, Brown, & Danielson, 1983).

Sheehan, Ostwald, and Rothenberger (1986) explored the perceptions of sexual responsibility of college students, finding that 91% of the students perceived contraception to be a shared responsibility. Consistent with White and Kellinger's findings, adolescents were unlikely to use contraception during their first intercourse, although at most recent intercourse, only 6% were not using contraception.

Fewer studies have focused on the contraceptive practices of adult women, but three studies (Lethbridge, 1991; Matteson, 1991; Swanson, 1988) have contributed a wealth of knowledge to our understanding of how women regulate their fertility and manage contraceptive use. Swanson described a concept of privatized discovery that typified the process of how contraceptive options are found and managed by men and women. Over time, and with repeated and private attempts, men and women learned to use and manage contraceptive options that suit their individual changing life circumstances. However, at any point in the process, factors can interfere. Incomplete knowledge, inexperience, or poor fit with a partner's experiences can frustrate management of contraception. If conditions remained stable, no need for change was identified; however, change in any conditions (e.g., new relationship, sexual practice, health or illness state) necessitated finding a new option. Matteson (1991) described a theory of advocating for self as a fertility-regulating process that women employ. Risks associated with five categories (personalizing pregnancy risk, exploring options, using an option, contending with ramifications of use, and contending with use-effectiveness rates) are balanced with the risks of pregnancy. Employing phenomenological methods, Lethbridge (1991) examined women's perceptions of their experience with contraceptive use over the course of their reproductive years. Thirty women of varying ethnicity and socioeconomic status described their experiences as contraceptive self-care that involved a central process, choosing and using contraception, and occurred within the context of three processes: forestalling pregnancy, assigning the burden of contraception, and negotiating with those who control contraception. Each process comprised specific themes. One theme identified was that of valuing sexual freedom or enjoying sexual relationships apart from the possibility of pregnancy.

Two researchers have explored contraception in specific population groups. Lethbridge (1991) described the contraceptive knowledge, methods, and consistency of contraceptive use by women of upper socioeconomic class. Women ($N = 83$) in this study were consistent users of their contraceptive method, had fewer unplanned pregnancies in their history than the general population, and used barrier methods predominantly. Women in Lethbridge's study were more knowledgeable about contraception than others tested with the same contraceptive knowledge instrument; women who had used more methods were most knowledgeable. The research of Wilkerson, Quillin, and Feetham (1994) explored how a serious life event, the birth of a child with a chronic health problem, alters sexual and marital relations. Mothers of healthy infants and those of infants who were placed on apnea monitors for at least 5 months after birth were surveyed about their contraceptive practices and sexual satisfactions. Mothers of children with a chronic health problem reported a significantly increased use of oral contraceptives over mothers of healthy infants. No statistically significant differences were found in the two groups' sexual satisfaction, although the mothers of healthy infants were slightly more satisfied. Findings that sexual satisfaction had decreased for both groups by 12 months supports findings discussed earlier (Ellis & Hewatt, 1985; Fischman et al., 1986).

Sexually Protective and Risky Behaviors

In the past decade, the epidemic of STDs and HIV/AIDS and the need for STD/AIDS prevention has sparked an explosion of research about women's sexual practices. This research has described women's knowledge of and attitudes toward risky sexual practices and their sexual risk behaviors and sexual protective practices. In addition, nursing research has begun to identify factors associated with or predictive of sexual protective and risk behaviors. Two populations predominate in this research: adolescents, particularly college students, and women presumed to have high-risk practices and who are usually low income and often minority. Several nurses, including Adeline Nyamathi, Loretta Sweet Jemmott, Jacqueline Flaskerud, and Colleen DiIorio, have developed programs of research that have made significant contributions to this body of knowledge.

Knowledge and Attitudes

Nurse researchers have developed a large body of knowledge regarding women's knowledge of STD and HIV/AIDS transmission and prevention, sexually protective practices, and behaviors that place women at risk for acquiring STDs. These researchers' study findings are often specific for age, ethnicity, and class and suggest ways in which educational programs can be tailored to fit specific groups of women.

Adolescents. Koniak-Griffin and associates (Koniak-Griffin, Nyamathi, Vasquez, & Russo, 1994) explored AIDS knowledge among young mothers. Using survey data from predominantly minority (African-American, Latinas) adolescent mothers, they found that the majority of participants had received information about AIDS in school and were able to identify popular misconceptions as false. However, a number of the adolescents had incorrect information about AIDS transmission, particularly perinatal transmission, and methods of prevention.

College students. Several studies have documented knowledge of STD prevention and knowledge about HIV in college students (Bridgers, Figler, Vaughan, & Sawin, 1990; DiIorio, Parsons, Lehr, Adame, & Carlone, 1993a, 1993b; Hale & Trumbetta, 1996; Jadack, Hyde, & Keller, 1995). College women report viewing AIDS as serious yet do not view themselves as susceptible and are uncertain if AIDS beliefs influence their contraceptive behaviors (Bridgers et al., 1990). DiIorio and associates (1993a, 1993b) documented that 689 college freshman were knowledgeable about the cause and transmission of AIDS but were less knowledgeable about medical aspects. Most knew that condoms were effective in preventing HIV transmission, but fewer could differentiate between the effectiveness of latex and nonlatex condoms. Hale and Trumbetta (1996) found that levels of knowledge about STD transmission were high, yet gaps in knowledge were identified. More than half of the 308 female college students in their study did not know that persons with an STD were at greater risk for contracting HIV during sexual intercourse and, similar to DiIorio's findings, almost 20% thought that latex and natural membrane condoms were equally protective against HIV transmission.

Adult women. Gender differences in knowledge about HIV in young adults has been examined as well (Jadack et al., 1995). In general, respondents had accurate knowledge regarding HIV transmission associated with various sexual behaviors and knowledge of HIV prevention. However, significant gender differences were identified, with men more likely to downplay the likelihood of transmission in comparison to women. Further, men rated animal skin condoms significantly less effective and the diaphragm as more effective in preventing transmission of HIV than did women.

As part of a study to evaluate a community-level HIV prevention program, information about lesbian and bisexual women's knowledge of HIV risk was obtained (Stevens, 1994). Women in this study appeared to believe that women who have sex with other women are at less risk for contracting HIV than are women who have sex with men. Further, a majority of the women were not knowledgeable about HIV prevention for women who had sex with women, and many had never thought about themselves and HIV. Respondents appeared to equate their exclusion from designated risk groups as evidence that they could not be infected.

High-risk women. Nyamathi and Flaskerud (Flaskerud & Nyamathi, 1989; Flaskerud & Rush, 1989; Flaskerud & Thompson, 1991; Nyamanthi, Bennett, Leake, Lewis, & Flaskerud, 1993) have contributed much to our understanding of impoverished minority and White women's AIDS-related knowledge and beliefs. Early research (Flaskerud & Nyamathi, 1989) suggested that Black women had more knowledge of AIDS than did Latinas and were more comfortable talking about AIDS; however, more recently, African-American women and Latinas were found to be equally knowledgeable in some areas of AIDS information (Nyamanthi, Bennett, Leake, Lewis, et al., 1993). At the same time, low-acculturated Latinas were less informed about modes of transmission. Beliefs about AIDS, health, and illness held by low-income White women and Black women have also been documented (Flaskerud & Rush, 1989; Flaskerud & Thompson, 1991), suggesting that these groups also have misconceptions about transmission. Early studies conducted by these research groups employed qualitative methods to better describe the full range of beliefs of low-income women about AIDS and its treatment; later research used a survey design.

Williams (1991), conducting a qualitative needs assessment of women at risk to acquire information needed to develop education programs for high-risk women, found that women perceived AIDS to be a serious personal health risk that necessitated sexual protective practices (condom use, reducing the number of sexual partners). However, they did not always believe that these practices would be effective and felt there were significant costs (partner rejection, disruption of established sexual relationships) associated with these behaviors.

Focus groups were used to explore injection drug users' (IVDUs') (male and female) knowledge of and attitudes toward safe sex (Weiss, Weston, & Quirinale, 1993). In this study, women IVDUs denied feeling vulnerable to acquiring HIV. Further, women respondents seemed more acquainted with STDs, particularly those that are primarily symptomatic in women, and more knowledgeable about different types of condoms than did men.

Risky Sexual Practices

Nurses have documented the risky sexual behaviors and protective sexual practices of wide variety of populations of women. The two major sexual risk-taking behaviors described in all studies were having unprotected sex (without use of a condom) and having multiple sexual partners. Studies by nurses have contributed information regarding women's experiences with condoms, including their perceptions and beliefs about condoms.

Adolescents. Koniak-Griffin and associates (Koniak-Griffin & Brecht, 1995; Koniak-Griffin et al., 1994) documented sexual practices among pregnant adolescents and young mothers. Using focus group and survey data from predominantly minority (African-American, Latina) adolescent (ages 12 to 20 years) women, they found a continuum of risk-taking practices ranging from multiple sex practices and drug and alcohol use to women who had had one or two partners and no history of substance use. The majority of women in each study were having unprotected sex. Factors that affected condom use for the study respondents included gender inequality, embarrassment, and personal preferences. Issues of personal safety in daily living, peer pressure, and emotion-focused coping also increased risk taking. Using data from a household probability sample of minority female youths (15 to 24 years old), Ford, Rubinstein, and Norris (1994) demonstrated that African-American females in Detroit, as compared to all U.S. minorities, had their first sexual experience earlier, were less likely to use a condom at first intercourse or currently, and thus might have higher-than-average vulnerability to HIV infection. Both African-American and Hispanic adolescent women did not use condoms with their most recent partner because they or their partner did not want to use condoms or because of specific problems with condoms. The most commonly noted problem was that a condom was not available.

College students. The sexually risky behaviors of college students have been documented in a number of studies (Bridgers et al., 1990; DiIorio et al., 1993a, 1993b; Hale & Trumbetta, 1996; Jadack et al., 1995; Sheahan, Coons, Seabolt, Churchill, & Dale, 1994). Risk-taking behaviors that have been identified include multiple sex partners (Hale & Trumbetta, 1996; Jadack et al., 1995), not knowing the partners' sexual history (Hale & Trumbetta, 1996; Jadack et al., 1995; Sheahan et al., 1994), no or inconsistent condom use (DiIorio et al., 1993a, 1993b; Hale & Trumbetta, 1996; Jadack et al., 1995; Jemmott & Jemmott, 1991) and initiation of sexual activity at an early age (DiIorio et al., 1993a, 1993b).

Young adult women. The sexual risk practices of different populations of young adult women have also been described by nurses. Prevalent factors documented in women attending hospital ambulatory clinics, community centers, and family planning clinics included sexual activity with persons at high risk for AIDS and multiple sex partners (Lauver, Armstrong, Marks, & Schwartz, 1995) and a history of STDs (Lauver et al., 1995). Military women also reported multiple partners and little or no condom use, as well as relationships of less than 6 months (Abel, Adams, & Stevenson, 1994). Marion (1990) documented that White, well-educated, divorced or separated women generally did not use condoms, even with casual partners.

At-risk women. Nyamathi and associates have described risky sexual behaviors of impoverished, minority women (Nyamathi, Bennett, & Leake, 1995; Nyamathi, Lewis, Leake, Flaskerud, & Bennett, 1995), finding that higher percentages of African-American women and highly acculturated Latinas report having a history of STDs, more than one sex partner, and accepting money for sex than do low-acculturated Latinas (Nyamathi, Bennett, Leake, Lewis, et al., 1993). Further, young, impoverished, minority women were more likely to have multiple sex partners. In general, African-American women were more likely to report having multiple partners and unprotected sex than were Latinas (Nyamathi, Lewis, et al., 1995), compared to all U.S. minorities.

Preventive Behaviors

No studies of the sexual protective practices of adolescents conducted by nurses were identified.

College students. Although college students employed a variety of sexual protective practices to reduce risk, the percentages of students who used these strategies was not high. Strategies reported included discussing STD history with a sexual partner (Sheahan et al., 1994), limiting sexual partners or having a monogamous relationship and/or getting to know their partners (Bridgers et al., 1990). Condom use to prevent disease transmission and abstinence to reduce risk were less-frequently-used measures (Bridgers et al., 1990; Jemmott & Jemmott, 1991).

Adult women. As in adolescent women, young adult women's preventive behavior rates of consistent condom use and HIV testing were low (Lauver et al., 1995). Older women, women who were one of a couple, and women of color were least likely to use condoms consistently; low-risk women were less likely to have had HIV tests (Lauver et al., 1995). In contrast, Swanson, Dibble, and Trocki (1995) found that 98% of their sample of adult women with genital herpes had used a condom at some time; however, less than 75% used condoms to prevent herpes.

Many studies have documented reasons why women do not use condoms. Reasons given include assumed safety of partner (Hale & Trumbetta, 1996; Jadack et al., 1995), greater concern with pregnancy (Hale & Trumbetta, 1996; Jadack et al., 1995), spontaneity or lack of planning (Hale & Trumbetta, 1996; Jadack et al., 1995), unavailability of condom (Ford et al., 1994; Hale & Trumbetta, 1996; Jadack et al., 1995), and low perception of risk (Lauver et al., 1995; Marion, 1990). High-risk African-American women were more likely to report barriers in using, discussing, and obtaining condoms; Latinas were more likely to report partner's dislike of condoms (Nyamathi, Lewis, et al., 1995).

Factors associated with risky sexual practices. Nurse researchers have built on factors identified with risky sexual behaviors and contributed much to our understanding of the factors that influence women's use or nonuse of sexual protective practices. Furthermore, nurses have provided information on those factors that do not influence sexual behaviors. In some studies, qualitative methods have been used to explore the experiences of women whose behaviors place them at risk for contracting STDs and HIV. Other studies have quantified the extent of the relationships between selected factors and risky practices.

Redfern and Hutchinson (1994) described women's experiences of repetitively contracting STDs. Themes important to women that emerged from in-depth interviews with 8 women as well as stories and anecdotes from one author's clinical practice were the power and significance of heterosexual relationships and idealized sexual encounters and relationships with men. Themes of powerlessness, stigma, and victimization pervaded the interviews. Women described using condoms early in relationships, stopping when they felt safe, and then contracting an STD. Negative reactions to condom use were described, including partner reactions. Women in this study believed that STDs were an inevitable part of women's lives and often due to an inherent characteristic of women rather than behavior of men or women.

Kinsey (1994) explored the lifestyle choices and HIV/AIDs risk appraisals of 105 urban childbearing women living in a city with a high incidence of AIDS cases. Analysis of data from personal and survey interviews, self-administered questionnaires, focus groups, and chart reviews revealed distinct differences between the risk appraisal of professionals and women's personal risk assessments. Women gauged their HIV risk by determining availability—the likelihood of the frequency of occurrence of the event—and deciding because their partner was monogamous or tested negative that they were not at risk. New information—someone close to them acquiring HIV or knowledge of partner infidelity—necessitated a revision of risk. Women distanced themselves from risk by testing negative and acknowledging that HIV/AIDS existed but was someone else's sickness. New information was used when it supported existing belief of low risk and discounted when it did not. Women might have a succession of sexual partners in a short time period but did not personalize the likelihood of increased HIV risk.

Nyamathi and Lewis (1991) have provided information about the beliefs of 66 African-American women at risk for HIV infection. A theme identified from focus groups was powerlessness. The risk of unprotected sex with multiple partners was real, yet concern about AIDS did not exist, as worries over daily survival and children took precedence. For many of the women, indiscriminant sex was simply a risk one took. Feeling of loss of control expressed by all but 6 of the women prevented them from changing their life situations. An additional barrier to changing one's circumstances was low self-esteem.

The effects of psychological factors on sexual behaviors has been examined by nurses. Marion's (1990) finding that women's ability to insist on condom use with a partner was significantly related to condom use in her divorced and separated respondents suggested that feelings of self-efficacy were an important psychological factor in the use of sexual protective practices. Further, two other studies have noted the beneficial effects of perceived self-efficacy on a woman's ability to practice safer sex behaviors (Hale & Trumbetta, 1996; O'Leary, Goodhart, Jemmott, & Boccher-Lattimore, 1992). Stronger perceptions of self-efficacy to engage in safer sex practices have significantly predicted safer sex behaviors in college women (O'Leary et al., 1992); perceived general self-efficacy and specific self-efficacy for condom use and communication were associated with lowered behavioral risk for STDs in adult women (Hale & Trumbetta,

1996). Jemmott, Jemmott, Spears, Hewitt, and Cruz-Collins (1992) found that Black adolescent women receiving an intervention designed to increase perceived self-efficacy and favorable expectancies about the hedonistic consequences of using condoms reported greater intention to use condoms than did those receiving one of two control interventions. Nyamathi (1991) demonstrated that high-risk women who were high in self-esteem and stronger in sense of coherence reported significantly fewer high-risk behaviors. In contrast, other researchers found no differences in self-esteem in 105 military women with or without chlamydia (Abel, Adams, & Stevenson, 1994).

The relationship of perceived susceptibility to or risk for STD and HIV/AIDs to sexual practices has been documented in several studies. Women's perception of increased susceptibility or risk was related to decreased risky practices in adult women (Hale & Trumbetta, 1996) and increased risk reduction behaviors in college women (Bridgers et al., 1990). In contrast, DiIorio and colleagues (1993a) found no relationship between perceived susceptibility and safer sex practices in women college freshmen in general; perceived susceptibility did differentiate sexually active from nonsexually active White college women freshmen.

The relationship of selected sociodemographic characteristics and sexual practices has also been examined. Koniak-Griffin and Brecht (1995) found ethnicity (African American) and current pregnancy status strongly predicted having had multiple sexual partners. A history of STD infection was strongly related to increased condom use in separated and divorced women (Marion, 1990), yet Redfern and Hutchinson (1994) found that their respondents who had repetitively contracted STDs associated condom use with pregnancy prevention rather than STD prevention. Women who use or abuse substances are less likely to practice safer sex. A history of marijuana use predicted having multiple partners in pregnant adolescents and young mothers (Koniak-Griffin & Brecht, 1995); poor women who had multiple sexual partners were less likely to be in drug programs and more likely to share needles and be sexually involved with men who used intravenous drugs (Nyamathi, Lewis, et al., 1995).

Another factor related to sexual practices investigated by nurses is social referents. Marion (1990) found that partners who favored condoms were associated with increased use of condoms by divorced and separated women. Communication with partners also increases condom use (Strader, Beaman, & McSweeny, 1992). In another study, Sheahan and colleagues (1994) found that only one third of women with a diagnosis of chlamydia discussed with their partners either their own or partner's sexual history. In a related study, Jemmott and Jemmott (1991) found that attitudes of mothers and sexual partners of 103 Black college women respondents were predictive of intention to use condoms.

Nurse researchers have also found that women's positive attitudes toward condoms (Jemmott & Jemmott, 1991) and negative experiences with condoms (Norris & Ford, 1994) influenced women's intention to use condoms. Further research has established that White college students who are not sexually active have a forward-looking perspective, differentiating them from sexually active White college students, who live in the present (DiIorio et al., 1993b).

Studies by nurses have also added to the growing evidence that knowledge is not sufficient to change sexual behaviors. For example, DiIorio and associates (1993a) documented that knowledge of AIDS, misconceptions about AIDs, and knowledge of safer sex practices were not related to implementing safer sex practices or decreasing risky behaviors in college women. Nor was AIDS knowledge a predictor of intention to use condoms in Black inner-city college women (Jemmott & Jemmott, 1991). Similarly, Koniak-Griffin and Brecht (1995) did not find AIDS knowledge to be a significant predictor of high-risk sexual behavior.

Interventions to Decrease Risk

Nurses have begun to test interventions designed to decrease sexually risky practices among women. Jemmott and colleagues (Jemmott & Jemmott, 1992; Jemmott, Jemmott, Spears, et al., 1992) tested whether a social cognitive theory AIDS prevention intervention would increase intention to use condoms among sexually active inner-city Black adolescents. Women who received the social cognitive intervention reported greater intention to use condoms than did women in an information-alone intervention or women in a general health promotion intervention. In a second study, women scored higher in intention to use condoms, AIDS knowledge, expectancies regarding condom use, and self-efficacy after a social cognitive intervention than before.

Peer educator-based interventions have been found to be effective in prompting interest in HIV prevention information and intent to change behavior in lesbian and bisexual women (Stevens, 1994). Group education about HIV risks, transmission, and prevention, coupled with

individual interviews within which information about HIV prevention, was provided. Findings from this study legitimated HIV prevention efforts that are culturally and community specific.

Other Studies

Nursing Practice

Numerous studies of nurses' knowledge and attitudes toward their own and their patients' sexuality were conducted in the 1970s (Hott & Ryan-Merritt, 1982) and 1980s. Typically, the subjects of these studies were convenience samples of nursing students, faculty, or administrators. Most studies employed descriptive, survey, or ex post facto designs; a few incorporated quasi-experimental or experimental designs with pre- and posttests administered (Hott & Ryan-Merritt, 1982). More recently, nurse researchers have focused on what current practice is related to sexuality.

Knowledge and Attitudes

Studies of nursing students in the 1980s suggested that although their knowledge of human sexuality was comparable to other health profession students and nonmedical undergraduate and graduate students, nursing students possessed significantly more conservative attitudes toward human sexuality (Kuczynski, 1980; Roy, 1983). Hacker's findings that undergraduate and graduate nursing students expressed much discomfort regarding patients' sexuality supported these findings (Hacker, 1984). In contrast, nursing students were found to have favorable attitudes toward sexually active older persons (Damroch, 1982; Quinn-Krach & Van Hoozer, 1988) and to be knowledgeable regarding sexuality in the aged (Quinn-Krach & Van Hoozer, 1988). Further, ethnicity and age of nursing students affected attitudes toward and knowledge of sexuality in the aged; older students had more positive attitudes toward the elderly and were more knowledgeable about sexuality in the aged than younger students; Asian students held more negative attitudes and were less knowledgeable than Caucasian nursing students (Quinn-Krach & Van Hoozer, 1988). Practicing nurses have also been found to be lacking in knowledge of human sexuality (Woleski-Wruble, 1991). In a related study of nurse educators, Randal (1989) documented negative attitudes toward and inaccurate knowledge about lesbians. Collectively, these findings suggested that nurses continue to have a need for additional knowledge in selected areas of human sexuality and, further, that it is not enough to include a course in human sexuality in the nursing curriculum, as knowledge does not necessarily change attitudes.

Current Practice Related to Sexuality

Nurse researchers have asked whether nurses address patients' sexual health care needs, and what factors influence current nursing practice related to sexuality. Research has documented that although staff nurses believe addressing sexual health care is important (Woleski-Wruble, 1991), few address sexual concerns with their clients (Matocha & Waterhouse, 1993). The only activities related to sexuality that were performed with regularity by a sample of 155 practicing, registered nurses from a variety of practice settings were the client-initiated activities of listening to client concerns and answering their questions about sexuality (Matocha & Waterhouse, 1993). Research has indicated that nurses were more likely to include sexuality in their practice if they worked in a hospital area in which sexuality was particularly relevant (e.g., obstetrics), if they believed they had responsibility for discussing sexual concerns, and if they felt knowledgeable and comfortable discussing sexuality (Lewis & Dphil, 1994; Matocha & Waterhouse, 1993). Reasons why nurses do not address their patients' sexual concerns have also been investigated. Kautz, Dickey, and Stevens (1990) documented that nurses perceived patients as too ill and too anxious to discuss sexual concerns and that the sexual concerns of patients were minor problems of low priority. Lewis and Dphil (1994) found no relationship between knowledge of and attitudes toward sexuality and nursing practice, but Matocha and Waterhouse (1993) found that nurses' perceived knowledge, comfort, and responsibility and practice area were useful predictors of the extent of nurses' practice related to sexuality. Matocha and Waterhouse (1993) asked whether continuing education on sexuality would alter nursing practice related to sexuality. Darst (1988) found that a short-term sex education training program had no significant effect on sex knowledge, had no significant effect on sex education or counseling skills, and did not affect outcomes for disabled, heterosexual clients' sexual functioning. The cumulative findings of these studies suggest that nurses do not consistently address sexuality concerns of their clients and that knowledge and skills have inconsistent effects on their ability to provide sexual health care.

Methodological Issues

Orienting Framework and Conceptualization

Many of the studies of normative experiences and clinical interruptions did not articulate an orienting perspective or conceptual model. In contrast, many of the studies of health promotion and disease prevention were grounded in an orienting framework. Common frameworks used in studies of contraceptive research were the Health Belief Model and Health Promotion Model and Piaget's cognitive framework. Studies of sexual protective practices and risk sexual behaviors also used the Health Belief Model, as well as the Theory of Reasoned Action or frameworks based on the Social Cognitive Theory.

Many different conceptualizations of sexuality have been used by nurses conducting research about women's sexuality. All too often, narrow definitions of sexuality that equated sexuality with sexual functioning were employed rather than a broader conceptual definition. In general, more comprehensive views of sexuality were found in those studies that used a qualitative research design. One of few studies employing quantitative methods that defined sexuality broadly, incorporating physical and emotional aspects, was that conducted by White and colleagues (1994). A similar dilemma was seen in studies of contraception, with inconsistent use or differing conceptual definitions of contraceptive practices.

Research Design

Although the majority of the studies reviewed here employed a descriptive or comparative quantitative research design, use of qualitative methods by number of researchers (Bernhard, 1992; Kearney et al., 1994; Lethbridge, 1991; Swanson, 1988; Teets, 1990) add rich detail to knowledge of the effects of clinical interruptions on women's sexuality and women's use of contraception. Nurses employed both qualitative and quantitative methodologies in their studies of sexually protective or risky behaviors. Qualitative methods, such as focus groups and in-depth unstructured interviews, have provided much information about the context in which women are able to institute sexual protective practices.

Ethical issues involved in the conduct of sexuality research affect the nature, quality, and quantity of the research and must be meticulously addressed. Nurses conducting sexuality research must be cognizant of professional, public, and political attitudes that can affect selection of research problems and access to subjects. Informed consent and confidentiality, although certainly not unique to research on sexuality, necessitate a greater attention and sensitivity to subject risk.

Sample

Some of the studies employed ethnically diverse samples, but this was not the case universally. Many of the respondents of adolescent female sexuality were multiracial, including African-American, Hispanic, and White adolescents. DeSantis and Thomas (1987) focused specifically on cultural differences among Cuban and Haitian immigrants. In contrast, Tucker (1989) focused only on Black females, stating that "Black adolescents are particularly at risk for an unplanned pregnancy" (p. 393). In contrast, postpartum samples were White, middle-class, and small and ethnically diverse Canadian.

Often, the ethnicity of the sample was not reported. For example, no information was provided on the ethnicity of the women in studies of aging and sexuality. Ethnicity data were reported in some studies of clinical interruptions (Bernhard, 1992; Henderson et al., 1995; Kearney et al., 1994; LeMone, 1993; Watts, 1982, 1994) and was not stated in the majority of the studies, making it difficult to determine clinical generalizability of study findings. Information on the ethnicity of respondents was always given for the studies of health promotion and disease prevention. The majority of the samples in quantitative studies of women's sexuality were of convenience; only one study of clinical interruptions reported using a random sample (White et al., 1994).

Measurement

Perhaps reflecting the lack of conceptual definitions of women's sexuality, no standard definitions of sexual functioning, sexual satisfaction, or sexual activity were found. Different instruments to measure aspects of sexuality were used in every study of normative experiences and clinical interruptions reviewed.

Although a few studies of sexuality and clinical interruptions used previously developed or standard instruments (Bernhard, 1992; Henderson, Boyd, & Whitmore, 1995), many of the researchers developed questionnaires for a specific study. A few of the researchers who developed an instrument reported strict attention to psychometric development (Bernhard, 1992; Pollack, 1993). Watts (1982) developed the Sexual Functioning Questionnaire for use in her study of sexuality and hyperten-

sion. This instrument was used in her later study with diabetic women (Watts, 1994) and in the development of the Sexual Adjustment Questionnaire (Waterhouse & Metcalfe, 1986). Similarly, although many of the contraceptive studies included similar or the same variables (e.g., contraceptive knowledge, cognitive level, contraceptive use), all studies operationalized them differently, and no common instruments were employed.

Recognition of the need for tools to assess the effect of illness and health problems on sexuality is seen in the study conducted by Waterhouse and Metcalfe (1986). These nurses developed and tested a questionnaire designed to assess sexual adjustment in cancer patients. The instrument consists of three parts, dealing with present sexuality and sexuality prior to diagnosis, and is intended for use only with cancer patients.

More recent studies (Wilkerson et al., 1994) used standard instruments to operationalize some variables (i.e., use of the Feetham Family Functioning Survey to measure family functioning).

Although sexually protective or risky behaviors were rarely defined conceptually, almost all studies defined sexual protective practices as consistent condom use and/or limiting the number of sexual partners and risky behaviors as inconsistent or no condom use and/or multiple sexual partners. However, studies differed in how inconsistent condom use and multiple partners were quantified and what number of partners was equated with increased risk. Further, the time periods associated with measurement of safe or risky practices differed among studies. Thus comparison of findings is made more difficult.

Gaps

The majority of research on women and sexuality has been problem focused. No research or descriptions of "normal" women's sexuality as women define, describe, and experience it was located. This is a particularly important gap, given the emphasis in women's health and nursing research on understanding women's lives from women's own perspectives and understanding the contexts within which experiences occur and develop. Also needed is information on the diversity of women's experiences of sexuality in their normal lives (Bernhard, 1993). Further, little or no attention has been paid to sexual practices of women using contraception. This information is critical to those making clinical practice recommendations to women, as choice of a contraceptive method is intimately linked to one's sexual behaviors.

With the exception of studies of women's risky sexual behaviors and sexual protective practices, only a few of the studies of women's sexuality reviewed contained an orienting framework or theoretical perspective. Inconsistent use of or differing conceptual definitions in studies make comparison of findings difficult, and thus less reliance can be placed on the accumulated weight of similar findings.

Descriptive studies of women's sexuality have not paid consistent attention to issues of ethnicity and class. For example, studies of adolescent sexuality do not provide much information on the experiences of White, middle-class girls, and ethnicity has not been recorded in studies of aging women and sexuality. Ethnicity and class have received more attention from nurse researchers documenting risky sexual behaviors, but gaps are also found. Less information is available on the practices and behaviors of White, middle-class women. Further, only one study of all the ones reviewed included Asian women in its sample.

No consistent definition of sexual activity (e.g., vaginal intercourse, masturbation) or standardization of measurement were found in the reported research studies. Further, no biological measurements of sexual experiences or activity were used in nursing research on women and sexuality.

Recommendations for Advancing Science to Guide Nursing Practice

Nurse researchers can take the lead in describing the sexual experiences of women of all classes and eth-

nicities. Research is needed that pays attention to the contexts of women's lives in which sexual behavior, practices, and activities occur and how these contexts affect sexual expression, activity, and sexuality.

Nursing research has accumulated a considerable body of knowledge that can be used to decrease women's risk of acquiring STDs and HIV. Risky practices and preventive behaviors have been well described for many different populations of low-risk and high-risk women, specifically adolescents, college students, and impoverished minority women, especially IVDUs. Factors associated with risky practices and the use of preventive behaviors have been identified for many of these populations of women. It is time for nurses to develop culturally specific interventions and test them in different populations of women.

Less information has been generated about risky practices and preventive behaviors of adult women, especially middle-aged and older women, and low-risk women in general. Additionally, no studies of women prisoners' risky practices and preventive behaviors have been published. Additional descriptive research is needed in these areas.

The body of published nursing research findings about women and their sexuality can potentially be used to inform nursing practice with women throughout their sexual lives. This knowledge base can be enhanced by attention to the measurement issues and gaps noted previously. Continued research and subsequent development of this knowledge base has important implications for understanding women's sexual practices and functions, life cycle experiences and the development of health promotion and disease prevention strategies, and illness or health-problem-related interventions.

References

Abel, E., Adam, E., & Stevenson, R. (1994). Self-esteem, problem solving, and sexual risk behavior among women with and without chlamydia. *Clinical Nursing Research, 3*(4), 353-370.

Bernhard, L. A. (1992). Consequences of hysterectomy in the lives of women. *Health Care for Women International, 13,* 281-291.

Bernhard, L. A. (1993). Women's sexuality. In B. J. McElmurry & R. S. Parker (Eds.), *Annual review of women's health* (pp. 67-93). New York: National League for Nursing Press.

Bridgers, C., Figler, K., Vaughan, S., & Sawin, K. J. (1990). AIDS beliefs in young women: Are they related to AIDS risk-reduction

behavior? *Journal of the American Academy of Nurse Practitioners, 2*(3), 107-112.

Bullough, B., David, M., Whipple, B., Dixon, J., Allgeier, E. R., & Drury, K. C. (1984, March). Subjective reports of female orgasmic explusion of fluid. *Nurse Practitioner, 9*(3), 55-56, 58-59.

Coker, A. L., Richter, D. L., Valois, R. F., McKeown, R. E., Garrison, C. Z., & Vincent, M. L. (1994). Correlates and consequences of early initiation of sexual intercourse. *Journal of School Health, 64*(9), 372-377.

Cooper, H. M. (1984). *The integrative research review.* Beverly Hills, CA: Sage.

Coray, G. M. (1991). *A descriptive study of biopsychosocial correlates of adolescent female sexual activity in a multicultural population.* Unpublished doctoral dissertation, University of California, San Francisco.

Damroch, S. P. (1982). Nursing students' attitudes toward sexually active older persons. *Nursing Research, 31*(4), 252-255.

Darling, C. A., Davidson, J. K., & Conway-Welch, C. (1990). Female ejaculation: Perceived origins, the Grafenberg spot/area, and sexual responsiveness. *Archives of Sexual Behavior, 19*(1), 29-47.

Darst, E. H. (1988). *Effect of sex education on nurses' skills and clinical outcomes with disabled patients.* Unpublished doctoral dissertation, University of Missouri–Kansas City.

DeSantis, L., & Thomas, J. T. (1987). Parental attitudes toward adolescent sexuality: Transcultural perspectives. *Nurse Practitioner, 12*(8), 43-44, 46, 48.

DiIorio, C., Parsons, M., Lehr, S., Adame, D., & Carlone, J. (1993a). Factors associated with use of safer sex practices among college freshmen. *Research in Nursing and Health, 16,* 343-350.

DiIorio, C., Parsons, M., Lehr, S., Adame, D., & Carlone, J. (1993b). Knowledge of AIDS and safer sex practices among college freshmen. *Public Health Nursing, 10*(3), 159-165.

Ellis, D. J., & Hewat, R. J. (1985). Mothers' postpartum perceptions of spousal relationships. *Journal of Obstetric, Gynecologic and Neonatal Nursing, 14*(2), 140-146.

Fischman, S. H., Rankin, E. A., Soeken, K. L., & Lenz, E. R. (1986). Changes in sexual relationships in postpartum couples. *Journal of Obstetric, Gynecologic and Neonatal Nursing, 15*(1), 58-63.

Flaskerud, J. H., & Nyamathi, A. M. (1989). Black and Latina women's AIDS related knowledge, attitudes, and practices. *Research in Nursing and Health, 12,* 339-346.

Flaskerud, J. H., & Rush, C. E. (1989). AIDS and traditional health beliefs and practices of Black women. *Nursing Research, 38*(4), 210-215.

Flaskerud, J. H., & Thompson, J. (1991). Beliefs about AIDS, health, and illness in low-income White women. *Nursing Research, 40*(5), 266-271.

Fogel, C. I. (1995). Common symptoms. In C. I. Fogel & N. F. Woods (Eds.), *Women's health care.* Thousand Oaks, CA: Sage.

Ford, K., Rubinstein, S., & Norris, A. (1994). Sexual behavior and condom use among urban, low-income, African-American and Hispanic youth. *AIDS Education and Prevention,6*(3), 219-229.

Froelicher, E. S., Kee, L. L., Newton, K. M., Lindskog, B., & Livingston, M. (1994). Return to work, sexual activity, and other activities after acute myocardial infarction. *Heart and Lung, 23*(5), 423-435.

Gloeckner, M. R. (1984) Perceptions of sexual attractiveness following ostomy surgery. *Research in Nursing and Health, 7,* 87-92.

Hacker, S. S. (1984, Winter). Students' questions about sexuality: Implications for nurse educators. *Nurse Education, 9*(4), 28-31.

Hale, P. J., & Trumbetta, S. L. (1996). Women's self-efficacy and sexually transmitted disease preventive behaviors. *Research in Nursing and Health, 19,* 101-110.

Henderson, D. J., Boyd, C. J., & Whitmore, J. (1995). Women and illicit drugs: Sexuality and crack cocaine. *Health Care for Women International, 16,* 113-124.

Hott, J. R., & Ryan-Merrit, M. (1982). A national study of nursing research in human sexuality. *Nursing Clinics of North America, 17*(3), 429-447.

Hughes, C. B., & Torre, C. (1987). Predicting effective contraceptive behavior in college females. *Nurse Practitioner, 12*(9), 44, 46, 48-59, 53-54.

Jadack, R. A., Hyde, J. S., & Keller, M. L. (1995). Gender and knowledge about HIV, risky sexual behavior, and safer sex practices. *Research in Nursing and Health, 18,* 313-324.

Jemmott, J. B., Jemmott, L. S., Spears, H., Hewitt, N., & Cruz-Collins, M. (1992). Self-efficacy, hedonistic expectancies, and condom-use intentions among inner-city Black adolescent women: A social cognitive approach to AIDS risk behavior. *Journal of Adolescent Health, 13*(6), 512-519.

Jemmott, L. S., & Jemmott, J. B. (1991). Increasing condom-use intentions among sexually active Black adolescent women. *Nursing Research, 40*(5), 273-279.

Jemmott, L. S., & Jemmott, J. B. (1992). Applying the Theory of Reasoned Action to AIDS risk behavior: Condom use among Black women. *Nursing Research, 41*(4), 229-234.

Kautz, D. D., Dickey, C. A., & Stevens, M. N. (1990). Using research to identify why nurses do not meet established sexuality nursing care standards. *Journal of Nursing Quality Assurance, 4*(3), 69-78.

Kearney, M., Murphy, S., & Rosenbaum, M. (1994). Learning by losing: Sex and fertility on crack cocaine. *Qualitative Health Research, 4*(2), 142-162.

Kinsey, K. K. (1994). "But I know my man!" HIV/AIDS risk appraisals and heuristical reasoning patterns among childbearing women. *Holistic Nursing Practice, 8*(2), 79-88.

Koniak-Griffin, D., & Brecht, M. L. (1995). Linkages between sexual risk taking, substance use, and AIDS knowledge among pregnant adolescents and young mothers. *Nursing Research, 44*(6), 340-346.

Koniak-Griffin, D., Nyamathi, A., Vasquez, R., & Russo, A. A. (1994). Risk-taking behaviors and AIDS knowledge: Experiences and beliefs of minority adolescent mothers. *Health Education Research, 9*(4), 449-463.

Krueger, J. C., Hassell, J., Goggins, D. B., Ishimatau, T., Pablico, M. R., & Tuttle, E. J. (1979). Relationship between nurse counseling and sexual adjustment after hysterectomy. *Nursing Research, 28*(3), 145-150.

Kuczynski, H. J. (1980). Nursing and medical students' sexual attitudes and knowledge. *Journal of Obstetric, Gynecologic and Neonatal Nursing, 9*(6), 339-342.

Lamb, M. A., & Sheldon, T. A. (1994). The sexual adaptation of women treated for endometrial cancer. *Cancer Practice, 2*(2), 103-113.

Lauver, D., Armstrong, K., Marks, S., & Schwartz, S. (1995). HIV risk status and preventive behaviors among 17,619 women. *Journal of Obstetric, Gynecologic and Neonatal Nursing, 24*(1), 33-39.

LeMone, P. (1991). *Transforming: Patterns of sexual function in adults with insulin-dependent diabetes mellitus.* Unpublished doctoral dissertation, University of Alabama at Birmingham.

LeMone, P. (1993). Human sexuality in adults with insulin-dependent diabetes mellitus. *Image: The Journal of Nursing Scholarship, 25*(2), 101-105.

Lethbridge, D. J. (1991). Choosing and using contraception: Toward a theory of women's contraceptive self-care. *Nursing Research, 40*(5), 276-280.

Lewis, S., & Dphil, R. B. (1994). Nurses' knowledge of and attitudes towards sexuality and the relationship of these with nursing practice. *Journal of Advanced Nursing, 20,* 251-259.

Marcy, S. A., Brown, J. S., & Danielson, R. (1983). Contraceptive use by adolescent females in relation to knowledge, and time and method of contraceptive counseling. *Research in Nursing and Health, 6,* 175-182.

Marion, L. N. (1990). *Risk reduction in sexual behaviors of divorced and separated women.* Unpublished doctoral dissertation, University of Illinois at Chicago.

Matteson, P. S. (1991). *Advocating for self: A grounded theory of women's process of fertility regulation.* Unpublished doctoral dissertation, Boston College, Boston.

Matocha, L. K., & Waterhouse, J. K. (1993). Current nursing practice related to sexuality. *Research in Nursing and Health, 16,* 371-378.

Norris, A. E., & Ford, K. (1994). Association between condom experiences and beliefs, intentions, and use, in a sample of urban, low-income, African-American and Hispanic youth. *AIDS Education and Prevention, 6*(10), 27-39.

Nyamathi, A. M. (1991). Relationship of resources to emotional distress, somatic complaints, and high-risk behaviors in drug recovery and homeless minority women. *Research in Nursing and Health, 14,* 269-277.

Nyamathi, A. M., Bennett, C., & Leake, B. (1995). Predictors of maintained high-risk behaviors among impoverished women. *Public Health Reports, 110*(5), 600-606.

Nyamathi, A. M., Bennett, C., Leake, B., Lewis, C., & Flaskerud, J. (1993). AIDS-related knowledge, perceptions, and behaviors among impoverished minority women. *American Journal of Public Health, 83*(1), 65-71.

Nyamathi, A. M., & Lewis, C. E. (1991). Coping of African-American women at risk from AIDS. *Women's Health Inventory, 1*(2), 53-62.

Nyamathi, A. M., Lewis, C., Leake, B., Flaskerud, J., & Bennett, C. (1995). Barriers to condom use and needle cleaning among impoverished minority female injection drug users and partners of drug users. *Public Health Reports, 110*(2), 166-172.

O'Leary, A., Goodhart, F., Jemmott, L. S., & Boccher-Lattimore, D. (1992). Predictors of safer sex on the college campus: A social cognitive analysis. *Journal of the Association of College Health, 40,* 254-263.

Pollack, L. E. (1993). Self-perceptions of interpersonal and sexual functioning in women with mood disorders: A preliminary report. *Issues in Mental Health Nursing, 14,* 201-218.

Portonova, M., Young, E., & Newman, M. A. (1984). Elderly women's attitudes toward sexual activity among their peers. *Health Care for Women International, 5,* 289-298.

Quinn-Krach, P., & Van Hoozer, H. (1988). Sexuality and the attitudes and knowledge of nursing students. *Journal of Nursing Education, 27*(8), 359-363.

Randall, C. E. (1989). Lesbian phobia among BSN educators: A survey. *Journal of Nursing Education, 28*(7), 302-306.

Redfern, N., & Hutchinson, S. (1994). Women's experiences of repetitively contracting sexually transmitted diseases. *Health Care for Women International, 15,* 423-433.

Rhodes, M. L. (1990). *Social and psychosocial factors related to pregnancy status and sexual practices of adolescent females ages 12-18.* Unpublished doctoral dissertation, State University of New York at Buffalo.

Roy, J. H. (1983). A study of knowledge and attitudes of selected nursing students toward human sexuality. *Issues in Health Care of Women, 4,* 127-137.

Sachs, B. (1985). Contraceptive decision-making in urban, Black female adolescents: Its relationship to cognitive development. *International Journal of Nursing Studies, 22*(2), 117-126.

Shah, H. S. (1989). *Psychosocial adjustment, self-concept, and sexual satisfaction of women with diabetes.* Unpublished doctoral dissertation, Boston University, Boston.

Sheahan, S. L., Coons, S. J., Seabolt, J. P., Churchill, L., & Dale, T. (1994). Sexual behavior, communication, and chlamydial infections among college women. *Health Care for Women International, 15,* 275-286.

Sheehan, M. K., Ostwald, S. K., & Rothenberger, J. (1986). Perceptions of sexual responsibility: Do young men and women agree? *Pediatric Nursing, 12*(1), 17-21.

Steinke, E. E. (1988). Older adults' knowledge and attitudes about sexuality and aging. *Image: The Journal of Nursing Scholarship, 20*(2), 93-95.

Steinke, E. E. (1994). Knowledge and attitudes of older adults about sexuality in ageing: A comparison of two studies. *Journal of Advanced Nursing, 19,* 477-485.

Stevens, P. E. (1994). HIV prevention education for lesbians and bisexual women: A cultural analysis of a community intervention. *Social Science and Medicine, 39*(11), 1565-1578.

Strader, M. K., Beaman, M. L., & McSweeney, M. (1992). Effects of communication with important social referents on beliefs and intentions to use condoms. *Journal of Advanced Nursing, 17,* 699-703.

Sullivan, J. F. (1989). *The relationship of age, level of cognitive development, future time perspective, parenthood motivation, and perception of invulnerability to contractive risk-taking behavior in female adolescents.* Unpublished doctoral dissertation, Adelphi University, Garden City, NY.

Swanson, J. M. (1988). The process of finding contraceptive options. *Western Journal of Nursing Research, 10*(4), 492-503.

Swanson, J. M., Dibble, S. L., & Trocki, K. (1995). A description of the gender differences in risk behaviors in young adults with genital herpes. *Public Health Nursing, 12*(2), 99-108.

Teets, J. M. (1990). What women talk about: Sexuality issues of chemically dependent women. *Journal of Psychosocial Nursing, 28*(12), 4-7.

Tucker, S. K. (1989). Black adolescents' source, quantity, and quality of sex related information. *Journal of the National Black Nurses Association, 3*(2), 29-40.

Tucker, S. K. (1990). Adolescent patterns of communication about the menstrual cycle, sex, and contraception. *Journal of Pediatric Nursing, 5*(6), 393-400.

Waterhouse, J., & Metcalfe, M. C. (1986). Development of the Sexual Adjustment Questionnaire. *Oncology Nursing Forum, 13*(3), 53-59.

Watts, R. J. (1982). Sexual functioning, health beliefs, and compliance with high blood pressure medications. *Nursing Research, 31*(5), 278-283.

Watts, R. J. (1994). Sexual function of diabetic and nondiabetic African American women: A pilot study. *Journal of the National Black Nurses Association, 7*(1), 60-69.

Weiss, S. H., Weston, C. B., & Quirinale, J. (1993). Safe sex? Misconceptions, gender differences and barriers among injection drug users: A focus groups approach. *AIDS Education and Prevention, 5*(4), 279-293.

White, J. E., & Kellinger, K. G. (1989). Teenagers' perceptions of unplanned adolescent pregnancies and oral contraceptive use. *Journal of the American Academy of Nurse Practitioners, 1*(2), 55-62.

White, M. J., Rintala, D. H., Hart, K., & Fuhrer, M. J. (1994). A comparison of the sexual concerns of men and women with spinal cord injuries. *Rehabilitation Nursing Research, 3*(2), 55-61.

Whitley, N. (1978). The first coital experience of one hundred women. *Journal of Obstetric, Gynecologic and Neonatal Nursing, 7*(4), 41-45.

Wilkerson, S., Quillin, S., & Feetham, S. (1994). Contraceptive practices before conception and after the birth of a child with a chronic health problem. *Health Care for Women International, 15,* 43-51.

Williams, A. B. (1991). Women at risk: An AIDS educational needs assessment. *Image: The Journal of Nursing Scholarship, 23*(4), 208-213.

Winter, E. S., Ashton, D. J., & Moore, D. L. (1991). Dispelling myths: A study of PMS and relationship satisfaction. *Nursing Research, 16*(5), 34-45.

Woleski-Wruble, A.C. (1991). *Staff nurse opinion of the importance of addressing patient sexual health care.* Unpublished doctoral dissertation. Columbia University Teachers College, New York.

Young, E. W., Koch, P. B., & Bailey, D. (1989). Research comparing the dyadic adjustment and sexual functioning concerns of diabetic and nondiabetic women. *Health Care for Women International, 10,* 377-394.

29

CLINICAL NURSING RESEARCH ON BATTERED WOMEN AND THEIR CHILDREN

A Review

Jacquelyn Campbell
Barbara Parker

Introduction

This review of clinical nursing research on battered women and their children is written as an update of the review of nursing research on the same topic covering nursing research published through 1991 (Campbell & Parker, 1992). The research covered in that review is summarized in Table 29.1. This chapter begins with a brief summary of that review and an overview of the state of the science on battering in general; delineates the inclusion and exclusion criteria for the current research; describes the nature and extent of the clinical problem of battering, the history of nursing involvement, and theoretical perspectives that have been used in examining the

535

TABLE 29.1. Summary of Nursing Research Prior to 1992 on Abused Women and Their Children

Author, Year	N	Description of Subjects	Research Design	Major Variables
Brendtro and Bowker, 1989	1,000	Self-reported abused women: 146 interviewed, 854 mailed questionnaires	Survey, descriptive	Helpfulness of informal help sources and health care providers
Bullock, McFarlane, Bateman, and Miller, 1989	793	Clients in Planned Parenthood clinic	Chart review, correlational	Prevalence of abuse
Bullock and McFarlane, 1989	589	300 private hospital postpartum patients, 289 public hospital patients, Anglo-American, Hispanic, African-American, Asian	Post-hoc correlational descriptive	Abuse, birth weight, smoking, alcohol use, prenatal care, prior abortions, maternal complications, hospital
Campbell, 1981, 1992	111	73 women killed, 28 men killed by female partner	Homicide record review	History of abuse, alcohol intoxication, circumstances of homicide
Campbell, 1986a	192	Women in shelter support groups	Qualitative thematic analysis	Male partner control, damaged self-esteem (body image), alternatives for ending violence, decision-making process, seeking and giving affirmation
Campbell, 1986b	79	Battered women from community	Interview, instrument development	Risk factors for homicide
Campbell, 1989a	193	97 battered women, 96 not-battered women, community sample	Interview, standardized instruments	Depression, self-esteem, physical symptoms of stress, attributions
Campbell, 1989b	79	Battered women from community	Interview, standardized instruments	Sexual abuse, severity and frequency of violence, self-esteem, body image
Campbell and Alford, 1989	115	Sexually abused battered women in shelters	Questionnaire	Types of sexual abuse, physical health problems
Campbell, Poland, Waller, and Ager, 1992	488	Postpartum women, African American, Anglo-American	Short answer, interview	Abuse during pregnancy, adequacy of prenatal care, social support, substance abuse
Drake, 1982	12	5 Anglo-American, 12 African-American self-identified abused women, shelter and nonshelter residents	Interview, ex post facto, exploratory	History of abuse, interactions with health care providers
Foster, Veale, and Fogel, 1989	12	Women imprisoned for killing abusive male partners	Interview, qualitative analysis	Demographics, description of abusive episodes, use of resources
Helton, McFarlane, and Anderson, 1987	292	Randomly selected pregnant women from public and private clinics, Latino, African American, Anglo-American	Interview, descriptive	Physical abuse, demographic data, medical history
Henderson, 1989	8	Women in a Canadian transition house	Series of interviews, qualitative analysis	Social support, stages of recovery process
Hoff, 1990	9,131	9 abused women, 131 members of women's network	Descriptive, qualitative	Values, social support
Humphreys, 1991	50	Children of battered women in shelter	Interviews, descriptive	Worries about their mothers
Kerouak, Taggert, Lescop, and Fortin, 1986	130	Canadian women in shelters and their children	Descriptive, comparative	Biological, psychological and social health status of women and children
Kurz, 1987	104	Battered women in emergency departments, emergency department staff	Observation of interactions between the woman and staff, descriptive	Attitudes of staff toward battered women

TABLE 29.1. *Continued*

Author, Year	N	Description of Subjects	Research Design	Major Variables
Landenburger, 1988, 1989	30	Abused women from shelter and respondents to advertisement	Interview, qualitative, descriptive	Index of Spouse Abuse, stages of entrapment and recovery
Lia-Hoagberg, Knoll, Swaney, Carlson, and Mullett, 1988	130	65 women with low birth weight infants, 65 women with normal birth weight infants, low income, African American, Native American, Anglo-American	Retrospective record review, descriptive, comparative	Birth weight, use of street drugs, physical and emotional abuse, childhood experiences of woman
Lichtenstein, 1981	28	Abused women responding to newspaper advertisement	Descriptive	Reasons for staying in or leaving relationship, experiences with medical and legal system
Mahon, 1981	11	Abused women from victim advocacy program	Descriptive, comparative to instrument norms	Psychological traits
Parker and Schumacher, 1977	50	Women at a legal aid bureau, 20 battered women, 30 not battered	Interviews, descriptive, correlational, comparative	Abuse, violence in family of origin, abuser's education, ability to terminate abusive relationship
Rose and Saunders, 1986	231	145 staff nurses, 86 physicians	Ex post facto mailed survey	Attitudes toward women, beliefs about abuse
Shipley and Sylvester, 1982	122	69 registered nurses, 51 physicians	Survey	Prior contact with victims of abuse, entry point into the health care system
Stuart, Laraia, Ballenger, and Lydiard, 1990	145	30 women with bulimia, 15 women with major depression, 100 women with no history of psychiatric illness	Descriptive, correlational, comparative	Family violence, victimization inventory, memory of childhood experiences
Tilden and Shepard, 1987	22	Staff nurses from an emergency department	Time series, chart review	Testing interview protocol
Torres, 1987, 1991	50	Abused women in shelters, 25 Hispanic Americans, 25 Anglo-Americans	Interview, descriptive, comparative	Severity of abuse, cultural differences, decision to leave the relationship
Trimpey, 1989	36	Battered women in support groups	Descriptive, comparisons with instrument norms	Anxiety (state and trait), self-esteem
Ulrich, 1991	51	Formerly battered women	Open-ended interviews, descriptive	Reasons for leaving an abusive relationship
Westra and Martin, 1981	20	Shelter residents 2.5 to 8 years, Anglo-American, Hispanic, African American, mixed ethnicity	Descriptive, comparisons with instrument norms	McCarthy Scale of children's attitudes, preschool behavior questionnaire, neurological examination, medical history, pregnancy history
Weingourt, 1990	53	Women in treatment for primary depression or anxiety	Semi-structured interview, descriptive comparative	Abuse (adult and child), sexual assault (adult and child)

issue both in nursing and other disciplines; and then proceeds with the actual review. The review is divided into the following sections: instrument development research, abuse during pregnancy, health (physical and mental) effects of battering, behavior of battered women, homicide and battering, model testing, intervention studies, and the children of battered women (health effects,

behavior, and interactions with their mothers). Each section includes a synthesis of the findings in that area as well as an overall methodological critique and specific study evaluation. The conclusion of the chapter provides an overall assessment of the state of the science, including the strengths and weaknesses of the nursing body of knowledge, depiction of gaps in that base, and identification of both types and specific studies needed in the future.

Summary of Review of Nursing Research, 1981-1991

Our first review concluded that nursing research had made a substantial contribution to the body of knowledge on battered women and their children in general, especially in the area of abuse during pregnancy. There was also a recognition that nursing's contribution had been primarily in the area of women and children's responses (physical, mental, and behavioral) to battering rather than causation (with the exception of the early exemplary identification of risk factors by Parker & Schumacher, 1977). In addition, the contribution of nursing was considered noteworthy because of its activist and/or feminist (woman-centered) assumptions and stance. To substantiate that conclusion, there was evidence of (a) close collaboration with shelters for abused women, (b) particular concern for the safety of women and their children, (c) a general concern for the empowerment of women as part of the research process as well as in the use of research results, (d) documentation of battered women's and their children's strengths as well as problems, and (e) an assumption that the locus of responsibility for battering was both the individual perpetrator and our societal structures and attitudes that facilitate or fail to sufficiently sanction or prevent the battering of female partners. There was also a beginning (but ahead of the field in general) inquiry into and sensitivity to cultural effects on women's responses to battering (e.g., Torres, 1987, 1991).

However, there were methodological shortcomings in terms of relatively small sample sizes and unsophisticated methodologies in some of the studies. There were very few studies testing nursing interventions or nursing (or other) theories. There was also a lack of studies systematically documenting the kinds of health problems battered women may demonstrate in comparison with other women and how and if battering compromises appropriate use of health care services. A scattering of studies in many different directions impeded the accumulation of nursing knowledge in specific areas. However, many of the study findings were corroborated by findings from other disciplines.

In summary, the findings in the first decade (primarily 1981-1991) of nursing research in the area of battered women and their children can be summarized as documenting a significant prevalence of abused women in a variety of health care settings (emergency, primary care, prenatal), with a range of physical and mental health care problems from the abuse (e.g., chronic pain, depression) and a general lack of identification by health care professionals (Campbell & Parker, 1992). Battered women's perception of less than adequate care given by professionals in health care settings was supported by attitude studies showing paternalistic and somewhat blaming attitudes of nurses, although these were less than those of physicians (King & Ryan, 1989; Rose & Saunders, 1986; Shipley & Sylvester, 1982). The earlier studies of abuse during pregnancy, importantly, established that there were significant proportions of women abused during pregnancy, a higher prevalence than many other complications of pregnancy such as toxemia (e.g., Helton, McFarlane, & Anderson, 1987). Few risk factors for abuse during pregnancy were found other than abuse prior to pregnancy, but depression, anxiety, and substance abuse were identified as correlates (Campbell, Poland, Waller, & Ager, 1992). Marital rape and homicide risk were two specific areas of multiple nursing investigations, documenting particular health problems (Campbell, 1986a, 1992; Campbell & Alford, 1989; Weingourt, 1990). Battered women, especially those sexually abused, were also documented by several nursing research efforts to have low self-esteem (e.g., Campbell, 1989a, 1989b; Mahon, 1981; Trimpey, 1989). There was also substantiation of significant strengths of battered women, indication of normal processes of grieving and recovering, leaving battering relationships as a process, and cultural and social support influences on responses to battering (e.g., Campbell, 1989; Hoff, 1990; Landenburger, 1989; Ulrich, 1991). Landenburger (1989) used grounded theory to develop a theory of entrapment and recovery from an abusive relationship that was later extended to the basis for clinical nursing intervention (yet to be tested) (Campbell, Ulrich, Campbell, Sheridan, & Landenburger, 1993; Landenburger, 1993).

The only experimental intervention study from the first review was a test of a training program for emergency room nurses that showed a significant increase in appropriate identification and documentation of battered women in the experimental group (Tilden & Shepard, 1987). This remains the only such experimental design study and is supported by other discipline intervention studies (e.g., McLeer & Anwar, 1989). The nursing research on the children of battered women was extremely limited at that juncture (as was true in other fields) but included documentation of these children having more health problems than other children (Kerouac, Taggart, Lescop, & Fortin, 1986; Westra & Martin, 1981).

Inclusion Criteria for Review

This review includes only published research; that is, publications based on systematic collection and analysis of qualitative and/or quantitative data. The studies were published from 1991 (if not included in the earlier review) through the end of 1996, plus a few studies that should have been included in the earlier review but not found until later. For the most part, this body of work has been published in journals, but a few original research book chapters and books reporting research have been included. A MEDLINE search was conducted for research in nursing journals. In addition, a hand search was conducted of the four major interdisciplinary research journals (*Journal of Family Violence, Journal of Interpersonal Violence, Violence and Victims,* and *Violence Against Women*) for articles by authors or coauthors identifying themselves as nurses or from a school of nursing.[1] Reference lists for nursing-authored articles in other journals and word of mouth was also used to identify additional studies. Finally, there was an oral solicitation at the 1995 Nursing Network on Violence Against Women International Conference, the major nursing conference on the issue. To facilitate the use of this review, an overview of the studies included is summarized in Table 29.2.

Overview of Battering as a Clinical Nursing Problem

Battering of female partners can be defined as repeated physical and/or sexual assault within a context of coercive control (Campbell & Humphreys, 1993). This definition allows for the inclusion of "dating" violence in adolescence and adulthood, as well as domestic violence between unmarried cohabitants, including same sex couples. It also includes the important sexual abuse that occurs for at least 40% to 45% of physically battered women (Campbell, 1989b) and acknowledges the emo-

tional abuse, threats, and coercive control in other areas of the woman's life (finances, social relationships, etc.) that are so important in understanding the dynamics of abusive relationships. At least 1.8 million women report abuse in this country, and most experts agree that the true figures are at least 3 to 4 million (Straus & Gelles, 1990).

It is clear from both nursing and other discipline research that battered women make up a significant proportion (from 8% to 25%) of women in any (illness- or wellness-focused) health care setting (Campbell & Parker, 1992) and use (mental and physical) health care services more than other women (Zung, Broadhead, & Roth, 1993). It is also clear that battering constitutes a significant risk for a variety of health care problems, including chronic pain, chronic irritable bowel syndrome, pelvic inflammatory disease, substance abuse, depression, post-traumatic stress disorder (PTSD), sexually transmitted diseases, and complications of pregnancy (low birth weight infants) (Hamberger, Saunders, & Hovey, 1993; Gielen, O'Campo, Faden, Kass, & Xue, 1994; Gleason, 1993; Parker, McFarlane, & Soeken, 1994). Thus the designation of battering as a significant health problem, first declared by former Surgeon General Everett Koop in 1985 (U.S. Department of Health and Human Services [USDHHS], 1991b), and reiterated in *Healthy People 2000: National Health Promotion and Disease Prevention Objectives* (USDHHS, 1991a), was supported as specifically a nursing concern by an American Academy of Nursing resolution in 1991. The children of battered women also have more health problems than other children and use managed health care services more often than controls (Kerouac et al., 1986; Zung et al., 1993). One of the most important aspects of battering as a clinical nursing problem is the potential for nursing to make significant primary and secondary prevention initiatives, as well as those on a tertiary level (Campbell & Humphreys, 1993). Because battering usually (although not always) increases in severity and frequency over time, identification and intervention with battered women, soon after the first abusive incident, will decrease the incidence and severity of subsequent health problems and possible homicide or suicide.

Nursing has been involved in efforts to enhance the health, safety, and well-being of battered women, supporting and supplementing the efforts of battered women advocates, since the beginning of the establishment of wife abuse shelters in the 1970s. A significant cadre of nurses was involved in the Surgeon General's Workshop on Family Violence in 1985, the first official recognition of the problems of wife (and elder) abuse as *health* prob-

TABLE 29.2.   Summary of Research on Abuse to Women, 1992-1996

Author, Year	N	Description of Subjects	Research Design	Major Variables
Attala, 1994	400	Clients in WIC program	Ex post facto, descriptive, correlational	Physical abuse, social and health histories
Attala, Hudson, and McSweeney, 1994	140	90 abused women in crisis center, 50 nursing students	Validation of instrument (PASPH and PASNP)	Partner Abuse Scales, history of abuse
Attala, Oetker, and McSweeney, 1995	243	Female nursing students	Descriptive, correlational study	Physical and nonphysical abuse, demographics, nursing students
Bokunewicz and Copel, 1992	18	Emergency nurses	One-group, pretest-posttest	Family violence curriculum, health care providers' views about abuse
Campbell, Pliska, Taylor, and Sheridan, 1994	123	74 battered women, 49 battered women's advocates	Survey	Perceptions of shelter advocates and battered women re: ED treatment
Campbell, Miller, Cardwell, and Belknap, 1994	114	Women having relationship problems	Longitudinal, interview, standardized instruments	Learned helplessness models, relationship status, predictors of continued abuse
Campbell, Oliver, and Bullock, 1993	51	51 battered women from community	Qualitative, in-depth interview	Women's perceptions of reasons for abuse during pregnancy, frequency
Campbell, Campbell, King, Parker, and Ryan, 1994	504	African-American women from public prenatal clinics, postpartum units, newspaper ads, posters	Factor structure analysis, instrument development	Ethnicity of abused women, validity of abuse instruments
Counts, Brown, and Campbell, 1992	14	Non-Western cultures	Primary ethnographic data	Western social science theories, wife beating, mutual violence
Henderson, 1990	8	Abused women in transition house	Qualitative, semi-structured interview	Abused women's decisions, perceptions of children's needs
Henderson, 1993	9	Mothers who had left abusive relationships	Phenomenological, interview	Abused women's decisions, perception of children's needs
Humphreys, 1995b	25	Battered women's shelter residents	Ethnographic interview, observations	Abused women's worries about their children, responses to these worries
Humphreys, 1991	50	Children living at battered women's shelters	Descriptive, qualitative, semistructured interview	Abuse, children's worries about their mothers
Humphreys, 1995a	50	Mothers at battered women's shelters	Semistructured interview guides	Abused mothers, patterns of dependent care, perceptions of hazards to children
Langford, 1996	30	Abused women	Interview, grounded theory	Ability to predict impending violence
Limandri and Tilden, 1996	241 + 9	Registered nurses	Survey and interview	Decision-making processes in assessing for abuse
McFarlane, Parker, and Soeken, 1995	1,203	414 African-American, 412 Hispanic, 377 White pregnant patients at prenatal clinics	Stratified, prospective cohort analysis	Frequency, severity, perpetrator of abuse, homicide risk factors
McFarlane, Parker, and Soeken, 1996a	1,203	414 African American, 412 Hispanic, 377 White pregnant patients at prenatal clinics	Prospective, stratified, cohort analysis	Abuse, pregnancy, low birth weight risk factors, ethnic differences
McFarlane, Parker, and Soeken, 1996b	1,203	African-American, Hispanic, Caucasian pregnant women	Prospective cohort analysis	Smoking, substance use, abuse, and overweight
Merritt-Gray and Weurst, 1995	13	Survivors of abuse in rural eastern Canada	Interview	Reclaiming self, breaking-free strategies to counteract abuse
Newman, 1993	7	Abused women in shelters, women attending shelter counseling sessions	Qualitative interview, observation	Abuse, giving up, helplessness, fear of unknown, shelter support, self-blame, social supports
Parker, McFarlane, Soeken, Torres, and Campbell, 1993	691	Pregnant women, 31% teenage	Prospective cohort analysis, interview, screening	Abuse, pregnancy, teenagers, assessment, nursing intervention

TABLE 29.2.   *Continued*

Author, Year	N	Description of Subjects	Research Design	Major Variables
Parker, McFarlane, Soeken, Torres, and Campbell, 1993	691	African-American, Hispanic, White pregnant teenage, adult women	Interview, instruments, descriptive, correlation	Abuse in pregnancy, age of victim
Parker, McFarlane, and Soeken, 1994	1,203	African-American, Hispanic, pregnant White urban females	Interview, record review, prospective analysis	Abuse, pregnancy, maternal complications, birth weight, age differences
Ratner, 1993	406	Married women living with partner	Survey, descriptive	Incidence of wife abuse, type of abuse, reported mental health status, alcohol dependence
Ratner, 1995	406	Married women reached by phone	Cross-sectional telephone survey	Wife abuse, state of marriage, injuries sustained, psychiatric morbidity, alcoholism, interactions with health care providers, level of education
Rodriguez, 1989	50	Battered women in urban domestic violence shelter	Descriptive survey	Abuse, demographics, perceived health needs, role of nurse
Sampselle, Petersen, Murtland, and Oakley, 1992	940	Pregnant women in private nurse midwifery or MD practice	Secondary analysis of survey data	Prevalence of abuse education
Tilden et al., 1994	1,588	Practicing clinicians in 6 disciplines	Survey	Clinicians' experience with and attitudes toward family violence, clinicians' recognition of abuse, intervention with victims
Varvaro, 1991	23	Battered women in resident community support group	Interview, descriptive, content analysis	Abused support group, grief process
Varvaro and Palmer, 1993	43	Abused women seeking care, reporting abuse in EDs	Instrument development, descriptive	Abused women, self-efficacy needs
Varvaro and Lasko, 1993	25	Women reporting abuse as cause of injuries in EDs	Interview	Types of injuries resulting from abuse, assessment questions, treatment and prevention of domestic violence

NOTE: ED = emergency department.

lems. The Nursing Network on Violence Against Women (NNVAW) was founded in 1986 and expanded by adding the word "International" in 1994 to reflect a growing international contingent. The stated aims of the organization are to end violence against women, empower battered women, and change the health care system to be more responsive to the needs of abused women and their children. The NNVAWI holds a national conference biannually, produces a newsletter, and maintains a mailing and expertise list available to persons looking for nursing expertise in the issue. The NNVAWI is concerned with both clinical and research issues related to violence against women; it has grown tremendously over the past 10 years in terms of membership, policy influence, and research sophistication. The NNVAWI has been a national force in supporting the Violence Against Women

Act, passed by Congress as part of the Crime Bill in 1994; as a consulting body to the Centers for Disease Control in its intentional injury control work; and in the drafting of the violence and abuse sections of *Healthy People 2000,* as well as in various nursing efforts to confront the problem.

Another influence on policy and clinical practice from nursing has been through the American Academy of Nursing (AAN) Expert Panel on Nursing (Campbell, Anderson, et al., 1993). The AAN's 1993 conference topic was violence, with a book of abstracts subsequently published (AAN, 1993) and selected overview papers from that conference also recently published (Glittenberg, Babich, & Campbell, 1995). The Canadian Nurses Association (1992) has been particularly active in the abuse arena, publishing the excellent *Clinical Guidelines for Nurses.* The Emergency Nursing Association, the Association of Women's Health, Obstetrical and Neonatal Nursing, and the American College of Nurse-Midwives (which has developed a curriculum; see Paluzzi & Slattery, 1996) have also taken significant action to address battering as a nursing problem.

In the research realm, the Nursing Research Consortium on Violence and Abuse (NRCVA) is a group of approximately 14 nurses actively engaged in research on violence against women. The consortium has been meeting since 1986 to assist members in the development of research proposals, conduct qualitative analysis of data, evaluate instruments, and share data and research ideas. The membership has changed over the years, with some members choosing to disaffiliate and with the addition of new members. Several studies have been conducted by groups within the consortium (McFarlane and Parker; Campbell, Campbell, King, Ryan, and Torres), and several research articles have been published. The consortium developed and distributed the Abuse Assessment Screen (AAS), a clinical screening instrument that has been used in numerous research studies. This has facilitated more consistent reporting and the ability to make comparisons between studies. In addition, the consortium developed a "safety protocol" for research on abuse of women (Parker, Ulrich, et al., 1990). This article, included as a protocol in applications to Institutional Review Boards (IRBs), has facilitated researchers in obtaining IRB approval from committees by suggesting a comprehensive approach to protecting the safety of abused women participating in research.

Theoretical Perspectives

The research addressing the battering of female partners has been interdisciplinary since its beginning. The first research was psychiatric case studies, closely followed by an epidemiological nursing study (Parker & Schumacher, 1977); several descriptive studies from social work, women's studies, and psychology; historical studies from feminist orientations; and the first national random survey from sociology. Anthropology, law, criminal justice, and nursing joined the earlier disciplines during the 1980s, with public health and medicine making significant contributions starting in the late 1980s.

Theoretical perspectives used for research can be divided into those addressing causation and those addressing women's responses. Sociology, criminal justice, anthropology, some psychological perspectives, and public health have primarily addressed causation. Two primary schools of thought have been sociological systems and stress, primarily represented by Straus and Gelles (1990), and feminist theoretical models emphasizing the role of patriarchal societal arrangements in the causation of woman abuse, first delineated with research support by Dobash and Dobash (1979). Both general models have included social learning theory as a partial explanation (although given various degrees of importance) for intergenerational transmission of violence. Ethnopsychological thought, emphasizing the role of the evolutionary advantage of male sexual proprietariness with violence used to enforce that prerogative when necessary, has been applied to woman abuse most systematically by Wilson and Daly (Wilson, Johnson, & Daly, 1995). Anthropologists have emphasized cultural and community influences, with theoretical schemas advanced most recently by Levinson (1989) and Counts, Brown, and Campbell (1992; 1999). Public health studies have been primarily atheoretical, endeavoring to identify risk factors for abuse as well as the risk that abuse presents for various health consequences.

The other groups of theories that have been used to explain women's responses to battering have been primarily psychological. The earliest theories used in this regard were psychoanalytic, but these have been generally discredited. Lenore Walker's cycle of violence and application of Seligman's learned helplessness theories dominated such research in the 1980s, but trauma response theory (Herman, 1992) has become more widely used in the 1990s. Campbell's (1989a) original cross-sectional study found multivariate analysis support for both a grief and a learned helplessness model of response to battering, but both her follow-up study of the same sample (Campbell, Miller, Cardwell, & Belknap, 1994) and Hoff's (1990) ethnographic study failed to support a learned helplessness application.

Nursing research has been primarily atheoretical also, although Campbell (1986a, 1989a; Campbell, Miller, et al., 1994) and Humphreys (1995a, 1995b) have continued to use Orem's (1995) Theory of Self-Care as a basis of their investigations into the health, concerns, and behavior of battered women and their children. Ulrich (1991) operates from Gilligan and colleagues' theory of self in relationships. Landenburger (1989) has developed a nursing theory of response from her grounded theory study. Most nursing investigations have proceeded from a feminist stance, as previously explicated. However, a feminist theory of battering is not ordinarily formally operationalized, primarily because of its more usual use in explaining causation. Counts, Brown, and Campbell (1992; 1999) found support for a modified version of feminist theories of causation of battering from primary anthropological data.

Although nursing research based on nursing theories is crucial in developing specific nursing knowledge related to battering, midrange nursing theory probably has the most promise for guiding testable nursing interventions, the most pressing need clinically. Except for Landenburger's (1989) work, the development of midrange nursing theory either by deduction or induction has yet to be undertaken in published work. This is a critical need for continued advancement of this area of research.

Synthesis and Evaluation of Clinical Nursing Research: Methodology

There are several important methodological issues that are similar to those in other areas of nursing research; some are unique to woman abuse. Methodological strengths of the body of nursing research include use of a variety of both qualitative and quantitative methods, inclusion of ethnic minorities in most samples and analysis for ethnic influences, and careful attention to measurement. There continues to be a need for more longitudinal research, but there have been three longitudinal nursing studies, two prospective studies during pregnancy (Curry, 1998; Parker, McFarlane, & Soeken, 1994), and one of not-pregnant battered women (Campbell et al., 1994). One of the methodological issues in longitudinal research is how to identify the current status of abuse with battered women and the ever-changing status of the relationship over time. A related challenge is balancing concern about study attrition with concerns about the woman's safety, an issue at least partly addressed by Rumptz, Sullivan, Davidson, and Basta's (1991) publication of strategies to minimize attrition with battered women.

Most of the nursing research efforts on abused women in the health care system are descriptive studies with small convenience samples. Exceptions include Tilden et al. (1994) and Ratner's (1993) work, which was population based, and the McFarlane and Parker program of research, which has used large clinical samples. All approaches are needed and, indeed, complement each other. Population-based studies are especially useful for determining risk factors and general sequelae of abuse, and, although they are more generalizable, they are still specific to the area (state, community) from which the sample was drawn. Clinical samples are more appropriate for in-depth examination of particular health problems and/or populations.

An additional methodological issue that is not unique to research on violence against women is reliance on secondary sources for basic "statement of the problem" information. Frequently, literature reviews of research publications contain statistical or numerical statements with multiple references, none of which are data-based publications. Unfortunately, there are several statements appearing frequently in our literature that repeat misleading conclusions made elsewhere by a faulty or incomplete interpretation of data. This does a disservice to our credibility as a scientific discipline. An example in the field of violence against women is the continued reference to the relationship between abuse during pregnancy and infant birth anomalies. This relationship has never been documented and yet is often repeated. Similarly, as there have been no longitudinal studies of women before and during pregnancy, we have not documented that "pregnancy causes an increase in violence [or is a risk factor for violence]," another frequently stated assumption. There has also been much misinterpretation of the extent of battered women in emergency departments (EDs) because of inappropriate generalizations, confusion and/or varying interpretations of incidence and prevalence terminology, and a variety of denominators being used in calculations.

Operationalization

One of the major methodological problems in research on violence against women is the issue of measurement. There are several research investigations in the area of measurement of abuse that will be reviewed in the context of an overall review of instrumentation on this body of knowledge.

In considering measurement issues, it is important to differentiate between *clinical* indicators or screening instruments that can readily identify a woman as abused and *research* or intensity instruments to measure violence severity, frequency, types, and sequela. The research instruments assume the person filling out the instrument is abused, and if used as a screen, may miss some abused women who are reluctant to define themselves as abused and are offended by the emphasis on the

Within the last year, have you ever been hit, slapped, kicked, or otherwise physically hurt by someone?   YES   NO

If YES, by whom (circle all that apply)

    Husband   Ex-husband   Boyfriend   Stranger   Other   Multiple

Total number of times _____

Since you've been pregnant, have you been hit, slapped, kicked, or otherwise physically hurt by someone?   YES   NO

If YES, by whom (circle all that apply)

    Husband   Ex-husband   Boyfriend   Stranger   Other   Multiple

Total number of times _____

Mark the area of injury on body map:

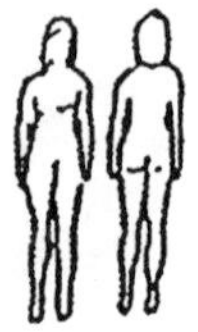

Score each incident according to the following scale: SCORE
1 = Threats of abuse including use of a weapon   _____
2 = Slapping, pushing, no injuries and/or lasting pain   _____
3 = Punching, kicking, bruises, cuts and/or continuing pain   _____
4 = Beating up, severe contusions, burns, broken bones   _____
5 = Head injury, internal injury, permanent injury   _____
6 = Use of weapon, wound from weapon   _____
(If any of the descriptions for the highest number apply, use the higher number.)

Within the last year, has anyone forced you to have sexual activities?   YES   NO

If YES, by whom (circle all that apply)

    Husband   Ex-husband   Boyfriend   Stranger   Other   Multiple

Total number of times _____

Figure 29.1. Abuse Assessment Screen

very negative descriptions of their relationship. Therefore, for most clinical studies, it is preferable to initially identify a woman as abused or not using a simple clinical screen, such as the Abuse Assessment Screen (AAS) (Figure 29.1). This facilitates rapid assessment as well as consistent definitions. Research instruments could then be used to document the level of frequency, severity, and type of abuse (i.e., physical, sexual, emotional, financial). Because of the importance of this issue, we review the instruments being used most often, beginning with the clinical instrument, followed by a description of research instruments.

The Abuse Assessment Screen (see Figure 29.1), was developed by the NRCVA, based on work first published by Helton (1986) and Helton, McFarlane, and Anderson (1987). This five-question screen has been used extensively as a clinical screening tool as well as a measure to identify abused women in comparative studies. The AAS includes one question for pregnant women and can easily be adapted for nonpregnant women by eliminating this question. The AAS has been published in several articles (McFarlane & Parker, 1994; Parker, McFarlane,

& Soeken, 1994), with notations that readers are encouraged to copy and use the instrument. Figure 29.2 is the Mexican-American Spanish translation of the instrument, which has been validated through back-translation processes. The psychometric properties of the AAS have recently been published, facilitating further use as a screening instrument for research (Soeken, McFarlane, Parker, & Lominak, 1996). In that assessment of the AAS, an ethnically stratified sample of 280 pregnant women who reported abuse on the AAS were compared with a random sample of 280 women not reporting abuse. Test-retest reliability with two subsamples of 48 and 40 women in this study was .83 and .975, respectively. Discriminant group validity was established by comparing the scores of the two groups of women on the Index of Spouse Abuse (ISA), the violence subscales of the Conflict Tactics Scale (CTS), and the Danger Assessment (DA). Significant differences ($p < .01$) were found between the two groups on all measures, indicating that the AAS was able to differentiate between abused and not-abused women. Construct validity was supported by significant and moderately strong correlations with all three

(Circule SI o NO por cada question)

Durante el año pasado, ha sido golpeada, bofeteada, pateada, o dañada   SI   NO
físicamente por alguien?

   Esposo   Ex-esposo   Amigo   Estraño   Otro

Número de veces _____

Desde el embarazo, ha sido golpeada, bofeteada, pateada, or dañada físicamente por alguien?   SI   NO

Si la respuesta es SI, por quien. (Circule todos los que se apliquen)

   Esposo   Ex-esposo   Amigo   Estraño   Otro

Número de veces _____

Marque las areas de daño en el mapa del cuerpo:

En el diagrama anatómico, marque/marca las partes de su (tu) cuerpo que han sido lastimadas   SCORE 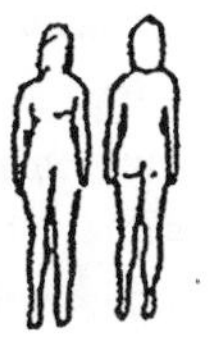
1 = amenazas de maltrato (abuso) que incluyen el uso de un arma
2 = golpes, empujones sin lesiones fçsicas o dolor permanente
3 = moquestes (puñetazos), patadas, moretones, haridas, y/o dolor continuo
4 = molida a palos, contusiones severas, quemaduras, fractures de huesos
5 = lesiones (heridas) en la cabeza, lesiones internas, lesiones permanentes
6 = uso de armas, herida por arma

Durante el año pasado, ha sido forzada a tener actividades sexsuales?   SI   NO

Si la respuesta es SI, por quien. (Circule todos los que se apliquen)

   Esposo   Ex-esposo   Amigo   Estraño   Otro

Número de veces _____

Figure 29.2. Abuse Assessment Screen: Spanish-Language Version

research instruments (McFarlane, Parker, Soeken, & Bullock, 1992).

A measurement issue in the use of this instrument is inconsistency in its use. Some researchers only use one or two questions from the AAS; others use the entire instrument. Additional inconsistencies include the use of the AAS as part of a self-report medical history filled out by patients, rather than a face-to-face interview. This discrepancy has resulted in a wide range of reported incidences of abuse. This reporting difference based on how the AAS was administered was studied by McFarlane, Christoffel, Bateman, Miller, and Bullock (1991), who found that 8% of women self-reported abuse on a standard medical intake form, but when asked the same questions by a health care provider, 29% of a comparable group of women reported abuse.

Instrument Development and Validation Research

Early research on domestic violence relied heavily on the Conflict Tactics Scale (CTS; Straus & Gelles,

1990). This instrument measures the frequency and severity of tactics used in disagreements. There is considerable support for validity of the instrument, and it has been used widely, which allows comparability amongst studies. Concerns with this instrument were that it omitted the extent of injury, self-defense, sexual assault, and emotional degradation. In addition, the CTS did not take into account that most men have greater strength than most women, self-defense (who first used violence and/or escalated the violence), and men's tendency to underestimate the extent of their violence. Therefore, the scale has been challenged in terms of reliability and validity for measuring the full nature of intimate battering. However, the scale has advantages as a telephone survey because it places violence in a normative context.

The Index of Spouse Abuse (Hudson & McIntosh, 1981) is a 30-item summated self-report scale to measure the magnitude of physical (ISA-P) and nonphysical (ISA-NP) abuse. The internal consistency reliability (coefficient alpha) for the instrument as a whole has been measured at .95. For the subscales, the reliability was .89 for the ISA-P and .93 for the ISA-NP (McFarlane, Parker,

& Soeken, 1995). In 1990, the instrument's developer replaced the instrument with the Partner Abuse Scale Physical (PASH) and Non-physical (PASNP). Currently, both instruments are in use.

Recently, Campbell, Campbell, King, Parker, and Ryan (1994) reported an important nursing study determining the reliability and factor structure of the ISA with a sample of 504 African-American women. Campbell found 3 factors with the African-American sample, compared with the original 2 reported by Hudson and McIntosh. The new factor identified with this sample reflected behaviors of an extremely controlling and iso7lating nature. Campbell interprets this phenomena by using the work of Oliver (1989), which indicates that "when black males engage in violence against black females, it is because they have defined the situation as one in which the female's actions constitute a threat to their manhood" (p. 265). This study further documented the importance of conducting and reporting separate instrument reliability and validity assessments for different ethnic groups and paying attention to ethnic group representation and analysis in both developing and choosing a measurement instrument.

Attala, Hudson, and McSweeney (1994) also conducted a nursing research validation study of the new version of the ISA, called the Partner Abuse Scale (PAS), with separate Physical (PASPH) and Nonphysical (PASNP) subscales. A sample of 90 known abused women in a wife abuse shelter were compared with 50 associate degree-level nursing students. Discriminant group validity was supported. Interestingly, although meeting the criteria for shelter admission, 27% of the shelter women did not identify themselves as physically abused. Using the cut scores suggested by Attala, 60% of those women met the criteria for physical abuse. This suggests that either the women underestimated their abuse (the author's interpretation) or the suggested cut score is too low, although the percentage of false negative classifications rises to 13.5% and above at higher cutoff scores. Internal consistency of both versions of the instrument were high (> .94) in both samples. Convergent construct validity was minimally supported by significant moderately strong positive correlations with two other infrequently used instruments measuring stress and general contentment but no other instruments measuring abuse. More than 80% of both the sheltered and control women (98%) were Anglo-American, precluding conclusive reliability or validity for women of color. There were other significant demographic differences (education, income, and number of children) between the two

groups, weakening confidence placed on the discriminate group validity findings.

The Severity of Violence Against Women (SVAW) is a recently developed 46-item instrument that measures the frequency of partner symbolic violence; threats of mild, moderate, and serious violence; and actual mild, moderate, serious, and sexual violence (Marshall, 1992). Some nursing researchers are finding this instrument to be a useful measure to define specific types of violence.

Continuing work on the development of the Danger Assessment (DA) instrument to determine homicide risk for battered women was reported by Campbell (1995). Although several small- and intermediate-size studies indicate preliminary support for reliability and construct validity, factor-analytic, predictive, or criterion-related validity studies have yet to be conducted. The author concluded that the instrument has adequate support for research and for use as a clinical intervention whereby the woman determines her own degree of risk based on the instrument. Expert prediction of the degree of risk based on this instrument score is as yet premature. The author also maintains that it is critical to include the calendar portion of this instrument to facilitate the woman's remembrance and counteract the normal minimization that many battered women employ.

Three nursing research instruments that are in the beginning stages of development are Varvaro's (Varvaro & Lasko, 1993) Self-Efficacy in Battered Women, Sheridan's (Campbell, McKenna, Torres, Sheridan, & Landenburger, 1993) HARRASS instrument, and Taylor's (1994) Woman Abuse instrument. All have initial support for reliability and validity, are undergoing further development, and may be appropriate for future investigations.

Synthesis and Evaluation of Clinical Nursing Research: Clinical Findings

Clinical areas of significant nursing research include investigations of women's physical, emotional, and behavioral responses to battering; some foundational work for intervention testing; and studies of the children of battered women. However, the area where nursing research has made the most significant clinical contribution is abuse during pregnancy.

▰ *Abuse During Pregnancy*

A program of research on battering during pregnancy was initiated by Anne Helton in conjunction with Elizabeth Anderson, Judith McFarlane, and Linda Bullock in the 1980s, as described in the earlier review section (Campbell & Parker, 1992). This endeavor has continued, with several initiatives by Judith McFarlane and Barbara Parker establishing the importance and legitimacy of nursing research and clinical interventions in the area of abuse to pregnant women. Thanks in great part to that ongoing research, the March of Dimes, the Centers for Disease Control (CDC), and the American College of Obstetrics and Gynecology (ACOG) have all identified battering during pregnancy as a serious health care problem. The CDC funded two major studies on abuse during pregnancy by Drs. McFarlane and Parker. In addition, the National Institute for Nursing Research funded a retrospective case control study on battering during pregnancy and birth weight in five different ethnic groups (Campbell, Torres, et al., in press). These studies built on prior work and contain both supplementary and replication components to develop a significant body of nursing knowledge in this area.

The first McFarlane and Parker study of 1,203 African American, Hispanic, and Caucasian pregnant women established a rate of abuse during pregnancy of 16%. The incidence of abuse during pregnancy found was similar to Curry (1998), who found a rate of 17%. McFarlane, Parker, and associates (McFarlane, Parker, & Soeken, 1996a; Parker, McFarlane, & Soeken, 1994) found that an additional 25% of women were beaten during the year prior to the pregnancy, making them highly at risk for further abuse after pregnancy (demonstrated by Gielen, O'Campo, et al., 1994) as well as subject to the atmosphere of threat and coercive control that accompanies physical violence (McFarlane, Parker, & Soeken, 1995; Parker & McFarlane, 1995, 1996). The Parker and McFarlane studies were also important in documenting an even greater proportion of pregnant adolescents being abused than adult women by boyfriends and, to a lesser extent, by other family members, a finding especially relevant for practitioners working with this group of young women (McFarlane, Parker, & Soeken, 1996a).

Both Curry (1998) and Parker et al. (Parker, McFarlane, & Soeken, 1994; McFarlane, Parker, & Soeken, 1996a) demonstrated a relationship between abuse and subsequent low birth weight (LBW) of the infant (a finding first reported in nursing research by Bullock & McFarlane, 1989). McFarlane and Parker found that, for the aggregate sample, abuse during pregnancy was a significant ($p < .05$) risk for LBW as well as low maternal weight gain, infections, anemia, smoking, and use of alcohol or drugs (Parker, McFarlane, & Soeken, 1994). Curry (1998) also found the rate of LBW infants born to abused women was significantly greater than those of not-abused women (8.2% versus 4.4%) in her sample of 403 urban low-income women. Although this connection has not been found in other research (e.g., Gielen, O'Campo, et al., 1994), the studies not detecting the relationship have found a lower prevalence of abuse and may therefore be less valid.

The Parker and McFarlane (McFarlane, Parker, & Soeken, 1996a; Parker, McFarlane, & Soeken, 1994; Parker, McFarlane, Soeken, Torres, & Campbell, 1993) study also documented a significant relationship between experiencing abuse and entering prenatal care in the third trimester (perhaps partially explaining the LBW finding). In contrast, Attala, Hudson, et al.'s (1994) study of WIC women (fully described later) did not support the hypothesis that abused pregnant women start their prenatal care later than those not abused or the hypothesis that abused women would have suffered more pregnancy "losses" (miscarriages, abortions, stillbirths, and neonatal deaths). Yet, because that research report did not clarify whether the interpersonal violence and pregnancy involved were contiguous, it is difficult to evaluate the validity of those findings.

The relationship between the use of substances (alcohol, street drugs, tobacco) during pregnancy and abuse has been well documented. Campbell, Poland, et al. (1992) found that violence during pregnancy was positively related to drug and alcohol abuse during pregnancy ($r = -.27, p < .01$) in a postpartum sample of 900 primarily poor African-American women in an urban area. Similarly, McFarlane, Parker, and Soeken (1996b) found that significantly more abused African-American and Caucasian pregnant women smoked and used alcohol or illicit drugs during pregnancy than not-abused women. As a triad, physical abuse, smoking, and alcohol or illicit drug use were significantly related to birth weight ($F = 30.19, p < .001$).

Using a combination of data from several studies, Campbell, Soeken, McFarlane, and Parker (1998) demonstrated an association of abuse during pregnancy and risk of homicide using the Danger Assessment instrument. Although the different sampling techniques used in the studies threaten the validity of the conclusions, this analysis, taken in conjunction with two different population-based studies showing homicide to be the current leading cause of maternal morbidity (maternal death during labor, delivery, or the immediate postpartum period) in New York City and Chicago, underscore the need to consider risk of homicide in pregnant abused women (Dannenberg et al., 1995; Fildes, Reed, Jones, Martin, & Barrett, 1992).

Campbell, Oliver, and Bullock (1993) conducted a latent content analysis of qualitative data from 51 battered women who had been pregnant by their abuser. Approximately one half were not abused during pregnancy (although they were abused prior to pregnancy and/or later in the relationship). The women abused during pregnancy were more severely and frequently abused and had incurred more severe injury than those who were not abused during pregnancy, but they did not differ on demographic characteristics. For those abused during pregnancy, the women's perceptions of the motivation of the abuser were grouped into four categories: (a) jealousy of infant (the woman's attention to the unborn child) (18.5%); (b) apparent anger at the infant, most often because the abuser thought the baby was another man's (15%); (c) pregnancy related but not anger against the infant (e.g., the woman was sick and not as attentive to him or was uninterested in sex) (15%); and (d) pregnancy did not seem to have anything to do with his motivation ("business as usual") (46%). Although limited by a small sample and the bias of the woman's interpretation of her partner's motives, the study gives some indication of why prior population-based studies (Gelles, 1988) demonstrated that controlling for age eliminated the apparent increased incidence of abuse during pregnancy. The Campbell, Oliver, et al. (1993) study suggests that differing patterns of abuse may present more risk during pregnancy for some women; for others, pregnancy is a protective period. The study also has important clinical implications in terms of increased risk for serious abuse when women are abused during pregnancy and probable additional increased risk for child abuse for women abused during pregnancy when the motivation is anger at or jealousy of the unborn child.

In a small focus group study (two focus groups of 12 women each) of battered women in shelters, preliminary evidence of the relationship between relationship abuse and unintended pregnancy was documented (Campbell, Pugh, Campbell, & Visscher, 1995). Women described five major themes related to this issue: (a) male partner control of contraception and pregnancy decisions, with women often becoming pregnant to try to appease violent men; (b) relentless and unpredictable abuse; (c) lack of consistency in the partner's relationship with the woman

and with offspring; (d) abusive partner investment in a strict traditional gender role definition of manhood that cut across the seven different ethnic groups represented, including not being responsible for day-to-day child care and not using condoms; and (e) considerable maternal and infant morbidity as a result of the abuse. Although severely limited by the small and nonrepresentative sample, the study suggested several theoretical links between unintended pregnancy and abuse deserving further investigation. It also provided support for the findings of another qualitative study (Campbell, Oliver, et al., 1993) that severe abuse during pregnancy can be motivated by the husband's (unfounded) suspicion that the baby does not belong to him and support for nursing and non-nursing recent findings that battered women are at risk for STDs because of their abuser's common refusal to use condoms (Eby, Campbell, Sullivan, & Davidson, 1995; Gielen, O'Campo, et al., 1994).

A different approach to the study of abuse in pregnancy was undertaken by Sampselle, Petersen, Murtland, and Oakley (1992), who used survey data to compare the amounts of reported abuse between women who choose to obtain prenatal care from a certified nurse midwife or a physician. They found a much lower rate of reported abuse than any other study, which they attributed to the method of data collection (2 questions on a written questionnaire given on the first visit). Additionally, the questions asked about experiences of abuse rather than specific violent incidents. As noted previously, these issues have resulted in apparent inconsistencies in reporting. However, Sampselle et al. were able to determine that a woman who selected a nurse midwife for care had a higher reported rate of past abuse. Additionally, as this was a relatively affluent population, the study provides further evidence that abuse is not restricted to women in lower socioeconomic classes.

Women's Responses to Battering

As in the prior published review (Campbell & Parker, 1992), the literature on women's responses to battering is divided into physical (health), psychological, and behavioral responses to being abused in an intimate relationship.

Physical Health Effects of Abuse

Nursing research has continued to document the mental and physical health effects from abuse but, unfortunately, has primarily done so with small descriptive studies using convenience samples; medical research has begun to conduct predictive correlational investigations using comparison groups and large samples (e.g., McCauley et al., 1995). An exception from this trend is Ratner's (1993, 1995) random-digit telephone survey of 406 married (including common law) adult female residents of Alberta, Canada. Using the CTS as a screen, she found a 10.6% incidence rate (similar to U.S. and other Canadian region rates), with abuse associated with women being younger, separated or divorced, low combined partner income, and male partner unemployment, similar to U.S. national statistics (Bachman & Saltzman, 1995). Abused women were significantly more likely than those not abused to have visited an emergency department; to have been hospitalized; and to have been in contact with public health nurses, psychiatrists, and psychologists in the prior year. Frequency of headaches and backaches was also associated with abuse, suggesting the possibility of head and back injuries. This was a well-designed study using established instruments, random sampling, and with an excellent (at 78.7%, higher than most telephone surveys) response rate. It was only limited by the use of the original CTS, which, although an excellent screening instrument because of its normative context, fails to measure sexual or emotional abuse, severity of injury, or differentiate tactics used in self-defense. Some of the more recent modifications of the CTS improve on one or all of these aspects but are less validated.

In emergency department settings, both Varvaro and Lasko (1993) and Campbell, Pliska, et al. (1994) corroborated other findings that the majority of injuries to known battered women seeking care in the ED are to the face, head, back, and neck; that contusions and soft tissue injuries are the most common types of injury; that many women were not referred to any services for the abuse; and that more than half had a negative ED experience. Also useful for clinical identification of battered women was that the second highest proportion of injuries were to multiple body locations (Varvaro & Lasko, 1993). Campbell, Pliska, et al. (1994) found that the majority of their sample of shelter women seen in the ED had been seen multiple times. They also found that 28.6% of the women of color believed that racism had affected their treatment in the ED; almost half felt that their insurance status (Medicaid) negatively affected their treatment. Both samples had approximately equal proportions of White women and women of color (primarily African American) and had a relatively low average income. Both studies were limited by their small sample size, sampling technique, and descriptive analysis. The findings of these

studies, that battered women present in emergency settings with a wide variety of physical and mental health problems and demographic characteristics, support the need to instigate universal screening of women for battering in health care settings.

In an ex post facto, descriptive, correlational study (Attala, Hudson, et al., 1994) tested hypotheses about abuse and health problems in a sample of 400 women (75% Anglo-American; 18% African American; 30% pregnant) from a midwestern WIC clinic. All women were approached consecutively over a 2-month period, and less than 1% refused participation. Thirty-one percent had experienced some physical abuse, primarily from husbands or boyfriends (11% of those abused named their mother as the perpetrator). The higher the score on the abuse scale, the more substances women used during pregnancy and during the prior month whether pregnant or not, the more health problems were present, and the fewer the social contacts with friends or family during the prior month. Self-perceived abuse and medical conditions were the strongest predictors of seriousness of abuse, explaining 30% of the variance. The study could have been strengthened by separating out the effects of partner and nonpartner violence; however, the results are still important in further corroborating the link between abuse and health problems in general and substance abuse specifically and the need for abuse assessments in a variety of health-related settings. The substance abuse and partner violence link has now not only been demonstrated in nursing research of pregnant and nonpregnant abused women but also independently in investigations of drug-abusing women (Boyd & Mast, 1983).

Rodriguez (1989) employed a descriptive design to document health problems of battered women. The majority of her sample of 50 shelter residents was Mexican American, making this the first study to examine health problems from abuse in nonpregnant Hispanic women. Also important from this study was the women's perception of a link between hypertension, menstrual problems, chronic back pain, and hysterectomies with battering, a relationship also found in other studies (e.g., Goldberg & Tomlanovich, 1985; Ratner, 1993). The majority of the women in Rodriguez' sample had never been to the emergency room for injuries, a finding supported in other research and indicative of the need for assessment for abuse in primary care and other settings.

Also employing a shelter sample, Eby et al. (1995) interviewed 110 women (half Anglo-American, 42% African American, 5.5% Latina, and 4% Native American) about their experiences, specifically with partner sexual abuse (using a 3-item scale) as well as physical violence and resultant physical health problems. Approximately 27% of the sample reported at least one type of sexual abuse, and 63% had experienced physical violence in the prior 6 months. Thus, approximately 43% of these physically abused women were also experiencing sexual abuse, a percentage congruent with previous nursing (and other discipline) research on marital rape (e.g., Campbell, 1989b; Campbell & Alford, 1989; Weingourt, 1985). Ninety-nine percent of the women reported at least one problematic physical health symptom during the past 6 months, the most common of which were feeling low in energy, sleep problems, and headaches. More than half of the women felt that most of their symptoms (especially sleeping problems, pains in heart or chest, heart pounding, and headaches) were a result of the abuse. Pelvic pain was the most frequently experienced gynecological symptom, with pain of intercourse most often attributed to abuse. There were moderate to high (.50 to .58) correlations between frequency and severity of physical and sexual abuse and physical symptoms, with those sexually as well as physically abused having significantly more symptoms than those "only" physically abused. The study also demonstrated the risk of battered women for STDs and exposure to HIV/AIDS, as has other-discipline research (Gielen, Faden, O'Campo, Kass, & Anderson, 1994). However, this study was remarkable in its demonstration of the link to this exposure through sexual assault as well as batterers' frequent refusals to wear condoms (also supported by Campbell, Pugh, et al., 1995). In fact, when men insist on unprotected sex against the woman's wishes, this can be considered an aspect of sexual abuse.

Psychological Responses

In a mental-health-related report of her population-based study of Canadian women, Ratner (1993) found that the abused women were significantly more depressed, had more physical symptoms of stress, had more anxiety and insomnia, and exhibited more social dysfunction than those not abused, with physical violence having a stronger effect than psychological abuse in all aspects. Physically abused women were eight times more likely to be alcohol dependent. Although most of these findings have been documented elsewhere, they have seldom been from population-based samples, and the insomnia finding has not been reported previously. This finding has important clinical nursing implications and

supports the importance of trauma theory and PTSD inquiries.

Also supporting the above and other nursing research findings of depression in battered women (e.g., Attala, Oetker, & McSweeney, 1995; Campbell, 1989a; Campbell, Pliska, et al., 1994; Campbell, Poland, et al., 1992), Campbell, Kub, Belknap, and Templin (1997) found 39% of a volunteer community sample of 164 battered women in the moderate to severe or severe depression categories on the Beck Depression Inventory, categories that would qualify for a psychiatric diagnosis of severe depression. Daily hassles (everyday stressors), self-care agency, childhood physical violence, and relationship physical violence (measured with the ISA), were significant predictors (in descending order of magnitude) of depression by multiple regression analysis, explaining a total of 44% of the variance. Interestingly, relationship nonphysical (emotional and sexual) abuse, childhood or adolescent sexual abuse (familial or nonfamilial), tangible resources (education, occupation, income) and ethnicity were *not* significant predictors of depression. The study was limited by nonpopulation-based, noncomparison-group sampling and a failure to measure PTSD, a variable with increasing importance, especially as a potential source of the widely documented depression of battered women.

Behavioral Responses

Nursing researchers have continued to examine the behavior of battered women, understanding that leaving the abusive relationship is a process involving many attempts and greatly influenced by (a) the batterer's behavior; (b) the safety and support available to her from the community in the form of shelter resources, the criminal justice system, and the health care system; (c) the degree of support from her family and friends; (d) financial support job opportunities and/or a humane temporary assistance program; and (e) individual personality characteristics or resources (Campbell & Humphreys, 1993; Landenburger, 1993). In that regard, Sheridan (Campbell, Ulrich, et al., 1993) has developed an instrument to measure harassment by the batterer after the woman has left him, an experience that the majority of battered women report and one that includes acts designed to obstruct her from keeping or getting a job and/or keep her from getting custody of the children, as well as physical and emotional abuse.

Campbell, Miller, et al. (1994), in a longitudinal study of abused women, found that the majority of the 51 battered women who returned for a follow-up interview were able to leave the abusive relationship or manage to make the violence end, with most of the data supporting a relatively healthy process of responding to abuse. The study also demonstrated that women often (23% of non-battered women) go from a nonabusive (troubled) relationship to a violent relationship (either by the same partner or a new partner), a different trajectory than is often assumed. Using discriminant function analysis, there were no predictive factors identified for continuing relationship violence for either the battered or nonbattered (but having serious relationship problems) comparison group ($N = 65$) in terms of the woman's personal characteristics (ethnicity, education, family income, childhood physical or sexual abuse, prior abusive relationship, self-care agency, self-esteem, depression, physical symptoms) or the frequency and severity of relationship violence (measured by the CTS). These findings were not supportive of a learned helplessness theory of response to battering. Community characteristics were not measured. The study was also limited by a high attrition rate (38%), in part related to the difficulties in following battered women over time while protecting their safety.

In a related qualitative study, using content analysis combined with a quantitative measure, Ulrich (1991) documented six "releases" that a sample of 50 women perceived as helping them the most in leaving an abusive relationship. An unusual finding in this study was Ulrich's careful delineation of which particular social support was especially important for each release (allowing easy deduction of clinical implications). The releases were (a) a lack of choice when the abuser let go; (b) the woman's interpretation that the relationship was over, in which condition family affirmation was most important; (c) personal dreams, a condition for which friends caring was crucial; (d) personal faith, when shelter or support group understanding was the most salient; (e) fear; and (f) personal growth, for which other professional support was most important. Ulrich also found that women who attributed leaving to their own efforts scored higher on a measure of self-esteem than did women who found external events, persons, or agencies most important in being able to leave. Unfortunately, Ulrich's (1991) report did not give full details of the research design, making evaluation of the study difficult.

Langford (1996) used grounded theory to describe how battered women develop sophisticated knowledge and response patterns to their partner's abuse. The women were able to identify specific changes in their partner's eyes, speech, and tone of voice, as well as other specific signs of impending violence. The women responded to these signs with a variety of strategies to avoid the violence temporarily, if not permanently. Langford concluded that policies and nursing care need to acknowledge the women's sophisticated knowledge of their partners, powers of observation, creativity within severely limited options, and their ability to control their emotional and behavioral reactions. An important component of all of these studies describing battered women's responses to abuse are the continued assessment and description of the women's strengths and abilities, a perspective not always pursued in research from other disciplines.

Merritt-Gray and Wuest (1995) presented a much more complete description of their well-designed feminist grounded theory study of women's process of leaving the relationship. The approach used the analysis of two separate interviews (for validation and theoretical sampling) of 13 Canadian women and then the analysis of interviews of seven more women to further develop the theory. The investigators have thus far reported on only the first stage of the process they identified: counteracting abuse. This conceptualization is different from other qualitative studies of woman abuse (e.g., Landenburger, 1989) in that women's resistance to abuse from the beginning of the violence is stressed. However, many of the other findings are similar; for instance, a substage of relinquishing parts of the self similar to Landenburger's descriptions of loss of self. With the convergence of these qualitative nursing studies, clinical nursing interventions with battered women should begin to recognize that there are identifiable stages of the abusive relationship and its dissolution and that in-depth interventions should be stage specific.

Children of Abused Women

The majority of abused women are also mothers. Several nursing studies have examined the special concerns of battered women as mothers and those of their children. These have included studies assessing the influence on the children of witnessing violence and studies documenting the special concerns of abused women regarding their children. It is particularly appropriate that nursing examine and appreciate the importance of these issues for battered women in their decisions about how to deal with the abuse and how to address health issues.

Humphreys (1991) interviewed 50 children, 10 to 17 years old, at five shelters in Michigan. Humphreys described two types of concerns: potential hazards and actual health hazards. Potential hazards included their fears when the mother was late in returning from work or when they knew their father was "mad." Actual hazards were identified by more than half of the sample regarding the abuse, such as actually witnessing the violent event. Additional actual concerns included fears regarding pregnancy complications for their mothers or other illnesses.

In a similar vein, Henderson (1993) noted a sense of sadness and powerlessness permeating the lives of a small sample of children of abused women. She also found that they accepted violence as a means of conflict resolution and were apparently unaware of alternative methods of handling anger.

Mothers who experience violence, like all mothers, intervene to protect their children from the hazards of life. For abused women, however, these hazards also include potential violence from the abusive partner. The children of abused women can be injured inadvertently or in attempts to protect their mother. Several nurses have undertaken research documenting the unique concerns that abused mothers have for their children. The most consistent finding in these studies is that the mothers' worries about their children significantly influence their behaviors and decisions, including decisions to leave the abusive relationship (Henderson, 1990, 1993; Humphreys, 1995b; Torres, 1991; Ulrich, 1991, 1994).

Humphreys (1995a) interviewed 50 abused mothers in shelters to identify patterns of dependent care. Humphreys identified three major patterns of dependent care: prevention, protection, and removal. Preventive dependent care activities included buying nutritious foods and not allowing drugs in the home. Protection care was reported by 72% of the women and included behaviors such as placating the abuser, establishing good habits and routines for their children, and physically protecting their children from abuse by their partner. Removal activities were primarily composed of physically seeking sanctuary elsewhere.

Henderson (1990, 1993) conducted two qualitative studies on abused women in Canadian shelters. She found that concerns about the children were a major factor in decision making and that options open to childless women were unavailable to women with children, as there was a need for continued contact with the children's fathers (1990). The mothers noted that their children had enormous unmet needs that they felt inadequately prepared to meet. The mothers also noted that dealing with their children was the most difficult aspect of the time following separation from the abuser (1993). Similarly, Humphreys (1995b) found that abused women's worries

about their children were keeping the children safe and creating order out of disorder.

Recently, Eriksen and Henderson (1998) compared the responses of abused women in shelters to their children's responses. They found major discrepancies between what the women believed their children had observed and what the children themselves reported. Most women were unaware of the extent of their children's knowledge about the violence.

The studies of children of abused mothers have been conducted using primarily qualitative methodology, providing a rich source of in-depth information about the experience, perceptions, and context of abuse. Future nursing research in this area can build on this beginning development of issues with further qualitative and quantitative studies, especially those using comparison groups of children from nonabusive homes. Additional needed studies will include longitudinal designs to study the long-term implications of abusive environments and the children's trajectory of healing and recovery.

Nursing Helpfulness, Attitudes, and Training

Using a written questionnaire, Hamilton and Coates (1993) examined the perceived helpfulness and use of professional services by a volunteer clinical sample of 270 Canadian abused women, primarily employed, single parents. Social workers were the professionals from whom help was sought the most often for all three types of relationship abuse, with physicians second (emotional abuse) or third (after police for physical and sexual abuse) and nurses in the bottom third of the list of 13 professionals. Nurses were contacted by 27% of the women for emotional abuse (with a perceived 59% helpfulness rating), 15% of women for physical abuse (67% helpfulness), and 11% of women for sexual abuse (45% helpfulness). The helpfulness ratings of nurses were similar to those of physicians, except for sexual abuse where the scores were much lower. Important clinically were the findings that for all three kinds of abuse, "listened respectfully and took me seriously" and "believed my story" were deemed the most helpful responses by professionals. Other helpful responses were "helping me see my strengths" (emotional and sexual), "helping me understand the effects on my children" (emotional and physical), and "helping me see I was in danger" and "figure out ways of making my present situation safer" (physical abuse only), with referrals helpful but endorsed by a much smaller number of women. Unhelpful responses to all three kinds of abuse reflected a lack of attentiveness, disbelief, and/or a failure to treat the situation seriously (especially for sexual abuse). The study was limited by its purely descriptive analysis and nonrepresentative, although large, sample.

In a well-designed study, Tilden and associates (1994) surveyed a random sample of three groups of professionals from six disciplines (dentists and dental hygienists, nurses and physicians, and psychologists and social workers) about their basic professional educational content on child, spouse, and elder abuse, with response rates ranging from 69% to 83% (Tilden et al., 1994). Subjects with more education on the topic more commonly suspected abuse in their patients. Spouse abuse was the most frequently suspected and elder abuse the least suspected across groups. Nurses were in the middle range of disciplines (below psychologists and social workers, above the dental professions, and about the same as physicians) in rates of identification and educational content, except for elder abuse. Nurses had the highest identification rate and the most educational content (along with social workers) in terms of physical elder abuse. The majority of nurses (86.7%) saw themselves as having as much responsibility in terms of family violence as other clinical problems but, like the other professionals, had little confidence in the effectiveness of current family violence laws. In a later extension of this research (Limandri & Tilden, 1996), the authors used interviews and surveys to explore nurses' reasoning in the assessment of family violence. The nurses reported that the major advantage for identifying victims of abuse was to provide safety to the victim and prevent further abuse. Equally compelling, however, was the nurses' concerns that they could be wrong in their assessment and do greater harm than good. The reasoning process used by most nurses was to seek a dynamic balance of what was good for the client, family, and community and of the nurses' professional obligations.

Three quarters of the nurses had educational content on child abuse, but only 44% reported such content in spouse abuse, a low percentage supported by Yam's (1995) data. Nurses picked consultation as their most frequent choice of intervention rather than direct discussion with the patient (or family) in all three kinds of family violence in the Tilden et al. (1994) survey, a less optimal intervention choice also supported by Yam (1995) and earlier nursing research (King & Ryan, 1989).

Although not published as a full research report (and therefore difficult to evaluate), Yam's (1995) article reported data from a survey of 52 emergency room nurses:

49% preferred a medical model approach of helping wife abuse victims (wherein the client is viewed as weak or ill, not held responsible but expected to be passive and compliant, and the professional is responsible for solving the problem). A significantly higher proportion of nurses who had themselves been abused (20% of the sample), compared to nurses who had not, preferred an empowerment model of helping abused women. There was a small but significant negative correlation between endorsement of the medical model and number of victims identified by the nurse. Both prior nursing research (King & Ryan, 1989) and medical research (Warshaw, 1989) point out the limitations in use of the medical model with battered women. Additionally, all of the research on the subject has been limited by sampling (convenience, one setting, small numbers) and a lack of multivariate and comparison analysis.

A pilot, single group, pre- and posttest design study of a 60-minute training program including a videotape of abusive scenarios for 18 randomly selected emergency department nurses was conducted by Bokunewicz and Copel (1992). There was a significant increase in attitude scores using a previously validated instrument and improvement in the scores of 17 of the 18 participants. The study was severely limited by the design and a low participation rate (less than half of those who originally agreed to participate), resulting in a subsequent small sample size. There is also the issue of whether or not attitude change actually reflects behavior change. However, the generally positive results further substantiate the well-designed experimental investigation done earlier by Tilden and Shepherd (1987), demonstrating that training of ED nurses in domestic violence can not only improve attitudes but actually increase identification rates of abused women. This finding has also been obtained by medical researchers, although the gain in identification rates was not sustained over time (McLeer & Anwar, 1989).

A survey of 243 BSN and AD nursing students (approximately half in each group) (Attala, Oetker, et al., 1995) is the first published study of the prevalence of abuse among nurses or nursing students. Using Hudson's Partner Abuse Scales (Physical and Nonphysical), there was an 8% prevalence of current physical abuse, not significantly different from national estimates. An 18.9% prevalence of nonphysical abuse was found. Significant positive (but weak) correlations were found between physical abuse and the Index of Clinical Stress and General Contentment Scale (measuring depression); stronger (moderate) correlations were found between nonphysical abuse and the same instruments. However, this finding may have been related to the lower base rate (more skewed distribution) of the physical abuse (a common methodological problem in domestic violence research), and no statistical adjustments were attempted. Unfortunately, multivariate analysis was not conducted, making it difficult to determine if differences in abuse between the BSN and AD students were related to other demographic differences between the two groups.

Culture-Related Research

Nursing research included some of the first efforts to address issues of cultural influences on battering (e.g., Torres, 1987). There have been several clinical articles addressing nursing care of battered women that take culture into account (e.g., Campbell, McKenna, et al., 1993) and also detail suggested (not yet tested) nursing care specific to various cultural and geographic groups (Bohn, 1993; Campbell, D. W., 1998; Fishwick, 1993; Rodriguez, 1993; Torres, 1991). In addition, McFarlane, Parker, Soeken, and Bullock (1992) specifically examined the prevalence, frequency, and severity of abuse during pregnancy in three different cultural groups and found the prevalence of abuse to be significantly lower among Hispanic women. Abuse severity was lowest among African-American couples. Campbell and her colleagues (Campbell, Miller, et al., 1994; Campbell, Kub, et al., 1997) have investigated the influence of ethnicity (African American versus Anglo) on depression and subsequent violence in battered women and found no effects. As reported above, Campbell, Campbell, et al. (1994) found that the Index of Spouse Abuse was as reliable and had as much support for construct validity among African-American women as among Anglo women but that the factor structure for the instrument was different, suggesting that African-American women may perceive their abuse differently. These results overall indicate the importance of continuing to include ethnicity as a variable in nursing research on battering and to report similarities in findings as well as differences.

Taking another approach, Counts, Brown, and Campbell (1992; 1999) used primary ethnographic evidence collected from 14 different societies worldwide, representing a range of geographic locations, industrialization, household arrangements, and degree of spousal violence to examine evidence supporting the theoretical stances about battering from Western social sciences. Although the feminist (or patriarchal) theoretical premises received considerable support, there were several aspects

brought into question. The review suggested that all forms of violence against women could not be considered as aspects of the same phenomenon and that status of women is an extremely complex, multifaceted phenomenon that may have a curvilinear rather than a direct relationship with wife battering. The review also demonstrated the importance of societal influences on individual couples. In that study, wife *beating* (occasional, nonescalating, without serious or permanent injury, and seen as ordinary by most members of the culture) was differentiated from wife *battering* (continuing, usually escalating, potentially injurious pattern of physical violence within a context of coercive control). Factors found that discouraged the escalation of wife *beating* to *battering* across societies included community-level sanctions against battering and sanctuary for beaten wives enacted in culturally specific and appropriate forms.

Intervention Studies

Using a nominal group process, Attala and De Frank (1991) identified priority health needs in one wife abuse shelter as (a) access to health care, (b) health education, (c) health problem prevention, (d) reducing gender bias in health care, and (e) supportive services and health supplies. Critical health care issues identified included prenatal care, access to medical care for both urgent and chronic conditions, hearing and vision screening, mental health counseling services, and family planning services. Process evaluation of subsequent implementation of nurse practitioner-provided health services was carried out and reported as successful, but actual data were not presented. Although severely limited by a nonexperimental design and presentation as a clinical report rather than as a formal research report, the study demonstrates nursing's ongoing concern and opportunities for providing health care in shelters and one model for planning and evaluating that care.

Another pilot study for an intervention was reported by Varvaro and Palmer (1993). Using a new self-efficacy scale specific to battered women, the investigators found preliminary reliability support (Cronbach's alpha = .88) and convergent construct validity in a small convenience sample of 43 currently or formerly abused women in the ED. However, there are problems in interpretation of the findings regarding comparisons of the currently and formerly battered women and items indicating lower or higher self-efficacy. The findings from the study were used to design nursing interventions based on women's answers to the items, a clinically useful approach. A very preliminary test of those interventions was conducted with six Anglo-American battered women in a support group setting. A pre- and posttest single-group design study resulted in a significant mean increase on the self-efficacy instrument with each woman. Obviously severely limited by lack of a control group (ideally randomly assigned), this study shows sufficient evidence to mount a larger clinical trial of the intervention (especially given the small sample size and resultant lack of power, the finding of significance warrants further investigation). However, the study shows an appropriate beginning of the progression of the launch of an intervention trial, a development seriously needed by nursing (and other discipline) research in this field (National Research Council, 1996).

A third descriptive, small, participant-observation study of group process with battered women was also conducted (Dimmitt & Davila, 1995). Replicating a prototype described in earlier nursing literature (Campbell, 1986b), these investigators used thematic analysis of the group process and found the same themes (control by the abusive partner, damaged self-esteem, exploring alternatives, decision making, and affirmation) replicated with the addition of themes of morality, nurturance, fear of intimacy, self-doubt, sociability, intelligence, trust, and fear of mental illness. Although the investigators concluded that the study supported both the earlier intervention and findings, these numerous additional themes cast some doubt on the replicability of the earlier work. In addition, a single-group design such as this can be considered as only preliminary to a true intervention evaluation. However, the replicability of the intervention in another site with a different ethnic mix of participants lays a beginning foundation for a true test of the intervention.

A clinical trial intervention study tested a nursing intervention for abused pregnant women (Parker, McFarlane, Soeken, Silva, & Reel, 1999). In the study, 132 abused pregnant women received three counseling sessions designed to reduce further abuse. A comparison group of 67 abused women were offered a wallet-size card listing community resources for abuse. Women in both groups were followed at 6 months and 12 months postdelivery. Using repeated measures MANCOVA with entry scores as a covariate, there was significantly less violence reported by women in the intervention group than by women in the comparison group. This intervention model has been published by the March of Dimes (McFarlane & Parker, 1994) and is available for all health care professionals. Future research endeavors on vio-

lence against women need to further refine and test this intervention, as well as developing and testing additional models of interventions.

Summary of Findings and Clinical Implications

In conclusion, nursing research has contributed significantly to the field of violence against women. In the area of abuse during pregnancy, nursing research has, in many respects, led the field, including documentation of a higher prevalence of abuse during pregnancy (16% to 17%) than other studies (see review by Gazmararian et al., 1996). This is probably related to the use of primarily face-to-face nurse-conducted interviews using an appropriate clinical screen (rather than a research instrument). The program of research of McFarlane and Parker and their associates has contributed greatly to the clinical documentation of abuse during pregnancy, investigation of outcomes of abuse during pregnancy, and beginning tests of intervention for abuse.

The documentation of successful screening for battered women in prenatal and other health settings through clinical nursing research has been an extremely important part of an interdisciplinary (primarily nursing, medicine, and public health) body of clinical research on the topic (e.g., Gielen, O'Campo, et al., 1994; Hamberger et al., 1993; McCauley et al., 1995). Findings from both abuse during pregnancy studies and other health-related studies in nursing and other disciplines suggest that universal screening of all women (including adolescents) for intimate partner abuse at *each* health care system encounter needs to become routine nursing practice because of (a) the change in abuse status over time (during pregnancy, before and after versus during pregnancy, and throughout the woman's life) (Campbell, Miller, et al., 1994; McFarlane, Parker, Soeken, & Bullock, 1992), (b) the variety of physical and mental health problems (most often *without* injury) battered women experience, and (c) the lack of personal or demographic characteristics that can identify women more likely to be abused (Hotaling & Sugarman, 1990; Page-Adams & Dersch, 1998) or likely to continue in battering relationships (Campbell, Miller, et al., 1994).

Supported findings from nursing research also include the link of abuse during pregnancy and LBW (Parker, McFarlane, & Soeken, 1994) and abuse during pregnancy and substance abuse (McFarlane, Parker, & Soeken, 1996a) (also strongly supported and further explicated in samples of not-battered women by Eby et al.,

1995, and Ratner, 1993). Depression has also been substantiated as a significant mental health problem of battered women, both in nursing and other discipline research (Campbell, Kub, & Rose, 1996). Noteworthy physical health problems found across studies (both population based and clinical) are headaches, backaches, STD risk, and sleeping problems (Eby et al., 1995; Ratner, 1993, 1995). Descriptive clinical studies have suggested important health-related effects such as unintended pregnancy, PTSD, and neurological problems. Most of these findings have been substantiated by research from other disciplines, strengthening the weight of their clinical implications. The often smaller descriptive and/or qualitative nursing studies have added depth and/or been precursors to the larger studies in other disciplines. Many of the findings from descriptive nursing studies have yet to be fully investigated in larger studies, offering rich opportunities for further work.

Related studies of nursing attitudes and practices about abuse taken as a whole suggest that nurses are underused as a resource for battered women and, although perceived as more helpful than not, too often use a medical rather than empowerment model approach to intervention. Basic and continuing nursing education is needed to improve knowledge, attitudes, and behavior regarding battered women. One of the studies reviewed (Attala, Oetker, et al., 1995) indicates a prevalence of abuse within nursing students in one midwestern city similar to the prevalence among American women overall, suggesting the need for nursing faculty to be alert for signs of abuse among students.

Studies of the children of battered women and their mothers' concerns about them suggest another important area for nursing assessment and intervention. A few nursing researchers have addressed this area, but more study is needed specific to physical and mental health effects and potential interventions in the health care setting. Researchers from other disciplines are also addressing this area, supporting the idea that children of battered women have significant problems but not solving the issue of the extent to which these problems are related to the stresses of shelter living (see Attala, Oetker, et al., 1995, for a review). Nursing has been in the forefront in one aspect of this area by addressing the reciprocity between abused mothers and their children but has not yet tested specific health care system interventions to address their health needs.

To further advance the body of nursing knowledge about battered women and their children, the strengths of nursing research, with its attention to culture and ethnicity, its use of both qualitative and quantitative data, and its strong clinical grounding and advocacy positions, need to be continued. Further longitudinal, comparison-group and large-sample studies are needed, especially those that further develop and test midrange nursing theory and/or further document and investigate health consequences of abuse for both mothers and children and/or build on existing nursing research. Most critical is the need for the testing of nursing and interdisciplinary interventions with battered women and their children. The field of violence-against-women research, especially in the health care setting, is recognized as both ready for and needing tested interventions (Crowell & Burgess, 1996). In terms of clinical nursing research, these interventions can draw on already completed studies and formulated theory. Tested interventions could demonstrate the value of nursing care in making the health care system both a form of sanctuary and a secondary, as well as tertiary, prevention site in the field of woman abuse.

Note

1. It is sometimes difficult to tell the disciplinary affiliation from the allowable designations in many of the interdisciplinary journals. Some nursing authors may not realize the importance of carefully designating their affiliation (at least as the address) as a school of nursing or department of nursing if licensure letters are not allowed. The hand search revealed only two nursing-authored articles in the four journals searched from the past 5 years, suggesting that nursing researchers are concentrating their efforts in nursing (or medical or public health) journals at this point. This concentration has both advantages (in terms of making sure that fellow nurses use the body of knowledge) and disadvantages (in terms of continuing the relative invisibility of the important nursing research contributions in the interdisciplinary body of knowledge on battering).

References

American Academy of Nursing. (1993). *Violence: Nursing debates the issues.* Washington, DC: Author.

Attala, J. M. (1994). Risk identification of abused women participating in a women, infants, and children program. *Health Care for Women International, 15,* 587-597.

Attala, J. M., & DeFrank, V. (1991). Identifying health needs in a shelter population. *Response, 79*(14), 2, 16-18.

Attala, J. M., Hudson, W. W., & McSweeney, M. (1994). A partial validation of two short-form partner abuse scales. *Women and Health, 21*(2/3), 125-139.

Attala, J. M., Oetker, D., & McSweeney, M. (1995). Partner abuse against female nursing students. *Journal of Psychosocial Nursing, 33*(1), 17-24.

Bachman, R., & Saltzman, L. E. (1995). *Violence against women: Estimates from the redesigned survey.* Washington, DC: U.S. Department of Justice.

Bohn, D. K. (1993). Nursing care of Native American battered women. In J. Campbell (Ed.), *AWHONN'S clinical issues in perinatal and women's health nursing* (pp. 424-436). Philadelphia: Lippincott.

Bokunewicz, B., & Copel, L. C. (1992). Attitudes of emergency nurses before and after a 60-minute educational presentation on partner abuse. *Journal of Emergency Nursing, 16*(1), 24-27.

Boyd, C., & Mast, D. (1983). Addicted women and their relationships with men. *Journal of Psychosocial Nursing and Mental Health Services, 21*(2), 10-13.

Brendtro, M., & Bowker, H. L. (1989). Battered women: How can nurses help. *Issues in Mental Health Nursing, 10,* 169-180.

Bullock, L., & McFarlane, J. (1989). The birthweight/battering connection. *American Journal of Nursing, 89*(9), 1153-1155.

Bullock, L., McFarlane, J., Bateman, L., & Miller, V. (1989). The prevalence and characteristics of battered women in a primary care setting. *Nurse Practitioner, 14*(6), 47-55.

Campbell, D. W. (1998). Providing effective interventions for African American battered women: Afrocentric perspectives. In J. Campbell (Ed.), *Empowering survivors of abuse: Health care for battered women, and their children* (pp. 229-240). Thousand Oaks, CA: Sage.

Campbell, D. W., Campbell, J. C., King, C., Parker, B., & Ryan, J. (1994). The reliability and factor structure of the Index of Spouse Abuse with African-American battered women. *Violence and Victims, 9,* 259-274.

Campbell, J., & Humphreys, J. (1993). *Nursing care of survivors of family violence.* St. Louis: Mosby.

Campbell, J., Kub, J., & Rose, L. (1996). Depression in battered women. *Journal of the American Medical Women's Association, 51*(3), 106-110.

Campbell, J., Kub, J., Belknap, R. A., & Templin, T. (1997). Predictors of depression in battered women. *Violence Against Women, 3*(3), 271-293.

Campbell, J., McKenna, L., Torres, S., Sheridan, D., & Landenburger, K. (1993). Nursing care of abused women. In J. Campbell & J. Humphreys (Eds.), *Nursing care of survivors of family violence* (pp. 248-299). St. Louis: Mosby.

Campbell, J., Miller, P., Cardwell, M., & Belknap, R. (1994). Relationship status of battered women over time. *Journal of Family Violence, 9,* 99-111.

Campbell, J., Soeken, K., McFarlane, J., & Parker, B. (1998). Risk factors for femicide among pregnant and nonpregnant battered women. In J. Campbell (Ed.), *Empowering survivors of abuse: Health care for battered women and their children* (pp. 90-97). Thousand Oaks, CA: Sage.

Campbell, J. C. (1981). Misogyny and homicide of women. *Advances in Nursing Science, 3*(2), 67-85.

Campbell, J. C. (1986a). Nursing assessment for risk of homicide with battered women. *Advances in Nursing Science, 8*(4), 36-51.

Campbell, J. C. (1986b). A survivor group for battered women. *Advances in Nursing Science, 8*(2), 13-20.

Campbell, J. C. (1989a). A test of two explanatory models of women's responses to battering. *Nursing Research, 38,* 18-24.

Campbell, J. C. (1989b). Women's responses to sexual abuse in intimate relationships. *Women's Health Care International, 8,* 335-347.

Campbell, J. C. (1992). "If I can't have you, no one can": Power and control in homicide of female partners. In J. Radford & D.E.H. Russell (Eds.), *Femicide: The politics of woman killing* (pp. 99-113). New York: Twayne.

Campbell, J. C. (Ed.). (1995). *Assessing dangerousness.* Newbury Park, CA: Sage.

Campbell, J. C., & Alford, P. (1989). The dark consequences of marital rape. *American Journal of Nursing, 89,* 946-949.

Campbell, J. C., Anderson, E., Fulmer, T. L., Girourd, S., McElmurray, B., & Raff, B. (1993). Violence as a nursing priority: Policy implications. *Nursing Outlook, 41*(1), 89-92.

Campbell, J. C., Oliver, C., & Bullock, L. (1993). Why battering during pregnancy? *AWHONN'S Clinical Issues, 4*(3), 343-349.

Campbell, J. C., & Parker, B. (1992). Review of nursing research on battered women and their children. In J. Fitzpatrick, R. Taunton, & A. Jacox, *Annual review of nursing research* (Vol. 10, pp. 77-94). New York: Springer.

Campbell, J. C., & Parker, B. (1996). Battered women and their children: A review and policy recommendations. In B. J. McElmurry & R. Parker (Eds.), *Annual review of women's health* (Vol. 3, pp. 259-281). New York: National League for Nursing Press.

Campbell, J. C., Pliska, M. J., Taylor, W., & Sheridan, D. (1994). Battered women's experiences in emergency departments: Need for appropriate policy and procedures. *Journal of Emergency Nursing, 20,* 280-288.

Campbell, J. C., Poland, M., Waller, J., & Ager, J. (1992). Correlates of battering during pregnancy. *Research in Nursing and Health, 15,* 219-226.

Campbell, J. C., Pugh, L. C., Campbell, D., & Visscher, M. (1995). The influence of abuse on pregnancy intention. *Women's Health Issues, 5*(4), 214-223.

Campbell, J. C., Torres, S., Ryan, J., King, C., Campbell, D., Stallings, R., & Fuchs, S. C. (1998). Physical and nonphysical abuse and other risk factors for low birthweight among term and preterm babies: A multiethnic case control study. *American Journal of Epidemiology.*

Campbell, J. C., Ulrich, Y., Sheridan, D., Campbell, D., & Landenburger, K. (1993). Nursing care of abused women. In J. Campbell & J. Humphreys (Eds.), *Nursing care of survivors of family violence.* St. Louis: Mosby.

Canadian Nurses Association. (1992). *Family violence: Clinical guidelines for nurses.* Ottawa, ON: National Clearinghouse on Family Violence, Health and Welfare Canada.

Counts, D., Brown, J., & Campbell, J. C. (1992). *Sanctions and sanctuary: Cultural analysis of the beating of wives.* Boulder, CO: Westview.

Counts, D., Brown, J., & Campbell, J. C. (1999). *To have to hit: Cultural perspectives on wife-beating.* Champaign, IL: University of Illinois Press.

Crowell, N., & Burgess, A. (Eds.). (1996). *Understanding violence against women.* Washington, DC: National Academy Press.

Curry, M. A. (1998). Stress related to domestic violence during pregnancy and infant birthweight. In J. Campbell (Ed.), *Empowering survivors of abuse: Health care for battered women and their children* (pp. 98-108). Thousand Oaks, CA: Sage.

Dannenberg, A. L., Carter, D. M., Lawson, H. W., Ashton, D. M., Dorfman, S. F., & Graham, E. H. (1995). Homicide and other injuries as causes of maternal death in New York City, 1987 through 1991. *American Journal of Obstetrics and Gynecology, 172,* 1557-1564.

Dimmitt, J., & Davisla, Y. R. (1995). Group psychotherapy for abused women: A survivor group prototype. *Applied Nursing Research, 8*(1), 3-7.

Dobash, R. E., & Dobash, R. P. (1979). *Violence against wives.* New York: Free Press.

Drake, V. K. (1982). Battered women: A health care problem in disguise. *Image: The Journal of Nursing Scholarship, 14,* 40-47.

Eby, K., Campbell, J. C., Sullivan, C., & Davidson, W. (1995). Health effects of experiences of sexual violence for women with abusive partners. *Women's Health Care International, 16,* 563-576.

Eriksen, J., & Henderson, A. (1998). Diverging realities: Abused women and their children. In J. Campbell (Ed.), *Empowering survivors abuse: Health care for battered women and their children* (pp. 138-155). Thousand Oaks, CA: Sage.

Fildes, J., Reed, L., Jones, N., Martin, M., & Barrett, J. (1992). Trauma: The leading cause of maternal death. *Journal of Trauma, 32,* 643-645.

Fishwick, N. (1993). Nursing care of rural battered women. In J. Campbell (Ed.), *AWHONN'S clinical issues in perinatal and women's health nursing* (pp. 441-448). Philadelphia: Lippincott.

Foster, L. A., Veale, C. M., & Fogel, C. I. (1989). Factors present when battered women kill. *Issues in Mental Health Nursing, 10,* 273-284.

Gazmararian, J. A., Lazorick, S., Spitz, A., Ballard, T., Saltzman, L., & Marks, J. (1996). Prevalence of violence against pregnant women. *Journal of the American Medical Association, 275*(24), 1915-1920.

Gelles, R. J. (1988). Violence and pregnancy: Are pregnant women at greater risk of abuse? *Journal of Marriage and the Family, 50,* 841-847.

Gielen, A. C., Faden, R. R., O'Campo, P., Kass, N., & Anderson, J. (1994). Women's protective sexual behaviors: A test of the health belief model. *AIDS Education and Prevention, 6*(1), 1-11.

Gielen, A. C., O'Campo, P. J., Faden, R. R., Kass, N. E., & Xue, X. (1994). Interpersonal conflict and physical violence during the childbearing years. *Social Science and Medicine, 39,* 781-787.

Gleason, W. J. (1993). Mental disorders in battered women: An empirical study. *Violence and Victims, 8,* 53-68.

Glittenburg, J., Babich, K., & Campbell, J. C. (Eds.). (1995). *Violence: A plague upon the land.* Washington, DC: American Academy of Nursing.

Goldberg, W. G., & Tomlanovich, M. C. (1985). Domestic violence victims in the emergency department. *Journal of the American Medical Association, 251,* 3259-3264.

Hamberger, L. K., Saunders, D. G., & Hovey, M. (1993). Prevalence of domestic violence in community practice and rate of physician inquiry. *Family Medicine, 24,* 283-287.

Hamilton, B., & Coates, J. (1993). Perceived helpfulness and use of professional services by abused women. *Journal of Family Violence, 8,* 313-324.

Helton, A. S. (1986). The pregnant battered woman. *Response, 9*(1), 22-23.

Helton, A. S., McFarlane, J., & Anderson, E. T. (1987). Battered and pregnant: A prevalence study. *American Journal of Public Health, 77,* 1337-1339.

Henderson, A. (1990, June/September). Children of abused women: Their influences on their mother's decisions. *Canada's Mental Health, 38,* 10-13.

Henderson, A. (1993). Abused women's perceptions of their children's experiences. *Canada's Mental Health, 41*(1), 7-10.

Henderson, D. A. (1989). Use of social support in a transition house for abused women. *Health Care for Women International, 10*(1), 61-73.

Herman, J. (1992). *Trauma and recovery.* New York: Basic Books.

Hoff, L. A. (1990). *Battered women as survivors.* London: Routledge.

Hotaling, G. T., & Sugarman, D. B. (1990). A risk marker analysis of assaulted wives. *Journal of Family Violence, 5,* 1-3.

Hudson, W. W., & McIntosh, S. R. (1981). The assessment of spouse abuse: Two quantifiable dimensions. *Journal of Marriage and the Family, 43,* 873-885.

Humphreys, J. (1991). Children of battered women: Worries about their mothers. *Pediatric Nursing, 17*(4), 342-345.

Humphreys, J. (1995a). Dependent care by battered women: Protecting their children. *Health Care for Women International, 16*(1), 9-20.

Humphreys, J. (1995b). The work of worrying: Battered women and their children. *Scholarly Inquiry for Nursing Practice: An International Journal, 9*(2), 126-145.

Kerouac, S., Taggart, M. E., Lescop, J., & Fortin, M. F. (1986). Dimensions of health in violent families. *Health Care for Women International, 7,* 413-426.

King, M. C., & Ryan, J. (1989). Abused women: Dispelling myths and encouraging intervention. *Nurse Practitioner, 14*(5), 47-58.

Kurz, D. (1987). Emergency department responses to battered women: Resistance to medicalization. *Social Problems, 34,* 501-513.

Landenburger, K. (1988). Conflicting realities of women in abusive relationships. *Communicating Nursing Research, 21,* 15-20.

Landenburger, K. (1989). A process of entrapment in and recovery from an abusive relationship. *Issues in Mental Health Nursing, 3,* 209-227.

Landenburger, K. (1993). Exploration of women's identity: Clinical approaches with abused women. In J. Campbell (Ed.), *AWHONN'S clinical issues in perinatal and women's health nursing* (pp. 378-384). Philadelphia: Lippincott.

Langford, D. R. (1996). Predicting unpredictability: A model of women's processes of predicting battering men's violence. *Scholarly Inquiry for Nursing Practice, 10*(4), 371-385.

Levinson, D. (1989). *Family violence in cross cultural perspective.* Newbury Park, CA: Sage.

Lia-Hoagberg, B., Knoll, K., Swaney, S., Carlson, G., & Mullett, S. (1988). Relationship of street drug use, hospitalization, and psychosocial factors to low birthweight among low income women. *Birth, 15*(1), 8-13.

Lichtenstein, V. R. (1981). The battered woman: Guidelines for effective nursing intervention. *Issues in Mental Health Nursing, 3,* 237-250.

Limandri, B. J., & Tilden, V. P. (1996). Nurses' reasoning in the assessment of family violence. *Image: The Journal of Nursing Scholarship, 28*(3), 247-252.

Mahon, L. (1981). Common characteristics of abused women. *Issues in Mental Health Nursing, 3,* 137-157.

Marshall, L. (1992). Development of the Severity of Violence Against Women Scale. *Journal of Family Violence, 17*(2), 103-121.

McCauley, J., Kern, D. E., Kolodner, K., Dill, L., Schroeder, A. F., DeChant, H., Ryden, J., Bass, E., & Derogatis, L. (1995). The "battering syndrome": Prevalence and clinical characteristics of domestic violence in primary care internal medicine practices. *Annals of Internal Medicine, 123*(110), 737-746.

McFarlane, J., Christoffel, K., Bateman, L., Miller, V., & Bullock, L. (1991). Assessing for abuse: Self report versus nurse interview. *Public Health Nursing, 8,* 245-250.

McFarlane, J., & Parker, B. (1994). *Abuse during pregnancy: A protocol for prevention and intervention.* White Plains, NY: March of Dimes.

McFarlane, J., Parker, B., & Soeken, K. (1995). Abuse during pregnancy: Frequency, severity, perpetrator and risk factors of homicide. *Public Health Nursing, 12*(5), 284-289.

McFarlane, J., Parker, B., & Soeken, K. (1996a). Abuse during pregnancy: Associations with maternal health and infant birth weight. *Nursing Research, 45*(1), 37-42.

McFarlane, J., Parker, B., & Soeken, K. (1996b). Physical abuse, smoking, and substance use during pregnancy: Prevalence, interrelationships and effects on birthweight. *Journal of Obstetric, Gynecologic and Neonatal Nursing, 25*(4), 313-320.

McFarlane, J., Parker, B., Soeken, K., & Bullock, L. (1992). Assessing for abuse during pregnancy: Severity and frequency of injuries and associated entry into prenatal care. *Journal of the American Medical Association, 267,* 2370-2372.

McLeer, S. V., & Anwar, R.A.H. (1989). Education is not enough: A systems failure in protecting battered women. *Annals of Emergency Medicine, 18*(6), 651-653.

Merritt-Gray, M., & Wuest, J. (1995). Counteracting abuse and breaking free: The process of leaving revealed through women's voices. *Health Care for Women International, 16,* 399-412.

National Research Council. (1996). *Evaluation of family violence interventions.* Washington, DC: National Academy Press.

Newman, K. D. (1993). Giving up: Shelter experiences of battered women. *Public Health Nursing, 10*(2), 108-113.

Oliver, W. (1989). Sexual conquest and patterns of Black-on-Black violence: A structural-cultural perspective. *Violence and Victims, 4,* 257-274.

Orem, D. (1995). *Nursing concepts of practice* (5th ed.). New York: McGraw-Hill.

Page-Adams, D., & Dersch, S. (1998). Physical and nonphysical abuse against women: Assessing prevalence in a hospital setting. In J. Campbell (Ed.) *Empowering survivors of abuse: Health care for battered women and their children* (pp. 204-213). Thousand Oaks, CA: Sage.

Paluzzi, P. A., & Slattery, L. (1996). *No woman deserves to hurt: Domestic violence education for health care providers.* Washington, DC: American College of Nurse-Midwives.

Parker, B., McFarlane, J., & Soeken, K. (1994). Abuse during pregnancy: Effects on maternal complications and birthweight in adult and teenage women. *Obstetrics and Gynecology, 84,* 323-328.

Parker, B., McFarlane, J., Soeken, K., Silva, C., & Reel, S. (1999). Testing an intervention to prevent further abuse to pregnant women. *Research in Nursing and Health.*

Parker, B., McFarlane, J., Soeken, K., Torres, S., & Campbell, D. (1993). Physical and emotional abuse in pregnancy: A comparison of adult and teenage women. *Nursing Research, 42,* 173-178.

Parker, B., & Schumacher, D. (1977). The battered wife syndrome and violence in the nuclear family of origin: A controlled pilot study. *American Journal of Public Health, 67*(8), 760-761.

Parker, B., Ulrich, Y., Bullock, L., Campbell, D., Campbell, J., King, C., Landenburger, K., McFarlane, J., McKenna, L., & Torres, S. (1990). A protocol of safety: Research on abuse of women. *Nursing Research, 39*(4), 248-250.

Ratner, P. A. (1993). The incidence of wife abuse and mental health status in abused wives in Edmonton, Alberta. *Canadian Journal of Public Health, 84*(4), 246-249.

Ratner, P. A. (1995). Indicators of exposure to wife abuse. *Canadian Journal of Nursing Research, 27*(1), 31-46.

Rodriguez, R. (1989). Perception of health needs by battered women. *Response, 12*(4), 22-23.

Rodriguez, R. (1993). Violence in transience: Nursing care of battered migrant women. *AWHONN's Clinical Issues, 4*(3), 437-440.

Rose, K., & Saunders, D. G. (1986). Nurses' and physicians' attitudes about women abuse: The effects of gender and professional role. *Health Care for Women International, 7,* 427-438.

Rumptz, M. H., Sullivan, C. M., Davidson, W. S., & Basta, J. (1991). An ecological approach to tracking battered women over time. *Violence and Victims, 6*(3), 237-244.

Sampselle, C. M., Petersen, B. A., Murtland, T. L., & Oakley, D. J. (1992). Prevalence of abuse among pregnant women choosing certified nurse-midwife or physician providers. *Journal of Nurse-Midwifery, 37*(4), 269-273.

Shipley, S. B., & Sylvester, D. C. (1982). Professionals' attitudes toward violence in close relationships. *Journal of Emergency Nursing, 8*(2), 88-91.

Soeken, K., Parker, B., McFarlane, J., & Lominak, M. C. (1996). The Abuse Assessment Screen: A clinical instrument to measure frequency, sever-

ity, and perpetrator of abuse against women. In J. Campbell (Ed.), *Beyond diagnosis: Changing the health care response to battered women and their children.* Newbury Park, CA: Sage.

Straus, M. A., & Gelles, R. J. (Eds.). (1990). *Physical violence in American families: Risk factors and adaptations to family violence in 8,145 families.* New Brunswick, NJ: Transaction.

Stuart, G., Laraia, M., Ballenger, J., & Lydiard, R. (1990). Early family experiences of women with bulimia and depression. *Archives of Psychiatric Nursing, 4,* 43-52.

Taylor, W. K. (1994). *Development of the woman abuse screening tool.* Unpublished doctoral dissertation, Rush University, Chicago, IL.

Tilden, V. P., & Shepard, P. (1987). Increasing the rate of identification of battered women in an emergency department: Use of a nursing protocol. *Research in Nursing and Health, 10,* 209-215.

Tilden, V. P., Schmidt, T. A., Linardi, B., Chioda, G. T., Garland, M. J., & Loveless, P. A. (1994). Factors that influence clinician's assessment and management of family violence. *American Journal of Public Health, 84*(4), 628-633.

Torres, S. (1987). Hispanic-American battered women: Why consider cultural differences? *Response, 10*(3), 20-21.

Torres, S. (1991). A comparison of wife abuse between two cultures: Perceptions, attitudes, nature and extent. *Issues in Mental Health Nursing, 12,* 113-131.

Trimpey, M. L. (1989). Self-esteem and anxiety: Key issues in an abused women's support group. *Issues in Mental Health Nursing, 10,* 297-308.

Ulrich, Y. (1991). Women's reasons for leaving abusive spouses. *Women's Health Care International, 12,* 465-473.

Ulrich, Y. C. (1994). What helped most in leaving spouse abuse: Implications for interventions. In J. Campbell (Ed.), *AWHONN'S clinical issues in perinatal and women's health nursing* (pp. 385-390). Philadelphia: Lippincott.

U.S. Department of Health and Human Services. (1991a). *Healthy People 2000: National health promotion and disease prevention objectives.* Washington, DC: U.S. Department of Health and Human Services, Public Health Service.

U.S. Department of Health and Human Services. (1991b). *Third national injury control in the 1990's.* Washington, DC: Author.

Varvaro, F. F. (1991). Using a grief response assessment questionnaire in a support group to assist battered women in recovery. *Response, 13*(4), 12-15.

Varvaro, F. F., & Lasko, D. L. (1993). Physical abuse as cause of injury in women: Information for orthopaedic nurses. *Orthopaedic Nursing, 12*(1), 37-41.

Varvaro, F. F., & Palmer, M. (1993). Promotion of adaptation in battered women: A self-efficacy approach. *Journal of the American Academy of Nurse Practitioners, 5*(6), 264-270.

Warshaw, C. (1989). Limitations of the medical model in the care of battered women. *Gender & Society, 3,* 506-517.

Weingourt, R. (1985). Wife rape: Barriers to identification and treatment. *Journal of Psychotherapy, 39*(2), 187-192.

Weingourt, R. (1990). Wife rape in a sample of psychiatric patients. *Image: The Journal of Nursing Scholarship, 22,* 144-147.

Westra, B., & Martin, H. (1981). Children of battered women. *Maternal-Child Nursing Journal, 10,* 41-54.

Wilson, M., Johnson, H., & Daly, M. (1995). Lethal and nonlethal violence against wives. *Canadian Journal of Criminology, 37,* 331-362.

Yam, M. (1995). Wife abuse: Strategies for a therapeutic response. *Scholarly Inquiry for Nursing Practice, 9,* 147-158.

Zung, W., Broadhead, E., & Roth, M. E. (1993). Prevalence of depressive symptoms in primary care. *Journal of Family Practice, 37,* 337-344.

PART
IIG

OLDER ADULTS
Health and Illness Issues

Patricia G. Archbold

The next 50 years will bring an unprecedented increase in the number and relative percentage of elders (persons 65 years of age and older) in the United States and throughout the world. Worldwide, the number of elders is projected to increase so that by the year 2020 there will be more than 690 million, with 460 million in developing countries (World Health Organization, 1997). Although many future elders will be healthy and able to function independently in their environments, others will experience age-related changes and chronic illnesses that interfere with their abilities to function in daily activities. As the projected demographic changes have become more widely known and understood, there has been more urgency for research directed toward preventing and treating the complex health problems of older people. Nurses have contributed, and are continuing to contribute, to the knowledge base in this important area.

Much research in gerontological nursing is rooted in the framework of person-environment fit. Gerontological

nursing interventions, in general, are designed to reduce the demands (press, stress) of the environment within which elders live or to enhance the elders' physical, cognitive, or emotional capacities in some way. The three chapters in this section are focused on important person and environment variables. Because person and environment continuously interact, the chapter divisions are not completely discrete: Chapter 32 is focused mainly on environment; Chapters 30 and 31 are focused mainly on aspects of person that are particularly important in gerontological nursing. The authors have done an excellent job of synthesizing a complex and diverse literature.

In Chapter 30, "Activities of Daily Living: Factors Related to Independence," Roberts focuses on person factors related to independence in activities of daily living. She provides an overview of three models developed to explain independence and dependence in function and a brief summary of empirical indicators of functional limitations. Research findings on performance of daily activities are synthesized in terms of the relationship

561

among functional limitations and disability; physical, psychological, and environmental factors related to functional limitations; and related concepts (e.g., decision making). The chapter concludes with an analysis of nursing practice issues related to functional independence and the identification of directions for research.

In Chapter 31, Beck, Cronin-Stubbs, Buckwalter, and Rapp summarize the literature related to the three most common mental health problems in older adults: delirium, dementia, and depression. The theoretical bases for identifying these clinical problems and for various nursing intervention strategies are described. In addition, research findings related to clinical nursing approaches to managing delirium, dementia, and depression are reviewed.

In Chapter 32, "Supportive and Nonsupportive Care Environments for the Elderly," Phillips and Ayres provide an overview of person-environment theories, then a synthesis of research findings regarding the environment and person-environment fit that are relevant to nursing practice. Most of the work in this area has been done in nursing homes. Investigators have focused on the physical environment in relation to specific problems (e.g., agitation, wandering), the social environment (e.g., communication, control), and the structural and organizational environment (e.g., the characteristics of the staff). This chapter concludes with a summary of research evaluating facilitative environments (those designed to promote function) such as special care units.

Researchers have noted that the aged are heterogeneous in phenomena such as behavior, attitudes, income, experience, health, and function, among others. Some of this heterogeneity is predictable in that it is based on "cohort membership." Some of it is unpredictable in that it is based on individual differences. Heterogeneity of the older population in this country will increase with predicted changes in the ethnic composition of the population. Gerontological nursing research and practice is based on an understanding of older "populations," as well as on the highly individual nature of the aging and illness experience of elders.

In the coming decades, predicted demographic shifts will mean that the practice of most nurses will incorporate older people. Indeed, unless morbidity patterns change markedly, the majority of health and medical care services will be provided to this group. Families and other nonprofessional caregivers, under the guidance of a nurse, will probably give much of the direct care. The chapters that follow provide an analysis of the current knowledge base in three important areas of gerontological nursing and point to research that is needed to become "ready" to care for the increasing numbers of elders who will access our health care system in the future.

Reference

World Health Organization. (1997). *World health report 1997: Conquering suffering, enriching humanity.* Geneva, Switzerland: Author.

30

ACTIVITIES OF DAILY LIVING
Factors Related to Independence

Beverly L. Roberts

Both the number and the proportion of elderly adults in the population are projected to increase through the 21st century. The increase is expected to be associated with greater prevalence of chronic disease and dependence in performing daily activities. Independence in daily activities related to personal care (ADLs), and in instrumental tasks (IADLs) related to caring for the home and to activities outside the home, is crucial for remaining in the community. Elderly adults with dependence in IADLs and some ADLs more frequently receive informal care from friends and family, as well as formal services (Hing & Bloom, 1990). With higher rates of dependence, the rates of institutionalization and death rise (Hirsch, Sommers, Olsen, Mullen, & Winograd, 1990; Manton, 1988). Thus, the increasing numbers of elderly adults at risk of dependence in daily

activities related to chronic illness and aging raise important social and personal issues related to the costs of health care and home care services and the quality of life.

Because nurses assist individuals in responding to disease and the effects of aging, knowledge development in factors that contribute to independence in daily activities is integral to guide nursing assessment and intervention. Two diagnoses developed by the North American Nursing Diagnosis Association (NANDA) address dependency self-care deficit and impaired home maintenance; others are factors that contribute to dependence (e.g., impaired mobility and thought process altered). Before nurses can intervene to promote maximum independence in daily activities and resolve factors contributing to dependence, they require knowledge about the efficacy of interventions.

In this chapter, the definitions and empirical indicators of daily activities and related concepts are examined, and research findings are reviewed within the framework of existing theory. Few nurse researchers have focused research on the maintenance of independence in performing daily activities by elderly adults, and much of this research was conducted by other disciplines. An exhaustive review of the literature is not possible within the confines of this chapter. Thus research that is instrumental in developing middle-range theory is highlighted.

Theoretical Approaches

Concepts and Definitions

Activities of daily living are defined as those tasks required for personal care and management of household tasks and provision of food and shelter; they refer to personal care (bathing, dressing, eating, toileting, and transferring). Although there is consensus on the definition of IADLs, the specific activities included in them vary (e.g., managing money, household cleaning, and preparing meals). There is no theory of activities of daily living, but ADLs are included as a dimension of conceptualizations of *functional health, functional limitation,* and *disability.* However, these terms, which are often used interchangeably, have not always been consistent with theoretical definitions used to guide research. This conceptual confusion has hindered the development of measures and theoretical models.

Functional health has been viewed as a requirement for independent living (Hogue, 1984), as functional impairment or limitation in body systems necessary for independence in daily activities (Nagi, 1991), or as functional decline in which the individual becomes dependent in daily activities (e.g., Landefeld et al., 1995). The latter two terms, *impairment* and *decline,* are more commonly used in recent research. Functional impairment or limitation has been defined as social limitations represented by dependence in activities of daily living (Johnson & Wolinsky, 1993) or as dependence in the performance of daily activities, independent of a social context (e.g., Landefeld et al., 1995). Nagi (1991) defines functional limitation at the level of the whole person, not specific body systems, and he defines impairments at the systems level. For example, the inability to walk a mile is a functional limitation, but poor gas exchange in the alveoli, which limits the distance walked, is an impairment. Nagi (1991) defines disability as an inability to perform socially defined roles, such as daily tasks (ADLs and IADLs) that are directly affected by functional limitations. In contrast, the World Health Organization (WHO) (1980) definition includes these activities in the definition of handicap. Finally, frailty is defined as reduced physiological reserves and capacity to engage in social roles (Buchner, Beresford, Larson, LaCroix, & Wagner, 1992; Lawton, 1991) and practical daily activities (Brown, Renwick, & Raphael, 1995), but this definition is the same as Nagi's definition of disability. Moreover, frailty is conceptualized as inevitable decline and is hypothesized to be associated with vulnerability to loss of independence in daily activities, morbidity, and death. In most models, activities of daily living show the number or degree to which people are dependent, and the nomenclature reflects this. However, the conceptual definitions also allow for variation in the degree of difficulty in performing tasks, not just dependence (Verbrugge & Jette, 1994).

This confusion in terms and theoretical definitions has led to differing measurement strategies and has precluded systematic development of theory. In spite of this, a few middle-range theories provide a structure for interpreting results and heuristic guidance to future research and theory development. The ability to live safely and independently is of paramount importance to society and elderly adults, thus the discussion of theoretical models and underlying factors focuses on independence in the performance of daily activities whether it is termed functional health (Hogue, 1984), functional status (Leidy, 1994), functional limitation (Johnson & Wolinsky, 1993), disability (Nagi, 1991), or handicap (WHO, 1980). Because of the conceptual clarity of Nagi's (1991) model and its widespread use to guide research, his definitions of functional limitation, disability, and impairment are used in this chapter. Thus, functional limitation refers to the inability to function at the level of the whole person (e.g., getting up from a chair or climbing stairs), as distinct from underlying impairments in anatomy, physiology, or psychological function (termed impairment) and from the effects on dependence in performing daily activities (termed disability).

Theoretical Models

Most research to date has been atheoretical, or the measures of concepts and relationships have not been consistent with the conceptual model used. The models reviewed here reflect the multiplicity of causal factors related to daily activities for independent living. They include Hogue's (1984) model of functional health, which depicts the interplay between environmental factors and personal competencies on functional health but also includes cognitive appraisal of these as influencing functional health. Nagi's (1991) model of disability is both conceptually clear and useful in explaining past research findings and guiding research; it also includes the notion of thresholds at which change in subsequent concepts occurs. The disablement process model (Verbrugge & Jette, 1994) includes risk factors for impairments, functional limitations (making a distinction between upper and lower body), and disability, as well as external and internal factors that affect these.

Models without theoretical development (e.g., functional decline and frailty) and those lacking conceptual and theoretical clarity and consistency are not described. For example, the WHO (1980) model of disability was intended as a taxonomy of disability, and it lacks conceptual clarity and theoretical consistency, hindering operationalization of the concepts and their interrelationships (Grimby, Finnstam, & Jette, 1988; Nagi, 1991). The model of Johnson and Wolinsky (1993) lacks conceptual clarity between functional limitations (ADLs and IADLs) and disability (e.g., some measures reflect cognitive impairment and not disability), and perceived health is used as a proxy for functional limitations. This association has not been found consistently nor should it be theoretically expected (Crimmins, 1996). The model of functional status (Leidy, 1994) includes new nomenclature and concepts that are based on inadequate review of existing nomenclature, theory, and measurement issues.

Hogue's Model of Functional Health

Hogue's (1984) model of functional health is an extension of person-environment fit theory in which functional health is an outcome of the interplay among environmental factors, personal competencies, cognitive appraisal of both, and coping/adaptation. Personal competencies are intrinsic to the individual and include biological (e.g., ejection fraction or aerobic capacity), cognitive, and psychological factors (e.g., depression or anxiety). Environmental factors are external to the person and include physical features of the environment, medications, social support, and others. The model includes cognitive appraisal and coping/adaptation that are consistent with recent descriptions of their importance in

functional limitations and disability (Avlund, Davidsen, & Schultz-Larsen, 1995). Cognitive appraisal is an evaluative judgment of physical competencies and the environment. Coping/adaptation is conceptually less clear because it can be both a state or a process. However, coping/adaptation is useful in that it reflects active mechanisms that people use to react to the environment and modify the effects of personal competencies and the environment on functional health. In spite of a lack of conceptual clarity in the definition of functional health used in this model, the separation of environment from personal competencies and the addition of cognitive appraisal and coping/adaptation provide a useful theoretical structure for evaluating research findings and new directions for theory and research.

Nagi's Model of Disability

Nagi's (1991) model of disability depicts the factors and relationships that affect independence in the performance of roles and daily tasks. Pathology is defined as factors that disrupt normal processes or return to a normal state (e.g., stroke, schizophrenia); it leads to impairment, defined as physiological, psychological, or anatomical abnormalities (e.g., denervation, hyperglycemia). Functional limitations are observed at the level of the whole person (e.g., inability to rise from a chair or pick up a penny from the floor) and can lead to disability. Although frequently limited to ADLs and IADLs (Verbrugge, 1990; Verbrugge & Jette, 1994), disability can include hobbies, job, outside chores, and social interchange. This model does not include other factors related to impairment, functional limitation, and disability, such as a sedentary lifestyle, body mass, or smoking. Integral to the relationships among pathology, impairment, functional limitations, and disability is the notion of a threshold at which changes occur; that is, a certain amount of change in causal factors must occur before changes in subsequent ones emerge. Hence, not all impairments lead to functional limitations, which may not lead to disability. Moreover, different patterns of impairment and functional limitations may be associated with different types of disability. Although not well developed in this model, the definition of the situation by the individual, which is consistent with Hogue's concept of cognitive appraisal, affects disability, as do the definition of the situation by others and characteristics of the environment. These latter concepts represent an interplay of physical, psychological, social, and environmental factors, which have the potential to add to the explanatory power of the model.

Disablement Model

Verbrugge and Jette (1994) propose a model of disablement that is an extension of Nagi's model. They suggest that disability is the result of the interplay between personal capabilities and the environment, which is consistent with Hogue's (1984) model. The disablement process reflects the temporal interrelationships among the concepts in the Nagi model and poses new relationships of risk factors to impairments and of the effects of extraindividual and intraindividual factors to functional limitation. Extraindividual factors are outside the individual and are therefore consistent with environment in Hogue's model. They include medical care (e.g., physical therapy or health education); medications and therapeutic regimens (e.g., bed rest, exercise); external supports (e.g., assistive devices, home care); and structural, physical, and social environment (e.g., lighting, pollution). Intraindividual factors are within the person and are consistent with personal competencies in Hogue's model. They include lifestyle and behavior (e.g., exercise, rest), psychosocial attributes and coping (e.g., social support groups, a confidante, or locus of control) and activity accommodations (e.g., how frequently tasks are done). A logical inconsistency in the disablement model is the inclusion of social support in intraindividual factors and not extraindividual factors.

In the models of Hogue, Nagi, and Verbrugge and Jette, multiple factors are viewed as affecting independence in daily activities. Cognitive appraisal of the environment and personal competencies is not well developed in Hogue's or Nagi's models and is not included in the disablement model. However, cognitive appraisal may make significant contributions to elderly adults' decisions about what and how they perform daily activities, and it has the potential to explain differences in independence in activities between individuals who have the same functional limitations. Moreover, threshold in Nagi's model has the potential to explain why some elderly adults do not exhibit functional limitations with impairments or do not have disability in the presence of functional limitations. For example, muscle strength may be low for two individuals, but only one may experience dependence in ADLs. The multifactorial models of Hogue and Nagi, however, are most helpful in understanding the complexity and the patterns in the effects of underlying factors on functional limitations that in turn

affect independence in daily activities. The disablement model provides additional understanding of the role of risk factors on impairments and the role of intraindividual and extraindividual factors in the development of impairment, functional limitation, and disability.

Empirical Indicators

An exhaustive review of measures of functional limitation and disability is not possible in this chapter. Examples of measures will be used to illustrate the issues related to operationalization. For a summary of measures, refer to the reviews by others (e.g., Kane & Kane, 1981; Rubenstein, Schairer, Wieland, & Kane, 1984).

Functional Limitation

Multi-item scales of functional limitation, for example, include the Arthritis Impact Measurement Scale (AIMS) (Meenan, Gertman, & Mason, 1980), Medical Outcome Health Survey (McHorney, Ware, & Raczek, 1993), Functional Independence Measure (Ottenbacher et al., 1994), and Physical Performance and Mobility Examination (Winograd et al., 1994). To measure functional limitations in the upper extremities, timed performance of motor tasks requiring fine motor control (opening and closing doors with different handles and latches) has been used (Williams & Hornberger, 1984). Although some measures have been developed specifically for elderly adults or persons with certain disease conditions, many contain the same or similar items. For example, the 12-minute walk has been used to assess functional limitations in persons with chronic obstructive pulmonary disease (Larson et al., 1996), and the 6-minute walk has been used in persons with cardiovascular disease (Peeters & Mets, 1996). Some measures contain items relating to independence in daily tasks (e.g., AIMS) that bias the measurement of functional limitations. Further, the measurement of functional limitations has sometimes been confused with measures of underlying physical and cognitive impairments (e.g., Johnson & Wolinsky, 1993). For example, the Performance-Oriented-Mobility Assessment (Tinetti, 1986) has two subscales. The Balance subscale measures a physical impairment; the Gait subscale measures a functional limitation integral to mobility.

Single-item measures have been used as indicators of the dimensions of functional limitations. Some items from the Tinetti (1986) Balance subscale have been used as single indicators of functional limitations (e.g., arising from a chair, bending down, or reaching up). Other single-item measures include the Get Up and Go test, the distance walked in 6 minutes, and walking speed (Nevitt, Cummings, Kidd, & Black, 1989). These latter items measure separate physical impairments, such as balance or muscle strength, from functional limitations.

Self-report has been used to measure functional limitation, but the quality of the data depends on the accuracy of the perceptions of respondents. These measures can be biased by cognitive impairment, social desirability, or minimization of impairments. Thus, self-report measures have respondent bias but may more accurately depict what the elderly person actually does than objective measures.

Observation has been thought to be less biased, or as biased, as self-report. Elderly adults may be able to perform a task but may not do so in their daily lives because of environmental obstacles, inaccurate perceptions of their capabilities, pain, the influence of others, or availability of informal support. Hence, both objective and self-report measures should be used because they provide different types of information about functional limitations and have different limitations.

Disability

Hierarchical relationships between ADLs and IADLs suggest that they represent a continuum of the same construct (Johnson & Wolinsky, 1993; Spector, Katz, Murphy, & Fulton, 1987). ADLs are hierarchically structured according to the development of complex motor tasks: eating, continence, transfer, going to the bathroom, dressing, and bathing (Spector et al., 1987). IADLs are more complex tasks than ADLs because they are more dependent on cognitive and physical capabilities (Johnson & Wolinsky, 1993). Although ADLs and IADLS have often been treated separately, they are highly related (Chappell & Badger, 1989; Strain, 1991), and a summative measure of these is appropriate. However, understanding the functional limitations that contribute to each activity may require treating each task separately.

ADLs measures have been used widely in research with elderly adults and have been used to identify active life expectancy characterized by independence (Katz, Branch, et al., 1983). The Katz ADL scale (Katz, Ford, Moskowitz, Jackson, & Jaffe, 1963) is the most frequently used instrument. The response categories in the original instrument were dichotomous (dependent or independent). To increase the variability of scores and sen-

sitivity of the instrument, other response schemes have been used. To be consistent with Nagi's definition, the response categories should represent difficulty in performing the tasks, not dependence (Verbrugge & Jette, 1994). No matter the responses used, this instrument has good reliability and validity. Other measures of ADLs include information obtained by self-report (e.g., the elder, caregiver, or health professional) or observations of performance. Glick and Swanson (1995) separated the tasks included in ADLs into those primarily dependent on the upper body and those primarily dependent on the lower body. For example, upper body tasks include brushing teeth and washing the face. In contrast, lower body measures include motor functions integral to independence (e.g., standing balance, turning, and getting up from a chair), but these tasks are not aspects of disability but functional limitations. Last, some measures, such as the Performance Test of ADL (Kruiansky & Gurland, 1976), also contain items measuring IADLs.

IADLs comprise household tasks (e.g., making meals and housekeeping) and others required to access resources (e.g., phoning, shopping). Although there is consensus in the definition of IADLs, there is not consensus about the tasks necessary for independent living, and no widely accepted measure of IADLs has emerged. However, the most often used measure is the Older American Resource Services (OARS) (Fillenbaum & Smyer, 1981).

Observation and self-report have been used to measure ADLs and IADLs. Concerns about bias in self-report measures led to the development of observational instruments (e.g., Loewenstein et al., 1989; Skurla, Rogers, & Sunderland, 1988). The limitations and advantages of self-report and observation described for functional limitation are also applicable to ADLs and IADLs. However, self-report measures may be less sensitive to early changes in these activities; observational measures may be more sensitive (Ruben, Siu, & Kimpau, 1992), but the psychometric properties of observational measures have not been found to be superior (Myers, Holliday, Harvey, & Hutchinson, 1993).

Proxies have provided information on ADLs and IADLs, but their ratings and those of the older adult have not been consistent. Discrepancies between them cannot be resolved (Rubenstein et al., 1984), but Magaziner, Simonsick, Kashner, and Hebel (1988) found significant discrepancy only for severely cognitively impaired adults; small discrepancies were found when the proxies were 65 years or older, a sibling or spouse, and lived with the person and provided assistance. The self-reports of elderly adults were more highly related to observed measures than those of families and physicians (Elam et al., 1989). Hence, the elderly adult, if cognitively intact, may be the most accurate source of information.

Synthesis of Research

Performance of daily activities is dependent on a complex interplay of physical, psychological, social, and environmental factors that are integral to the decisions elderly adults make about whether and how they engage in activities. Older age has been consistently associated with functional limitations (e.g., holding objects, lifting weights, stooping, or standing) (Jette & Branch, 1981), as well as greater dependence in daily activities (e.g., Jette & Branch, 1981; Jette, Branch, & Berlin, 1990; Palmore, Nowlin, & Wang, 1985); being female has sometimes been associated with disability (Palmore et al., 1985; Seeman, Charpentier, et al., 1994). However, these demographic characteristics are not amenable to intervention, and they may be explained by gender differences in functional limitations and impairments (e.g., postural stability or muscle strength) or by the impact of disease. Hence, research on these variables is not reviewed here. Rather, the focus of this chapter is on research related to impairments, functional limitation, and disability. Research on physical factors (postural stability, gait, and muscle strength) related to functional limitations and their impact on daily activities is reviewed first because, in some studies and in a large sample of elderly adults ($N = 9,704$), these have been found to be significantly associated with independence in daily activities even when age, gender, and disease status were controlled (Ensrud et al., 1994). Although these physical factors and functional limitations may be a consequence of disease, they are more proximate factors related to disability and may have an effect on disability irrespective of disease. Physical factors and functional limitations are also more amenable to nursing intervention than the treatment of disease. Next, psychological, social, and environmental factors are discussed. Although there is no known research on decisions that elderly adults make regarding performing daily activities, the possible effects of these on independence in these activities will be discussed, using research about cognitive appraisal of physical abilities and risk for falls, as well as coping strategies. Risks for falls is included in this section be-

cause a fall reflects a loss of independence in safe ambulation. Potential interventions and those assessed in research are identified throughout this section.

Relationship Between Functional Limitations and Disability

A relationship of functional limitations to disability has not always been found and may be explained by the measures used. Most investigators (e.g., Hughes, Dunlop, Edelman, Chang, & Singer, 1994; Palmore et al., 1985) have used summary measures of functional limitations and have not considered that functional limitations of the upper and lower extremities, concepts in the disablement model, may have differential effects on disability. Upper body function (e.g., grasping or reaching) has been associated with performance of ADLs (Jette, Branch, & Berlin, 1990; Lawrence & Jette, 1996); lower body function (e.g., arising from a chair or bending down to pick up an object) has been associated with IADLs (Lawrence & Jette, 1996; Wolinsky, Callahan, Fitzgerald, & Johnson, 1993). Moreover, advanced IADLs, which require cognitive capabilities (e.g., managing money, preparing meals, or using the phone), are distinctly different from other dimensions (Johnson & Wolinsky, 1993; Wolinsky & Johnson, 1991), but all dimensions are interrelated (Wolinsky et al., 1993).

Considerable heterogeneity in disability has been found among elderly adults. Even when dependent in some activities of daily living, elderly adults may regain independence (Branch, Katz, Kniepmann, & Papsidero, 1984; Manton, 1988) or may become more dependent (Wolinsky et al., 1993). Functional limitations are associated with a decline in independence in ADLs and IADLs (Guralnik, Ferrucci, Simonsick, Salive, & Wallace, 1995; Harris, Kovar, Suzman, Kleinman, & Felman, 1989; Jette et al., 1990; Lawrence & Jette, 1996; Palmore et al., 1985). However, improvement and decline may have different correlates. For example, improvement has been associated with less functional limitation at baseline and a small loss of independence from baseline to the next measurement; decline in independence in daily activities has been associated with demographic characteristics and disease when functional limitations have not been measured (Crimmins & Saito, 1993). Decline in independence in one daily activity can be associated with decline in other activities, but, over time, the patterns of independence in daily activities may differ; that is, independence in one activity may be offset by dependence in other activities (Crimmins & Saito, 1993). The importance of separating functional limitations from disability can be demonstrated by looking at the effects of exercise. Although the frequency of physical activity (currently or in the past) is associated with greater independence in ADLs and IADLs (e.g., Harris, Dunlop, Edelman, Chang, & Singer, 1994; Mor et al., 1989), this can be accounted for by improvements in upper and lower body functional limitations (Lawrence & Jette, 1996).

Physical Factors Related to Functional Limitation

Gait

Although gait requires movement of the whole body, control of body position during movement, as indicated by characteristics of gait and responses to postural perturbations, is essential for mobility and independence in daily activities (Hu & Woollacott, 1995). Hence, characteristics of gait are consistent with the definition of functional limitation. Most research has evaluated the effects of gait on falls (loss of independence in walking and transferring). Patterning of stepping (Clark, Lord, & Webster, 1993) and decreases in toe and heel clearance during the swing phase of gait have been related to falls or altered responses to stepping over obstacles (Chen, Ashton-Miller, Alexander, & Schultz, 1991). Last, greater anteroflexion of the upper torso during gait moves the center of gravity forward over the base of support and reduces the distance the foot can be moved forward, which can reduce stride length (Tideiksaar, 1995). Gait speed and stride length have also been found to predict recovery of mobility (Friedman, Rickmond, & Basket, 1988), reflecting their importance in everyday activities.

Postural responses to perturbations are less effective among elderly adults than among young adults (e.g., Luchies, Alexander, Schultz, & Ashton-Miller, 1994; Manchester, Woollacott, Zederbauer-Hylton, & Martin, 1989), and these responses have been associated with falls among older adults (e.g., Wolfson, Whipple, Amerman, & Kleinberg, 1986). However, the relationship between responses to perturbations and independence in activities of daily living has not been established. Although several characteristics of gait are important to the elderly person's ability to engage in daily activities, more

research needs to be done to link gait characteristics to independence in these activities.

Physical activity has been associated with greater independence in daily activities, but little research has examined the effects of exercise on these activities. However, some findings support the potential positive effects of exercise on gait. For example, aerobic walking has been associated with greater toe and heel clearance, greater percentage of time in single-stance phase of gait, and slower gait speed, all of which indicate better neuromotor control of gait (Roberts, Srour, Woollacott, & Tang, 1994). Muscle-strengthening exercise increased gait velocity (Topp, Mikesky, Wigglesworth, Holt, & Edwards, 1993) and reduced the use of assistive devices for ambulation (Fiatarone et al., 1990). In contrast, Tai Chi reduced gait velocity (Wolf et al., 1996). Differences in the results of these interventions may be attributable to the type of gait used (usual, slowest, or highest), the gait characteristics measured, and the differing effects of each type of exercise on impairment, functional limitation, and disability.

Postural Stability

Postural stability is integral to the performance of activities of daily living and is manifested in the ability to maintain a stable posture, whether upright or sitting. Poor postural stability has been associated with falls (e.g., Clark, Lord, & Webster, 1993; Pescatello & Judge, 1995; Robbins et al., 1989), and greater postural stability has been associated with fewer limitations in ADLs among institutionalized elderly adults (Roberts & Wykle, 1993). Although no investigator has assessed the effects of increasing postural stability on independence in ADLs and IADLs, aerobic exercise (e.g., Roberts, 1989; Roberts, Srour, Mansour, Palmer, & Wagner, 1994b), Tai Chi (e.g., Tse & Bailey, 1992), and balance training (e.g., Wolf et al., 1996) have all had significant positive effects on postural stability.

Muscle Strength

A few days of inactivity and immobility reduce muscle strength, with muscles of the lower extremities showing the greatest loss (Tideiksaar, 1995). The strength of these muscles is integral to functional limitations (e.g., arising from a chair or for the stabilization of the knee during walking and standing) and to independence in ambulation, transfers, and toileting (aspects of activities of daily living) (Roberts, 1993). For example, greater strength of the quadriceps was associated with less time to walk a known distance and arise from a chair (Fiatarone et al., 1990). Greater strength of the knee flexors and extensors was related to walking farther before exhaustion (Ades, Ballor, Ashikaga, Utton, & Nair, 1996), and greater strength of hip extensors was associated with independence in getting up from a chair (Kaufman, 1983).

Although the effect of muscle strength on independence in daily activities has yet to be determined, strength of the plantar and dorsal flexors of the ankle has been found to be lower in elderly adults who fell (Whipple, Wolfson, & Amerman, 1987). Other investigators have described a potential threshold in strength where dependence in daily activities begins (Cress, Questad, et al., 1995). Because muscle strength is lower in women than in men (e.g., Frontera, Hughes, Lutz, & Evans, 1991; Vandervoort & McComas, 1986), the greater dependence in ADLs and IADLs found in women may be related to gender differences in strength.

Strength training and aerobic exercise involving the lower extremities have been associated with increases in muscle strength. In a study of high-intensity strength training in nursing home residents, Fiatarone and associates (1990) found that this intervention decreased the use of assistive devices and increased distances walked (also found by Schilke, Johnson, Housh, & O'Dell, 1996). Independence in ambulation is requisite for some ADLs and most IADLs, and muscle strengthening interventions have the potential to increase independence in daily activities, but more research is needed in this area.

With declines in muscle strength, greater activation of existing muscle fibers is required to get up from a chair, climb stairs, or walk to the kitchen (Pescatello & Judge, 1995). Thus, an activity that may have required 25% of maximal strength may now require 70%. Although elderly adults may be capable of doing the activity, Pescatello and Judge (1995) hypothesize that they may perceive a task as too demanding and be less likely to perform it or more likely to request assistance with it. However, the relationships among strength and perceptions of difficulty during a task and independence in this task have not been established.

Psychological Factors

Cognitive Impairment

Most research results suggest a relationship between cognitive impairment and dependence in daily activities, whether instrumental or related to self-care (e.g., Hill,

Backman, & Fratiglioni, 1995; Teri, Borson, Kiyak, & Yamagishi, 1989), no matter whether measured by self-report or objective assessment (Skurla, Rogers, & Sunderland, 1988). Cognitive impairment also predicts subsequent dependence in ADLs (e.g., Moritz, Kasl, & Berman, 1995). Cognitive impairment was the strongest predictor of dependence in ADLs and IADLs, and visuoperception explained a significant amount of additional variance in dependence (Hill et al., 1995). These findings suggest that sensory factors associated with cognitive impairments may be important to independence but these factors have not been identified. Interventions that decrease cognitive impairment should also increase independence in ADLs and IADLs.

Depression

Depression has been associated with poor physical health and with an increased risk of development of dependence in ADLs, even when physical function was controlled (Bruce, Seeman, Merrill, & Blazer, 1994). Depression has been related to IADLs (heavy home chores, housekeeping, and carrying a bundle) and functional limitations (walking a mile and climbing stairs) (Guccione et al., 1994). A possible explanation for these findings is that depression may limit what a person is willing to do or that the restriction of activity often found with depression may reduce physical competencies related to activities of daily living (Bruce et al., 1994). These hypotheses deserve further exploration.

Environmental Factors

Environments of Care

Although nursing home residents are likely to experience functional limitations, the trajectory of changes in function has not been adequately studied. In a study of long-stay elderly persons (residence of 100 days or more), slight improvement or maintenance of independence in ADLs was found from admission to 1 year later (Gillen, Spore, Mor, & Freiberger, 1996). Although this sample did not include persons residing in the facility more than a year, the findings suggest that functional decline is not inevitable and that subgroups of elderly adults may have different trajectories. These results support the findings by others that even those who have a long stay in the nursing home have heterogeneous trajectories of dependence (Manton, Liu, & Cornelius, 1985).

During hospitalization, more than 60% of elderly patients have some loss of independence in ADLs and IADLs (Campion, Jette, & Berkman, 1983). Elderly patients who are dependent in some IADLs and up to three ADLs are at high risk of dependency in ADLs during hospitalization, which may continue after discharge (Hing & Bloom, 1990). Little is known about the trajectory of changes in independence in daily activities during and after hospitalization, and even less is known about the underlying factors that affect recovery after discharge. Moreover, in spite of clinical evidence of dependence in ADLs, nurses did not identify self-care deficit as a nursing diagnosis and may not have intervened to promote independence (Roberts, Anthony, Madiger, & Pabst, in press). Hospitalization is associated with acute illness or serious exacerbation of chronic conditions, so the primary focus is prevention and resolution of life-threatening conditions, and the current short length of stays may preclude adequate attention to factors affecting independence in daily activities. Patients are now discharged "sicker and quicker," thus interventions to promote independence may now be priorities in home care services and short-term rehabilitation programs in long-term care facilities and hospitals.

Even elderly adults living independently in the community experience dependence in IADLs and ADLs. As noted above, cognitive impairment (e.g., Moritz et al., 1995), functional limitations in the lower and upper extremities (e.g., Guralnik et al., 1995) and depression (e.g., Bruce et al., 1994) have been associated with dependence. Functional limitations and hazards in the home have been associated with falls (Northridge, Nevitt, Kelsey, & Link, 1995). Elderly adults at home may remain independent because of environmental factors and social support that differ from the environment and support found in a hospital or nursing home (Roberts & Fitzpatrick, 1994). More longitudinal studies are needed to describe the trajectory of independence in ADLs and IADLs and related factors.

The progressively lowered stress threshold model, in which environmental demands are consistent with elders' physical and cognitive abilities, has been used in nursing homes to reduce disruptive behavior in cognitively impaired adults (Hall & Buckwalter, 1987), and it holds promise for developing interventions to reduce dependency and improve behavior in other settings. Special care units consistent with the model significantly improved social behavior but not ADLs (Swanson, Maas, & Buckwalter, 1994). This model may also apply to care-givers, who are part of the environment. For example, greater caregiver expectations of the resident's independence in daily activities was related to greater independence (e.g., Langer & Rodin, 1976), and behavior management to encourage residents to do self-care increased independence in ADLs (Blair, 1995).

Social Support

Social support has been associated with dependence in activities of daily living (e.g., Bowling, Farquhar, & Grundy, 1994; Seeman, Charpentier, et al., 1994). This support has usually been conceptualized as provision of tangible support, although emotional support has also been identified. Among nursing home residents, dependence in self-care tasks was greater when nursing personnel provided assistance with these activities than when the residents were encouraged to do them themselves (e.g., Langer & Rodin, 1976). In community-dwelling elders, Roberts, Anthony, Matejczyk, and Moore (1994) found that men and women mobilized social support differently in response to difficulties in mobility, ADLs, and household IADLs. In women, greater mobility was associated with greater tangible support and, to a lesser extent, to greater emotional support, but in men these relationships were very small. Also, men had much larger associations of emotional support to household IADLs and ADLs. Similarly, instrumental and emotional support were associated with subsequent dependence in ADLs for men but not women (Seeman, Bruce, & McVay, 1996). Perhaps, the availability of social support and the willingness of persons in the social network to provide assistance encourages elderly adults to avail themselves of this assistance even when they are capable of performing the task independently. These findings, however, suggest that social support may have negative effects, and the responses of men and women to it may also differ.

Decision Making

Performance of daily activities is dependent on complex interrelated environmental, physical, psychological, and social factors that affect decisions elderly adults make about when and how to engage in daily activities. Integral to these decisions is the person's appraisal of the adequacy of personal competencies and environmental factors. These decisions may explain why elderly adults can perform ADLs and IADLs but self-report dependence in them.

In cognitively intact adults, the congruence between functional competence and the appraisal of competence may be low. For example, Roberts (1989) found a moderate relationship between observed and perceived postural stability; others found small to moderate associations between perceived and observed physical function (Cress, Questad, et al., 1995). Hence, perceptions of functional competencies and environmental hazards may not be consistent with actual abilities and environmental factors. Moreover, fear of falling, an appraisal of the risk of this event, was found to increase disability because elders restricted their activities (e.g., Tinetti, Mendes de Leon, Doucette, & Baker, 1994). Hence, behavior based on inaccurate perceptions may place a person at greater risk for dependence.

Self-efficacy, a type of cognitive appraisal, is the perceived confidence to perform certain behaviors and is related to actual performance of them (Bandura, 1986). Self-efficacy is context specific and is not generalizable to other domains of behavior. The most widely studied falls in self-efficacy have been related to reduced participation in activities (e.g., Tinetti et al., 1994). Moreover, low self-efficacy was associated with decline in independence in ADLs, although high self-efficacy was not associated with greater independence (Mendes de Leon, Seeman, Baker, Richardson, & Tinetti, 1996). The latter findings are consistent with the hypothesis that self-efficacy has the greatest effect on the probability of performing behaviors when these behaviors are threatened or challenged, such as in disability (Bandura, 1989). Although elders make decisions about engaging in daily activities, the effects of these decisions on daily tasks and the effect of self-efficacy on independence has yet to be explored. Yet, these decisions may be as important as the factors described above, and they have the potential to explain why some elders are dependent in certain daily activities in spite of physical and psychological capabilities to perform the activities safely. The information used in making these decisions and the congruence between actual and perceived functional capacities needs to be explored. Research is needed to understand this decision-making process and to develop interventions to assist elderly adults in making choices that allow them to be as independent as is possible in daily activities.

Coping

The congruence between actual and perceived impairments, functional limitations, and factors in the environment relevant to safe mobility are not only crucial to the person's decision to move about but also to the manner in which it is done. For example, a person who perceives functional limitations may be more vigilant about environmental hazards and take additional precautions during movement, such as holding onto furniture, a hypothesis supported by a case history (Fried, Herdman, Kuhn, Rubin, & Turano, 1991). These actions may reduce the person's risk of dependence or falls below the risk that exists when extra vigilance and precautions are not used. Although these compensatory strategies in the presence of functional limitations and impairment have been noted, little research has explicated their role within a multifactorial model of disability.

Clinical Practice Issues and Directions for Research

Assessment

An understanding of the multiple factors associated with functional limitation and the threshold of limitations where dependence in daily activities occurs will provide direction for assessment. Although cardiovascular disease and arthritis have been associated with greater dependence in daily activities (e.g., Guccione et al., 1994; Harris, Kovar, et al., 1989), a large proportion of elderly adults have these diseases and yet are not dependent in ADLs and IADLs. Hence, disease alone is not a sensitive indicator of functional limitation or disability. However, a subgroup of people with more advanced disease will have functional limitations associated with walking, bending, and stooping; a smaller proportion of this group will also be dependent in some daily activities.

The large body of research focused on the physical factors related to functional health should be extended to identify the simultaneous contributions of many factors and determine the thresholds where decrements in these factors are associated with declines in independence in daily tasks. Thresholds of physical and psychological impairment and functional limitations have the potential to be more sensitive and specific in identifying elderly adults at risk for dependence than disease alone. For example, Stern and associates (1996) found that cognitive impairment preceded dependence in ADLs and IADLs, and this relationship was not based on the timing of changes but on the level of cognitive impairment. Although research on thresholds is rudimentary at best, future investigations should focus on measures that can be used in clinical practice and the development of norms.

All too often, investigators have treated elderly adults as a homogeneous group contrary to the great heterogeneity in this population related to aging, disease, history of physical activity, and life circumstances. The factors associated with functional limitation and disability will differ even among people with similar pathologies. The pattern of functional limitations and disability may also vary in different pathologies and impairments, which may require differing interventions. For example, elderly adults with osteoarthritis in the knees and those with chronic heart failure may not be able to walk a mile or climb a flight of steps. Although the functional limitations are similar, the contributing underlying pathologies and impairments differ, and the appropriate interventions to reduce functional limitations also differ. Also, different functional limitations may be associated with different types of disability. For example, functional limitations of the lower extremities are more strongly associated with dependence in IADLs than they are with limitations in the upper extremities (Lawrence & Jette, 1996; Jette et al., 1990).

Assessment strategies require an understanding of the multiplicity of environmental, physical, and psychological factors related to functional limitations and dependence. Assessment strategies and norms for thresholds and their assessment developed through research should be clinically relevant and feasible. Last, the role of decisions that elderly adults make about whether and how they will engage in daily behaviors has been ignored but has important implications for assessment beyond that related to impairments, functional limitations, and disability.

▦ Interventions

Most interventions reviewed above or suggested by research results have focused on one or a limited number of impairments, functional limitations, and disability, but the most effective ones will probably focus on multiple underlying factors. For example, interventions have included outpatient geriatric assessment and management (Boult et al., 1994), nursing protocols in an acute care unit for elders (Landefeld et al., 1995), and a nurse-managed clinic to reduce functional limitations and disability (Evans, Yurkow, & Siegler, 1995). Most multidimensional interventions are costly, and their effects have been small to modest at best. Hence, the cost of the intervention (time, personnel, and money) must be weighed against its benefits. The development of such interven-

tions requires an understanding of the factors contributing to functional limitations and dependence, and identifying those most likely to benefit from the interventions requires being able to identify those at high risk. Gaining insight into risks for disability and functional limitation, and thresholds in factors related to these, will require studying subpopulations of elderly adults who are expected to have reduced capabilities in certain areas. Knowledge of underlying risk factors can then be used to identify those at highest risk and to provide direction to develop interventions targeted to specific risk factors. Hence, interventions can be targeted to those elders who would benefit most, which is very important when interventions are costly and time consuming for the health care provider and elderly adult or are associated with significant risk. Because large changes in underlying factors may be needed before any change is possible in complex tasks of daily living, knowledge of thresholds where rapid decline in independence occurs is needed to target interventions to those factors contributing the most to this decline and to persons at greatest risk. The effects of interventions on underlying impairments and functional limitations may be significant, but the effects on disability may be smaller and may emerge only when effects are large enough to overcome thresholds in impairments and functional limitations.

Interventions may be most beneficial for the moderately and severely functionally impaired who have little room to deteriorate further and may be nearer thresholds for dependence in activities than those with little or no impairments. For example, a nurse-managed outpatient service for moderately impaired elderly adults focuses on assessment and interventions to increase independence in daily activities (Evans et al., 1995). In nursing home residents, a walking program increased mobility (Koroknay, Werner, Cohen-Mansfield, & Braun, 1995), and chair exercises improved rising from a chair and decreased dependency in activities (McMurdo & Rennie, 1993). However, more research is needed to determine if some subgroups are so impaired that they receive little or no benefits from an intervention.

Functional limitations and disability can arise from sources other than pathology, so other factors amenable to change should be the focus of interventions. For example, high body mass and frequency of walking a mile were predictors of functional limitations (Lawrence & Jette, 1996). Hence, a weight loss intervention and exercise may be able to reduce impairments and functional limitations. An understanding of the role of cognitive appraisal of the environment and personal competencies and coping may lead to different interventions than considered thus far.

Directions for Research

Although there is a large body of research on disability, functional limitations, and the physical and cognitive factors integral to these, only recently has research examined the relationship of appraisal of capabilities to functional limitation, much less their role in daily activities. Although research identifying thresholds where functional limitations and dependency occur is even less developed, this research may be very fruitful in identify-

ing elderly adults at high risk for loss of independence in daily activities and in understanding the complexity of underlying factors in the performance of functional tasks and dependency. As persons dependent in daily activities are more likely to be institutionalized and receive costly formal services, those at high risk of dependency may need to be the focus of future research and development of interventions. A subgroup of the elderly who should be targeted are those elders with functional limitations who have not yet developed dependency. Although a considerable body of knowledge has been developed about activities of daily living and related impairments and functional limitations, there are several areas in need of more research. However, nurse researchers must ensure that the knowledge generated is applicable to practice.

References

Ades, P. A., Ballor, D. L., Ashikaga, T., Utton, J. L., & Nair, K. S. (1996). Weight training improves walking endurance in healthy elderly persons. *Annals of Internal Medicine, 124,* 568-572.

Avlund, K., Davidsen, M., & Schultz-Larsen, E. (1995). Changes in functional ability from ages 70 to 75. *Journal of Aging and Health, 7,* 254-282.

Bandura, A. (1986). *Social foundations of thought and action: A social cognitive theory.* Engelwood Cliffs, NJ: Prentice Hall.

Bandura, A. (1989). Human agency in social cognitive theory. *American Psychologist, 44,* 1175-1184.

Blair, C. E. (1995). Combining behavior management and mutual goal setting to reduce physical dependency in nursing home residents. *Nursing Research, 44,* 160-165.

Boult, C., Boult, L., Murphy, C., Ebbitt, B., Luptak, M., & Kane, R. L. (1994). A controlled trial of outpatient geriatric evaluation and management. *Journal of the American Geriatrics Society, 42,* 465-470.

Bowling, A., Farquhar, M., & Grundy, E. (1994). Associations with changes in level of functional ability: Results from a follow-up survey at two and a half years of people aged 85 years and over at baseline interview. *Ageing and Society, 14,* 53-73.

Branch, L. G., Katz, S., Kniepmann, K., & Papsidero, J. A. (1984). A prospective study of functional status among community elders. *American Journal of Public Health, 74*(3), 266-268.

Brown, I., Renwick, R., & Raphael, D. (1995). Frailty: Constructing a common meaning, definition and conceptual framework. *International Journal of Rehabilitation Research, 18,* 93-102.

Bruce, M. L., Seeman, T. E., Merrill, S. S., & Blazer, D. G. (1994). The impact of depressive symptomology on physical disability: MacArthur studies of successful aging. *American Journal of Public Health, 84,* 1796-1799.

Buchner, D. M., Beresford, S.A.A., Larson, E. B., LaCroix, A. Z., & Wagner, E. H. (1992). Effects of physical activity on health status in older adults II: Interventional studies. *Annual Review of Public Health, 13,* 469-488.

Campion, E. W., Jette, A., & Berkman, B. (1983). An interdisciplinary geriatric consultation service: A controlled trial. *Journal of the American Geriatrics Society, 31,* 792-796.

Chappell, N. L., & Badger, M. (1989). Social isolation and well-being. *Journals of Gerontology: Social Sciences, 44,* S169-S176.

Chen, H. C., Ashton-Miller, J. A., Alexander, N. B., & Schultz, A. B. (1991). Stepping over obstacles: Gait patterns of healthy young and old adults. *Journals of Gerontology: Medical Sciences, 46,* M196-203.

Clark, R. D., Lord, S. R., & Webster, I. W. (1993). Clinical parameters associated with falls in an elderly population. *Gerontology, 39,* 117-123.

Cress, M. E., Questad, K. A., Esselman, P. E., Schwartz, D. B., Buchner, D. B., & De Lateur, B. J. (1995). Physical functional reserve in independent elders [abstract]. *The Gerontologist, 35,* 164.

Cress, M. E., Schechtman, K. B., Mulrow, C. D., Fiatarone, M. A., Gerety, M. B., & Buchner, D. M. (1995). Relationship between physical performance and self-perceived physical function. *Journal of the American Geriatrics Society, 43,* 93-101.

Crimmins, E. M. (1996). Mixed trends in population health among older persons. *Journals of Gerontology: Social Sciences, 51B,* S223-S225.

Crimmins, E. M., & Saito, Y. (1993). Getting better and getting worse. *Journal of Aging and Health, 5,* 3-36.

Elam, J. T., Beaver, T., El Derwi, D., Applegate, W. B., Graney, M. J., & Miller, S. T. (1989). Comparison of sources of functional report with observed functional ability of frail older persons [abstract]. *The Gerontologist, 29*(Suppl.), 30A.

Ensrud, K. E., Nevitt, M. C., Yunis, C., Cauley, J. A., Seeley, D. G., Fox, K. M., & Cummings, S. R. (1994). Correlates of impaired function in older women. *Journal of the American Geriatrics Society, 42,* 481-489.

Evans, L. K., Yurkow, J., & Siegler, E. L. (1995). The CARE program: A nurse managed collaborative outpatient program to improve function of frail older people. Collaborative assessment and rehabilitation for elders. *Journal of the American Geriatrics Society, 43,* 1155-1160.

Fiatarone, M. A., Marks, M. S., Ryan, N. D., Meredith, C. N., Lipsitz, L. A., & Evans, W. J. (1990). High-intensity strength training in nonagenarians: Effects on skeletal muscle. *Journal of the American Medical Association, 263,* 3029-3034.

Fillenbaum, G. G., & Smyer, M. A. (1981). The development, validity and reliability of the OARS multidimensional functional assessment questionnaire. *Journals of Gerontology, 36,* 428-434.

Fried, L. P., Herdman, S. J., Kuhn, K. E., Rubin, G., & Turano, K. (1991). Preclinical disability: Hypotheses about the bottom of the iceberg. *Journal of Aging and Health, 3,* 285-300.

Friedman, P. J., Rickmond, D. E., & Basket, J. J. (1988). A prospective trial of serial gait speed as a measure of rehabilitation in the elderly. *Age and Ageing, 17,* 227-235.

Frontera, W., Hughes, V., Lutz, K., & Evans, W. (1991). A cross-sectional study of muscle strength and mass in 45- to 78-yr-old men and women. *Journal of Applied Physiology, 67,* 644-650.

Gillen, P., Spore, D., Mor, V., & Freiberger, W. (1996). Functional and residential status transitions among nursing home residents. *Journals of Gerontology: Medical Sciences, 51A,* M29-M36.

Glick, O. J., & Swanson, E. A. (1995). Motor performance correlates of functional dependence in long-term care residents. *Nursing Research, 44,* 4-8.

Grimby, G., Finnstam, J., & Jette, A. (1988). On the application of the WHO handicap classification in rehabilitation. *Scandinavian Journal of Rehabilitation Medicine, 20,* 93-98.

Guccione, A. A., Felson, D. T., Anderson, J. J., Anthony, J. M., Zhang, Y., Wilson, P.W.J., Kelly-Hayes, M., Wolf, P. A., Kreger, B. E., & Kannel, W. B. (1994). The effects of specific medical conditions on the functional limitations of elders in the Framingham study. *American Journal of Public Health, 84,* 351-358.

Guralnik, J. M., Ferrucci, L., Simonsick, E. M., Salive, M. E., & Wallace, R. B. (1995). Lower-extremity function in persons over the age of 70 years as a predictor of subsequent disability. *New England Journal of Medicine, 332,* 556-561.

Hall, G. R., & Buckwalter, K. C. (1987). Progressively lowered stress threshold: A conceptual model for care of adults with Alzheimer's disease. *Archives of Psychiatric Nursing, 1,* 399-406.

Harris, S. L., Dunlop, D., Edelman, P., Chang, R. W., & Singer, R. H. (1994). Impact of joint impairment on longitudinal disability in elderly persons. *Journals of Gerontology: Social Sciences, 49,* S291-S300.

Harris, T., Kovar, M. G., Suzman, R., Kleinman, J. C., & Felman, J. J. (1989). Longitudinal study of physical ability in the oldest-old. *American Journal of Public Health, 79,* 698-702.

Hill, R. D., Backman, L., & Fratiglioni, L. (1995). Determinant of functional abilities in dementia. *Journal of the American Geriatrics Society, 43,* 1092-1097.

Hing, E., & Bloom, B. (1990). *Vital health statistics, series 13.* Hyattsville, MD: National Center for Health Statistics.

Hirsch, C. H., Sommers, L., Olsen, S., Mullen, L., & Winograd, C. H. (1990). The natural history of functional morbidity in hospitalized older patients. *Journal of the American Geriatrics Society, 38,* 1296-1303.

Hogue, C. C. (1984). Falls and mobility in late life: An ecological model. *Journal of the American Geriatrics Society, 32,* 858-861.

Hu, M., & Woollacott, M. (1995). Characteristic patterns of gait in older persons. In B. S. Spivack (Ed.), *Evaluation and management of gait disorders* (pp. 167-185). New York: Marcel Dekker.

Hughes, S. L., Dunlop, D., Edelman, Chang, R. W., & Singer, R. H. (1994). Impact of joint impairment on longitudinal disability in elderly persons. *Journal of Gerontology, 49*(6), S291-S300.

Jette, A. M., & Branch, L. G. (1981, November). The Framingham Disability Study: II. Physical disability among the aging. *American Journal of Public Health, 71*(11), 1211-1216.

Jette, A. M., Branch, L. G., & Berlin, J. (1990). Musculoskeletal impairments and physical disablement among the aged. *Journals of Gerontology: Medical Sciences, 45,* M203-M208.

Johnson, R. J., & Wolinsky, F. D. (1993). The structure of health status among older adults: Disease, disability, functional limitation and perceived health. *Journal of Health and Social Behavior, 34,* 105-121.

Kane, R. A., & Kane, R. L. (1981). *Assessing the elderly: A practical guide to measurement.* Lexington, MA: Lexington Books.

Katz, S., Branch, L. G., Branson, M. H., Papsidero, J. A., Beck, J. C., & Greer, D. S. (1983). Active life expectancy. *New England Journal of Medicine, 309,* 1218-1224.

Katz, S., Ford, A. D., Moskowitz, R. W., Jackson, B. A., & Jaffe, M. W. (1963). Studies of illness in the aged, index of ADL: Standardized measure of biological and psychosocial function. *Journal of the American Medical Association, 185,* 914-919.

Kaufman, T. (1983). Association between hip extension strength and standup ability in geriatric patients. *Physical and Occupational Therapy in Geriatrics, 1,* 39-41.

Koroknay, V. J., Werner, P., Cohen-Mansfield, J., & Braun, J. V. (1995). Maintaining ambulation in the frail nursing home resident: A nursing administered walking program. *Journal of Gerontological Nursing, 21*(11), 18-24.

Kruiansky, J., & Gurland, B. (1976). The performance test of activities of daily living. *International Journal of Aging and Human Development, 7,* 343-352.

Landefeld, C. S., Palmer, R., Kowal, J., Kresevic, D., Fortinsky, R. H., & Kowal, J. (1995). A randomized trial of care in a hospital medical unit especially designed to increase functional outcomes of acutely ill older patients. *New England Journal of Medicine, 332,* 1338-1344.

Langer, E. J., & Rodin, J. (1976). The effects of choice and enhanced personal responsibility for the aged: A field experiment in an institutional setting. *Journal of Personality and Social Psychology, 34,* 191-198.

Larson, J. L., Covey, M. K., Vitalo, C. A., Alex, C. G., Patel, M., & Kim, M. J. (1996). Reliability and validity of the 12-minute distance walk in patients with chronic obstructive pulmonary disease. *Nursing Research, 45,* 203-210.

Lawrence, R. H., & Jette, A. M. (1996). Disentangling the disablement process. *Journals of Gerontology: Social Sciences, 51,* S173-S182.

Lawton, M. P. (1991). A multidimensional view of quality of life in frail elders. In J. E. Birren, J. C. Rowe, & D. E. Deutchman (Eds.), *The concept and measurement of quality of life in the frail and elderly* (pp. 4-27). San Diego: Academic Press.

Leidy, N. (1994). Functional status and the forward progress of merry-go-rounds: Toward a coherent analytical framework. *Nursing Research, 43,* 196-202.

Loewenstein, D. A., Amigo, E., Duara, R., Guterman, A., Hurwitz, D., Berkowitz, N., & Eisdorfer, C. (1989). A new scale for the assessment of functional status in Alzheimer's disease and related disorders. *Journals of Gerontology: Psychological Sciences, 44,* P114-P121.

Luchies, C. W., Alexander, N. B., Schultz, A. B., & Ashton-Miller, J. (1994). Stepping responses of young and old adults to postural disturbances: Kinematics. *Journal of the American Geriatrics Society, 42,* 506-512.

Magaziner, J., Simonsick, E. M., Kashner, T. M., & Hebel, J. R. (1988). Patient-proxy response comparability on measures of patient health and functional status. *Journal of Clinical Epidemiology, 41,* 1065-1074.

Manchester, D., Woollacott, M., Zederbauer-Hylton, N., & Martin, O. (1989). Visual, vestibular and somatosensory contributions to balance control in older adult. *Journals of Gerontology: Medical Sciences, 44,* M118-127.

Manton, K. G. (1988). A longitudinal study of functional change and mortality in the United States. *Journals of Gerontology: Social Sciences, 43,* S153-S161.

Manton, K. G., Liu, K., & Cornelius, E. S. (1985). An analysis of the heterogeneity of U.S. nursing home patients. *Journals of Gerontology, 40,* 34-46.

McHorney, C. A., Ware, J. E., & Raczek, A. E. (1993). The MOS 36-item short-form health survey (SF-36): II. Psychometric and clinical tests of validity in measuring physical and mental health constructs. *Medical Care, 31,* 247-263.

McMurdo, M. E., & Rennie, L. (1993). A controlled trial of exercise by residents of old people's homes. *Age and Ageing, 22,* 11-15.

Meenan, R. F., Gertman, P. M., & Mason, J. H. (1980). Measuring health status in arthritis: The Arthritis Impact Measurement Scales. *Arthritis and Rheumatism, 23,* 146-152.

Mendes de Leon, C. F., Seeman, T. E., Baker, D. I., Richardson, E. D., & Tinetti, M. E. (1996). Self-efficacy, physical decline, and change in functioning in community-living elders: A prospective study. *Journals of Gerontology: Social Sciences, 51B,* S183-S190.

Mor, V., Murphy, J., Masterson-Allen, S., Willey, C., Razmpour, A., Jackson, M. E., Greer, D., & Katz, S. (1989). Risk of functional decline among well elders. *Journal of Clinical Epidemiology, 42,* 895-904.

Moritz, D. J., Kasl, S. V., & Berman, L. F. (1995). Cognitive functioning and the incidence of limitations in activities of daily living in an elderly community sample. *American Journal of Epidemiology, 141,* 41-49.

Myers, A. M., Holliday, P. J., Harvey, K. A., & Hutchinson, K. S. (1993). Functional performance measures: Are they superior to self-assessments? *Journals of Gerontology: Medical Sciences, 48,* M196-M206.

Nagi, S. Z. (1991). Disability concepts revisited. In A. M. Pope and A. R. Tarlov (Eds.), *Disability in America: Toward a national agenda for prevention* (pp. 309-327). Washington, DC: National Academy Press.

Nevitt, M. C., Cummings, S. R., Kidd, S., & Black, D. (1989). Risk factors for recurrent non syncopal falls: A prospective study. *Journal of the American Medical Association, 261,* 2663-2668.

Northridge, M. E., Nevitt, M. C., Kelsey, J. L., & Link, B. (1995). Home hazards and falls in the elderly: The role of health and functional status. *American Journal of Public Health, 85,* 509-515.

Ottenbacher, K. J., Mann, W. C., Granger, C. V., Tomita, M., Hurren, D., & Charvat, B. (1994). Inter-rater agreement and stability of functional assessment in the community-based elderly. *Archives of Physical Medicine and Rehabilitation, 75,* 1297-1301.

Palmore, E. B., Nowlin, J. B., & Wang, H. S. (1985). Predictors of function among the old-old: A 10-year follow-up. *Journals of Gerontology, 40,* 244-250.

Peeters, P., & Mets, T. (1996). The 6-minute walk as an appropriate exercise test in elderly patients with chronic heart failure. *Journals of Gerontology: Medical Sciences, 51A,* M147-M151.

Pescatello, L. S., & Judge, J. O. (1995). The impact of physical activity and physical fitness on functional capacity in older adults. In B. S. Spivack (Ed.), *Evaluation and management of gait disorders* (pp. 325-339). New York: Marcel Dekker.

Robbins, A. S., Rubenstein, L. Z., Josephson, K. R., Schulman, B. L., Osterweil, D., & Fine, G. (1989). Predictors of falls among elderly people: Results of two population based studies. *Archives of Internal Medicine, 149,* 1628, 1633.

Roberts, B. L. (1989). The effects of walking on balance among elders. *Nursing Research, 38,* 180-182.

Roberts, B. L. (1993). Is a stay in an intensive care unit a risk for falls? *Applied Nursing Research, 6,* 135-136.

Roberts, B. L., Anthony, M., Madigan, E., & Pabst, S. (in press). Congruence between clinical indicators and nursing diagnoses. *Nursing Diagnosis.*

Roberts, B. L., Anthony, M. K., Matejczyk, M., & Moore, D. (1994). The relationship of social support to functional limitations, pain and well-being among men and women. *Journal of Women and Aging, 6,* 3-19.

Roberts, B. L., & Fitzpatrick, J. J. (1994). Margin in life among hospitalized and non-hospitalized elderly persons. *International Journal of Nursing Studies, 31,* 573-582.

Roberts, B. L., Srour, M. I., Mansour, J. M., Palmer, R. M., & Wagner, M. B. (1994). The effects of a 12-week aerobic walking program on postural stability. In K. Taguchi, M. Igarashi, & S. Mori (Eds.), *Vestibular and neural front* (pp. 215-218). New York: Elsevier.

Roberts, B. L., Srour, M. I., Woollacott, M. H., & Tang, P. F. (1994). The effects of a 12-week aerobic walking program on gait of healthy elderly. In K. Taguchi, M. Igarashi, & S. Mori (Eds.), *Vestibular and neural front* (pp. 295-298). New York: Elsevier.

Roberts, B. L., & Wykle, M. (1993). Falls among institutionalized elderly. *Journal of Gerontological Nursing, 19*(5), 13-20.

Ruben, D. B., Siu, A. L., & Kimpau, S. (1992). The predictive validity of self-report and performance-based measures of function and health. *Journals of Gerontology, 47,* M106-M110.

Rubenstein, L. Z., Schairer, C., Wieland, G. D., & Kane, R. (1984). Systematic bias in functional status assessment of elderly adults: Effects of different data sources. *Journals of Gerontology: Medical Sciences, 39,* 686-691.

Schilke, J. M., Johnson, G. O., Housh, T. J., & O'Dell, J. R. (1996). Effects of muscle-strength training on the functional status of patients with osteoarthritis of the knee joint. *Nursing Research, 45,* 68-72.

Seeman, T. E., Bruce, M. L., & McVay, G. J. (1996). Social network characteristics and onset of ADLs disability: MacArthur studies of successful aging. *Journals of Gerontology: Social Sciences, 51B,* S191-200.

Seeman, T. E., Charpentier, P. A., Berkman, L. F., Tinetti, M. E., Guralnick, J. M., Albert, M., Blazer, D., & Rowe, J. W. (1994). Predicting changes in physical performance in a high-functioning elderly cohort: MacArthur studies of successful aging. *Journals of Gerontology: Medical Sciences, 49,* M97-M108.

Skurla, E., Rogers, J. C., & Sunderland, T. (1988). Direct assessment of activities of daily living in Alzheimer's disease: A controlled study. *Journal of the American Geriatrics Society, 36,* 97-103.

Spector, W. D., Katz, S., Murphy, J. B., & Fulton, J. P. (1987). The hierarchical relationship between activities of daily living and instrumental activities of daily living. *Journal of Chronic Disease, 40,* 481-489.

Stern, Y., Liu, X., Albert, M., Bandt, J., Jacobs, D. M., Castillo-Castaneda, C., Marder, K., Bell, R., Sano, M., Bylsma, F., LaFleche, G., & Tsai, W. (1996). Application of a growth curve approach to modeling the progression of Alzheimer's disease. *Journals of Gerontology: Medical Sciences, 51A,* M179-M184.

Strain, L. A. (1991). Use of health services in later life: The influence of health beliefs. *Journals of Gerontology: Social Sciences, 46,* S143-S150.

Swanson, E. A., Maas, M. L., & Buckwalter, K. C. (1994). Alzheimer's residents' cognitive and functional measures: Special and traditional care unit comparison. *Clinical Nursing Research, 3,* 27-41.

Teri, L., Borson, S., Kiyak, H. A., & Yamagishi, M. (1989). Behavioral disturbance, cognitive dysfunction, and functional skill: Prevalence and relationship to Alzheimer's disease. *Journal of the American Geriatrics Society, 37,* 109-116.

Tideiksaar, R. (1995). Falls in older persons. In B. S. Spivack (Ed.), *Evaluation and management of gait disorders* (pp. 243-266). New York: Marcel Dekker.

Tinetti, M. E. (1986). Performance-oriented assessment of mobility problems in elderly patients. *Journal of the American Geriatrics Society, 34,* 119-126.

Tinetti, M. E., Mendes de Leon, C. F., Doucette, J. T., & Baker, D. I. (1994). Fear of falling and fall-related efficacy in relationship to functioning among community-living elders. *Journals of Gerontology: Medical Sciences, 49,* M140-M147.

Topp, R., Mikesky, A., Wigglesworth, J., Holt, W., & Edwards, J. E. (1993). The effect of a 12-week dynamic resistance strength training program on gait velocity and balance of older adults. *Gerontologist, 33,* 501-506.

Tse, S. K., & Bailey, D. M. (1992). Tai Chi and postural control in the well elderly. *American Journal of Occupational Therapy, 46,* 295-300.

Vandervoort, A. A., & McComas, A. J. (1986). Contractile changes in opposing muscles of the human ankle joint with aging. *Journal of Applied Physiology, 61,* 361-367.

Verbrugge, L. M. (1990). The iceberg of disability. In S. M. Stahl (Ed.), *Longevity: Health and health care in later life* (pp. 55-75). Newbury Park, CA: Sage.

Verbrugge, L. M., & Jette, A. M. (1994). The disablement process. *Social Science and Medicine, 38,* 1-14.

Whipple, R. H., Wolfson, L. I., & Amerman, P. M. (1987). The relationship of knee and ankle weakness to falls in nursing home residents: An isokinetic study. *Journal of the American Geriatrics Society, 35,* 13-20.

Williams, M. E., & Hornberger, J. C. (1984). A quantitative method of identifying older persons at risk for increasing long term care services. *Journal of Chronic Disease, 37,* 705-711.

Winograd, C. H., Lemsky, C. M., Nevitt, M. C., Nordstrom, T. M., Stewart, A. L., Miller, C. J., & Bloch, D. A. (1994). Development of a physical performance and mobility examination. *Journal of the American Geriatrics Society, 42,* 743-749.

Wolf, S. T., Barnhart, H. X., Kutner, N. G., McNeely, E., Coogler, C., Xu, T., & Atlanta FICSIT Group. (1996). Reducing frailty and falls in older persons: An investigation of Tai Chi and computerized balance training. *Journal of the American Geriatrics Society, 44,* 489-497.

Wolfson, L. I., Whipple, R., Amerman, P., & Kleinberg, A. (1986). Stressing the postural response: A quantitative method for testing balance. *Journal of the American Geriatrics Society, 34,* 845-850.

Wolinsky, F. D., Callahan, C. M., Fitzgerald, J. F., & Johnson, R. J. (1993). Changes in functional status and the risks of subsequent nursing home placement and death. *Journals of Gerontology: Social Sciences, 48,* S93-S101.

Wolinsky, F. D., & Johnson, R. J. (1991). The use of health services by older adults. *Journals of Gerontology: Social Sciences, 47,* S304-S312.

World Health Organization. (1980). *International classification of impairment, disabilities and handicaps.* Geneva, Switzerland: Author.

MANAGING COGNITIVE IMPAIRMENT AND DEPRESSION IN THE ELDERLY

Cornelia K. Beck
Diane Cronin-Stubbs
Kathleen C. Buckwalter
Carla Gene Rapp

In this chapter, we offer a critical assessment of the state of nursing research involving delirium, dementia, and depression. We review the definitions, theoretical bases, and differential diagnoses for each disorder, followed by a discussion of the interventions for these prevalent disorders in older adults. We then critique the

AUTHORS' NOTE: The authors gratefully acknowledge the contributions of Dr. Lori Frank and Dr. Neale Chumbler, postdoctoral fellows at the John L. McClellan Veterans Administration HSR&D Field Program; Theresa Vogelpohl, Project Director; and Valorie Shue, Research Assistant, at the University of Arkansas for Medical Sciences College of Nursing; Mary Lynn Piven and Virginia Cruz, University of Iowa College of Nursing doctoral students; and Andrew J. Straub, Rush University College of Nursing graduate student, to the development of this chapter. This chapter is dedicated to Dr. Beverly A. Baldwin, mentor, colleague, and friend.

cited studies for strengths and weaknesses and, finally, offer suggestions for future research.

Descriptions and Theoretical Bases of Delirium

Delirium, also known as *acute confusion* or *acute confusional state* (ACS), is a relatively common and reversible type of cognitive impairment often seen in hospitalized or institutionalized older adults. Incidence and prevalence rates for ACS vary from 0% to 80%, most often reported to range from 20% to 50% (Foreman, 1989, 1991; Francis, Martin, & Kapoor, 1990; Lipowski, 1984; Rockwood, 1989; Schor et al., 1992; Seymour, Henschke, Cape, & Campbell, 1980; Williams, Campbell, Raynor, Musholt, et al., 1985). The wide variation in these rates may result from differences in definitions and measurement of ACS, along with other methodological issues.

Several researchers have explored risk factors or predictors of ACS. The most commonly reported factor is dementia (Francis et al., 1990; Kuroda et al., 1990; Rockwood, 1989; Schor et al., 1992; Seymour et al., 1980; Williams, Raynor, Musholt, et al., 1985). Another predictor is age, with increasing rates in those more than 65 years old and the highest incidence in those 80 years and older (Levkoff, Safran, Cleary, Gallop, & Phillips, 1988; Rockwood, 1989; Schor et al., 1992; Williams, Raynor, Musholt, et al., 1985). Limited social contact and male gender also may be risk factors (Foreman, 1989; Schor et al., 1992).

Research suggests that ACS is related to metabolic disturbances, fluid and electrolyte imbalances, drug toxicity, and sensory and environmental disturbances (Francis et al., 1990); neurological and cardiovascular disease (Kuroda et al., 1990); congestive heart disease (Rockwood, 1989); and severity of illness (Francis et al., 1990; Rockwood, 1989). Research also indicates that the alleviation of ACS results in "usually . . . paralleled improvement in the arterial oxygen and carbon dioxide partial pressures, and . . . acid-base status" (Rockwood, 1989, p. 152).

Foreman (1991) addressed prediction of ACS from a slightly different conceptual base. When specifically trying to describe the phenomenon in cognitive and behavioral terms, he found ACS had multiple dimensions (cognition, orientation, perception, motoric behavior, and higher integrative functions), which accounted for little of the variance. These findings suggest that examining a patient's ability to focus and maintain attention is the most useful method to quickly assess ACS (Foreman, 1991).

Historically, delirium has been the medical and psychological label used to describe this acute, confusional type of cognitive impairment. The American Psychiatric Association's (APA's) *Diagnostic and Statistical Manual of Mental Disorders, Fourth Edition (DSM-IV)* (1994) defines delirium as:

A. Disturbance of consciousness (i.e., reduced clarity of awareness of the environment) with reduced ability to focus, sustain, or shift attention.

B. A change in cognition (i.e., memory deficit, disorientation, language disturbance) or the development of a perceptual disturbance that is not better accounted for by a preexisting, established, or evolving dementia.

C. The disturbance develops over a short period of time (usually hours to days) and tends to fluctuate during the course of the day. (p. 142)

Delirium has associated features such as sleep-wake cycle disturbances and altered psychomotor behavior. Also, persons with delirium may attempt to attack others, escape (often resulting in falls), remove medical equipment (intravenous lines), or make verbalizations (screaming, cursing, moaning).

Delirium has been categorized as postoperative, seen especially in patients with hip fractures (Bowman, 1992; Gustafson, Brannstrom, Berggren, et al., 1991; Gustafson, Brannstrom, Norberg, Bucht, & Winblad, 1991); originating during acute or intensive care (Inaba-Roland & Maricle, 1992; Kroeger, 1991; Tess, 1991); or nocturnal, also known as sundown syndrome (Beel-Bates & Rogers, 1990; Bliwise & Lee, 1993; Evans, 1987).

Lipowski (1984, 1989) advanced the idea of subtypes of delirium. The *DSM-IV* contains two of these subtypes (hyperactive and hypoactive). The common hyperactive delirium features agitation, constant motion, and verbalizations. In contrast, hypoactive delirium involves inaction, withdrawal, sluggishness, and limited verbalizations that are often slow and wavering (Lipowski, 1984, 1989). A third subtype is mixed; the patient fluctuates unpredictably between the two extremes.

Although the definitions of ACS and delirium (especially the hyperactive variant) usually include agitation, one study found that less than half of the delirious patients developed agitation (Francis et al., 1990). Foreman's research (1991) implies that agitation occurs less frequently than previously assumed. He suggests that the agitation does not represent ACS itself and has an underlying cause. In fact, hyperactivity may indicate sympathetic nervous system overactivity; hypoactivity may indicate metabolic toxicity (Lipowski, 1989).

Tripp-Reimer (1995) sees delirium as a small area of specific symptoms and behaviors within ACS. Physicians generally do not recognize "delirium" until the *DSM-IV* criteria are met. Nurses, who tend to have closer contact with patients, often identify more subtle changes in cognition, attention, and behavior. Thus, it appears that nurses may identify ACS earlier than physicians do because it may have milder symptoms than those of delirium. For clarity, this discussion uses the label ACS.

The majority of those who study ACS have conceptualized it using the APA *Diagnostic and Statistic Manual of Mental Disorders, Third Edition (DSM-III)* criteria (Brannstrom, Gustafson, Norberg, & Winblad, 1991; Gustafson, Brannstrom, Berggren, et al., 1991; Gustafson, Brannstrom, Norberg, et al., 1991; Kroeger, 1991; Neelon, Champagne, McConnell, Carlson, & Funk, 1992; Schor et al., 1992). Other investigators have used the APA's *Diagnostic and Statistic Manual of Mental Disorders, Third Edition–Revised (DSM-III-R)*, or the International Classification of Disease (ICD) code criteria (Inaba-Roland & Maricle, 1992; Liptzin et al., 1991). Still others devised definitions with a wide range of symptoms (Batt, 1989; Bowman, 1992). The inability of researchers to agree on a definition inhibits knowledge development about ACS.

The study of ACS also needs further theoretical development, even though Neelon et al. (1992) offer a model of three patterns to guide understanding of and interventions for ACS. The first pattern appears when persons have low cognitive reserve (are "cognitively restricted") and react easily to sensory-environmental changes. The second pattern ("physiologic instability") emerges from pathological changes in physiological function. The third pattern arises from biochemical functioning ("metabolic instability") and stems from pharmacologically or metabolically induced toxicity (Foreman, 1993; Neelon & Champagne, 1992).

ACS requires early assessment and intervention because it appears to develop early during hospitalization. Compared to patients without ACS, patients with ACS tend to have longer lengths of stay (approximately 1½ times), increased hospital charges (Francis et al., 1990; Levkoff et al., 1988; Rockwood, 1989), higher mortality rates, and higher probability of being discharged to a long-term institution (Francis et al., 1990; Levkoff et al., 1988). Thus, early and sustained intervention could reap great cost savings.

Descriptions and Theoretical Bases of Dementia

Dementia refers to a set of symptoms and behavioral patterns seen in particular neurological diseases of older adults. The etiologies of dementia are varied, but the resulting cognitive, emotional, and behavioral deficits are similar. Reports of Alzheimer's disease (AD), the most prevalent form of the irreversible dementias, indicate that AD affects from 1.6% to 15.3% of those over age 65 and from 7.1% to 47.2% of those over age 80 (Rockwood & Stadnyk, 1994). The symptoms are manifestations of neuropathological and neurophysiological brain changes. Other irreversible dementias include the second major cause of dementia, multi-infarct dementia, and the less prevalent Pick's, Creutzfelt-Jacob, Huntington's, and forms of Parkinson's disease. The type of cognitive impairment differs depending on the disease entity, the stage of the disease, comorbid conditions, and individual factors.

Experts have divided the symptoms of dementia into two groups: primary (those of a physiological or biological nature) and secondary (those of a behavioral nature). The primary symptoms refer to cognitive impairments affecting memory, speech, language, judgment, visual-spatial and perceptive motor skills, and personality. The secondary symptoms include functional difficulties and disruptive behaviors.

The *DSM-IV* (1994) defines dementia as:

A. The development of multiple cognitive deficits manifested by both:

1. memory impairment (impaired ability to learn new information or to recall previously learned information)
2. one (or more) of the following cognitive disturbances:
   a. aphasia (language disturbance)
   b. apraxia (impaired ability to carry out motor activities despite intact motor function)
   c. agnosia (failure to recognize or identify objects despite intact sensory function)
   d. disturbance in executive functioning (i.e., planning, organizing, sequencing, abstracting)

B. The cognitive deficits in criteria A1 and A2 each cause significant impairment in social or occupational functioning and represent a significant decline from a previous level of functioning.

C. The course is characterized by gradual onset and continuing cognitive decline. (p. 129)

Interventions for both groups of symptoms include pharmacological approaches prescribed mainly by medical researchers. A discussion of their theoretical bases is beyond the scope of this chapter. Thus, this chapter focuses only on nonpharmacological interventions for older adults with dementia (OADs) that help them deal with cognitive loss, functional decline, and behavioral problems, interventions that come from a variety of disciplines and theoretical perspectives. Other pertinent research involves caregivers of OADs and health service use.

Theoretical bases for cognitive interventions. Interventions for the cognitive symptoms come from an information psychology perspective (Grasel, 1994). Researchers have relied on the notion of the brain as a "mental muscle," which needs exercise to retain abilities, or the notion of maximizing remaining cognitive skills through cognitive prosthetics or classical conditioning.

Camp et al. (1993) have proposed a heuristic classification scheme described in a 2×2 matrix for memory interventions. One dimension of the matrix addresses the use of internal versus external mnemonics, and the other addresses the use of explicit (effortful or conscious) versus implicit (automatic or unconscious) learning. In normal older populations, most memory interventions, such as mental imagery, fall within the explicit-internal cell of the matrix. They require much cognitive effort and involve the conscious use of internal storage devices to retain or retrieve information. Older adults with early to middle dementia may benefit from interventions in the explicit-external cell, such as memory wallets that take advantage of relatively automatic cognitive processes resulting from much practice and experience (Bourgeois, 1992). Neuropsychological literature suggests that some memory systems operate unconsciously or automatically or both (implicit memory, indirect memory, procedural memory). AD patients seem to retain motor and verbal priming (implicit or procedural memory functions). Priming involves the facilitation of performance or retrieval of information after exposure and can occur even when an individual is unaware of prior exposure (McKitrick, Camp, & Black, 1995). Ecologically-based

tasks using familiar stimuli have maintained memory and other cognitive functions (Quayhagen & Quayhagen, 1989).

Classical conditioning is another promising avenue for intervention. Camp et al. (1993) have trained OADs to remember specific pieces of information using the technique of spaced retrieval, which involves recalling information at increasingly longer time intervals.

Using adaptation and information processing theory, Rosswurm (1990) found that OADs could improve their ability to match single-dimensional stimuli of color and geometric shapes when they only had to choose from four examples and could repeat the tasks. This suggests that OADs do have the potential to improve in the early states of perceptual processing, which leads to storage in short-term memory (30 seconds). Short-term memory filters information into long-term memory, where one may store it indefinitely and retrieve it for higher level cognitive functions. If persons inaccurately process information in the early stages, deficits most likely will occur in late stages.

In summary, studies on memory have provided direction for interventions that capitalize on and support the OADs' remaining cognitive abilities. The heterogeneity of cognitive losses means that researchers must individualize interventions to specific cognitive disabilities. Likewise, the intraindividual variability in susceptibility to memory training is considerable in AD. External mnemonics and implicit learning seem to have the most potential as neuropsychological rehabilitation approaches. However, although older adults without cognitive deficits can benefit from memory training programs, no one has documented any long-term benefits of such programs for those with dementia. At best, they can slow the progression of the disease (Backman, 1992). Even less data support the notion of the brain as a "mental muscle."

Theoretical bases for functional interventions. When developing interventions to retain functional ability in OADs, researchers have used several conceptual approaches. Ajuriagguerra et al. (in Auer, Sclan, Yaffee, & Reisberg, 1994) observed more than 25 years ago that decline in OADs approximates a reversal of Piaget's developmental stages. By studying similarities between the functional development of a normal child and the apparent reversal of that process in AD, Matteson, Linton, Barnes, Cleary, and Lichtenstein (1996) found that decreasing cognition did indeed match decline in Piaget's stages.

In the progressively lowered stress threshold model, it is proposed that decreasing tolerance of stressful stimuli partly causes functional decline (Hall, Gerdner, Zwycart-Stauffacher, & Buckwalter, 1995). Learning to recognize antecedents of secondary behavioral symptoms facilitates planning of care that prevents dysfunctional episodes.

Leidy's (1994) conceptualization of functional ability has provided a framework for standardizing vocabulary and clarifying critical elements of functional status. This framework defines functional status by its dimensions: functional capacity, functional performance, capacity utilization, and functional reserve. Researchers could use this framework to study measures of functional capacity and capacity utilization in preparation for intervention studies that address functional performance and functional reserve.

Heacock, Walton, Beck, and Mercer (1991) reconceptualized disability to include both cognitive and physical deficits and expanded the related concept of rehabilitation using a behavioral approach that provides OADs with specific prompts needed to support remaining abilities and immediate reinforcers to reward desired behaviors. They also stressed that the type of caregiver assistance plays an important role in maintaining the OAD's self-care ability. One instrument, the Beck Dressing Performance Scale (Beck, 1988), documents the amount of caregiver assistance needed to compensate for cognitive deficits and physical disabilities that limit dressing performance. Based on task analysis, the instrument identifies component steps of the activity, which improves sensitivity to detect change in OADs and provides additional avenues for intervention (Beck, 1988) in contrast to other instruments that use a global approach. Further research is needed to apply this approach with other ADLs.

In summary, theorists have eschewed the notion that OADs cannot respond to therapy and now believe that their functional deficits may be reversible. These functional deficits often represent excess disability caused by medications, depression, lack of motivation, social isolation, inappropriate assistance, or physical illness. Researchers are developing interventions that address excess disability and use a cognitive disability perspective to match the level of caregiver assistance with the patients' remaining cognitive abilities to optimize functional performance.

Theoretical bases for interventions to decrease troublesome behaviors. Although many investigators have evaluated interventions to decrease the behaviors that are troublesome to caregivers of OADs, most have a weak theoretical base. Researchers need to reframe their approach from one that views these behaviors as disruptive to caregivers to one that attempts to understand the meaning of these behaviors to OADs. Algase et al. (1996) have proposed such a framework. They have reconceptualized problem behaviors as the OADs' most integrated and meaningful response to stimuli, given the limitations imposed by their condition; preserved strengths of their basic abilities and personality; and preserved constraints, challenges, or supports offered by their environment. Terming these *need-driven, dementia-compromised behaviors,* the authors suggest that this perspective will promote better understanding of the behaviors and targeting of interventions to the needs of OADs.

Validation therapy (Feil, 1993), which focuses on the emotional and psychological consequences of short-term memory loss, has come closest to attempting to understand patients' behaviors from their perspectives. With this interactive technique, the goal of communicating with OADs to ease distress and restore self-worth supersedes the goal of making them grasp reality. It assumes that OADs' behaviors and speech have an underlying meaning and that the returns to the past are to resolve unfinished conflicts by expressing undisclosed feelings. In practice, the therapist validates what OADs say rather than correcting factual errors to have a meaningful conversation on important issues to people (Morton & Bleathman, 1991).

Simulated presence theory has also guided interventions from OADs' perspectives and holds that an established caregiver is the primary source of stability for OADs. Based on the hypothesis that replication of a caregiver's presence may comfort the OAD, simulated presence therapy (SPT) consists of a personalized audiotape composed of a family member's side of a telephone conversation and soundless spaces for the OAD's responses. SPT may comfort the OAD because it introduces family and prompts pleasant memories (Woods & Ashley, 1995).

In summary, most studies use a broad person-environment framework. However, they need to more specifically describe these behaviors, their potential etiologies, and consequent interventions.

Theoretical bases for caregiver interventions. Families provide a significant amount of care to elders with AD (Dillehay & Sandys, 1990; Montgomery, Karl, & Borgatta, 1988). Caregiving can cause depression, anxiety, increased risk of physical illness, and restrictions on time or activities for the caregivers (Montgomery et al., 1988; Mullan, 1993). Recognition of the profound, and sometimes overwhelming, physical and emotional strains for caregivers has stimulated pioneering research on interventions to assist caregivers. Zarit and Teri label the current work the "first generation" of studies (1992; cited in Bourgeois, Schulz, & Burgio, 1996).

Theoretical origins include stress-coping theory (Folkman & Lazarus, 1991; Lazarus & Folkman, 1991), separation-individuation (Mahler, Pine, & Bergman, 1994), support theory (Barrera & Ainlay, 1983), social learning and conditioning (Bandura, 1969), and problem-solving (D'Zurilla, 1988). Irvin and Acton (1997) have used modeling and role-modeling theory to test the stress-mediating effects of perceived support and self-worth. Their data substantiate the importance of affiliated-individuation as a mediator of stress.

In general, early research on caregiver support groups has evolved into research on counseling, respite services, and skills training, services that have multiplied over the last 20 years. The field is shifting from case and observational studies to experimental research.

Theoretical bases for health services use. Family members link the OADs to health and community-support services (Mullan, 1993). Thus, a theoretical framework of health service use must include the characteristics of caregivers as well as OADs. Only within the past decade have researchers explored the predictors of service use.

The current theoretical framework for examining services consists primarily of two models. The first employs an adapted version of the Andersen-Newman model by collecting data on the OAD and caregiver. This model views the use of services as a function of predisposing factors or personal characteristics (i.e., the propensity of individuals to use services, most often operationalized by age, gender, education, marital status, and previous illnesses), enabling factors (i.e., circumstances or individual characteristics that can hinder or facilitate service use, such as availability of family resources or awareness of services), and need factors (i.e., objectively and subjectively assessed needs, including perceived health status and number of diagnoses) (Chappell & Blandford, 1987; Penning, 1995; Stephens, 1993). Overall, most of these studies have two shortcomings. First, most of these studies do not use OADs as the unit of analysis. In other words, OADs are not respondents of the study and do not provide information about themselves. Instead, the family caregivers render such information. Second, when operationalizing the need factors, most of these studies, except for the Bass, Looman, and Ehrlich study (1992), do not ascertain the OADs' level of cognitive impairment.

The second framework builds on the original Andersen-Newman framework by placing the decision to use services within a stress framework (Cohler, Groves, Borden, & Lazarus, 1989; Mullan, 1993; Pearlin, Mullan, Semple, & Skaff, 1990) in the broader context of the caregivers' lives (Mullan, 1993). The stress framework offers insight into the caregivers' decision-making process to accept or reject services (Stephens, 1993; Wan, 1989). In the stress framework, the caregivers' primary stressors are the AD adults' need factors, which place demands on them to provide care (Mullan, 1993; Pearlin et al., 1990). Mullan (1993) summarizes a typical scenario: "Caregivers must evaluate the patient needs, assess their own capacities to provide appropriate care, and then set up a strategy for dealing with these primary stressors" (pp. 242).

The stress framework also considers the impact of secondary strains such as role overload, anger, depression, and family conflict on caregivers (Mullan, 1993). As these strains increase, caregivers may reevaluate their resources and reformulate caregiving strategies that may include caring for the patient alone, sharing the responsibilities with others, seeking formal services, or electing to institutionalize (Mullan, 1993; Noelker & Bass, 1989). Equally important, however, these secondary strains may lead caregivers to seek help for themselves from a trained professional. When caregivers turn to formal services, the stress model considers seven features (Mullan, 1993): (a) background characteristics (e.g., gender or education), (b) economic resources (e.g., income or economic strain), (c) caregiving context (e.g., relationship of caregiver to patient, informal help and service use), (d) social resources (e.g., instrumental assistance and emotional support), (e) physical health of the patient and caregiver, (f) primary stressors (e.g., patient characteristics that demonstrate need for assistance), and (g) secondary strains.

The original and adapted versions of the Andersen-Newman framework, as well as the stress framework, exclude some characteristics that have influenced service use in past studies (e.g., see Mullan, 1993; Ward, Sherman, & LaGory, 1984). These include knowledge of available services and how to access them, cost of services, acceptability of using formal care, and beliefs of families about using formal services rather than performing the assistance themselves.

In summary, a broad stress framework has guided most of the research on OADs' caregivers. However, other theoretical approaches are beginning to contribute to this research and may eventually converge into a broader common framework.

Descriptions and Theoretical Bases of Depression

Depression refers to "a syndrome that includes a constellation of physiological, affective, and cognitive manifestations" (National Institutes of Health Consensus Development Panel on Depression in Late Life [NIH], 1992, p. 1019). In older adults, depression varies in symptoms, age of onset, and clinical course. Late-onset depression is associated with cognitive impairment, cerebral atrophy, medical comorbidity, and mortality. Suicide rates in older adults are more than twice that of the general population (Schneider, 1995). Major depression requires immediate treatment; subsyndromal depression (or depressive symptoms that do not meet standardized diagnostic criteria) is more prevalent (15% of community-dwelling older adults) and potentially more important to older adults' functional status and quality of life.

Depression in nursing homes and other institutions is highly prevalent (affecting up to 50% of frail, medically compromised residents) and is related to lack of resources and staff trained to recognize and treat depression (NIH, 1992). About 13% of residents develop new episodes of major depression in a 1-year period, and another 18% develop new depressive symptoms (NIH, 1992), which can increase risks of comorbid medical conditions and major depressive episodes.

Geropsychiatric disorders often remain unrecognized, misdiagnosed, or mistreated, leading to high comorbidity, increased health care costs, unnecessary suffering, and diminished quality of life (Buckwalter, 1992; Heston et al., 1992). Failure to recognize and treat depression in late life can lead to increased health care use, longer hospital stays, lack of compliance with treatment, and mortality. Lack of treatment may occur because the signs and symptoms of depression in the elderly differ from those in the young (Gomez & Gomez, 1993) or because of ageism, negative reimbursement systems, reluctance to seek psychiatric care, the tendency to believe that physical ills rather than emotional problems are causing the distress, insufficient numbers of health care providers trained or interested in psychogeriatrics, and the failure of many primary care practitioners to recognize somatic complaints as masking depression.

The goals of treatment include decreasing symptoms, the risk of relapse and recurrence, mortality, and health costs and enhancing quality of life and general health status (Schneider, 1995). In general, more severe depression (with melancholia, delusions, suicidal idea-

tion, or concomitant medical illness) requires more intensive treatment. Approaches to care include biological and psychosocial therapies. Biological approaches include pharmacotherapy and electroconvulsive therapy (ECT). Prevalent psychosocial approaches include cognitive, behavioral, integrated cognitive-behavioral, and brief psychodynamic therapy and interpersonal psychotherapy. Cognitive therapy is based on the premise that depression results from self-deprecatory thinking that one can interrupt by identifying erroneous "self-talk" and substituting self-affirming and realistic thinking patterns. Behavioral therapy holds that a loss of positive reinforcers may cause depression and that changes in behavior can lead to a change in thinking and feeling. Integrated cognitive-behavioral therapy combines correcting negative "self-talk" with the behavioral strategies of reinforcing alternative thinking patterns. Brief psychodynamic therapy holds that unresolved, intrapsychic conflicts from early life cause emotional distress. Interpersonal psychotherapy focuses on patients' relationships to significant others, as social disruptions increase the risk of depression. The above psychotherapies stem from psychopathological theories, but supportive psychotherapy is "eclectic" and focuses on what seems to make the patient feel and function better. Supportive psychotherapy can involve evaluating patients' psychosocial strengths and weaknesses and helping them make choices that increase their functional capacity. These therapies effectively treat depression in family caregivers of medically ill older adults (Gallagher-Thompson & Steffen, 1994).

Research shows convergence in the efficacy of cognitive, behavioral, and interpersonal approaches for the acute treatment of depression. However, researchers do not know about the long-term effectiveness of these approaches (Agency for Health Care Policy and Research: Depression Guideline Panel [AHCPR], 1993; Schneider, 1995). A recent meta-analysis of 17 studies confirmed that psychosocial treatments were "highly" efficacious for treating both major and less severe depressive disorders of older adults but that there was "no clear superiority" of any psychotherapy in treating geriatric depression (Scogin & McElreath, 1994, p. 72). Others have found the efficacy of psychotherapies in severe depression to be equivocal (Schneider, 1995) due to the heterogeneity of depressive disorders (Schneider, 1995) and the lack of conceptual clarity in defining depression.

Clinicians regard combined therapeutic approaches (e.g., antidepressant medications and psychotherapy) as the standard of care. Improvement rates exceed those of no treatment or placebo. Although these strategies remain inadequately evaluated in the elderly, nortriptyline and interpersonal therapy (Reynolds et al., 1992) and cognitive-behavioral therapy combined with desipramine (Gallagher-Thompson & Thompson, 1994) helped elderly outpatients. The relative contributions of each approach are unknown (Schneider, 1995). Most studies for clinical practice used cognitive or cognitive-behavioral frameworks derived from Beck's (1976) theory. Those that evaluated reminiscence therapy used Butler's (1963) concept of life review, and Campbell (1992) used nursing theory.

Clinical Nursing Research Approaches for Delirium

The study of ACS has much conceptual vagueness and little theoretical work. Despite this, researchers have applied or developed a number of instruments to assess ACS. The Mini-Mental State Examination (Folstein, Folstein, & McHugh, 1975) is the most used and helps identify persons with mental status impairment, but it inaccurately assesses ACS.

Several other investigator-designed tools include the Confusion Assessment Method (Inoye et al., 1990), the Clinical Assessment of Confusion (Vermeersch, 1992), the Delirium Rating Scale (Trzepacz, Baker, & Greenhouse, 1988), and the NEECHAM Confusion Scale (Neelon & Champagne, 1992). These tools attempt to assess behaviors and symptoms of ACS through observation. Some studies have addressed their validity and reliability. Foreman (1993) points out that many of these tools rely on clinical judgment; measure behaviors not exclusive to ACS, thus limiting their specificity; have high response burdens; or take too much time to learn or administer. No instrument assesses the temporal aspect of ACS, so some researchers suggest using repeated measures of an established tool.

The cornerstone of intervention for ACS is prompt and appropriate assessment (Brannstrom et al., 1991; Champagne & Wiese, 1992; Gustafson, Brannstrom, Norberg, et al., 1991; Kroeger, 1991; Williams, Ward, & Campbell, 1988). Once providers identify ACS, they must recognize and treat the associated or underlying causes as well as provide appropriate nursing care (Champagne & Wiese, 1992).

To decrease ACS post-operatively in older adults with hip fractures, Gustafson, Brannstrom, Berggren, et al. (1991) used the following interventions: expediency in timing of surgery postinjury, preoperative assessment,

treatment of existing congestive heart failure and thrombosis prophylaxis, oxygen therapy during and after surgery, specific anesthesia, and postoperative assessment and treatment for any medical complications. These interventions decreased the incidence, severity, and duration of ACS (Gustafson, Brannstrom, Berggren, et al., 1991). Other physiological interventions have attempted to increase activity and mobility, prevent elimination problems, manage medications, and treat dehydration (Seymour et al., 1980; Wanich, Sullivan-Marx, Gottlieb, & Johnson, 1992; Williams, Holloway, et al., 1979).

Foreman (1993) reviewed the literature on reasons and interventions for patients' medication noncompliance without making a critical appraisal. Questions remain about the characteristics of patients who comply with medication treatments and how nurses and patients can collaboratively promote adherence. This would help older adults, for whom side effects and polypharmacy are particularly hazardous.

Many nursing researchers have examined the effect of environmental and psychosocial-interactional interventions in patients with ACS. Common psychosocial-interactional interventions included subtle reorientation, informing patients about their care and explaining treatment, helping patients feel in control, encouraging friends or family to visit, promoting family involvement in care planning, early discharge planning, and planned recreational activities (McCrone, 1991; Voelkel, 1978; Wanich et al., 1992; Williams, Campbell, Raynor, Mlynarczyk, & Ward, 1985).

Environmental interventions have included use of clocks or watches, presence of a calendar, watching television, staying in a private room, providing continuity of care, correcting sensory deficits, limiting numbers of nursing staff, lighting to help decrease sensory deprivation, and having families bring items from home (Wanich et al., 1992; Williams, Campbell, Raynor, Mlynarczyk, et al., 1985; Williams, Holloway, et al., 1979). Neelon and Champagne's (1992) model seems to support these psychosocial-interactional and environmental interventions.

Clinical Nursing Research Approaches for Dementia

Interventions for dementia concentrate on delaying the progressive decline of cognitive and behavioral symptoms and reducing caregiver stress.

Organizations' reports. The Alzheimer's Association Medical and Scientific Advisory Board treatment committee outlined the state of knowledge on managing the behavioral disturbances of AD. The committee's report summarized the thinking on agitation, assault and aggression, screaming, wandering, and depression (apathy, withdrawal) (Teri et al., 1992). Bourgeois et al. (1996) have provided a comprehensive review of interventions for AD patients' caregivers. Most studies demonstrate caregiver satisfaction with the intervention but offer little evidence of other positive outcomes for either the caregiver or the OAD in terms of coping skills, prevention of psychological disturbances, increase in support systems, and improvement in ability to care for self (Toseland & Rossiter, cited in Bourgeois et al., 1996).

Basic research. Therrien, a nurse researcher, has conducted basic research to elucidate wayfinding behaviors (how one finds one's way) of persons with hippocampal lesions. The hippocampus is essential to spatial memory and navigation in humans and other animals. Using rats with surgically induced hippocampal damage, she simulated large-scale space with external cueing (cognitive mapping) or with a single movable cue for guiding navigation. She demonstrated that rats with left-sided or bilateral hippocampal damage were slower at wayfinding that was dependent on cognitive mapping when she moved the goal than were controls or those with right-sided damage (Holden & Therrien, 1993). Practice with single-cue navigation prior to injury improved relearning of single-cue wayfinding postsurgery (Holden & Therrien, 1989). These studies help nurses understand the need for exploratory activity and wayfinding in humans with hippocampal damage.

Nursing research on biological therapies. Souder (1996a) is examining the relationship between neuroimaging and functional performance in OADs. Specifically, she is exploring the relationship of specific Instrumental Activities of Daily Living (IADLs) requiring visuospatial ability to physiological status of the right parietal lobe as identified by single photon emission computed tomography (SPECT) to answer this question: What is the predictive value of right parietal lobe perfusion as measured by SPECT and of performance on selected neurocognitive tests on IADL performance in AD? In addition, Souder is examining whether SPECT can predict (a) ADL performance in AD better than neurocognitive tests and (b) future areas of dysfunction identified by reassessment 18 months later (Souder, 1996b).

Nursing research on nonbiological therapies. Very little nursing research has been focused on memory training or cognitive rehabilitation with OADs. Beck, Heacock, Mercer, Thatcher, and Sparkman (1988) observed a significant improvement in memory in hospitalized OADs with moderately severe dementia after cognitive skills remediation training. Friedman and Tappen (1991) found a connection between walking behavior and increased communication in a two-group study. The first group walked and talked; the second only talked. Communication performance considerably improved for the first group.

Nursing studies on promoting functional performance in OADs have focused on either teaching functional skills to OADs in a group setting (Tappen, 1994) or teaching family or formal caregivers to match the level and type of assistance with the remaining abilities of OADs (Beck et al., 1995; Heacock, Mayhew, Souder, O'Sullivan, & Chastain, 1995; Heacock, Garrett, & Mayhew, 1996). Some investigators have addressed a number of ADLs concurrently (Blair, 1995; Josephsson, Backman, Borell, Bernspang, et al., 1993; Josephsson, Backman, Borell, Nygard, & Bernspang, 1995; McEvoy & Patterson, 1986; Reichenbach & Kirchman, 1991; Tappen, 1994); others have focused exclusively on bathing (A. Hurley, personal communication, 1996; Sloane et al., 1995; Whall, Gillis, Yankou, Booth, & Beel-Bates, 1992), dressing (Beck, 1993a, 1993b; Beck & Baldwin, 1992; Beck, Heacock, Mercer, Walls, et al., 1997; Beck, Heacock, Mercer, Walton, & Shook, 1991; Beck, Heacock, Rapp, & Mercer, 1993; Heacock, Mayhew, et al., 1995), or eating (Coyne, 1990; Nolen & Garrard, 1988; Osborn & Marshall, 1993; Rosswurm, 1989; Van Ort & Phillips, 1992). Still another has addressed the self-efficacy of caregivers in promoting functional performance (Heacock, Mayhew, et al., 1995).

Using a group approach, Tappen (1994) compared a targeted program of skill training in the basic ADLs; a more traditional general stimulation program that used adult games, music, and conversation; and regular nursing home care. She found significant differences. In general, the greatest improvement occurred in the skill training group, modest improvement in the stimulation group, and decline in the control group. Blair (1995) showed that staff education in mutual goal setting and operant behavioral management had a positive effect on OADs' self-care behaviors.

Van Ort and Phillips (1992) found that nursing assistants (NA) do not encourage self-feeding behavior other than frequent verbal prompts to open the mouth. Osborn and Marshall (1993) demonstrated that OADs in nursing homes were capable of significantly more independence in feeding when NAs used graded assistance techniques.

Using behavioral strategies matched to OADs' types of cognitive disability, Beck, Heacock, Mercer, Walls, et al. (1997) showed a decrease in assistance from formal caregivers during OAD dressing after 6 weeks of intervention. This clinically relevant improvement in dressing occurred without a clinically relevant increase in caregiver time.

A report of a consensus conference on bathing OADs (Sloane et al., 1995) provides an excellent summary of this research. In addition, Whall demonstrated that physically aggressive behaviors occurred most often during care procedures, especially the shower or bath. Caregivers moderated aggression by changing the social environment (slower paced caregiving) or the physical environment (introducing stimuli meaningful to the patient) and using desserts as reinforcers (Whall et al., 1992).

Generally, studies promoting functional performance have concluded that many OADs can increase functioning when caregivers provide the appropriate environmental prosthetics and levels of assistance. However, improvement in one ADL does not necessarily generalize to other ADLs and may depend on the context in which the skill training occurs. The level of caregiver self-efficacy also plays a role in the outcome.

Nursing studies that have addressed disruptive behaviors in OADs can be organized around the approaches used to manage the behaviors. Woods and Ashley (1995) reported in a feasibility study that 81.5% of 27 OADs showed positive responses to simulated presence therapy (SPT). The OADs responded differently to SPT based on the type of behavior they exhibited. In a subsequent study of nine OADs, problem behaviors improved 91% of the time. Other nursing studies generally found music effective in reducing agitated behaviors (Gerdner & Swanson, 1993; Sambandham & Schirm, 1995; Tabloski, McKinnon-Howe, & Remington, 1995).

Quayhagen et al. (1995) investigated the impact over time of an active cognitive stimulation intervention implemented by family caregivers at home on the cognitive and behavioral functioning of OADs. The OADs in the experimental group improved in cognitive and behavioral performance, but improvements dissipated over time. Those in the control group worsened and those in the placebo group remained the same. This work demonstrates the value of remediation interventions for OADs despite the trajectory of cognitive decline.

Clinical Nursing Research Approaches for Depression

Interventions target remission of prevalent depression, restoration of premorbid functioning, and prevention of incident and recurrent depression. An expert panel commissioned by the AHCPR from diverse health care disciplines, including nursing, conducted a synthesis of clinical knowledge and research on treating depression. Medications, psychotherapy, or both can treat depression successfully (AHCPR, 1993). For outpatients with moderate or severe major depression, the panel concluded that over half experienced relief of depressive symptoms with an initial trial of antidepressants, individuals responded to medications differently, and no one antidepressant was more effective than another.

In another synthesis of research, the NIH Consensus Development Panel (NIH, 1992) identified strong evidence from randomized placebo-controlled trials that antidepressants are more effective than placebo controls in treating acute depression. In older adults, a positive response to antidepressants requires 6 to 12 weeks of therapy (NIH, 1992). Clinicians are prescribing the newer antidepressants (e.g., bupropion, fluoxetine) because they have fewer cardiovascular and anticholinergic side effects and may thus decrease the incidence of falls and fractures (AHCPR, 1993; NIH, 1992; Schneider, Martinez, & Lebowitz, 1993).

Moreover, we have limited understanding of "failure to thrive" syndromes, mostly in institutionalized older adults who fail to respond to traditional antidepressant therapies. Studies of starved animals that do not respond biochemically to antidepressants suggest some important clues for understanding and treating anorexia and failure to thrive in older adults, but this research is in its early stages (Katz, 1995).

Lack of medication compliance is a leading predictor of poor outcomes of pharmacotherapy (NIH, 1992). Approximately 70% of patients fail to take 25% to 50% of their medications due to undesirable side effects. Strong evidence suggests that patient and family education can improve adherence to treatment (AHCPR, 1993).

Community-dwelling elderly are often isolated, lack economic and social resources, and require in-home care and outreach services. A meta-analysis of 58 studies provided evidence for the cost-effectiveness of outpatient mental health treatment. The largest cost offset occurred in decreased inpatient costs (Mumford, Schlesinger, Glass, Patrick, & Cuerdon, 1984).

Patients over 60 constitute the largest group receiving electroconvulsive therapy (ECT), despite a high relapse rate. Short-term efficacy of ECT has occurred with severely symptomatic older adults. These older adults are suicidal and psychotically depressed with somatic delusions, psychomotor retardation, vegetative signs, and early insomnia. Severe medical disorders (cardiopulmonary) or cognitive impairment and concurrent psychotropic medication usage often preclude the use of ECT with the elderly (AHCPR, 1993; Blazer, 1989; Gomez & Gomez, 1992; NIH, 1992).

Most nursing studies have focused on evaluating the efficacy of structured group therapy formats, and the majority of those used cognitive or cognitive-behavioral frameworks or approaches with various results (Abraham, Niles, Thiel, Siarkowski, & Cowling, 1991; Campbell, 1992; Emmerson, Pugh, Wright, Bolton, & Hoskins, 1992; Hughes, 1991; Pollack, 1991; Scanland & Emershaw, 1993; Zerhusen, Boyle, & Wilson, 1991). Scanland and Emershaw (1993) compared the effects of reality orientation and validation therapy groups on mental (cognition and affect) and functional status in elderly nursing home residents and found no differences in pre- or posttest scores for either approach. In contrast, Zerhusen et al. (1991) demonstrated greater improvement in depression scores of nursing home residents who received cognitive group therapy instead of music group therapy.

Other nursing studies evaluated the efficacy of guided imagery, therapeutic touch, music therapy, massage, or reminiscence therapies (Lappe, 1987; Leja, 1989; Rowlands, 1984; Tourangeau, 1988; Quinn & Strelkauskas, 1993; Zerhusen et al., 1991). Reminiscence or life review therapies received more consistent support, perhaps because reminiscence therapy helped older adults accomplish developmental tasks. Studies that compared cognitive therapies with alternative approaches, such as focused visual imagery, had mixed results. Abraham, Neundorfer, and Currie (1992) found that none of their three approaches reduced depressive symptoms. However, focused visual imagery improved cognition in mildly to moderately cognitively impaired nursing home residents more than cognitive-behavioral therapy and education-discussion groups.

In a rare placebo-controlled study of the efficacy of individual therapy, Campbell (1992) used cognitive therapy techniques, standardized protocols, and trained nursing staff to promote reduction of depressive symptoms in well elderly who resided in low-income high-rise apartments. The active ingredients of the intervention are difficult to identify because Campbell used a combination of therapies.

Combinations of biological and psychosocial therapies may synergistically relieve late-life depression. For example, as part of the Gospel Oak depression study, Waterreus, Blanchard, and Mann (1994) evaluated the efficacy of a comprehensive pharmacotherapy and eclectic psychosocial treatment package delivered by a community psychiatric nurse. Although the nurse monitored the dose-effect of each intervention by timing it, analyzing the effects of each approach separately and in combination, under controlled conditions, would have revealed the critical active ingredients of the multifaceted program. Replicating the study with multiple experimenters randomly assigned to specific psychological interventions would control for experimenter effects.

Strengths and Weaknesses in the Science

Strengths and weaknesses of studies on cognitive impairment (delirium and dementia) and depression have many similarities. Thus, we discuss them simultaneously and note differences.

Inadequate congruence between theoretical and operational definitions threatens the construct validity of the research base. Definitions across the studies did not consistently control for diagnosis, types of cognitive impairment, or levels of depressive disorders. In caregiver studies, Bourgeois et al. (1996) observed that although researchers refer to a particular theoretical perspective as a basis for the intervention, they rarely design truly theoretically based studies. Each theoretical area has its own history of empirical research, and, in most cases, researchers did not use this research in the design and analysis of caregiver intervention studies.

Researchers have established construct validity in models of memory interventions and behavioral approaches for increasing functional performance for dementia and in models of psychotherapy for depression. Recent examples include classification schemes for memory interventions (Camp et al., 1993) and algorithms for promoting functional independence (Beck, Heacock, Rapp, et al., 1993). Depression models integrate (a) group process phases (Clark & Vorst, 1994), (b) cognitive and cognitive-behavioral approaches with reminiscence and life review (Campbell, 1992; Leszca, 1990), and (c) cognitive-behavioral approaches with level of patient functioning (Pollack, 1991). Although reminiscence is congruent with older adults' developmental tasks, cognitive approaches with OADs remain invalidated. Construct validity of group psychotherapy would be enhanced by testing approaches that are less cognitive and more supportive in subsets of OADs.

Most studies give only brief descriptions of their subjects and the intervention, which threatens construct validity. They do not examine characteristics of the caregiver (level of caregiver distress or relationship to the patient) or the patient (impairment level), which may determine what treatment works for which clients. For example, a daughter caring for an impaired parent might have different needs and responses than a caregiving spouse would (Bourgeois et al., 1996). Neundorfer (1991) pointed out that subject selection problems may unduly influence findings in the caregiver literature, particularly when outcomes are physical and emotional health, and subjects are recruited from help-seeking situations. Failure to adequately describe the content of the intervention itself prohibits replication. Bourgeois et al. (1996) note that most current research focuses on outcomes and methodology, with little attention to therapeutic *process*. Therapeutic process refers to the mechanism of the intervention, a function of intensity (the amount and duration of the service) and integrity (the match between the actual intervention and the planned intervention).

Researchers studying depression need to better specify and operationalize the studies' unit of analysis, details of protocols, and adherence criteria and provide adequate doses of the interventions (Stewart & Archbold, 1992). Also, not all studies attend to the integrity of the intervention; monitoring the implementation would address this shortcoming both by providing a more precise picture of the intervention and by specifying crucial implementation details, such as the intervention agent. These problems limit the generalizability of this work.

Threats to statistical conclusion validity in the research base ensued from diagnostically mixed samples (samples inadequate from which to draw significant differences or associations), and unreliable methods for implementing and monitoring treatments and measuring outcomes. This may reflect a lack of psychometrically

rigorous tools that specifically and sensitively measure constructs, treatments, and outcomes germane to older adults. Generally, individual studies excluded psychometric information about the reliability and validity of the measures. Exceptions included Abraham's (1991) longitudinal results on the utility of the Geriatric Depression Scale and the Hopelessness Index with frail elderly. Many studies used established measures; others relied on monitoring patients' charts or using clinicians' judgments. The science needs objective, congruent measures of treatments and outcomes. Because researchers can only demonstrate cause-and-effect relationships between treatments and outcomes longitudinally (not cross sectionally), they need to develop measures that detect relatively small changes over time.

Differences in intervention implementation and caregiver's and patient's history probably result in varied responses to interventions. Gerontology requires acknowledging the influence of each person's history. Given that individuals tend to become more heterogeneous with increasing age (Schaie & Willis, 1993), research would be strengthened by attending to individual differences, like best timing for intervention and best match of caregiver with intervention type. In caregiver research, numerous factors may influence intervention effectiveness, including length of time in caregiving role and level of patient's behavioral impairment.

Threats to internal validity in the research base resulted from attrition (often due to mortality), intervention dose effect issues, and lack of control for alternative explanations of the outcomes through random assignment. In addition, matching patients or using selected covariates (e.g., medications, comorbid physical illnesses, cognitive impairment) would enhance the design. Finally, nonstandardized administration of the treatments or outcome measures may have compromised the validity of the studies. Many nursing home studies, for example, rely on overworked, undertrained staff to collect data and implement sophisticated protocols. Many instruments rely on proxy observations, which may invalidly report the older adult's subjective state, or self-report of depression, which may be unreliable in OADs. In addition, measures may lack the sensitivity to detect changes in patients' symptom severity and frequency.

In summary, lack of internal validity (Cook & Campbell, 1979) or the inability to randomly select participants from representative samples of the older adult population threatened validity of the research base. Investigators have used groups comprising heterogeneous populations, lacked assurance that all therapists applied the treatment systematically and consistently to all patients, and found little maintenance of treatment effects.

Recommendations for Advancing the Science in This Field of Study

The state of the science may be related to the threats to validity in the research base. A priori attention to construct validity would contribute to external validity; a priori attention to statistical conclusion validity would foster the internal validity of the studies' results (Cook & Campbell, 1979). Researchers can strengthen claims of treatment efficacy by attending closely to the methodological quality of research, particularly the validity of the interventions and the study's design.

Scientific and methodological attention is needed to more precisely specify clinical inclusion criteria (e.g., diagnostic subtypes). For example, better knowledge of cognitive deterioration in the normal elderly would help provide correct diagnostic distinction between physiological aging and dementia.

Theoretical and operational definitions of targeted symptoms, treatments, and outcomes would facilitate research, too. Leidy's (1994) conceptualization of functional performance could be applied to OADs. Similarly, a reconceptualization of disruptive behaviors within a well-specified person-environment framework would help illuminate the meaning of these behaviors and strengthen interventions.

Also needed are randomized, placebo-controlled designs and psychometrically established and clinically useful measures. For example, developing instruments to gather information from the OADs on important people, places, and events in the past has potential therapeutic value.

Further, researchers must devise specific, age-associated, objective criteria for evaluating changes in outcomes directly attributable to interventions and comprehensive and diverse methods of assessing treatments and their implementation; must specify length and intensity of treatment; and must establish outcomes. Too few nursing intervention studies have developed integrative reviews that employ quantitative techniques, such as meta-analysis, to determine the effect size of particular

approaches. In dementia research, outcome measures that detect changes in well-being and affect need development. It is also important to identify the particular aspects of the treatment that contributed to its effect. For example, in dementia research to promote functional performance, did the prompting, the reinforcement, the practice itself, an increase in physical activity, the social setting, or a combination of these factors contribute to the treatment effect?

Ideally, independent, double-blinded raters (blinded to the study's purposes and subjects' membership in treatment and control groups) and direct observations of studies' variables would corroborate paper-and-pencil measures. Cognitive training researchers cannot use placebo training; thus tests including a control group that has not undergone training still provide the most valid results (Grasel, 1994). Memory training and aids for OADs need to ameliorate everyday memory problems, improve daily skills, and prompt natural reinforcement from others (Bourgeois, 1993). To decrease depressive symptoms, a priori evaluation of participants' cognitive status would enhance the internal validity of cognitive and cognitive-behavioral studies.

Other specific recommendations for research include nursing interventions to help older adults meet their spiritual needs (Nelson, 1990), enhance resourcefulness and optimism (i.e., teaching the use of positive self-statements, problem solving, creative visualization, and cognitive restructuring) (Zauszniewski, 1994), and enhance group psychotherapy to promote or restore mental health by viewing developmental characteristics of later life as "natural resources" (Reed, 1991). Similarly, existential psychotherapeutic approaches focusing on freedom, isolation, meaninglessness, and death warrant more rigorous examination (McDougall, 1995).

More replication studies, using diverse but well-defined samples and settings, would strengthen nursing's knowledge base in effective interventions for cognitive impairment and depression and enhance the external validity of extant interventions. "Nearly all randomized controlled treatment trials in elderly depressed individuals to date have been conducted in the otherwise medically healthy" (AHCPR, 1993, p. 100). Therefore, effective interventions require replication in more heterogeneous groups of depressed older adults in more diverse settings. Including covariates, such as comorbid medical and neuropsychiatric illnesses, would better represent the population of older adults with late-life depression. In dementia research, the influence of a variety of factors on response to treatment deserves further attention. These factors include gender; education; racial, ethnic, and cultural background; socioeconomic status; social risk factors and social support; environmental context; stressful life events; religious orientation and self-transcendence; and personal traits, such as hope, hardiness, and learned resourcefulness. Related to caregiver research, the study of Quayhagen et al. (1995) discusses the importance of studying gender differences; we cannot assume equivalence of experiences and responses.

The available literature suggests that biological, psychological, and social factors underlie the onset of both cognitive impairment and depression in later life. Both cognitive impairment and depression can be associated with medical illness and with each other. Their interaction can interfere significantly with assessment, response to treatment, and adherence to treatment regimens and can amplify the disability, pain, and treatment refusal associated with general medical disorders. Therefore, researchers must test and evaluate algorithms for treating coexisting medical conditions and responses to treatment. For example, up to 60% of AD patients have specific visual deficits, which include decreased depth perception, contrast sensitivity, and color discrimination, especially of blue hues. Such visual deficits may be highly related to functional disability (Cronin-Golomb, 1995; Cronin-Golomb, Corkin, & Growdon, 1995). In depression research, the interaction of multiple determinants in both the onset and outcomes of depression in older adults needs consideration (Kurlowicz, 1993), which supports the need for interdisciplinary research with nurses playing a more pivotal investigative role than they have to date.

The lack of posttreatment follow-up of older adults with depression and their vulnerability to relapse and recurrence, medical comorbidity, medication side effects, and the prevalence of polypharmacy require research in all settings on cost-effective follow-up strategies and educational approaches. For those receiving ECT, the efficacy of perioperative care strategies needs investigation. Likewise, involving OADs' families in training may reduce levels of anxiety in a stressful and demanding situation and facilitate continued training after the study. The former benefit has considerable theoretical relevance (Backman, 1992).

Patients, family members, and caregivers need to help identify meaningful and useful clinical outcomes. For example, Neundorfer (1991) demonstrated that the meaning of the situation to the caregiver, including appraisals of stress and coping, can explain caregiver outcomes more completely than can the severity of dementia. Qualitative research may be particularly useful in exploring the experience's meaning (Kuhlman, Wilson, Hutchinson, & Wallhagen, 1991). Also, researchers must make allowances for unanticipated effects. For example, social support may have both negative and positive consequences for the caregiver (Kuhlman et al., 1991). During the experimental design, the potential for multiple, and even conflicting, effects should receive attention. Researchers must consider the practicality of the intervention in light of caregivers' responsibilities. Particularly in dementia research, the characteristics of the caregiver or intervener are important variables. For example, OADs' performance may decline with a stranger but improve with someone they know. The OADs may also prefer, and respond to, the quality of a voice or the way someone approaches them. The intervener must find the right channel of communication to elicit optimal performance (Auer et al., 1994).

As interventions for OADs are applied in the clinical setting, it is critical that clinicians' assessments accurately distinguish between apparent and real cognitive deficits and identify the patient's preferred activities and goals. Testing for functional performance needs to involve real-life tasks, and the training must be generalized to real-life situations. Other important areas that researchers have yet to sufficiently address and that are thus important for clinicians to consider in implementing interventions are identifying the characteristics of patients who are most likely to benefit from the treatment, the intensity of the treatment needed, and the amount of maintenance treatment needed to prevent decline.

Because nurses are responsible for patient teaching and supervising patients' medication regimes, more research is needed on the efficacy of innovative teaching strategies and promoting physiological stability and compliance with treatment regimens. Given older adults' diverse physical changes, shrinking social networks, and unstable living arrangements, nurse researchers need to compare strategies across diverse social systems and methods of health care delivery.

Advanced nurse practitioners in primary care settings are in key positions to evaluate the usefulness and effectiveness of the guidelines for managing depression developed by AHCPR. More studies of particularly vulnerable groups of depressed older adults (e.g., nursing home, homeless, and terminally ill patients) are needed. Culture and ethnicity strongly influence how patients and their families seek assistance for mental illnesses, comply with medications, and respond to treatments, so nurses need to consider cohort differences in designing and evaluating nursing interventions.

Summary

The two most prevalent mental illnesses, cognitive impairment (delirium and dementia) and depression, for older adults prevent them from functioning optimally and diminish their quality of life. For the past 25 years, nurse researchers have conducted studies to determine these illnesses' risk factors, etiologies, and subtypes. They have also developed and tested interventions to treat them. However, much work remains. Nurse researchers need to develop standardized definitions, validate theoretical frameworks, and operationalize constructs with objective, congruent measures of treatment and outcomes. They also need to replicate intervention studies on dementia and depression in controlled environments, synthesize and meta-analyze the results, translate them into clinical practice, and confirm their utility by clinicians to provide evidence of the interventions' effectiveness. This pioneering work has provided the foundation for the science, which now must advance in a more systematic direction toward the 21st century.

References

Abraham, I. L. (1991). The Geriatric Depression Scale and Hopelessness Index: Longitudinal psychometric data on frail nursing home residents. *Perceptual and Motor Skills, 72*(3), 875-880.

Abraham, I. L., Neundorfer, M. M., & Currie, L. J. (1992). Effects of group interventions on cognition and depression in nursing home residents. *Nursing Research, 41*(4), 196-202.

Abraham, I. L., Niles, S. A., Thiel, B. P., Siarkowski, K. I., & Cowling, W. R. (1991). Therapeutic group work with depressed elderly. *Nursing Clinics of North America, 26*(3), 635-650.

Agency for Health Care Policy and Research: Depression Guideline Panel. (1993). *Depression in primary care: Vol. 2. Treatment of major depression* (AHCPR Pub. No. 93-0551). Washington, DC: U.S. Government Printing Office.

Algase, D. L., Beck, C., Kolanowski, A., Whall, A., Berent, S., Richards, K., & Beattie, E. (1996). Need-driven dementia-compromised behavior: An alternative view of disruptive behavior. *American Journal of Alzheimer's Disease, 11*(6), 10, 12-19.

American Psychiatric Association. (1994). *Diagnostic and statistical manual of mental disorders* (4th ed.). Washington, DC: Author.

Auer, S. R., Sclan, S. G., Yaffee, R. A., & Reisberg, B. (1994). The neglected half of Alzheimer disease: Cognitive and functional concomitants of severe dementia. *Journal of the American Geriatrics Society, 42*(12), 1266-1272.

Backman, L. (1992). Memory training and memory improvement in Alzheimer's disease: Rules and exceptions. *Acta Neurologica Scandinavica, 139*(Suppl.), 84-89.

Bandura, A. (1969). *Principles of behavior midification.* New York: Holt, Rinehart & Winston.

Barrera, M., & Ainlay, S. L. (1983). The structure of social support: A conceptual and empirical analysis. *Journal of Community Psychology, 11*(2), 133-143.

Bass, D. M., Looman, W. J., & Ehrlich, P. (1992). Predicting the volume of health and social services: Integrating cognitive impairment into the modified Andersen framework. *The Gerontologist, 32*, 33-43.

Batt, L. J. (1989). Managing delirium: Implications for geropsychiatric nurses. *Journal of Psychosocial Nursing and Mental Health Services, 27*(5), 22-25.

Beck, A. T . (1976). *Cognitive therapy and the emotional disorders.* New York: International Universities Press.

Beck, C. (1988). Measurement of dressing performance in persons with dementia. *American Journal of Alzheimer's Care and Related Disorders and Research, 3*(3), 21-25.

Beck, C. (1993a, July). *Promoting functional independence in the cognitively impaired elderly.* Paper presented at the Annual Summer Series on Aging, University of Kentucky, Lexington.

Beck, C. (1993b, November). *Improving behavior in cognitively impaired elderly.* Paper presented at the Gerontological Society of America 46th Scientific Meeting, New Orleans, LA.

Beck, C., & Baldwin, B. (1992). *Reducing disruptive behavior in demented elderly.* Grant R01 NA10321, National Institutes of Health, National Institute on Aging.

Beck, C., Heacock, P., Mercer, S. O., Thatcher, R., & Sparkman, C. (1988). The impact of cognitive skills remediation training on persons with Alzheimer's disease or mixed dementia. *Journal of Geriatric Psychiatry, 21*(1), 73-78.

Beck, C., Heacock, P., Mercer, S. O., Walls, R. C., Rapp, C. G., & Vogelpohl, T. S. (1997). Improving dressing behavior in cognitively impaired nursing home residents. *Nursing Research, 46*(3), 126-132.

Beck, C., Heacock, P., Mercer, S., Walton, C. G., & Shook, J. (1991). Dressing for success: Promoting independence among cognitively impaired elderly. *Journal of Psychosocial Nursing and Mental Health Services, 29*, 30-35, 39-40.

Beck, C., Heacock, P., Rapp, C. G., & Mercer, S. O. (1993). Assisting cognitively impaired elders with activities of daily living. *American Journal of Alzheimer's Care and Related Disorders and Research, 8*(6), 11-20.

Beel-Bates, C. A., & Rogers, A. E. (1990). An exploratory study of sundown syndrome. *Journal of Neuroscience Nursing, 22*(1), 51-52.

Biegel, D. E., Bass, D. M., Schulz, R., & Morycz, R. (1993). Predictors of in-home and out-of-home service use by family caregivers of Alzheimer's disease patients. *Journal of Aging and Health, 5*, 419-438.

Blair, C. E. (1995). Combining behavior management and mutual goal setting to reduce physical dependency in nursing home residents. *Nursing Research, 44*(3), 160-165.

Blazer, D. (1989). Depression in the elderly. *New England Journal of Medicine, 320,* 164-166.

Bliwise, D. L., & Lee, K. A. (1993). Development of Agitated Behavior Rating Scale for discrete temporal observations. *Journal of Nursing Measurement, 1*(2), 115-124.

Bourgeois, M. S. (1992). Evaluating memory wallets in conversations with persons with dementia. *Journal of Speech and Hearing Research, 35,* 1344-1357.

Bourgeois, M. S. (1993). Effects of memory aids on the dyadic conversations of individuals with dementia. *Journal of Applied Behavior Analysis, 26*(1), 77-87.

Bourgeois, M. S., Schulz, R., & Burgio, L. (1996). Interventions for caregivers of patients with Alzheimer's disease: A review and analysis of content, process, and outcomes. *International Journal of Aging and Human Development, 43*(1), 35-92.

Bowman, A. M. (1992). The relationship of anxiety to development of postoperative delirium. *Journal of Gerontological Nursing, 18*(1), 24-30.

Brannstrom, B., Gustafson, Y., Norberg, A., & Winblad, B. (1991). ADL performance and dependency on nursing care in patients with hip fractures and acute confusion in a task allocation care system. *Scandinavian Journal of Caring Sciences, 5*(1), 3-11.

Buckwalter, K. C. (1992). *Geriatric mental health nursing: Current and future challenges.* Thorofare, NJ: Slack.

Butler, K. (1963). The life review: An interpretation of reminiscence in the aged. *Psychiatry, 26,* 65-76.

Camp, C. J., Foss, J. W., Stevens, A. B., Reichard, C. C., McKitrick, L. A., & O'Hanlon, A. M. (1993). Memory training in normal and demented elderly populations: The E-I-E-I-O Model. *Experimental Aging Research, 19,* 277-290.

Campbell, J. M. (1992). Treating depression in well older adults: Use of diaries in cognitive therapy. *Issues in Mental Health Nursing, 13,* 9-29.

Champagne, M. T., & Wiese, R. A. (1992). Research on cognitive impairment: Implications for practice. In S. G. Funk, E. M. Tornquist, M. T. Champagne, & R. A. Wiese (Eds.), *Key aspects of elder care: Managing falls, incontinence and cognitive impairment* (pp. 340-346). New York: Springer.

Chappell, N. L., & Blandford, A. A. (1987). Health service utilization by elderly persons. *Canadian Journal of Sociology, 12,* 195-215.

Clark, W. G., & Vorst, V. R. (1994). Group therapy with chronically depressed geriatric patients. *Journal of Psychosocial Nursing and Mental Health Services, 32*(5), 9-13.

Cohler, B. J., Groves, L., Borden, W., & Lazarus, L. (1989). Caring for family members with Alzheimer's disease. In E. Light & B. D. Lebowitz (Eds.), *Alzheimer's disease treatment and family stress: Directions for research* (pp. 50-105). Rockville, MD: U.S. Department of Health and Human Services.

Cook, T. D., & Campbell, D. T. (1979). *Quasi-experimentation: Design and analysis issues for field settings.* Boston: Houghton Mifflin.

Coyne, M. L. (1990). The effect of directed verbal prompts and positive reinforcement on the level of eating independence of elderly nursing home clients with dementia. *Dissertation Abstracts International, 50*(8), 3396B.

Cronin-Golomb, A. (1995). Vision in Alzheimer's disease. *The Gerontologist, 35*(3), 370-376.

Cronin-Golomb, A., Corkin, S., & Growdon, J. H. (1995). Visual dysfunction predicts cognitive deficits in Alzheimer's disease. *Optometry and Vision Science, 72*(3), 168-176.

Dillehay, R. C., & Sandys, M. R. (1990). Caregivers for Alzheimer's patients: What we are learning from research. *International Journal of Aging and Human Development, 30,* 263-285.

D'Zurilla, T. J. (1988). Problem-solving therapies. In K. S. Dobson (Ed.), *Handbook of cognitive-behavioral therapies* (pp. 85-135). New York: Guilford.

Emmerson, C., Pugh, M., Wright, S., Bolton, L., & Hoskins, A. (1992). Fighting depression. *Nursing Times, 88*(17), 60-62.

Evans, L. (1987). Sundown syndrome in institutionalized elderly. *Journal of the American Geriatrics Society, 35,* 101-108.

Feil, N. (1993). *The validation breakthrough: Simple techniques for communicating with people with Alzheimer's-type dementia.* Baltimore, MD: Health Professions.

Folkman, S., & Lazarus, R. S. (1991). Coping and emotion. In A. Monat & R. S. Lazarus (Eds.), *Stress and coping: An anthology* (3rd ed., pp. 207-227). New York: Columbia University Press.

Folstein, M. F., Folstein, S. E., & McHugh, P. R. (1975). "Mini-mental state": A practical guide for grading the cognitive status of patients for the clinician. *Journal of Psychiatric Research, 12,* 189-198.

Foreman, M. D. (1989). Confusion in the hospitalized elderly: Incidence, onset, and associated factors. *Research in Nursing and Health, 12,* 21-29.

Foreman, M. D. (1991). The cognitive and behavioral nature of acute confusional states. *Scholarly Inquiry for Nursing Practice: An International Journal, 5*(1), 3-16.

Foreman, M. D. (1993). Acute confusion in the elderly. *Annual Review of Nursing Research, 11,* 3-30.

Francis, J., Martin, D., & Kapoor, W. N. (1990). A prospective study of delirium in hospitalized elderly. *Journal of the American Medical Association, 263*(8), 1097-1101.

Friedman, R., & Tappen, R. M. (1991). The effect of planned walking on communication in Alzheimer's disease. *Journal of the American Geriatrics Society, 39*(7), 650-654.

Gallagher-Thompson, D., & Steffen, A. M. (1994). Comparative effects of cognitive-behavioral and brief psychodynamic therapies for depressed family caregivers. *Journal of Consulting and Clinical Psychology, 62,* 543-549.

Gallagher-Thompson, D., & Thompson, L. (1994). Psychotherapy with older adults in theory and practice. In B. Bongar & L. Beutler (Eds), *Foundations of psychotherapy: Theory, research and practice.* New York: Oxford University Press.

Gerdner, L. A., & Swanson, E. A. (1993). Effects of individualized music on confused and agitated elderly patients. *Archives of Psychiatric Nursing, 7*(5), 284-291.

Gomez, G. E., & Gomez, E. A. (1992). The use of antidepressants with elderly patients. *Journal of Psychosocial Nursing and Mental Health Services, 30*(11), 21-26.

Gomez, G. E., & Gomez, E. A. (1993). Depression in the elderly. *Journal of Psychosocial Nursing and Mental Health Services, 31*(5), 28-33.

Grasel, E. (1994). Non-pharmacological intervention strategies on aging processes: Empirical data on mental training in "normal" older people and patients with mental impairment. *Archives of Gerontology and Geriatrics 4*(Suppl.), 91-98.

Gustafson, Y., Brannstrom, B., Berggren, D., Ragnarsson, J. I., Sigaard, J., Bucht, G., Reiz, S., Norberg, A., & Winblad, B. (1991). A geriatric-anesthesiologic program to reduce acute confusional states in elderly patients treated for femoral neck fractures. *Journal of the American Geriatrics Society, 39*(7), 655-662.

Gustafson, Y., Brannstrom, B., Norberg, A., Bucht, G., & Winblad, B. (1991). Underdiagnosis and poor documentation of acute confusional states in elderly hip fracture patients. *Journal of the American Geriatrics Society, 39*(8), 760-765.

Hall, G. R., Gerdner, L., Zwycart-Stauffacher, M., & Buckwalter, K. C. (1995). Principles of nonpharmacological management: Caring for people with Alzheimer's disease using a conceptual model. *Psychiatric Annals, 25*(7), 432-440.

Heacock, P., Garrett, A., & Mayhew, P. (1996). *Intervention for caregiver dementia client dyads.* Grant R01 NR03302, National Institutes of Health, Nursing Research Institute.

Heacock, P., Mayhew, P., Souder, E., O'Sullivan, P., & Chastain, J. D. (1995). Intervention for caregiver-dementia client dyads [abstract]. *The Gerontologist, 35*(Special Issue 1), 222.

Heacock, P., Walton, C., Beck, C., & Mercer, S. (1991). Caring for the cognitively-impaired: Reconceptualizing disability and rehabilitation. *Journal of Gerontological Nursing, 17*(3), 22-26.

Heston, L. L., Garrard, J., Makris, L., Kane, R. L., Cooper, S., Dunham, T., & Zelterman, D. (1992). Inadequate treatment of depressed nursing home elderly. *Journal of the American Geriatrics Society, 40*, 1117-1122.

Holden, J. E., & Therrien, B. (1989). The effects of hippocampal damage on adaptation to novelty in rats. *Journal of Neuroscience Nursing, 21*(1), 38-41.

Holden, J. E., & Therrien, B. (1993). Cue familiarity reduces spatial disorientation following hippocampal damage. *Nursing Research, 42*(6), 338-343.

Hughes, C. P. (1991). Community psychiatric nursing and the depressed elderly: A case for using cognitive therapy. *Journal of Advanced Nursing, 16*, 565-572.

Inaba-Roland, K. E., & Maricle, R. A. (1992). Assessing delirium in the acute care setting. *Heart and Lung, 21*(1), 48-55.

Inoye, S. K., van Dyck, C. H., Alessi, C. A., Balkin, S., Siegal, A., & Horowitz, R. I. (1990). Clarifying confusion: The confusion assessment method. A new method for detection of delirium. *Annals of Internal Medicine, 86*, 40-46.

Irvin, B. L., & Acton, G. J. (1997). Stress, hope, and well-being of women caring for family members with Alzheimer's disease. *Holistic Nursing Practice, 11*(2), 69-79.

Josephsson, S., Backman, L., Borell, L., Bernspang, B., Nygard, L., & Ronnberg, L. (1993). Supporting everyday activities in dementia: An intervention study. *International Journal of Geriatric Psychiatry, 8*, 395-400.

Josephsson, S., Backman, L., Borell, L., Nygard, L., & Bernspang, B. (1995). Effectiveness of an intervention to improve occupational performance in dementia. *Occupational Therapy Journal of Research, 15*(1), 36-49.

Katz, I. (1995, September 10). *Depression in the elderly.* Paper presented at the Long Term Care Conference, Minneapolis Geriatric Research Education and Clinical Center, Minneapolis, MN.

Kroeger, L. L. (1991). Critical care nurses' perceptions of the confused elderly patient. *Focus on Critical Care, 18*(5), 395-400.

Kuhlman, G. J., Wilson, H. S., Hutchinson, S. A., & Wallhagen, M. (1991). Alzheimer's disease and family caregiving: Critical synthesis of the literature and research agenda. *Nursing Research, 40*(6), 331-337.

Kurlowicz, L. H. (1993). Social factors and depression in late life. *Archives of Psychiatric Nursing, 7*(1), 30-36.

Kuroda, S., Ishizu, H., Ujike, H., Otsuki, S., Mitsusuke, K., Chuda, M., & Yamamoto, M. (1990). Senile delirium with special reference to situational factors and recurrent delirium. *Acta Medica Okayama, 44*(5), 267-272.

Lappe, J. M. (1987). Reminiscing: The life review therapy. *Journal of Gerontological Nursing, 13*(4), 12-16.

Lazarus, R. S., & Folkman, S. (1991). The concept of coping. In A. Monat & R. S. Lazarus (Eds.), *Stress and coping: An anthology* (3rd ed., pp. 189-206). New York: Columbia University Press.

Leidy, N. K. (1994). Functional status and the forward progress of merry-go-rounds: Towards a coherent analytical framework. *Nursing Research, 43*(4), 196-202.

Leja, A. M. (1989). Using guided imagery to combat postsurgical depression. *Journal of Gerontological Nursing, 15*(4), 7-11.

Leszca, M. (1990). Towards an integrated model of group psychotherapy with the elderly. *International Journal of Group Psychotherapy, 40*(4), 379-399.

Levkoff, S. E., Safran, C., Cleary, P. D., Gallop, J., & Phillips, R. S. (1988). Identification of factors associated with the diagnosis of delirium in elderly hospitalized patients. *Journal of the American Geriatrics Society, 36*, 1099-1104.

Lipowski, Z. (1989). Delirium in the elderly patient. *New England Journal of Medicine, 320*(9), 578-582.

Lipowski, Z. J. (1984). Acute confusional states (delirium) in the elderly. In M. O. Albert (Ed.), *Clinical neurology of aging* (pp. 277-297). New York: Oxford University Press.

Liptzin, B., Levkoff, S. E., Cleary, P. D., Pilgrim, D. M., Reilly, C. H., Albert, M., & Wetle, T. T. (1991). An empirical study of diagnostic criteria for delirium. *American Journal of Psychiatry, 148*(4), 454-457.

Mahler, M. S., Pine, F., & Bergman, A. (1994). Stages in the infant's separation from the mother. In G. Handel & G. G. Whitchurch (Eds.), *The psychosocial interior of the family* (4th ed., pp. 419-448). New York: Aldine deGruyter.

Matteson, M. A., Linton, A. D., Barnes, S. J., Cleary, B. L., & Lichtenstein, M. L. (1996). The relationship between Piaget and cognitive levels in persons with Alzheimer's disease and related disorders. *Aging, 8*(1). 61-69.

McCrone, S. H. (1991). Resocialization group treatment with confused institutionalized elderly. *Western Journal of Nursing Research, 13*(1), 30-45.

McDougall, G. J. (1995). Existential psychotherapy with older adults. *Journal of the American Psychiatric Association, 1*(1), 16-21.

McEvoy, C. L., & Patterson, R. L. (1986). Behavioral treatment of deficit skills in dementia patients. *The Gerontologist, 26*, 475-478.

McKitrick, L. A., Camp, C. J., & Black, F. W. (1995). Prospective memory intervention in Alzheimer's disease. *Journals of Gerontology: Psychological Sciences, 47*(5), P337-P343.

Montgomery, R.J.V., Karl, K., & Borgatta, E. (1988). The influence of cognitive impairment on service use and caregiver response. *Journal of Applied Social Science, 13*, 142-169.

Morton, I., & Bleathman, C. (1991). The effectiveness of validation therapy in dementia: A pilot study. *International Journal of Geriatric Psychiatry, 6*, 327-330.

Mullan, J. T. (1993). Barriers to the use of formal services among Alzheimer's caregivers. In S. H. Zarit, L. I. Pearlin, & K. W. Schaie (Eds). *Caregiving systems: Informal and formal helpers* (pp. 241-316). Hillsdale, NJ: Lawrence Erlbaum.

Mumford, E., Schlesinger, H. J., Glass, G. V, Patrick, C., & Cuerdon, B. A. (1984). A new look at evidence about reduced cost of medical utilization following mental health treatment. *American Journal of Psychiatry, 141*, 1145-1158.

National Institutes of Health Consensus Development Panel on Depression in Late Life. (1992). Diagnosis and treatment of depression in late life. *Journal of the American Medical Association, 268*(8), 1018-1024.

Neelon, V. J., & Champagne, M. T. (1992). Managing cognitive impairment: The current bases for practice. In S. G. Funk, E. M. Tornquist, M. T. Champagne, & R. A. Wiese (Eds.), *Key aspects of elder care: Managing falls, incontinence and cognitive impairment* (pp. 239-250). New York: Springer.

Neelon, V. J., Champagne, M. T., McConnell, E., Carlson, J., & Funk, S. G. (1992). Use of the NEECHAM confusion scale to assess acute confusional states of hospitalized older patients. In S. G. Funk, E. M. Tornquist, M. T. Champagne, & R. A. Wiese (Eds.), *Key aspects of elder care: Managing falls, incontinence and cognitive impairment* (pp. 278-289). New York: Springer.

Nelson, P. B. (1990). Intrinsic/extrinsic religious orientation of the elderly: Relationship to depression and self-esteem. *Journal of Gerontological Nursing, 16*(2), 29-35.

Neundorfer, M. M. (1991). Coping and health outcomes in spouse caregivers of persons with dementia. *Nursing Research, 40*(5), 260-265.

Noelker, L. S., & Bass, D. M. (1989). Home care for elderly persons: Linkages between formal and informal caregivers. *Journal of Gerontology, 44,* 63-70.

Nolen, N. R., & Garrard, J. (1988). Predicting dependent feeding behaviors in the institutionalized elderly. *Journal of Nutrition for the Elderly, 7,* 17-25.

Osborn, C. L., & Marshall, M. J. (1993). Self-feeding performance in nursing home residents. *Journal of Gerontological Nursing, 19*(3), 7-14.

Pearlin, L. I., Mullan, J. T., Semple, S. J., & Skaff, M. M. (1990). Caregiving and the stress process: An overview of concepts and their measures. *The Gerontologist, 30,* 583-594.

Penning, M. J. (1995). Health, social support, and the utilization of health services among older adults. *Journal of Gerontology, 50,* 330-339.

Pollack, L. E. (1991). Problem-solving group therapy: Two inpatient models based on level of functioning. *Issues in Mental Health Nursing, 12,* 65-80.

Quayhagen, M. P., & Quayhagen, M. (1989). Differential effects of family-based strategies on Alzheimer's disease. *The Gerontologist, 29*(2), 150-155.

Quayhagen, M. P., Quayhagen, M., Corbeil, R. R., Roth, P. A., & Rodgers, J. A. (1995). A dyadic remediation program for care recipients with dementia. *Nursing Research, 44*(3), 153-159.

Quinn, J. F., & Strelkauskas, A. J. (1993). Psychoimmunologic effects of therapeutic touch on practitioners and recently bereaved recipients: A pilot study. *Advances in Nursing Science, 15*(4), 13-26.

Reed, P. (1991). Toward a nursing theory of self-transcendence: Deductive reformulation using developmental theories. *Advances in Nursing Science, 13*(4), 64-77.

Reichenbach, V. R., & Kirchman, M. M. (1991). Effects of a multi-strategy program upon elderly with organic brain syndrome. In E. D. Taira (Ed.), *The mentally impaired elderly* (pp. 131-151). Binghamton, NY: Haworth.

Reynolds, C. F., Frank, E., Perel, J. M., Imber, S. D., Cornes, C., Morycz, R. K., Mazumdar, S., Miller, M. D., Pollock, B. G., Rifai, A. H., Stack, J. A., George, C. F., Houck, P. R., & Kupfer, D. J. (1992). Combined pharmacotherapy and psychotherapy in the acute and continuation treatment of elderly patients with recurrent major depression: A preliminary report. *American Journal of Psychiatry, 149,* 1687-1692.

Rockwood, K. (1989). Acute confusion in elderly medical patients. *Journal of the American Geriatrics Society, 37,* 150-154.

Rockwood, K., & Stadnyk, K. (1994). The prevalence of dementia in the elderly: A review. *Canadian Journal of Psychiatry, 39,* 253-257.

Rosswurm, M. A. (1989). Assessment of perceptual processing deficits in persons with Alzheimer's disease. *Western Journal of Nursing Research, 11*(4), 458-468.

Rosswurm, M. A. (1990). Attention-focusing program for persons with dementia. *Clinical Gerontologist, 10*(2), 3-16.

Rowlands, D. (1984). Therapeutic touch: Its effects on the depressed elderly. *Australian Nurses Journal, 13*(11), 45-52.

Sambandham, M., & Schirm, V. (1995). Music as a nursing intervention for residents with Alzheimer's disease in long-term care. *Geriatric Nursing, 16*(2), 79-83.

Scanland, S. G., & Emershaw, L. E. (1993). Reality orientation and validation therapy. *Journal of Gerontological Nursing, 19*(6), 7-11.

Schaie, K. W., & Willis, S. L. (1993). Age difference patterns of psychometric intelligence in adulthood: Generalizability within and across ability domains. *Psychology and Aging, 8*(1), 44-55.

Schneider, L. S. (1995). Efficacy of clinical treatment for mental disorders among older persons. In M. Gatz (Ed.), *Emerging issues in mental health and aging* (pp. 19-72). Washington, DC: American Psychological Assocation.

Schneider, L. S., Martinez, R. A., & Lebowitz, B. D. (1993). Clinical psychopharmacology research in geriatrics: An agenda for research. *International Journal of Geriatric Psychiatry, 8,* 89-93.

Schor, J. D., Levkoff, S. E., Lipsitz, L. A., Reilly, C. H., Cleary, P. D., Rowe, J. W., & Evans, D. A. (1992). Risk factors for delirium in hospitalized elderly. *Journal of the American Medical Association, 267*(6), 827-831.

Scogin, F., & McElreath, L. (1994). Efficacy of psychosocial treatments for geriatric depression: A quantitative review. *Journal of Consulting and Clinical Psychology, 62*(1), 69-74.

Seymour, D. G., Henschke, P. J., Cape, R.D.T., & Campbell, A. J. (1980). Acute confusional states and dementia in the elderly: The role of dehydration volume depletion, physical illness and age. *Age and Aging, 9*(3), 137-146.

Sloane, P. D., Rader, J., Barrick, A. L., Hoeffer, B., Dwyer, S., McKenzie, D., Lavelle, M., Buckwalter, K., Arrington, L., & Pruitt, T. (1995). Bathing persons with dementia. *The Gerontologist, 35*(5), 672-678.

Souder, E. (1996a). *SPECT and spatial neurocognitive predictors of IADLs in AD.* Grant R03 NR03814, National Institutes of Health, Nursing Research Institute.

Souder, E. (1996b). *The relationship of ADLS, neuropsychological test data and SPECT perfusion patterns.* Clinical Mental Health Academic Award K107 MH01115-01A1, National Institutes of Health, National Institute of Mental Health.

Stephens, M.A.P. (1993). Understanding barriers to caregivers' use of formal services: The caregiver's perspective. In S. H. Zarit, L. I. Perlin, & K. W. Schaie (Eds.), *Caregiving systems: Informal and formal helpers* (pp. 261-272). Hillsdale, NJ: Lawrence Erlbaum.

Stewart, B. J., & Archbold, P. G. (1992). Nursing intervention studies require outcome measures that are sensitive to change: Part one. *Research in Nursing and Health, 15,* 477-481.

Tabloski, P. A., McKinnon-Howe, L., & Remington, R. (1995, March/April). Effects of calming music on the level of agitation in cognitively impaired nursing home residents. *Alternative Medicine Journal, 2*(2), 27-33.

Tappen, R. M. (1994). The effect of skill training on functional abilities of nursing home residents with dementia. *Research in Nursing and Health, 17*(3), 159-165.

Teri, L., Rabins, P., Whitehouse, P., Berg, L., Reisberg, B., Sunderland, T., Eichelman, B., & Phelps, C. (1992). Management of behavior disturbance in Alzheimer disease: Current knowledge and future directions. *Alzheimer Disease and Associated Disorders, 6*(2), 77-88.

Tess, M. M. (1991). Acute confusional states in critically ill patients: A review. *Journal of Neuroscience Nursing, 23*(6), 398-402.

Tourangeau, A. (1988). Group reminiscence therapy as a nursing intervention: An experimental study. *AARN Newsletter, 44*(8), 17-18.

Tripp-Reimer, T. (1995). *Annual report (no. 2): Iowa-Veterans Affairs Nursing Research Consortium.* Iowa City: College of Nursing, University of Iowa.

Trzepacz, P. T., Baker, R. W., & Greenhouse, J. (1988). A symptom rating scale for delirium. *Psychiatry Research, 23,* 89-97.

Van Ort, S., & Phillips, L. (1992). Feeding nursing home residents with Alzheimer's disease. *Geriatric Nursing: The American Journal of Care for the Aging, 13*(5), 249-253.

Vermeersch, P. E. (1992). Clinical assessment of confusion. In S. G. Funk, E. M. Tornquist, M. T. Champagne, & R. A. Wiese (Eds.), *Key aspects of elder care: Managing falls, incontinence and cognitive impairment* (pp. 251-262). New York: Springer.

Voelkel, D. (1978). A study of reality orientation and resocialization groups with confused elderly. *Journal of Gerontological Nursing, 4*(3), 1-8.

Wan, T. (1989). The behavioral model of health-care utilization by older people. In M. Ory & K. Bond (Eds.), *Aging and health care: Social science and policy perspectives* (pp. 54-76). London: Routledge.

Wanich, C. K., Sullivan-Marx, E., Gottlieb, G. L., & Johnson, J. C. (1992). Functional status outcomes of a nursing intervention in hospitalized elderly. *Image: The Journal of Nursing Scholarship, 24*(3), 201-207.

Ward, R. A., Sherman, S. R., & LaGory, M. (1984). Informal networks and knowledge of services for older persons. *Journal of Gerontology, 39,* 216-223.

Waterreus, A., Blanchard, M., & Mann, A. (1994). Community psychiatric nurses for the elderly: Well tolerated, few side-effects and effective in the treatment of depression. *Journal of Clinical Nursing, 3,* 299-306.

Whall, A. L., Gillis, G. L., Yankou, D., Booth, D. E., & Beel-Bates, C. A. (1992). Disruptive behavior in elderly nursing home residents: A survey of nursing staff. *Journal of Gerontological Nursing, 18*(10), 13-17.

Williams, M. A., Campbell, E. B., Raynor, W. J., Jr., Mlynarczyk, S. M., & Ward, S. E. (1985a). Reducing acute confusional states in elderly patients with hip fractures. *Research in Nursing and Health, 8,* 329-337.

Williams, M. A., Campbell, E. B., Raynor, W. J., Jr., Musholt, M. A., Mlynarczyk, S. M., & Crane, L. F. (1985). Predictors of acute confusional states in hospitalized elderly patients. *Research in Nursing and Health, 8,* 31-40.

Williams, M. A., Holloway, J. R., Winn, M. C., Wolanin, M. O., Lawler, M. L., Westwick, C. R., & Chin, M. H. (1979). Nursing activities and acute confusional states in elderly hip-fractured patients. *Nursing Research, 28*(1), 25-35.

Williams, M. A., Ward, S. E., & Campbell, E. B. (1988). Confusion: Testing versus observation. *Journal of Gerontological Nursing, 14*(1), 25-30.

Woods, P., & Ashley, J. (1995). Simulated presence therapy: Using selected memories to manage problem behaviors in Alzheimer's disease patients. *Geriatric Nursing, 16*(1), 9-14.

Zarit, S., & Teri, L. (1992). Interventions and services for family caregivers. In K. W. Schaie & M. Powell Lawton (Eds.), *Annual review of gerontology and geriatrics* (Vol. 11, pp. 287-310). New York: Springer.

Zauszniewski, J. A. (1994). Potential sequelae of family history of depression: Identifying family members at risk. *Journal of Psychosocial Nursing, 32*(9), 15-21.

Zerhusen, J. D., Boyle, K., & Wilson, W. (1991). Out of the darkness: Group cognitive therapy for depressed elderly. *Journal of Psychosocial Nursing and Mental Health Services, 29*(9), 16-21.

32

SUPPORTIVE AND NONSUPPORTIVE CARE ENVIRONMENTS FOR THE ELDERLY

Linda R. Phillips
Martha Ayres

A central goal of gerontological nursing is to assist elders to optimize or preserve functional abilities in the face of age-related changes and illness and its long-term consequences. Many factors that influence reaching this goal are person related. For example, although many controversies exist (such as whether age-related changes are a natural consequence of aging or induced externally and whether these changes should be interpreted in terms of decline or *growth;* e.g., Birren & Bengston, 1988), there is no argument that elders experience physical and, to some degree, psychological and cognitive changes that have an impact on their self-care abilities. Similarly, there is no argument that, compared to younger people, elders have a greater predisposition to acute and chronic illness and to the long-term, potentially disabling effects of these illnesses. Understanding person-related factors is instructive for creating interventions to meet the goal of gerontological nursing, but evidence

suggests other factors play a part as well. An elder's functional limitations are not always directly proportional to either the severity of illness or the apparent threat to physical capabilities, which has given rise to the concepts of imposed disability and premature decline (Dawson, Kline, Wiancko, & Wells, 1986). Therefore, considering person-related factors alone is not sufficient for creating interventions to meet the goal.

To some degree, the functional abilities of all individuals are dependent on the person, the environment, and the person-environment interaction. Young people function ably because their environment is designed to support their capabilities. In other words, a balance is maintained between the person's ability to manipulate the environment and the degree of difficulty inherent in the environment. For the elderly, the situation can be quite different. The elder's capabilities may change, but this does not necessarily mean there is a concomitant

599

change in the environment. Further, an environment designed to support function in the young may actually impede function in the elderly. Although many of the person-related factors associated with being older are unchangeable, environment-related factors have great potential for modification. Thus, although the concepts of environment and person/environment interaction can be virtually ignored in many subspecialties within nursing, in gerontological nursing they are central.

The purpose of this chapter is to describe the gerontological nursing research that focuses on environment and the person-environment interaction. The first part of the chapter creates the theoretical context for the research by exploring conceptualizations of environment both within and outside of nursing. The second part focuses on selected research studies of supportive and nonsupportive environments for the elderly.

Conceptualizing Environment

Environment is at once a simple yet complex concept. On the one hand, it is easy to use the dictionary definition of environment: an individual's physical surroundings. On the other hand, many theorists inside and outside of nursing have recognized that environments are composed of more than physical objects and atmosphere (i.e., air, temperature, etc.). For example, Nightingale's (1859/1992) theory of nursing dealt in detail with the physical environment, including the nurse as a part of the patient's environment. Rogers' (1994) theory of unitary human beings identified both persons and environments as energy fields without boundaries that are in constant interaction and exchange. Outside of nursing, the field of environmental psychology is devoted to the study of the relationship between the individual and his or her environment and the way the interaction between individual and environment affects behavior (Lawton, Windley, & Byerts, 1982). Architects and sociologists are also interested in the interaction of person and environment. These disciplines have had a profound influence on the way in which environment has been conceptualized and studied within the field of gerontological nursing. It has affected the ways environment and supportive environment have been defined in nursing research, the environmental attributes that have been studied, and the ways nurses have conceptualized using environmental manipulation as an intervention for the elderly.

Definitions of Environment and Supportive Environment

Most theorists agree that environment is a multidimensional concept. Wolanin and Phillips (1981) discuss the environment of elders, specifically the assessment of the environment of confused elders, in terms of two dimensions: the personal/social environment, which consists of the people in the elder's environment and the degree of interaction between them, and the physical environment, which begins where the physical body of the individual ends. From these authors' point of view, the responsibility of the nurse in establishing a facilitative or supportive environment consists of both changing the environment to allow the elder to be successful within it and assisting the elder to change and adapt to his or her environment in light of personal capabilities. The degree to which negative interactions between elders and environments are changed to positive interactions (either through changes in the environment or changes in the elder or both) is the degree to which the elder-environment relationship is supportive or nonsupportive.

Lawton (1982) identified four dimensions of environment. The *personal* environment is composed of the significant others in the elder's life, such as family, friends, and others with whom the elder interacts directly. The *suprapersonal* environment consists of the characteristics (e.g., race, age, financial status) of the individuals surrounding the elder. From Lawton's point of view, the elder living in a nursing home has a significantly different suprapersonal environment than an elder living in a neighborhood with families of different ages or an elder living in a retirement community. The *social* environment is determined by the norms and values of the elder's community and culture. Finally, the *physical* environment is the nonsocial aspect of the environment in which the elder lives. Lawton's premise is that an individual's behavior is a function of the individual, the environment, and the interaction between the two. Supportive environments are those in which the demands of the elder's needs are balanced by the ability of the environment to meet the needs.

Kolcaba (1991) incorporates the environment into her taxonomy of comfort, including the physical, social, psychospiritual, and environmental context. The physical context refers to the physical sensations experienced by the individual, and the psychospiritual context refers to self-awareness, ranging from self-concept and self-esteem to spirituality and the individual's relationship to a higher being. The social and environmental contexts are the equivalents of physical and social environments as defined by Wolanin and Phillips (1981) and Lawton (1982). For Kolcaba (1991), supportive environment is defined by the presence and degree of comfort the elder experiences in navigating and occupying the environment.

Cookman (1996) offers a slightly different view of environment as it applies to elders. He proposes that components of environments constitute attachment objects for elders. Within this context, he asserts that the environments of elders are composed of people, places, things, companion animals, and ideas and beliefs and that elders have attachments to and interactions with each of these. He believes that Lawton's concept of environmental press (described later) takes on new meaning when the conceptualization of environment is expanded beyond the notion of physical environment and when changes in any of the five dimensions are viewed in terms of loss of attachment objects or as changes in the elder's relationship to attachment objects. He believes that human-environment interactions are central to growth throughout the life span and that understanding the nature of these environmental connections is central to our understanding of health in aging.

Environmental Attributes

Hiatt (1982) describes the attributes of environment as related to the functional needs of the elderly. The attributes she addresses are visual environments, auditory environments, movement and mobility, continence, boredom, orientation to place, social needs and privacy, and size and configuration of the physical environment. She addresses these attributes on the microenvironmental level, such as lighting levels, acoustics, room size, and arrangement, and also on the macroenvironmental level, which includes those characteristics of the physical and social environment that permit interaction. Similar to Lawton (1982), Wolanin and Phillips (1981), Kolcaba (1991), and many other scholars who have influenced the study of gerontological nursing (e.g., Dawson, Wells, & Kline, 1993; Hall & Buckwalter, 1987), Hiatt works from the premise that the environment and its attributes can be manipulated to promote or support optimal functioning of the elderly individual.

Four environmental attributes are considered by Wolanin and Phillips (1981): intensity, complexity, pattern, and relevance. *Intensity* is defined in terms of the strength or magnitude of the environmental characteristic. For example, temperature is a characteristic of the physical environment, and degree of heat or cold would be considered an attribute. *Complexity* is the number

of characteristics impinging on the individual at any given time within a given environment. For example, a supermarket, where there are many different objects and people together in a confined space, has a higher level of complexity than a bedroom, where there are fewer objects and people. *Pattern* relates to predictability and regularity of the environmental characteristics. On a nursing unit, for example, meals, rounds, shift changes, and medication administration routines provide a certain predictability and, therefore, a certain kind of meaning for the individuals occupying the nursing unit. In contrast, in an emergency room, there is little routine or predictability and, consequently, little pattern. *Relevance* refers to the meaning individuals attach to the various aspects of the environment. My living room occupied by family and familiar objects has great meaning, hence relevance for me, whereas when I am with a casual friend in the waiting room of a physician's office, the room has little relevance. Wolanin and Phillips' premise is that one strategy for creating a supportive environment for the elderly is the manipulation of the environmental attributes.

The classic work of Goffman (1961) provides another viewpoint on the attributes of environments that has influenced gerontological nursing research. Goffman describes the attributes of total institutions. Nursing homes fall under the category of institutions that are established for the care of like individuals considered incapable of self-care yet who present no threat to the community. Included in Goffman's other categories are prisons, mental institutions, hospitals, schools, and the military. It is his position that the study of one type of institution provides insights into the qualities of all others. The first attribute he ascribes to institutions is that within an institution all activities occur in a single place and under a single authority, as opposed to the general community in which individuals live, work, and play in several different places. Second, he believes that in institutions all activities involve the participation of other individuals with similar characteristics and circumstances, all of whom are treated in a like manner. Included in this attribute is the presence of two distinct groups within the institution: the "inmates" and those designated to care for or supervise them. Third, according to Goffman, all activities within an institution are scheduled, including personal activities such as sleeping, waking, eating, and bathing. Finally, activities in institutions are structured to further the goals of the institution, not the individual. Comparing a nursing home to a prison may be threatening to individuals who provide care to residents, but such a comparison can sensitize caregivers and administrators to the effect of institutional polices that may make life easier for the staff but limit the freedoms of an already option-deprived group. The attributes of institutional environments as described by Goffman have greatly influenced nursing research on the use of restraints in elders.

Use of Environments by Nurses as Intervention

Within nursing, environmental interventions can be grouped in two broad categories: (a) environment used as therapy and (b) manipulation of the environment to affect behavior. Both of these approaches have driven gerontological nursing research.

Environment as therapy. The use of environment as therapy, also known as therapeutic milieu, has its origins in psychiatric care. Gunderson (1978) proposed that the therapeutic milieu has five functions or processes: containment, support, structure, involvement, and validation. Within gerontological nursing, Taft, Delaney, Seman, and Stansell (1993) have modified Gunderson's model of therapeutic milieu to apply to dementia care.

Gunderson believed *containment* has the purpose of preventing psychiatric patients from harming themselves. Taft and colleagues modified this process to address the threats to safety and well-being of individuals with dementia that might lead to harm resulting from cognitive deficits, agitation, and the physical deficits involved with dementia.

Support was defined by Gunderson as a social process in which the patient is made to feel secure, safe, and comfortable, and conscious effort is made by staff to enhance the patient's self-esteem. Within the dementia care model proposed by Taft and colleagues, the same goal is present but achieved through the support of personal choice, reminiscence, communication, family interaction and involvement, and support of staff by administration.

Structure within the Gunderson model consisted of a series of behavioral strategies such as contracting, privilege systems, and token economies. Gunderson used structure to establish a routine, predictable system that would make the patient feel safe and promote the therapeutic effect of changing behaviors identified as maladaptive. Although strategies such as contracting may be inappropriate for persons with dementia, staff can still use structure to regulate the social environment through predictable activities and routines. The routine gives the individual temporal landmarks throughout the

day. The model proposed by Taft and colleagues also specifies enough flexibility in the structure to accommodate the individual's needs and wishes. Structure of the physical environment is accomplished through control of environmental stimulation, orienting cues such as physical landmarks or color codes, minimizing confusing cues (e.g., such as an open wastebasket next to a toilet with the lid closed), and maintaining a home-like and comfortable environment.

Involvement processes assist and promote active attention to and interaction with the environment. For the psychiatric population, this involves rounds in the unit, participation in unit activities, and the like. For individuals with dementia, involvement processes consist of meaningful activities, meaningful relationships, and role modeling by staff.

The final process described by Gunderson is *validation*, defined as affirmation of a patient's individuality through individual therapy, one-to-one interaction with staff, recognized right to privacy, and so on, provided in an atmosphere of acceptance. For the individual with dementia, the loss of the self is often an integral part of the disease process. Therefore, validation also involves maintaining the sense of self for as long as possible through personal items, cuing, and use of the other therapeutic processes. The use of the therapeutic milieu process model in the care of individuals with dementia requires manipulation of both the physical and the psychosocial environment. This model has been the basis of many studies of the use of the environment as therapy with elderly persons with dementia.

Manipulation of the environment as nursing intervention. One particularly influential theory outside of nursing and several nursing theories form the basis for research conducted on environmental manipulation as nursing intervention. Lawton's (1982) theory of person-environment relations is the theory outside of nursing that has been particularly influential. The concepts of competence and environmental press are key components of this theory. *Competence* consists of the overlapping and interacting processes of biological health, sensory and perceptual capacities, motor skill, cognitive capacity, and ego strength. The assessment of competence is multidimensional. *Environmental press* is any element within the elder's environment that results in behavior. Lawton and Nahemow (1973) define environmental press in normative terms, requiring empirical evidence to demonstrate the relationship between a stimulus and behavioral outcome before the stimulus is considered environmental press. The perception of the elder determines whether environmental press is positive or negative. The final component of the competence-environmental press relationship is adaptability of the elder, which assumes that the higher the competence of the individual, the higher the ability of that individual to adapt to negative environmental press. Lawton's conception of environmental press states that mild to moderate levels of environmental press result in activity that is labeled in the *zone of maximal performance potential*. In contrast, low levels of environmental press result in inactivity and passivity, labeled the *zone of maximal comfort*. This is considered to be a negative state, although maladaptive behavior does not result until extreme levels of understimulation are present. Lawton's use of the word *comfort* in a negative context is in direct opposition to the majority of the nursing literature, which defines comfort in terms of a goal for independent nursing intervention (e.g., Kolcaba, 1991, 1995), but important notions in his model are that high levels of environmental press result in the inability of the elder to respond in adaptive or functional ways, and low levels of environmental press can lead to premature decline and excessive disability.

The concept of comfort and the controversy in its definition and conceptualization are important to understand within the context of nursing research on environmental manipulation. Kolcaba's (1991, 1992, 1995) analysis and resulting taxonomy of the concept of comfort is highly applicable to the subject of supportive environments for the care of the elderly if the presence and degree of comfort is used as an outcome for intervention studies in nursing. Kolcaba (1991) developed a taxonomy of comfort in which three senses of comfort (ease, relief, transcendence) are experienced in four contexts (physical, psychospiritual, psychosocial, environmental). In applying the comfort taxonomy to gerontological nursing, Kolcaba (1995) uses (a) the concept of facilitative environment, with its psychological and physical dimensions (Wolanin & Phillips, 1981); (b) the concept of excess disability as a temporary condition related to an existing disability resulting from interaction with a nonsupportive environment (Schwab, Rader, & Doan, 1985); and (c) the concept of optimum function when using a baseline of function with the elder in a state of comfort. The apparently opposing use of the concept of comfort by Lawton and Kolcaba demonstrates the complexity of the concept. If the comfort of the elder results in inactivity or lethargy, this is potentially harmful both

physiologically and psychologically. At the other end of the continuum is the presence of discomfort, which is also harmful physiologically and psychologically. In research, the issue of comfort has not been well addressed, but the need to consider the issues in the design and testing of nursing interventions involving environmental manipulations is apparent.

The effect of Lawton's work can be seen in three nursing models that have served as the basis for gerontological nursing research. These are Dawson, Wells, and colleagues' (1993) model of enablement nursing process, Hall and Buckwalter's (1987) progressively lowered stress threshold model, and Roberts and Algase's (1988) model of person-environment interaction.

The enablement nursing process model (Dawson, Wells, et al., 1993) focuses on the function of nurses in the regulation of environmental press as it relates to the competence and behavior of the individual with cognitive impairment. Within this model, the concept of excess disability is also used. When the individual with cognitive impairment does not use his or her abilities, disability beyond the actual disability ensues. Understimulation, or low environmental press, allows this. Another consequence of low environmental press is the occurrence of inappropriate behavior in the elder's attempt at self-stimulation. High levels of environmental press in individuals with dementia can result in agitation or withdrawal if the level of press is greater than the individual's level of competence. Dawson and colleagues advocate the design of interventions based on an assessment of the individual's level of competence through identification of abilities, assessment of the individual's environment, and comparison of the individual's abilities to the degree of environmental press.

The progressively lowered stress threshold model (PLST) (Hall & Buckwalter, 1987) used the concept of environmental press as the basis for structuring special care units for individuals with dementia. According to the PLST model, individuals with dementia have a declining ability to accommodate themselves to the demands of the environment. The stress caused by declining capacity to meet the demands of both environmental and internal stimuli results in behavior that is progressively dysfunctional and finally catastrophic in nature. The use of the term *stress,* which denotes a negative stimulus and response, as opposed to "press" as presented by Lawton, which has the potential for both positive and negative response, reflects the declining competence of the population for whom the PLST model was developed. Catastrophic behavior is defined as a sudden behavioral reaction that is disproportionate to the stimulus or stimuli. The PLST model advocates control of environmental stimuli, with the goal of reducing the incidence of catastrophic behavior.

The person-environment interaction model (Roberts & Algase, 1988) also describes the behavior of elders with dementia by focusing on the interaction between person and environment. The premise of these authors is that behavior is determined by the meaning an individual ascribes to his or her situation. Meaning is derived through an appraisal process involving input from multiple sources (sensory function, mobility, memory, context of past and present personal experience, and environmental legibility). Environmental legibility, a key concept in their model, refers to the quality, quantity, and stability of the cues within the environment. Cues can be both physical and social in nature, and they are conveyed by physical presence (e.g., the color of the walls) as well as verbal and nonverbal communication. Cues can be meaningful and relevant to the individual or irrelevant, creating only noise and distraction. Stability refers to predictability, the degree to which cues provide information about what will happen next. Stability varies along the dimensions of degree and frequency, and changes in either of these can disrupt the stability of the pattern. Roberts and Algase believe three types of behavior represent disruptions in the person-environment interaction: repetitive behavior, which may be the individual's attempt to "anchor" him- or herself or increase sensory input; catastrophic reactions, which occur when pattern is disrupted; and situationally inappropriate behaviors, which suggest the individual is misinterpreting some portion of the environmental input during the appraisal process. Interventions for changing behavior that flow from this model suggest manipulation of the environment in four different areas: physical cues (creating redundant cues and reducing or eliminating irrelevant ones), social cues (clear communication focused on reducing ambiguity and creating relevance), physical stability (preserving physical continuity and reducing change), and social stability (preserving continuity of individuals and continuity of daily routine).

These models have greatly influenced literature about clinical care of elders, particularly those with dementia, and have provided the background for many of the studies of environments and environmental manipulation as a nursing intervention for the elderly. The next section presents an overview of the studies of supportive environments for the elderly.

State of the Science: Supportive and Nonsupportive Environments for the Elderly

The notion that environments for the elderly can either be facilitative (designed to allow an elder to be successful within it in light of personal capabilities) or nonfacilitative (in which aspects of the environment inhibit success) has been around for many years. Generally, in nursing no controversy exists about whether environment is a factor worthy of study. Nevertheless, environment is the metaparadigm concept in nursing that has been most neglected in our research, even in studies of the elderly. Interest in studying the effects of environment or the person-environment interaction on patient outcomes is relatively recent, and, even in these more recent studies, environment is usually studied either secondarily or indirectly because the primary purpose of studies is usually the person-related factors involved in various problems of the elderly. This incongruity is interesting given that person-related factors are often uncontrollable and amenable only to indirect manipulation, whereas the environment is often easily manipulated and is, in general, under the direct control of the nurse.

The next sections discuss studies that have directly or indirectly considered environment as a factor influencing the outcomes of nursing practice. Most attention is given to studies conducted in long-term care facilities because these represent the bulk of the research, although some studies have been conducted in other locations (e.g., adult care homes, home care). Four types of environment are considered: physical environments, social environments, structural environments, and facilitative environments. The studies discussed represent an extensive but not exhaustive review. They were selected because they were relatively recent and identifiable through computerized or pedigree literature searches. Some, but not all, studies were done by nurses.

Studies of Physical Environments for the Elderly

Studies of physical environments for the elderly have mostly been problem-focused. Problem-focused studies are those that target a particular difficulty that either creates a care dilemma, represents a hazard, or represents a real or inferred discomfort for the elderly client. The environment-related problems that have received the most research attention are agitation and confusion, sundowning, wandering, safety and falls, and restraints.

Agitation, Confusion, and Sundowning

Agitation, a behavioral state characterized by inappropriate vocal or motor activity that is not explained by the elder's needs or confusion (Cohen-Mansfield, 1986); *confusion,* a term used by nurses to denote "a constellation of client behaviors including inattention and memory deficits, inappropriate verbalizations, disruptive behavior, noncompliance, and failure to perform activities of daily living" (Wolanin & Phillips, 1981, p. 2); and *sundowning,* a state manifested by "disruptive and unusual behavioral demonstrated by the elderly client during the late afternoon and early evening hours" (Wallace, 1994, p. 164) have been concepts of concern to gerontological nurses for some time. Although each of these has unique aspects, they are considered together here because of their common behavioral—physical and verbal—manifestations. A significant amount of nursing research has focused on describing these problems and their antecedents and consequences. In addition, some studies have focused on developing and testing instruments for measuring agitation and confusion (e.g., the NEECHAM Confusion Scale, Neelon, Champagne, Carlson, & Funk, 1996; Cohen-Mansfield Agitation Inventory, Cohen-Mansfield, Marx, & Rosenthal, 1989; Pittsburgh Agitation Scale, Rosen et al., 1994; Confusion Inventory, Evans, 1987; Ryden Aggression Scale, Ryden, 1988; Behavior Inventory, Winger, Schirm, & Stewart, 1987; Disruptive Behavior Scale, Beck, Baldwin, Heithoff, & Cuffel, 1990). Much of this work is summarized in Gerdner and Buckwalter's (1994) excellent review article, which identifies the antecedents as cognitive impairments, psychiatric disorders, and internal and external stimuli resulting in situational anxiety, sensory impairment, physical disorders, and pharmacological effects. Environmental factors as antecedents to agitation are included in the Gerdner and Buckwalter (1994) review under external and internal stimuli. Not only studies cited in that review (e.g., Cohen-Mansfield, Marx, et al., 1989; Cohen-Mansfield, Marx, & Rosenthal, 1990; Cohen-Mansfield, Werner, & Marx, 1990; Marx, Werner, & Cohen-Mansfield, 1989; Ryden, Bossenmaier, & McLachlan, 1991) but also others (e.g., Nilsson, Palmstierna, & Wistedt, 1988; Rossby, Beck, & Heacock, 1992) document the relationship between care activities (e.g., bathing, meals, toileting) and increased agitation. Jackson and colleagues (1989) and Spector and Jackson (1994) docu-

mented the relationship between incontinence and disruptive behavior. In addition, Spector and Jackson (1994) found that severity of cognitive impairments, ADL (activities of daily living) dysfunction, and mobility are associated with disruptive behavior. Chrisman, Tabar, Whall, and Booth (1991) investigated the environment as an antecedent to agitation, and the data showed that agitated behavior could be precipitated by both environmental stimulation (i.e., the presence of another agitated person in the environment or being encouraged to participate in an activity when the patient expressed a desire to be alone) and lack of environmental stimulation. The findings also suggested that communication patterns (also considered as an environmental factor) influence manifestations of agitation. Various explanations for the mechanisms underlying these relationships have been advanced. For example, Boettcher (1983) suggests that agitation may be caused by the client's need to feel free from physical intrusion and invasion of personal space. Rossby and colleagues (1992) suggest that the mechanism may also be either need deficit or blocked goal attainment. Whatever the mechanics, however, it is fairly clear that intrusive care activities and other environmental factors are associated with increased agitation.

Confusion has been studied by several nurse researchers, including, for example, Foreman (1989, 1991, 1993) and Neelon and Champagne (1992). Person-related, research-based assessment protocols and environmental interventions tested for confusion are described in Chapter 31.

Evans (1987) conducted a study of sundowning in which she sought to describe the phenomenon, examine its prevalence, and identify psychosocial, physiological, and environmental factors associated with it. Among the 89 subjects observed, 11 were identified as sundowners, as characterized by increased restlessness and verbal behavior as evening approached. The sundowners had greater mental impairment than the nonsundowners. Of the psychosocial factors studied by Evans, only two (in addition to mental impairment) were significant. Sundowners had a shorter length of stay in the facility, and more of them had had a recent room transfer. They were also observed to have few visitors and to engage in few activities. Of the physiological factors studied, three were significant. Sundowners had more medical diagnoses than nonsundowners. Sundowners tended to have a strong urine odor in the evening. Sundowners were also awakened more in the evening hours than nonsundowners. Although not significant, 8 of 11 sundowners had a decrease in diastolic blood pressure in the evening on one or both observation days, and four had lower oral temperatures in the evening on one study day. Evans posited that given the strong urine odor, decreased diastolic blood pressure, and altered temperature, dehydration as a cause of possible sundowning cannot be ignored. Evans studied two environmental factors: mean light intensity change and restraint use. Neither was different between the two groups. Overall, sundowners were more likely to be in restraints than nonsundowners, but the use did not increase in the evening. No demographic variables were related to sundowning.

Beel-Bates and Rogers (1990) conducted a descriptive study of sundowning to compare behaviors of institutionalized women with and without dementia. Between 1:30 and 4:30 p.m. and 6:30 and 8:30 p.m., subjects were observed for 5 to 10 minutes every 30 minutes; between 4:00 and 6:00 p.m., subjects were observed every 15 minutes. Observation focused on 5 verbal behaviors (quiet, talking to others, talking to self, calling out, and screaming) and 8 skeletal motor activities (sleeping, sitting quietly, eating, ADL, sitting fidgeting, roaming, pacing, and attempts to escape from the unit). Higher numerical scores were given to activities that interfered with nursing care. Data were graphed for analysis. Activity between the groups differed between 4:00 and 6:30 p.m., with demented subjects increasing their activity and nondemented subjects decreasing their activity. Anecdotal data suggest that sundowning may be related to social cues and light illumination, but these were not tested.

A variety of interventions have been tested for the problems of confusion, agitation, and sundowning, and many of these are reviewed in an article by Beck and Shue (1994). Some interventions have been strictly person-focused, with no attention given to the environment. Examples include studies of the effects of therapeutic touch (e.g., Gagne & Toye, 1994; Snyder, Egan, & Burns, 1995a); hand massage (e.g., Snyder, Egan, et al., 1995a, 1995b); relaxation therapy (e.g., Gagne & Toye, 1994); presence (e.g., Snyder, Egan, et al., 1995a); exercise (Meddaugh, 1986); and the SERVE intervention, which is a combination of group intervention, exercise, and relaxation (Schwab et al., 1985).

Other studies have considered the effects of environment-focused interventions to reduce agitation or confusion. For example, relaxing music administered at meals and other times has been studied by Bright (1986); Cohen-Mansfield, Werner, and Marx (1990); Gerdner and Swanson (1993); and Goddaer and Abraham (1994). In general, music has been shown to reduce the amount of agitation as well as the range of agitated behaviors, in-

cluding a reduction in screaming. Mayers and Griffin (1990) used stimulus items (e.g., mechnical items, "adult toys," or both) to determine if they could be used to reduce agitation. Their findings suggest that such items provide distraction, hold the resident's attention, and reduce agitation and combativeness.

In a study of assaultive and combative resident behavior, Negley and Manly (1990) used observation to determine the location of the bulk of patient assaults on the staff. Data showed that most assaults occurred while patients were in transit to meals. By centralizing services on the unit and reducing the number of transits, assaults were effectively reduced. Hussian and Brown (1987) studied a variety of environmental techniques (e.g., attentional cues such as symbols and tape and perceptual cues such as grid patterns) on the disruptive behavior of dementia patients. The environmental cues provided some "control" over the disruptive behaviors being studied. One study (Satlin, Volicer, Ross, Herz, & Campbell, 1992) investigated the effect of light as an environmental variable on sundowning. In this study, residents were exposed to bright light pulses during the evening hours (between 7 and 9 p.m.). Residents were observed for sleep-wake cycle disturbances, activity, and sundowning behavior. Results showed an improvement in 8 of the 10 residents and an association between the severity of symptoms at baseline and response to the therapy.

Still other intervention studies of agitation, confusion, and sundowning have targeted the interaction between the person and the environment, usually through education of the nursing staff. For example, Feldt and Ryden (1992) trained nursing assistants in the management of aggressive behavior. Although this study yielded data suggesting that the capabilities of the nursing assistants were improved, effectiveness of the interventions for reducing agitation or confusion was not documented. Wallace (1994) implemented a training program for nursing assistants that involved a standardized set of interventions for the management of sundowning. Results suggested that the training program was effective for reducing the number of disruptive behaviors displayed by the residents 2 weeks later.

Similarly, Maxfield, Lewis, and Cannon (1996) designed an educational intervention for nursing staff to prevent aggressive behavior during bathing and grooming. The intervention had four components: helping staff examine the approaches customarily used, introducing new models of behavior, demonstrating how to apply the new methods with practice, and follow-up. The new models taught included recognition (helping staff recognize how cognitively impaired individuals might perceive bathing and grooming), empathy (helping staff understand the elderly person's feelings), support (helping staff alter approaches and schedules to support a person's needs), prevention (learning strategies for de-escalating aggression), enhancement (helping staff be creative when helping patients use their own abilities), caring (helping staff to display their concern for a patient's needs and preferences), and taking time (allowing time for therapeutic interactions to occur). One month later, results showed a significant drop in the amount of aggression patients showed during bathing and grooming. In addition, there was a drop in use of PRN medications during bathing and a drop in staff injuries. Although this was not the test of an environmental intervention per se, aspects of the environmental context of care were considered along with the psychosocial context of care.

Likewise, Hoeffer, Rader, McKenzie, Lavelle, and Stewart (1997) studied strategies for reducing physical and verbal aggression during bathing. Their intervention focused on changing the psychosocial environment of bathing and modifying the function, frequency, and form of bathing. Their results showed that aggression could be reduced, making bathing less distressing to residents and nursing assistants as well.

Beck and Shue (1994) suggest that although some of the well-documented consequences of disruptive behavior relate to endangerment of residents (e.g., physical harm, increased use of chemical and physical restraints, stress, fright, and frustration and social isolation), other consequences relate to endangerment of staff. These consequences include injury from assault, burnout, absenteeism, and turnover. Some nursing research has attempted to elicit staff's perceptions of these problems. For example, Whall, Gillis, Yankou, Booth, and Beel-Bates (1992) surveyed staff (RNs and LPNs) to determine their perceptions of disruptive behavior in nursing home residents. The most frequent behavior identified by staff was hitting and slapping. The next most frequently listed behaviors were verbal aggression, screaming, and pacing or wandering. Staff's most frequently identified interventions for these behaviors were verbal discussion, followed by chemical restraints, physical restraints, time out, and touch. Rantz and McShane (1994, 1995) asked the staff (certified nursing assistants, nurses, other health care workers) to describe their experiences working with chronically confused residents in nursing homes. Using focus groups, they elicited information about frequently occurring behaviors of confused residents and interventions for disruptive behavior. Rantz and McShane (1994)

sorted responses into four categories (verbal behavior disturbances, such as screaming and yelling; fear-related behavior disturbances, such as anxiety, fear, and anger; wandering behavior disturbances, such as restlessness, pacing, and getting lost; and behaviors related to level of awareness of time, day, and place). The interventions identified by staff fell into four categories: interpreting reality, maintaining normalcy, meeting basic needs, and managing behavior disturbances. It is interesting in this research that behaviors that threatened harm to the staff, such as hitting, were not identified by staff. Although compared to the Whall and colleagues (1992) study, a richer and wider variety of nursing interventions for dealing with the problems was identified, as in the Whall study, almost no interventions were identified that focused on modifying the environment as a primary method for intervention.

Wandering

Definitions of wandering vary. It has been described as aimless locomotion, as pacing, and as hazardous ambulation. In addition, some investigators have identified specific verbal expressions as part of the definition (e.g., expressions of looking for lost objects, being lost, or wanting to go home). Part of the problem with definition is that whether locomotion is interpreted as wandering or not depends to some degree on the ability of the observer to identify the intent of the individual being observed, and part of identifying intent lies in the communication ability of the individual being observed. In addition, whether the behavior is seen as healthy and essential exercise or disruptive behavior depends on a number of contextual factors (e.g., size of space available, density of the population, staff time needed to find those who are "lost," presumed or documented etiology of the behavior, etc.). For example, Algase (1992a, 1992b) suggests progressive social withdrawal may be one possible etiology for wandering. Within this framework, wandering is a negative behavior, one that requires intervention directed at increasing social interaction and improving social skills. Decreasing wandering is a primary goal. On the other hand, Algase (1992a, 1992b) also posits, as Monsour and Robb's (1982) study suggests, that wandering may be a strategy used by certain individuals to reduce stress. Within this framework, wandering is a positive behavior, one that may require intervention so access of the wanderer to certain restricted areas is decreased but certainly not intervention to reduce or eliminate the behavior. Despite these difficulties, a number of studies of wandering have been conducted, including those that have sought to describe the behavior and the wanderers and those that have sought to test interventions for wandering.

A number of studies have sought to identify how wanderers are different from nonwanderers. For example, Snyder, Rupprecht, Pyrek, Brekhus, and Moss (1978) showed that wanderers displayed more complexity and range of locomotion than nonwanderers. Compared to nonwanderers, wanderers had significantly more involvement in nonsocial behavior and lower cognitive function. The authors suggested that possible correlates of wandering were person-focused factors, such as lifelong patterns of coping with stress, previous work roles, and search for security. Similarly, in the Monsour and Robb (1982) study, compared to nonwanderers, wanderers had more active premorbid lives, more stressful life events, customarily dealt with stress by motor activities (taking a walk), and had more motorific lifestyles when young.

Cohen-Mansfield, Werner, Marx, and Freedman (1991) also studied differences between wanderers and nonwanderers. Their results suggested that cognitive impairment was the variable most related to pacing (the term they used for wandering). Some other differences were evident as well: For example, pacers were more frequently separated or divorced, had experienced a previous life-threatening situation, and had never relocated prior to admission to the nursing home. In a second study of only pacers, Cohen-Mansfield, Werner, Marx, and Freedman (1991) found that pacing was most frequent during nonmeal time periods and occurred more frequently in open areas such as corridors, not in close proximity to others. Several environmental variables were also related to pacing. More pacing occurred when there was no noise or low-level noise, and less pacing occurred in the dark.

Dawson and Reid (1987) based their study of wanderers on reports of nursing staff. Two categories of behavior differentiated wanderers from nonwanders: hyperactivity (good social skills, better hearing, less withdrawal, good gait) and cognitive deficits (speech and reading difficulties, incontinence, transitory disorientation, and inability to know when they were lost). In the Algase (1992b) study, wanderers differed from nonwanderers in terms of abstract thinking, language, judgment, and spatial skills. Algase suggests that wanderers are heterogeneous in regard to cognitive impairments, which suggests that different etiologies account for the various types of wandering observed.

Martino-Saltzman, Blasch, Morris, and McNeal (1991) conducted a very interesting study in which the behavior of wanderers and nonwanderers was continuously videotaped for 50 days. Analysis showed very different patterns of locomotion for the two groups. Although the majority of travel in both groups was direct (going from one place to another without diversion), nonwanderers showed more direct travel and slightly more pacing, whereas wanderers showed more lapping (repetitive travel characterized by circling a large area) and slightly more random travel. Based on these categorizations, the results showed that nonwanderers had more travel efficiency. Further analysis showed that travel efficiency was related to severity of dementia. For those with moderate dementia, travel efficiency was high during the day and decreased in the evening. For those with severe dementia, travel efficiency remained low all day. No other variables, including drugs, were related to travel efficiency.

Matteson and Linton (1996) observed 49 residents with dementia to identify the behavioral and physiological characteristics of wanderers. Their data showed that subjects were agitated or restless only 2% of the time. About half of the residents, however, were observed to be pacing or agitated at some time during the observations. Subjects were less active at night than during the day, and agitation and restlessness occurred more frequently during the day. Physical restraints, however, were most commonly used in the evening. Almost half the subjects were taking a psychotropic drug at the time of the study, but there was no relationship between psychotropic medication use and time spent standing and pacing or amount of agitation. There was a significant inverse relationship between time spent wandering and systolic blood pressure and a significant inverse relationship between oxygen saturation and time spent lying in bed. The researchers discussed the importance of environmental interventions for wandering, but these variables were not considered as part of the study.

A number of studies have compared wanderers to nonwanderers under preexisting conditions (e.g., a protected unit) or have tested interventions for wandering. For example, Cornbleth (1977) compared wanders and nonwanderers residing on and off protected care units. The wanderers showed greater range of locomotion on protected units, whereas nonwanderers showed greater range of locomotion off the unit. As a result, Cornbleth suggests interventions designed for wanderers (protected units) may be detrimental to the well-being of nonwanderers.

Several environmental interventions for wandering have been tested. For example, Rosswurm, Zimmerman, Schwartz-Fulton, and Norman (1986) tested an intervention centered on providing controlled environmental stimuli and group activity. The goal of the intervention was to make an activity room more interesting and easier for wanderers to access than other patients' rooms. The researchers altered the environment in the room by changing the furniture, altering the colors, and adding flowers, an aquarium, and music. An example of altering the environment outside the activity room was putting environmental cues on the rooms so patients could identify their own space. The planned group activity was conducted three times a week and included exercise, walks, dancing, games, and pet therapy. The intervention worked as predicted. Residents spent more time in the activity room and less time in other resident's rooms. In addition, there was a decrease in daytime sleeping, an increase in walking, a noticeable increase in staff-subject interactions, and a positive change in resident social behavior.

Hussian and Brown (1987) addressed the problem of elopement (undetected exit from a unit) using different grid patterns created with masking tape at exit doors. Although all grids were effective, the most effective was a series of eight horizontal strips ending 57.2 cms from the door. The researchers cautioned that grids did not stop one person who never looked at the floor when walking. Namazi, Rosner, and Calkins (1989) also studied the effect of visual barriers on elopement through a fire door. They created a number of different conditions: some grid patterns on the floor, different-colored cloth strips placed across the door hiding the door knob, painting the doorknob the same color as the door, and placing a special doorknob cover on the doorknob that required a certain sequence of action to make it possible to open the door. The most effective strategy for decreasing elopement was a cloth barrier that covered the doorknob. The color of the cloth was irrelevant. The problem of elopement was also addressed by Negley, Molla, and Obenchain (1990). This group studied the effect of an electronic monitoring system for alerting nursing staff when patients entered the monitored area and the door was opened. The system was effective for alerting nurses, and the need to retrieve patients remained very low even when the door was unlocked. The authors, however, cautioned that the system would not keep a resident on the unit who was determined to leave.

It is important to mention that almost all studies of wandering include some consideration of the environ-

ment in the discussion section. For example, Cornbleth (1977), McGrowder-Lin and Bhatt (1988), and Cherry and Rafkin (1988) all suggest the creation of walking courts and use of structured walking programs as interventions for wandering. Modification of the environment to use barriers to reduce access to certain spaces, use of colors, placement of furniture, layout of the facility, noise, and staffing are all issues considered in discussion sections. Interestingly enough, actual tests of the effects of these interventions are absent from the literature.

Safety and Falls

Many studies of falls have focused on describing the problem and the risk factors involved in an effort to know how to target interventions. Person-related risk factors have been identified in many studies. For example, falls have been shown to be associated with (a) *advanced age* (Craven & Bruno, 1986; Exton-Smith, 1977; Gross, Shimamoto, Rose, & Frank, 1990; Lucht, 1971; Margulec, Librach, & Schadel, 1970; Perry, 1982; Prudham & Evans, 1981; Sheldon, 1960; Wild, Nayak, & Isaacs, 1981); (b) *being female* (Colling & Park, 1983; Exton-Smith, 1977; Gryfe, Amies, & Ashley, 1977; Kalchthaler, Bascan, & Quintos, 1978; MacQueen, 1977; Morris & Isaacs, 1980; Prudham & Evans, 1981; Sheldon, 1960); (c) *severity of illness* (Lucht, 1971; Morris & Isaacs, 1980; Perry, 1982; Prudham & Evans, 1981; Rodstein, 1964; Sehested & Severin-Nielsen, 1977; Sheldon, 1960; Waller, 1974); (d) *impaired mental function* (Feist, 1978; Gross et al., 1990; Kippenbrock & Soja, 1993; Prudham & Evans, 1981; Wild et al., 1981); (e) *having the diagnosis of cerebral vascular accident* (CVA) (e.g., Colling & Park, 1983; Gross et al., 1990; Mayo, Korner-Bitensky, Becker, & Georges, 1989); (f) *having mobility limitations* (Berry, Fisher, & Lang, 1981; Flemming & Pendergast, 1993; Gross et al., 1990; Kalchthaler et al., 1978; Perry, 1982; Wild et al., 1981); (g) *incontinence* (Garcia et al., 1988; Mayo et al., 1989; Walshe & Rosen, 1979); and (h) *drugs,* including psychotropics, sedatives, diuretics, and anticonvulsives (Blumenthal & Davie, 1980; Colling & Park, 1983; Feist, 1978; Kalchthaler et al., 1978; Mayo et al., 1989; Prudham & Evans, 1981; Walshe & Rosen, 1979). Wolf-Klein and colleagues (1988) provided data that most patients have more than one person-related factor that can be associated with their falling. In addition, falls have been associated with certain care activities such as transferring and walking (Craven & Bruno, 1986;

Fleming & Pendergast, 1993; Myers et al., 1989; Rodstein, 1964).

Several environment-related risk factors have also been associated with falls, including the presence of environmental hazards (Craven & Bruno, 1986; Fine, 1959; Fleming & Pendergast, 1993; Louis, 1983; Lucht, 1971; Lynn, 1980; Sheldon, 1960; Walshe & Rosen, 1979) and the use of assistive devices, most particularly wheelchairs (e.g., Berry et al., 1981; Catchen, 1983; Feist, 1978; Fleming & Pendergast, 1993; Myers et al., 1989; Rodstein, 1964). Fleming and Pendergast (1993) found that over 50% of the falls in their study were associated with environmental factors such as furniture, walkers, floor finish, stairs, footwear, vehicles, bath or toilet, and wheelchairs. In the Myers and colleagues (1989) study, half of the fractures, injurious falls, and total falls involved at least one piece of equipment (most frequently wheelchairs), suggesting the importance of the environment as a risk factor for falls. The place in the environment where most falls occur has also been studied. The patient's room or bedside is the most dangerous place for falls (Colling & Park, 1983; Fleming & Pendergast, 1993; Gross et al., 1990; Myers et al., 1989).

Environmental patterns and issues in the structural environment have also been associated with falls. For example, Kalchthaler and colleagues' (1978) data showed a relationship between shift change and falls. The studies by Fine (1967), Jarvinen and Jarvinen (1968), Morris and Isaacs (1980), and Louis (1983) showed a relationship between falls and times when units had least staffing. Kalchthaler and colleagues' (1978) study showed that falls were most numerous when staffing was very low (fewer than three staff members) or very high (more than six staff members). The relationship between more staff and more falls was also found by Sehested and Severin-Nielson (1977) and Tutuarima, deHaan, and Limburg (1993).

Another environmental pattern that has been explored for its relationship to falls has been time of day. The results of these studies have been quite mixed (e.g., Catchen, 1983; Colling & Park, 1983; Feist, 1978; Fleming & Pendergast, 1993; Gross et al., 1990; Myers et al., 1989; Tutuarima et al., 1993; Walshe & Rosen, 1979). One reason for these mixed results is that different sites have been studied (e.g., community versus long-term care facilities versus acute care settings). But even within one setting—for example, long-term care facilities— there is little consistency in results. In a unique study, Harris (1989) studied the relationship of falls to organizational factors (leadership of charge nurse, primary work group cohesion, and job involvement) and staff at-

titudes (attitude toward elderly and job expectations). She found these aspects of the structural environment accounted for 25% of the variance in falls in a Veterans Administration population.

Interventions for falls have also been studied. Some interventions have targeted reducing the fall or fall and injury rate in a specific setting; others have tackled the more complex problem of preventing falls in elderly populations. Several institution-based studies targeting fall reduction have been reported. For example, Innes and Turman (1983) reported on a quality assurance program focused on falls. The program had patient-related interventions, such as assessment of individual risk, frequent rounds, and informing patients of staff expectations regarding getting out of bed, and environment-related interventions, including a variety of strategies such as attention to safety (no-skid wax, carpets on hard surfaces, nonskid slippers, night lighting, orange sticker on the door of those at high risk) and arranging the environment so the patient could meet his or her needs without undue effort (e.g., arrangement of call lights, television controls, lowering noise levels). Evaluation showed that the program reduced the number of falls by half.

Kustaborder and Rigney (1983) designed an intervention for falls that involved alteration of the physical environment (signal cords) and the social environment (alterations in staffing, rules about leaving high-risk clients alone in the bathroom, and a buddy system for staff relief during breaks and meals). Implementation of the program produced no effect on the number of falls, even though the nursing staff was consistent in implementation of the interventions. The authors suggested that lack of effectiveness was related to the philosophy of care in the rehabilitation center, which valued patient independence. Nurses were unwilling to jeopardize patient independence even if it meant a reduction in patient accidents. Kilpack, Boehm, Smith, and Mudge (1991) reported on a research utilization project that involved implementing a fall prevention program on the neuroscience and oncology-renal units of an acute care hospital. The intervention included the identification of research-based risk factors and research-based interventions, staff education, and consciousness-raising efforts (by, for example, posting the rate of falls in comparison to the rate last year, etc.). Over a period of 1 year, there was a reduction in patient fall rates on the demonstration units in spite of an overall increase in patient fall rates in the hospital as a whole. Nurses reported using a wide variety of research-based interventions for preventing patient falls. It was not clear, given the nature of the project, however, whether it was the consciousness-raising activities or the research-based interventions that actually made the difference in reducing fall rates.

Meddaugh, Friedenberg, and Knisley (1996) conducted a study to determine the effect of using treaded slipper socks at night on all residents in one special care unit. The intervention was designed to target one particular type of fall—that caused by elders getting up at night to go to the bathroom, being incontinent on the way to the bathroom, and slipping in their own urine. After implementation, there was an overall reduction in falls by 9%; only one of these falls was caused by slipping in urine (prior to institution of the intervention, eight such falls were documented). Six months later, the intervention was still being implemented and no falls were related to patients slipping in urine.

Population-based fall prevention programs is the other category of intervention studies currently appearing in the literature. Most of these studies employ a multidimensional view of fall prevention that includes environmental manipulation along with other intervention targets. For example, Edwards, Cere, and LeBlond (1993) implemented a falls prevention program based on self-efficacy in the areas of medication management, environmental safety, use of assistive devices, exercise and strength training, and referrals to community resources. The intervention was implemented in four seniors' apartment buildings in Canada. Seniors with multiple risk factors tended to agree to a follow-up home visit by a public health nurse. During the home visit, the public health nurse tailored interventions to match risk profiles. Overall, the response to the clinic was positive, but few elders (23.7%) indicated they actually planned to make the changes in lifestyle or environment recommended by the nurse.

El-Faizy and Reinsch (1994) investigated the effect of an in-home environmental assessment for reduction of fall risk. Subjects were recruited from senior centers and centers were randomly assigned to treatments. Subjects in both treatment and control groups received an in-home assessment ($n = 14$ in each group). No safety information was provided to those in the control group, but those in the intervention group were shown the hazardous conditions in their home, given suggestions for changing them, and provided with fall-prevention posters. Phosphorescent tape was provided to mark the stairs. Results showed that although participants acknowledged safety hazards and concerns, few were able or willing to make the changes necessary to take care of the hazard. The authors attributed some reluctance to change to denial of the problems associated with aging and some to the eco-

nomic and logistical problems involved in making home modifications. In addition, their data suggested that the environment, as a major causative factor in falls, has less significance with advancing age, when most falls are related to health and health problems.

Frailty and Injuries: Cooperative Studies of Intervention Techniques (FICSIT) is a series of studies funded in multiple sites by the National Institutes of Health (NIH) to study fall prevention from a multidimensional, multidisciplinary perspective. Reports of these projects are just beginning to appear in the literature, and, for the most part, results are not yet available. Some of these studies focus exclusively on the person-related risk factors associated with increased frailty and age, and the interventions focus on exercise (Buchner et al., 1993; Wolf, Kutner, Green, & McNeely, 1993; Wolfson et al., 1993) and exercise and nutrition (Fiatarone et al., 1993). Wallace, Ross, Huston, Kundel, and Woodworth (1993) are testing the use of a protective garment for reducing hip fractures among individuals at high risk for falls; that is, those who have previously had a hip fracture, those with Parkinson's disease, poststroke patients in rehabilitation, individuals institutionalized with dementing illness, and other frail individuals with a history of falls.

Other studies in the FICSIT trials take a more comprehensive view of fall prevention and include consideration of environmental factors. For example, the Biobehavioral-Environmental Model of Falls designed by Hornbrook, Stevens, and Wingfield (1993) contained five elements: physical structure (strength, joints, senses), physiological function (balance, reaction time, proprioception), behavior (risk taking, preventive behaviors), environment (gradient of surface, texture of surface, lighting), and outcomes (falls, injuries, use of medical care). The Seniors' Program for Injury Control and Intervention (SPICE) focused attention on each of these components, using a behavioral self-management approach. The intervention was administered in a group format over a 4-month period and involved eleven 90-minute sessions. The study targeted individuals over age 65 living in the community at higher than average risk for falls. The study population included those enrolled in Kaiser Permanente's Northwest Region HMO (Hornbrook, Stevens, Wingfield, Hollis, et al., 1994). Subjects were randomly assigned to the minimal-treatment control or the intervention group. Both groups received risk and home assessments along with consumer safety pamphlets. For those in the intervention group, support was given to remove home hazards, and subjects were given technical and financial advice. Intervention group members also participated in four weekly, 90-minute group meetings led by a health behavioralist and physical therapist. During meetings, participants developed action plans for addressing risk factors and risky behaviors and participated in exercise programs to increase strength, range of motion, and proprioception. Both groups demonstrated a reduction in falls, with those in the intervention group demonstrating the greatest reduction. The intervention also reduced the probability of falling and the average number of falls among fallers during the 23-month follow-up period. Unfortunately, although the intervention was effective for total falls, a similar effect was not seen for serious falls (those requiring medical care, resulting in a fracture, hospitalization, or both). The authors suggest that this negative finding may be the result of reporting biases or the very small number of serious falls seen during the study period. The authors also suggest that the exercise was the most effective aspect of the intervention.

The Yale FICSIT site also used a multidimensional approach to fall prevention. Their protocol had an assessment and an intervention phase. Both phases focused on physical problems (e.g., postural hypotension, medications), home safety, environmental hazards, physical frailty (e.g., gait, transfers, balance, strength, etc.), and foot problems. During the assessment phase, a nurse practitioner and a physical therapist performed in-home assessments. Based on the assessments, targeted risk factors were identified, number of visits for subjects were prescribed, and interventions for treatment subjects were planned. Individuals were randomly assigned either to receive a social visit or to be included in the risk abatement protocol. The risk abatement protocol was administered by a nurse practitioner and a physical therapist during home visits.

The FICSIT trials represent an enormous investment in time and effort for the purpose of reducing fall risk among the elderly, and they are likely to yield some very interesting and useful results. In general, the major focus of these studies is on patient-related factors associated with falls, with much less attention paid to the environmental risk factors, although some studies include consideration of home hazards and home safety as a part of the interventions.

Restraints

Restraints are externally imposed devices designed to limit or control the behavior of elderly individuals in specific situations, such as wandering, confusion and agi-

tation, sundowning, and preventing falls and accidents. Restraints may be physical (mechanical) or chemical, but most research has focused on the use of physical or mechanical devises. In general, a very extensive research base exists describing the *incidence and prevalence* of, *antecedents* to (factors that render an individual high risk for the use of restraints), *consequences* of, and *rationale given by health care workers for the use* of physical restraints. Evans and Strumpf have published two excellent state-of-the-science papers (1989, 1990) that summarize research in these four areas and explore some of the ethical and legal issues involved in restraint use. Since the Evans and Strumpf reviews, other studies (e.g., Macpherson, Lofgren, Granieri, & Myllenbeck, 1990; Magee et al., 1993; Mion, Frengley, Jakovcic, & Marino, 1989; Murray, Mulvihill, White, & Libow, 1992; Tinetti, Liu, & Ginter, 1992; Werner, Cohen-Mansfield, Braun, & Marx, 1989) have added to our knowledge about many of these same issues. For example, Magee and colleagues (1993) studied many of the factors considered by previous investigators but also considered the relationship of restraint use to staffing patterns and prescriptions for psychotropic drugs. They also described the relationship between restraint use and diagnoses (medical and nursing). Tinetti, Liu, and Ginter (1992) related the use of restraints to serious injuries associated with falls.

Also included in the Evans and Strumpf (1989, 1990) research reviews were studies that considered nurses' knowledge about alternatives to restraint and studies of strategies for managing behavior that might otherwise lead to restraint. Since their review, this body of research has expanded somewhat. In addition, two other content areas related to restraints have appeared in the literature: evaluations of patient and system outcomes associated with introduction of policies requiring the release of restraints and studies of attitudes of family members to the application of restraints.

Evaluations of outcomes. Some of the studies, case studies, and anecdotal reports evaluating patient and system outcomes of policies requiring the release of restraints result from long-term care facilities' attempts to comply with the 1987 Omnibus Budget Reconciliation Act (OBRA) regulations that prohibit the routine use of physical restraints in long-term care facilities. Some of this literature, however, predates the OBRA regulations.

Two very interesting reports, for example, predate the OBRA regulations by many years. The first was conducted by Snellgrove and Flaherty (1975). This anecdotal report, which included empirical data, involved the implementation of "attitude therapy" as a strategy for reducing restraint use for psychiatric patients (some of whom were old). Attitude therapy was an environmental intervention that involved restructuring the ward environment so treatment team members used a consistent attitude toward particular patients. The attitudes were prescribed during a staff meeting the patient attended and included friendliness, passive friendliness, matter-of-fact, no demand, and kind firmness. Prescriptions were based on the patient's behavior. Following implementation, the authors reported a marked decrease in restraint use (no significance tests were reported). The authors believed the changes were due to a decrease in aggressive and assaultive behavior on the part of the patients.

The second study was conducted by Davidson, Hemingway, and Wysocki (1984). It involved a sample of individuals with mental retardation, some of whom were old. The intervention, which targeted the social and structural environment, was an extensive policy change about the use of seclusion, physical restraints, and chemical restraints instituted by the administrator. Use of all three types of restraints was monitored continuously, and staff were provided with feedback about their success in decreasing restraint use. Data were prepared so each individual unit was compared to all other units in the facility. In addition, staff were informed that data would be routinely shared with next of kin, mental health advocates, courts, the recipient rights office, and the state department of mental health. Over the 3 years of the study there was a marked reduction in seclusion hours, restraint hours, and psychotropic drug use. In addition, there were no noticeable escalations in patient problem behaviors or mean injuries of employees per month. The authors believed there was an actual decrease in patient aggressive and assaultive behavior, as well as an increase in patient learning and patient responsiveness to programming.

Many of the studies that have evaluated changes since implementation of the OBRA regulations have sought to document patient outcomes, particularly with regard to falls. Many of these studies do not describe any specific interventions other than policy change (an intervention targeting the structural environment). For the most part, outcomes with regard to decreased restraint use, falls, and serious injury rates have been positive (e.g., Bloom & Braun, 1991; Cutchins, 1991; Mitchell-Pedersen, Edmund, Fingerote, & Powell, 1985; Powell, Mitchell-Pederson, Fingerote, & Edmund, 1989; Shadlen, 1991; Suprock, 1990). Some have shown no change in number of staff (e.g., Bloom & Braun, 1991), which has been interpreted as showing that such a policy can be imple-

mented without increasing staff size. Some other studies have documented other outcomes, including improved sleep and decreased pressure sores (e.g., Bloom & Braun, 1991) and decreased agitation and increased wandering (Suprock, 1990).

For the most part, the studies identified are the result of natural experiments (the introduction of a policy change). The Werner, Cohen-Mansfield, Koroknay, and Braun (1994) study is in another category in that it was designed as a prospective intervention study to evaluate the effect of staff instruction in combination with policy change. Between baseline measurement and removal of restraints, all staff received instruction on environmental care alternatives to restraints, alterations in nursing care (e.g., flexible scheduling), involvement in structured activities (e.g., distraction and exercise), physiological alternatives (e.g., pain relief, sensory aids), and psychosocial alternatives (e.g., companionship, therapeutic touch, active listening, behavior modification). The researchers attempted to match restrained with nonrestrained residents, but matching was difficult, and at baseline, groups were significantly different for cognitive impairment, ADL impairment, number of falls (nonrestrained fell more), and pressure sores (restrained had more). Data were analyzed by three groups: the never restrained, the formerly restrained, and the still restrained. Results showed cognitive functioning of the still-restrained group was significantly lower than the never-restrained or formerly restrained groups. For ADL function, there were no significant differences. Residents in the never-restrained group improved in ambulation over time, but residents in other two groups decreased in ambulation (particularly those in the still-restrained group). Those in the never-restrained group had significantly less incontinence. Levels of agitation in the formerly restrained group decreased. For falls, pressure sores, and involvement in activities, there were no differences for any group.

The Morse and McHutchion (1991) study is an interesting example of a naturalistic experiment. It was an observational study, involving continuous videorecording of two patients for 1 week with restraints and 1 week without restraints. Results showed that when restraints were released, nurses spent less time with clients, but frequency of surveillance increased. For one client, there was a major difference in sleeping position with and without restraint (the other clients' positions were seriously limited because of pain). For one patient, there was an increase in moderate motor and "awake and still" behaviors and a decrease in minor motor behavior (restlessness). The other was seriously ill with cancer and showed no similar differences.

In general, studies show positive outcomes as a result of releasing restraints, although the positive outcomes are not unequivocal. The range of outcomes measured, however, has been quite limited (mostly falls and injury rates), and few replications have been conducted documenting other types of outcomes. In addition, most studies have been descriptive, focusing only on the effect of policy change, and have not included systematic tests of interventions. Most interventions have not been environmental in nature.

Nurses' knowledge and attitudes about restraints and alternatives to restraint. A few studies have considered what nurses and nursing staff know about restraints and alternatives to restraints as well as the restraints and alternatives they actually use. For example, Stilwell (1991) surveyed a random sample of nurses in Maryland to determine what they knew about restraint use. Most reported very little formal or continuing education about restraints. Most said there were alternatives to restraints, but few alternatives except drugs were actually identified by the nurses. Most believed minor injuries or outcomes (e.g., depression) happened as a result of restraints, but very few believed major injury or death were possible adverse consequences of restraints.

Janelli, Kanski, Scherer, and Neary (1992) studied attitudes of staff toward restraint use. Over half of the nurses said they followed orders to put on restraints but usually had someone else (another staff member) do it. Only about half said they tried other approaches first. Over half felt the nursing home was legally responsible for resident safety even if the measures required to maintain safety jeopardized resident dignity. Nursing staff performed fairly well on a knowledge test about restraint use included in the questionnaire.

Janelli, Kanski, and Neary (1994) surveyed 159 nursing homes to determine restraint use, reasons for restraints, knowledge of alternatives, alternatives actually used, and factors related to decreased reliance since OBRA. Factors related to decreased restraint use included support from administration, education of all staff members, reassessment of residents, cooperation of physicians, and involvement of patients' families. Although nurses could list alternatives to restraint, only two of the top four alternatives identified were actually being used. These were an ambulation program and frequent assistance to the bathroom.

Jagella, Tideiksaar, Mulvihill, and Neufeld (1992), in a letter to the editor, reported on an efficacy study of staff and family attitudes about using alarm devices instead of restraints. Staff reported that they used alarm devices to eliminate restraints in residents who had had prior falls and to prevent falls in those who were at risk. Most staff and family members believed alarm devices were effective, but almost half of the staff identified problems with alarm devices, including false alarms and malfunctioning, increased work for staff, excessive cost, and lack of established criteria for use. Some staff members noted residents' fear about using alarms and their abilities to disarm the devices.

In general, although few in number and nonrepresentative, these results show serious gaps in nursing staff's knowledge about alternatives to restraints and in their actual use of alternatives. An overriding issue appears to be lack of staff to implement some of the alternatives and the need for administrative support before successful restraint release programs can be implemented.

Studies of strategies for managing behavior that might otherwise lead to restraint. Overall, the literature is replete with excellent clinical articles describing strategies for managing behavior that might otherwise lead to use of restraints (e.g., Blakeslee, Goldman, Papougenis, & Torrell, 1991; Brower, 1991; Coberg, Lynch, & Mavretish, 1991; Conely & Campbell, 1991; Cutchins, 1991; Eigsti & Vrooman, 1992; English, 1989; Kallmann, Denine-Flynn, & Blackburn, 1992; Masters & Marks, 1990; McHutchion & Morse, 1989; Mion & Mercurio, 1992; Rader & Donius, 1991; Sloane, Papougenis, & Blakeslee, 1992). Many of the interventions described involve environmental manipulation of some kind. In general, however, it is extremely important to note that, although some of these clinical articles rely on data-based studies designed for other purposes (e.g., the reduction of wandering), no systematic tests exist of nursing interventions (environmental or otherwise) designed specifically to reduce restraint use.

Attitudes of family members to the application of restraints. Almost no research exists in this area, with one notable exception. Newbern and Lindsey (1994) used a qualitative approach and constant comparative analysis to explore the reactions of wives to the restraint of their husbands ($N = 6$). The major theme identified was the symbolism of restraints as finality or loss of hope. Several minor themes were also discovered. These included control (the need the wives had to occasionally release restraints while they were in the room and the pleasure they derived from seeing the nursing staff allowing their husbands to wander), denial (the wives' need to keep the restraining devices covered), and anger at nursing staff for using restraints and degradation (feelings that the presence of the restraint degraded their husbands). In addition, the wives reported the need for emotional support from staff and gratitude that staff allowed them some latitude in manipulating the restraints. Studies of this type are an interesting and potentially productive area of inquiry.

Studies of Social Environments

Studies of social environments for the elderly most often respond to problems of communication and control, often in relation to quality of life in the nursing home setting. The primary characteristic of the studies reviewed here is the idea that individualized care is the key element of any intervention.

Individualized care is defined by Happ, Williams, Strumpf, and Burger (1996) as "an interdisciplinary approach which acknowledges elders as unique persons and is practiced through consistent caring congruent with past patterns and individual preferences" (pp. 7-8). The maintenance of the elder's individual identity, personal relationships, participation in care, and opportunities for making personal choices is the goal for individualized care of frail elders (Happ et al., 1996). Activities that nondependent individuals take for granted, such as bathing and eating, can become problematic for nursing home residents, especially those with cognitive impairment. The principle of individualized care can minimize difficulties, whereas care determined solely by institutional policy and staff-determined or task-oriented care planning can result in catastrophic behavior (e.g., Maxfield et al., 1996; Rader, Lavelle, Hoeffer, & McKenzie, 1996).

Knowledge of the elder's individual patterns of behavior is the basis for decision making and planning care (Evans, 1996), as well as determining the ability of the professional or nonprofessional caregiver to respond to a particular need of a frail or cognitively impaired elder. Maxfield and colleagues (1996) describe an intervention study in which nursing home staff were trained to recognize and understand cognitively impaired elders' responses to caregiving situations, supportive responses to elder behaviors, and how to individualize these responses.

The training included nursing assistants, LPNs, and RNs. New knowledge was applied specifically to the problem of aggressive, catastrophic behaviors associated with bathing and grooming. The result was an increase in caregiver knowledge, a decrease in incidents of aggression, and a decrease in the use of PRN medications prior to bathing. In addition, the administrative staff reported there was a decrease in time required to bathe residents due to the decrease in aggressive behaviors and that there was a decrease in complaints received from the staff with regard to assignments for resident baths. It is important to note that the administration was highly supportive of the intervention program, giving aides the authority to alter care plans and bathing schedules to accommodate individual resident needs. Rader and colleagues (1996) provide additional support for this method of intervention, pointing out that often administrative policies and unit cultures exert pressure on aides to complete their bathing assignments in a certain amount of time and require that the established bathing routine be followed regardless of the needs of the elder. Rader and colleagues also point out there are multiple methods of maintaining personal hygiene. The decisions of whether to use a bathtub, a shower, a towel bath, when to bathe, how often to bathe, and so on should be based on the needs of the elder, and this is determined by understanding what makes the bathing experience comfortable for the elder.

Communication

Communication is an aspect of the social environment that is the subject of research in long-term care environments. Research on the types of interactions that occur between elderly nursing home residents and their caregivers indicates that much communication is task focused (Gibb & O'Brien, 1990; Jones & van Amelsvoort Jones, 1986) and controlling (Hewison, 1995; Lanceley, 1985). Kaakinen (1992) explored the implicit rules of communication as perceived by nursing home residents. As with the majority of social gerontological research, only cognitively intact elders participated in this qualitative study. A role-play method of data collection was used in which the elders were asked to respond to the researcher as though she were a new resident in the nursing home asking about the home rules. Following a script, the researcher focused the residents on their perceptions of rules about talking. Perceived communication taboos included complaining (59%), talking about loneliness (54%), talking about death (61%), and talking to the opposite sex (45%). The most frequently reported communications beliefs reported by residents participating in the study included ignoring confused residents (50%), ignoring residents with hearing impairment (29%), talking with residents who talk with you (43%), and either fear of talking (28%) or lack of desire to talk (28%). Twenty-eight percent of the elders interviewed stated that they used silence for control, which is especially significant in a context in which control is often at a minimum. The results of the study demonstrate that talk among nursing home residents is constrained based on the perceptions and beliefs of cognitively intact residents.

Studies of communication between elder nursing home residents and caregivers support Kaakinen's (1992) findings about silence in the nursing home setting. Armstrong-Esther and Browne (1986) found that staff are less likely to interact with confused residents. This is especially significant in light of the finding of (a) Kaakinen (1992) that cognitively intact residents have an implicit rule of ignoring confused residents, (b) Campbell and Linc's (1996) finding that family members are most disturbed by symptoms of cognitive deterioration, and (c) the strength of negative emotional reactions in response to the behavior of cognitively impaired residents found in relation to the willingness of cognitively intact residents to live in the same unit (Levesque, Cossette, & Potvin, 1993).

Salmon (1993) instituted reality orientation groups as an intervention to increase nurse-resident interaction. Results showed that interactions outside of the reality orientation groups were almost exclusively task oriented. Additional testing to explore the relationship of staff attitudes to the frequency and duration of interaction found that there was only a minimal relationship. Findings revealed that nurses who were observed in behaviors that were classified recreational were the least sensitive to the emotional needs of the unit residents. No positive relationship between attitude and behavior was detected. This is supported by Woods and Cullen (1983), who found that the attitudes of nurses were not as influential on the quality of nurse-resident interaction as the degree of task orientation of the facility. This has implications for educational interventions that target ageist attitudes of nursing home staff as the mediators of quality of elder caregiving. However, this does not imply that educational interventions are ineffective.

The Penn State Nursing Home Intervention Project (Smyer, 1995) developed and instituted an intervention project based on the education of nursing assistants to improve job performance. Although this project was very similar to the educational interventions addressed in the previous section, the project failed. The intervention increased the knowledge of the aides, but there was no significant improvement in job performance. The researchers concluded that the critical error was not including the supervisors in the intervention process, and that the success of any intervention is dependent on the support of the institution's organizational culture. Cooperation of the entire staff is identified as important in all cited successful intervention studies. The need to include all members of the staff in educational interventions is also supported by Cox, Kaeser, Montgomery, and Marino (1991), who observed that although the nursing assistants participating in the implementation of the Quality of Life Nursing Care (QLNC) Model may have benefited indirectly from the education received by the licensed staff, the outcomes might have been greater if the nursing assistants had been included in the educational programs. The QLNC Model was developed to plan care based on the individual needs of nursing home residents.

Kihlgren, Norberg, Brane, Engstrom, and Melin (1993) had positive results following an educational program targeting communication in conjunction with training on improving the quality of morning care of elders with severe cognitive impairment. The activity of morning care was expanded from the task-oriented approach that has, strictly, hygiene and neatness as its goal to include activities that promoted the elder's sense of integrity. At the first data collection time, the experimental unit had a significant increase in the frequency and quality of interaction during morning care, as shown by increased verbal interaction, increased frequency of orienting (use of name, time, place, etc.) and aesthetic (appearance) comments, and increased control and choice during care. Positive resident outcomes were an increase in attempts to engage in verbal communication, increased levels of orientation, and increased cooperation. The increase in verbalization, however, had a twofold effect in that there were an increase in power struggles and an increase in negative verbal comments and opinions on the part of the residents. At the second data collection, the findings remained essentially the same.

Communication among families of nursing home residents is also a topic of research. From the perspective of individualized care, attention to the excess disabilities of cognitively impaired elders, especially communicative abilities, can have the effect of increasing the quality of family relations (Brody, Kleban, Lawton, & Silverman, 1971). The difficulties of having a family member in long-term care is an accepted fact for gerontological nurses. The guilt and ambivalence involved in nursing home placement is well documented (see Johnson, 1990; Krammer, 1994; Matteson, 1989). The involvement of the family as a part of the care of an elderly nursing home resident is essential for counteracting the characteristics of the "total institution" (Goffman, 1961), specifically, the characteristic of social isolation from the world outside the confines of the nursing home. Families are a source of essential information about the elder's identity, particularly if that resident is cognitively impaired (Harvath et al., 1994; Rowles & High, 1996). Campbell and Linc (1996) describe an intervention program that, following a qualitative needs assessment, initiated a series of family support group meetings. As requested in the needs assessment, the meetings consisted of education on aging, skills training that enabled them to participate in care, communication with and expectations of staff, and the opportunity to express feelings and receive support. In response to problems discussed by family members, the group facilitators, rather than intervening, discussed constructive methods of problem solving. The response was strongly positive to the extent that the meetings were increased from the original weekly format to biweekly. The support groups also continued after the conclusion of the research.

Pet therapy is another type of communication that occurs within the social domain. The benefits of pet therapy in special populations is supported by research. Calvert (1988) found that nursing home residents who had high levels of interaction with pets had lower levels of loneliness as compared to residents who had low levels of interaction. The use of pets on home visits by volunteers had the effect of significantly decreasing blood pressure and heart rate (Harris, Rinehart, & Gerstman, 1993) and generating positive comments by the elders about looking forward to the visits. The use of pet therapy in an Alzheimer's unit also revealed positive effects of both having a dog as a weekly visitor and as a resident on the unit. There was an increase in social interaction, and the presence of the dog acted as a catalyst for interaction between the residents and their families and with the staff (Kongable, Buckwalter, & Stolley, 1989).

Fick (1993) demonstrated the positive effect of a pet on the achievement of group therapy goals in a Veterans Affairs (VA) nursing home. The presence of a pet has been shown to ease the discomfort and awkwardness felt by volunteers, providing a focus and purpose for visits (Savishinsky, 1992). The involvement of elders who either previously owned pets or expressed a desire for the presence of an animal was a key factor in the success of

interactions with caregivers (Kongable, Buckwalter, et al., 1989), suggesting that the use of pet therapy as an intervention must be carefully considered based on the individualized needs of the elder. Similarly, the occurrence of negative reactions to the dog placed in residence emphasizes the need to carefully monitor resident reactions to pets to prevent incidents of this type resulting in harm to the animal. In addition, the need for planning and the cooperation of the administration and the caregiving staff is essential when instituting a pet therapy program. Even though Kongable, Stolley, and Buckwalter (1990) found positive reactions when surveying nursing home staff and administration, the concerns of cost and time required to care for the animal and the risk of animal-associated falls or infections were expressed as concerns that had to be satisfactorily addressed for the program to be successful. Within the framework of environmental press, the presence of a pet provides a catalyst for interaction, serving as a topic of conversation, a point of connection, a trigger for reminiscence. The animal is also a source of physical contact and comfort, as well as a source of unconditional positive regard, as pets do not appear to care about physical or mental impairment.

Control

Control, or autonomy, for elders in a long-term care environment is of particular interest to gerontological nurses. The principle of individualized care is essential to this aspect of elder care. Bowsher and Gerlach (1990) studied well-being in institutionalized elders and found that maintenance of feelings of well-being in institutionalized elders was related to the elders' ability to maintain their expected levels of control. The implications are that interventions related to this finding would involve care that is individualized and based on thorough assessment of both baseline abilities of the elder and the elder's expected level of control.

Cox and colleagues (1991) found that when a program of individualized care was instituted in which individual needs of the institutionalized elder were the goal of care, the attitudes of staff toward resident control and autonomy improved. The improvement in the attitudes of nonlicensed staff were less positive than those of licensed staff, though they were still significant. This may be attributed to the fact that only the licensed staff were included in the educational program.

Ryden (1985) found that the expectations of nursing home elders and their caregivers for amount of control were congruent, with 60% of both groups responding that the elders had sufficient power and autonomy. This is in contrast to the administrators, of whom 70% responded that the elders should have more power. Compared to administrators, the caregivers also perceived elders to be more competent, but only 43% of the elders were perceived by caregivers as competent. This may be the explanation for the findings that activities of daily living (dressing, toileting, eating, grooming) were all controlled by the caregivers. The significance of this finding is supported by Cohen (1988), who states that the perception of decreasing competence in elders is responsible for decreased autonomy because there are decreased levels of expectation and estimations of potential. Cohen states that elders may also have this perception. If this is the case, then Ryden's (1985) assertion (that institutionalized elders are passive and placed at the bottom of the institutional hierarchy) has merit. A final observation made by Ryden, and reinforced by Rodin (1986), is that part of autonomy is the choice of the elder not to make choices but that choices should be offered at a level of complexity appropriate to the elder's capabilities.

▬ *Structural and Organizational Environment*

The power of the administrative structure and the organizational culture of a nursing home over both the elder resident and the nursing home staff is agreed upon in the literature. The concept of individualized care noted above is replete with warnings that administrative support is a prerequisite to the success of a program of individualized care (see especially Cox et al., 1991; Smyer, 1995).

The Institute of Medicine (1986) found that unskilled staff provide 71% of the care in the average nursing home. Nursing assistants providing this care are typically female, have not graduated from high school, are making about minimum wage, come from low-income families, and receive poor benefits. Waxman, Carner, and Berkenstock (1984) found that turnover of nursing assistants in seven Philadelphia nursing homes ranged from 5.2% to 75.8%. The highest turnover rate (75.8%) was reported by a nursing home that employed students as aides over the summer months. The data on nursing assistant satisfaction show that a more controlling administrative environment results in lower satisfaction, but the ability to participate in planning of patient care and make suggestions that are acted upon can result in lower turnover (Brannon, Cohn, & Myer, 1990; Caudill, 1989;

Waxman et al., 1984). Waxman and colleagues (1984) found that the satisfaction received as a result of helping others was the most positive response on the satisfaction scale used (Minnesota Satisfaction Scale).

The Tellis-Nayak and Tellis-Nayak (1989) ethnographic study of nursing assistants and the contrasts of their home and work cultures illustrated the difficulties of adaptation and coping that the majority of nursing assistants encounter. The nursing assistants interviewed were all from low socioeconomic groups and were coping with minimal resources (low pay, poor benefits, and minimal training in their job), as well as with difficulties in their personal lives). Tellis-Nayak and Tellis-Nayak believe that the conflicting messages of some long-term care institutions of caring and homelike atmosphere versus their devaluing of the nursing assistants through low salaries, poor benefits, and demeaning attitudes toward the functions they fulfill leave nursing assistants to function in an intolerable environment. They suggest that the institutional culture of the nursing home needs to place a higher value on nursing assistants by developing management policies that support commitment and satisfaction as well as productivity.

Increasing support is accumulating for the use of advanced practitioners in the long-term care setting. For example, Joel and Patterson (1990) state that an autonomous nursing staff is key to restraint reduction, and research shows that advanced practice nurses and nurses with master's degrees perform with the most autonomy (Schutzenhofer & Musser, 1994). Administrators surveyed about their perceptions regarding nurse practitioners revealed that they were very positive about the role of the geriatric nurse practitioner as a role model, resource person, and change agent in the movement away from the medical model. In addition, use of geriatric nurse practitioners resulted in (a) faster response to health problems, (b) assessments that were comprehensive and complete, and (c) an increase in the time spent with residents (Melillo, 1992). The primary difficulties identified with the incorporation of geriatric nurse practitioners into the long-term care health team is the role confusion caused by conflicts between clinical and administrative roles, lack of role definition, and reimbursement issues (Aaronson, 1992). As stated by Mezey (1990), with the increase in the age and acuity of institutionalized elders, a combination of skill levels within the nursing staff, including the presence of geriatric nurse practitioners, may well be the determinant of quality care, as demonstrated by a decrease in physical and chemical restraints and improved management of wandering and aggressive behaviors. Increasing registered nurse staffing is also supported by research by Munroe (1990) in which higher quality care was directly related to a higher RN:LVN ratio.

Studies of Facilitative Environments

For the purpose of this chapter, studies of facilitative environments have two basic characteristics. First, they are designed to promote function rather than simply to decrease the frequency of a problem. Second, they use a multidimensional approach that involves manipulating more than one aspect of the environment simultaneously. Almost all of these studies have focused either on dementia care units (as a total therapeutic entity) or on providing care to individuals who have dementia.

Special Care Units

Ohta and Ohta (1988) conducted an analysis of published and unpublished reports describing the characteristics of special care units (SCUs) for dementia. They identified elements believed to make SCUs different from other units in long-term care facilities, as well as some issues about the way these elements operate to create a great deal of heterogeneity among units. Common elements included the focus of resident care (focus on promoting function and minimizing memory and behavioral problems), environmental design (small units, special environmental features, and interesting wandering spaces), staff-to-resident ratios (higher than other units), consistency of staffing, staff training (focus on special care of residents with dementia), individually tailored care plans to promote function and social skills, and special admission and discharge criteria. As Ohta and Ohta (1988) note, however, the ways in which these are implemented can be quite different, and, in some situations, the "special" unit is not very different from other units in the facility. In addition, units can differ markedly in whether they focus on benefiting the resident as a primary focus or on protecting other residents in the facility from those who have dementia.

Henderson (1994) conducted an ethnographic study of SCUs. The study involved questionnaires, interviews with staff, and on-site participant observation. His findings, which focused on the perspectives of care staff, confirmed many of the commonalities Ohta and Ohta iden-

tified from the literature. The major themes he identified included the concept of "specialness," expansion of behavior management skills, expansion of staff role boundaries, and a uniquely structured environment and work effort differential in which staff in SCUs viewed their working situation as different from others in the institution and vice versa. He also identified factors that contribute to failure to build an SCU culture, including staff turnover, floating staff to the unit from other units, and having staff in the SCUs working on more than one unit, which usually occurred during the night shift.

Despite the popularity of SCUs, very few studies have evaluated the effect of creating this kind of a special environment. Some of the issues involved in doing such research and the issues of instituting such units are discussed by Berg and colleagues (1991). Of the few studies available, results are mixed. Holmes and colleagues (1990) studied SCU residents and non-SCU residents in four facilities. The characteristics of the residents differed (SCU residents were more impaired cognitively, behaviorally, and functionally), but during a 6-month measurement period, no beneficial or deleterious effects were found in dementia, arousal, disorientation, depression, disturbing behavior, mood, sleep disorders, range of motion, or visual impairments. Holmes and colleagues (1990) concluded from their data that differences between residents in SCUs and others were trivial and nonsignificant. In a letter to the editor, Chan, Ouslander, and Osterweil (1992) provided data collected from individuals in an SCU and individuals in other areas in the facility. Their measurement timeframe was 2 years. Results showed no significant differences between the residents for number of acute hospitalizations, number of acute visits by physicians or nurse practitioners, or number of visits for infections. The authors concluded that few clinically important differences exist between individuals treated in SCUs and others.

Swanson, Maas, and Buckwalter (1993) used a quasi-experimental pretest-posttest design to examine the effects of an SCU on the incidence of catastrophic and other behaviors. In the original design, subjects were to be matched for age and cognitive status and then randomly assigned to (a) the SCU treatment, (b) a traditional unit, or (c) a control group to replace those lost from the experimental or control group. Because of attrition, the randomization could not be maintained throughout the study. Results showed that subjects in the SCU treatment group had fewer catastrophic reactions or mood changes over the 12-month period. There was also an increase in unscheduled activities that involved interactions with staff for those on the SCU. For those in the control group, there was a decrease in unscheduled activities involving interactions with staff.

The question of whether SCUs, as a total effort to create a facilitative environment for individuals with dementia, are effective is still largely unanswered. It is important to note the heterogeneity of these units and the lack of theoretical models underlying the care and care philosophies (the notable exception is Buckwalter's work) and failure to determine what the important outcome variables are. In the Holmes and colleagues (1990) study, for example, it is difficult to know if improvement in the parameters measured over the period chosen (6 months) is a realistic expectation. Similarly, there is little reason to believe that SCUs should reduce or change the medical outcomes studied by Chan et al. (1992). Answers about outcomes should be forthcoming soon in the literature.

Nursing Interventions for Supporting Function and Self-Care

Manipulation of the physical and social (and sometimes even the structural) environment is at the heart of almost all reported nursing interventions for elders designed to support function and self-care and prevent excess disability and premature decline. Most literature addressing support of function has focused on the ADL and self-care problems of persons with dementia, but some has focused on the generally disabled population in long-term care. Some of it has considered promoting function in general, whereas other literature has focused on improving the ability to perform only one specific ADL (e.g., feeding, dressing, grooming, etc.). Both categories of literature are considered in the following discussion.

Improving global function. Improving global function has been the focus of numerous theoretical and anecdotal accounts in the nursing literature and some of the formal studies. In 1988, Beck and Heacock published an excellent review article that analyzed the available literature base and proposed nursing interventions based on the literature. Their review considered five aspects of care for persons with dementia: communication, the physical dimension of care (oral hygiene, nutrition, sleep, bowel and bladder function, and safety), the emotional dimension of care (sexual behavior, anxiety, catastrophic reactions, anger and aggressive behavior, and depression), the cog-

nitive dimension of care (sensation, perception, motor behavior, orientation and memory, and wandering), and the social dimension of care (environment, social interaction and suspiciousness and paranoia). The extensive bibliography includes research conducted by nurses and others, as well as theoretically-based accounts. Manipulation of the social environment through behavioral and other structured approaches and manipulation of the physical aspects of the environment are fundamental to the interventions proposed by Beck and Heacock (1988).

In another article, Danner, Beck, Heacock, and Modlin (1993) identified studies in communication, motor skills memory, and procedural learning and translated the findings of these studies into nursing interventions designed to improve function in persons with dementia. The interventions proposed are strongly rooted in manipulation of the social environment through structured communication, behavioral techniques such as cuing and repetition, and manipulation of the physical environment through altering sensory input.

Beck and Heacock (1988) stress that the majority of nursing interventions for improving function have not been tested formally through research. Since 1988, a few tests of nursing interventions in this area have appeared in the literature. For example, Tappen (1994) reported on an experimental study designed to compare the effects of skill training, a traditional stimulation approach, and regular care on the ability of persons with dementia to perform activities of daily living. Subjects were randomly selected from a nursing home population and randomly assigned to one of the three groups. All subjects were selected because they had a chart diagnosis of dementia. Subjects in two of the three groups received group-based interventions. Functional skills training involved providing opportunities for practicing all basic ADL, including toileting, eating, bathing, dressing, grooming, standing, and walking. Verbal prompting, physical demonstration, and positive reinforcement supported and guided practice. The amount of guidance given was based on the individual's abilities. General stimulation involved group activities that stimulated interaction and cognitive function, including dominoes, bowling, group discussion, music, and simple relaxation. Both interventions focused on manipulation of the social environment. In both intervention groups, the intervention was applied for 2.5 hours a day, 5 days a week, for 20 weeks. Results showed that individuals in the skill-training group showed a rather large increase in basic ADL, individuals in the general stimulation group showed a modest increase, and those in the regular care group showed a decline. Results lend support to the supposition that ADL can be improved in individuals with dementia and that structured nursing interventions to improve function and prevent excess disability can be effective.

Blair (1995) conducted a quasi-experimental study in which three nursing homes were randomly assigned to one of three treatments: a combination of behavior modification and mutual goal setting (Condition 1), mutual goal setting only (Condition 2), and routine nursing care (Condition 3). Nursing home residents who were completely dependent on staff for morning self-care but had previously done these activities and were considered by staff as capable, and those who were cognitively intact, were targeted in sample selection. Staff were taught to administer the interventions. Staff involved in Condition 1 received 1 hour of training every day for 2 weeks. Staff involved in Condition 2 received 1 hour of training on 2 days of 2 weeks, as did staff involved in Condition 3. Training for staff in Condition 3 focused on follow-up goal attainment only. Following training, staff spent 6 weeks focusing on helping residents reacquire skills, then 16 weeks focusing on helping residents maintain progress. Results showed that residents in Condition 1 showed significant improvement over residents in Conditions 2 and 3. Significant differences also existed between those in Conditions 2 and 3. Subjects in both Conditions 1 and 2 improved with the intervention, but scores of those in Condition 2 declined at Time 3, whereas scores for those in Condition 1 were maintained. This study also provides support for the importance of manipulating the environment as a nursing intervention for improving function among nursing home residents.

Improving specific function. Research on the effect of environmental manipulation of ADL function, for example, grooming and feeding, has been conducted by nurses, as discussed in Chapters 30 and 31. Environmental interventions for incontinence have also been tested, as described below.

Among the institutionalized elderly, the problem of incontinence is of major importance. Two related but different concepts underlie this discussion: incontinence, which is a physiological event, and toileting, an activity of daily living involving certain behavioral and cognitive abilities and environmental supports. Unfortunately, it is agreed in the literature that the method of addressing incontinence in most nursing homes is not prevention and control but simply to change the elder following wetting.

According to the guidelines developed by the Agency for Health Care Policy and Research (AHCPR, 1992), the least invasive method of resolving incontinence should be used. For institutionalized elderly, an appropriate diagnostic evaluation should be performed to determine whether an incontinent resident could benefit from behavioral or pharmacological treatment rather than insertion of a catheter or allowing the incontinence to continue without active intervention. For a summary of the literature, the AHCPR (1992) guidelines provide a complete review of the research up to about 1991.

Aggressive intervention for incontinence in the institutionalized elderly requires alteration of the social and organizational environment of the institution itself. Behavioral interventions such as prompting and exercise regimens require an increase in staff time, as well as education and supervision. Freundl and Dugan (1992) studied the knowledge and attitudes of nursing home staff as well as the policies in the nursing homes in which the subjects were employed. The participating agencies reported multiple intervention methods for incontinence, but protocols were often absent. The subjects also lacked specific knowledge needed to intervene, although the level of knowledge increased with the educational level of the subject.

In the long-term care environment, impaired cognition and impaired mobility stand out as two of the characteristics associated with incontinence (Burgio, Jones, & Engel, 1988; Jirovec & Wells, 1990; Ouslander, Kane, & Abrass, 1982). Jirovec and Wells (1990) suggest that in elders with mobility impairment, the presence of incontinence may be an excess disability that is imposed by the nursing home environment and suggest that limiting restraint use, providing sufficient mobility assistance, and focusing efforts on maintenance of mobility should be a part of any incontinence protocol. The presence of cognitive deficits does not necessarily negate the potential effectiveness of a behavioral program. For instance, Schnelle and colleagues (1989) demonstrated that even among severely debilitated elders, a prompted voiding program significantly decreased the frequency of incontinence. Similarly, Jirovec (1991) found that when a toileting routine was developed based on an incontinent elder's pattern of wetting, a prompted voiding program was successful, but only if the program was consistently applied. Jirovec found that of the two nursing homes participating in the study, only one staff was intervening consistently, and this was the determinant of success of the toileting program. Likewise, in a sample of intermediate care residents, Kirkpatrick and Davies (1987) hypothesized that staff attitudes about use of pads and diapers as the most efficient method of dealing with incontinence was a primary barrier to the success of their study. Palmer, Bennett, Marks, McCormick, and Engel (1994) found that even when the sample of incontinent elders was cognitively impaired, administrative support, consistent supervision of nursing assistants implementing the toileting program, and the fact that there were administrative sanctions for missed toileting prompts were the keys to success. When staff were counseled concerning missed toileting checks, the primary reason was workload demand that necessitated either late or early checks. Ouslander and colleagues (1995) suggest that part of the solution is to establish a method of evaluation that allows staff to identify those residents most likely to benefit from behavior intervention if attitudinal and policy barriers to aggressive incontinence intervention are to be breached. A lack of immediate results is discouraging and frustrating to both staff and residents and may interfere with the success of toileting programs (Kirkpatrick & Davies, 1987).

Summary and Conclusions

There is an enormous body of literature in gerontological nursing that addresses the importance of the environment in providing care to older clients. There has been strong theoretical development in this area, and, to some degree, interventions proposed in the literature are linked to this theoretical base. This is particularly evident in the areas related to improving global function and specific function and to reducing certain problem behaviors, specifically confusion and agitation. In the areas of falls, wandering, restraints, and, to some degree, special care units, the links to the theoretical base are much less evident and, to a large extent, literature in this area is atheoretical. In addition, in many of the studies in these areas, environment is defined narrowly to include only aspects of the physical environment, with little attention given to the social and structural environments.

It is noteworthy that many of the interventions proposed in the gerontological nursing literature are research-based, and at least some studies have been conducted to test interventions involving environmental manipulation. This is particularly evident in the area of dementia care, where attention has been given to testing interventions involving both the physical and social environments.

The literature base on supportive environments reviewed for this discussion is extremely rich and diverse. Much of it is exciting because of its potential for improving the quality of care and quality of life of older adults as results are translated into practice. It also provides a very strong basis for entire lines of research for scientists in the future. The great potential evident in this literature, however, will only be realized under three conditions. First, although the importance of person-focused interventions cannot be ignored, focusing exclusively on person-focused interventions without simultaneously considering environmental impacts is likely to be disappointing as the results of studies are translated into gerontological nursing practice. Second, although the importance of the environmental context in the long-term care setting has been acknowledged in research, the environmental context of other care settings (e.g., acute care, home care, etc.) has largely been ignored. Studies must begin to focus on identifying the effects of the person-environment interaction in other settings and on testing person-focused interventions within the environmental context in other settings. Third, in gerontological nursing, conceptualizations of environment must be broad, and studies of the effect of environment must be theory based. The power of the social and structural environment on elders has been documented clearly in many studies, yet many times, if environment is considered at all, the measures focus on narrow facets of the physical environment. Environment is viewed as an accidental variable rather than as an integral part of the whole. Drawing on the strong theoretical base about the person-environment interaction that has evolved in gerontological nursing is essential for further development in the field.

References

Aaronson, W. E. (1992). Is there a role for physician extenders in nursing homes? *Journal of Long Term Care Administration, 20*(3), 18-22.

Agency for Health Care Policy and Research. (1992). *Urinary incontinence in adults.* Washington, DC: U.S. Department of Health and Human Services.

Algase, D. L. (1992a). A century of progress: Today's strategies for responding to wandering behavior. *Journal of Gerontological Nursing, 18*(1), 28-34.

Algase, D. L. (1992b). Cognitive discriminants of wandering among nursing home residents. *Nursing Research, 41*(2), 78-81.

Armstrong-Esther, C. A., & Browne, K. D. (1986). The influence of elderly patients' mental impairments on nurse-patient interactions. *Journal of Advanced Nursing, 11*(4), 379-387.

Beck, C., Baldwin, B., Heithoff, K., & Cuffel, B. (1990). *Disruptive behavior scale.* Unpublished manuscript, University of Arkansas for Medical Sciences, College of Nursing.

Beck, C., & Heacock, P. (1988). Nursing interventions for patients with Alzheimer's disease. *Nursing Clinics of North America, 23*(1), 95-124.

Beck, C. K., & Shue, V. M. (1994). Interventions for treating disruptive behavior in demented elderly people. *Nursing Clinics of North America, 29*(1), 143-155.

Beel-Bates, C. A., & Rogers, A. E. (1990). An exploratory study of sundown syndrome. *Journal of Neuroscience Nursing, 22*(1), 51-52.

Berg, L., Buckwalter, K. C., Chafetz, P. K., Gwyther, L. P., Holmes, D., Koepke, K. M., Lawton, M. P., Lindeman, D. A., Magaziner, J., Maslow, K., Morley, J. E., Ory, M. G., Rabins, P. V., Sloane, P. D., & Teresi, J. (1991). Special care units for persons with dementia. *Journal of the American Geriatrics Society, 39,* 1229-1236.

Berry, G., Fisher, R. H., & Lang, S. (1981). Detrimental incidents, including falls, in elderly institutional population. *Journal of the American Geriatrics Society, 29,* 322-324.

Birren, J. E., & Bengston, V. L. (1988). *Emergency theories of aging.* New York: Springer.

Blair, C. (1995). Combining behavior management and mutual goal setting to reduce physical dependency in nursing home residents. *Nursing Research, 44*(3), 160-165.

Blakeslee, J. A., Goldman, B. D., Papougenis, D., & Torell, C. A. (1991). Making the transition to restraint-free care. *Journal of Gerontological Nursing, 17*(2), 4-8.

Bloom, B., & Braun, J. (1991). Success with wanderers. *Geriatric Nursing, 12*(1), 20.

Blumenthal, M., & Davie, J. W. (1980). Dizziness and falling in elderly psychiatric outpatients. *American Journal of Psychiatry, 137,* 137.

Boettcher, E. G. (1983). Preventing violent behavior: An integrated theoretical model for nursing. *Perspectives in Psychiatric Care, 21*(2), 54-58.

Bowsher, J. E., & Gerlach, M. J. (1990). Personal control and other determinants of psychological well-being in nursing home elders. *Scholarly Inquiry for Nursing Practice, 4*(2), 91-108.

Brannon, D., Cohn, M. D., & Myer, M. A. (1990). Care giving as work: How nurse's aides rate it. *Journal of Long Term Care Administration, 18*(1), 10-14.

Bright, R. (1986). The use of music therapy and activities with demented patients who are deemed difficult to manage. *Clinical Gerontologist, 6*(2), 131-144.

Brody, E. M., Kleban, M. H., Lawton, M. P., & Silverman, H. A. (1971). Excess disabilities of mentally impaired aged: Impact of individualized treatment. *Gerontologist, 2,* 124-133.

Brower, H. T. (1991). The alternatives to restraints. *Journal of Gerontological Nursing, 17*(2), 18-22.

Buchner, D. M., Cress, M. E., Wagner, E. H., de Lateur, B. J., Price, R., & Abrass, I. B. (1993). The Seattle FICSIT/MoveIt study: The effect of exercise on gait and balance in older adults. *Journal of the American Geriatrics Society, 41,* 321-325.

Burgio, L. D., Jones, L. T., & Engel, B. T. (1988). Studying incontinence in an urban nursing home. *Journal of Gerontological Nursing, 14*(4), 40-45.

Calvert, M. M. (1989). Human-pet interaction and loneliness: A test of concepts from Roy's adaptation model. *Nursing Science Quarterly, 2*(4), 194-202.

Campbell, J. M., & Linc, L. G. (1996). Support groups for visitors of residents in nursing homes. *Journal of Gerontological Nursing, 22*(2), 30-35.

Catchen, H. (1983). Repeaters: Inpatient accidents among the hospitalized elderly. *Gerontologist, 23*(3), 273-376.

Caudill, M. (1989). Nursing assistant involvement in patient care planning pays off. *Nursing Management, 20*(5), 112Y-112Z, 112DD, 112FF.

Chan, A. S., Ouslander, J. G., & Osterweil, D. (1992). Placement of the demented elderly: Special versus usual care in a nursing home [Letter to the editor]. *Journal of the American Geriatrics Society, 40,* 640-641.

Cherry, D. L., & Rafkin, M. J. (1988). Adapting day care to the needs of adults with dementia. *Gerontologist, 28*(1), 116-120.

Chrisman, M., Tabar, D., Whall, A. L., & Booth, D. E. (1991). Agitated behavior in the cognitively impaired elderly. *Journal of Gerontological Nursing, 17*(12), 9-13.

Coberg, A., Lynch, D., & Mavretish, B. (1991). Harnessing ideas to research restraints. *Geriatric Nursing, 12*(3), 133-134.

Cohen, E. S. (1988). The elderly mystique: Constraints on the autonomy of the elderly with disabilities. *Gerontologist, 28*(Suppl.), 24-31.

Cohen-Mansfield, J. (1986). Agitated behaviors in the elderly: Preliminary results in the cognitively deteriorated. *Journal of the American Geriatrics Society, 34*(10), 722-727.

Cohen-Mansfield, J., Marx, M. S., & Rosenthal, A. S. (1989). A description of agitation in a nursing home. *Journal of Gerontology, 44*(3), M77-M84.

Cohen-Mansfield, J., Marx, M. S., & Rosenthal, A. S. (1990). Dementia and agitation in nursing home residents: How are they related? *Psychology and Aging, 5,* 3-8.

Cohen-Mansfield, J., Werner, P., & Marx, M. S. (1989). An observational study of agitation in agitated nursing home residents. *International Psychogeriatrics, 1,* 153-165.

Cohen-Mansfield, J., Werner, P., & Marx, M. S. (1990). Screaming in nursing home residents. *Journal of the American Geriatrics Society, 38,* 785-792.

Cohen-Mansfield, J., Werner, P., Marx, M. S., & Freedman, L. (1991). Two studies of pacing in the nursing home. *Journal of Gerontology, 46*(3), M77-M83.

Colling, J., & Park, D. (1983). Home, safe home. *Journal of Gerontological Nursing, 9*(3), 175-179.

Conely, L. G., & Campbell, L. A. (1991). The use of restraints in caring for the elderly: Realities, consequences and alternatives. *Nurse Practitioner, 16*(12), 48-52.

Cookman, C. (1996). Older people and attachment to things, places, pets, and ideas. *Image: The Journal of Nursing Scholarship, 28*(3), 227-231.

Cornbleth, T. (1977). Effects of a protected hospital ward area on wandering and nonwandering geriatric patients. *Journal of Gerontology, 32*(5), 573-577.

Cox, C. L., Kaeser, L., Montgomery, A. C., & Marion, L. H. (1991). Quality of life nursing care: An experimental trial in long-term care. *Journal of Gerontological Nursing, 17*(4), 6-11.

Craven, R., & Bruno, P. (1986). Teach the elderly to prevent falls. *Journal of Gerontological Nursing, 12*(8), 27-33.

Cutchins, C. H. (1991). Blueprint for restraint-free care. *American Journal of Nursing, 91*(7), 36-42.

Danner, C., Beck, C., Heacock, P., & Modlin, T. (1993). Cognitively impaired elders: Using research findings to improve nursing care. *Journal of Gerontological Nursing, 19*(4), 5-11.

Davidson, N. A., Hemingway, M. J., & Wysocki, T. (1984). Reducing the use of restrictive procedures in a residential facility. *Hospital and Community Psychiatry, 35*(2), 164-167.

Dawson, P., Kline, D., Wiancko, D. C., & Wells, D. (1986). Preventing excess disability in patients with Alzheimer's disease. *Geriatric Nursing, 7*(6), 298-301.

Dawson, P., & Reid, D. W. (1987). Behavioral dimensions of patients at risk of wandering. *Gerontologist, 27*(1), 104-107.

Dawson, P., Wells, D. L., & Kline, K. (1993). *Enhancing the abilities of persons with Alzheimer's and related dementias.* New York: Springer.

Edwards, N., Cere, M., & LeBlond, D. (1993). A community-based intervention to prevent falls among seniors. *Family and Community Health, 15*(4), 57-65.

Eigsti, D. G., & Vrooman, N. (1992). Releasing restraints in the nursing home. *Journal of Gerontological Nursing, 18*(1), 21-23.

El-Faizy, M., & Reinsch, S. (1994). Home safety intervention for the prevention of falls. *Physical and Occupational Therapy in Geriatrics, 12*(3), 33-49.

English, R. A. (1989). Implementing a non-restraint philosophy. *Canadian Nurse, 85*(3), 18-20, 22.

Evans, L. K. (1987). Sundown syndrome in institutionalized elderly. *Journal of the American Geriatrics Society, 35,* 101-108.

Evans, L. K. (1996). Knowing the patient: The route to individualized care. *Journal of Gerontological Nursing, 22*(3), 15-19.

Evans, L. K., & Strumpf, N. E. (1989). Tying down the elderly: A review of the literature on physical restraint. *Journal of the American Geriatrics Society, 37,* 65-74.

Evans, L. K., & Strumpf, N. E. (1990). Myths about elder restraint. *Image: The Journal of Nursing Scholarship, 22*(2), 124-128.

Exton-Smith, A. N. (1977). Clinical manifestations. In A. N. Exton-Smith & G. Evans (Eds.), *Care of the elderly: Meeting the challenges of dependency.* London: Academic Press.

Feist, R. R. (1978). A survey of accidental falls in a small home for the aged. *Journal of Gerontological Nursing, 4*(6), 15-17.

Feldt, K. S., & Ryden, M. B. (1992). Aggressive behavior: Educating nursing assistants. *Journal of Gerontological Nursing, 18*(5), 3-12.

Fiatarone, M. A., O'Neill, E. F., Doyle, N., Clements, K. M., Roberts, S. B., Kehayias, J. J., Lipsitz, L. A., & Evans, W. J. (1993). The Boston FICSIT study: The effects of resistance training and nutritional supplementation on physical frailty in the oldest old. *Journal of the American Geriatrics Society, 41,* 333-337.

Fick, K. (1993). The influence of an animal on social interactions of nursing home residents in a group setting. *American Journal of Occupational Therapy, 47*(6), 529-534.

Fine, W. (1959). An analysis of 277 falls in hospital. *Gerontological Clinics, 1,* 292.

Fine, W. (1967). Fits and falls. *Gerontologica Clinica, 9*(4), 270-284.

Flemming, B. E., & Pendergast, D. R. (1993). Physical condition, activity pattern, and environment as factors in falls by adult care facility residents. *Archives of Physical and Medical Rehabilitation, 74,* 627-630.

Foreman, M. D. (1989). Confusion in the hospitalized elderly: Incidence, onset, and associated factors. *Research in Nursing and Health, 21*(1), 21-29.

Foreman, M. D. (1991). The cognitive and behavioral nature of acute confusional states. *Scholarly Inquiry for Nursing Practice, 5*(1), 3-20.

Foreman, M. D. (1993). Acute confusion in the elderly. *Annual Review of Nursing Research, 11,* 3-30.

Freundl, M., & Dugan, J. (1992). Urinary incontinence in the elderly: Knowledge and attitude of long-term care staff. *Geriatric Nursing, 13*(2), 70-75.

Gagne, D., & Toye, R. C. (1994). The effects of therapeutic touch and relaxation therapy in reducing anxiety. *Archives of Psychiatric Nursing, 8*(3), 184-189.

Garcia, R. M., Cruz, M., Reed, M., Taylor, P. V., Sloan, G., & Beran, N. (1988). Relationship between falls and patient attempts to satisfy elimination needs. *Nursing Management, 19*(7), 80v-80x.

Gerdner, L. A., & Buckwalter, K. C. (1994). Assessment and management of agitation in Alzheimer's patients. *Journal of Gerontological Nursing, 20*(4), 11-20.

Gerdner, L. A., & Swanson, E. A. (1993). Effects of individualized music on confused and agitated elderly patients. *Archives of Psychiatric Nursing, 7*(5), 284-291.

Gibb, H., & O'Brien, B. (1990). Jokes and reassurance are not enough: Ways in which nurses relate through conversation with elderly clients. *Journal of Advanced Nursing, 15,* 1389-1401.

Goddaer, J., & Abraham, I. L. (1994). Effects of relaxing music on agitation during meals among nursing home residents with severe cognitive impairment. *Archives of Psychiatric Nursing, 8*(3), 150-158.

Goffman, E. (1961). *Asylums: Essays on the social situation of mental patients and other inmates.* Garden City, NY: Doubleday.

Gross, Y. T., Shimamoto, Y., Rose, C. L., & Frank. (1990). Monitoring risk factors in nursing home. *Journal of Gerontological Nursing, 16*(6), 20-25.

Gryfe, C. I., Amies, A., & Ashley, M. J. (1977). A longitudinal study of falls in an elderly population: I. Incidence and morbidity. *Age and Ageing, 6*(4), 201-210.

Gunderson, J. G. (1978). Defining the therapeutic processes in psychiatric milieus. *Psychiatry, 41,* 327-335.

Hall, G., & Buckwalter, K. (1987). Progressively lowered stress threshold: A conceptual model for care of adults with Alzheimer's disease. *Archives of Psychiatric Nursing, 1*(6), 399-406.

Happ, M. B., Williams, C. C., Strumpf, N. E., & Burger, S. G. (1996). Individualized care for frail elders: Theory and practice. *Journal of Gerontological Nursing, 22*(3), 7-14.

Harris, M. D., Rinehart, J. M., & Gerstman, J. (1993). Animal-assisted therapy for the homebound elderly. *Holistic Nursing Practice, 8*(1), 27-37.

Harris, P. B. (1989). Organizational and staff attitudinal determinants of falls in nursing home residents. *Medical Care, 27*(7), 737-749.

Harvath, T. A., Archbold, P. G., Stewart, B., Gadow, S., Kirschling, J. M., Miller, L., Hagan, J., Brody, K., & Schook, J. (1994). Establishing partnerships with family caregivers: Local and cosmopolitan knowledge. *Journal of Gerontological Nursing, 20*(2), 29-35.

Henderson, J. N. (1994). The culture of special care units: An anthropological perspective on ethnographic research in nursing home settings. *Alzheimer's Disease and Associated Disorders, 8*(1), S410-S416.

Hewison, A. (1995, May 24). Power of language in a ward for the care of older people. *Nursing Times, 91*(21), 32-33.

Hiatt, L. G. (1982). The importance of the physical environment. *Nursing Homes, 31*(5), 2-10.

Hoeffer, B., Rader, J., McKenzie, D., Lavelle, M., & Stewart, B. (1997). Reducing aggressive behavior during bathing cognitively impaired nursing home residents. *Journal of Gerontological Nursing, 23*(5), 16-23.

Holmes, D., Teresi, J., Weiner, A., Monaco, C., Ronch, J., & Vickers, R. (1990). Impacts associated with special care units in long-term care facilities. *Gerontologist, 30*(2), 178-183.

Hornbrook, M. C., Stevens, V. J., & Wingfield, D. J. (1993). Seniors' program for injury control and education. *Journal of the American Geriatrics Society, 41,* 309-314.

Hornbrook, M. C., Stevens, V. J., Wingfield, D. J., Hollis, J. F., Greenlick, M. R., & Ory, M. G. (1994). Preventing falls among community-dwelling older persons: Results from a randomized trial. *Gerontologist, 34*(1), 16-23.

Hussian, R. A., & Brown, D. C. (1987). Use of two-dimensional grid patterns to limit hazardous ambulation in demented patients. *Journal of Gerontology, 42*(5), 558-560.

Innes, E. M., & Turman, W. G. (1983). Evaluation of patient falls. *Quality Review Bulletin, 9*(2), 30-35.

Institute of Medicine, C.O.N.H.R. (1986). *Improving the quality of care in nursing homes.* Washington, DC: National Academy Press.

Jackson, M. E., Drugovich, M. L., Fretwell, M. D., Spector, W. D., Sternberg, J., & Rosenstein, R. B. (1989). Prevalence and correlates of disruptive behavior in the nursing home. *Journal of Aging and Health, 1*(3), 349-369.

Jagella, E., Tideiksaar, R., Mulvihill, M., & Neufeld, R. (1992). Alarm devices instead of restraints? [Letter to the editor]. *Journal of the American Geriatrics Society, 40*(2), 191.

Janelli, L. M., Kanski, G. W., & Neary, M. A. (1994). Physical restraints: Has OBRA made a difference? *Journal of Gerontological Nursing, 20*(6), 17-21.

Janelli, L. M., Kanski, G. W., Scherer, Y. K., & Neary, M. A. (1992). Physical restraints: Practice, attitudes and knowledge among nursing staff. *Journal of Long Term Care Administration, 20*(2), 22-25.

Jarvinen, K. A., & Jarvinen, P. H. (1968). Falling from bed as a complication of hospital treatment. *Journal of Chronic Diseases, 21*(5), 375-378.

Jirovec, M. M. (1991). Effect of individualized prompted toileting on incontinence in nursing home residents. *Applied Nursing Research, 4*(4), 188-191.

Jirovec, M. M., & Wells, T. J. (1990). Urinary incontinence in nursing home residents with dementia: The mobility-cognition paradigm. *Applied Nursing Research, 3*(3), 112-117.

Joel, L. A., & Patterson, J. E. (1990). Nursing homes can't afford cheap nursing care. *RN, 53*(4), 57-60.

Johnson, M. A. (1990). Nursing home placement: The daughter's perspective. *Journal of Gerontological Nursing, 16*(11), 6-11.

Jones, D. C., & vanAmelsvoort Jones, G.M.M. (1986). Communication patterns between nursing staff and the ethnic elderly in a long-term care facility. *Journal of Advanced Nursing, 11,* 265-272.

Kaakinen, J. R. (1992). Living with silence. *Gerontologist, 32*(2), 258-264.

Kalchthaler, T., Bascon, R. A., & Quintos, V. (1978). Falls in the institutionalized elderly. *Journal of the American Geriatrics Society, 26*(9), 424-428.

Kallmann, S. L., Denine-Flynn, M., & Blackburn, D. M. (1992). Comfort, safety, and independence: Restraint release and its challenges. *Geriatric Nursing, 13*(3), 143-148.

Kihlgren, M., Norberg, A., Brane, G., Engstrom, B., & Melin, E. (1993). Nurse-patient interaction after training in integrity promoting care at a long-term ward: Analysis of video-recorded morning care sessions. *International Journal of Nursing Studies, 30*(1), 1-13.

Kilpack, V., Boehm, J., Smith, N., & Mudge, B. (1991). Using research-based interventions to decrease patient falls. *Applied Nursing Research, 4*(2), 50-56.

Kippenbrock, T., & Soja, M. E. (1993). Preventing falls in the elderly: Interviewing patients who have fallen. *Geriatric Nursing, 14*(4), 205-209.

Kirkpatrick, M. K., & Davies, C. (1987). A bladder retraining program in a long-term-care facility. *Nursing Homes, 36*(4), 29-31.

Kolcaba, K. Y. (1991). A taxonomic structure for the concept of comfort. *Image: The Journal of Nursing Scholarship, 23*(4), 237-240.

Kolcaba, K. Y. (1992). The concept of comfort in an environmental framework. *Journal of Gerontological Nursing, 18*(6), 33-38.

Kolcaba, K. Y. (1995). The art of comfort care. *Image: The Journal of Nursing Scholarship, 27*(4), 287-289.

Kongable, L. G., Buckwalter, K. C., & Stolley, J. M. (1989). The effects of pet therapy on the social behavior of institutionalized Alzheimer's clients. *Archives of Psychiatric Nursing, 3*(4), 191-198.

Kongable, L. G., Stolley, J. M., & Buckwalter, K. C. (1990). Pet therapy for Alzheimer's patients: A survey. *Journal of Long Term Care Administration, 18*(3), 17-21.

Krammer, C. H. (1994). Stress and coping of family members responsible for nursing home placement. *Research in Nursing and Health, 17,* 89-98.

Kustaborder, M. J., & Rigney, M. (1983). Interventions for safety. *Journal of Gerontological Nursing, 9*(3), 159-162, 173, 182.

Lanceley, A. (1985). Use of controlling language in the rehabilitation of the elderly. *Journal of Advanced Nursing, 10,* 125-135.

Lawton, M. P. (1982). Competence, environmental press, and the adaptation of older people. In M. P. Lawton, P. G. Windley, & T. O. Byerts (Eds.), *Aging and the environment: Theoretical approaches* (pp. 33-59). New York: Springer.

Lawton, M. P., & Nahemow, L. (1973). Ecology and the aging process. In C. Eisdorfer & M. P. Lawton (Eds.), *The psychology of adult development and aging* (pp. 619-674). Washington, DC: American Psychological Association.

Lawton, M. P., Windley, P. G., & Byerts, T. O. (1982). An orientation to theory in environment and aging. In M. P. Lawton, P. G. Windley, & T. O. Byerts (Eds.), *Aging and the environment: Theoretical approaches* (pp. 1-7). New York: Springer.

Levesque, L., Cossette, S., & Potvin, L. (1993). Why alert residents are more or less willing to cohabit with cognitively impaired peers: An exploratory model. *Gerontologist, 33*(4), 514-522.

Louis, M. (1983). Falls and causes. *Journal of Gerontological Nursing, 9,* 144-156.

Lucht, U. (1971). A prospective study of accidental falls and resulting injuries in the home among elderly people. *Acta Socio-Medica Scandinavica, 3*(2), pp. 105-120.

Lynn, F. H. (1980, June). Incidents: Need they be accidents? *American Journal of Nursing,* pp. 1098-1101.

MacPherson, D. S., Lofgren, R. P., Granieri, R., & Myllenbeck, S. (1990). Deciding to restrain medical patients. *Journal of the American Geriatrics Society, 38,* 516-520.

MacQueen, I. A. (1977). *Home accidents in Aberdeen.* London: Livingston.

Magee, R., Hyatt, E. C., Hardin, S. B., Stratmann, D., Vinson, M. H., & Owen, M. (1993). Use of restraints in extended care and nursing homes. *Journal of Gerontological Nursing, 19*(4), 31-39.

Margulec, I., Librach, G., & Schadel, M. (1970). Epidemiological study of accidents among residents of homes for the aged. *Journal of Gerontology, 25*(4), 342-346.

Martino-Saltzman, D., Blasch, B. B., Morris, R. D., & McNeal, L. W. (1991). Travel behavior of nursing home residents perceived as wanderers and nonwanderers. *Gerontologist, 31*(5), 666-672.

Marx, M. S., Werner, P., & Cohen-Mansfield, J. (1989). Agitation and touch in the nursing home. *Psychological Reports, 64*(3, pt. 2), 1019-1026.

Masters, R., & Marks, S. F. (1990). The use of restraints. *Rehabilitation Nursing, 15*(1), 22-25.

Matteson, M. A., & Linton, A. (1996). Wandering behaviors in institutionalized persons with dementia. *Journal of Gerontological Nursing, 22*(9), 39-46.

Matteson, V. (1989). Guilt and grief when daughters place mothers in nursing homes. *Journal of Gerontological Nursing, 15*(7), 11-15.

Maxfield, M., Lewis, R., & Cannon, S. (1996). Training staff to prevent aggressive behavior of cognitively impaired elderly patients during bathing and grooming. *Journal of Gerontological Nursing, 22*(1), 37-43.

Mayers, K., & Griffin, M. (1990). The play project: Use of stimulus objects with demented patients. *Journal of Gerontological Nursing, 16*(1), 32-39.

Mayo, N. E., Korner-Bitensky, N., Becker, R., & Georges, P. (1989). Predicting falls among patients in a rehabilitation hospital. *American Journal of Physical and Medical Rehabilitation, 68*(3), 139-146.

McGrowder-Lin, R., & Bhatt, A. (1988). A wanderers lounge program for nursing home residents with Alzheimer's disease. *Gerontologist, 28*(5), 607-609.

McHutchion, E., & Morse, J. M. (1989). Releasing restraints: Nursing dilemma. *Journal of Gerontological Nursing, 15*(2), 16-21.

Meddaugh, D. I. (1986). Exercise-to-music for the abusive patient. *Clinical Gerontologist, 6*(2), 147-154.

Meddaugh, D. I., Friedenberg, D. L., & Knisley, R. (1996). Special socks for special people: Falls in special care units. *Geriatric Nursing, 17*(1), 24-26.

Melillo, K. D. (1992). Nurse practitioners in long-term care: Perceptions of DON's. *Journal of Long Term Care Administration, 20*(3), 13-17.

Mezey, M. (1990). GNP's on staff. *Geriatric Nursing, 11*(3), 145-147.

Mion, L. C., Frengley, J. D., Jakovcic, C. A., & Marino, J. A. (1989). A further exploration of the use of physical restraints in hospitalized patients. *Journal of the American Geriatric Society, 37,* 949-956.

Mion, L. C., & Mercurio, A. T. (1992). Methods to reduce restraints: Process, outcomes, and future directions. *Journal of Gerontological Nursing, 18*(11), 5-11.

Mitchell-Pedersen, L., Edmund, L., Fingerote, E., & Powell, C. (1985, October). Let's untie the elderly. *Quarterly Journal of Long-Term Care,* pp. 10-14.

Mohler, G. (1987). Falls: Can they be prevented? Are restraints the only solution? *Nursing Homes, 36*(4), 24-26.

Monsour, N., & Robb, S. S. (1982). Wandering behavior in old age: A psychosocial study. *Social Work, 27*(5), 411-416.

Morris, E. V., & Isaacs, B. (1980). Prevention of falls in a geriatric hospital. *Age and Ageing, 9,* 181-185.

Morse, J. M., & McHutchion, E. (1991). Releasing restraints: Providing safe care for the elderly. *Research in Nursing and Health, 14,* 187-196.

Munroe, D. J. (1990). The influence of registered nurse staffing on the quality of nursing home care. *Research in Nursing and Health, 13,* 263-270.

Murray, C., Mulvihill, M., White, H., Neufeld, R., & Libow, L. (1991). Nursing home characteristics which predict restraint use [abstract]. *Journal of the American Geriatrics Society, 39*(8), A71.

Myers, A. H., Baker, S. P., Robinson, E. G., Abbey, H., Doll, E. T., & Levenson, S. (1989). Falls in the institutionalized elderly. *Journal of Long Term Care Administration, 17*(4), 12-18.

Namazi, K. H., Rosner, T. T., & Calkins, M. P. (1989). Visual barriers to prevent ambulatory Alzheimer's patients from exiting through an emergency door. *Gerontologist, 29*(5), 699-702.

Neelon, V. J., & Champagne, M. T. (1992). Managing cognitive impairment: The current bases for practice. In S. G. Funk, E. M. Tornquist, M. T. Champagne, & R. A. Wiese (Eds.), *Key aspects of elder care: Managing falls, incontinence and cognitive impairment* (pp. 239-250). New York: Springer.

Neelon, V. J., Champagne, M. T., Carlson, J. R., & Funk, S. G. (1996). The NEECHAM Confusion Scale: Construction, validation, and clinical testing. *Nursing Research, 45*(6), 324-330.

Negley, E. N., & Manley, J. T. (1990). Environmental interventions in assaultive behavior. *Journal of Gerontological Nursing, 16*(3), 29-35.

Negley, E. N., Molla, P. M., & Obenchain, J. (1990). No exit: The effects of an electronic security system on confused patients. *Journal of Gerontological Nursing, 16*(8), 21-25.

Newbern, V. B., & Lindsey, I. H. (1994). Attitudes of wives toward having their husbands restrained. *Geriatric Nursing, 15*(3), 135-138.

Nightingale, F. (1992). *Notes on nursing.* Philadelphia: J. B. Lippincott. (Original work published 1859)

Nilsson, K., Palmstierna, T., & Westedt, B. (1988). Aggressive behavior in hospitalized psychogeriatric patients. *Acta Psychiatrica Scandinavica, 78*(2), 172-175.

Ohta, R., & Ohta, B. (1988). Special care units for Alzheimer's disease: A critical look. *Gerontologist, 28,* 803.

Ouslander, J. G., Kane, R. L., & Abrass, L. B. (1982). Urinary incontinence in elderly nursing home patients. *Journal of the American Medical Association, 248*(10), 1194-1198.

Ouslander, J. G., Schnelle, J. F., Uman, G., Fingold, S., Nigam, J. G., Tuico, E., & Bates-Jensen, B. (1995). Predictors of successful prompted voiding among incontinent nursing home residents. *Journal of the American Medical Association, 273*(17), 1366-1370.

Palmer, M. H., Bennett, R. G., Marks, J., McCormick, K. A., & Engel, B. T. (1994). Urinary incontinence: A program that works. *Journal of Long Term Care Administration, 22*(2), 19, 22-24.

Perry, B. C. (1982). Falls among elderly: Review of methods and conclusions of epidemiologic studies. *Journal of the American Geriatrics Society, 30,* 367.

Powell, C., Mitchell-Pedersen, L., Fingerote, E., & Edmund, L. (1989). Freedom from restraint: Consequences of reducing physical restraints in the management of the elderly. *Canadian Medical Journal, 141,* 561-564.

Prudham, D., & Evans, J. G. (1981). Factors associated with falls in the elderly: A community study. *Age and Aging, 10,* 141-146.

Rader, J., & Donius, M. (1991). Restraints in the 90's: Leveling off restraints. *Geriatric Nursing, 12*(2), 71-73.

Rader, J., Lavelle, M., Hoeffer, B., & McKenzie, D. (1996). Maintaining cleanliness: An individualized approach. *Journal of Gerontological Nursing, 22*(3), 32-38.

Rantz, M. J., & McShane, R. E. (1994). Nursing-home staff perception of behavior disturbance and management of confused residents. *Applied Nursing Research, 7*(3), 132-140.

Rantz, M. J., & McShane, R. E. (1995). Nursing interventions for chronically confused nursing home residents. *Geriatric Nursing, 16*(1), 22-27.

Roberts, B. L., & Algase, D. L. (1988). Victims of Alzheimer's disease and the environment. *Nursing Clinics of North America, 23*(1), 83-93.

Rodin, J. (1986). Aging and health: Effects of the sense of control. *Science, 233,* 1271-1276.

Rodstein, M. (1964). Accidents among aged: Incidence, causes and prevention. *Journal of Chronic Disability, 17,* 515-526.

Rogers, M. E. (1994). Nursing: Science of unitary, irreducible, human beings: Update 1990. In V. M. Malinski & E.A.M. Barrett (Eds.), *Martha E. Rogers: Her life and her work* (pp. 244-249). Philadelphia: F. A. Davis.

Rosen, J., Burgio, L., Kollar, M., Cain, M., et al. (1994). The Pittsburgh Agitation Scale: A user-friendly instrument for rating agitation in dementia patients. *American Journal of Geriatric Psychiatry, 2*(1), 52-59.

Rossby, L., Beck, C., & Heacock, P. (1992). Disruptive behaviors of a cognitively impaired nursing home resident. *Archives of Psychiatric Nursing, 6*(2), 98-107.

Rosswurm, M. A., Zimmerman, S. L., Schwartz-Fulton, J., & Norman, G. A. (1986). Can we manage wandering behavior? *Journal of Long Term Care Administration, 14*(2), 5-8.

Rowles, G. D., & High, D. M. (1996). Individualizing care: Family roles in nursing home decision-making. *Journal of Gerontological Nursing, 22*(3), 20-25.

Ryden, M. B. (1985). Environmental support for autonomy in the institutionalized elderly. *Research in Nursing and Health, 8,* 363-371.

Ryden, M. B. (1988). Aggressive behavior in persons with dementia in the community. *Alzheimer's Disease and Associated Disorders, 2,* 342-355.

Ryden, M. B., Bossenmaier, M., & McLachlan, C. (1991). Aggressive behavior in cognitively impaired nursing home residents. *Research in Nursing and Health, 14*(2), 87-95.

Salmon, P. (1993). Interactions of nurses with elderly patients: Relationship to nurses' attitudes and to formal activity periods. *Journal of Advanced Nursing, 18,* 14-19.

Satlin, A., Volicer, L., Ross, V., Herz, L. R., & Campbell, S. (1992). Bright light treatment of behavioral and sleep disturbances in patients with Alzheimer's disease. *American Journal of Psychiatry, 149*(8), 1028-1032.

Savishinsky, J. (1992). Intimacy, domesticity and pet therapy with the elderly: Expectation and experience among nursing home volunteers. *Social Science and Medicine, 34*(12), 1325-1334.

Schnelle, J. F., Traughber, B., Sowell, V. A., Newman, D. R., Petrilli, C. O., & Ory, M. (1989). Prompted voiding treatment of urinary incontinence in nursing home patients: A behavior management approach for nursing home staff. *Journal of the American Geriatrics Society, 37,* 1051-1057.

Schutzenhofer, K. K., & Musser, D. B. (1994). Nurse characteristics and professional autonomy. *Image: The Journal of Nursing Scholarship, 26*(3), 201-205.

Schwab, M., Rader, J., & Doan, J. (1985). Relieving the anxiety and fear in dementia in music, exercise, touch, and relaxation, administered in a group setting. *Journal of Gerontological Nursing, 11*(5), 8-11.

Sehested, P., & Severin-Nielsen, T. (1977). Falls by hospitalized elderly patients: Causes, prevention. *Geriatrics, 32*(4), 101-108.

Shadlen, F. (1991). Psychotropic drug utilization during interventions to reduce the use of physical restraints in a dementia and a long term care ward [abstract]. *Journal of the American Geriatrics Society, 39*(8), A62.

Sheldon, J. H. (1960). On the natural history of falls in old age. *British Medical Journal, 5214,* 1685.

Sloane, P. D., Papougenis, D., & Blakeslee, J. A. (1992). Alternatives to physical and pharmacologic restraints in long-term care. *American Family Physician, 45*(2), 763-769.

Smyer, M. (1995). Formal support in later life: Lessons for prevention. In L. A. Bond, S. J. Cutler, & A. Grams (Eds.), *Promoting successful and productive aging* (pp. 186-202). Thousand Oaks, CA: Sage.

Snellgrove, C. E., & Flaherty, E. L. (1975). An attitude therapy program helps reduce the use of physical restraints. *Journal of the American Geriatrics Society, 26*(3), 137, 140.

Snyder, L. H., Rupprecht, P., Pyrek, J., Brekhus, S., & Moss, T. (1978). Wandering. *Gerontologist, 18*(3), 272-280.

Snyder, M., Egan, E. C., & Burns, K. R. (1995a). Efficacy of hand massage in decreasing agitation behaviors associated with care activities in persons with dementia. *Geriatric Nursing, 16*(2), 60-63.

Snyder, M., Egan, E. C., & Burns, K. R. (1995b). Interventions for decreasing agitation behaviors in persons with dementia. *Journal of Gerontological Nursing, 21*(7), 34-40.

Spector, W. D., & Jackson, M. E. (1994). Correlates of disruptive behaviors in nursing homes. *Journal of Aging and Health, 6*(2), 173-184.

Stilwell, E. M. (1991). Nurses' education related to the use of restraints. *Journal of Gerontological Nursing, 17*(2), 23-26.

Sullivan-Marx, E. M. (1996). Restraint-free care: How does a nurse decide? *Journal of Gerontological Nursing, 22*(9), 7-14.

Suprock, L. A. (1990). Changing the rules. *Geriatric Nursing, 11*(6), 288-290.

Swanson, E. A., Maas, M. L., & Buckwalter, K. C. (1993). Catastrophic reactions and other behaviors of Alzheimer's residents: Special unit compared with traditional units. *Archives of Psychiatric Nursing, 7*(5), 292-299.

Taft, L. B., Delaney, K., Seman, D., & Stansell, J. (1993). Dementia care: Creating a therapeutic milieu. *Journal of Gerontological Nursing, 19*(10), 30-39.

Tappen, R. M. (1994). The effect of skill training on functional abilities of nursing home residents with dementia. *Research in Nursing and Health, 17,* 159-165.

Tellis-Nayak, V., & Tellis-Nayak, M. (1989). Quality of care and the burden of two cultures: When the world of the nurse's aide enters the world of the nursing home. *Gerontologist, 29*(3), 307-313.

Tinetti, M. E., Liu, W. L., & Ginter, S. F. (1992). Mechanical restraint use and fall-related injuries among residents of skilled nursing facilities. *Annals of Internal Medicine, 116,* 369-374.

Tutuarima, J. A., de Haan, R. J., & Limburg, M. (1993). Number of nursing staff and falls: A case-control study on falls by stroke patients in acute-care settings. *Journal of Advanced Nursing, 18,* 1101-1105.

Wallace, M. (1994). The sundown syndrome. *Geriatric Nursing, 15*(3), 164-166.

Wallace, R. B., Ross, J. E., Huston, J. C., Kundel, C., & Woodsworth, G. (1993). Iowa FICSIT trial: The feasibility of elderly wearing a hip joint protective garment to reduce hip fractures. *Journal of the American Geriatrics Society, 41,* 338-340.

Waller, J. (1974). Injury in the aged: Clinical and epidemiological implications. *New York State Journal of Medicine, 74,* 2200-2208.

Walshe, A., & Rosen, H. (1979). A study of patient falls from bed. *Journal of Nursing Administration, 9*(5), 31-35.

Waxman, H. M., Carner, E. A., & Berkenstock, G. (1984). Job turnover and job satisfaction among nursing home aides. *Gerontologist, 24*(5), 503-509.

Werner, P., Cohen-Mansfield, J., Braun, J., & Marx, M. S. (1989). Physical restraints and agitation in nursing home residents. *Journal of the American Geriatrics Society, 37,* 1122-1126.

Werner, P., Cohen-Mansfield, J., Koroknay, V., & Braun, J. (1994). The impact of a restraint-reduction program on nursing home residents. *Geriatric Nursing, 15*(3), 142-146.

Whall, A. L., Gillis, G. L., Yankou, D., Booth, D. E., & Beel-Bates, C. A. (1992). Disruptive behavior in elderly nursing home residents: A survey of nursing staff. *Journal of Gerontological Nursing, 18*(10), 13-17.

Wild, D., Nayak, U.S.L., & Isaacs, B. (1981). Prognosis of falls in old people at home. *Journal of Epidemiology Community Health, 35,* 200-204.

Winger, J., Schirm, V., & Stewart, D. (1987). Aggressive behavior in long-term care. *Journal of Psychosocial Nursing in Mental Health Services, 25*(4), 28-33.

Wolanin, M. O., & Phillips, L.R.F. (1981). *Confusion: Prevention and care.* St. Louis, MO: C. V. Mosby.

Wolf, S. L., Kutner, N. G., Green, R. C., & McNeely, E. (1993). The Atlanta FICSIT study: Two exercise interventions to reduce frailty in elders. *Journal of the American Geriatrics Society, 41,* 329-332.

Wolf-Klein, G. P., Silverstone, F. A., Basavaraju, N., Foley, C., Pascaru, A., & Ma, P.-H. (1988). Prevention of falls in the elderly population. *Archives of Physical Medicine and Rehabilitation, 69,* 689-691.

Wolfson, L., Whipple, R., Judge, J., Amerman, P., Derby, C., & King, M. (1993). Training balance and strength in the elderly to improve function. *Journal of the American Geriatrics Society, 41,* 341-343.

Woods, P. A., & Cullen, C. (1983). Determinants of staff behavior in long-term care. *Behavioral Psychotherapy, 11*(1), 4-17.

PART

IIH

ENVIRONMENTS FOR
OPTIMIZING CLIENT
OUTCOMES

Joyce A. Verran

The three chapters in this section examine nursing research that investigates the impact of nursing environments on outcomes for clients in a variety of settings. Environments have been broadly defined in these chapters to include both the internal and external context in which care is delivered; however, emphasis has been placed on the internal environment, or that context in which nurses practice that is believed to directly affect the clients served.

Much of the research in this area, no matter the setting, is in its infancy. Nursing has recognized for many years that context has an impact on care delivery. Most of the formal research has, however, examined the effect of context on staff and organizational outcomes rather than health status outcomes for clients. We have strong evidence from a number of studies that various aspects of context improve job satisfaction for nurses and increase the resources available to provide care (Verran, 1996). Unfortunately, limited work has been done on establishing links between contextual factors, staff outcomes or organizational outcomes, and client responses.

Because of this past emphasis, there are many gaps and inconsistencies in the knowledge base of how elements of the context in which nurses practice affect clients. All authors in the subsequent chapters address these gaps from the perspective of various settings and acuity levels.

In Chapter 33, Ingersoll and Mitchell review research that has been conducted about the context of acute care settings. Their review includes both intermediate and critical care levels of acuity and indicates that most of the current research in acute care areas is problem based rather than being grounded in theoretical perspectives. The authors make a strong plea for theory-based, scientifically rigorous research that allows for generalization of findings across settings and times. They further emphasize the need for consistent outcomes that cross settings of care and are sensitive to nursing service but of interest to multiple disciplines. The work of the American

Academy of Nursing's Expert Panel on Quality Health Care is cited as providing beginning work in this area (Mitchell, Heinrich, Moritz, & Hinshaw, 1997).

Chapter 34, by Brooten and Naylor, looks at the emerging research in a relatively new field of inquiry, that of transitional environments. The authors define transitional settings as those that provide short-term services to assist clients with a transfer from one acuity level of service to another. With this definition, work looking at outcomes attributable to home care, subacute settings, integrated health care systems, and community nursing case management becomes transitional. Most of the current research that may be termed community based really belongs in this area of transitional nursing rather than in a true community health perspective. Brooten and Naylor identify four issues influencing research. These issues involve the need to determine the length of service required by clients, the specific clients needing service, the level of providers necessary for the needed service, and the costs for the transitional services that are provided. Although issues exist, it is within the area of transitional nursing services that strong programs of research have emerged that provide evidence of the effect of nursing practice models on client outcomes. This is primarily evident in the research on the effect of advanced practice nurses on the outcomes achieved for clients in the transition from hospital to home.

Maas and Specht (Chapter 35) examine the research that has been done on context within long-term care settings, specifically, nursing homes. They note that the examination of context has received little attention from nurses researching the care given to the elderly, even though extensive databases are available for secondary analysis. Unfortunately, these databases are limited in the concepts included. This is particularly true in terms of contextual variables, as well as the specific client outcomes that would be influenced most by elements in the environment. Much of the work that has been done by nursing has involved the environmental concept of staffing ratios and mix and its effect on individual client outcomes. The authors contend that more work needs to address other elements of context as well as group level outcomes. Of the research examining nursing home environments, much of it has been grounded in the two theoretical perspectives of environmental effects on the elderly and the quality model of structure, process, outcomes.

Although the formal examination of the effect of environmental concepts on client outcomes is sparse and limited by lack of theory and incomplete programs of research, the potential for future investigations that support nursing practice is great. The authors of the following chapters provide guidance for further research needed to build and support this area of nursing science.

References

Mitchell, P. H., Heinrich, J., Moritz, P., & Hinshaw, A. S. (Eds.). (1997). Outcome measure and care delivery systems conference. *Medical Care 35*(suppl.), 11.

Verran, J. A. (1996). Quality of care, organization variables, and nurse staffing. In G. S. Wunderlich, F. A. Sloan, & C. K. Davies (Eds.), *Nursing staff in hospitals and nursing homes: Is it adequate?* (pp. 308-331). Washington, DC: National Academy Press.

33

ACUTE CARE ENVIRONMENTS

Gail L. Ingersoll
Pamela H. Mitchell

Early studies of acute care environments focused primarily on hospital characteristics that affect patient outcome (Verran & Mark, 1992). With the exception of a recent report by Aiken, Smith, and Lake (1994), large studies of patient outcome, defined most commonly as *mortality rate,* have focused on hospital and physician characteristics, with only a passing nod at factors associated with nurse performance (Hartz et al., 1989; Shortell & Hughes, 1988).

To determine the state of the science concerning the effect of nursing-related environments on patient outcomes, a comprehensive review of the nursing and health services literature was conducted for the years 1980 through 1995. Computer searches using nursing (CINAHL) and medical (MEDLINE) indexes were done. Citations within research reports were also tracked for identification of other studies.

Included in the review were studies of professional practice models and organizational environments in which the practice model or the acute care environment was the independent variable. In each case, patient outcome was the dependent variable, thereby eliminating studies in which the focus of the outcome was change in nurse attitude or behavior. Excluded also were reports in which descriptions of the study design or methods and findings were insufficient to allow for adequate assessment of scientific rigor.

In this chapter, the findings of that review are described and recommendations are made for future research. Conceptual and methodological issues associated with the studies are discussed, as is suitability of findings for application to clinical practice.

Theoretical Perspectives

Most of the studies of the effect of acute care environments on patient outcomes have been atheoretically driven. Some investigators have used previous research to guide the selection of variables and instruments, but few have identified any overarching framework for their approach to research questions, study design, or methods. Those studies that have been guided by theory have tended to use frameworks from disciplines other than nursing.

A number of nurse authors and experts have described the need for theory to guide both the development of acute care models and the evaluation of their effect on patient outcome. Newman (1990) has proposed a movement to a trilevel model of professional practice to improve care delivery practices and outcome. As of yet this model is untested; consequently, its effect on patient outcome is uncertain. Theorists have also proposed ways to guide the development of differentiated practice models according to nursing theory (Frederickson, 1991; Isenberg, 1991; Mitchell, 1991; Parse, 1991; Roy, 1991). Each of these, likewise, is untested.

Several other professional practice models have been proposed, but few have been evaluated for their effect on patient outcomes. Most reports simply describe the models and the strategies used to implement them, or they focus exclusively on employee response. When patient outcome is included, it is most often defined as *patient satisfaction* (McKenzie, Torkelson, & Holt, 1989). Although patient satisfaction (or, preferably, "patient perception of care delivery") is a reasonable indicator of environmental effect, the use of unreliable and invalid instruments is not. Only a few studies use instruments that have undergone more than the most basic assessments of reliability and validity.

One of the more widely studied conceptually driven acute care approaches involves the assessment of continuous quality improvement (CQI) and total quality management (TQM) programs on patient outcome. Most of the reports found in the literature, however, contain limited information about how the conceptual framework actually guided the conduct of the study. Instead, the CQI or TQM process is described as the approach used to monitor care delivery practices or problem-solving approaches.

In one TQM study in which a conceptual framework was identified by the authors, Shortell, O'Brien, et al. (1995) described using "variance theory" (p. 379) to identify factors that influence implementation of quality improvement activities and their perceived impact on human resources development, finances, and patient care outcomes. Although no information is provided about variance theory per se, the researchers did develop a framework for comparison of effect of independent vari-

ables (bed size, hospital culture, use of CQI/TQM, and implementation approach) on intervening (degree of quality improvement implementation) and dependent (perceived impact and clinical efficiency) variables. Further use of theory was evident in the statement of hypotheses and the selection of instruments. Use of the framework also allowed the authors to describe findings according to the framework proposed. The failure to clearly define variance theory and why it was selected is a limitation.

Clear descriptions of the conceptual models used to guide studies of acute care settings were included in reports by Mitchell, Shannon, Cain, and Hegyvary (1996); Mitchell, Armstrong, Simpson, and Lentz (1989); Koerner, Cohen, and Armstrong (1985); and Cassard, Weisman, Gordon, and Wong (1994). In the 1989 Mitchell, Armstrong, et al. study, the investigators reviewed several bodies of literature to develop a framework for determining whether positive nurse and patient outcomes were evident in favorable organizational structures and effective critical care nursing processes. Using information obtained from the literature, they examined a combination of organizational and care delivery unit structure and process indicators, as well as multiple organizational and clinical outcomes.

Mitchell and colleagues identified a unit level of organizational structure, which was characterized by degree of specialization, standardization of work, discretion over tasks, and expertise or professionalism (p. 220). These unit-level structures, in combination with the nature of the work, were expected to influence the unit-level organizational processes, which were subsequently reflected in organizational outcomes. Organizational processes and nature of work were expected to influence the clinical processes by which nursing care was delivered. These clinical processes were then expected to influence clinical and organizational outcomes and cost. Clinical outcomes and cost were also expected to be influenced by the patient's actual health status.

Mitchell, Armstrong, et al. (1989) used previous studies of acute care hospitals to guide the development of a framework for the study. These prior studies had found positive associations between organizational outcome and organizational climate and structure. Fewer findings were available concerning the relationship between positive clinical outcome and organizational structures or processes in critical care. As a result, Mitchell, Armstrong, et al. simultaneously measured the effect of organizational structures and processes on organizational *and* clinical outcomes. They also identified which clinical outcomes were likely to be influenced by nursing practice as opposed to other organizational factors. In subsequent work, they explored in multiple critical care units one component of this framework by using Van de Ven's Patterned Contingency Theory to test the relationship between use of a discretionary pattern of organizational process and structure and clinical and organizational outcomes (Mitchell, Shannon, et al., 1996).

In the Cassard et al. (1994) study, two theoretical bases were used to measure the effect of a professional practice model on patient care. These two theories were described by the researchers as contradictory. One theory, derived from the literature on self-managed groups, proposes that self-managed groups increase worker satisfaction and group effectiveness, thereby positively influencing patient care. The other theory, derived from the utility maximization view of human behavior, suggests that nurses work to maximize their financial return by working longer hours, keeping permanent staffing low, and avoiding use of purchased nursing services. These behaviors increase the potential for negative patient outcome. To account for the discrepancies in these hypotheses, the investigators used a null hypothesis approach to model testing.

The Mitchell et al. (Mitchell, Armstrong, et al., 1989; Mitchell, Shannon, et al., 1996) and the Cassard et al. (1994) studies highlight several issues common to organizational research in which nursing care delivery practices are evaluated for their effect on patient outcome. First, multiple theories are often required to describe and explain relationships among variables. Second, multiple methods are needed to capture information about the processes, structures, and outcomes associated with the environment under investigation. Third, theories and findings may conflict, leading to difficulty in interpreting results and comparing studies.

In a few studies, evaluation theories have been alluded to but minimally described. In one example, Carlson and Rosenqvist (1991) identified an organization, process, and outcomes framework for assessing the effect of a diabetes care program on patient outcome. Unfortunately, they never clarified how the model guided the selection of instruments to measure process and outcome components. In addition, they failed to identify how changes in the organization and the process were expected to result in changes in the outcome. According to Chen (1990), a necessary component of an evaluation theory is a description of both the structure of the program and the underlying causal mechanisms that clarify the relationships of the program components and imple-

mentation process to outcome. Without both, the theory is incomplete. In the case of the Carlson and Rosenqvist study, no information was provided about how the model was expected to produce a change in patient outcome nor why the variables were chosen to indicate evidence of positive effect. Consequently, the relationships between theory and research are unclear. As a result, the theory was never actually tested—so the findings provide no information about whether or not the intervention actually led to the effect seen.

The problem identified in the Carlson and Rosenqvist study is a common one in program evaluations, in which a model is introduced but no measure is included for ensuring that the model is introduced as intended. Without some indication of the extent and the configuration of the model implemented, there can be no assurance that what was introduced was consistent with what was theorized to produce the outcome. This measurement issue has been described as Type III evaluation error by Basch, Sliepcevich, Gold, Duncan, and Kolbe (1985). It occurs when something other than what was intended is introduced, when an insufficient amount of intervention is introduced, and when inappropriate measures are used to determine effect. In each case, the cause-effect relationship between the intervention and the outcome is uncertain.

Koerner et al. (1985) used systems theory to guide their study of the effect of a collaborative practice care delivery model on quality of patient care. They chose systems theory because of its usefulness for examining "the interrelatedness of specific organizational variables to patient outcomes" (p. 302). They organized their variables according to a model proposed by Jelinek (1967) in which organizational factors, workload factors, and environmental factors are defined. The collaborative practice model was identified as the organizational factor, with workload, personnel, physical facilities, and environment being controlled for through selection of comparable experimental and comparison units.

Quality of patient care was measured by a researcher-developed patient perception of care delivery and satisfaction with care survey. According to the authors, content validity was checked through review of items by experts and by pilot testing the instrument with well and ill elderly clients. Internal consistency was not established because items in the tool were not considered unidimensional and a summed score was not computed. A review of the items provided in the report suggests that most are unidimensional and could have been checked through comprehensive item to item and item to total scale correlations before computing coefficient alpha to test for internal consistency. Factor analysis of the scale also would have clarified whether the constructs identified for measurement (patient-provider interaction, quality of care, health education, knowledge of practitioners, and the environment of the unit) were indeed reflected by the items in the scale.

Because no differences were seen according to time post-model implementation (4, 8, and 12 months), data were combined and compared for experimental and comparison units. Findings indicated that collaborative practice units' patients were better able to identify the nurse and the physician who were primarily responsible for their care. They also perceived greater collaboration between care providers and greater involvement of selves and families in discharge planning. Knowledge of care providers was rated higher by experimental unit patients, although quality of care was not. Patients on both experimental and comparison units stated they received the type of care expected. Despite this, communication of needs, attainment of services by primary nurse, and services planned with individual patient in mind were rated higher on the experimental unit. Long-term effect is not identified, as final data collection occurred at 12 months post-model implementation.

A retrospective medical record review conducted as part of the study assessed for differences in average length of stay, average number of laboratory tests ordered, number of intravenous therapy days, number of cardiac arrests, number of deaths, number of transfers to intensive care, number of referrals to other care providers, and number of teaching plans and discharge plans completed. No differences were seen between units for any variables except number of patient teaching plans. In this case, the comparison unit had significantly more.

State of the Science

The nursing science concerning the effect of acute care settings on patient outcomes is in its infancy. Only recently have nurse researchers begun to conceptualize nursing care organizations as environments that can promote or hinder health outcomes. Prior to the 1980s, most research on nursing care organizations was either atheoretically driven or was linked to theories of personnel management and retention. As a result, this review draws heavily from work outside the discipline.

Nurse clinicians and managers in a variety of health care delivery organizations assume that organizational structures and processes (sometimes called organizational, contextual, or nonclinical variables) interact with disease-specific clinical treatments to influence patient care outcome (Crane, 1992; Verran & Mark, 1992). This assumption is often conveyed through the contention that nursing care "makes a difference" in patient outcomes. These care delivery elements comprise an environment that is assumed, but rarely tested, to contribute positively to healthy outcomes for patients in acute care settings. In fact, only one study demonstrates convincingly that nursing care delivery approach (as opposed to number or ratio of RNs) distinguishes among acute care hospitals with lower and higher mortality rates (Aiken et al., 1994).

Considerable evidence suggests that professional environments and opportunities to influence clinical care and work settings result in staff nurse satisfaction and decreased propensity to leave (Alexander, 1988; Blegen & Mueller, 1987; Dear, Weisman, Alexander, & Chase, 1982; Duxbury & Thiessen, 1979; Hinshaw & Atwood, 1983; Hinshaw, Smeltzer, & Atwood, 1987; Irvine & Evans, 1995; Packard & Motowildo, 1987; Price & Mueller, 1981; Weisman, 1981). Moreover, although longevity does not guarantee expertise, the potential for greater expertise is evident when nurses are experienced in their work (Benner, Tanner, & Chesla, 1992). As a result, better-functioning units are expected to retain experienced nurses and maintain a level of expertise necessary for optimal patient outcome.

Better outcomes, such as lower mortality rate and lower readmission rate to intensive care, are documented when nurses and physicians communicate effectively (Alt-White, Charns, & Strayer, 1983; Baggs, Ryan, Phelps, Richeson, & Johnson, 1992; Knaus, Draper, Wagner, & Zimmerman, 1986). Although no direct relationship has been found between information flow and communication with other units and patient care outcomes, newspaper reports of erroneously performed surgery and fatal medication errors are cited as examples of how poor communication and information flow influences hospital mortality (Altman, 1995; Navarro, 1955; Sharp, 1995).

The most commonly measured outcome indicators (morbidity, mortality, and adverse effect) are not particularly sensitive to differences in clinical delivery systems except when large samples are used (Verran, 1996). In addition, most health services and clinical outcomes research have focused on organizational structural variables such as size, ownership, professional credentialing, and reimbursement type. None of these allow for determination of the mechanisms by which these variables account for differences in outcomes (Flood, Scott, & Ewy, 1984a, 1984b; Hartz et al., 1989; Shortell & Hughes, 1988). Finally, most outcomes research in acute care settings has focused on treatment effects during a single episode of care. Consequently, the long-term effect of integrated systems of care on patient care outcomes is unknown (Fitzgerald, Freund, Hughett, & McHugh, 1993; Fowler, Cleary, Magaziner, Patrick, & Benjamin, 1994; Jones, 1993).

A literature review by the inter-PORT (Patient Outcomes Research Teams) work group on outcomes assessment noted that the few studies that do use multiple outcomes are unrepresentative and measure only short-term outcomes. They also lack appropriate control groups and fail to control such contextual variables as size, ownership, and professional credentialing (Fowler et al., 1994). Studies of hospital variations in mortality have focused on organizational-level structural variables such as size, ownership, and professional credentialing (Al-Haider & Wan, 1991; Flood et al., 1984a, 1984b; Hartz et al., 1989; Keeler et al., 1992; Krakauer et al., 1992; Shortell & Hughes, 1988) and have found that larger size, greater proportion of RNs, and greater volume of patients in specific diagnostic categories are associated with lower severity-adjusted mortality.

Some investigators have begun examining the specific organizational structures and processes that account for lower mortality in some hospitals or care units. Organizational or unit level inputs (e.g., degree of uncertainty) and structures and processes (e.g., formalization or standardization of protocols, and modes of communication and coordination) might be considered the nonspecific treatment effects of care delivery because direct linkages to outcomes such as morbidity, mortality, and adverse events can be postulated (Cassard et al., 1994; Fitzgerald et al., 1993; Flood & Scott, 1987; Knaus et al., 1986; Mitchell et al., 1996; Shortell, Zimmerman, et al., 1994).

Discretionary decision making, control over practice, and professional status of nurses has been found to result in lower severity-adjusted Medicare mortality rates (Aiken et al., 1994). Better-quality nursing surveillance, as an intermediate process variable, is predictive of lower severity-adjusted Medicare mortality (Kahn et al., 1990; Rubenstein, Chang, Keeler, & Kahn, 1992; Rubenstein, Kahn, et al., 1990). Another intermediate process variable, readmission to the ICU, is reduced when better collaboration exists between critical care nurses and resident physicians (Baggs & Ryan, 1990; Baggs et al., 1992).

Sample size appears to be an important dimension of these studies, however, because mortality, morbidity, and adverse events have not been shown to be sensitive to changes in organizational structure and process characteristics in smaller-sample studies (Cassard et al., 1994; Mitchell et al., 1996; Shortell, Zimmerman, et al., 1994; Taunton, Kleinbeck, Stafford, Woods, & Bott, 1994).

Long-term care delivery research, although not the focus of this review, is relevant in terms of outcome measures that might be appropriate for acute care settings as well. This literature has emphasized the effects of interdisciplinary teams on patient functioning, models of adult day care, home care with at-risk women and children, case management models, and use of innovations such as "swing" beds in rural hospitals (Olds & Kitzman, 1990; Rabiner, Stearns, & Mutran, 1994; Rothman, Hedrick, Bulcroft, Erdly, & Nickinovich, 1993; Schmitt, Farrell, & Heineman, 1988; Shaugnessy, Schlenker, & Kramer, 1990). No published studies were found concerning subacute care outcomes and long-term care environments.

Both demonstration projects and controlled trials have been reported for long-term agencies, but the samples are not sufficiently large (in terms of the number of organizations or caregiving units) to examine the specific organizational structure and process factors that distinguish better and worse client outcomes. Functional status measures, stabilization of cognitive and social function, and placement outcomes are used as frequently as morbidity and mortality outcomes in this population, with both adults and children.

Recommendations for Advancing the Science

Summary of Issues

The majority of reports of studies pertaining to acute care environments and patient outcome contain no description of the theory used to guide selection of variables or methodology. Moreover, several interventions introduced in acute care environments have been directed at workers rather than patients (Weisman, 1992). Consequently, the conceptual link to patient outcomes may not be evident. This is particularly problematic if the researchers fail to describe the link and the underlying theory that led to its connection.

Lack of theoretic framework has contributed to a proliferation of researcher-developed questionnaires and other outcome measurement instruments. These pose serious problems for the extension of science and limit comparisons of findings. They also restrict the interpretability of findings: No framework is available to explain how the variables conceptually hang together.

In addition, relatively little work has been published concerning the relationship between organizational factors and any patient outcome other than mortality. It may be that organizational features enhancing clinical care delivery and employee well-being have no effect on clinical outcomes. Plausible links exist between some organizational elements of care delivery (e.g., collaboration among providers, nursing surveillance of client well-being, and coordination of care) and extreme outcomes (e.g., mortality and morbidity), so this seems unlikely. Moreover, evidence for relationships between the environment and favorable perception of care delivery (an element of satisfaction), change in health status (positive health behaviors, achievement of optimal symptom relief), change in health-related quality of life, and achievement of attainable self-care support the existence of these relationships. Clinicians and administrators are convinced that such links exist but that the measures used are rare or insensitive to the impact of care delivery systems or patient outcomes.

Taken together, acute care studies are unclear about the extent to which nursing care environments influence patient outcomes. There is support in some studies, but not in others, that nursing surveillance, quality of working environment, and quality of interaction with other professionals distinguishes hospital mortality and complication rates. Relatively few studies have measured the more fine-grained patient outcome variables that are suggested to be more sensitive to variations in nursing practice, particularly over time. It is clear that some nursing care units are viewed as better places to work, as having higher-quality professional care and smoother communication. Whether these behaviors translate into a range of patient outcomes is unknown. Most of the work in this area is not reported in the literature and is known only through preliminary reports at conferences.

Given the apparent subtle effects of the care delivery environment, even extensive primary data collection in fewer than 100 settings may not be adequate to uncover relationships, let alone explicate the mechanisms by which change occurs. Work needs to be undertaken on two fronts: specifying outcomes that are more sensitive to the caregiving environment and routinely measuring those same outcomes as an ongoing part of caregiving in the continuum of settings where people receive care.

Recommendations for Future Directions

Hegyvary (1992) has stressed the need for metaparadigmatic research to test the effect of nursing interventions on patient outcomes. This recommendation can be extended to the environments where nurses intervene. Doing so, however, adds considerable complexity to the study. As demonstrated by Cassard et al. (1994), when multiple paradigms or theories are used, results may conflict with one another, depending on the theories selected and the measures used to observe effect. Because of the complex nature of acute care settings, the potential for conflicting hypotheses based on multiple theories is great.

An issue mentioned by Brooten and Naylor (1995) is the need for sufficient "nurse dose" to detect effect on patient outcome. This issue is especially relevant in light of the move by acute care settings to team focused care delivery approaches where the effect of the nurse is difficult to distinguish from others.

An additional need pertains to the untested theoretical premise about whether interventions initiated at the unit level or the organizational level are most effective. Although some authors have suggested that interventions be introduced at the organizational level to produce sufficient effect on patient outcomes (Dienemann & Gessner, 1992), there are no studies to substantiate that one approach is better than the other. As Ingersoll (1996) has noted, as long as administrative support is available, unit-level interventions appear to be equally effective as those instituted at the organizational level. Moreover, they may have a greater likelihood for full implementation; those living the experience have direct responsibility for seeing that the changes happen. There are also fewer bureaucratic barriers to overcome, meaning that fewer changes to the original model are required.

What is clearly needed in the future is a better set of outcome measures suitable for use in large sample studies. The American Academy of Nursing (AAN) Expert Panel on Quality Indicators has proposed such a set, based on the assumption that nursing care is an integral component of most health care delivery systems and is characterized by structures and processes that integrate functional, social, and physiological aspects of patient experiences during illness (Rosenthal et al., 1992). Therefore, outcome indicators for quality nursing care need to incorporate multiple aspects of patient response to presenting condition and care delivery—clinical, functional, financial, and perceptual (Hegyvary, 1991; Mitchell, 1995).

The AAN Expert Panel, at a working meeting in October 1994, proposed a set of five outcome measures that, if collected for all patient care encounters, would allow for a clearer determination of the impact of organizational factors on patient care outcomes. These outcome indicators seem likely to be more sensitive to differences

in care delivery than the current negative indicators (morbidity, mortality, adverse events). Moreover, there is some support in the literature for their use in detecting differences in care delivery. These indicator dimensions include health-related quality of life (HRQOL), symptom management to criterion, achievement of appropriate self-care, patient perception of being well cared for (often incorporated in patient satisfaction), and demonstration of health-promoting behaviors. This set of five outcomes is proposed in addition to the typical morbidity and mortality measures and would, ideally, be included in developing databases that allow for tracking outcomes over place and time for a defined episode of care (rather than in a specific place of care). In addition, costs can be attached to better describe the financial outcomes of care.

References

Aiken, L. H., Smith, H. L., & Lake, E. T. (1994). Lower Medicare mortality among a set of hospitals known for good nursing care. *Medical Care, 32,* 771-787.

Alexander, J. (1988). The effects of patient care unit organization on nursing turnover. *Health Care Management Review, 13*(2), 61-72.

Al-Haider, A., & Wan, T. (1991). Modeling organizational determinants of hospital mortality. *Health Services Research, 26,* 303-323.

Alt-White, A. C., Charns, M., & Strayer, R. (1983). Personal, organizational and managerial factors related to nurse-physician collaboration. *Nursing Administration Quarterly, 8*(1), 8-18.

Altman, L. K. (1995, May 31). Federal officials cite differences at Harvard hospital. *New York Times,* p. A16.

Baggs, J. G., & Ryan, S. A. (1990). Intensive care nurse-physician collaboration and nurse satisfaction. *Nursing Economics, 8,* 386-392.

Baggs, J. G., Ryan, S. A., Phelps, C. E., Richeson, J. F., & Johnson, J. E. (1992). The association between interdisciplinary collaboration and patient outcomes in medical intensive care. *Heart and Lung, 21,* 18-24.

Basch, C. E., Sliepcevich, E. M., Gold, R. S., Duncan, D. F., & Kolbe, L. J. (1985). Avoiding Type III errors in health education program evaluations: A case study. *Health Education Quarterly, 12,* 315-331.

Benner, P., Tanner, C., & Chesla, C. (1992). From beginner to expert: Gaining a differentiated clinical world in critical care nursing. *Advances in Nursing Science, 14*(3), 13-28.

Blegen, M. A., & Mueller, C. W. (1987). Nurses' job satisfaction: A longitudinal analysis. *Research in Nursing and Health, 10,* 227-237.

Brooten, D., & Naylor, M. D. (1995). Nurses' effect on changing patient outcomes. *Image: The Journal of Nursing Scholarship, 27,* 95-99.

Carlson, A., & Rosenqvist, U. (1991). Diabetes care organization, process, and patient outcomes: Effects of a diabetes control program. *Diabetes Educator, 17,* 42-48.

Cassard, S. D., Weisman, C. S., Gordon, D. L., & Wong, R. (1994). The impact of unit-based self-management by nurses on patient outcomes. *Health Services Research, 29,* 415-433.

Chen, H. T. (1990). *Theory-driven evaluations.* Newbury Park, CA: Sage.

Crane, S. C. (1992). A research agenda for outcomes research. In *Patient outcomes research: Examining the effectiveness of nursing practice* (NIH Pub. No. 93-3411, pp. 54-62). Bethesda, MD: Department of Health and Human Services.

Dear, M. R., Weisman, C. S., Alexander, C. S., & Chase, G. A. (1982). The effect of intensive care nursing on job satisfaction and turnover. *Heart and Lung, 11,* 560-565.

Dienemann, J., & Gessner, T. (1992). Restructuring nursing care delivery systems. *Nursing Economics, 10,* 253-258.

Duxbury, M. L., & Thiessen, V. (1979). Staff nurse turnover in neonatal intensive care units. *Journal of Advanced Nursing, 4,* 591-602.

Fitzgerald, J., Freund, D. A., Hughett, B., & McHugh, G. J. (1993). Influence of organizational components on delivery of asthma care. *Medical Care, 31*(3 Suppl.), MS61-MS73.

Flood, A., Scott, W. R., & Ewy, W. (1984a). Does practice make perfect? Part I: The relation between hospital volume and outcomes for selected diagnostic categories. *Medical Care, 22,* 98-114.

Flood, A., Scott, W. R., & Ewy, W. (1984b). Does practice make perfect? Part II: The relation between hospital volume and outcomes and other hospital characteristics. *Medical Care, 22,* 115-124.

Flood, A. B., & Scott, W. R. (1987). *Hospital structure and performance.* Baltimore: Johns Hopkins University Press.

Fowler, F. J., Cleary, P. D., Magaziner, J., Patrick, D. L., & Benjamin, K. L. (1994). Methodological issues in measuring patient care outcomes: The agenda of the work group on outcomes. *Medical Care, 32*(7 Suppl.), JS65-JS76.

Frederickson, K. (1991). Nursing theories—a basis for differentiated practice: Application of the Roy adaptation model in nursing practice. In I. E. Goertzen (Ed.), *Differentiating nursing practice: Into the twenty-first century* (pp. 41-44). Kansas City, MO: American Academy of Nursing.

Hartz, A. J., Krakauer, H., Kuhn, E. M., Young, M., Jacobsen, S. J., Gay, G., Muenz, L., Katzoff, M., Bailey, C., & Rimm, A. A.

(1989). Hospital characteristics and mortality rate. *New England Journal of Medicine, 321,* 1720-1725.

Hegyvary, S. T. (1991). Issues in outcomes research. *Journal of Nursing Quality Assurance, 5*(2), 1-6.

Hegyvary, S. T. (1992). Outcomes research: Integrating nursing practice into the world view. In *Patient outcomes research: Examining the effectiveness of nursing practice* (NIH Pub. No. 93-3411, pp. 17-24). Bethesda, MD: Department of Health and Human Services.

Hinshaw, A. S., & Atwood, J. R. (1983). Nursing turnover, stress and satisfaction: Models, measures and management. *Annual Review of Nursing Research, 1,* 133-153.

Hinshaw, A. S., Smeltzer, C. H., & Atwood, J. R. (1987). Innovative retention strategies for nursing staff. *Journal of Nursing Administration, 17*(16), 8-16.

Ingersoll, G. L. (1996). Organizational redesign: Effect on institutional and consumer outcomes. In J. Fitzpatrick & J. Norbeck (Eds.), *Annual review of nursing research* (pp. 121-143). New York: Springer.

Irvine, D. M., & Evans, M. G. (1995). Job satisfaction and turnover among nurses: Integrating research findings across studies. *Nursing Research, 44,* 246-252.

Isenberg, M. A. (1991). Insights from Orem's nursing theory on differentiating nursing practice. In I. E. Goertzen (Ed.), *Differentiating nursing practice: Into the twenty-first century* (pp. 45-49). Kansas City, MO: American Academy of Nursing.

Jelinek, R. C. (1967). A structural model for the patient care operation. *Health Services Research, 2,* 226-242.

Jones, K. R. (1993). Outcomes analysis: Methods and issues. *Nursing Economics, 11,* 145-152.

Kahn, K. L., Rogers, W. H., Rubenstein, L. V., Sherwood, M. J., Reinisch, E. J., Keeler, E. B., Draper, D., Kosecoff, J., & Brook, R. H. (1990). Measuring quality of care with explicit process criteria before and after implementation of the DRG-based prospective payment system. *Journal of the American Medical Association, 264,* 969-1973.

Keeler, E. B., Rubenstein, L. V., Kahn, K. L., Draper, D., Harrison, E. R., McGinty, M. J., Rogers, W. H., & Brook, R. H. (1992). Hospital characteristics and quality of care. *Journal of the American Medical Association, 268,* 1709-1714.

Knaus, W. A., Draper, E. A., Wagner, D. P., & Zimmerman, J. E. (1986). An evaluation of outcome from intensive care in major medical centers. *Annals of Internal Medicine, 104,* 410-418.

Koerner, B. L., Cohen, J. R., & Armstrong, D. M. (1985). Collaborative practice and patient satisfaction. *Evaluation & the Health Professions, 8,* 299-321.

Krakauer, H., Bailey, R., Skellan, K., Stewart, J., Hartz, A., Kuhn, E., & Rimm, A. (1992). Evaluation of the HCFA model for the analysis of mortality following hospitalization. *Health Services Research, 27,* 317-335.

McKenzie, C. B., Torkelson, N. G., & Holt, M. A. (1989). Care and cost: Nursing case management improves both. *Nursing Management, 20*(10), 30-34.

Mitchell, G. J. (1991). Distinguishing practice with Parse's theory. In I. E. Goertzen (Ed.), *Differentiating nursing practice: Into the twenty-first century* (pp. 55-58). Kansas City, MO: American Academy of Nursing.

Mitchell, P. H. (1995). The significance of treatment effects: Significance for whom? *Medical Care, 33*(4 Suppl.), AS280-AS285.

Mitchell, P. H., Armstrong, S., Simpson, T. F., & Lentz, M. (1989). American Association of Critical-Care Nursing demonstration project: Profile of excellence in critical care nursing. *Heart and Lung, 18,* 219-237.

Mitchell, P. H., Shannon, S. E., Cain, K., & Hegyvary, S. T. (1996). Critical care outcomes: Linking structures, processes, organizational and clinical outcomes. *American Journal of Critical Care, 5,* 353-363.

Navarro, M. (1995, April 14). Confidence shaken, hospital tries to bounce back after series of errors. *New York Times,* p. A6.

Newman, M. A. (1990). Toward an integrative model of professional practice. *Journal of Professional Nursing, 6,* 167-173.

Olds, D. L., & Kitzman, H. (1990). Can home visitation improve the health of women and children at environmental risk? *Pediatrics, 86,* 108-116.

Packard, J. S., & Motowildo, S. J. (1987). Subjective stress, job satisfaction and job performance of hospital nurses. *Research in Nursing and Health, 10,* 253-261.

Parse, R. R. (1991). Parse's theory of human becoming. In I. E. Goertzen (Ed.), *Differentiating nursing practice: Into the twenty-first century* (pp. 51-53). Kansas City, MO: American Academy of Nursing.

Price, J. L., & Mueller, C. W. (1981). A causal model of turnover for nurses. *Academy of Management Journal, 24,* 543-565.

Rabiner, D. J., Stearns, S. C., & Mutran, E. (1994). The effect of channeling on in-home utilization and subsequent nursing home care: A simultaneous equation perspective. *Health Services Research, 29,* 605-622.

Rosenthal, G. E., Halloran, E. J., Kiley, M., Pinkley, C., Landefeld, S., & the nurses of University Hospital of Cleveland. (1992). Development and validation of the Nursing Severity Index: A new method for measuring severity of illness using nursing diagnosis. *Medical Care, 30,* 1127-1141.

Rothman, M. L, Hedrick, S. C., Bulcroft, K. A., Erdly, W. W., & Nickinovich, D. G. (1993). Effects of VA adult day health care on health outcomes and satisfaction with care. *Medical Care, 31*(Suppl.), SS38-SS49.

Roy, C. (1991). Structure of knowledge: Paradigm, model, and research specifications for differentiated practice. In I. E. Goertzen (Ed.), *Differentiating nursing practice: Into the twenty-first century* (pp. 31-39). Kansas City, MO: American Academy of Nursing.

Rubenstein, L. V., Chang, B. L., Keeler, E. B., & Kahn, K. L. (1992). Measuring the quality of nursing surveillance activities for five diseases before and after implementation of the DRG-based prospective payment system. In *Patient outcomes research: Examining the effectiveness of nursing practice* (NIH Pub. No. 93-3411, pp. 39-53). Bethesda, MD: Department of Health and Human Services.

Rubenstein, L. V., Kahn, K. L., Reinisch, E. J., Sherwood, M. J., Rogers, W. H., Kamberg, C., Draper, D., & Brook, R. H. (1990). Changes in quality of care for five diseases measured by implicit review 1981 to 1986. *Journal of the American Medical Association, 264,* 1974-1979.

Schmitt, M. H., Farrel, M. P., & Heinemann, G. D. (1988). Conceptual and methodological problems in studying the effects of interdisciplinary geriatric teams. *The Gerontologist, 28,* 753-764.

Sharp, D. (1995, April 14-16). Error-ridden hospital loses accreditation. *USA Today,* pp. 1A, 3A.

Shaugnessy, P. W., Schlenker, R. C., & Kramer, A. M. (1990). Quality of long-term care in nursing homes and swing bed hospitals. *Health Services Research, 25,* 65-96.

Shortell, S. M., & Hughes, E.F.X. (1988). The effects of regulation, competition, and ownership on mortality rates among hospital inpatients. *New England Journal of Medicine, 318,* 1100-1107.

Shortell, S. M., O'Brien, J. L., Carman, J. M., Foster, R. W., Hughes, E.F.X., Boerstler, H., & O'Connor, E. J. (1995). Assessing the impact of continuous quality improvement/total quality management: Concept versus implementation. *Health Services Research, 30,* 377-401.

Shortell, S. M., Zimmerman, J. E., Rousseau, D. M., Gillies, R. R., Wagner, D. P., Draper, E. A., Knaus, W. A., & Duffy, J. (1994). The performance of intensive care units: Does good management make a difference? *Medical Care, 32,* 508-525.

Taunton, R. L., Kleinbeck, S. V., Stafford, R., Woods, C. Q., & Bott, M. J. (1994). Patient outcomes: Are they linked to registered nurse absenteeism, separation or work load? *Journal of Nursing Administration, 24*(Suppl.), 48-55.

Verran, J. A. (1996). Quality of care, organizational variables, and nurse staffing. In G. S. Wunderlich, F. A. Sloan, & C. K. Davies (Eds)., *Nursing staff in hospitals and nursing homes: Is it adequate?* (pp. 308-322). Washington, DC: National Academy Press.

Verran, J. A., & Mark, B. (1992). Contextual factors influencing patient outcomes individual/group/environment: Interactions and clinical practice interface. In *Patient outcomes research: Examining the effectiveness of nursing practice* (NIH Pub. No. 93-3411, pp. 121-142). Bethesda, MD: Department of Health and Human Services.

Weisman, C. S. (1981). Determinants of hospital nurse staff turnover. *Medical Care, 19,* 431-443.

Weisman, C. S. (1992). Nursing practice models: Research on patient outcomes. In *Patient outcomes research: Examining the effectiveness of nursing practice* (NIH Pub. No. 93-3411, pp. 112-120). Bethesda, MD: Department of Health and Human Services.

34

TRANSITIONAL ENVIRONMENTS

Dorothy Brooten
Mary Duffin Naylor

The science supporting environments that provide transitional care and that optimize outcomes is sparse and relatively recent. Although some empirical data are available, much of the reported literature is anecdotal, descriptive, and lacks reported outcomes. This chapter (a) defines transitional environments and the research issues that have arisen in the literature on transitional care, (b) describes the major current and emerging models of transitional care reported in the literature, and (c) summarizes gaps in the current science in this area and offers recommendations for future research.

Definitions and Issues

Transitional Environments

Transitional environments are those environments in which a transitional care service is provided. These services, however, are defined and implemented differently. Transition implies an in-between period. Therefore, the nature of transitional services is that they are not long-term services but temporary short-term services, which are different from long-term home care. Most commonly, transitional care refers to care and services required in the safe and timely transfer of patients from one level of care to another (e.g., acute to subacute), or from one type of health care setting to another (e.g., hospital to home) (Brooten, 1993). Therefore, transitional care environments may include the hospital, home, nursing home, rehabilitation center, home care agency, and hospice. Some authors differentiate subacute care from transitional care (Micheletti & Shlala, 1995; Robinson, Mead, & Boswell, 1995; Stahl, 1994); others use the terms interchangeably (Ellis & Mendlen, 1995; Heller & Walton, 1995; Hyatt, 1995). Those who do differentiate view subacute care as a unit or component of inpatient care in an acute care hospital, skilled nursing facility, or freestanding medical or rehabilitation center. Transitional services ideally end with normal functioning and recovery, functional independence, or stabilization of the patient's condition (Brooten, 1993).

Transitional services have increased exponentially over the past 15 years in response to changes in the delivery of health care services, mainly the shortening of hospital length of stay and the increase in acuity levels of patients cared for in sites outside hospitals. One indicator of the growth of transitional care services is the increase in the number of home care agencies from approximately 1,100 in 1963 to 17,561 in 1995 (National Association for Home Care [NAHC], 1995). In examining transitional care services that optimize patient outcomes, current issues affecting research include determining the nature and needed length of the service, the profile of patients who require the service, the type and level of providers needed, and costs for the services.

Determining the Nature and Needed Length of the Services

Features of transitional care include discharge planning from one site of care to another, coordination of postdischarge services needed in the new site of care, provision of in-home services on a short-term basis, and continued health care follow-up. The most important features of transitional services are continuity of care across sites of care, communication of the plan of care among the differing providers, and matching patient needs and the knowledge and skills of the care providers (Brooten, 1993).

Transitional care services most often begin with discharge planning from an acute care setting. Discharge planning should begin on the day of the patient's admission. This is essential in this time of very short hospital stays and increased patient acuity, for only then can services be projected and referrals made (Morrow-Howell & Proctor, 1994; Naylor, 1993; Prescott, Soeken, & Griggs, 1995). However, this appears to be an ideal. Currently, discharge planning is fragmented (Haddock, 1991; Prescott et al., 1995; Roe-Prior, Watts, & Burke, 1994). Often, discharge planning is conducted using protocols developed for use across all patient groups, with little or no modification to meet the needs of specific patient groups (Naylor, 1993). In addition, there is institutional variability in the criteria used to determine which patients receive more than cursory discharge planning and follow-up services (Prescott et al., 1995; Winograd, 1990). There is also institutional variability in the preparation and expertise of the persons conducting the discharge planning (Anderson & Helms, 1993; Findeis, 1994; Naylor, 1990; Prescott et al., 1995; Roe-Prior et al., 1994; Winograd, 1990). One panel of experts in the care of the elderly, for example, rated the quality of current planning for care after discharge as very poor. A study of over 900 Medicare-certified hospitals revealed that only 9% of elderly patients were discharged with plans for further care, and of that 9%, only half actually received the care (U.S. General Accounting Office [GAO], 1987).

The length of the transitional service should vary with the specific needs of the patient or group of patients. Currently, however, data are not available indicating the most effective and cost-efficient endpoint for receipt of these services with specific patient groups or subgroups. In today's era of health care cost containment, transitional services end with as much home care or service as is reimbursable.

Determining Which Patients Require Transitional Care Services

There is general agreement (nonempirically based) that vulnerable groups such as the elderly, the technologically dependent, the disabled, and some high-risk infants and children should receive transitional services (Berk & Berstein, 1985). Yet, as many researchers have noted, not everyone within these groups may need the full complement of services or services over the same length of time or with the same level and type of provider (Brooten, 1993; Patterson, Leonard, & Titus, 1992).

Research providing early hospital discharge and advanced practice nurse (APN) transitional services to women with unplanned cesarean births demonstrated that women who experienced infections required an average of 40 more minutes during home visits and 20 more minutes during hospitalization than women without infections. However, many women without infections also consumed much APN time during home visits and during telephone follow-up. This time was used teaching infant care and parenting and making referrals to community resources (Brooten, Knapp, et al., 1996).

Data to date suggest that not all hospitalized elderly are at risk for poor postdischarge outcomes. Many elderly and their families who receive effective preparation while in the hospital do quite well after discharge and do not require transitional care services. Naylor (1990) and Neidlinger, Scroggins, and Kennedy (1987) have demonstrated this. Research findings have helped to identify those patients who will require transitional care services. The group includes elderly with major mental and functional deficits, those without people who are able or willing to help them, and those with complex medical problems (Naylor, 1993).

Currently, decisions regarding which patients should receive transitional services are based on the patient's functional ability, available caretakers at home, ethnicity, geography, age, sociodemographics, previous hospitalizations, and technology dependence (Bakewell-Sachs & Porth, 1995; Corrigan & Martin, 1992; Gilmartin, 1994; Helberg, 1994; Prescott et al., 1995). The decision that a patient is in need of discharge planning and follow-up services is often based on a patient's ability to perform activities of daily living (Branch et al., 1988; Cox et al., 1990; Helberg, 1994; Kemper, 1992). There is, however, no uniform method used to evaluate a patient's functional ability during hospitalization.

Reed, Pearlman, and Buchner (1991) reported that the only two measures of functional ability consistently recorded on the medical record were ability to ambulate and orientation. In their study of 737 elderly discharged from 15 Illinois hospitals, Jones, Densen, and Brown (1989) found that 63% of elders with an identified deficit in one or more activity of daily living at the time of hospital discharge did not receive a referral for home services, and of these patients, 60% reported that no one at the hospital had asked them how they would be able to manage postdischarge. Prescott et al. (1995) reported that hospital personnel were fairly adept at identifying the most impaired patients in need of postdischarge services. However, clinicians failed to identify a subgroup of patients in need of transitional services who had less severe functional impairment but a greater number of diagnoses. Clearly, functional ability, although predictive of a patient's need for transitional services, should not be the only criterion used to make that determination.

Presence or absence of a family member, assumed to provide caretaking, is also often used to determine who receives transitional follow-up services. Living with someone frequently excludes the patient from receiving essential posthospital services. Furstenberg and Mezey's (1987) study, for example, reported that 94% of patients who lived alone were visited by a discharge planner, but only 40% of those who lived with someone else received a similar visit. One of the patients not visited was an 89-year-old woman who accurately reported that she lived with someone—her 91- and 93-year-old sisters, who clearly were not capable of providing her with postdischarge care.

Length of acute care stay may also determine who receives transitional services. Shorter lengths of acute care stays may result in staff having insufficient time to identify patients who would benefit from transitional services (Magilvy & Lakomy, 1991). Shorter acute care stays may also prevent staff from adequately preparing both the patient and family for postdischarge treatment. Several investigators have suggested links between readmissions to acute care hospitals with lack of adherence to therapeutic regimes due to inadequate patient education prior to discharge (Ghali, Kadakia, Cooper, & Ferlinz, 1988; Vinson, Rich, Sperry, Shah, & McNamara, 1990). Even when discharge teaching has been provided, patients may be too anxious to absorb the information or the quantity of information too overwhelming to absorb at one time (O'Brien & McCluskey-Fawcett, 1993). Ethnicity also had been a factor in who received what type of transitional services. Falcone, Bolda, and Leak (1991) reported that elderly Black patients were more likely to face a delay in hospital-to-nursing-home placement than White patients, even after controlling for the complexity of care required and the type of insurance coverage. The researchers suggest that the delay may be attributable to nursing home policies of "race matching" elders in semi-private rooms, in violation of anti-discrimination laws. Mui and Burnette (1994) reported that there were ethnic differences related to the use of in-home, community-based, and nursing home services. They found that White elders were more likely than African-Americans or Hispanics to use in-home and nursing home services. In contrast, African-Americans and Hispanics were more likely to rely on informal support networks and community-based services. Kemper (1992) found race to be the only important sociodemographic factor to have a large effect on the amount or type of home care used. African-Americans and Hispanics were more likely than White patients to depend on informal care, both resident and visiting, to meet home care needs. These ethnic differences in the use of transitional care services may reflect variations in acceptability of the services, awareness of availability of the services, and differences in accessibility for economic or geographic reasons.

As with other health care services, communication among providers of the service is an important factor in who receives adequate transitional services. A study evaluating the adequacy of the communication between a hospital's discharge planners and home health agencies found that patient records contained only slightly more than half the information deemed necessary to ensure continuity of patient care (Anderson & Helms, 1993). Significantly more patient data were communicated to the receiving agency when patient information was collected by a liaison nurse employed by the home care agency. The results of the study indicate that even when discharge planning occurs, essential information may not be relayed to the providers of the next level of service and may have a negative effect on patient outcomes. Similar findings have been reported by others (Harrington, Lynch, & Newcomer, 1993; Hazlett, 1989; Meara, Wood, Wilson, & Hart, 1992; Patterson et al., 1992; Williams, Greenwell, & Groom, 1992).

The type of health institution, insurer, and the patient's distance from care sites also influence which patients receive transitional care. In a national study designed to document the types and quantity of transitional care provided by psychiatric hospitals, Dorwart and Hoover (1994) reported that the provision of transitional care was inadequate and uneven. Urban psychiatric hospitals with residency programs were more likely than general hospitals to provide aftercare services and to use case management to ensure continuity of care. Others report that even when a service is available locally, insurers may dictate that care be received at a distant site and restrict access to certain providers and services (Fox, Wicks, & Newacheck, 1993; Harrington et al., 1993).

Determining Type and Level of Providers of Transitional Care

The providers of transitional care are as varied as the programs and services (Brooten, 1993; Schwartz, Blumenfield, & Perlman Simon, 1990), and there is disagreement in who should provide the care (Kornowski, 1995; Rich, 1995; Roselle & D'Amico, 1990). The work of Brooten (Brooten, Knapp, et al., 1994; Brooten, Kumar, et al., 1986; Brooten, Naylor, et al., 1995), Naylor (1994), and others (Thurber & DiGiamarino, 1992; York

et al., in press) using APNs to provide transitional care for high-risk groups has consistently demonstrated improved patient outcomes with reduced health care costs for the patient groups followed. Nurses specialize at the master's level; thus, use of a master's-prepared nurse specialist assumes that this nurse has advanced knowledge and skill in the care of the specific patient groups followed, an assumption that cannot be made of a nurse generalist. Using a master's-prepared nurse also avoids the great variability in preparation (Diploma, AND, BSN) of the nurse generalist. Master's-prepared nurse specialists with advanced knowledge and skills can function under general protocols needing less-detailed procedures, protocols, and direct supervision than do personnel with less preparation. Finally, the average annual salaries nationally of master's-prepared nurses in nonadministrative roles is only approximately $5,500 higher than that of a registered nurse (American Nurses Association, 1994). When this cost is divided among patients followed, the added cost is negligible. Whether master's-prepared nurse specialists are needed for all patient populations has yet to be tested (Brooten, Naylor, et al., 1995).

Patterson et al. (1992) reported that home care provided by professional nurses decreased the negative psychosocial impact on parents caring for medically fragile children at home, especially as the number of nursing hours increased. In this study, care by a home health aide was associated with a greater negative psychosocial impact on the family. Improved patient outcomes from home care provided by RNs has also been reported by Hazlett (1989) with ventilator-dependent children, by McCorkle (1994) and colleagues with oncology patients, and by Bull (1994) with elders.

Many authors (Katz, 1993; Landefeld, Palmer, Kresevic, Fortinsky, & Kowal, 1995; Rich, 1995; Sivak, Cordasco, & Gipson, 1983; Wong, 1991) have advocated a multidisciplinary model to implement discharge planning and assure the successful transition of patients from one level of care to another. However, this model is not routinely used in most institutions due to cost. Staff providing transitional care range from individuals with little health care training to master's-prepared nurses and include a variety of providers who offer specialized services such as respiratory therapy, physical therapy, occupational therapy, and social work. Transitional care is most successful using a multidisciplinary approach from the hospital to the many community agencies and resources needed by the patient and family. However, some member of the multidisciplinary team must coordinate the care.

Determining Costs for Transitional Care Services

Managed care and capitated reimbursement have changed the system of care delivery, the focus of care, and the window for examining patient outcomes and costs. Examining cost and outcome in one setting (e.g., hospital or home) provides one snapshot but fails to capture outcome and cost over a period of transitional care or over a period of insured care. In addition, cost and outcome data focused on one site of care fail to capture cumulative effects of system changes, such as those resulting from shortened hospital stay, on cost and outcomes in other sites of care or on the family unit. The issues in collecting valid and meaningful cost data across sites of care include what costs can be collected, whether they can be collected across all sites of care, and who is responsible for absorbing these costs.

What Costs Can Be Collected

Estimation of true costs of health care resources consumed in transitional care is problematic, and there are no perfect solutions. In some studies, charges are used as reasonably good proxies for resource costs. However, the health care market suffers from severe distortions, such that charges for services often have little relationship to resource costs. Various mechanisms have been used in studies to improve the validity of estimates of health care resource costs, including cost-to-charge ratios (subject to accounting artifacts and problems of aggregation), time and motion studies (limited by high cost of collecting information, sampling error, and generalizability of results), and costs estimates derived from managed care payments, which often consider only payer's costs.

A major issue in attempting to cost out transitional care is what should be included in calculating the cost and whether the investigators were able to cost out all the factors that should be included. Items commonly included in calculating costs include personnel time (salary and benefits), administrative costs, supplies, and indirect costs (space, heat, light). Costs for personnel time are often measured based on actual or average salary and fringe benefits for the personnel plus time involved for the task. This approach may work well when single personnel can be identified with tasks or similar types and levels of patient need. However, when a number of types and levels of staff are involved, such as in transitional care, cost allocation and association with specific outcomes becomes more difficult.

Charge data have been commonly used in studies as a proxy for the costs of hospital and physician care (Carey, 1996). Charges for hospitalization and physician services are obtained from patient bills acquired either through the hospital or agency or from patients themselves. In today's cost-cutting environment, however, many hospitals and agencies have become very resistant to providing patient bills, making the cost estimates for comparing types of transitional services difficult. Although charges are not the same as costs, they can serve as a reasonable proxy. Use of charge information is adequate to uncover *relative* changes in cost-in studies. Given the use of sensitivity analysis, this approach can provide adequate information to generate useful comparisons of study results.

The limitations of using charges as a proxy for costs should be acknowledged in studies on transitional care that use this method. Charges include both fixed and variable costs. Fixed costs may not fall as output is reduced. Furthermore, methods of cost allocation may fail to accurately assign costs to patients who were responsible for the consumption of specific resources.

Microcosting, a method considered superior to the use of charge information, has been used in few studies comparing transitional services. In this approach, specific data collection is undertaken for every element of resource consumed. Microcosting has been successfully employed in clinical situations that are very narrow and limited in scope, such as the study of the administration of one particular drug, but it is less feasible for studies that include costs of an entire hospital stay. The many aspects of cost to be evaluated, given most existing hospital cost-accounting systems and the resources required to perform such studies, make them prohibitive.

Resource units or health service resource use is another approach used to measure costs in studies of transitional care services. Here, all major health care resources consumed are collected and the various resource units converted to estimates of costs (Horn, Sharkey, Tracy, Horn, James, & Goodwin, 1996). Resources consumed include numbers of hospitalizations (length of stay and unit within the hospital), physician services, nursing services, allied professional services, ancillary services, postdischarge nursing, and vendor services. Costs are then summarized overall and by type of service and component. This approach allows evaluation of the impact of an intervention—for example, on total costs—and provides insight into how and where cost savings may be achieved.

Allowable insurer's costs (the allowable cost upon which payments by both insurer and patient are calculated) are often then used as proxies for costs to convert resource use to estimates of costs. Allowable costs based on national providers (e.g., Medicare) provide an enhanced level of generalizability for comparing study results. In today's era of health care cost containment, comparisons of the most efficient and cost-effective transitional care services are especially difficult given the differences in cost-accounting methods available for researchers in documenting health care costs across sites of care.

Finally, any evaluation of cost in transitional care must include examination of the shift in cost burden from hospitals and insurers to patients and families. As length of hospital stay has decreased, costs for care normally incurred by hospitals have shifted to the family unit. Nonreimbursable costs for supplies as well as caregiver time and loss of employment and leisure time are cost issues that should be captured and compared. Documented costs of home care have included increased utility bills with ventilator-dependent children, insufficient funds for home care services, loss of employment, and increased physical illnesses of family caretakers (Hazlett, 1989; Sevick et al. 1992).

In summary, although the costs for transitional services are calculated in some studies, indirect costs, such as prevention of rehospitalization, acute care visits, decreased employment, and burden on family caregivers, are less well documented. These data are important in examining the overall cost benefit or cost-effectiveness of transitional services.

Current and Emerging Models of Transitional Care

Home Health Care

The fastest growing site of transitional care services is home health care. Currently, several types of agencies provide home services: public agencies, operated by the state or local government; private not-for-profit agencies, freestanding and privately operated; proprietary agencies, freestanding and operated for profit; hospital-based agencies; and dedicated units or departments operated by a hospital. In the past, public health agencies were the major providers of home care. Since the revision of the Medicare home payment law in 1987, hospital-based and proprietary agencies have supplanted public health agencies (NAHC, 1995) as the largest providers of this service.

Expansion in home care is also a result of cost-containment efforts to substitute home care for acute care stays. With fewer acute care beds occupied, hospitals have entered the home care field both to provide a safety net for their patients and as another source of revenue (Keenan & Fanale, 1989; Stahl, 1995b). Some authors note differences in the patient population and services provided based on the type of home care agency. Public agencies are more likely to serve Medicare patients or the indigent. Proprietary agencies are more likely to serve the relatively well-insured. Hospital-based agencies substitute home care for inpatient days (Williams, 1991).

Home Health Care From Community Nursing Services

Community or public health nurses have historically provided home follow-up to high-risk patients with complex health needs. Their services are well known and accepted by the general public and health care providers. Nurses working within the community are also familiar with community resources, health care needs, and the values and culture of the community residents. Unfortunately, over the past 10 to 15 years, budget reductions of community nursing services have virtually eliminated home follow-up services to many patient groups. Programs focused on prevention and well child care, for example, were curtailed to provide services to more acutely ill patients, mainly elders, now discharged home earlier and still recovering (Bull, 1994; NAHC, 1995). More recently, however, services for less stable, more acutely ill newborns and pregnant and newly delivered women have been added (NAHC, 1995).

Current challenges for community nursing services include updating the specialty knowledge and skills of agency nurses with a generalist preparation, maintaining continuity of patient care from the hospital to the home, and providing sufficient services to maintain good patient outcomes while insurers are reimbursing for fewer services (Brooten, 1995). To provide service to a more high-risk group of patients, agencies have been providing continuing education for their nurses, using master's-prepared clinical nurse specialists and nurse practitioners with advanced practice skills as consultants (Zelle, 1995) or, in agencies with sufficient caseloads, hiring advanced practice nurses to provide direct care in the home. Attempts to improve continuity of care to high-risk groups have included predischarge hospital visits to patients by a community nurse and having a community liaison nurse on site in the hospital (Dawson, 1994). Some agencies now provide 7-days-a-week, 24-hour-a-day nurse coverage and expanded use of ancillary personnel, including homemaker-home health aides.

Hospital Home Care Services and HMO Follow-Up Services

As reimbursed length of stay for even high-risk patients decreases, hospitals' need for improved discharge planning and postdischarge home care services for these groups increases. Documented discharge planning is mandatory for hospitals, and many have hired discharge planners to facilitate earlier discharge. Some hospitals contract with community nursing services or independent home care agencies to provide home care services for their high-risk patients. An increasing number of hospitals are establishing their own home care services. In some instances, this home care is provided by existing hospital nursing staff from units where bed occupancy has decreased, thus reducing the numbers of nursing staff needed on the units. As Dahlberg and Koloroutis (1994) note, one of the greatest advantages of a hospital-based program is the internal availability of knowledgeable and skilled nursing staff. Physicians are more likely to refer patients to a program that is staffed with nurses they know and trust from the hospital setting (Dahlberg & Koloroutis, 1994). In other hospitals, home care services are provided by a nursing staff hired and managed by the hospital's home care department (Brooten, 1995).

HMOs have a clear financial incentive for discharging patients early and for preventing costly rehospitalizations. They have used case managers and nurses with specialty knowledge and skills to review patients' discharge and home care needs. Because realizing a profit is essential, the HMO approach has been one of minimal hospital length of stay and postdischarge services. Home follow-up services vary in number of visits provided, type of nurse provider (nurse generalist or specialist), and length of follow-up. More than the routine allowable number of home visits may be reimbursable for a patient, but this must be negotiated between provider and insurer.

Entrepreneurial Services

Over the past decade, many entrepreneurial groups have established services to provide home care to patients (Eaton, 1994). Usually these groups are not involved in discharge planning but do provide home care services on a fee-for-service or contractual basis. Services provided may be determined by the company's medical advisory board or by the contracting agency and reviewed and approved by the company's medical advisory board. Nurses providing services may be full-time employees or temporary nursing staff who may or may not have specialty preparation and skills in caring for the patient groups they are following.

Research Models of Transitional Services

Quality cost model of APN transitional care. Responding to national trends in earlier hospital discharge of vulnerable patient groups, an interdisciplinary model of transitional care (comprehensive discharge planning and home follow-up) delivered by advanced practice nurse (APN) specialists was developed by Brooten and colleagues in 1981 (Brooten, Brown, et al., 1988; Brooten, Kumar, et al., 1986) and has undergone further testing and refinement over the past 16 years (Brooten, Roncoli, et al., 1994; Hollingsworth, Cohen, Finkler, Rubin, & Morgan, in review; Naylor et al., 1994; Thurber & DiGiamarino, 1992; York et al., in press). The model uses master's-prepared APNs (clinical nurse specialists and nurse practitioners), for reasons of both quality and cost.

The model was originally designed to discharge patients early from the hospital by replacing a portion of hospital care with a comprehensive program of transitional care delivered by advanced practice nurse (APN) specialists whose speciality preparation matched the patient groups they followed. Transitional care was defined as comprehensive discharge planning developed for each specific patient group plus home follow-up care through the period of normally expected recovery or stabilization (Brooten, Brown, et al., 1988).

Using the model, patients are discharged early provided they meet a standard set of discharge criteria agreed upon by the physician and nurse specialist. Criteria include physical, emotional, and informational patient readiness for discharge and an environment supportive of convalescence at home. The APN prepares the patient for discharge and coordinates discharge planning with the patient, physician, hospital nursing staff, and, where appropriate, social service staff, community resource groups, and equipment vendors. The APN also coordinates or does patient teaching, helps establish a timeframe for the day of discharge, coordinates plans for medical follow-up, and makes referrals to community agencies where needed.

Following discharge, the APN specialist conducts a series of home visits and is also frequently in touch with patients and their families by telephone. The number and timing of home visits varies with the patient group being followed. APNs were available to patients and families by telephone from 8 a.m. to 10 p.m. Monday through Fridays and from 8 a.m. to noon on Saturday and Sundays. After 10 p.m. on weekdays and after noon on weekends, patients were asked to call their private physician or hospital emergency room should immediate care be needed (Brooten, Brown, et al., 1988).

The APNs assess and monitor the physical, emotional, and functional status of the patient, provide direct care where needed, assist in obtaining services or other resources available in the community, and provide group-specific as well as individual teaching, counseling, and support during the period of convalescence. If complications arise, the nurse specialist consults with the backup physician for a plan of immediate and most effective treatment.

The model was designed to provide data on the quality of care as reflected in patient outcomes, cost of care, and thorough documentation of nursing functions. It was developed for use with any patient population, from frail infants to frail elders. It was designed to provide data on physical and psychosocial patient outcomes, including mortality, morbidity (e.g., rehospitalizations, emergency room visits, incidence of infection), return of patients to normal activities, patient satisfaction with care, and outcomes important to specific patient groups.

The model was also constructed to provide data on the cost of transitional follow-up care by APN specialists, as compared to routine care and discharge. Cost data include charges for initial hospitalization, rehospitalizations and physician services, and in the early discharge group, it includes the cost of the services of the APN specialist as well as time lost from employment by family members who assume care of the patient during the period of early discharge (Brooten, Brown, et al., 1988).

Using a randomized clinical trial, the model was originally tested with very low birth weight (VLBW) (< 1500 gms) infants (Brooten, Kumar, et al., 1986). One group was discharged earlier from the hospital and received the APN intervention; a second group received usual care and discharge. Both groups were followed for 18 months postdischarge. Study results demonstrated no significant differences in infant outcomes (rehospitalizations, acute care visits, infant growth and development) between groups; however, there were significant cost savings in the early-discharge group of over $18,000 per infant.

The model was next tested with three high-volume, high-risk, and/or high-cost groups of women. In a ran-

domized clinical trial, women with unplanned cesarean births were enrolled following birth and followed for 8 weeks postpartum. Study results demonstrated that women receiving the APN intervention were able to be discharged a mean of 30.3 hours earlier ($p < .001$), had significantly greater satisfaction with care, had a significantly greater number of infants immunized, had a 29% reduction in health care costs, and no maternal rehospitalizations (vs. 3 in the control group). No significant differences were found between groups in maternal affect, self-esteem, and overall functional status (Brooten, Roncoli, et al., 1994).

In a randomized clinical trial with pregnant women with diabetes (gestation and pregestational) during pregnancy, women were followed from diagnosis to 8 weeks postpartum. In the APN intervention group, there were significantly fewer rehospitalizations ($p < .05$), fewer LBW infants (8.3% vs. 29%), and 38% lower total hospital charges than the control group. No significant differences were found between groups in outcomes of affect, self-esteem, return to function, satisfaction with care, and infant immunization (York et al., in press).

In the randomized trial with women with abdominal hysterectomy, women were followed from surgery to 8 weeks postdischarge. In the APN intervention group, women were able to be discharged a mean of 12 hours earlier, were significantly more satisfied with their care, and had a savings in health care costs of 6%. The number of acute care visits and rehospitalizations was similar for both groups, but the mean rehospitalization charges for the control group were $2,153, compared to $609 for the APN-followed group (Hollingsworth et al., in review).

In a randomized clinical trial of elders with cardiac medical and surgical DRGs, Naylor and colleagues (1994) tested the comprehensive discharge planning portion of the model without the home visit component. The intervention consisted of comprehensive discharge planning conducted by the APNs, APN hospital visits, and 2-week APN telephone follow-up. Study results demonstrated that in the APN intervention group, readmissions were significantly reduced for subjects with medical DRGs in the first 6 weeks, and postdischarge rehospitalization charges were reduced 20.5%, compared to the control group during this same period. There were no statistically significant differences in other patient and family outcomes.

Ongoing work by Naylor and colleagues is testing the full model, incorporating the home visit component with elders with common medical and surgical DRGs who are at high risk for poor outcomes. Ongoing work by Brooten and colleagues focuses on women with medically and socioeconomically high-risk pregnancies. This effort substitutes half of prenatal care normally delivered in the clinic or physician's office with prenatal care delivered in the woman's home by APNs. Pilot work by Medoff-Cooper is testing the model with earlier discharge of smaller, more vulnerable infants than those involved in the original work.

Subacute Care Units

Another rapidly growing transitional care setting is the subacute care unit (Stahl, 1994, 1995a). These units are designed to meet the needs of medically stable patients who no longer require acute care services but whose needs for licensed skilled nursing care exceed the abilities of skilled nursing facilities or nursing homes (Micheletti & Shlala, 1995; Stahl, 1994; Walsh, 1995). Patients referred to subacute care units include those who are technology dependent, those who require frequent respiratory or physical therapy, and those with complex nursing needs.

To serve these patients, existing hospital beds are being converted to subacute beds, free-standing subacute care hospitals are being established, and skilled nursing facilities are adding subacute units (Ellis & Mendlen, 1995; Micheletti & Shlala, 1995). The incentive for the establishment of these units is economic. Care is provided in a less expensive setting, hospital beds are freed up for acutely ill patients, and unoccupied hospital beds are converted into a revenue source (Ellis & Mendlen, 1995; Stahl, 1994).

In-hospital subacute care units have been reported to improve patient outcomes for selected patient populations, including the elderly (Brymer et al., 1995; Landefield et al., 1995), ill infants and children (Goldson, 1981; Grebin & Kaplan, 1995), and ventilator-dependent individuals (Gilmartin, 1994; Gracey, et al., 1995; Make, 1986). The success of the units has been partially attributed to a multidisciplinary approach. Not all of these reports are research based.

The concept for subacute care units builds upon the experience of transitional or step-down units, which have existed in many institutions for years. Transitional units have long been established for previously acutely ill newborns, cardiac patients, and so on, who now need less acute hospital care (Goldson, 1981; Whitby, 1983a,

1983b). Many of these transitional units have also served as sites where family members are taught postdischarge care of patients and serve as a point of postdischarge contact for patients and family members with questions and concerns. These services can facilitate home management of patients rather than transfer to other institutional facilities (MacLeod & Head, 1994).

Integrated Health Care Systems

Managed care has fueled the formation of integrated health care delivery systems providing all levels of service delivery, from acute care to home care, skilled nursing facilities, nursing homes, outpatient clinics, durable medical suppliers, and subacute care units (Heller & Walton, 1995; Stahl, 1995b). These systems provide "one-stop shopping" for managed care organizations. Theoretically, integrated systems provide continuity of care for patients by having them remain within the same health care delivery system (Frasca, 1986; Stahl, 1995b). Such systems also have the potential to coordinate health services and to have good communication between care providers in the various settings. Currently, despite the use of case management and other coordination mechanisms, much fragmentation of care across systems remains (Fox, 1993; Harrington et al., 1993).

Robinson et al. (1995) discussed the efforts of one center to provide continuity of care in a vertically integrated system that included an acute care hospital, a subacute ward, a nursing home unit, domiciliary care, ambulatory care, and extended care programs including adult day health care. The hospital hired hospital-based APNs to coordinate and plan care between the various care settings. The APNs were also responsible for collaborating with community-based home care agencies and nursing homes to which the patients were transferred. Provider communication and consultation reportedly improved, resulting in less duplication of services by providers from different disciplines. Hospital admissions and lengths of stay also decreased.

Nurse Case Management

Case management by nurses to coordinate the delivery of care to patients across settings may be an effective method of reducing fragmentation and improving patient and cost of care outcomes. One model of nurse case management was developed at Carondelet St. Mary's Hospital and Health Center to assist high-risk elderly in managing their health care and to access needed services in a timely and effective manner (Lamb, 1992). The professional nurse case manager (PNCM) is at the "hub" of the Nursing Network, the integrated system of nursing care at Carondelet St. Mary's (Ethridge & Lamb, 1989). Network components include acute care inpatient services, extended care or long-term care services, home care services, hospice, and ambulatory care services. Nurse case managers work with clients across acute and chronic care settings as well as in the home (Lamb, 1992) and are responsible for facilitating patient movement through the components of the Nursing Network (Etheridge & Lamb, 1989).

Research conducted with Carondelet St. Mary's clients revealed that elders who worked with a nurse case manager had greater confidence in self-care, had improved symptom management, and had less frequent use of hospital and emergency department services (Lamb, 1992). Analysis of cost data revealed that nurse case management also resulted in decreased length of stay as compared with non-case managed patients (Etheridge & Lamb, 1989).

Gaps and Recommendations

As noted earlier, transitional environments are a relatively new dimension in the continuum of health care services. Consequently, the gaps in science to support this increasingly important component of care are considerable, and many have been identified throughout this chapter. Additional research is needed to determine the nature, intensity, and length of transitional services needed to optimize patient and family outcomes; the profile of patients who would benefit most from these services; and the type and level of providers needed to deliver these services and the costs of the services. Continued study of existing and emerging models of transitional care is also necessary to determine which of these models achieve the highest quality, most cost-effective outcomes.

To date, research findings suggest that the core components of transitional care for patients discharged from hospital to home are comprehensive discharge planning and home follow-up. Further, study findings suggest that, for selected patient groups (or subgroups), discharge planning and home care protocols designed to meet their unique needs are more effective than the general protocols designed for all patients currently used by many hospitals and home care agencies. Targeted protocols should be derived from empirical data regarding the unique needs of specific patient groups and their caregivers after hospital discharge. Transitional care protocols should be based on an empirical understanding of the nature of the patients' and caregivers' needs (e.g., lack of knowledge, complexity of therapeutic regimen), strengths (e.g., supportive family) and/or barriers (e.g., language) to meeting needs, timing of needs (e.g., 24 hours after discharge), most cost-effective strategy to meet needs (e.g., telephone contact vs. home visit), and length of follow-up needed. Unfortunately, for many patient groups, this research base is limited. For these patient groups, research efforts should be focused first on identifying patients' and caregivers' needs and subsequently on the design and testing of interventions to meet these unique needs.

Rigorous testing of transitional care protocols is needed not only to determine the efficacy of the protocols but also to determine which patient groups (or subgroups) will benefit the most from these services. As noted earlier, evidence to date suggests that not all patient groups (or subgroups) require transitional services to achieve stabilization and/or functional recovery. An important scientific gap is the profile of patients who are at high risk for poor outcomes and for whom transitional care is essential. What is the constellation of sociodemographic, clinical, and health care system factors that contribute to these poor outcomes? Equally important is the need to identify the profiles of patients who are at low risk for poor outcomes and do not require transitional care services. Researchers have only begun to address these knowledge gaps. The design and testing of profiles to assess the relative risk of patients for positive and negative outcomes following a major change in health status (e.g., pregnancy or an episode of illness) is essential to advance the knowledge base related to transitional care.

Transitional care has only recently been incorporated into the health care system, so it is not surprising that little research has been conducted on the issue of access to these services. As noted earlier, there is some evidence to suggest that level of awareness about services, race, culture, ethnicity, economics, and geography are among the factors that may influence use of such services. Research is needed to identify factors that promote access and serve as barriers to transitional care. The relatively rich information base on factors influencing access to primary care services should be used to advance this important component of the transitional care research agenda.

A number of approaches have emerged to guide the delivery of transitional care services. Only a few of these, however, are research models of transitional care. There is a need for additional testing of existing models of transitional care, with particular attention to their effectiveness in responding to continued pressures within the health care system to further decrease lengths of stay and prevent the use of more costly health services, such as hospitals. Further, there is a need for studies that compare and contrast existing and emerging models of transitional care focusing on differences in both processes and outcomes of care. Knowledge generated from studies of these models would contribute to the on-going discussion and debate about which providers are most effective and efficient in coordinating transitional care services and providing continuity of care for patients and their caregivers. Study findings would also advance our understanding about effective ways to engage a multidisciplinary team of providers in transitional services. Finally, the knowledge generated from this research would help inform the processes of care that available data suggest

are important to positive patient outcomes: assessing, communicating, clinical decision making, teaching, collaborating, referring, monitoring, and evaluating.

There are a number of methodological issues that need to be considered as part of the recommended research agenda for transitional care. For example, what outcomes are important to examine in measuring the effectiveness of transitional services, and when and for how long should they be measured? The methodological issues related to the measurement of costs were explored earlier in this chapter. Because of the nature and length of the service, transitional care provides a unique opportunity to examine the contributions of different providers (i.e., processes of care) to patient and family outcomes. Brooten and colleagues are taking advantage of this opportunity by examining the relationship between APN functions and patient outcomes in the delivery of transitional care services to five different patient groups.

In summary, transitional care is emerging as a critical component of the U.S. health care system. At this stage in its evolution, opportunities abound for significant research contributions spearheaded by nurse scholars in advancing the knowledge base related to the needs of patients and caregivers during this phase of care and in the design and testing of clinical interventions and models of care to optimize outcomes while decreasing costs of care. *Carpe Diem!*

References

Anderson, M. A., & Helms, L. (1993). An assessment of discharge planning models: Communication in referrals for home care. *Orthopedic Nursing, 12*(4), 41-49.

American Nurses Association. (1994). *Today's registered nurse: Numbers and demographics.* Washington, DC: Author.

Bakewell-Sachs, S., & Porth, S. (1995). Discharge planning and home care of the technology-dependent infant. *Journal of Obstetric, Gynecologic and Neonatal Nursing, 24*(1), 77-83.

Berk, M., & Bernstein, A. (1985). Home health services: Some findings from the national medical care expenditure survey. *Home Health Care Services Quarterly, 6,* 13-23.

Branch, L. G., Wetle, T. T., Scherr, P. A., Cook, N. R., Evans, D. A., Hebert, L. E., Masland, E. N., Keough, M. E., & Taylor, J. O. (1988). A prospective study of incident comprehensive medical home care use among the elderly. *American Journal of Public Health, 78*(3), 255-259.

Brooten, D. (1993). Assisting with transitions from hospital to home. In S. Funk, E. Tornquist, M. Champagne, & R. Wiese (Eds.), *Key aspects of caring for the chronically ill: Hospital and home.* New York: Springer.

Brooten, D. (1995). Perinatal care across the continuum: Early discharge and nursing home follow-up. *Journal of Perinatal and Neonatal Nursing, 9*(1), 38-44.

Brooten, D., Brown, L., Munro, B., York, R., Cohen, S., Roncoli, M., & Hollingsworth, A. (1988). Early discharge and specialist transitional care. *Image: The Journal of Nursing Scholarship, 20*(2), 64-68.

Brooten, D., Knapp, H., Borucki, L., Jacobsen, B., Finkler, S., Arnold, L., & Mennuti, M. (1996). Early discharge and home care after unplanned cesarean birth: Nursing care time. *Journal of Obstetric, Gynecologic and Neonatal Nursing, 25*(7), 595-600.

Brooten, D., Kumar, S., Brown, L., Butts, P., Finkler, S., Bakewell-Sachs, S., Gibbons, A., & Delivoria-Papadapoulos, M. (1986). A randomized clinical trial of early discharge and home follow-up of very low birth weight infants. *New England Journal of Medicine, 315,* 934-939.

Brooten, D., Naylor, M., York, R., Brown, L., Roncoli, M., Hollingsworth, A., Cohen, S., Arnold, L., Finkler, S., Munro, B., & Jacobsen, B. (1995). Effects of nurse specialist transitional care on patient outcomes and cost: Results of five randomized trials. *American Journal of Managed Care, 1*(1), 35-41.

Brooten, D., Roncoli, M., Finkler, S., Arnold, L., Cohen, A., & Mennuti, M. (1994). A randomized clinical trial of early hospital discharge and home follow-up of women having cesarean birth. *Obstetrics and Gynecology, 84,* 832-838.

Brymer, C. D., Kohm, C. A., Naglie, G., Shekter-Wolfson, L., Zorzitto, M. L., O'Rourke, K., & Kirkland, J. L. (1995). Do geriatric programs decrease long-term use of acute care beds? *Journal of the American Geriatrics Society, 43,* 885-889.

Bull, M. J. (1994). Use of formal community services by elders and their family care givers 2 weeks following hospital discharge. *Journal of Advanced Nursing, 19,* 503-508.

Carey, T. (1996). Outcomes and costs of care for acute low back pain among specialties: Implications for managed care. *American Journal of Managed Care, 11*(4), 409-413.

Corrigan, J. M., & Martin, J. B. (1992). Identification of factors associated with hospital readmission and development of a predictive model. *Health Services Research, 27*(1), 81-101.

Cox, C. L., Wood, J. E., Montgomery, A. C., & Smith, P. C. (1990). Patient classification in home health care: Are we ready? *Public Health Nursing, 7*(3), 130-137.

Dahlberg, N.L.F., & Koloroutis, M. (1994). Hospital-based perinatal home-care program. *Journal of Obstetric, Gynecologic and Neonatal Nursing, 23*(8), 682-686.

Dawson, B. (1994). "Special care" in the community: Role of the community neonatal liaison sister. *Professional Nurse, 10*(2), 78-80.

Dorwart, R. A., & Hoover, C. W. (1994). A national study of transitional hospital services in mental health. *American Journal of Public Health, 84*(8), 1229-1234.

Eaton, D. G. (1994). Perinatal home care: One entrepreneur's experience. *Journal of Obstetric, Gynecologic and Neonatal Nursing, 23*(8), 726-730.

Ellis, S., & Mendlen, J. (1995). Teaming up with hospitals. *Provider, 21*(3), 35-36.

Etheridge, P., & Lamb, G. S. (1989). Professional nursing case management improves quality, access and cost. *Nursing Management, 20*(3), 30-35.

Falcone, D., Bolda, E., & Leak, S. C. (1991). Waiting for placement: An exploratory analysis of determinants of delayed discharges of elderly hospital patients. *Health Services Research, 26*(3), 339-374.

Findeis, A., Larson, J. L., Gallo, A., & Shekleton, M. (1994). Caring for individuals using home ventilators: An appraisal by family care givers. *Rehabilitation Nursing, 19*(1), 6-11.

Fox, H. B., Wicks, L. B., & Newacheck, P. W. (1993). Health maintenance organizations and children with special needs. A suitable match? *American Journal of the Disabled Child, 147*(5), 546-552.

Frasca, C., & Christy, M. W. (1986). Assuring continuity of care through a hospital-based home health agency. *Quality Review Bulletin, 12*(5), 167-171.

Furstenberg, A., & Mezey, M. (1987). Mental impairment of elderly hospitalized hip fracture patients. *Comprehensive Gerontology, 1,* 80-86.

Ghali, J. K., Kadakia, S., Cooper, R., & Ferlinz, J. (1988). Precipitating factors leading to decompensation of heart failure: Traits among urban Blacks. *Archives of Internal Medicine, 148,* 2013-2016.

Gilmartin, M. (1994). Transition from the intensive care unit to home: Patient selection and discharge planning. *Respiratory Care, 10*(4), 456-480.

Goldson, E. (1981). The family care center: Transitional care for the sick infant and his family. *Children Today, 10*(4), 15-20.

Gracey, D. R., Naessens, J. M., Viggiano, R. W., Koenig, G. E., Silverstein, M. D., & Hubmayr, R. D. (1995). Outcome of patients cared for in a ventilator-dependent unit in a general hospital. *Chest: The Cardiopulmonary Journal, 107*(2), 494-499.

Grebin, B., & Kaplan, S. (1995). Toward a pediatric subacute care model: Clinical and administrative features. *Archives of Physical Medicine and Rehabilitation, 76*(12 Suppl.), SC16-SC20.

Haddock, K. S. (1991). Characteristics of effective discharge planning programs for the frail elderly. *Journal of Gerontological Nursing, 17*(7), 10-14.

Haffey, W. J., & Welsh, J. H. (1995). Subacute care: Evolution in search of value. *Archives of Physical Medicine and Rehabilitation, 76*(12 Suppl.), SC2-SC4.

Harrington, C., Lynch, M., & Newcomer, R. J. (1993). Medical services in social health maintenance organizations. *Gerontologist, 33*(6), 790-800.

Hazlett, D. E. (1989). A study of pediatric home ventilator management: Medical, psychosocial, and financial aspects. *Journal of Pediatric Nursing, 4*(4), 284-294.

Helberg, J. L. (1994). Use of home care nursing resources by the elderly. *Public Health Nursing, 11*(2), 104-112.

Heller, J. F., & Walton, J. R. (1995). The postacute link. *RT: The Journal for Respiratory Care Practitioners, 8*(1), 153-155.

Hollingsworth, A., Cohen, S., Finkler, S., Rubin, M., & Morgan, M. (in review). A randomized trial of early hospital discharge and home follow-up discharge and home follow-up of women having hysterectomy.

Hyatt, L. (1995). The feds focus on subacute. *Nursing Homes, 44*(1), 11.

Jones, E. W., Densen, P. M., & Brown, S. D. (1989). Posthospital needs of elderly people at home: Findings from an eight-month follow-up study. *Health Services Research, 24*(5), 643-664.

Katz, K. S. (1993). Project Headed Home: Intervention in the pediatric intensive care unit for infants and their families. *Infants and Young Children, 5*(3), 67-75.

Keenan, J. M., & Fanale, J. E. (1989). Home care: Past and present, problems and potential. *Journal of the American Geriatrics Society, 37,* 1076-1083.

Kemper, P. (1992). The use of formal and informal home care by the disabled elderly. *Health Services Research, 27*(4), 421-451.

Kornowski, R., Zeeli, D., Averbuch, M., Finkelstein, A., Schwartz, D., Moshkovitz, M., Weinreb, B., Hershkovitz, R., Eyal, D., Miller, M., Levo, Y., & Pines, A. (1995). Intensive home-care surveillance prevents hospitalization and improves morbidity rates among elderly patients with severe congestive heart failure. *American Heart Journal, 129*(4), 762-766.

Lamb, G. S. (1992). Conceptual and methodological issues in nurse case management research. *Advances in Nursing Science, 15*(2), 16-24.

Landefeld, C. S., Palmer, R. M., Kresevic, D. M., Fortinsky, R. H., & Kowal, J. (1995). A randomized trial of care in a hospital medical unit especially designed to improve the functional outcomes of acutely ill older patients. *New England Journal of Medicine, 332*(20), 1338-1344.

MacLeod, F., & Head, D. (1994). Transitional care: Filling the gap for older patients. *Leadership in Health Services, 3*(6), 28-32.

Magilvy, J. K., & Lakomy, J. M. (1991). Transitions of older adults to home care. *Home Health Care Services Quarterly, 12*(4), 59-70.

Make, B. J. (1986). Long-term management of ventilator-assisted individuals: The Boston University experience. *Respiratory Care, 31*(4), 303-310.

McCorkle, R., Jepson, C., Malone, D., Lusk, E., Braitman, L., Buhler-Wilkerson, K., & Daly, J. (1994). The impact of posthospital home care on patients with cancer. *Research in Nursing and Health, 17,* 243-251.

Meara, J. R, Wood, J. L., Wilson, M. A., & Hart, M. C. (1992). Home from hospital: A survey of hospital discharge arrangements in Northamptonshire. *Journal of Public Health Medicine, 14*(2), 145-150.

Micheletti, J. A., & Shlala, T. J. (1995). Understanding and operationalizing subacute services. *Nursing Management, 26*(6), 49, 51-52, 54-56.

Morrow-Howell, N., & Proctor, E. (1994). Discharge destinations of Medicare patients receiving discharge planning: Who goes where? *Medical Care, 32*(5), 486-497.

Mui, A. C., & Burnette, D. (1994). Long-term care service use by frail elders: Is ethnicity a factor? *The Gerontologist, 34*(2), 190-198.

National Association for Home Care. (1995). *Basic statistics about home care 1995*. Washington, DC: Author.

Naylor, M. (1990). Comprehensive discharge planning for hospitalized elderly: A pilot study. *Nursing Research, 39*(3), 156-160.

Naylor, M., & Brooten, D. (1993). The roles and functions of clinical nurse specialists: State of the science. *Image: The Journal of Nursing Scholarship, 25*(2), 99-104.

Naylor, M., Brooten, D., Jones, R., Lavizzo-Mourey, R., Mezey, M., & Pauly, M. (1994). Comprehensive discharge planning for hospitalized elderly: A randomized clinical trial. *Annals of Internal Medicine, 120*(12), 999-1006.

Neidlinger, S. H., Scroggins, K., & Kennedy, L. M. (1987). Cost-evaluation of discharge planning for hospitalized elderly: The efficacy of a clinical nurse specialist. *Nursing Economics, 5*(5), 225-230.

Patterson, J. M., Leonard, B. J., & Titus, J. C. (1992). Home care for medically fragile children: Impact on family health and well-being. *Developmental and Behavioral Pediatrics, 13*(4), 248-255.

Prescott, P. A., Soeken, K. L., & Griggs, M. (1995). Identification and referral of hospitalized patients in need of home care. *Research in Nursing and Health, 18*, 85-95.

Reed, R. L., Pearlman, R. A., & Buchner, D. M. (1991). Risk factors for early unplanned hospital readmission in the elderly. *Journal of General Internal Medicine, 6*, 223-228.

Rich, M. W., Beckham, V., Wittenberg, C., Leven, C. L., Freedland, K. E., & Carney, R. M. (1995). A multidisciplinary intervention to prevent the readmission of elderly patients with congestive heart failure. *New England Journal of Medicine, 333*(18), 1190-1195.

Robinson, D. K., Mead, M. J., & Boswell, C. R. (1995). Inside looking out: Innovations in community health nursing. *Clinical Nurse Specialist, 9*(4), 227-229, 235.

Roe-Prior, P., Watts, R. J., & Burke, K. (1994). Critical care clinical specialist in home health care: Survey results. *Clinical Nurse Specialist, 8*(1), 35-40.

Roselle, S., & D'Amico, F. J. (1990). The effect of home respiratory therapy on hospital readmission rates of patients with chronic obstructive pulmonary disease. *Respiratory Care, 35*(12), 1208-1213.

Schwartz, P., Blumenfield, S., & Perlman Simon, E. (1990). The interim home care program: An innovative discharge planning alternative. *Health and Social Work, 15*, 152-160.

Sevick, M. A., Zucconi, S., Sereika, S., Puczynski, S., Drury, R., Marra, R., Mattes, P., & Taylor, J. (1992). Characteristics and health service utilization patterns of ventilator-dependent patients cared for within a vertically integrated health system. *American Journal of Critical Care, 1*(3), 45-51.

Sheikh, L., O'Brien, M., & McCluskey-Fawcett (1993). Parent preparation for the NICU to home transition: Staff and parent perceptions. *Children's Health Care, 22*(3), 227-239.

Sivak, E. D., Cordasco, E. M., & Gipson, W. T. (1983). Pulmonary mechanical ventilation at home: A reasonable and less expensive alternative. *Respiratory Care, 28*(1), 42-49.

Stahl, D. A. (1994). Subacute care: The future of health care. *Nursing Management, 25*(10), 34, 36, 38-40.

Stahl, D. A. (1995a). Maximizing reimbursement for subacute care. *Nursing Management, 26*(4), 16-19.

Stahl, D. A. (1995b). Integrated delivery system: An opportunity or a dilemma. *Nursing Management, 26*(7), 20, 22-23.

Thurber, F., & DiGiamarino, L. (1992). Development of a model of transitional care for the HIV positive child and family. *Clinical Nurse Specialist, 6*(3), 142-146.

U.S. General Accounting Office. (1987). *Post-hospital care: Discharge planners report increasing difficulty in planning for medicare patients* (GAO/PMED 87-5BR). Washington, DC: Author.

Vinson, J. M., Rich, M. W., Sperry, J. C., Shah, A. S., & McNamara, T. (1990). Early readmission of elderly patients with congestive heart failure. *Journal of the American Geriatrics Society, 38*, 1290-1295.

Walsh, M. B., & Wilhere, S.P.G. (1988). The future of teaching nursing homes. *Geriatric Nursing, 9*(6), 354-356.

Whitby, C. A. (1983a). Moving forward in neonatal care–transitional care. *Midwives Chronicle, 96*(1149, Suppl.), 17-18.

Whitby, C. A. (1983b). Transitional care of low birth weight infants. *Journal of Nurse-Midwifery, 28*(5), 25-26.

Williams, B. C., MacKay, S. A., & Torner, J. C. (1991). Home health care: Comparison of patients and services among three types of agencies. *Medical Care, 29*(6), 583-587.

Williams, E. I., Greenwell, J., & Groom, L. M. (1992). The care of people over 75 years old after discharge from hospital: An evaluation of timetabled visiting by health visitor assistants. *Journal of Public Health Medicine, 14*(2), 138-144.

Winograd, C. H. (1991). Targeting strategies: An overview of criteria and outcomes. *Journal of the American Geriatrics Society, 39*(Suppl.), 25S-35S.

Wong, D. L. (1991). Transition from hospital to home for children with complex medical care. *Journal of Pediatric Oncology Nursing, 8*(1), 3-9.

York, R., Brown, L. P., Samuels, P., Finkler, S., Jacobsen, B., Armstrong, C., Swank, A., & Robbins, D. (in press). A randomized clinical trial of early discharge and nurse specialist transitional home follow-up of high-risk childbearing women. *Nursing Research*.

Zelle, R. S. (1995). Follow-up of at-risk infants in the home setting: Consultation model. *Journal of Obstetric, Gynecologic and Neonatal Nursing, 24*(1), 51-55.

35

QUALITY OUTCOMES AND CONTEXTUAL VARIABLES IN NURSING HOMES

Meridean L. Maas
Janet P. Specht

There is increasing emphasis on measurement of resident outcomes to determine the effectiveness and quality of health care services. Substantial research, including nursing research, has focused on testing the effects of specific interventions on resident outcomes, but the study of the effects of context on quality outcomes has received little attention by nurse researchers. For nursing homes, the enactment of the Omnibus Budget Reconciliation Act (OBRA) in 1987 focused attention on specific outcomes for long-term care residents and mandated documentation that has facilitated health services research. Yet, context in nursing homes has been underassessed in nursing research, despite recognition of the importance of examining the effects of the context of nursing interventions on resident outcomes (Kayser-Jones, 1989; Verran & Mark, 1992).

There is clearly a need to study the relationship of context and quality in nursing homes. The study of context is critical because of the importance of quality of life for persons who live in long-term care institutions. The average length of stay in nursing homes is 2.9 years, compared to 5 days in a hospital (U.S. Department of Health and Human Services [USDHHS], 1989). The nursing home is not just a place where persons receive treatment. For many, it is a home and a way of life (Kane & Kane, 1988). The nursing home is often the only environment for its residents and thus exerts a powerful influence on the quality of residents' lives (Ryden, 1985). Interventions and processes alone do not account for quality of life. Quality of life, a meaningful resident outcome, is influenced by the nursing home routines, its programs and activities, its residents and staff, and its social and physical milieu. The environment within which processes occur, including the cultural climate; organizational structures; and the social relationships among residents, staff, and families, influences how processes are implemented and the extent to which desired outcomes are achieved.

Nursing homes are also highly subject to influences of the external environment; the nursing home industry is one of the most highly regulated in the United States. Regulations and reimbursement rates for care provided are politically sensitive issues. The average age, disability, illness acuity of persons, and sophistication of technology in nursing homes are increasing and expected to continue to increase into the 21st century (Maas, Buckwalter, & Specht, 1996). The demands for care are increasing, but there is concern that payment for nursing home services is taking too large a portion of federal and state budgets, and there are pressures to control this spending. Efforts to demonstrate quality outcomes for innovative care programs and environments are expected to intensify. Evaluation of the impact of reduced expenditures of resources on quality of care is a major issue and another compelling reason to examine the relationship of context and quality outcomes.

Organizational context is defined as social and physical characteristics of the internal and external environment of the focal organization (Duncan, 1972; Verran & Mark, 1992). The focal organization studied may be a nursing home, a resident care unit in a nursing home, or a corporation composed of several nursing homes. The internal environment includes structures and processes of the nursing home, such as ownership, size, staffing, and the social and physical milieu within the organization. Characteristics of the external environmental include social, political, legal, technological, demographic, cultural and economic contingencies that exist outside the boundaries of the nursing home (Maas & Mulford, 1989; Mulford, 1984).

Resident outcomes are states, behaviors, or perceptions that characterize individuals, groups, or aggregates of individuals who receive health care services from individual or organization providers (Maas, Johnson, & Moorhead, in press). Outcomes include the functional status of individual residents, aggregated resident outcomes, and characteristics of the nursing home's structures and processes such as cost and regulatory compliance. Organization outcomes characterize the performance of the organization as a whole, as opposed to outcomes that are characteristics of individual residents. Quality outcomes are consistent with the state of health care science and practice. In nursing home health services re-

search, quality outcomes that have received most attention can be grouped into five broad categories: use of health care resources, quality of life, resident function, morbidity and mortality, and regulatory compliance.

This chapter describes the theoretical perspectives and points of view that have been most influential in guiding nursing research of the relationship of contextual variables to resident outcomes in nursing homes. A synthesis of nursing science regarding nursing home context and resident outcomes is presented, including what is substantiated by research and remaining gaps in knowledge. Finally, recommendations for research needed to advance nursing science in the area are discussed.

Perspectives Used in Studies of Context and Resident Outcomes in Nursing Homes

Two dominant perspectives, (a) environmental effects on the elderly and (b) structure, process, and outcome dimensions of quality, have guided nursing studies of organizational context and resident outcomes in nursing homes. Although several variations have evolved, they tend to be a matter of differing emphases on groups of contextual variables included in one of the two dominant perspectives.

Theoretical strategies most often used to assist with understanding the effects of the institutional environment on older people include social ecological models and person-environment fit and interaction perspectives. All of these theoretical approaches view behaviors of elders as outcomes of interchanges with their environments (Kahana, 1982; Lawton, 1970, 1982; Moos, 1976, 1980). There are, however, some differences in how the theorists view the effect of environment on resident outcome. Moos (1980) focuses on the individual's ability to cope with the environment in determining outcome. Individual competence compared to environmental press or demands is emphasized by Lawton (1982); Kahana (1982) highlights aspects of personality and environmental demands. If the individual's coping, competence, or personality is adequate relative to the environment, positive behavioral responses result. As the individual's ability to cope declines, competence is impaired or personality does not fit the environment's demands, and undesirable behavioral outcomes occur.

Building on the social-ecological work of Lawton (1970, 1980, 1982) and Moos (1976) and Kahana's (1982) theory of person-environment interaction, Kayser-Jones (1989, 1991) described three major contextual aspects of the environment to be studied in long-term care institutions: physical characteristics, organizational climate, and psychosocial milieu. Components of physical characteristics identified by Kayser-Jones are architectural design, color, lighting, and space. Organizational climate includes policy, staffing, and financing of care. Norms, values, activities, philosophy, attitudes and beliefs of the caregivers, and personal interaction of all who are a part of the institution constitute the psychosocial milieu of the environment. Ryden (1985) drew on Lewin's equation of behavior as a function of characteristics of the person and the environment and Goffman's (1961) concept of the "total institution" as corrupting of individuals' autonomy to describe three important dimensions of the organization's internal environment: interpersonal environment, organizational environment, and physical environment. According to Ryden, attitudes, philosophy, practices of staff about choices and options for residents, and availability of administrators and their contact with residents make up the interpersonal environment. She described the organizational environment as mechanisms for enabling residents to exercise their rights, participate in care planning, participate on committees, control personal belongings, and leave and return to the organization as desired. Included in the physical environment are amount of personal space, privacy, ventilation, lighting, type of room, use of radio and television, and security for belongings.

According to Donabedian (1966), quality care is composed of the essential conceptual components of structure, process, and outcomes. Structure refers to physical and social attributes of the organization. Processes are the behaviors and activities of personnel in providing a service. Outcomes are the end products of a service. Donabedian views quality outcomes as the result of quality processes that are dependent on quality structures. In this view, poor outcomes are the result of omissions or substandard service by organizations or individual providers. To date, most studies have failed to demonstrate these theoretical linkages among structure, process, and outcome (Kurowski & Shaughnessy, 1985). Yet, without the linkages, outcomes cannot be used to determine quality or to design policy that will ensure quality (Vladek, 1988).

Health services researchers have for the most part used the Donabedian perspective to guide their studies of nursing home context and resident outcomes. Most often, but not always, using analysis of large secondary data sets, health services researchers focus on the nursing home organization as the unit of analysis and examine the relationship of external and internal organization context to aggregate resident outcomes. The emphasis is on prediction of resident outcomes from structure and process aspects of the nursing home context. Arising from a structural-functionalist perspective (Blau, 1975), but incorporating the notion of organizations as goal directed, semiopen systems (Thompson, 1967), health services researchers assume that certain internal and external environmental organizational structures and processes have positive functions and lead to quality resident outcomes. Outcomes studied tend to be the traditional rates of mortality, morbidity, and discharge, as well as some form of resource use, such as number of hospitalizations and physician visits. Although functional status and other measures of resident health status are used, these outcomes ordinarily characterize an aggregate of residents.

In contrast to health services research in other disciplines, nursing studies of nursing home context and resident outcomes have usually focused on the effects of the nursing home environment on outcomes for individual residents. Satisfaction with the nursing home, resident autonomy, life satisfaction, and disturbing behaviors are among the outcomes most often measured (Gould, 1992; Kolanowski, Hurwitz, Taylor, Evans, & Strumpf, 1994; Kruzich, Clinton, & Kelber, 1992; Ryden, 1985). Although few in number, most nursing studies are individual- or mixed- (organization and individual) level analyses; more studies by health services researchers in other fields tend to be organization-level analyses.

Nursing's perspective appears to be more concerned with the humanistic and internal aspects of the nursing home environment, such as the social and physical context and the adequacy of care staff. Most nursing studies emphasize the internal social environment (Gould, 1992; Kruzich et al., 1992; Ryden, 1985), perhaps because it is an aspect of the nursing home environment that has been neglected by traditional measures of structure and process reviewed by regulators. Other aspects of the internal organizational context of nursing homes examined in nursing studies are staffing, staff mix, turnover, ownership, percentage of Medicaid residents, and physical environment (Kane et al., 1989; Kolanowski et al., 1994; Kruzich et al., 1992). Most nursing studies have not examined the effects of the nursing home's external environment on resident outcomes. Outcomes of interest to nurse researchers focus on individual resident satisfaction, autonomy, and behaviors. Some nursing studies have tested the effects of environmental interventions on resident outcomes. Examples are Hall, Kirschling, and Todd (1986); Kongable, Buckwalter, and Stolley (1989); Maas and Buckwalter (1988); Maas, Buckwalter, et al. (1994); Swanson, Maas, and Buckwalter (1993); and Van Ort and Phillips (1995). Munroe (1990), most closely following the health services research approach, analyzed the relationships of resident case mix and the ratio of registered nurses (RNs) to licensed vocational nurses (LVNs) to number of nursing home health-related deficiencies at annual survey, with other organization structure and process characteristics (e.g., facility size, payer mix, and personnel turnover) as control variables.

Overall, nursing studies emphasize interventions to improve the care of individuals living in nursing homes; health services researchers in other fields design studies that more directly inform policy regarding reimbursement and regulatory issues. Health services researchers capitalize on the availability of large data sets, although the global outcomes that are readily available suffer from lack of measurement sensitivity, questionable quality of data sources, and weak equivalence between the research questions and the outcomes (Verran & Mark, 1992). Nursing research intends to inform policy and has the advantage of analyzing more sensitive outcomes for individuals, but it has the disadvantages of limitations of sample size and lack of replication.

In contrast, the health services view inclines toward a more medical-business orientation, emphasizing reimbursement, competition, and resource use aspects of context, as well as outcomes of adequacy of care and compliance with regulators at the aggregated organization level. Research by Munroe (1990) and Rantz, Mehr, Hicks, et al. (1996) are examples of nurse-directed health services research that bridge the two orientations. Clearly, both emphases and the associated strategies are needed to illumine the black box of the relationships of nursing home context to resident outcomes to inform practice and health policy.

Research in nursing home context and resident outcomes leaves a number of issues and questions unresolved. First, there is a paucity of nursing studies that examine the relationships among contextual variables and resident outcomes. Health services researchers in other fields tend to focus on global organizational characteristics but mostly ignore attributes of the nursing organization and systems of care delivery other than staffing. Both health services and nurse researchers have paid little attention to factors in the external organizational environment that may affect resident outcomes. As a result, there is a lack of empirical evidence as to the salient internal and external environmental variables that affect resident outcomes in nursing homes. Further, the use of global outcome measures leaves many questions unanswered as to the specific linkages among contextual and outcome variables. Many questions remain as to what outcomes reflect quality, what aspects of context affect quality outcomes, and what are the best measures of the variables.

Unlike health services researchers in other fields, few nurse researchers have conducted secondary analyses of national minimum data sets to describe linkages among nursing home context and resident outcomes. This is despite the recent interest in effectiveness research to inform health policy and the implementation of a national standardized long-term care minimum data set (LTC MDS) for nursing homes. The LTC MDS, however, does not contain standardized nursing data to describe and measure all diagnoses, interventions, and outcomes needed to assess nursing effectiveness. For example, there is no standardized measure of quality of life in the LTC MDS. Although some nursing home contextual variables are available from other standardized data sets, many of interest to nursing are not available, such as physical and social environment. The lack of measures of context and of resident outcomes that are sensitive to nursing interventions in large data sets constrains analysis of the effects of context and intervention on resident outcomes.

Many questions remain to be answered regarding the specific nursing home contextual variables that are related to quality resident outcomes. Of particular concern to nurses and health policy makers is the adequacy of nurse staffing numbers and mix for achieving quality resident outcomes in nursing homes (Wunderlich, Sloan, & Davis, 1996). The relationship of staff turnover to resident quality outcomes is also an issue. Answers are needed as to what resident outcomes are indicators of quality and what measures of outcomes are sensitive, reliable, and valid. Because nursing is the primary service and nursing staff make up the largest group of providers in nursing homes, an important question is whether or not resident outcomes more sensitive to nursing are needed to assess the relationship to context in addition to those outcomes that tend to be of more interest to other health services researchers.

Questions also remain about how to best measure nursing home contextual variables. Because about 70% of the residents in nursing homes are reported to have cognitive or behavioral impairments, these questions are especially important when resident perceptions are considered for data collection (Harrington, Thollaug, & Summers, 1995). The needs of all residents must be considered. The discovery of the contextual variables that are most conducive to the achievement of quality outcomes for residents who are cognitively impaired and behaviorally challenging are issues of particular significance to nursing.

A number of issues surround the relationship of quality resident outcomes to cost. Many fear that increased concerns about cost encourage lower standards for quality in a competitive, managed-care environment. Concern for cost can affect most nursing home contextual variables. Thus, how context, cost, and outcomes are interrelated is an important question. A critical issue for nursing is whether adequate nursing data will be available in local and large national data sets to allow nurse scientists to examine these questions from a nursing perspective to inform the field and influence health policy.

The State of the Science

Nursing research of nursing home context and resident outcomes is in an early stage of development. Although the findings in each of the reported studies document a relationship between some contextual variable and resident outcomes, there have not been enough studies to validate a relationship between specific contextual attributes and specific resident outcomes. Nursing studies have tended to focus on the impact of the internal environment on resident satisfaction outcomes. Yet these studies are not of a sufficient number to replicate observed relationships. The studies measure a variety of contextual variables, so it is difficult to summarize those that have examined a particular type of internal environmental context. Further, variables studied suffer from problems of semantic and conceptual clarity. For example, social environment is defined and measured in several different ways by researchers studying its relationship with resident outcomes.

Statistically significant relationships for psychosocial aspects of the internal environment and resident outcomes were documented by Gould (1992), Kruzich et al. (1992), and Ryden (1985). Each of the studies, however, measured different aspects of the psychosocial environment and different resident outcomes. Similarly, physical

environmental variables studied by Kolanowski et al., 1994; Kruzich et al., 1992; and Ryden, 1985 were found to be significantly related to resident outcomes, but the same variables or measures were not used for either the independent or dependent variables. Nurse staffing was the organizational variable most frequently found to be statistically significantly related to resident outcomes (Kane et al., 1989; Kolanowski et al., 1994; Kruzich et al., 1992; Munroe, 1990), but each researcher studied different aspects of staffing (e.g., staffing number, staff mix, staff-resident ratio, general nurse practitioner [GNP] presence) and different resident or organization outcomes (e.g., disturbing behaviors, resident satisfaction with nursing home, resource use, survey citations).

The internal and external validity of nursing studies that have tested the effects of environmental interventions on resident outcomes have tended to use small samples, weak designs, or a single site. Few are replications of previous studies. Research to study the effects of special care units on outcomes for residents with Alzheimer's disease (AD) is one exception. These studies have shown some consistency in findings that the specifically designed internal unit environment results in fewer resident disturbing and catastrophic behaviors, increased social interaction, decreased use of physical restraints, fewer injurious falls, and reduced use of psychoactive medications (Cleary, Price, Clamon, & Shullaw, 1988; Hall et al., 1986; Maas & Buckwalter, 1990; Swanson et al., 1993). Kongable et al. (1989) also found positive effects of an environmental intervention on social behaviors of residents with AD on a special care unit, although the intervention was the introduction of a pet (dog) onto the unit. Van Ort and Phillips (1995) introduced a contextual feeding intervention for residents with AD on a special care unit that resulted in improved resident self-feeding without extending the time required to eat.

More recently, there have been indications that nurse researchers are beginning to focus more on outcome effectiveness of nursing interventions while accounting for the effects of organizational contextual variables, although cost and cost-effectiveness have not been consistently examined. In general, the perspectives used by nurse scientists to study the relationship of contextual variables and resident outcomes have ignored contextual characteristics of the larger environment external to the nursing home.

Most nursing studies sampled a moderate number of residents, but relatively small numbers of nursing homes, compared to studies that analyze large national data sets. Most of the analyses were cross-sectional and used mixed- or individual-level analysis. In general, patient outcomes research continues to be unilevel, with the individual resident as the unit of analysis, rather than multilevel investigations of the relationship of organization context and patient outcomes (Hegyvary, 1992; Hughes & Anderson, 1994; McDaniel, 1990). More organization- and mixed-level analyses are needed in the study of nursing home context and resident outcomes, yet it is a strength of nursing studies that individual-level analysis has been largely retained for the dependent variable, resident outcomes.

Multisite nursing studies tended not to control for other contextual variables that might be related to the resident outcomes or to the contextual variables analyzed. If sites were matched, there was minimal description of how they were matched and on what variables. A strength of nursing studies, however, is that most included some controls for resident variables. There is a need for the development of a theory-based taxonomy of contextual variables that are expected to influence resident outcomes to assist researchers with the planning of more rigorous research strategies.

Although most of the nursing studies reviewed were based on some theoretical perspective, none presented a well-developed model to be tested. Most studies were cross-sectional and lacked a model with strong theoretical underpinning; thus the relationships documented between context and outcomes are often equally plausible in either direction. Clearly, more efforts must be devoted to the development and testing of theoretical models containing explicit linkages among contextual variables, resident characteristics, and resident outcomes. In addition, conceptual clarification of variables is needed to eliminate semantic vagueness, synonymity, and ambiguity so that measurement and comparison and replication of study findings are feasible.

Nursing studies that used aggregated measures of organization context did not test the reliability, validity, or adequacy of the measures at the aggregated level. Further, no discussion provided evidence that the referent for subjects who supplied the data was the group rather than the individual. Overall, in the limited number of reported studies of organizational context and resident outcomes, it is often difficult to determine exactly how the analyses were conducted; that is, whether the analysis is individual level, organization level, or mixed level. The tendency not to supply adequate detail contributes to a lack of clarity needed for complete understanding of the methods used. For example, complete regression tables with Ns and degrees of freedom and description of the presence or absence of multicollinearity among the independent variables are sometimes omitted. Most studies have not used multivariate procedures to assess the interrelationships of contextual and patient outcome variables.

A number of studies used resident perceptions to measure context. The instrument used most often to measure nursing home context was the Multiphasic Environmental Assessment Procedure (MEAP) (Lemke & Moos, 1987; Moos & Lemke, 1984) that elicits subjects' perceptions of seven dimensions of the internal environment. There is some question that resident perceptions are reliable and valid measures of context, as residents are dependent upon staff caregivers and the nursing home organization and may be reluctant to express negative views (Gould, 1992). The same question is of course relevant for the use of resident satisfaction to measure quality resident outcomes. To measure resident satisfaction, it is necessary to exclude more than half of the available subjects because of cognitive, language, or behavioral deficits. This makes resident satisfaction a less than useful outcome for assessing quality in nursing homes, although satisfaction of cognitively intact residents is an important aspect of quality. The exclusion of persons who have been in the facility less than 6 months is often done to avoid capturing dissatisfaction with a change in living environment. However, this exclusion also may inflate satisfaction by giving residents time to accept less than desirable circumstances in their living and care environments. In general, resident satisfaction measures are subject to inflation from social desirability. For this reason, it is important that investigators report the variation in resident satisfaction scores for the sample.

There has been a lack of research that examines how the relationship of nursing home context and resident outcomes may vary for residents of differing ethnicity, in different regions of the country, or for residents in rural versus urban nursing homes. Although one nursing study assessed differences among resident case-mix groups (Kruzich et al., 1992), many more studies are needed that compare the relationship of context and resident outcomes among a variety of resident populations.

In summary, the state of nursing science in the study of nursing home context and resident outcomes is in an early stage of development. The few studies reported have tended to focus on aspects of the internal organizational environment and its impact on quality-of-life issues. Most of the studies are individual-level analyses, with a few using mixed-level units of analysis. Nurse researchers have tended to use a small number of nursing home sites with moderate-size resident samples, and most have not conducted analyses at the organizational level with large, national data sets. Issues pertaining to measurement of independent and dependent variables and to extending the study of relationships among context and outcomes to more ethnically diverse populations have not been addressed. Largely due to the small number of studies and methodological limitations, many questions remain unanswered. Several recommendations are set forth in an effort to highlight the important efforts needed to advance the science in the field.

Advancing Nursing Science in Nursing Home Context and Resident Outcomes

The inclusion of standardized nursing data in national minimum data sets would assist nurse scientists to analyze the relationship of context and resident outcomes in nursing homes. Availability of these data in large clinical and national minimum data sets would enable cross-sectional and longitudinal analyses of the effects of contextual variables on nursing-sensitive outcomes. The LTC MDS data set provides the opportunity for some of this but does not include standardized nursing data or nurse provider information. Further, the LTC MDS and other uniform data sets do not include all nursing organizational contextual variables needed for optimal analysis of questions of interest to nurses. There is a need for standardized nursing minimum data elements in national LTC minimum data sets, including data elements that describe attributes of the nursing organization context, such as turnover and job satisfaction (Huber, Delaney, Crossley, Mehmert, & Ellerbe, 1992). The nursing community should unite in actions to gain the inclusion of standardized nursing data in the LTC MDS and other national minimum data sets.

Collaborative research of nurse scientists and health services researchers in other fields is recommended to advance the study of nursing home context and resident outcomes. Health services researchers in other disciplines would benefit from the nursing perspective regarding contextual variables that affect resident quality of life. The nursing perspective is clearly important because nursing is the primary service in nursing homes. Nurse

scientists would benefit from the health services research tradition of the use of large national data sets and macrolevel analysis, including more attention to factors in the external organization environment that may influence resident outcomes. There is a need, however, for more work to assess the reliability and validity of secondary data and aggregated measures.

Research by Rantz, Mehr, Conn, et al. (in press) is an example of the interdisciplinary research that is needed to unravel the linkages among nursing home contextual variables and quality resident outcomes. Using cross-sectional and longitudinal secondary analyses of the LTC MDS and the Health Care Financing Administration's Federal On-line Survey and Certification Annual Reports (OSCAR) for all Missouri nursing homes, the Rantz research team is examining the relationships among nursing home context (e.g., staffing, ownership, social environment), interventions (e.g., processes of care), and indicators of quality outcomes (Rantz, Mehr, Conn, et al., in press).

Much work is needed to gain greater conceptual clarity of contextual and quality resident outcome variables to enhance the adequacy of measurement and comparison across studies. More qualitative studies are recommended to explore quality outcomes from the residents' perspectives. Alternatives to measures of resident satisfaction should be sought, along with measures that capture quality outcomes for the cognitively impaired. Measures of context other than resident perceptions need to be developed.

Nurse scientists should conduct more replication studies to increase confidence in specific findings or to provide evidence that some findings are not valid. As nursing studies of nursing home context and resident outcomes increase, the use of integrative reviews and meta-analysis will be important to synthesize findings and focus continued research. Meta-analytic studies may be warranted now if unpublished reports and dissertations are available to include. Combining nursing and other health services research on nursing home context and resident outcomes for meta-analysis may also be warranted.

More nursing research that tests the effects of interventions on resident outcomes must take greater care in accounting for nursing home context. A larger number of sites is needed for multisite studies to enable the assessment of interaction effects of sites characterized by specific contexts. When the strategy is to control the effects of organization context by matching, more precise equivalence of theory-based contextual variables that are expected to affect resident outcomes must be accomplished and described in greater detail in published reports.

Finally, nurse scientists should make a priority of the development of theoretical models that include the salient nursing home contextual variables that affect resident outcomes. Sound theoretical models that have been tested and revised are required to focus and increase the efficiency of research efforts and to enhance the accumulation of knowledge in the field. More important, models that can be systematically tested and revised will speed the identification and advancement of contextual factors that produce quality resident outcomes.

Conclusion

Substantiated findings of nursing studies of context and resident outcomes in nursing homes are limited to some evidence that social and physical context and staffing are related to quality resident outcomes. Findings that are most substantiated are that (a) greater nursing-staff-to-resident and greater registered-nurse-to-unlicenced-nursing-staff ratios are positively related to quality resident outcomes, and (b) specially designed physical and psychosocial environments result in improved outcomes for residents with Alzheimer's disease and related disorders. However, many gaps remain in what is known in this important area of nursing science, primarily due to the lack of well-developed theoretical models and the small number of studies conducted. Only some of the nursing home contextual variables that may be related to resident outcomes have been examined, and fewer still have been included in replication studies. Although nurse researcher interest in the relationship of context to individual resident responses is a strength, more multisite studies are needed, and more opportunities for nursing investigations using large national data sets should be sought. Nurse researcher collaboration with health services researchers in other disciplines is strongly encouraged to broaden the conceptual and methodological approaches used by each to study the effects of nursing home context on resident outcomes.

Overall, most nurse scientists have shown little interest in the effects of context on nursing home resident outcomes. With the rapid changes taking place in health care delivery systems, alternative provider patterns, and the continued emphasis on cost-effective care, questions regarding the relationship of organization context and resident outcomes are of increasing interest. Thus, to inform nursing practice and health care policy, it is vitally important that nurse researchers examine the influence of context, along with interventions, on resident outcomes.

References

Blau, P. (1975). *Approaches to the study of social structure.* New York: Free Press.

Cleary, A. F., Price, M., Clamon, C., & Shullaw, G. (1988). A reduced stimulus unit: Effects on patients with Alzheimer's disease and related disorders. *Gerontologist, 28,* 511-514.

Donabedian, A. (1966). Evaluating the process of medical care. *Milbank Quarterly, 44,* 166-206.

Duncan, R. (1972). Characteristics of organizational environments and perceived environmental uncertainty. *Administrative Science Quarterly, 17,* 313-327.

Goffman, E. (1961). *Asylums.* Garden City, NY: Anchor.

Gould, M. T. (1992). Nursing home elderly: Social-environmental factors. *Journal of Gerontological Nursing, 18*(8), 3-20.

Hall, G., Kirschling, M., & Todd, S. (1986, May/June). Sheltered freedom: An Alzheimer's unit in an ICF. *Geriatric Nursing, 7,* 132-137.

Harrington, C., Thollaug, S. C., & Summers, P. R. (1995, August). *Nursing facilities, staffing, residents, and facility deficiencies, 1991-93.* Paper prepared for the Health Care Financing Administration, University of California, San Francisco.

Hegyvary, S. T. (1992). Outcomes research: Integrating nursing practice into the world view. In *Patient outcomes research: Examining the effectiveness of nursing practice* (NIH Pub. No. 93-3411, pp. 17-24). Rockville, MD: National Institutes of Health.

Huber, D., Delaney, C., Crossley, J., Mehmert, M., & Ellerbe, S. (1992). An nursing management minimum data set: Significance and development. *Journal of Nursing Administration, 22*(7/8), 35-40.

Hughes, L. C., & Anderson, R. A. (1994). Issues regarding aggregation of data and nursing systems research. *Journal of Nursing Measurement, 2*(1), 79-101.

Kahana, E. (1982). A congruence model of person-environment interaction. In M. P. Lawton, P. G. Windley, & T. O. Byerts (Eds.), *Aging and the environment: Theoretical approaches* (pp. 97-121). New York: Springer.

Kane, R. L., Garrard, J., Skay, C. L., Radosevich, D. M., Buchanan, J. L., McDermott, S. M., Arnold, S. B., & Kepferle, L. (1989). Effects of a geriatric nurse practitioner on process and outcome of nursing home care. *American Journal of Public Health, 79*(9), 1271-1277.

Kane, R., & Kane, R. (1988). Long term care: Variations on a quality assurance theme. *Inquiry, 25,* 132-146.

Kayser-Jones, J. (1989). The environment and quality of life in long term care institutions. *Nursing and Healthcare, 10*(3), 124-130.

Kayser-Jones, J. (1991). The impact of environment on the quality of care in nursing homes: A social-psychological perspective. *Holistic Nursing Practice, 5*(3), 29-38.

Kolanowski, A., Hurwitz, S., Taylor, L. A., Evans, L., & Strumpf, N. (1994). Contextual factors associated with disturbing behaviors in institutionalized elders. *Nursing Research, 43*(2), 73-79.

Kongable, L. G., Buckwalter, K. C., & Stolley, J. M. (1989). The effects of pet therapy on the social behavior of institutionalized Alzheimer's clients. *Archives of Psychiatric Nursing, 3*(4), 191-198.

Kruzich, J. M., Clinton, J. F., & Kelber, S. T. (1992). Personal and environmental influences on nursing home satisfaction. *The Gerontologist, 32*(3), 342-350.

Kurowski, B. D., & Shaughnessy, P. W. (1985). The measurement and assurance of quality. In R. J. Vogel & H. C. Palmer (Eds.), *Long-term care: Perspectives from research and demonstrations.* Rockville, MD: Aspen.

Lawton, M. P. (1970). Assessment, integration, and environments for the elderly. *The Gerontologist, 10,* 38-46.

Lawton, M. P. (1980). *Environment and aging.* Monterey, CA: Brooks/Cole.

Lawton, M. P. (1982). Competence, environmental press, and the adaptation of older people. In M. Lawton, P. Windley, & T. O. Byerts (Eds.), *Aging and the environment: Theoretical approaches* (pp. 33-59). New York: Springer.

Lemke, S., & Moos, R. H. (1987). Measuring the social climate of congregate residences for older people: The Sheltered Care Environment Scale. *Psychology and Aging, 2,* 20-29.

Maas, M., & Buckwalter, K. (1988). Evaluation of a special Alzheimer's unit: Baseline data. *Journal of Applied Nursing Research, 1*(1), 41.

Maas, M., & Buckwalter, K. (1990). *Evaluation of a special Alzheimer's unit* (final report). Rockville, MD: NIH National Center for Nursing Research.

Maas, M., Buckwalter, K., & Specht, J. (1996). Nursing staff and quality of care in nursing homes. In G. Wunderlich, F. Sloan, & C. Davis (Eds.), *Nursing staff in hospitals and nursing homes: Is it adequate?*(Institute of Medicine Report, pp. 361-452). Washington, DC: National Academy Press.

Maas, M., Buckwalter, K., Swanson, E., Specht, J., Hardy, M., & Tripp-Reimer, T. (1994, November/December). The caring partnership: Staff and families of persons institutionalized with Alzheimer's disease. *Journal of Alzheimer's Disease and Related Disorders, 9*(6), 21-30.

Maas, M., Johnson, M., & Moorhead, S. (in press). Classification of nursing-sensitive patient outcomes. *Image: The Journal of Nursing Scholarship.*

Maas, M., & Mulford, C. (1989). *Structural adaptation of organizations: Issues and strategies for nurse executives.* Redwood City, CA: Addison-Wesley.

McDaniel, C. (1990). Nursing administration research as a paradigm reflection. *Nursing and Healthcare, 11,* 191-193.

Moos, R. H. (1976). *The human context: Environmental determinants of behavior.* New York: Wiley-Interscience.

Moos, R. H. (1980). Specialized living environments for older people: A conceptual framework for evaluation. *Journal of Social Issues, 39*(2), 75-94.

Moos, R. H., & Lemke, S. (1984). *Multiphasic environmental assessment procedure: Supplementary manual.* Palo Alto, CA: Veterans Administration and Stanford University Medical Center.

Mulford, C. (1984). *Interorganizational relations: Implications for community development.* New York: Human Sciences.

Munroe, D. J. (1990). The influence of registered nurse staffing on the quality of nursing home care. *Research in Nursing and Health, 8,* 263-270.

Rantz, M., Mehr, D., Conn, V., Hicks, L. L., Porter, R., Madsen, R. W., Petroski, G. S., & Maas, M. (in press). Assessing quality of nursing home care: The foundation for improving resident outcomes. *Journal of Nursing Care Quality.*

Rantz, M., Mehr, D., Hicks, L., Conn, V., Porter, R., Madsen, R., Petroski, G., Maas, M., Zimmerman, D., & Givens, B. (1996). *MDS quality indicator comparative feedback intervention to improve Missouri nursing home resident outcomes.* Unpublished manuscript, University of Missouri–Columbia.

Ryden, M. (1985). Environmental support for autonomy in the institutionalized elderly. *Research in Nursing and Health, 8,* 363-371.

Swanson, E., Maas, M., & Buckwalter, K. (1993). Catastrophic reactions and other behaviors of Alzheimer's residents: Special unit compared with traditional units. *Archives of Psychiatric Nursing, 7*(5), 292-299.

Thompson, J. D. (1967). *Organizations in action.* Philadelphia: McGraw-Hill.

U.S. Department of Health and Human Services. (1989). *The National Nursing Home Survey: 1985 summary for the United States* (DHHS Pub. No. 89-1758). Hyattsville, MD: Author.

Van Ort, S., & Phillips, L. R. (1995). Nursing interventions to promote functional feeding. *Journal of Gerontological Nursing, 21*(10), 6-14.

Verran, J. A., & Mark, B. (1992). Contextual factors influencing patient outcomes, individual/group/environment: Interactions and clinical practice interface. In *Patient outcomes research: Examining the effectiveness of nursing practice* (NIH Pub. No. 93-3411, pp. 121-143). Rockville, MD: National Institutes of Health.

Vladek, E. C. (1988). Quality assurance through external controls. *Inquiry, 25,* 100-107.

Wunderlich, G. S., Sloan, F. A., & Davis, C. K. (1996). *Nursing staff in hospitals and nursing homes: Is it adequate?* Washington, DC: National Academy Press.

AUTHOR INDEX

SUBJECT INDEX

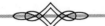

ABOUT THE EDITORS

Ada Sue Hinshaw, PhD, RN, FAAN, is Professor and Dean at the University of Michigan School of Nursing. She was the founding Director of the National Institute of Nursing Research (NINR) at the National Institutes of Health (NIH) from 1987 to 1994. Prior to her term at NINR, Dr. Hinshaw held a joint appointment for 12 years as Professor and Director of Nursing Research at the University of Arizona College of Nursing and Associate Director of Nursing for Research at the Department of Nursing, University Medical Center. She received her BS from the University of Kansas, her MS from Yale University, and her MA and PhD in sociology from the University of Arizona. Her honors include Nurse Scientist of the Year (ANA Council of Nurse Researchers), Elizabeth McWilliams Miller Award for Excellence in Research (Sigma Theta Tau, International) and Health Leader of the Year (U.S. Public Health Service Corps). She has received several honorary doctoral degrees. She is a member of the Institute of Medicine of the National Academy of Sciences and a Fellow in the American Academy of Nursing.

Suzanne L. Feetham, PhD, RN, FAAN, is Professor, Harriet Werley Research Chair, College of Nursing, at the University of Illinois at Chicago. Formerly, she was Chief Officer of Planning, Analysis and Evaluation (1990-1996) and Deputy Director (1993-1996), National Institute of Nursing Research, National Institutes of Health. She also served part-time as Professor of the Associated Faculty of the University of Pennsylvania School of Nursing. She conducts a program of research with children with health problems and their families that includes the development of the Feetham Family Functioning Survey (FFFS). Developed in the mid-1970s, the FFFS has been translated into five languages and used in research in several countries. She is recognized for her landmark publications on the conceptual and methodological issues in research of families. She is a Fellow of the American Academy of Nursing.

Joan L. F. Shaver, PhD, RN, FAAN, is Professor and Dean, College of Nursing, University of Illinois at Chicago. She holds a PhD in Physiology and Biophysics and an advanced practice degree in nursing. She has been a Fellow of the American Academy of Nursing since 1988 and currently serves on the Governing Council. She and her team have been studying sleep problems in women for nearly two decades and were among the first to study sleep problems as a part of menopause. She has had NIH NCNR/NINR funding since 1984, and her current work addresses sleep and sleep-related hormone output in fibromyalgia, using a multidisciplinary team of investigators. She has published her work in sleep, medical, and nursing journals. She was at the University of Washington until 1996, where she codirected the Center for Women's Health Research in the School of Nursing with Dr. Nancy Woods.

ABOUT THE CONTRIBUTORS

Patricia G. Archbold, DNSc, RN, FAAN, is the El-nora E. Thomson Distinguished Professor at the School of Nursing, Oregon Health Sciences University, and Adjunct Investigator at the Center for Health Research at Kaiser Permanente. Her research focuses on family care for frail elders and on methods that home health nurses and health care systems can use to better serve elders and their families. She is actively involved in preparing gerontological nurse researchers and clinicians in the graduate programs of the university.

Martha Ayres, MSN, RN, received her BSN and MSN from Kent State University School of Nursing. Her clinical expertise is in critical care and community nursing, with a focus on gerontology. After receiving her master's degree, she was a clinical instructor at Kent State University School of Nursing for 2 years before leaving to pursue doctoral study. At present, she is a doctoral student at the University of Arizona College of Nursing and works as a research associate on a National Institute of Aging grant studying the abuse of aging caregivers. She is currently funded by an Institutional National Research Service Award for predoctoral study of community-based intervention through the University of Arizona College of Nursing. The focus of her research is family caregiving of individuals with dementia.

Cornelia K. Beck, PhD, RN, FAAN, is Professor, College of Nursing and Department of Psychiatry and Be-havioral Sciences, University of Arkansas for Medical Sciences, Little Rock. She received her PhD in nursing from Texas Women's University, Denton, in 1978. She has edited a textbook, *Psychiatric Nursing—A Holistic Life-Cycle Approach,* has written extensively in the area of mental health care of the older adult, and has conducted research with cognitively impaired elderly since 1984. She is the recipient of multiple research grants from the NIH and various foundations.

Dorothy A. Brooten, PhD, RN, FAAN, is the John Burry, Jr. Professor in Nursing and Dean of the Research and Graduate Studies, Frances Payne Bolton School of Nursing, Case Western Reserve University. For 17 years, she and her colleagues have been developing, testing, and refining a model of transitional care delivered by master's-prepared advanced practice nurses (APNs). The model, developed for use with high-risk, high-cost groups of patients, was initially tested with low birth weight infants. The model, which includes comprehensive discharge planning, home visits, and on-call availability of APNs who have physician back-up, has been tested with seven high-risk patient groups and has demonstrated improved outcomes and reduced costs.

Nancy J. Brown, PhD, RN, FAAN, is Associate Professor and Chair, Division of Community, Health Systems, and Policy, University of Colorado Health Sciences Center School of Nursing, Denver. She received her PhD in Education Administration, with a cognate in nursing, from the University of Denver in 1989; her MS in community health nursing from Arizona State University; and her BSN from Ball State University in Muncie, Indiana. Her research has focused on health promotion and disease prevention in a variety of populations, including migrant farmworkers and those living in proximity to a nuclear weapons clean-up site. Other research interests include disadvantaged and at-risk populations, community analysis, and community-based interventions and outcomes. She was inducted into the American Academy of Nursing in 1998.

Kathleen C. Buckwalter, PhD, RN, FAAN, is Associate Provost for Health Sciences, University of Iowa. She is also Distinguished Professor of Nursing, Associate Director of the Gerontological Nursing Interventions Research Center at the College of Nursing, and serves as Director of the University's Center on Aging. She conducts research on issues affecting mental health services and community-based care for chronically ill older persons and their caregivers, and she has written extensively in this field. She is editor of the *Journal of Gerontological Nursing* and serves on numerous review committees, editorial boards, and advisory groups. She received her BSN (1971) and MA (1976) from the University of Iowa and her PhD (1980) from the University of Illinois at Chicago. She completed postdoctoral training in geriatric mental health through the National Institute of Mental Health.

Mary E. Burman, PhD, RN, FNP, CS, is Associate Professor and Coordinator, Family Nurse Practitioner Program, University of Wyoming, Laramie. She received her BSN from the University of Minnesota and her master's degree and PhD from the University of Michigan. She is a family nurse practitioner in a private practice. She has been involved in a number of research projects focusing on rural health and rural health care, specifically on the impact of chronic illness on families living in rural areas.

Jacquelyn Campbell, PhD, RN, FAAN, is currently Anna D. Wolf Endowed Professor and Associate Dean for Doctoral Education Programs and Research at Johns Hopkins University School of Nursing, with a joint appointment in the School of Hygiene and Public Health. She is Principal Investigator of five NIH, DOD, or CDC major funded research studies on battering and author or coauthor of more than 80 publications on the

subject. These include the books *Nursing Care of Survivors of Family Violence, Sanctions and Sanctuary, Assessing Dangerousness, Drawing the Line,* and *Empowering Survivors of Abuse: Health Care for Battered Women and Their Children.* She has worked with wife abuse shelters and policy-related committees on domestic violence for more than 15 years.

Diane Cronin-Stubbs, PhD, RN, FAAN, is Professor, Rush University College of Nursing, and Research Scientist, Rush Institute for Healthy Aging, Chicago. She recently completed a Clinical Mental Health Academic Award, National Institute of Mental Health (KO7 MH00953), in which the clinical and research emphases were the research-based care of older adults with depression and cognitive impairment. She is currently investigating the separate and synergistic effects of depressive symptoms, cognitive impairment, and social networks on change in disability status among community-living older adults.

Molly C. Dougherty, PhD, RN, FAAN, the Frances Hill Fox Professor of Nursing at the University of North Carolina at Chapel Hill, is a specialist in women's health and aging and editor of *Nursing Research.* She holds BSN, MN, and PhD (Anthropology) degrees from the University of Florida in Gainesville. For 14 years she was the principal investigator on NIH grants related to urinary incontinence and aging women; the findings from these awards inform her chapter, coauthored with Linda Jensen. She and her colleagues have published over 50 research-based articles and chapters on the research they have conducted.

Betty Ferrell, PhD, RN, FAAN, has been in oncology nursing for 21 years and has focused her clinical expertise and research on pain management and quality of life. She is Research Scientist at the City of Hope National Medical Center in Duarte, California. She was a member of the Expert Panel on Pain for the Agency of Health Care Policy and Research (AHCPR) and was Cochair of the Task Force on "Pain in the Elderly" for the International Association for the Study of Pain from 1994-1996. Currently, she is Chairperson of the Southern California Cancer Pain Initiative and is on the NIH-National Advisory Council for Nursing Research. She has written three books: *Cancer Pain Management* (1995), a text on *Suffering* (1995), and a text on *Pain in the Elderly* (1996).

Catherine Ingram Fogel, PhD, RNC, FAAN, is Professor in the School of Nursing at University of North Carolina at Chapel Hill, with a clinical practice in women's health care. She is an advocate for women's health care, especially vulnerable women such as prisoners. She is nationally recognized as an expert on the health and health care of incarcerated women. Her research has focused on women prisoners and improving their health status. Her publications on women's health, including *Health Care of Women* (1980), *Women's Health Care* (with Nancy Fugate Woods; 1995), and *Sexual Health Promotion* (with Diane Lauver; 1990) have had a major impact on nursing practice with women.

Catherine L. Gilliss, DNSc, RN, CS, FAAN, is currently Dean and Professor at Yale University School of Nursing and Senior Fellow, University of California, San Francisco, Center for the Health Professions. A graduate of Duke University, she holds an MSN in psychiatric-mental health nursing from the Catholic University of America and a DNSc from the University of California, San Francisco. Her scientific interests include the family and chronic illness. She has coedited two volumes on family nursing: *The Nursing of Families* (with Suzanne Feetham, Susan B. Meister, and Janice Bell) and *Toward a Science of Family Nursing* (with B. Highley, B. Roberts and I. Martinson). She was a member of the National Institutes of Health, National Institute of Nursing Research, Nursing Sciences Review Committee from 1994 to 1997 and is currently Chair of the Study Section.

Joanne S. Harrell, PhD, RN, FAAN, is Professor and Director, Center for Research on Preventing and Managing Chronic Illness in Vulnerable People. She is also Principal Investigator of the Interdisciplinary Cardiovascular Health in Children and Youth (CHIC) Study, which has been funded by NINR since 1990. She received her PhD in nursing from the University of Texas at Austin in 1984.

Margaret Heitkemper, PhD, RN, FAAN, received a BSN (magna cum laude) degree from Seattle University in 1973; a master's in nursing degree with specialty in gerontological nursing in 1975 from the University of Washington, Seattle; a PhD from the Department of Physiology and Biophysics, University of Illinois Medical Center, Chicago, in 1981. She has been a member of the University of Washington School of Nursing faculty since 1981 and is currently Professor and Chairperson of the Department of Biobehavioral Nursing and Health Systems. Her research is in the area of gastrointestinal symptoms in women.

Suzanne Bakken Henry, DNS, RN, FAAN, is Associate Professor, Department of Community Health Systems, School of Nursing, University of California, San Francisco.

Martha N. Hill, PhD, RN, FAAN, is Professor and Director, Center for Nursing Research, Johns Hopkins University School of Nursing. She holds joint appointments in the School of Hygiene and Public Health and the School of Medicine. She was President of the American Heart Association from 1997 to 1998. She is a Fellow in the American Academy of Nursing. She received her BSN from Johns Hopkins University, her master's degree from the University of Pennsylvania, and her PhD in behavioral sciences from the Johns Hopkins University School of Public Health. She is internationally known for her work, research, and consultation in preventing and treating hypertension, particularly among the population of young, urban, African-American men. She has published extensively and served on numerous review panels and boards, including the World Health Organization's Patient Education Program and the Coordinating Committee of the National High Blood Pressure Education Program.

Diane Holditch-Davis, PhD, RN, FAAN, is Professor and Chair, Department of Children's Health, University of North Carolina, Chapel Hill, School of Nursing. She has a BSN from Duke University and an MS in parent-child nursing and a PhD in developmental psychobiology from the University of Connecticut. She is a Fellow in the American Academy of Nursing and received the 1993 Association of Women's Health, Obstetric, and Neonatal Nurses Award for Excellence in Research. She has conducted research on the development of sleep-wake states in premature infants, developmental outcomes of high-risk infants, and parenting of premature or medically fragile infants and after infertility of maternal HIV.

William L. Holzemer, PhD, RN, FAAN, is Professor and Chair, Department of Community Health Systems, School of Nursing, University of California, San Francisco.

Gail L. Ingersoll, EdD, RN, FAAN, is Associate Dean for Nursing Research and Director, Doctoral Program, Vanderbilt University School of Nursing. She holds the Julia Eleanor Chenault Chair as Professor of Nursing in Practice, Education, and Research. Following completion of a master's degree in nursing and a doctoral degree in higher education administration at the University of Rochester, she was awarded a 2-year postdoctoral research fellowship as a Robert Wood Johnson Clinical Nurse Scholar, which she completed at the University of Pennsylvania School of Nursing. She has conducted a number of studies pertaining to health systems redesign and patient outcomes.

Ada Jacox, PhD, RN, FAAN, is Professor and Associate Dean for Research at Wayne State University. From 1990 to 1995 she was Professor of Nursing at Johns Hopkins University School of Nursing, where she was also the Independence Foundation Chair in Health Policy and Director of the Doctoral Program. In 1994 she received the Alumni of the Year award from Wayne State University College of Nursing, and in 1992 she received the Maryland Nurses' Foundation Leadership award. Her recent research interests include cancer pain guidelines, determinants of nursing care costs and patient outcomes, and evaluation of cost-effectiveness of drug therapies. She has written over 125 publications, including *Pain: A Sourcebook for Nurses and Other Health Professionals* (1977).

Susan Janson, DNSc, RNC, FAAN, is Professor of Nursing and Adjunct Professor of Medicine at the University of California, San Francisco. As a nationally and internationally known expert in asthma patient education and management, she served on the National Heart, Lung and Blood Institute Expert Panels that wrote *Guidelines for the Diagnosis and Management of Asthma*. She is actively engaged in funded asthma research, teaches in the adult nurse practitioner master's program and the doctoral nursing program, and sees patients in a weekly clinic for patients with pulmonary disease. She has published numerous data-based and review articles and book chapters on asthma and dyspnea associated with pulmonary disease.

Linda L. Jensen, RN, BCIAC, has been employed as Clinical Research Director for 13 colon and rectal surgeons for the last 16 years. Their practice includes an affiliation with the University of Minnesota as well as a large private practice. Although she is responsible for coordinating all clinical research, her main focus is on fecal incontinence. This includes patient assessment, biofeedback, clinical studies, and experimental surgical procedures. She has presented at numerous nursing and physician conferences and has authored many papers on fecal incontinence.

Marcia Gruis Killien, PhD, RN, FAAN, is currently Professor and Chair, Department of Family and Child Nursing, University of Washington. She also serves as Director, Research Development and Dissemination Core, Center for Women's Health Research, University of Washington, and is a member of the Expert Panel on Women's Health of the American Academy of Nursing. Her program of research has focused on the interface between women's work and family lives, especially during the childbearing years, and the impact of women's employment on their own and their family's health.

Kathleen A. Knafl, PhD, is Professor, Department of Maternal Child Nursing, and Executive Associate Dean, College of Nursing, University of Illinois, Chicago. She serves as director of the college's graduate program and is responsible for its Office of Research Facilitation. Her research interests focus on family response to childhood illness and disability. She has been especially interested in developing the concept of normalization to understand how families adjust to the challenges of chronic illness.

Ada M. Lindsey, PhD, RN, FAAN, is Dean and Professor, College of Nursing, University of Nebraska Medical Center. She has been a member of the American Academy of Nursing since 1980 and served on the Governing Council from 1987 to 1989. She has served as a consultant to schools of nursing, presented research and invitational papers nationally and internationally, published studies related to breast and lung cancer, and served on editorial boards and as reviewer of professional journals. Her research leadership includes her service as a member (from 1987 to 1991) of the Sigma Theta Tau International Research Committee. She was appointed to serve (from 1997 to 2001) as a member of the National Advisory Council for Nursing Research, NIH, NINR.

Juliene G. Lipson, PhD, RN, FAAN, is nurse-anthropologist and Professor, School of Nursing, University of California, San Francisco. She has taught psychiatric, community health, and international and cross-cultural nursing since 1976. Her ethnographic research since 1982 has been on Middle Eastern and Afghan immigrants and refugees and on Bosnian and Russian refugees and culturally competent nursing care. She has published 36 journal articles, 12 book chapters, and four books, including *Self-Care Nursing in Multi-Cultural Context* and *Culture and Nursing Care: A Pocket Guide,* which received an *American Journal of Nursing* Book of the Year award.

Carol J. Loveland-Cherry, PhD, RN, FAAN, is Professor and Director, Division of Health Promotion and Risk Reduction Programs, University of Michigan School of Nursing, Ann Arbor. She has been a member of the faculty at the University of Michigan since 1984. She received her BSN in 1964 and her MPH in 1974 from the University of Michigan. Her PhD is in nursing from Wayne State University, Detroit, MI (1982). She is Principal Investigator on two National Institutes of Health research grants: the Altering Family Norms Regarding Adolescent Alcohol Misuse study, funded by the National Institute on Drug Abuse Alcoholism, and the School and Family Based Adolescent Drug Abuse Prevention study, funded by the National Institute on Drug Abuse. The program of research focuses on the development and testing of community-based interventions to decrease adolescents' skills. She has served as the university's Senate Assembly representative from the School of Nursing since 1990 and was elected as Vice Chair of the Senate Advisory Committee on University Affairs (SACUA), beginning in May 1997. She is an active member of several professional organizations, including the American Nurses Association, ANA Council of Nurse Researchers, American Public Health Association, Michigan Public Health Association, National Council on Family Relations, Society for Research on Alcohol, Sigma Theta Tau, and Midwest Nursing Research Society.

Sally Lechlitner Lusk, PhD, RN, FAAN, is Professor, Community Health Nursing, and Director, Occupational Health Nursing, School of Nursing, University of Michigan. She has made presentations and published book chapters and articles regarding health promotion and disease prevention in the worksite. Her own program of research on promoting the use of personal protective equipment to prevent disease, primarily hearing protection devices to prevent noise-induced hearing loss, is well established, with funding from

NIH and NIOSH. With support from UAW-GM, she has begun to identify nonauditory effects of noise exposure at work. As a result of her program of research, she received the 1998 Distinguished Contributor to Research in the Midwest award from MNRS. She participated in NINR's second conference on research priorities for nursing research and the NINR Priority Expert Panel on Community Based Models and currently serves on NIH grant review panels. She is also Section Editor for Linking Practice and Research in the *American Association of Occupational Health Nurses Journal* and a reviewer for several other journals.

Meridean L. Maas, PhD, RN, FAAN, is Professor and Chair, Adult and Gerontological Nursing Area Studies, University of Iowa College of Nursing. She is also Senior Associate Director, Office of Research, College of Nursing, and Consultant to the University of Missouri–Columbia Sinclair School of Nursing Office of Research. Her research interests include the effects of organizational and other environmental contextual variables on nursing practice and patient outcomes; testing the effects of nursing interventions on outcomes for persons with Alzheimer's and related dementias, their family members, and staff caregivers; and clinical testing of standardized patient outcomes that are responsive to nursing interventions. Since 1997, she has published a regular column, "Nursing Outcomes Accountability," in the *Journal of Nursing Outcomes Management.* Other recent publications include "Special Care Units for Persons With Alzheimer's Disease: Only for a Privileged Few?" (with J. Specht, K. Weiler, and B. Turner, in the *Journal of Gerontological Nursing,* 1998) and *Nursing Outcomes Classification* (with M. Johnson, 1997).

Mary MacVicar is Professor Emeritus at The Ohio State University. She earned her BS in Nursing from the University of Colorado, Boulder. She earned her MS in Nursing, a MA in Sociology, and PhD in Medical Sociology/Disability Rehabilitation from The Ohio State University. She is especially interested in cancer rehabilitation and symptom management through the use of aerobic exercise. She was Principal Investigator on R01s from both NCI and NCNR examining the use of aerobic exercise in cancer, and was co-investigator on an NINR funded R01 examining the role of aerobic exercise in HIV infected adults. She remains active in cancer rehabilitation and assisting investigators with grant preparation.

Joan K. Magilvy, PhD, RN, FAAN, is Professor in the Environmental Contexts and Outcomes Division of the University of Colorado Health Sciences Center School of Nursing. She is also Program Director of the PhD program in nursing. She received her BSN from the University of Cincinnati, her MS in community health nursing from Northern Illinois University, and her PhD in nursing from the University of Colorado. Her program of research is focused on rural health services for older adults and community-based interventions and outcomes. Other research interests are qualitative research designs, chronicity, and disability studies. She is a Fellow in the American Academy of Nursing.

Marilyn A. McCubbin, PhD, RN, FAAN, is Professor, School of Nursing, and a Fellow with the Center for Family Studies and the University of Wisconsin Comprehensive Cancer Center, and Nursing Core Discipline Chief with the Pediatric Pulmonary Center at the University of Wisconsin–Madison. She is a coauthor of the Resiliency Model of Family Stress, Adjustment, and Adaptation that has been used as the theoretical framework for research on normative and nonnormative family transitions in the United States and internationally. She has also developed instruments to measure aspects of family functioning such as family hardiness, family problem-solving communication, and parental coping with children's chronic illness. Her research on family resiliency and adaptation in children's chronic and life-threatening illness has been funded by the National Institute for Nursing Research and private foundations.

Barbara S. Medoff-Cooper, PhD, RN, FAAN, is Professor and Director, Center for Nursing Research, School of Nursing, University of Pennsylvania. She has been investigating neurodevelopment of the preterm infant for the past two decades. Included in her program of research is the development of the the Early Infancy Temperament Questionnaire with Drs. William Carey and Sean McDevitt, the study of brain metabolism postintraventricular hemorrhage in preterm infants, and nutritive sucking as an index of neurobehavioral maturation. She has received funding from the NIH through the National Institute of Nursing Research and the Heart, Lung and Blood Institute. Using this NIH funding, her interdisciplinary research team is developing the instrumentation necessary to use sucking patterns as a neonatal screening tool.

Susan B. Meister, PhD, RN, FAAN, is a member of Harvard's Working Group of Early Life and Adolescent Health Policy. As Director of Health Services Research, Children's Hospital, San Diego, she was the first Director of the California Association of Children's Hospitals' six-hospital project to quantify clinical resource consumption in children's hospitals. She was Principal Investigator of a joint project of Children's Hospital in San Diego and Children's Memorial Hospital in Chicago; the project tested the impact of innovations in care for children with chronic illnesses. She has served on technical advisory panels for the Health Care Financing Administration. Her research focuses on child health policies.

Afaf I. Meleis, PhD, DrPS (Hon), FAAN, is a nurse and medical sociologist who was educated in Egypt and in the United States. She is Professor, Department of Community Health Systems, University of California, San Francisco. Her research interests are in the relationship between women's multiple roles, their life transitions, their health and immigration, and marginalization and health. She has conducted collaborative research projects in these areas in the United States, Brazil, Columbia, Mexico, Egypt, and Kuwait. She established the Mid-East Study of Immigrants' Health and Adjustment (SIHA) Project in the UCSF School of Nursing.

Ellen Sullivan Mitchell, PhD, RN, ARNP, is Associate Professor, College of Nursing, University of Washington. She received her MN from the University of Florida in 1967 and her PhD in Nursing Science from the University of Washington in 1986. She is currently the coordinator of the Women's Primary Care Nurse Practitioner Program at the University of Washington, as well as coinvestigator of two women's health research programs. In 1993, she received the Distinguished Teaching award. Her primary interests in research, teaching, and clinical practice are in the areas of primary health care of women and expertise in problems related to the menstrual cycle. Her broad focus is on biopsychosocial factors that affect the health of women within the context of cyclic changes across the menstrual cycle. Specific research has addressed symptom experiences related to the menstrual cycle and menopause

Pamela H. Mitchell, PhD, RN, FAAN, is Professor of Biobehavioral Nursing and Health Systems, Elizabeth S. Soule Distinguished Professor of Health Promotion,

Associate Dean for Research, and Adjunct Professor, Department of Health Service, University of Washington. She holds an MS from the University of California, San Francisco, and a PhD in health care systems ecology from the University of Washington. Her practice and research are in clinical neuroscience and critical care nursing, with expansion into studying care delivery systems as they affect clinical outcomes. She is a member of scientific review panels for the National Center for Research Resources, a reviewer for the Health Quality Research Panel, AHCPR, a member of the American Academy of Nursing Expert Panel on Quality Care, and an investigator in the Center for Cost and Outcomes Research at the University of Washington.

Patricia Moritz, PhD, RN, FAAN, is Associate Professor, Community, Health Systems, and Policy Division; Associate Dean for Research; and Director, Center for Nursing Research, University of Colorado Health Sciences Center, Denver. Her research is focused on demonstrating the effect of nursing on clinical outcomes and on the interactive effects of health care delivery and nursing systems. Specific interests include decision making, chronicity as a clinical model, rural health, practice-based research strategies, clinical evaluation, and health policy.

Carolyn L. Murdaugh, PhD, RN, FAAN, is Professor and Associate Dean for Research, University of South Carolina, Columbia. She was Intramural Scientist, National Institute of Nursing Research, 1991 to 1995; prior to her NINR appointment, she was a member of the faculty at the University of Arizona from 1981 to 1991. In Arizona she was Director of Clinical Research, College of Nursing, and Director of Nursing Research, University Medical Center. She received her BS and MS degrees from the University of California, San Francisco, and her PhD degree from the University of Arizona. She is a Fellow in the American Academy of Nursing and the American Heart Association Council on Cardiovascular Nursing. Her research focuses on quality of life outcomes in chronic illness and healthcare system outcomes.

Mary Naylor, PhD, RN, FAAN, holds the Killebrew Term Chair and is Associate Professor at the University of Pennsylvania School of Nursing. From 1986-1988 she served as Associate Dean and Director of Undergraduate Studies. She earned both her PhD and MSN from the University of Pennsylvania. Her BSN is from

Villanova University. She is also a Senior Fellow of the University of Pennsylvania's Leonard Davis Institute of Health Economics. Since 1989, she has led an interdisciplinary program of research designed to improve outcomes and reduce costs of care for vulnerable community-based elders. To date, she and her reserch team have completed two NINR-funded randomized clinical trials focusing on discharge planning and home follow-up of high risk elders by advanced practice nurses. A third NINR-funded study "Home Follow-Up of Elders Hospitalized With Heart Failure" is ongoing.

Ellen Olshansky, DNSc, RN-C, is Associate Professor at Duquesne University School of Nursing in Pittsburgh, Pennsylvania, where she recently relocated after serving as Associate Professor at the University of Washington School of Nursing. She has conducted several research studies on infertility, focusing on emotional responses of both men and women and on women's experiences of pregnancy and parenting after infertility. She is currently conducting a study, funded by NINR, on "Depression in Previously Infertile New Mothers," and on another study, funded byDuquesne University, on "Experiences of Menopause in Women With a History of Infertility." She has worked as a counselor for individuals and couples who are experiencing infertility and as a support group leader for Resolve, an infertility support and information organization.

Barbara Parker, PhD, RN, FAAN, is Professor of Nursing and Director of the Doctoral Program and Center for Nursing Research at the University of Virginia. She is currently President of the Nursing Network on Violence Against Women, International, and has conducted several studies on violence against women with Dr. Judith McFarlane of Texas Women's University. The first study documented the frequency and severity of violence against pregnant women and resulting maternal and infant outcomes. The second study tested a nursing intervention for abuse with pregnant women in urban (Houston) and rural (Virginia) populations. With a longitudinal design, all women are followed throughout pregnancy and until the infant is 12 months old. Both studies have been funded by the International Injury Division of the Centers for Disease Control. She has published over 45 articles and book chapters on violence against women.

Nola J. Pender, PhD, RN, FAAN, is Associate Dean for Research, School of Nursing, University of Michigan. She has been funded by the National Institute of Nursing Research for a program of research testing the predictive power of the health promotion model for health-promoting lifestyles and exercise among adults and adolescents. She and her colleagues developed the Health Promoting Lifestyle Profile. She directs the Child and Adolescent Health Behavior Research Center and chaired the NINR Expert Panel on Health Promotion for Older Children and Adolescents. She is Past President, Midwest Nursing Research Society and American Academy of Nursing.

Linda R. Phillips, PhD, RN, FAAN, graduated from the University of Pittsburgh and the University of Arizona. She is presently Professor and Associate Dean for Research at the University of Arizona College of Nursing. She has served on the Internal Review Group for the National Institute of Nursing Research and is Vice President of the Board of Directors of Handmaker Jewish Services for the Aged. She has been awarded the Sigma Theta Tau International Founders Award for Excellence in Research. The unifying theme of her research is caregiving dynamics and the nature of the social processes involved in care. Particular interest areas have included the dynamics of family caregiving, elder abuse, and institutional care for demented and confused elders. She is currently funded by the National Institute of Aging to study caregiver abuse among Anglos and Mexican Americans.

Carla Gene Rapp, MNSc, CRRN, RN, is currently a doctoral candidate, Teaching Assistant, and Research Assistant, University of Iowa College of Nursing. She is pursuing a PhD in nursing care of the aged, with a cognate in cognition and its impairment. Her research interests include agitation and aggression, acute confusion and delirium, and cognitive impairment. She holds a bachelor's degree in nursing, with a second major in gerontology, and a Master's of Nursing Science with specializations in gerontological nursing and nursing administration. She is certified in rehabilitation nursing. She speaks and has been published in the areas of aging, neurology, rehabilitation, and cognitive impairment.

Beverly L. Roberts, PhD, RN, FAAN, is Associate Professor and Associate Dean of Academic Programs at Frances Payne Bolton School of Nursing at Case Western Reserve University, Senior Faculty Associate of the University Center of Aging and Health, and a Fellow of the Gerontological Society of America. Her research focuses on healthy and physically and chronically ill older adults. She continues to assess the efficacy of exercise (aerobic exercise and muscle-strengthening exercise) on independence in activities of daily living and related factors. She is replicating these studies in Korea.

Barbara Smith, PhD, RN, FAAN, is Professor and Mario O'Koren Endowed Chair at the Unversity of Alabama School of Nursing at Birmingham. She earned her BSN and MSN from Case Western University in nursing and public health nursing and her PhD from Ohio State University in exercise physiology. Her special interests include using various types of exercise to improve functional capacity and life quality in chronically ill special populations. She is a Fellow in the American Academy of Nursing, The American College of Sports Medicine, and the American Association of Cardiovascular and Pulmonary Rehabilitation. She has had NINR funding to examine an after-school program of aerobic exercise to reduce cardiovascular disease risk factors in African American children. She is currently completing a study examining the use of aerobic exercise training for symptom management in HIV and has plans to explore the effects of aerobic and resistive exercise in HIV-infected adults on body composition, energy balance, and fatigue. She is a member of the NINR Initial Review Group and the ANF Research Review Committee.

Janet P. Specht, PhD, RN, is a 1996 graduate of the University of Iowa, with a doctorate in nursing with emphasis in nursing administration. She is currently Clinical Associate Professor in Nursing at the University of Iowa in the Adult and Gerontological Area Studies and is also Health Research Scientist at the Iowa City VA Medical Center, where she is working on the evaluation of the use of telemedicine between acute and long-term care. In addition, she is the developer and owner of a community-supported living facility for persons with dementia, in partnership with Dr. Meridean Maas. Her research interests include practice models to promote professional nursing practice; diagnosis, interventions, and outcomes for older persons with urinary incontinence; and care of persons with dementia and their families. An overarching research interest has been the influence of the environment in each of these areas of research. Recent publications include two articles coauthored with Dr. Maas, "Shared Governance in Nursing: What Is Shared, Who Governs and

Who Benefits?" (in *Current Issues in Nursing,* 4th edition), and "Special Care Units for Persons with Alzheimer's Disease: Only for a Privileged Few?" (*Journal of Gerontological Nursing,* 1998).

Barbara J. Speck, PhD, RN, earned her PhD from the University of North Carolina at Chapel Hill School of Nursing in 1997 and is currently Assistant Professor, University of Louisville, School of Nursing. During her doctoral program, she worked on the Cardiovascular Health in Children and Youth Study for 3½ years. She worked with Dr. Joanne Harrell and the multidisciplinary team of investigators in all phases of the study, particularly in instrument development and testing psychometric properties of the Youth Health Survey, the major self-report questionnaire of the longitudinal, school-based study. Her research interests are health promotion and disease prevention behaviors, and she is currently involved in research on the maintenance of regular physical activity in working women. With M. J. Gilmer, C. B. Bradley, Joanne S. Harrell, and M. Belyea, she wrote "The Youth Health Survey: Reliability and Validity of an Instrument for Assessing Cardiovascular Health Habits in Adolescents" *(Journal of School Health,* 1996).

Elaine Stashinko, PhD, RN, is Assistant Professor at the School of Nursing at The Johns Hopkins University, Baltimore, Maryland.

Frederick Suppe, PhD, is Professor of Philosophy in the Philosophy Department and the History and Philosophy of Science Program, University of Maryland, College Park. He has taught theory development in the PhD nursing programs at the University of Maryland and Johns Hopkins University. He is strongly committed to the view that philosophy of science should be firmly grounded in scientific practice, and he has made active participation in science, including nursing sciences and interaction with scientists, a staple of his career and a key source of insight about the nature of science. He has published 9 books and more than 100 articles, including "The Structure of Scientific Theory," "The Scientific Conception of Theories," and "Scientific Realization."

Kristen M. Swanson, PhD, RN, FAAN, is currently Associate Professor of Family and Child Nursing at the University of Washington. She received her BS in nursing from the University of Rhode Island, her master's

in adult health and illness nursing from the University of Pennsylvania, and her PhD in psychosocial nursing from the University of Colorado. She also completed an individually awarded NSRA 2-year postdoctoral fellowship at the University of Washington with Dr. Kathryn Barnard. She is a Fellow of the American Academy of Nursing. Her research is on the topics of caring and pregnancy loss; her most recent research has been focused on the effects of caring on women's well-being subsequent to miscarriage.

Diana Taylor, PhD, RN, NP, FAAN, nurse practitioner, educator, and researcher, is Associate Professor, Family Health Care Nursing Department, and was formerly Director of the Women's Primary Care Program, the first women's health training program in California (founded in 1970). She has focused much of her clinical and research work on the understanding of the biopsychosocial and lifespan factors that affect the health and illness experience within the context of cyclic changes across the menstrual cycle. She is principal investigator of an NIH-funded study of the effectiveness of nonpharmacological treatments for women's symptom experience and the co-principal investigator of a longitudinal study of midlife women's health across three ethnic groups. A member since 1984, she coauthored, with Nancy Woods, the 1987 SMCR Conference Proceedings, *Menstruation, Health and Illness* (1991).

Toni Tripp-Reimer, PhD, RN, FAAN, is currently Professor of Nursing and Anthropology and Associate Dean for Research, University of Iowa. She received a BSN from the University of Maryland/Walter Reed Army Institute of Nursing in 1969 and MSN in adult/gero and psych/mental health and MA and PhD (1977) in anthropology from Ohio State University. She has been a member of the University of Iowa Faculty of Nursing and Anthropology since 1977. Her research area is in intercultural nursing; her current focus is cultural issues in patient education.

Joyce A. Verran, PhD, RN, FAAN, is Professor, College of Nursing, University of Arizona, where she also serves as Interim Director for the Nursing Systems Division. She received her PhD in clinical nursing research from the University of Arizona. Her clinical experience has been primarily in nursing services administration in acute care settings. Her program of research involves nursing systems in terms of practice patterns and models of care delivery and their affect on staff, organizational, and client outcomes. This research has involved ambulatory, acute care, and community settings.

Clarann Weinert, SC, PhD, RN, FAAN, is Professor, Montana State University College of Nursing, Bozeman, and a Sister of Charity of Cincinnati. She received a BSN from the College of Mount St. Joseph on the Ohio, an MS in nursing from Ohio State University, and an MA and PhD in sociology from the University of Washington. She has been active in rural theory development and has written and spoken widely on the topic of rural health and rural nursing. She has conducted research related to rural families managing chronic illness and is published in the areas of social support and instrument development.

Nancy Fugate Woods, PhD, RN, FAAN, is Dean, School of Nursing, University of Washington. She received a BSN from the University of Wisconsin, Eau Claire, in 1968, a Master of Nursing degree from the University of Washington in 1969, and a PhD in epidemiology from the University of North Carolina, Chapel Hill, in 1978. Since the mid-1970s, she has provided leadership in the development of women's health as a field of study in nursing science. In collaboration with colleagues at the University of Washington, in 1989 she established the Center for Women's Health Research, focusing on women's health across the lifespan. Her current research focuses on midlife women, their health, and health-seeking behavior patterns. She is currently involved in projects focusing on menopause, including women's decisions about using hormone replacement therapy. She has been active in professional organizations, having served as President of the American Academy of Nursing and the Society for Menstrual Cycle Research and as a member of the National Advisory Council on Nursing Research of the National Center for Nursing Research, NIH. She recently received the American Nurses Foundation Distinguished Contribution to Nursing Research award and was elected to the Institute of Medicine, National Academy of Sciences.